DATE DUE

5-3-19	

PRINTED

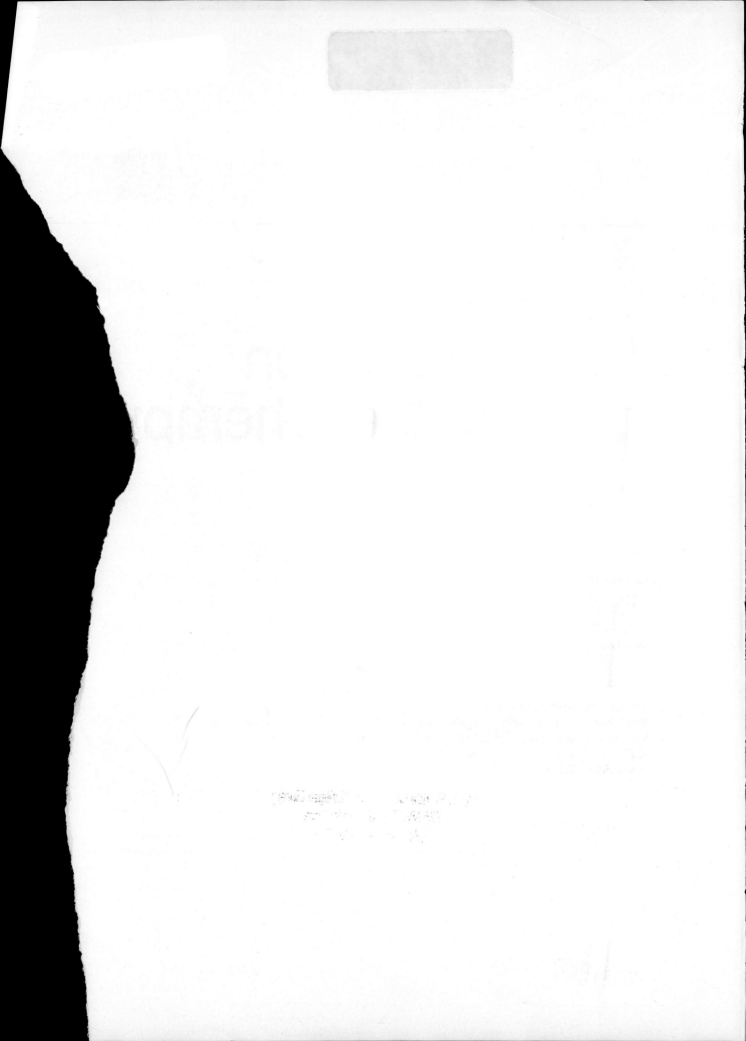

11th EDITION

Williams'
Essentials
of Nutrition
and Diet Therapy

Eleanor D. Schlenker, PhD, RD
Professor and Extension Specialist
Department of Human Nutrition, Foods, and Exercise
College of Agriculture and Life Sciences
Virginia Polytechnic Institute and State University
Blacksburg, Virginia

Joyce Gilbert, PhD, RD
Professor and Executive Director
Department of Family and Consumer Sciences
College of Health and Human Development
California State University, Northridge
Northridge, California

North Florida Community College Library
325 NW Turner Davis Drive
Madison, FL 32340

3251 Riverport Lane
St. Louis, Missouri 63043

WILLIAMS' ESSENTIALS OF NUTRITION & DIET THERAPY,   ISBN: 978-0-323-18580-6
ELEVENTH EDITION
Copyright © 2015 by Mosby, an imprint of Elsevier Inc.
Copyright © 2011, 2007, 2003, 1999, 1994, 1990, 1986, 1982, 1978, 1974 by Mosby, Inc.,
an affiliate of Elsevier Inc.

Library of Congress Cataloging-in-Publication Data
Schlenker, Eleanor D., author.
  Williams' essentials of nutrition and diet therapy / Eleanor D. Schlenker, Joyce Gilbert. — Eleventh edition.
      p. ; cm.
  Essentials of nutrition and diet therapy
  Preceded by Williams' essentials of nutrition and diet therapy / Eleanor D. Schlenker, Sara Long Roth.
10th ed. c2011.
  Includes bibliographical references and index.
  ISBN 978-0-323-18580-6 (pbk. : alk. paper)
  I. Gilbert, Joyce, author.   II. Title.   III. Title: Essentials of nutrition and diet therapy.
  [DNLM: 1. Nutritional Physiological Phenomena.   2. Diet Therapy.   3. Nutritional Sciences–methods. QU 145]
  RM216
  613.2–dc23
                                                                    2014027630

Director, Traditional Education: Kristin Geen
Content Development Management: Jean Sims Fornango
Senior Content Development Specialist: Danielle M. Frazier
Publishing Services Manager: Deborah Vogel
Project Manager: Brandilyn Flagg
Designer: Renee Duenow

Printed in China

Last digit is the print number: 9   8   7   6   5   4   3   2   1

Working together
to grow libraries in
developing countries

www.elsevier.com • www.bookaid.org

Marianna K. Baum, PhD, MS, RD
Professor
Department of Dietetics & Nutrition
R. Stempel College of Public Health and
Social Work
Florida International University
Miami, Florida
Chapter 24 Acquired Immunodeficiency
Syndrome (AIDS)

Adriana Campa, PhD
Associate Professor
Florida International University
Miami, Florida
Chapter 24 Acquired Immunodeficiency
Syndrome (AIDS)

Pamela Charney, PhD, RD, CHTS-CP
Program Chair, Healthcare Technology and
Management
Bellevue College
Bellevue, Washington
Chapter 19 Nutrition Support: Enteral and
Parenteral Nutrition

Dorothy Chen-Maynard, PhD, RD
Program Coordinator, Nutrition and Food
Sciences
California State University, San Bernardino
San Bernardino, California
Chapter 20 Gastrointestinal Diseases

Irene Hatsu, PhD
Assistant Professor
The Ohio State University
Columbus, Ohio
Chapter 24 Acquired Immunodeficiency
Syndrome (AIDS)

Allan Higginbotham, PhD, RD
Private Practice Dietitian and Corporate
Wellness Consultant
Birmingham, Alabama
Chapter 15 The Complexity of Obesity:
Beyond Energy Balance

Beth Kunkel, PhD, RD
Professor Emeritus
Department of Food, Nutrition and
Packaging Services
Clemson University
Clemson, South Carolina
Chapter 25 Cancer

Ritamarie Little, MS, RD
Associate Director, Marilyn Magaram
Center for Food Science, Nutrition and
Dietetics
Faculty, Department of Family and
Consumer Sciences
California State University, Northridge
Northridge, California
Chapter 16 Nutrition Assessment and
Nutrition Therapy in Patient Care

Staci Nix, MS, RD, CD
Assistant Professor
University of Utah
Salt Lake City, Utah
Chapter 14 Nutrition and Physical Fitness

**Sharon M. Nickols-Richardson,
PhD, RD**
Professor and Head
Department of Food Science and Human
Nutrition
University of Illinois, Urbana-Champaign
Champaign, Illinois
Chapter 11 Nutrition During Pregnancy
and Lactation
Chapter 12 Nutrition for Normal Growth
and Development

Melody Anacker, MS, RD, LN
Instructor and Didactic Program Director
Montana State University
Bozeman, Montana

Sandra Blair, MS, RN
Associate Professor of Nursing
LaGrange College—BSN Program
LaGrange, Georgia

Cindy Fitch, PhD, RD
Extension Professor
West Virginia University Extension Service
Families and Health Programs
Morgantown, West Virginia

Mary M. Flynn, PhD, RD, LDN
Associate Professor of Medicine (Clinical)
Brown University
Providence, Rhode Island

Kathleen Gould, EdD, MA, RD, LDN
Clinical Assistant Professor
Department of Health Science
Towson University
Towson, Maryland

Anita K. Reed, RN, MSN
Department Chair Adult and Community
    Health Practice
Saint Joseph's College/St. Elizabeth School
    of Nursing
Rensselaer, Indiana

Katheryn Swyden, MS, RD, LD
PhD Candidate
Department of Allied Health
The University of Oklahoma Health
    Sciences Center
Oklahoma City, Oklahoma

Lanette E. Tanaka MSN, RN
Assistant Teaching Professor
College of Nursing
University of Missouri—St. Louis
St. Louis, Missouri

Eric Vlahov, PhD
Professor
Department of Health Science and Human
    Performance
The University of Tampa
Tampa, Florida

Kim Webb, RN, MN
Retired Nursing Chair
Ponca City, Oklahoma

Through ten highly successful editions, this nutrition textbook has presented a sound approach to student learning and clinical practice in the health professions. It provides both a strong research base and a person-centered approach to the study and application of nutrition in human health. We have appreciated the suggestions and positive reception of this text by users in colleges, community colleges, and clinical settings throughout the United States and in other parts of the world. We welcome a new co-author to this edition, Dr. Joyce Gilbert, who brings her extensive background and experience as an author, an educator, and a clinician to the preparation of the eleventh edition.

New discoveries in nutrition science and its application to human health are the basis of rapidly evolving protocols in both public health and clinical care. Evidence-based practice rather than dependence on custom or prior learning has become the standard for decision-making. As the science base in biology, biotechnology, and health is expanding, new arenas of practice include nanotechnology, nutrigenomics, and functional foods. Recent changes in the U.S. population are creating new challenges for the health professional. The Advisory Committee to the 2010 Dietary Guidelines for Americans noted that for the first time in history, our population cannot be considered "healthy," based on the prevalence of obesity and growing chronic disease. Our population is also becoming older and more diverse in culture and ethnicity. These observations carry implications for the health professionals of the future and their formal preparation for working in community, clinical, or industry settings. The health professionals of the future must deal creatively with the realities of chronic disease. They must develop a framework of understanding of the needs of the aging population and ethnic and cultural food patterns that differ from their own. The worldwide epidemic of obesity, diabetes, and related chronic disease, fueling the rise in health care costs, is bringing new attention to delivery of health care and disease prevention strategies. Public interest and concern with nutrition and health are increasing, although consumers often depend on less reliable sources of information. New technology and the Internet offer unlimited opportunities for meaningful nutrition and health intervention programs, despite the appearance of false advertising and misleading health information. Nutrition has become prominent in the marketplace promoting functional foods and expanding product lines. Such changes present both opportunities and challenges for the future health professional.

This new edition reflects these far-reaching changes. We continue to be guided by a commitment to sound nutrition principles rooted in basic science and their application to human health and well-being. We have built on previous editions to produce this new book—updated and rewritten, with our new design and format—to meet the changing needs of students, faculty, and practitioners in the health professions.

NEW TO THIS EDITION

To accommodate the demands of a rapidly emerging science and an increasingly diverse society, the entire text has been updated. Changes and additions based on input from many teachers, students, and clinicians have been incorporated to increase its usefulness.

Chapter Changes

With the retirement of Dr. Sue Rodwell Williams, the founder and primary author of the first eight editions of this textbook, we continue to share responsibility for the preparation of this new edition. Part 1, *Introduction to Human Nutrition,* provides the foundation in nutrition science, as applied to human nutrition needs in Part 2, *Community Nutrition and the Life Cycle.* Part 3, *Introduction to Clinical Nutrition,* describes the nutrition care process for meeting the nutritional needs associated with specific illnesses and conditions and the application of medical nutrition therapy. Our continuing contributors include Dr. Sharon M. Nickols-Richardson, who prepared Chapter 11, "Nutrition During Pregnancy and Lactation," and Chapter 12, "Nutrition for Normal Growth and Development." Staci Nix, author of *Williams' Basic Nutrition & Diet Therapy,* contributed Chapter 14, "Nutrition and Physical Fitness," and Dr. Allan Higginbotham revised Chapter 15, "The Complexity of Obesity: Beyond Energy Balance." We also welcome five new contributors to this edition. Ritamarie Little prepared Chapter 16, "Nutrition Assessment and Nutrition Therapy in Patient Care," and Pamela Charney, Chapter 19, "Nutrition Support: Enteral and Parenteral Nutrition." Dr. Dorothy Chen-Maynard completed Chapter 20, "Gastrointestinal Diseases," Dr. Adriana Campa, Dr. Hatsu, and Dr. Baum contributed Chapter 24, "Acquired Immunodeficiency Syndrome (AIDS);" and Dr. Beth Kunkel prepared Chapter 25 "Cancer."

New material has been incorporated throughout this edition, reflecting recent research findings and clinical treatment therapies. Examples include new roles for traditional nutrients such as vitamin D, updates on the transmission and treatment of acquired immunodeficiemcy syndrome (AIDS), and recent attention to the glycemic index with representative food values. Health promotion with strategies for implementation is a recurring theme throughout the text, and students are encouraged to look for the *Health Promotion* heading in each chapter for special information to assist with nutrition education in a variety of settings. Full coverage of the U.S. Department of Agriculture and U.S. Department of

Health and Human Services health initiatives including MyPlate, the Dietary Guidelines for Americans, and Healthy People 2020 includes goals, practice standards, and application and usefulness to health promotion. Nutrient density is given a new emphasis as a means to address current deficiencies within the U.S. population. We also provide an overview of the newly proposed Nutrition Label. The chapters on energy balance and obesity provide readers with a comprehensive review of this public health problem including proposed contributing factors such as sleep deprivation. Interventions to stem the advance of the obesity epidemic, including new regulations for school breakfast and lunch that limit kcalories and emphasize fruit, vegetables and whole grains, and current activity recommendations for children are presented. The chapter on nutrition and physical performance includes emerging research pertaining to protein and fluid needs, dietary supplements, and the benefits of exercise on risk factors for cardiovascular disease and diabetes. Chapter 10 as revised takes a public health approach to nutrition and well-being, providing a framework for developing and marketing community nutrition and health intervention programs with attention to needs assessment, implementation, and evaluation.

Feature boxes addressing contemporary issues in nutrition and health have been continued and updated. Each chapter includes an example of *Evidence-Based Practice*, guiding students through the critical thought process and reinforcing this concept for future use in the practice setting. The *Complementary and Alternative Medicine (CAM)* boxes—found in all chapters in Part 3—review and evaluate new therapies relevant to chapter topics. *Focus on Culture* boxes introduce students to the concept of cultural competence and the particular nutritional deficiencies, health problems, and appropriate interventions pertinent to various cultural, ethnic, racial, and age-groups. *Focus on Food Safety* boxes alert readers to food safety issues with a particular nutrient, age-group, or medical condition. *Perspectives in Practice* boxes provide practical elements for nutrition education that students will find helpful in their future roles. Tools available for download from government or other reputable public sites have been included. "Websites of Interest" connect students with truthful Internet resources, useful in finding answers to patient inquiries. "Further Readings and Resources" from the research and professional literature enable further inquiry in a topic of interest.

PERSONAL APPROACH

The person-centered approach that has been a hallmark of previous editions continues to be emphasized in this new edition. The authors and contributors write in a personal style using materials and examples from personal research and clinical experience. Scientific knowledge is presented in human terms as a tool to develop practical solutions to individual problems.

Illustrations and Design

Numerous illustrations, anatomic figures, graphic line drawings, and photographs, most in full color, enhance the overall design and help students better understand the concepts and clinical practices presented.

Enhanced Readability and Student Interest

Continuing attention has been given to enhancing readability and enlivening the text stylistically with use of boxes, illustrations, and recurring themes that capture student interest and assist in comprehension. New material has been added, and remaining sections have been rewritten. Recent advances in basic and clinical science are explained and applied. Issues of public and professional controversy pertinent to students' future practice are examined.

Learning Aids Within the Text

This eleventh edition continues to include many aids that assist student learning.

Chapter Openers

To alert students to the content of each chapter and draw them into its study, each chapter opens with a preview of chapter topics and their relevance to professional practice. An outline of the major chapter headings is also included on this page.

Key Terms

Key terms important to the student's understanding and application of the chapter content are presented in two steps. First, they are identified in orange type in the body of the text. Then, these terms are grouped and defined in boxes in the lower corners of the pages close to their mention. This dual-level approach to vocabulary development greatly improves the overall study and usefulness of the text.

Pedagogy Boxes

Perspectives in Practice, Focus on Culture, Complementary and Alternative Medicine (CAM), Focus on Food Safety, and *Evidence-Based Practice:* These special features throughout the text introduce supplemental material, an introduction to chapter-related issues or controversies, a deeper look at chapter topics, or a practical application of a nutrition concept. These interesting and motivating studies help the student comprehend the importance of scientific thinking and develop sound judgment and openness to varied points of view.

Case Studies

In Parts 2 and 3 realistic case studies provide opportunities for problem solving, applying the information learned to practical situations in nutrition care. Each chapter contains at least one case with questions for analysis, decision-making, and intervention. These case studies help students apply principles of community nutrition and medical nutrition therapy to individuals and groups they will meet in their clinical assignments.

Chapter Summaries

To assist students in drawing the chapter material together as a whole, each chapter concludes with a summary of the key concepts presented and their significance or application. The student can then return to any part of the chapter for repeated study and clarification as needed.

Review Questions

To help students think critically about key components of the chapter and apply them to community and patient needs or problems, review questions conclude each chapter. Review questions may require the student to seek information or perspective beyond what is found in the text using the scientific literature, the popular literature, community meal or public health programs, or retail food stores.

Chapter References

A strength of this text is the documentation of the topics presented, drawn from a wide selection of pertinent journals. To provide immediate access to all references cited in the chapter text, a full list is given at the end of each chapter rather than collected at the end of the book.

Further Readings and Resources

In addition to referenced material from the text, an annotated list of suggestions for further reading is provided at the end of each chapter. These selections extend or apply the text material according to student needs or special interests. The annotations improve their usefulness by identifying the pertinent topics of the reference. Also included is a list of reliable websites for further reference and study.

Appendixes

The appendixes found in the text and on the Evolve web site contain reference tools and guidelines in learning and practice. These include Choose Your Foods: Food Lists for Diabetes (ed 7) and extended tables for calculating Body Mass Index. A table of common conversions between metric and British measurement systems is included for student review. A summary of Cultural Dietary Patterns and Religious Dietary Practices, including both foods eaten and foods avoided within each food group, assists in meal planning with specific ethnic, racial, or religious groups. A summary of federal food assistance programs funded and supervised by the U.S. Department of Agriculture and the Administration on Aging, useful for future patient referral, describes the target audience, guidelines for participation, and food resources provided.

Supplementary materials available on Evolve

Our Evolve website is designed to provide supplemental online learning opportunities to complement the material in the book. The Evolve website contains sections for both instructor and student resources. The material was prepared by experienced nutrition writer, editor, and project coordinator Gill Robertson, MS, RD.

Instructor Resources

- **NEW!** TEACH for Nurses
- Extensive Test Bank of about 1200 NCLEX-style multiple-choice examination questions
- Image Collection of approximately 100 images from the text
- PowerPoint presentations for each chapter, each containing approximately 20 to 30 text slides to guide classroom lecture
- Audience response questions, approximately 4 per chapter

Student Resources

- 250 Study questions with instant feedback
- Case Studies (1 to 3 per chapter)
- Flashcards (5 to 10 per chapter)
- This food database contains over 5000 foods in 18 different categories: Baby Food, Baked Goods, Beverages, Breads/Grains and Pasta, Breakfast Foods/Cereals, Dairy and Eggs, Fats and Oils, Fruits and Vegetables, Meats and Beans, Nuts and Seeds, Frozen Entrees and Packaged Foods, Restaurant Chains–Fast Foods, Restaurant Chains–Other, Seafood and Fish, Snacks and Sweets, Soups, Supplements, and Toppings and Sauces.
- A complete listing of more than 150 activities—daily/common, sporting, recreational, and occupational—is included in the *Detailed Energy Expenditure* section.
- The profile feature allows users to enter and edit the intake and output of an unlimited number of individuals, and the weight management planner helps outline healthy lifestyles tailored to various personal profiles.
- In addition to foods and activities, features include an ideal body weight (IBW) calculator, a basal metabolic rate calculator to estimate total daily energy needs, and sample diets with nutrition recommendations for a variety of conditions.

ACKNOWLEDGMENTS

A textbook of this size is never the work of just authors and contributors. It develops into the planned product through the committed hands and hearts of a number of persons who bring their specialized skills and expertise to its completion. It would be impossible to name all of the individuals involved, but several groups deserve special recognition.

First, the authors are grateful to the reviewers, who gave their valuable time and skills to strengthen the manuscript:

Second, we are indebted to Elsevier and the many persons there who had a part in this extensive project. We especially thank our director of nutrition publications, Kristin Geen, whose skills and support have always been invaluable; and our senior content development specialist, Danielle Frazier, whose creative and energetic talents helped shape the book's pages. We also thank our production project manager, Brandilyn Flagg, for essential guidance; and our book designer, Renee Duenow, who helped to bring a new look to this eleventh edition. To our marketing managers and the many fine Elsevier sales representatives throughout the country, we owe great appreciation for their help in ensuring the book's success with users.

Eleanor D. Schlenker
Blacksburg, Virginia
Joyce Gilbert
Northridge, California

CONTENTS

Introduction to Human Nutrition

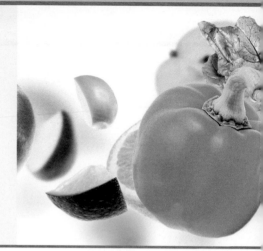

CHAPTER

1

Nutrition and Health

Eleanor D. Schlenker

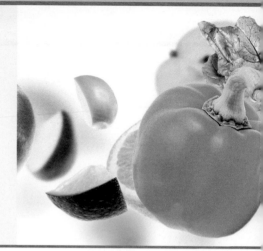 EVOLVE WEBSITE

http://evolve.elsevier.com/Williams/essentials/

A mother is told that her 11-year-old son, who is overweight and sedentary, will likely develop type 2 diabetes before he reaches the age of 18. A 23-year-old pregnant woman whose sister delivered a low-birth-weight baby is worried that this may happen to her. A 62-year-old man has been told by his doctor that he has hypertension and is at risk of a stroke. The 2010 Dietary Guidelines Advisory Committee noted that for the first time in our history, the U.S. population could not be described as healthy. Nearly two-thirds of all Americans are overweight or obese, the prevalence of type 2 diabetes is reaching epidemic proportions, and even adolescents are being diagnosed with heart disease. Statisticians predict that today's youth will be the first generation to have a shorter life expectancy than their parents. The key to successful intervention is a healthy lifestyle with nutrition as the cornerstone. A diet higher in fruits, vegetables, and whole grains, and lower in calories, sugar, and fat could help the 11-year-old boy lower his body fat and disease risk. Appropriate food choices support a successful pregnancy. A healthy diet with attention to sodium and potassium can lower the need for medications to control cardiovascular risk.

In this chapter we begin our study of nutrition and human health and see how these principles apply to the U.S. population. Current knowledge in nutrition reflects our growing understanding of the relationship between food, health, and well-being. Government agencies and institutions charged with reducing chronic disease and containing health care costs are giving attention to what people eat. Access to a safe and wholesome food supply for all people must be our goal.

NEW CHALLENGES FOR HEALTH PROFESSIONALS

Our society is constantly changing, including health care and how it is delivered. The problem of overweight points to the need for lifestyle education and the availability of affordable and healthy food. The Internet and smart phones have changed the way we deliver information and help consumers distinguish between appropriate and problematic information sources. The rise in life expectancy brings rapid shifts in population demographics with growing cohorts of older individuals and a greater need to address prevention and treatment of chronic disease. These changes will continue to affect your future practice as a health professional.

The Obesity Epidemic

The growing prevalence of obesity is a major health problem across the globe. Countries previously facing food shortages and underweight are now experiencing increasing overweight.[1] Current food and lifestyle patterns have influenced obesity statistics across the U.S. (Figure 1-1). In 2000, no state had an obesity prevalence of 30% or more; by 2010, 12 states

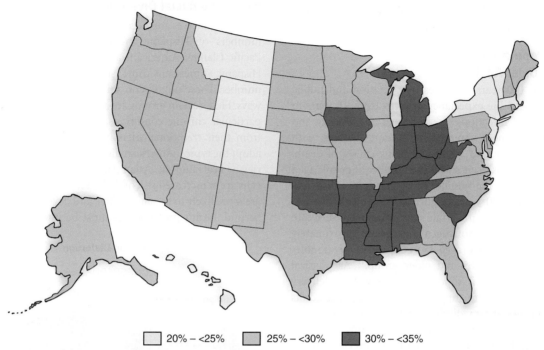

FIGURE 1-1 Prevalence of self-reported obesity among U.S. adults in 2012. Note that no state had an obesity prevalence of less than 20%. Thirteen states had an obesity prevalence of 30% or higher. (Obesity is defined as a body mass index of 30 or higher.) (Map from the Behavioral Risk Factor Surveillance System, Centers for Disease Control and Prevention: *Overweight and Obesity. Adult Obesity Facts,* Atlanta, Ga, U.S. Department of Health and Human Services. from: <http://www.cdc.gov/obesity/data/adult.html>. Retrieved September 8, 2013.)

Legend: 20% – <25%   25% – <30%   30% – <35%

had reached this level.[2] Seventy-four percent of men and 64% of women are overweight or obese,[3] and 32% of children aged 2 and over are either overweight or at risk for becoming overweight.[4] Among men, overweight or obesity is more likely to occur in middle age (ages 40 to 59); among women it is more common in older age (over age 60).[3] Children over the age of 5 are at greater risk of being overweight than pre-schoolers.[4] The rise in type 2 diabetes has paralleled the rise in obesity, such that 20.9 million people have been diagnosed, more than triple the number in 1990,[5] and it is estimated that another 7 million are undiagnosed.[6] However, the good news is that body weight appears to be leveling off in both children[4] and adults.[3]

Our environment, which promotes the consumption of **energy-dense** foods while providing limited need or opportunity for energy expenditure, has been referred to as "obe-sogenic," and contributes to the obesity problem.[7,8] In contrast to earlier times when humans survived as "hunter-gatherers," we now have a plentiful supply of good-tasting, high-calorie food, with little physical activity required to obtain it. The ever-present vending machine, special offers of two ham-burgers for the price of one, and accessible food at all sporting and most social events all contribute to excessive food intake (Box 1-1). Portions served at fast-food restaurants are two to five times larger than those offered 20 years ago,[9] and food served at home often equals three to four times the serving size referred to in meal planning guides (Figure 1-2). Most people increase their energy intake when more food is

served,[10] adding to the potential for overeating at "all you can eat" food outlets.

As energy intake has risen, energy expenditure has dropped. For many children, television or video games have replaced active outdoor games, and they ride rather than walk to school. Rural localities and new residential developments lack sidewalks, and many neighborhoods are unsafe for walking. Collaborative efforts among government agencies,

KEY TERMS
overweight A body weight above the average weight for a person of that sex and body height; this measurement does not distinguish between body fat and body muscle.
hypertension Medical term to describe high blood pressure; dietary and lifestyle interventions can help to lower blood pressure and reduce dependence on antihypertensive medications.
obese An excessive accumulation of body fat.
type 2 diabetes A form of diabetes mellitus usually occurring in middle or older age; results from impaired insulin secretion or body resistance to insulin action resulting in elevated blood glucose levels; often associated with overweight or obesity and a sedentary life style.
energy dense Term used to describe the relative kcalorie content of a particular food; an energy-dense food may also be nutrient dense if it is a good source of essential nutrients.

schools, community planners, and health professionals will be required to solve these problems.

Shifts in Population
Number of Older Adults

Over the past 100 years, advances in sanitation and public health have raised life expectancy at birth from 45 years to nearly 80 years.[11] Infectious diseases, such as influenza and pneumonia, have been replaced by chronic diseases, with heart disease, cancer, and stroke as leading causes of death. As life expectancy has risen, so has the number of people aged 65 and over. In fact, the number of older adults will nearly double in the next 20 years (Figure 1-3),[11] and this carries implications for health care. While average annual health care spending is $2739 for persons aged 25 to 44, it approximately doubles to $5511 for those aged 45 to 64, and nearly doubles again to $9744 in the 65 and older group.[12] As physical changes bring about loss in function, innovative food delivery systems will be needed to support homebound older adults in the community and medically compromised older adults in long-term care facilities. Intervention programs emphasizing appropriate food and activity patterns directed toward young and middle-aged adults can slow this development of chronic disease and ensuing disability.

BOX 1-1   FACTORS CONTRIBUTING TO INCREASED FOOD INTAKE

- Media advertising of high-sugar and high-calorie foods
- Constant access to vending machines selling high-sugar drinks and high-fat snacks
- More meals eaten away from home
- All-you-can-eat restaurant buffets
- Larger portion sizes both at home and in restaurants
- Continuous snacking
- "Supersizing": larger portions costing only a fraction more than a smaller portion

---

Ethnic and Racial Diversity

As a nation we are becoming increasingly diverse.[13] The numbers of Hispanic Americans, Asian Americans, and Pacific Islander Americans are increasing at rapid rates, and Hispanic Americans now surpass African Americans in number. These population shifts affect health care in several ways. First, certain groups are at increased risk for developing particular chronic conditions, especially if they move away from their traditional diets high in plant-based foods and adopt the typical American diet higher in **kilocalories** (kcalories or kcal) and fat. Asian Americans and Hispanic Americans are at increased risk of diabetes,[14] and African Americans are more likely to be salt sensitive and develop hypertension.[14] Second, health professionals must be knowledgeable about

Portion Distortion

CHEESEBURGER

20 Years Ago	Today
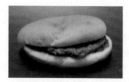	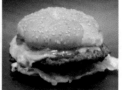
260 calories	850 calories

FIGURE 1-2 Change in portion size of common foods. Over the past 20 years, portion sizes have almost tripled. A hamburger and roll that supplied 260 kcal in earlier years may now contain 850 kcal. Visit the website of the National Heart, Lung and Blood Institute (http://hp2010.nhlbihin.net/portion/keep.htm) to view other food items that have changed in size and kcalories. Take the quiz to see how many minutes you would need to exercise to burn the extra kcalories. (Concept from U.S. Department of Health and Human Services, National Heart, Lung and Blood Institute, Obesity Education Initiative: *Keep an eye on portion size,* Bethesda, Md., 2004, U.S. Government Printing Office.)

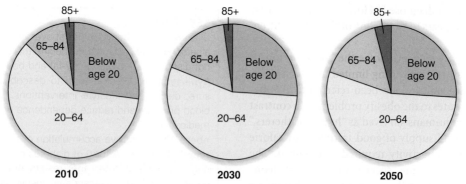

FIGURE 1-3 Projected increases in the number of persons aged 65 and older and 85 and older. Between 1900 and 2010, this age cohort grew from 3 million to 40 million and currently makes up 13% of the total population. By 2030, the group aged 65 and older is expected to number 72 million and represent almost 20% of the general population. By 2050, 19 million people will be age 85 or older. (From Federal Interagency Forum on Aging-Related Statistics: *Older Americans 2012: Key indicators of well-being,* Federal Interagency Forum on Aging-Related Statistics, Washington, D.C., 2012, U.S. Government Printing Office.)

FOCUS ON CULTURE

How Did Our Food Patterns Become So Diverse?

Food provides the nutrients that sustain life, but for most of us this is not the reason we eat what we do. Food habits—what we eat and when we eat it—have evolved over thousands of years. In all cultures and societies, various factors have influenced food habits.

Agriculture: Available land for crops or animals led to patterns emphasizing plant or animal foods. Cattle require land for grazing, along with water resources. Although parts of Europe were well-adapted to raising cattle or pigs, other areas were better suited to goats and sheep for meat and milk. Feta cheese made from sheep or goat's milk is common in Greece and Turkey.

The cereal or grain of a particular region influenced daily meals. Rice, indigenous to Southeast Asia, is served at every meal in traditional Chinese, Japanese, Hmong, and Cambodian households, much the same as bread is in the American diet. Because animal foods are limited, the Asian pattern combines a small amount of meat or fish with vegetables and rice for stew-like dishes. Maize or field corn along with rice are the traditional cereals in regions of the U.S. and Central and South America. Dishes made from corn—corn bread, corn cake, tortillas, cornmeal mush, and popcorn—were dietary staples among Native Americans. Corn is the basic grain in Mexican meals, with bread taking the form of tortillas, flat cakes baked on a hot griddle. Recognizing the differences between the Mexican food pattern, which emphasizes corn and beans, and the Puerto Rican food pattern, which relies on rice, tropical fruits, and vegetables, is important when working with Latino families.

Climate: When people raised all of their own food, the growing season and amount of rainfall defined what they ate. Root vegetables such as potatoes and cold-hardy cabbage, carrots, and apples were common in northern Europe because they could be stored in a root cellar to sustain families over the winter. In contrast, grains and legumes, along with a bountiful supply of fresh produce, provided the plant base of the healthful Mediterranean diet. Olives, olive oil, and dates remain important foods in Mediterranean cultures. The Caribbean region with its extended growing season is known for its tropical fruits and starchy vegetables. These foods are often imported for sale in street markets in U.S. cities with large populations from that region.

Proximity to water: Populations living near water included fish or seafood in their daily diet. The typical Japanese meal includes grilled, broiled, or pan-cooked fish or shellfish, along with steamed rice. The French-American (Cajun) foods common to southeast Louisiana, with seafood as a base, are strongly flavored and spicy, and served over rice.

Religion: Religious beliefs define not only what appropriate foods are, but also when they may be eaten. The dietary laws of Judaism are defined in the *Rules of Kashruth* and foods selected and prepared accordingly are called *kosher,* from the Hebrew word meaning *fit* or *proper.* Jewish law governs how animals are slaughtered, and the process must be supervised by a rabbi. For strict Orthodox believers, meat and milk may not be combined, and two sets of dishes and cooking utensils are required—one for serving meat and the other for dairy. Many traditional Jewish foods such as matzo, a type of unleavened bread, relate to observances commemorating significant events in Jewish history.

Muslim dietary laws come from the Quran. As in Judaism, pork is forbidden. Certain foods, including figs, olives, dates, honey, milk, and buttermilk, are believed to have special spiritual and physical value. In the ninth month of the Islamic calendar, Muslims celebrate Ramadan, a 30-day period of daylight fasting during which no food or beverages are eaten from dawn to sunset; a special meal is served after sundown.

Various foods brought to the U.S. by particular ethnic and cultural groups have joined the mainstream of American foods. Bagels, a traditional Jewish food, sushi from Japan, and olive oil from the Mediterranean are commonly used by many Americans. A balance between the old and the new preserves one's heritage and health.

For lists of specific foods from each food group common to particular ethnic and religious groups, see Appendix D.

Bibliography

Goody CM, Drago L, editors: *Cultural food practices*, Chicago, Ill., 2010, Diabetes Care and Education Dietetic Practice Group, American Dietetic Association.

Kittler PG, Sucher KP: *Cultural foods: traditions and trends,* Belmont, Calif., 2000, Wadsworth/Thomson Learning.

the eating patterns and favorite foods of various racial, ethnic, and cultural groups if they are to help these families develop meal plans that will be accepted and implemented.[13] Working with diverse groups can require language training. About one in five families in the U.S. speak a language other than English at home; within this group, over half speak Spanish.[15]

KEY TERM

kilocalorie   The general term *calorie* refers to a unit of heat measure and is used alone to designate the *small calorie.* The *large calorie,* 1000 calories or kilocalorie, is used in the study of metabolism to avoid the use of very large numbers in calculations.

The Focus on Culture box, "How Did Our Food Patterns Become So Diverse?" introduces factors influencing food patterns. Appendix D "Cultural Dietary Patterns and Religious Dietary Practices" will help begin your study of cultural and ethnic foods.

New Products in the Marketplace

Researchers have found that various foods contain naturally occurring substances other than nutrients that promote health. These foods are known as *functional foods. Phytochemicals* (plant chemicals) found in fruits, vegetables, and whole grains appear to have cancer-fighting properties.[16] Dark chocolate, often considered a food to be avoided, is now known to contain flavonoids, phytochemicals that help to control blood pressure.[17] Public interest in nutrients and other substances believed to influence health has prompted the food industry to develop new foods that meet this demand. Plant sterols that help lower blood cholesterol levels are being added to margarine; orange juice has become an alternative source of calcium and vitamin D to prevent bone loss. Conversely, "energy drinks" with added herbs and stimulants are being marketed to replace water or other healthy beverages. As more products claiming health benefits enter the marketplace, the task of helping consumers make appropriate choices will fall to the health professional.

Genes in Nutrition and Health

The Human Genome Project, an international project to map the human genetic code, is helping scientists learn how diet and the environment influence our genes (nutrigenomics), and how these interactions influence our survival. The study of nutrigenetics concentrates on how even slight variations in our genetic code affect our nutrient needs, susceptibility to particular diseases, and response to our environment.[18] A gene is a DNA sequence that can be translated into a protein, and bioactive components in food influence its expression. Nutrients such as essential fatty acids and vitamin A are bioactive; phytochemicals also act in this way. Individuals with different genes react differently to particular phytochemicals, and while an increased intake can have a positive effect on one person, it may not benefit another.[19] This likely contributes to why research studies looking at nutrient requirements have different results, as particular individuals will differ in their requirement for a specific nutrient.[20] Gene–nutrient interactions also influence response to nutritional interventions. For individuals with a specific genetic alteration, changes in the amounts and types of dietary fat may effectively lower their elevated blood LDL (low-density lipoprotein) cholesterol, but for others the intervention will have no biological effect.[18]

The study of nutrigenetics can help us learn why certain people cannot produce the enzyme lactase needed to break down the lactose in milk, or why individuals with celiac disease have an immune response to certain proteins in wheat flour. The study of nutrigenomics will help us understand how particular substances in functional foods, such as tomatoes or green tea, influence various chronic diseases. In the future, a young man may seek information from a genetic screening service about variations in his genetic code that will increase his risk of chronic disease and then take this report to his health professional who will use computer software to generate personalized dietary advice to help avoid these conditions.[21] Currently, we are able to make general recommendations regarding disease prevention for individuals whose family history or medical diagnoses put them at risk, but we still have a lot to learn before we can prepare individualized diets based on one's genetic code. Consumers should avoid commercial companies that offer genetic screening and are not associated with a legitimate health care facility.[22]

Nutrition Misinformation

Consumer surveys indicate that the majority of Americans (91%) believe they have some control over their health, and 72% believe that food and nutrition play the greatest role.[23] However, 75% of consumers rely on media outlets including the Internet as their major sources of health and nutrition information, and only half use medical sources.[24] A Google search for "nutrition listservs" yielded over 100,000 sites,[25] but it is likely that many of these writings are not reviewed by nutrition experts. Internet sites marketing herbs, drugs, and health devices are not monitored by government regulatory agencies and often contain misleading information. Reputable food companies provide helpful facts about the nutrient content of their products, but commercial sites devoted to sales often post misleading health claims. Internet sites maintained by government agencies, universities, state extension services, and medical facilities provide evidence-based information and should be the first source for public information on foods, nutrition, and health. At the close of each chapter in this text is a list of recommended websites for consumers or health professionals seeking additional information.

THE SCIENCE OF NUTRITION

Nutrition builds on two areas of science. The life sciences of biochemistry and physiology tell us how nutrition relates to our physical health and body function. The behavioral sciences help us understand how nutrition is interwoven with our psychosocial needs. Both aspects are at work in our lives.

Human organisms are highly complex groupings of chemical compounds constantly at work in an array of reactions that sustain life. Nutrients participate in and help control these chemical reactions. Various physiologic systems integrate the activities of millions of functioning cells, uniting them into a functioning whole. This highly sensitive internal control is called homeostasis.

We also have social and emotional qualities rooted in our earliest awareness. Eating patterns and attitudes toward food develop over a lifetime based on the influences of our primary family and friends, ethnic or cultural group, community, nation, and world. How we perceive food, what we choose to eat, why we eat what we do, and the ways in which we eat are all integral to human nutrition.

Working Definitions

Nutrition means *to nourish* and encompasses the food people eat and how it enriches their lives physically, socially, and personally. From the moment of conception until death, an appropriate supply of food supports optimal growth and maturation and mental and physical well-being. Good nutrition promotes health and reduces the risk of adverse conditions ranging from low birth weight to obesity to cardiovascular disease. Food supplies the energy to carry out body functions, such as inhaling and exhaling, maintaining body temperature, and engaging in physical activity. Food also nourishes the human spirit. We all have our particular "soul foods," comfort foods that connect us to our family and provide a sense of psychological and emotional well-being.

To study nutrition, we need to define the terms that describe this body of knowledge and the health professionals who work within it. *Nutrition* refers to the food people eat and how it nourishes their bodies, whereas nutrition science defines the nutrient requirements for body maintenance, growth, activity, and reproduction. Dietetics is the health profession with primary responsibility for the practical application of nutrition science throughout the life cycle in health and disease. The registered dietitian (RD) or registered dietitian nutritionist (RDN) is the nutrition expert on the health care team, and in collaboration with the physician and nurse, carries the major responsibility for a patient's nutritional care. Public health nutritionists focus on disease prevention and oversee programs that serve high-risk groups in the community such as pregnant teens or older adults, assessing needs, and applying interventions. RDs cooperate with school nurses to teach weight-management classes for children and parents, assist day care providers in planning menus and snacks, or help clients at fitness centers improve their body composition or athletic performance.

Functions of Food and Nutrients

Food serves as the vehicle for bringing nutrients into the body; however, the specific chemical compounds and elements in food—the nutrients—are the substances the body needs. No one particular food or food combination is required to ensure health. The human race has survived for centuries on a wide variety of foods, depending on what was available and what the culture designated as appropriate. Approximately 50 nutrients are known to be essential to human life and health, although countless other elements and molecules are being studied and may be found to be essential. The identification of essential nutrients is especially important when developing liquid formulas for feeding critically ill patients.

Essential nutrients include the macronutrients (carbohydrates, fats, and proteins), the micronutrients (vitamins and minerals), and water. The macronutrients supply energy and build tissue, whereas the micronutrients, needed in much smaller amounts, form specialized structures and regulate body processes. Water is the additional and often-forgotten nutrient that sustains all life systems. The sum of all the chemical reactions occurring in the body that use nutrients is referred to as metabolism. The first section of this text defines the essential nutrients; later chapters describe how they participate in growth, maturation, aging, and diet interventions in health and disease.

Nutrients have three general functions, as follows:
1. To provide energy
2. To build and repair body tissues and structures
3. To regulate the metabolic processes that maintain homeostasis.

Energy

All three of the macronutrients—carbohydrate, fat, and protein—can be used for energy, although carbohydrate and fat are the preferred energy sources.

Carbohydrates. Dietary carbohydrates—starch and sugars—are the primary sources of fuel for heat and energy. Glucose, the breakdown product of dietary carbohydrate, is the energy currency of the body. *Glycogen* is the storage form of carbohydrate available for quick energy when glucose is needed. Each gram of carbohydrate when metabolized in the body yields 4 kilocalories (kcalories or kcal), known as its fuel factor. In a well-balanced diet for a healthy person, 45% to 65% of total kcalories come from carbohydrate.[26] The majority of these kcalories should be obtained from complex carbohydrates (starch), with a smaller amount from simple carbohydrates (sugars). Another form of complex carbohydrate, known as *fiber,* does not yield energy but has other important body functions. Although the general public uses the word *calorie* to refer to the energy value of food, nutritionists use the technical term *kilocalorie.* As noted later in this chapter, MyPlate (ChooseMyPlate .gov), the food guidance system developed for the general public, and the *Dietary Guidelines for Americans* use the term *calorie* when indicating the energy value of foods or meals.

Fats. Dietary fats from either animal or plant sources provide an alternate or storage form of energy. Fat is a more concentrated fuel than carbohydrate, with a fuel factor of 9, yielding 9 kcal/g. Most nutrition experts recommend that fats supply no more than 20% to 35% of total kcalories.[26] Fats contain the essential fatty acids required for life and health. Saturated fats are a less healthy form of fat; therefore, the majority of our fat intake should be unsaturated.

Proteins. The primary function of protein is tissue building, although it can be used for energy if needed. The body draws on dietary or tissue protein for energy when the fuel supply from carbohydrates and fats is not sufficient to meet body needs. Protein yields 4 kcal/g, making its fuel factor 4. Protein can provide 10% to 35% of total kcalories in a well-balanced diet for healthy people.[26]

Tissue Building and Repair

Protein is the primary nutrient for building and maintaining body tissues. Vitamins and minerals are used in smaller amounts in the structure of specialized tissues.

Protein. Proteins are broken down into amino acids, the building blocks for body growth and repair. Body tissues are constantly being broken down and rebuilt to ensure growth and maintenance of body structure. Proteins also form vital substances such as enzymes and hormones that regulate body systems.

Minerals. Minerals help build tissues with very specific functions. The major minerals—calcium and phosphorus—give strength to bones and teeth. The trace element iron is a component of hemoglobin and binds oxygen for transport to cells and carbon dioxide for return to the lungs.

KEY TERMS

nutrigenomics The study of the effects of nutrients and other bioactive substances found in food on genes, body proteins, and metabolites.

nutrigenetics The study of the effect of an individual's particular genetic make-up on metabolic and physiologic functions, including nutrient requirements and risk of certain diseases.

homeostasis State of dynamic equilibrium within the body's internal environment, a balance achieved through the control of various interrelated physiologic mechanisms.

nutrition The sum of the processes involved in taking in food, releasing the nutrients it contains, and assimilating and using these nutrients to provide energy and maintain body tissue.

nutrition science The body of scientific knowledge developed through controlled research that relates to all aspects of nutrition—national, international, community, and clinical.

dietetics The science related to the nutritional planning and preparation of foods and diets.

registered dietitian (RD) or registered dietitian nutritionist (RDN) A health professional who has completed an accredited academic program and a minimum of 1200 hours of postbaccalaureate-supervised practice and has passed the National Registration Examination for Dietitians administered by the Commission on Dietetic Registration of the Academy of Nutrition and Dietetics.

public health nutritionist A health professional who has completed an academic program in nutrition and a graduate degree (MPH or DrPH) in a school of public health accredited by the Council on Education for Public Health, and supervises the nutrition component of public health programs in county, state, national, or international community settings.

nutrients Substances in food that are essential for energy, growth, normal body function, and maintenance of life.

essential nutrients Substances that cannot be made by the body and must be supplied in food. These include essential fatty acids, essential amino acids for making protein, vitamins, and minerals.

macronutrients The three energy-yielding nutrients: carbohydrate, fat, and protein.

carbohydrate Nutrient class that includes starch, sugar, and fiber; starch should be the major source of energy in the diet; sugar and starch have a fuel factor of 4 kcal/g; fiber is an indigestible form of carbohydrate.

fat Nutrient providing a concentrated form of energy (yields 9 kcal/g); stored in the body as adipose tissue as an energy reserve; supplies essential fatty acids in the diet.

protein Nutrient that contains nitrogen and essential amino acids; amino acids serve as building blocks for forming body tissues, enzymes, and hormones; fuel factor is 4 kcal/g.

micronutrients The two classes of non-energy-yielding elements and compounds—minerals and vitamins; these nutrients regulate and control cell metabolism and are components of specialized body structures.

metabolism The sum of all the biochemical and physiologic processes by which the body grows and maintains itself (anabolism), breaks down and reshapes tissue (catabolism), and transforms energy to do its work. Products of these reactions are called *metabolites*.

fuel factors The number of kcalories that 1 g of a nutrient yields when completely oxidized; the fuel factor is 4 for carbohydrate and protein, 9 for fat, and 7 for alcohol. Fuel factors are used in computing the energy values of foods and diets (e.g., 10 g of fat yields 90 kcal).

Vitamins. Vitamins are complex molecules needed in very minute amounts but are essential in certain tissues. Vitamin C produces the intercellular ground substance that cements tissues together and prevents tissue bleeding. Vitamin A in the rods and cones of the eye is needed for vision in dim light.

Metabolic Regulation

Specific vitamins and minerals are necessary for enzyme activities responsible for a host of chemical reactions. Water provides the appropriate environment for these reactions to occur.

Minerals. Minerals serve as cofactors in controlling cell metabolism. One example is iron, which controls the enzyme actions in the cell mitochondria that produce and store high-energy compounds.

Vitamins. Many vitamins are components of cell enzyme systems. They govern reactions that produce energy and synthesize important molecules. For example, thiamin controls the release of energy for cell work and vitamin B_{12} is needed for the synthesis and maturation of red blood cells.

Water. Water forms the blood, lymph, and intercellular fluids that transport nutrients to cells and remove waste. Water also functions as a regulatory agent, providing the fluid environment in which all metabolic reactions take place.

Nutrient Interrelationships

An important principle in nutrition is *nutrient interaction*. It has the following two parts:

1. Individual nutrients participate in many different metabolic functions; for some functions a nutrient has a primary role, and for others, it has a supporting role.
2. No nutrient ever works alone.

Intimate and ongoing metabolic relationships exist among all the nutrients and their metabolites. Although we look at each nutrient individually to simplify our study, they do not exist that way in the body. Nutrients are always working together within an integrated whole, providing energy, building and rebuilding tissue, and regulating metabolic activities. This synergy and interaction among nutrients is important in carrying out body functions and is sometimes overlooked when we examine the effects of one nutrient at a time.[27]

Nutritional Status

The nutritional health of an individual is known as his or her *nutritional status* and describes how well nutrient needs are being met. Nutritional status is influenced by living situation, social and economic factors, available food, food choices, and state of health. *Nutritional status* differs from *dietary status*. Evaluating nutritional status requires a combination of dietary, biochemical, **anthropometric**, and clinical measurements (Box 1-2), whereas dietary status focuses only on what foods are being consumed and their nutrient content. It is important to know not only what an individual is eating, but also whether the body is absorbing and making use of those nutrients. This helps us distinguish between a *primary nutrient deficiency* and a *secondary nutrient deficiency*. A primary nutrient deficiency is caused by insufficient dietary intake of a particular nutrient or nutrients. A secondary nutrient deficiency is the result of poor absorption or metabolism of a nutrient caused by an interfering substance, a disease or condition, or an elevated requirement. Blood nutrient levels can help identify a nutrient deficiency or a nutrient excess brought about by overuse of highly fortified foods or dietary supplements, although this is not true for all nutrients. Body weight for height and other anthropometric measurements provide estimates of the proportion of body fat versus lean body mass. An evaluation of nutritional status usually includes related conditions associated with food and nutrient intake, such as diabetes and obesity, or osteoporosis and calcium.[28] Clinical and biochemical parameters included in a nutritional assessment are discussed in detail in Chapter 16; however, when describing the individual nutrients we will refer to the current status of the U.S. population based on the methods listed in Box 1-2.

Optimal Nutrition

Individuals with optimal nutritional status have neither a deficiency nor an excess of nutrients. Nutrient stores are at the upper end of the normal range. Evidence of optimal nutrition includes appropriate weight for height and good muscle development and tone. The skin is smooth, and the eyes are clear and bright. Appetite, digestion, and elimination are normal. Well-nourished persons are more likely to be alert, both mentally and physically. They are not only meeting their day-to-day needs, but also maintaining appropriate nutrient stores to resist disease and support body function in times of stress.

Undernutrition

Undernutrition takes various forms ranging from marginal nutritional status to the emaciated famine victim. Persons with *marginal nutritional status* are meeting their minimum day-to-day nutritional needs but lack the nutrient stores to cope with any added physiologic or metabolic demand arising from injury or illness, pregnancy, or growth spurt. Marginal nutritional status results from poor eating habits, stressful environments, or insufficient resources to obtain appropriate types or amounts of food.

Current U.S. food trends add to the risk of marginal nutritional status or undernutrition among all age groups. Money spent for food away from home has increased, while money spent for food eaten at home has decreased by almost half.[29] Meals away from home, especially those obtained at fast-food restaurants, tend to be high in fat, sodium, and added sugar, but limited in calcium, fiber, whole grains, fruits, and green, yellow, and orange vegetables. Foods contributing the most kcalories to the diets of persons ages 2 and over are grain-based desserts (cookies, cake, doughnuts, and granola bars), followed by yeast breads, chicken and chicken-mixed dishes, sugar-sweetened soft drinks, and pizza.[29] Sugar-sweetened soft drinks and fruit drinks supply almost half of the added sugar in the U.S. diet, and sugar intakes are $2\frac{1}{2}$ times higher than recommended in the 2010 *Dietary Guidelines for Americans*. Added sugar contributes 316 kcal per day to the average diet and is believed by some nutrition experts to be a major contributor to the obesity epidemic and rise in type 2 diabetes.[30] Despite an abundance of kcalories, most Americans are deficient in calcium, vitamin D, fiber, and potassium.[29]

Public health nutritionists describe the American diet as energy rich but nutrient poor. Although persons with less-than-optimal intakes of micronutrients may not suffer from overt malnutrition, they are at greater risk of physical illness than those who are well nourished. The body can

---

BOX 1-2   USEFUL MEASUREMENTS FOR EVALUATING NUTRITIONAL STATUS

Dietary Intake
- Where and when food is eaten
- Use of dietary or nutritional supplements
- Money available for food and other food resources
- Special diet, if any
- Facilities for cooking and storing food

Biochemical Measurements
- Blood protein levels
- Blood lipid levels
- Blood vitamin levels

Anthropometric Measurements (Body Measurements)
- Body weight for height (body mass index)
- Skinfold thicknesses
- Waist circumference

Clinical Evaluation
- Skin
- Hair
- Eyes

KEY TERMS

amino acid   An acid containing the essential element nitrogen in the chemical group NH_2. Amino acids are the structural units of protein and the building blocks of body tissue.

synthesize   The action of forming new compounds in the body for use in building tissues or carrying out metabolic or physiologic functions.

metabolites   Any substance produced by metabolism or by a metabolic process.

anthropometric   Measurement of the human body to determine height, weight, skinfold thickness, or other dimensions that help to estimate the relative proportion of body fat and body muscle; these measurements are used to evaluate health status and risk of chronic disease.

adapt to marginal nutrient intake but any added physiologic stress that calls on nutrient stores will result in overt malnutrition.

Overt Malnutrition

When nutrient intake is insufficient to meet day-to-day needs and nutrient stores are depleted, signs of malnutrition begin to appear. Limited-resource individuals and families often have diets lacking in food quantity or quality. When asked about their food supply, approximately 14.9% of U.S. households (17.9 million) reported some level of food insecurity during the preceding 12 months, meaning they were uncertain of having or being able to acquire a sufficient amount of food for all members of their family.[31] Single-parent families, families with incomes below the poverty line, and African-American and Hispanic families are most at risk. Even if energy needs are met, foods high in micronutrients—fruits, vegetables, and whole grains—may not be accessible based on the money available[32] or location of stores that offer healthy and affordable options.[33]

Hunger influences the health of all ages and sexes, but the most vulnerable are infants, children, pregnant women, and older adults. Toddlers from families that are food insecure are more likely to have only fair or poor health, be at greater risk of hospitalization for health problems, or show deficits in cognitive development.[34,35] Children with chronically inadequate diets often develop iron-deficiency anemia, with reduced resistance to infection and low energy. Women who are poorly nourished in pregnancy are more likely to have a low-birth-weight infant. Homeless and limited-resource families have low intakes of fruits and vegetables that supply important micronutrients,[36] and these foods are in short supply at many food pantries.[37]

Malnutrition also exists among hospitalized patients and residents of long-term care facilities. Both prescription and over-the-counter medications can diminish appetite or interfere with the absorption of nutrients that are consumed. Tests or surgery requiring a prior period of fasting interfere with meals and food intake. Hypermetabolic diseases such as congestive heart failure or cancer increase energy requirements and lead to nutrient depletion and weight loss. Cytokines, secreted by the immune system in response to infection and chronic disease, interfere with the efficient use of nutrients, resulting in loss of body protein, loss of body weight, and impaired nutritional status if illness is prolonged. Among older adults, even aggressive nutrition intervention cannot always reverse these negative effects.[38]

Overnutrition

Overnutrition takes various forms. Excessive energy intake coupled with low physical activity leads to unwanted weight gain and elevated health risks for conditions such as metabolic syndrome.[39] Overnutrition also occurs with excessive intakes of micronutrients from overuse of dietary supplements. Inappropriate amounts of particular vitamins or minerals damage tissues and interfere with the absorption and metabolism of other essential nutrients. Herbal preparations, growing in popularity, carry the potential for harmful interactions with nutrients or medications.

Nutrient Density

A major factor in nutritional health is the *nutrient density* of the diet. This term refers to the relative nutrient content of a food in relation to its energy content. A nutrient-dense food contributes vitamins, minerals, essential fatty acids, and/or protein to the diet in addition to kcalories. A food that is not nutrient dense adds kcalories but lacks other nutrients. As described in Table 1-1, a hamburger made from lean ground beef supplies protein and many vitamins and minerals, although it adds some fat. Fruits and vegetables high in vitamins and minerals and low in kcalories are nutrient dense. In contrast, a doughnut high in kcalories adds primarily

TABLE 1-1	NUTRIENT DENSITY OF VARIOUS FOODS* BLUE DOTS INDICATE AT LEAST 10% OF THE DRI; RED DOTS EQUAL 50% OR MORE OF THE DRI[†]					
	ORANGE JUICE (1 cup)	GLAZED DOUGHNUT 3-IN DIAM (1)	BEEF PATTY PAN BROILED (3 oz)	BAKED BEANS CANNED, NO SALT ADDED (1 cup)	SWEET POTATO, CANNED, MASHED (1/2 cup)	MILK—1% FAT (1 cup)
Kcalories	117	192	197	266	124	118
Fat (g)	—	10	12	1	<1	3
Protein	—	—	♦	♦	—	♦
Fiber	—	—	—	♦	♦	—
Vitamin A	—	—	—	—	♦	♦
Vitamin C	♦	—	—	—	♦	—
Folate	♦	—	—	♦	—	—
Vitamin B₆	♦	—	♦	♦	♦	♦
Calcium	♦ (if fortified)[‡]	—	—	♦	—	♦
Iron	—	—	♦	♦	♦	—

Source: U.S. Department of Agriculture, Agricultural Research Service: USDA National Nutrient Database for Standard Reference, Release 26, 2013. Nutrient Data Laboratory Home Page: <http://www.ars.usda.gov/nutrientdata>.
*Calculations based on DRI values for men ages 19 to 50
[†]Foods supplying at least 10% of the DRI are considered a good source of that nutrient
[‡]Orange juice is not a good source of calcium unless this nutrient has been added

sugar and fat, and sugar-sweetened soft drinks add only kcal-ories. These foods we consider to be "empty calories" as they contribute no essential nutrients. Many Americans who are overweight or obese exhibit undernutrition because the foods they consume are not nutrient dense.

NUTRITION POLICY AND NATIONAL HEALTH PROBLEMS

Diet, Health, and Public Policy

Public policy refers to the laws, regulations, and government programs surrounding a certain topic. Nutrition policies are concerned with food guidance for the public, nutrition stan-dards for government food programs, and the health and well-being of the population. Recently, nutrition policy has focused on obesity and related chronic disease. In Chapter 9 we will discuss food safety regulations and nutrition labeling, which are other examples of public policy.

Development of Nutrition Policy

Until about 1950, government policies and programs were intended to eradicate hunger and malnutrition. Nutrient deficiency diseases such as rickets and pellagra still existed in various regions of the United States. A law passed in the 1930s mandated the addition of vitamin D to milk as a measure against rickets, and the enrichment of grains with thiamin, riboflavin, niacin, and iron began sometime later to address the problems of pellagra and anemia. The development of the School Nutrition Program with policies for free and reduced-cost lunches was a response to existing hunger among chil-dren and adolescents. By the 1980s, however, the focus had shifted to overnutrition as new research linked dietary habits to the growing prevalence of cardiovascular disease. Congres-sional committees began to discuss the role of government in setting dietary guidelines to improve health.

The first major policy report issued by the U.S. govern-ment linking nutrition and chronic disease was the *Surgeon General's Report on Nutrition and Health*[40] released in 1988. This report established the connection between the typical American diet high in fat and salt and morbidity and early death from cardiovascular disease. In 1989 the Food and Nutrition Board of the Institute of Medicine issued another extensive report, *Diet and Health: Implications for Reducing Chronic Disease Risk.*[41] Their conclusions agreed with the Surgeon General and people were advised to (1) reduce total fat to 30% or less of total kcalories, (2) reduce saturated fat and cholesterol, (3) increase fiber and complex carbohy-drates, (4) avoid excessive sodium and protein, and (5) main-tain appropriate levels of calcium.

Healthy People 2020

In 1990, the United States Department of Health and Human Services (USDHHS) introduced the public health initiative Healthy People 2000 that established science-based, national objectives for promoting health. These objectives are updated every 10 years using a process that invites input from both health professionals and consumers and builds on the progress made in the decade prior.[42] Healthy People 2020 includes many nutrition-related goals pertaining to dietary intake, maternal and child health, and management of chronic disease (see examples in Box 1-3).[43,44] The Healthy People 2020 website contains the current status, projected goal, and ideas for related community programs for each objective.[43]

HEALTH PROMOTION

Healthy People 2020,[42] the National Institutes of Health,[45] and nonprofit health groups such as the American Heart Associa-tion[46] are encouraging population approaches to health pro-motion to reach more people with important health messages. Such approaches include the use of media such as public service announcements and newspapers, package labeling, school programs, worksite programs, and community

> **BOX 1-3 EXAMPLES OF NUTRITION-RELATED TARGETS FROM HEALTHY PEOPLE 2020***
>
> - Increase the contribution of total vegetables to the diets of individuals aged 2 and older from 0.8 cups equivalent per 1000 calories to 1.1 cups equivalent per 1000 calories.
> - Reduce consumption of calories from added sugars from 15.7% of total calories to 10.8% of total calories in the diets of individuals aged 2 and older.
> - Increase the proportion of infants who are breast-fed at 6 months from 43.5% to 60.6%.
> - Reduce the proportion of U.S. households reporting **food insecurity** from 14.6% to 6.0%.
> - Reduce the proportion of adults aged 18 years and older with hypertension from 30% to 27% (10% reduction).

Data from United States Department of Health and Human Services: *Healthy People 2020: 2020 Topics and Objectives,* Washington, D.C., 2013, U.S. Department of Health and Human Services. at: <http://www.healthypeople.gov/2020/default.aspx>. Accessed on August 19, 2013.
*Baseline levels estimated from available government surveys and statistics

> **KEY TERMS**
> **food insecurity** Households that at times during the previ-ous year were uncertain of having enough food or were unable to acquire enough food to meet the needs of all their members because they had insufficient money or other resources for food
> **anemia** A condition of abnormally low blood hemoglobin level caused by too few red blood cells or red blood cells with low hemoglobin content
> **nutrient dense** Term used to describe a food that is a good source of at least one essential nutrient as well as providing kcalories
> **empty calories** Term used to describe foods high in kcalo-ries that are sources of solid fats, added sugar, or alcohol but low in essential nutrients

programs sponsored by local coalitions, health facilities, and other health groups. The most effective community programs involve several activities that reach a broad base of consumers and reinforce the messages in various ways. Several of the Healthy People 2020 objectives pertain to childhood obesity, and schools are well positioned to reach children and families with in-school and after-school activities.

A comprehensive school program could include the school nutrition program, school nurse, teachers, parents, parent-teachers association, and local health care professionals as follows:

- *School food service:* Review menus to conform to current guidelines limiting fat, sodium, and sugar, and emphasize fruits, vegetables and whole grains; offer fruit or cereal-based treats for dessert; provide fresh fruit as a snack.
- *School art department:* Sponsor a student contest for posters or displays that "advertise" healthy cafeteria options or encourage students to drink water rather than sugar-sweetened beverages.
- *School health/physical education curriculum:* Discuss healthy eating and ways to limit kcalorie intake if you are gaining unwanted weight; support physical activities that are feasible for students who are obese; set up an after-school walking club.
- *Parent/teacher organization:* Have a local health professional speak about childhood overweight and intervention strategies; review fund-raising policies and determine whether sales items or vending machine contents are in balance with child obesity prevention.
- Engage the local hospital or health groups in sponsoring a walking event for the community at large with emphasis on "getting in the game" rather than how far or how fast a participant can walk. Make step counters available to encourage continued walking.

Health promotion must be ongoing and advance a consistent message across the community. Programs are most successful if they stress specific goals relating to food or activity, rather than overall healthy living.[46] Just as poor eating and activity patterns develop over time, so must intervention be a continuing process. As a health professional, look for other programs and individuals with similar goals with whom you can partner to maximize your impact on community health.[47] (We will learn more about organizing community interventions in Chapter 10.)

NUTRITION GUIDES FOR FOOD SELECTION

For the past 100 years government agencies have been issuing food guides to help Americans meet their nutritional needs. The underlying assumptions have been influenced by emerging nutrition science, as well as social, political, and economic events, including wars and national emergencies. Their focus also shifted from preventing undernutrition to controlling chronic diseases related to overnutrition. These guides are of three types: (1) nutrition standards, (2) dietary guidelines, and (3) food guides. Each has a different purpose and target audience.

Nutrition Standards
Dietary Reference Intakes

Most countries have standards for nutrient intakes of healthy people according to age and sex. Health professionals use these standards in making decisions about the nutritional health of individuals and groups. In the U.S., these nutrient and energy standards are called the Dietary Reference Intakes (DRIs), and include several categories of recommendations.[48] Each category within the DRIs has a different purpose and use for the health professional. Each of these terms is described below:

- *Dietary Reference Intakes (DRIs):* The U.S. framework of nutrient standards that provide reference values for use in planning and evaluating diets for healthy people. The DRIs include the recommended dietary allowance, the adequate intake, the tolerable upper intake level, and the estimated average requirement.
- *Recommended Dietary Allowance (RDA):* The average daily intake of a nutrient that will meet the requirement of 97% to 98% (or two standard deviations of the mean) of healthy people of a given age and sex. The RDAs were established and are reviewed periodically by an expert panel of nutrition scientists; they are amended as needed based on new research findings. RDAs have been set for carbohydrate, protein, essential fatty acids, and most vitamins and minerals. When planning diets the RDA serves as an intake goal.
- *Adequate Intake (AI):* A suggested daily intake of a nutrient to meet body needs and support health. The AI is used when there is not sufficient research available to develop an RDA but the nutrient appears to have a strong health benefit. The AI serves as a guide for intake when planning diets.
- *Tolerable Upper Intake Level (UL):* The highest amount of a nutrient that can be consumed safely with no risk of toxicity or adverse effects. The UL is used to evaluate the nutrient content of dietary supplements or review total nutrient intake from food and supplements. Intakes exceeding the UL usually result from concentrated supplements, not food.
- *Estimated Average Requirement (EAR):* The average daily intake of a nutrient that will meet the requirement of 50% of healthy people of a given age and sex. The EAR is used to plan and evaluate the nutrient intakes of groups rather than individuals.
- *Acceptable Macronutrient Distribution Range (AMDR):* The AMDR guides the division of kcalories among carbohydrate, fat, and protein in ranges supportive of health; carbohydrate should provide 45% to 65% of total kcalories, fat should provide 20% to 35% of total kcalories, and protein should provide 10% to 35% of total kcalories.

The DRIs for vitamins, minerals, and macronutrients can be found on the inside front cover and first page of this text. Note there are two age categories for persons over age 50, directing our attention to the changes in nutrient requirements as we age.

The first set of DRIs, replacing earlier RDAs, was released in 1997. They provided new standards for calcium, phosphorus, magnesium, and vitamin D and emphasized the role of these nutrients in bone health.[49] Since then, DRIs have been established for the B-complex vitamins (1998)[50]; antioxidant nutrients and carotenoids (2000)[51]; vitamins A and K and the trace minerals (2001)[52]; energy, the energy-yielding macronutrients, and fiber (2002)[26]; and electrolytes and water (2004).[53] The DRIs for calcium and vitamin D were revised again in 2010, based on new evidence indicating increased needs for bone health.[54]

The nutrient standards of Canada and Great Britain are similar to those of the U.S. Developing countries use standards set by the United Nations Food and Agriculture Organization (FAO).

Dietary Guidelines

Dietary guidelines are the second type of nutrition guide. First published in 1980, the *Dietary Guidelines for Americans* (DGA) expressed the growing concerns of government agencies about the health of the American people. The *Dietary Guidelines* (1) provide the basis for nutrition messages and consumer materials developed by government agencies, and (2) give direction to government programs involving food and nutrition, such as Head Start, school meals, and nutrition programs for older adults. By law the *Guidelines* are updated every 5 years and represent a cooperative effort between the USDHHS, the federal agency concerned with health, and the U.S. Department of Agriculture (USDA), the federal agency concerned with food. For each update an advisory panel of experts is charged with the responsibility of reviewing the current guidelines and identifying needed changes based on new nutrition science or population needs.[55]

The Advisory Committee appointed to develop the *Dietary Guidelines* released in 2010 was presented with a differing environment from committees of past years and developed the following approaches to their task[56]:

- *Health status of the U.S. population*: The health status of the American public has deteriorated. Barely one third of adults are normal weight and type 2 diabetes is reaching epidemic proportions. Although kcalorie intake has been relatively stable over the past 10 years,[57] the majority of the population is low in several important nutrients.[29] Thus, the 2010 *Guidelines* were prepared for an unhealthy American public as compared to previous editions directed toward all healthy persons ages 2 and over.
- *Use of evidence-based research*: The 2010 Advisory Committee relied on the most current scientific and medical research available that they accessed through a Web-based electronic system known as the Nutrition Evidence Library (NEL). Maintained by the USDA, the NEL provides a framework for experts to evaluate the amount and type of research available on a particular topic and see how it was carried out.[58,59] The dietary recommendations the Advisory Committee developed using the NEL were based on studies with real people who had benefited from the interventions described. (Visit the NEL website at www.nel.gov and see the Evidence-Based Practice box, "Evidence-Based Practice: How Do I Use It?" to learn more about this concept.)

- *Focus on the total diet*: The 2010 *Guidelines* help people integrate energy and nutrient recommendations into an overall food pattern that meets their cultural, religious, and personal preferences.[29] Diet patterns include the Mediterranean diet (associated with lower risk of cardiovascular disease), the DASH diet (Dietary Approaches to Stop Hypertension), and lacto-ovo-vegetarian and vegan patterns that meet nutrient needs.[60] Consumers are urged to take responsibility for what they eat: read labels, ask questions when eating out, and choose wholesome ingredients when cooking at home. Learning to cook and preparing more of their own food enables individuals to better control their fat, sodium, and kcalories.
- *Balance between energy intake and physical activity*: The 2010 *Dietary Guidelines*, along with the 2008 *Physical Activity Guidelines for Americans*, emphasize daily physical activity and encourage parents to plan family events that reflect active living.[61]
- *Partnerships between health professionals, government agencies, food processors, and community leaders*: Adoption of healthy food practices by the American public will require a change in the food environment at home, at school, at the workplace, and in the community.[29] Consumers need access to fresh produce and healthy choices when eating away from home. Food processors must review the kcalorie, sugar, solid fat, and sodium content of their packaged foods.[29,62] Community leaders must consider the locations of sidewalks, trails, and parks that provide accommodations for walking and other physical activity. We must develop a plan to enable all Americans to eat well, be physically active, and maintain good health and function.

2010 Dietary Guidelines Recommendations

A complete summary of the 2010 *DGA* recommendations are found in Box 1-4, but several important dietary concepts are described below:

1. Substitute lower calorie, nutrient-dense foods for refined grains and snack foods high in solid fat and sugar (SoFAS). Move to a more plant-based diet by adding fruits, vegetables, whole grains, peas, and beans. These foods, along with fat-free, low-fat, or reduced-fat dairy products, will raise intakes of potassium, calcium, fiber, and vitamin D, now inadequate in many American diets.[29]
2. The minerals sodium and potassium are known to have opposite effects on blood pressure, with potassium blunting the blood-pressure-raising effect of sodium. The 2005 *DGA*[63] recommended a sodium intake of no more than 2300 mg/day (the UL for sodium) for the general population, but noted that hypertensive individuals, African Americans, and middle-aged and older individuals would benefit from reducing their intakes to 1500 mg/day or less (the AI for sodium). Because these groups now

EVIDENCE-BASED PRACTICE

How Do I Use It?

How will you, as a practicing professional, seek out information when developing a nutrition care plan for your patient? Will it be based on what you learned in clinical rotations or what has been the long-term protocol in your facility, or what you learned in your nutrition class? Over time, new evidence becomes available and new practice standards are developed. How do you stay up-to-date on new findings?

The new paradigm in health care is evidence-based practice: using current research and published findings to make appropriate decisions. Successful evidence-based practice requires that you keep current on new standards of practice, carry out planned protocols to evaluate new methods or programs, and share your outcomes with others.

Evidence-based practice is a three-step process, as follows:

- *Identify the problem:* What is the question that you need to answer? Are you developing a new treatment protocol and need some guidance? Are you planning a community health education program and want to learn how you can evaluate it? Do you need some new ideas on how to motivate pregnant teens to consume a healthy diet?
- *Review the evidence:* Search for studies in your professional journals that address this question and critically evaluate what you find. How many patients or clients participated? What was the time period of the study? What types of information did the researchers collect? Were the research participants and circumstances similar to yours? Based on the outcomes of the studies you find, are there some things that you will try to do differently to achieve a better outcome?
- *Implement the findings:* Following your review of the existing information, develop and implement a plan for your patients or group. Be sure to include an evaluation component so that you can rate the outcome and success of your plan. When you have completed your project and compiled your results, share them with other professionals at your facility and at local or state professional meetings. Was your plan successful or what would you do differently next time? We all learn from each other, and sometimes an intervention that was not successful can help others avoid similar outcomes.

Nutrition and health experts have developed formal systems for evaluating research evidence. Evidence may be rated as good or strong, fair, limited, or supported only by opinion. These rating scales are used in review articles published in professional journals and on reputable websites maintained by government agencies and professional societies. Make use of these systems in your decision-making process.

Examples of evidence-based approaches to nutrition and health issues are as follows:

Academy of Nutrition and Dietetics: Position paper of the Academy of Nutrition and Dietetics: use of nutritive and non-nutritive sweeteners. *J Acad Nutr Diet* 112(5):739, 2012.

National Institutes of Health, Office of Dietary Supplements: *Herbs at a Glance.* 2012. at: <http://nccam.nih.gov/health/herbsataglance.htm>. Accessed on February 13, 2013.

United States Department of Agriculture: *Nutrition Evidence Library.* 2013. at: <www.nel.gov>. Accessed on February 13, 2013.

Van Horn L, McCoin M, Kris-Etherton PM, et al: The evidence for dietary prevention and treatment of cardiovascular disease. *J Am Diet Assoc* 108:287, 2008.

Bibliography

Gray GE, Gray LK: Evidence-based medicine: applications in dietetic practice. *J Am Diet Assoc* 102:1263, 2002.

Laramee SH: Evidence-based practice: a core competency for dietetics. *J Am Diet Assoc* 105:333, 2005.

Vaughan LA, Manning CK: Meeting the challenges of dietetic practice with evidence-based decisions. *J Am Diet Assoc* 104:282, 2004.

comprise a major proportion of U.S. adults, the Advisory Committee recommended a goal of 1500 mg/day of sodium for the general population. However, given the current high sodium content of food in the marketplace and the taste perception of the general public, the decrease from 2300 mg to 1500 mg will need to occur gradually over time. Because blood pressure-related atherosclerotic disease begins in childhood, both children and adults must lower their sodium intake.[29]

3. All population groups are encouraged to consume two servings of seafood each week to obtain important fatty acids, selecting from fish low in mercury content.

Note that many of the dietary recommendations of 2010, along with goals for physical activity, promote heart health,[64] and if implemented can reduce the prevalence of overweight and chronic disease.

To provide consumers with practical advice that they can use every day, USDA has developed seven short messages that summarize the important concepts of the 2010 *Dietary Guidelines* (Box 1-5). These messages are part of an ongoing multimedia publicity campaign by state and local agencies, so watch for them in your community.

Food Guides

Food guides are intended to help individuals with day-to-day meal planning. They provide a practical interpretation of nutrition standards and dietary guidelines that are useful in daily food selection. Most food guides group foods based on their nutrient content and recommend a certain number of servings from each group. The most commonly used food group guides are the USDA MyPlate (ChooseMyPlate.gov), developed to accompany the 2010 *Dietary Guidelines for Americans,* and *Choose Your Foods: Food Lists for Diabetes* from the American Diabetes Association and the American Dietetic Association (now the Academy of Nutrition and Dietetics). These guides classify foods differently and serve different purposes.

BOX 1-4 DIETARY GUIDELINES FOR AMERICANS 2010—KEY RECOMMENDATIONS

Balancing Calories to Manage Weight

- Prevent and/or reduce overweight and obesity through improved eating and physical activity behaviors.
- Control total calorie intake to manage body weight. For people who are overweight or obese, this will mean consuming fewer calories from food and beverages.
- Increase physical activity and reduce time spent in sedentary behaviors.
- Maintain appropriate calorie balance through each stage of life: childhood, adolescence, adulthood, pregnancy and breast-feeding, and older age.

Foods and Food Components to Reduce

- Reduce daily sodium intake to less than 2300 milligrams (mg) and further reduce intake to 1500 mg among persons who are 51 and older and those of any age who are African American or have hypertension, diabetes, or chronic kidney disease. The 1500 mg recommendation applies to about half of the U.S. population, including children, and the majority of adults.
- Consume less than 10% of calories from saturated fatty acids by replacing them with monounsaturated and polyunsaturated fatty acids.
- Consume less than 300 mg per day of dietary cholesterol.
- Keep trans fatty acid consumption as low as possible by limiting foods that contain synthetic sources of trans fats, such as partially hydrogenated oils, and by limiting other solid fats.
- Reduce the intake of calories from solid fats and added sugars.
- Limit the consumption of foods that contain refined grains, especially foods that contain solid fats, added sugars, and sodium.
- If alcohol is consumed, it should be consumed in moderation—up to one drink per day for women and two drinks per day for men—and only by adults of legal drinking age.*

Foods and Nutrients to Increase

Individuals should meet the following recommendations as part of a healthy eating pattern while staying within their calorie needs.

- Increase vegetable and fruit intake.
- Eat a variety of vegetables, especially dark-green and red and orange vegetables and beans and peas.
- Include at least half of all grains as whole grains. Increase whole-grain intake by replacing refined grains with whole grains.

- Increase intake of fat-free or low-fat milk and milk products such as milk, yogurt, cheese, or fortified soy beverages.[†]
- Choose a variety of protein foods, which include seafood, lean meat and poultry, eggs, beans and peas, soy products, and unsalted nuts and seeds.
- Increase the amount and variety of seafood consumed by choosing seafood in place of some meat and poultry.
- Replace protein foods that are higher in solid fats with choices that are lower in solid fats and calories and/or are sources of oils.
- Use oils to replace solid fats where possible.
- Choose foods that provide more potassium, dietary fiber, calcium, and vitamin D, which are nutrients of concern in American diets. These foods include vegetables, fruits, whole grains, and milk and milk products.

Recommendations for Specific Population Groups

Women capable of becoming pregnant:

- Choose foods that contain heme iron, which is more readily absorbed by the body, additional iron sources, and enhancers of iron absorption, such as vitamin C-rich foods.[‡]
- Consume 400 micrograms (mcg) per day of synthetic folic acid (from fortified foods and/or supplements) in addition to food forms of folate from a varied diet.[§]

Women who are pregnant or breast-feeding:

- Consume 8 to 12 oz of seafood per week from a variety of seafood types.
- Due to their high methyl mercury content, limit white (albacore) tuna to 6 oz per week and do not eat the following four types of fish: tilefish, shark, sword fish, or king mackerel.
- If pregnant, take an iron supplement as recommended by an obstetrician or other health care provider.

Individuals age 50 years and older:

- Consume foods fortified with vitamin B_{12}, such as fortified cereals or dietary supplements.

Building Healthy Eating Patterns

- Select an eating pattern that meets nutrient needs over time at an appropriate calorie level.
- Account for all foods and beverages consumed and assess how they fit within a total healthy eating pattern.
- Follow food safety recommendations when preparing and eating foods to reduce the risk of foodborne illness.

Source: U.S. Department of Agriculture and U.S. Department of Health and Human Services: *Dietary Guidelines for Americans, 2010* (Policy Document), ed 7, Washington, D.C., 2010, U.S. Government Printing Office. Can be accessed at: <http://www.cnpp.usda.gov/DGAs2010 -PolicyDocument.htm>.
*Women who are pregnant or breast-feeding should refrain from drinking alcoholic beverages.
[†]Soy beverages includes products that may be marketed as soy milk.
[‡]Includes adolescent girls.
[§]"Folic acid" is the synthetic form of the nutrient whereas "folate" is the form found naturally in foods.

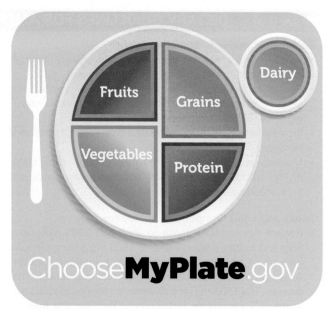

FIGURE 1-4 MyPlate (ChooseMyPlate.gov) The MyPlate food icon was developed by the USDA as part of an overall communication initiative to help consumers implement the 2010 *Dietary Guidelines for Americans*. MyPlate uses a familiar mealtime setting to remind us to eat healthfully and include appropriate amounts of each of the five food groups. (From U.S. Department of Agriculture, Center for Nutrition Policy and Promotion: *MyPlate [ChooseMyPlate.gov]*, Washington, D.C., 2010. from: <http://www.choosemyplate.gov>. Retrieved July 10, 2012.)

USDA Food Guides

The USDA issued its first food guide in the 1940s, and food guides evolved over time into various formats and shapes.[65] The Food Guide Pyramid, modified to MyPyramid in 2005, was the graphic used from 1992 to 2010 to encourage healthy eating.[66] Although the MyPyramid icon was recognized by the majority of Americans, it was viewed as complicated and difficult to interpret. The relative amount of food to be eaten from each food group was expressed by the width of that section of the pyramid. Consumer interviews, focus groups, and media articles established the need for a new icon that was simple and easy to put into action.[67]

MyPlate (ChooseMyPlate.gov)

MyPlate (Figure 1-4), the icon released in 2010, illustrates the five major food groups using a familiar mealtime visual—a place setting.[68] Food groups join foods with similar nutrient content, and to include more foods similar in nutrients, several food groups were renamed. The MyPyramid Meat and Beans group was renamed the Protein Group and the MyPyramid Milk group was renamed the Dairy group. The general themes of MyPlate (ChooseMyPlate.gov) are (1) eat smaller portions, and (2) choose lower calorie, nutrient-dense foods. Cover half of your plate with fruits and vegetables, add smaller amounts of protein foods and grains, and include a dairy food or similar calcium source. (Table 1-2 describes the nutrients supplied by each food group.)

In contrast to the MyPyramid graphic, which tried to include everything that consumers needed to know to select a healthy diet, MyPlate is intended to remind consumers to eat healthfully but is not expected to work alone in changing behavior.[68] The MyPlate icon is one piece of an overall communication initiative that includes easy-to-read fact sheets, daily meal plans, sample menus, recipes, and strategies for improving food intake (see www.ChooseMyPlate.gov). The interactive feature, SuperTracker, allows consumers to set personal goals and develop individualized daily food plans based on their age, sex, and level of physical activity.[69] Over 800,000 individuals became registered users of the SuperTracker within 6 months of its launch.[70]

Successful implementation of any food and activity plan as found on SuperTracker requires an understanding of serving size and physical activity levels, but both concepts are poorly understood by the general public. Consumers tend to think of a serving size as what they choose to eat[71] or "what I have on my plate," and this confusion contributes to weight gain.[72-74] MyPlate (ChooseMyPlate.gov) gives food amounts in household measures allowed at various kcalorie levels (Table 1-3). Each food plan defines the number of empty calories that can be used for solid fats, added sugars, or alcohol (if appropriate); however, these empty calories, based on age, sex, and physical activity are quite limited. Note that the 2000-kcal food plan (Figure 1-5) allows only 260 empty calories—the equivalent of two chocolate chip cookies.

Materials on the ChooseMyPlate.gov website offer advice on how to divide the ingredients of mixed dishes such as pizza into the appropriate food group portions. Consumers might be encouraged to measure their food servings for several meals to establish what standard serving sizes look

TABLE 1-2 — MAJOR NUTRIENTS SUPPLIED BY THE MYPLATE FOOD GROUPS

FOOD GROUP	MAJOR NUTRIENTS*	SERVING EQUIVALENTS
Fruits (color code red)	Vitamin C Folate Potassium Fiber	1 cup raw or cooked fruit or 1 cup 100% fruit juice or $\frac{1}{2}$ cup dried fruit equals 1 cup from the fruit group
Vegetables (color code green)	Vitamin A Vitamin C Vitamin E Vitamin B_6 Folate Potassium Fiber	1 cup raw or cooked vegetables or 1 cup vegetable juice or 2 cups raw leafy greens equal 1 cup from the vegetable group
Grains (color code deep orange) Enriched grains	Thiamin Riboflavin Niacin Folate Iron	1 slice of bread, 1 oz ready-to-eat cereal (about 1 cup cereal flakes), $\frac{1}{2}$ cup cooked rice, pasta, or cooked cereal, 1 tortilla (6-inch diameter) or 1 pancake (5-inch diameter) equals 1 oz from the grains group
Whole grains	Zinc, magnesium, and fiber in addition to the nutrients in enriched grains	
Protein foods (color code purple)	Protein Thiamin Riboflavin Niacin Vitamin B_6 Vitamin B_{12}† Iron Zinc Vitamin E (nuts)	1 oz lean meat, poultry, or seafood, 1 egg, 1 Tbsp peanut butter, $\frac{1}{4}$ cup cooked dry beans or peas, or $\frac{1}{2}$ oz nuts or seeds equals 1 oz from the protein foods group
Dairy (color code blue)	Protein Vitamin A Riboflavin Vitamin B_{12} Calcium Phosphorus Magnesium	1 cup milk, 1 cup yogurt, 1 cup fortified soy or rice beverage, $1\frac{1}{2}$ oz natural cheese (e.g., cheddar) or 2 oz processed cheese (e.g., American) equals 1 cup from the dairy group
Other important food components		
Oils (Not a food group but oils supply essential nutrients)	Vitamin E Linoleic acid‡ Alpha-linolenic acid‡	Includes vegetable, nut, and fish oils and soft vegetable oil table spreads that have no trans fats (Equivalents differ according to source)

Data from Dietary Guidelines Advisory Committee, 2005: *Report of the Dietary Guidelines Advisory Committee on the Dietary Guidelines for Americans 2005,* Beltsville, Md., 2004, U.S. Department of Agriculture, Agricultural Research Service, and U.S. Department of Agriculture and U.S. Department of Health and Human Services: *Dietary Guidelines for Americans, 2010* (Policy Document), ed 7, Washington, D.C., 2010, U.S. Government Printing Office.
*Each of the food groups is a major source of the nutrients listed but also adds smaller amounts of other nutrients to the daily diet.
†Vitamin B_{12} is found only in animal foods.
‡Linoleic acid and alpha-linolenic acid are the essential fatty acids.

TABLE 1-3 — USDA FOOD INTAKE PATTERNS FOR DIFFERENT CALORIE LEVELS

For all food groups and grain subgroups, amounts given represent average daily intake for that calorie level; for vegetable and protein subgroups amounts given represent intake per week at that calorie level. All foods are assumed to be nutrient dense and prepared without added fats, sugar, or salt. Solid fats and sugars may be added up to the calorie limit defined in the table.

CALORIE LEVEL	1000	1200	1400	1600	1800	2000	2200	2400	2600	2800	3000	3200
Fruits*	1 cup	1 cup	$1\frac{1}{2}$ cups	$1\frac{1}{2}$ cups	$1\frac{1}{2}$ cups	2 cups	2 cups	2 cups	2 cups	$2\frac{1}{2}$ cups	$2\frac{1}{2}$ cups	$2\frac{1}{2}$ cups
Vegetables†	1 cup	$1\frac{1}{2}$ cups	$1\frac{1}{2}$ cups	2 cups	$2\frac{1}{2}$ cups	$2\frac{1}{2}$ cups	3 cups	3 cups	$3\frac{1}{2}$ cups	$3\frac{1}{2}$ cups	4 cups	4 cups

Continued

TABLE 1-3   USDA FOOD INTAKE PATTERNS FOR DIFFERENT CALORIE LEVELS—cont'd

CALORIE LEVEL	1000	1200	1400	1600	1800	2000	2200	2400	2600	2800	3000	3200
Dark-green vegetables	½ cup/wk	1 cup/wk	1 cup/wk	1½ cups/wk	1½ cups/wk	1½ cups/wk	2 cups/wk	2 cup/wk	2½ cups/wk	2½ cups/wk	2½ cups/wk	2½ cups/wk
Red and orange vegetables	2½ cups/wk	3 cups/wk	3 cups/wk	4 cups/wk	5½ cups/wk	5½ cups/wk	6 cups/wk	6 cups/wk	7 cups.	7 cups/wk	7½ cups/wk	7½ cups/wk
Beans and peas (legumes)	½ cups/wk	½ cups/wk	½ cups/wk	1 cups/wk	1½ cups/wk	1½ cups/wk	2 cups/wk	2 cups/wk	2½ cups/wk	2½ cups/wk	3 cups/wk	3 cups/wk
Starchy vegetables	2 cups/wk	3½ cups/wk	3½ cups/wk	4 cups/wk	5 cups/wk	5 cups/wk	6 cups/wk	6 cups/wk	7 cups/wk	7 cups/wk	8 cups/wk	8 cups/wk
Other vegetables	1½ cups/wk	2½ cups/wk	2½ cups/wk	3½ cups/wk	4 cups/wk	4 cups/wk	5 cups/wk	5 cups/wk	5½ cups/wk	5½ cups/wk	7 cups/wk	7 cups/wk
Grains‡	3 oz-eq	4 oz-eq	5 oz-eq	5 oz-eq	6 oz-eq	6 oz-eq	7 oz-eq	8 oz-eq	9 oz-eq	10 oz-eq	10 oz-eq	10 oz-eq
Whole grains	1½ oz-eq	2 oz-eq	2½ oz-eq	3 oz-eq	3 oz-eq	3 oz-eq	3½ oz-eq	4 oz-eq	4½ oz-eq	5 oz-eq	5 oz-eq	5 oz-eq
Enriched grains	1½ oz-eq	2 oz-eq	2½ oz-eq	2 oz-eq	3 oz-eq	3 oz-eq	3½ oz-eq	4 oz-eq	4½ oz-eq	5 oz-eq	5 oz-eq	5 oz-eq
Protein foods§	2 oz-eq	3 oz-eq	4 oz-eq	5 oz-eq	5 oz-eq	5½ oz-eq	6 oz-eq	6½ oz-eq	6½ oz-eq	7 oz-eq	7 oz-eq	7 oz-eq
Seafood	3 oz/wk	5 oz/wk	6 oz/wk	8 oz/wk	8 oz/wk	8 oz/wk	9 oz/wk	10 oz/wk	10 oz/wk	11 oz/wk	11 oz/wk	11 oz/wk
Meat, poultry, eggs	10 oz/wk	14 oz/wk	19 oz/wk	24 oz/wk	24 oz/wk	26 oz/wk	29 oz/wk	31 oz/wk	31 oz/wk	34 oz/wk	34 oz/wk	34 oz/wk
Nuts, seeds, soy products	1 oz/wk	2 oz/wk	3 oz/wk	4 oz/wk	4 oz/wk	4 oz/wk	4 oz/wk	5 oz/wk	5 oz/wk	5 oz/wk	5 oz/wk	5 oz/wk
Dairy‖	2 cups	2½ cups	2½ cups	3 cups	3 cups	3 cups	3 cups	3 cups	3 cups	3 cups	3 cups	3 cups
Oils¶	15 g	17 g	17 g	22 g	24 g	27 g	29 g	31 g	34 g	36 g	44 g	51 g
Maximum SoFAS# Kcal (% of kcal)	137 (14%)	121 (10%)	121 (9%)	121 (8%)	161 (9%)	258 (13%)	266 (12%)	330 (14%)	362 (14%)	395 (14%)	459 (15%)	596 (19%)

Source: U.S. Department of Agriculture and U.S. Department of Health and Human Services: *Dietary Guidelines for Americans, 2010* (Policy Document), ed 7, Washington, D.C., 2010, U.S. Government Printing Office. Can be accessed at: <http://www.cnpp.usda.gov/DGAs2010-PolicyDocument.htm>.

*Fruits: All fresh, frozen, canned, and dried fruits and fruit juices, e.g., oranges and orange juice, apples and apple juice, bananas, grapes, berries, melon, raisins.

†Vegetables:
- Dark-green vegetables: All fresh, frozen, and canned dark-green leafy vegetables and broccoli, cooked or raw, e.g., broccoli; spinach; romaine; collard, turnip, and mustard greens.
- Red and orange vegetables: All fresh, frozen, and canned red and orange vegetables, cooked or raw, e.g., tomatoes, red peppers, carrots, sweet potatoes, winter squash, and pumpkin.
- Beans and peas (legumes): All cooked beans and peas, e.g., kidney beans, lentils, chickpeas, and pinto beans. Does not include green beans or green peas. (Also note listing under protein foods.)
- Starchy vegetables: All fresh, frozen, and canned starchy vegetables, e.g., white potatoes, corn, green peas.
- Other vegetables: All fresh, frozen, and canned other vegetables, cooked or raw, e.g., iceberg lettuce, green beans, and onions.

‡Grains
- All whole grains: All whole-grain products and whole grains used as ingredients, e.g., whole-wheat bread, whole-grain cereals and crackers, whole-grain pasta, oatmeal, and brown rice.
- Enriched grains: All enriched refined-grain products and enriched refined grains used as ingredients, e.g., white breads, enriched grain cereals and crackers, enriched pasta, white rice.

§Protein foods: All meat, poultry, seafood, eggs, nuts, seeds, and processed soy products. Meat and poultry should be lean and low-fat and nuts should be unsalted. Beans and peas are part of this group, as well as the vegetable group, but should be counted in one group only.

‖Dairy: All milks, including lactose-free and lactose-reduced products and fortified soy beverages, yogurt, frozen yogurt, dairy desserts, and cheese. Most choices should be fat-free or low-fat. Cream, sour cream, and cream cheese are not included due to their low calcium content.

¶Oils: All vegetable, nut, and fish oils and soft vegetable oil table spreads (margarine) that have no trans fats.

#SoFAS: Calories from solid fats and added sugars. The limit for SoFAS is the calories remaining in each food pattern after specifying the food amounts needed from each food group. SoFAS calories are lower in the 1200-, 1400-, and 1600-calorie food patterns than in the 1000-calorie food pattern because the nutrient goals are higher in the higher calorie patterns requiring more calories be used for nutrient-dense foods from the various food groups.

oz-eq: ounce-equivalents; quantity equivalents for each food group can be found in Table 1-2.

Vegetables	Fruits	Grains	Dairy	Protein Foods
Eat more red, orange, and dark-green veggies like tomatoes, sweet potatoes, and broccoli in main dishes. Add beans or peas to salads (kidney or chickpeas), soups (split peas or lentils), and side dishes (pinto or baked beans), or serve as a main dish. Fresh, frozen, and canned vegetables all count. Choose "reduced sodium" or "no-salt-added" canned veggies.	Use fruits as snacks, salads, and desserts. At breakfast, top your cereal with bananas or strawberries; add blueberries to pancakes. Buy fruits that are dried, frozen, and canned (in water or 100% juice), as well as fresh fruits. Select 100% fruit juice when choosing juices.	Substitute whole-grain choices for refined-grain breads, bagels, rolls, breakfast cereals, crackers, rice, and pasta. Check the ingredients list on product labels for the words "whole" or "whole grain" before the grain ingredient name. Choose products that name a whole grain first on the ingredients list.	Choose skim (fat-free) or 1% (low-fat) milk. They have the same amount of calcium and other essential nutrients as whole milk, but less fat and calories. Top fruit salads and baked potatoes with low-fat yogurt. If you are lactose intolerant, try lactose-free milk or fortified soymilk (soy beverage).	Eat a variety of foods from the protein food group each week, such as seafood, beans and peas, and nuts as well as lean meats, poultry, and eggs. Twice a week, make seafood the protein on your plate. Choose lean meats and ground beef that are at least 90% lean. Trim or drain fat from meat and remove skin from poultry to cut fat and calories.
For a 2,000-calorie daily food plan, you need the amounts below from each food group. To find amounts personalized for you, go to ChooseMyPlate.gov.				
Eat 2½ cups every day **What counts as a cup?** 1 cup of raw or cooked vegetables or vegetable juice; 2 cups of leafy salad greens	**Eat 2 cups every day** **What counts as a cup?** 1 cup of raw or cooked fruit or 100% fruit juice; ½ cup dried fruit	**Eat 6 ounces every day** **What counts as an ounce?** 1 slice of bread; ½ cup of cooked rice, cereal, or pasta; 1 ounce of ready-to-eat cereal	**Get 3 cups every day** **What counts as a cup?** 1 cup of milk, yogurt, or fortified soymilk; 1½ ounces natural or 2 ounces processed cheese	**Eat 5½ ounces every day** **What counts as an ounce?** 1 ounce of lean meat, poultry, or fish; 1 egg; 1 Tbsp peanut butter; ½ ounce nuts or seeds; ¼ cup beans or peas

Cut back on sodium and empty calories from solid fats and added sugars

Look out for salt (sodium) in foods you buy. Compare sodium in foods and choose those with a lower number.

Drink water instead of sugary drinks. Eat sugary desserts less often.

Make foods that are high in solid fats—such as cakes, cookies, ice cream, pizza, cheese, sausages, and hot dogs—occasional choices, not every day foods.

Limit empty calories to less than 260 per day, based on a 2,000 calorie diet.

Be physically active your way

Pick activities you like and do each for at least 10 minutes at a time. Every bit adds up, and health benefits increase as you spend more time being active.

Children and adolescents: get 60 minutes or more a day.

Adults: get 2 hours and 30 minutes or more a week of activity that requires moderate effort, such as brisk walking.

USDA U.S. Department of Agriculture • Center for Nutrition Policy and Promotion
August 2011
CNPP-25
USDA is an equal opportunity provider and employer.

FIGURE 1-5 MyPlate (ChooseMyPlate.gov) Mini-poster: What's on your plate, a daily food plan providing 2000 calories. Consumers can access a daily food plan based on their age, sex, and level of physical activity at http://www.choosemyplate.gov/supertracker-tools/daily-food-plans .html. (From U.S. Department of Agriculture, Center for Nutrition Policy and Promotion: *MyPlate (ChooseMyPlate.gov) Mini-poster, What's on your plate, 2000-calorie daily food plan, CNPP 25*, Washington, D.C., 2011. from: <http://www.choosemyplate.gov/downloads/mini_poster_English _final.pdf>. Retrieved July 10, 2012.)

like. Figure 1-6 presents a simple tool that is easily downloaded from the USDHHS website and carried in a wallet or backpack to help with serving size.

Estimating activity level—sedentary, low active, or active—is also difficult, given that most of us think we are more physically active than we really are. MyPlate (ChooseMyPlate.gov) and SuperTracker materials offer suggestions for measuring your minutes of physical activity. As we see in Figure 1-5, adults are directed to obtain at least 2½ hours of physical activity per week, and children need 60 minutes of physical activity every day. Walking is a good way to get started for those who have been sedentary. (We will learn more about estimating level of activity in Chapter 8.)

Nutrition messages that are easy to understand, tailored to specific audiences, and make use of existing technology require the combined efforts of communication experts working side by side with nutrition scientists. Government agencies and nutrition educators must join forces to produce practical resources in formats and languages appropriate to all segments of our society.[55,75]

Food Lists for Meal Planning

The *Food Lists for Diabetes* (formerly called the *Exchange Lists*) were introduced in 1950 by the American Diabetes Association and the American Dietetic Association as a meal-planning tool for people with diabetes. The *Food Lists* group foods based on macronutrient content and equivalent energy values, making this tool useful for planning any diet in which control of carbohydrate, fat, protein, and total kcalories is the goal. Because the foods in each list are equal to one

SERVING SIZE CARD:
Cut out and fold on the dotted line. Laminate for longtime use.

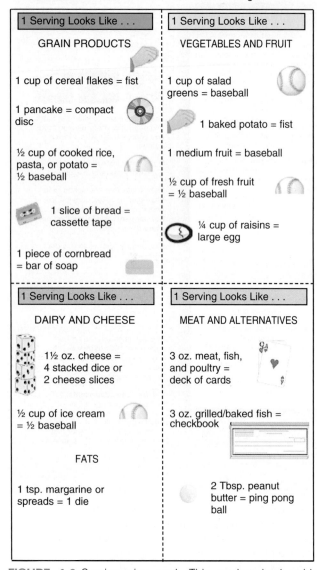

FIGURE 1-6 Serving size card. This pocket-sized guide can be useful when choosing serving sizes at home or when eating out. (From U.S. Department of Health and Human Services, National Heart, Lung and Blood Institute, Obesity Education Initiative: *Keep an eye on portion size,* Bethesda, Md., 2004. from: <http://hp2010.nhlbihin.net/portion/servingcard7.pdf>. Retrieved July 29, 2013.)

another when eaten in the portions indicated, items can be freely interchanged within each list, and food values and kcalories remain constant. The freedom of choice within groups to exchange within groups promotes increased variety and satisfaction with meals and snacks.

The most recent edition of the *Choose Your Foods: Food Lists for Diabetes* is found on the Evolve site.[76] Foods are arranged into the following three groups:

1. *Carbohydrates:* includes starches (grains, starchy vegetables, crackers, snacks, and legumes), fruits, milk, sweets, and nonstarchy vegetables.

2. *Proteins:* includes animal protein foods arranged by fat content (lean, medium fat, and high fat) and plant-based proteins
3. *Fats:* includes both animal and plant fats arranged by degree of saturation—unsaturated (monounsaturated and polyunsaturated) and saturated.

Serving sizes and macronutrient content for combination foods, fast foods, and free foods are also provided. Use of the *Food Lists* in helping people with diabetes control their carbohydrate intake is discussed in Chapter 22.

A SAFE AND HEALTHY FOOD SUPPLY

Food safety is an important public health priority and included in the Healthy People 2020 initiatives.[43] Foodborne illness arising from microbial contamination and sometimes incorrectly referred to as "food poisoning" is common and costly, yet preventable.[77] The Centers for Disease Control and Prevention (CDC) estimates that each year about 1 in 6 Americans (48 million people) get sick; 128,000 are hospitalized; and 3000 die of foodborne illness. The actual number of individuals who get sick from contaminated food is likely higher, as many cases go unreported when people attribute their symptoms to a "stomach virus" or the flu and do not seek medical care. Symptoms of foodborne illness include diarrhea, nausea, and stomach upset and cramping, and in most cases victims feel better in 1 or 2 days. However, in young children, older adults, and patients with compromised immune systems, foodborne pathogens result in severe dehydration, fever, hospitalization, and even death. Careful washing of fresh produce, especially leafy vegetables; thorough cooking of poultry and raw meat; avoiding raw eggs (including not tasting batters containing raw eggs)[78]; and always washing your hands before eating and cooking help prevent foodborne illness. Proper food handling should be included in any comprehensive nutrition education program. In Chapter 9 we explore these topics in greater depth.

PERSONAL PERCEPTIONS OF FOOD

What Do I Usually Eat

Each of us develops ways of eating based on our ethnic or cultural background, religious beliefs, family habits, socioeconomic status, health status, geographic location, and personal likes and dislikes. However, the growing ethnic and cultural diversity in our society has brought about a greater intermingling of foods and ideas about food. How people perceive themselves in relation to food and food patterns plays a role in their attitudes toward food and personal eating behavior.

A simple way to get an idea of your own food pattern is to look at what you actually eat. See the Perspectives in Practice box, "My Personal Food Patterns: Do They Need Improvement?" for directions on keeping a food diary. Keeping a record of everything you eat and drink for a day, noting the time, place, any related activity, and people with you provides insight to your true relationship with food.

PERSPECTIVES IN PRACTICE

My Personal Food Patterns: Do They Need Improvement?

Before we can help others make healthy food choices, we need to help ourselves. What do you usually eat? Do you eat regular meals or snack most of the time? Do you make an effort to choose nutritious foods or eat whatever is around? This activity provides an opportunity to evaluate your personal food and nutrient intake.

- To get started, keep a detailed record of everything you eat and drink for 3 days: 2 weekdays and 1 weekend day. List the type and amount of food in household measures (e.g., cups, tablespoons, or dimensions), how it was prepared, and brand name, if applicable. Be specific: was your milk nonfat, 1% fat, 2% fat, or whole? Include butter, margarine, salad dressings, condiments, and additions to coffee or tea. When you have completed your record, consider the following:
- What social or emotional factors influenced your food choices? Where and when did you eat? Were you alone or with someone? How did you feel at the time?

- Using MyPlate (ChooseMyPlate.gov), compare your intake with the number of servings and portion sizes recommended for your age, sex, and level of physical activity. Did you have too many or too few servings from any of the food groups?
- Using the Nutritrac software available on the Evolve website, evaluate your intakes of macronutrients and micronutrients. Are your kcalories partitioned appropriately? How do your intakes compare with the DRIs for your age and sex?
- Now that you have thought about it, how do you view your diet? Do you have food behaviors that you should modify to promote good health? Do you feel good about certain nutrient categories for which you are meeting current recommendations? If improvements are needed, develop a plan for making changes over time that are consistent with your lifestyle and resources and can be sustained.

Most of us eat by habit, according to where we are and what is available, rather than by serious thought or plan. Evaluating food and beverage intake using MyPlate (ChooseMyPlate. gov) to determine the appropriate kcalorie intake and food servings is a means of rapid dietary assessment.

Nutritional Analysis by Nutrients and Energy Values

A comprehensive nutritional analysis of food intake is accomplished using a computer-assisted nutrient analysis program, as found on the Evolve website that accompanies your text. A computer-assisted program enables you to evaluate individual intakes of vitamins and minerals, protein, specific fats, fiber, and energy as compared with the DRIs. Government agencies use such analyses to evaluate dietary information obtained in national surveys and to identify nutrition problems among various age, sex, or ethnic groups.

TO SUM UP

The role of nutrition in human health continues to evolve in response to our changing society and food supply. As available food increased and the physical activity required in daily living decreased, overweight and obesity emerged as major health problems worldwide. Discovery of new substances in plant foods that are beneficial to health led to the definition of functional foods and recommendations for their use. Despite the accessibility of nutrient-dense foods, many American diets are high in sugar and fat, compromising nutritional status. Children and adults who are chronically undernourished as a result of illness, disease, or inadequate food resources are more vulnerable to poor growth, infection, and nutrition-related diseases. Resources developed by government agencies are helpful in planning and evaluating the nutrient intakes of all population groups. The Dietary Reference Intakes (DRIs) intended for use by health professionals provide the foundation for the *Dietary Guidelines for Americans* and MyPlate (ChooseMyPlate.gov), which offer practical guidance for family meal planning. Together, these materials build a framework for public policy that directs state and federal nutrition programs and health messages reaching people of all ages.

QUESTIONS FOR REVIEW

1. Visit the U.S. Obesity Trends website of the Centers for Disease Control and Prevention at http://www.cdc.gov/obesity/data/adult.html and scroll down to the state maps and overweight/obesity statistics. What is the prevalence of obesity and overweight in your state as compared with the national average? How has it changed

over the past 5 to 10 years? Review the PowerPoint slide program that illustrates national increases in obesity over the past 20 years.

2. What are the two major fields of science that provide the foundation for the study of nutrition? What does each contribute to our understanding of human nutrition needs?

3. What is the difference between the terms *nutrition* and *dietetics?* Describe three possible activities of nutrition-related professionals.

4. Compare the four levels of nutritional status: optimal nutrition, marginal nutrition, malnutrition, and overnutrition. In what community or clinical situations might you expect to find individuals representing each of these conditions and what physical or clinical signs would you use to identify them?

5. What are the six major nutrient groups? What is the primary function of each?

6. What are the various categories within the DRIs? What is the purpose of each?

7. Compare nutrient standards, dietary guidelines, and food guides: (a) list an example of each, (b) the intended audience (professional or consumer), (c) the type of information included, and (d) a professional situation in which you would use it.

8. Visit the Healthy People 2020 website at www.healthypeople.gov/ and look for a nutrition or health issue of interest. Review the suggested community-based interventions for that objective and develop an intervention that would be applicable to your community and target audience.

9. Visit the Nutrition Evidence Library of the U.S. Department of Agriculture at www.nel.gov. Choose a topic of interest and review the studies and evidence that is described there. Do you agree with the experts' evaluation? Has your opinion changed as to the effectiveness of the intervention or treatment based on what you read? Why?

10. Research the food patterns of a cultural or ethnic group different from your own. Using MyPlate (http://www.choosemyplate.gov), develop a 1-day menu for a child or adult in that group using foods common to their daily pattern.

REFERENCES

1. Popkin BM: What can public health nutritionists do to curb the epidemic of nutrition-related noncommunicable disease? *Nutr Rev* 67(Suppl 1):S79, 2009.

2. Centers for Disease Control and Prevention: *Overweight and obesity. Data and statistics. Adult obesity facts,* Atlanta, Ga., 2012, Centers for Disease Control and Prevention. at: <http://www.cdc.gov/obesity/data/adult.html>. Accessed on September 8, 2013.

3. Flegal KM, Carroll MD, Kit BK, et al: Prevalence of obesity and trends in the distribution of body mass index among US adults, 1999-2012. *JAMA* 307(5):491, 2012.

4. Ogden CL, Carroll MD, Kit BK, et al: Prevalence of obesity and trends in body mass index among US children and adolescents, 1999-2010. *JAMA* 307(5):483, 2012.

5. Centers for Disease Control and Prevention: *Diabetes data and trends. Number (in millions) of civilian, noninstitutionalized persons with diagnosed diabetes, United States, 1980-2011,* Atlanta, Ga., 2011, National Center for Chronic Disease Prevention and Health Promotion, Centers for Disease Control and Prevention, Division of Diabetes Translation. at: <http://www.cdc.gov/diabetes/statistics/prev/national/figpersons.htm>. Accessed on January 25, 2013.

6. Centers for Disease Control and Prevention: *National diabetes fact sheet: national estimates and general information on diabetes and prediabetes in the United States, 2011,* Atlanta, Ga., 2011, U.S. Department of Health and Human Services, Centers for Disease Control and Prevention. at: <http://www.cdc.gov/diabetes/pubs/pdf/ndfs_2011.pdf>. Accessed on August 19, 2013.

7. Chaput JP, Doucet E, Tremblay A: Obesity: a disease or a biological adaptation? An update. *Obes Rev* 13:681, 2012.

8. Frank LD, Saelens BE, Chapman J, et al: Objective assessment of obesogenic environments in youth. Geographic information system methods and spatial findings from the Neighborhood Impact on Kids Study. *Am J Prev Med* 42(5):e47, 2012.

9. Ledikwe JH, Ello-Martin JA, Rolls BJ: Portion sizes and the obesity epidemic. *J Nutr* 135:905, 2005.

10. Piernas C, Popkin BM: Food portion patterns and trends among U.S children and the relationship to total eating occasion size, 1977-2006. *J Nutr* 141:1159, 2011.

11. Federal Interagency Forum on Aging-Related Statistics: *Older Americans 2012: Key indicators of well-being,* Washington, D.C., 2012, U.S. Government Printing Office.

12. Henry J Kaiser Family Foundation: *Health Care Costs: A Primer. Key Information on Health Care Costs and Their Impact, Publ 7670-03,* Menlo Park, Calif., 2012. at: <http://kaiserfamilyfoundation.files.wordpress.com/2013/01/7670-03.pdf>. Accessed on January 25, 2013.

13. United States Census Bureau: *Statistical Abstract of the United States,* ed 131, Washington, D.C., 2012. at: <http://www.census.gov/compendia/statab/>. Accessed on August 19, 2013.

14. Goody CM, Drago L: *Cultural Food Practices, American Dietetic Association (now the Academy of Nutrition and Dietetics),* Chicago, Ill., 2010, Diabetes Care and Education Dietetic Practice Group.

15. United States Bureau of Census: *Selected social characteristics in the United States, 2011 American Community Survey 1-year estimates, American FactFinder, DP02,* Washington, D.C., 2011, U.S. Department of Commerce. at: <http://factfinder2.census.gov/faces/tableservices/jsf/pages/productview.xhtml?pid=ACS_11_1YR_DP02&prodType=table>. Accessed on January 25, 2013.

16. American Dietetic Association: Position of the American Dietetic Association: functional foods. *J Am Diet Assoc* 109:735, 2009.

17. Djousse L, Hopkins PN, North KE, et al: Chocolate consumption is inversely associated with prevalent coronary

heart disease: The National Heart, Lung, and Blood Institute Family Heart Study. *Clin Nutr* 30:182, 2011.

18. DeBusk R: The role of nutrition genomics in developing an optimal diet for humans. *Nutr Clin Prac* 25:627, 2010.

19. Ferguson LR: Nutrigenomics approaches to functional foods. *J Am Diet Assoc* 109:452, 2009.

20. Zeisel SH: Nutritional genomics: defining the dietary requirement and effects of choline. *J Nutr* 141(3):531, 2011.

21. Hesketh J: Personalised nutrition: how far has nutrigenomics progressed? *Eur J Clin Nutr* 67(5):430, 2013.

22. Annes JP, Giovanni MA, Murray MF: Risks of presymptomatic direct-to-consumer genetic testing. *N Engl J Med* 363:12, 2010.

23. Kapsak WR, Rahavi ER, Childs NM, et al: Functional foods: consumer attitudes, perceptions, and behaviors in a growing market. *J Am Diet Assoc* 111(6):804, 2011.

24. Wellman NS, Borra ST, Schleman JC, et al: Trends in news media reporting of food and health issues. *Nutr Today* 46(3):123, 2011.

25. Rowe S, Alexander N: Nutrition communications in the new age (revisited). *Nutr Today* 46(4):178, 2011.

26. Food and Nutrition Board, Institute of Medicine: *Dietary Reference Intakes for energy, carbohydrate, fiber, fat, fatty acids, cholesterol, protein, and amino acids, (macronutrients),* Washington, D.C., 2002, National Academies Press.

27. Jacobs DR, Gross MD, Tapsell LC: Food synergy: an operational concept for understanding nutrition. *Am J Clin Nutr* 89(Suppl):1543S, 2009.

28. Kuczmarski MF, Kuczmarski RJ: Nutrition monitoring in the United States. In Shils ME, Shike M, Olson J, editors: *Modern nutrition in health and disease,* ed 10, Baltimore, Md., 2006, Lippincott Williams & Wilkins.

29. United States Department of Health and Human Services and Agriculture: *Report of the Dietary Guidelines Advisory Committee on the Dietary Guidelines for Americans, 2010,* Washington, D.C., 2010, Center for Nutrition Policy and Promotion, U.S. Department of Agriculture. at: <http://www.cnpp.usda.gov/DGAs2010-DGACReport.htm>. Retrieved November 12, 2012.

30. Malik VS, Popkin BM, Bray GA, et al: Sugar-sweetened beverages and risk of metabolic syndrome and type 2 diabetes. *Diabetes Care* 33(11):2477, 2010.

31. United States Department of Agriculture: *Food security in the U.S. Key statistics and graphics,* Washington, D.C., 2012, Economic Research Service. at: <http://www.ers.usda.gov/topics/food-nutrition-assistance/food-security-in-the-us/key-statistics-graphics.aspx#.Uhqt3BYaWNM>. Accessed on August 13, 2013.

32. Zizza CA, Duffy PA, Gerrior SA: Food insecurity is not associated with lower energy intakes. *Obesity* 16:1908, 2008.

33. Jiao J, Moudon AV, Ulmer J, et al: How to identify food deserts: measuring physical and economic access to supermarkets in King County, Washington. *Am J Public Health* 102(10):e32, 2012.

34. Cook JT, Frank DA, Levenson SM, et al: Child food insecurity increases risks posed by household food insecurity to young children's health. *J Nutr* 136:1073, 2006.

35. American Dietetic Association: Position of the American Dietetic Association: food insecurity in the United States. *J Am Diet Assoc* 110:1368, 2010.

36. Robaina KA, Martin KS: Food insecurity, poor diet quality and obesity among food pantry participants in Hartford, CT. *J Nutr Educ Behav* 45(2):159, 2012.

37. Gany F, Bari S, Crist M, et al: Food insecurity: limitations of emergency food resources for our patients. *J Urban Health* 90(3):552, 2013.

38. Morley JE, Thomas DR, Wilson MM: Cachexia: pathophysiology and clinical relevance. *Am J Clin Nutr* 83:735, 2006.

39. Richard C, Couture P, Desroches S, et al: Effect of the Mediterranean diet with or without weight loss on markers of inflammation in men with metabolic syndrome. *Obesity* 21(1):51, 2013.

40. U.S. Department of Health and Human Services, Public Health Service: *The Surgeon General's report on nutrition and health,* PHS Publication No. 88-50210. Washington, D.C., 1988, U.S. Government Printing Office.

41. Food and Nutrition Board, Institute of Medicine: *Diet and health: implications for reducing chronic disease risk,* Washington, D.C., 1989, National Academies Press.

42. U.S. Department of Health and Human Services: *Healthy People 2010: Final review,* Washington, D.C., 2011, National Center for Health Statistics, Centers for Disease Control and Prevention. at: <http://www.cdc.gov/nchs/healthy_people/hp2010/hp2010_final_review.htm/>. Accessed on July 16, 2012.

43. U.S. Department of Health and Human Services: *Healthy People 2020: 2020 Topics and Objectives,* Washington, D.C., 2013, U.S. Department of Health and Human Services. at: <http://www.healthypeople.gov/2020/default.aspx>. Accessed on August 19, 2013.

44. Brown DW: The dawn of Healthy People 2020: a brief look back at its beginnings. *Prev Med* 48:94, 2009.

45. U.S. Department of Health and Human Services: *Local We Can!®,* Bethesda, Md., 2012, Community Programs, National Heart, Lung and Blood Institute. at: <http://www.nhlbi.nih.gov/health/public/heart/obesity/wecan/partner-with-us/local-community-programs.htm>. Accessed on August 19, 2013.

46. Mozaffarian D, Afshin A, Benowitz NL, et al: Population approaches to improve diet, physical activity, and smoking habits: a scientific statement from the American Heart Association. *Circulation* 126:1514, 2012.

47. Jain A, Langwith C: Collaborative school-based obesity interventions: Lessons learned from 6 southern districts. *J Sch Health* 83:213, 2013.

48. Food and Nutrition Board, Institute of Medicine: *Dietary Reference Intakes [DRI]. The essential guide to nutrient requirements,* Washington, D.C., 2006, National Academies Press.

49. Food and Nutrition Board, Institute of Medicine: *Dietary Reference Intakes for calcium, phosphorus, magnesium, vitamin D, and fluoride,* Washington, D.C., 1997, National Academies Press.

50. Food and Nutrition Board, Institute of Medicine: *Dietary Reference Intakes for thiamin, riboflavin, niacin, vitamin B_6, folate, vitamin B_{12}, pantothenic acid, biotin, and choline,* Washington, D.C., 1998, National Academies Press.

51. Food and Nutrition Board, Institute of Medicine: *Dietary Reference Intakes for vitamin C, vitamin E, selenium, and carotenoids,* Washington, D.C., 2000, National Academies Press.

52. Food and Nutrition Board, Institute of Medicine: *Dietary Reference Intakes for vitamin A, vitamin K, arsenic, boron, chromium, copper, iodine, iron, manganese, molybdenum, nickel, silicon, vanadium, and zinc,* Washington, D.C., 2001, National Academies Press.

53. Food and Nutrition Board, Institute of Medicine: *Dietary Reference Intakes for water, potassium, sodium, chloride, and sulfate,* Washington, D.C., 2004, National Academies Press.

54. Food and Nutrition Board, Institute of Medicine: *Dietary Reference Intakes for calcium and vitamin D,* Washington, D.C., 2011, National Academies Press.

55. Rowe S, Alexander N, Almeida NG, et al: Translating the Dietary Guidelines for Americans 2010 to bring about real behavior change. *J Am Diet Assoc* 111:28, 2011.

56. Van Horn L: Development of the 2010 US Dietary Guidelines Advisory Committee Report: Perspectives from a registered dietitian. *J Am Diet Assoc* 110:1638, 2010.

57. Wright JD, Wang C-Y: *Trends in intake of energy and macronutrients in adults from 1999-2000 through 2007-2008,* Data Brief, No 49. Atlanta, Ga., 2010, National Center for Health Statistics. at: <http://www.cdc.gov/nchs/data/databriefs/db49.htm>. Accessed on August 19, 2013.

58. Spahn JM, Lyon JMG, Altman JM, et al: The systematic review methodology used to support the 2010 Dietary Guidelines Advisory Committee. *J Am Diet Assoc* 111:520, 2011.

59. U.S. Department of Agriculture: *USDA's Nutrition Evidence Library (NEL),* Washington, D.C., 2010, U.S. Department of Agriculture. at: <www.nel.gov>. Accessed February 13, 2013.

60. United States Department of Health and Human Services, United States Department of Agriculture: *Dietary guidelines for Americans (Policy Document), 2010,* ed 7, Washington, D.C., 2010, U.S. Government Printing Office. at: <http://www.cnpp.usda.gov/DGAs2010-PolicyDocument.htm>. Accessed on January 25, 2013.

61. Kapsak WR, Edge MS, White C, et al: Putting the Dietary Guidelines for Americans into action: behavior-directed messages to motivate parents—phase I and II observational and focus group findings. *J Acad Nutr Diet* 113(2):196, 2013.

62. Rowe S, Alexander N, Almeida N, et al: Food science challenge: translating the Dietary Guidelines for Americans to bring about real behavior change. *J Food Sci* 76(1):R29, 2011.

63. U.S. Department of Health and Human Services, U.S. Department of Agriculture: *Dietary guidelines for Americans 2005,* ed 6, Washington, D.C., 2005, U.S. Government Printing Office. at: <http://www.health.gov/dietaryguidelines/dga2005/document/>. Accessed on February 13, 2013.

64. Flock MR, Kris-Etherton PM: Dietary Guidelines for Americans 2010: Implications for cardiovascular disease. *Curr Atheroscler* 13:499, 2011.

65. U.S. Department of Agriculture: *A brief history of USDA food guides,* Washington, D.C., 2011, Center for Nutrition Policy and Promotion. at: <http://www.choosemyplate.gov/food-groups/downloads/MyPlate/ABriefHistoryOfUSDAFoodGuides.pdf>. Accessed on February 13, 2013.

66. U.S. Department of Agriculture: *Archived MyPyramid materials,* Washington, D.C., 2010, Center for Nutrition Policy and Promotion. at: <http://www.choosemyplate.gov/print-materials-ordering/mypyramid-archive.html>. Accessed on February 13, 2013.

67. U.S. Department of Agriculture: *Development of 2010 Dietary Guidelines for Americans. Consumer messages and new food icon. Executive summary of formative research,* Washington, D.C., 2011, Center for Nutrition Policy and Promotion. at: <http://www.choosemyplate.gov/food-groups/downloads/MyPlate/ExecutiveSummaryOfFormativeResearch.pdf>. Retrieved on July 19, 2011.

68. Post R, Haven J, Maniscalco S: Commentary: Putting MyPlate to work for nutrition educators. *J Nutr Educ Behav* 44:98, 2012.

69. Post R, Maniscalco S, Herrup M, et al: The MyPlate message chronicles: What's new on MyPlate? A new message, redesigned web site, and Super Tracker debut. *J Acad Nutr Diet* 112:18, 2012.

70. Post RC, Haven J, Chang S, et al: The MyPlate message chronicle: one year and counting! *J Acad Nutr Diet* 112(9):1314, 2012.

71. U.S. Department of Health and Human Services, National Heart, Lung and Blood Institute: *Keep an Eye on Portion Distortion,* Bethesda, Md., 2013, U.S. Department of Health and Human Services. at: <http://hp2010.nhlbihin.net/portion/keep.htm>. Accessed on February 13, 2013.

72. Wansink B, van Ittersum K: Portion size me: downsizing our consumption norms. *J Am Diet Assoc* 107:1103, 2007.

73. Academy of Nutrition and Dietetics: Position paper of the Academy of Nutrition and Dietetics: Total diet approach to healthy eating. *J Acad Nutr Diet* 113(2):307, 2013.

74. Duffey KJ, Popkin BM: Energy density, portion size, and eating occasions: contributions to increased energy intake in the United States, 1977-2006. *PLoS Med* 8(6):e1001050, 2011.

75. Rowe S, Alexander N: Communicating Dietary Guidelines to a balking public. *Nutr Today* 44:81, 2009.

76. Academy of Nutrition and Dietetics, American Diabetes Association: *Choose your foods: food lists for diabetes,* ed 7, New York, 2014, Academy of Nutrition and Dietetics, American Diabetes Association.

77. Centers for Disease Control and Prevention: Estimating foodborne illness: an overview, 2013. at: <http://www.cdc.gov/foodborneburden/estimates-overview.html#trends>. Accessed on February 13, 2013.

78. Painter JA, Hoekstra RM, Ayers T, et al: Attribution of foodborne illnesses, hospitalizations, and deaths to food commodities by using outbreak data, United States, 1998-2008. *Emerg Infect Dis* 19(3):407, 2013.

FURTHER READINGS AND RESOURCES

Readings

Academy of Nutrition and Dietetics: Position of the Academy of Nutrition and Dietetics: total diet approach to healthy eating. *J Acad Nutr Diet* 113:307, 2013.

[This review helps us understand the importance of the overall food pattern, not just one day or one meal.]

Klurfeld DM: What do government agencies consider in the debate over added sugars? *Adv Nutr* 4(2):257, 2013.

[Dr. Klurfeld reviews the trends in added sugar intake and the health implications for the American public.]

Reilly PR, DeBusk RM: Ethical and legal issues in nutritional genomics. *J Am Diet Assoc* 108:36, 2008.

[When it becomes possible to customize nutrition intervention based on an individual's genetic code, there are various issues that will need to be considered.]

Slavin J: Dietary Guidelines. Are we on the right path? *Nutr Today* 47(5):245, 2012.

[This nutrition expert raises questions about the 2010 Dietary Guidelines and provides suggestions for change when the 2015 Guidelines are developed.]

U.S. Department of Agriculture, Center for Nutrition Policy and Promotion: *An evidence-based approach to reviewing the science on nutrition and health, Nutrition Insight 38*, Alexandria, Va., 2008, U.S. Government Printing Office. from: <http://www.cnpp.usda.gov/Publications/NutritionInsights/Insight38.pdf>. Retrieved on August 19, 2013.

[This publication provides a helpful summary on why we need to apply an evidence-based approach to our practice and gives an example of the process.]

U.S. Department of Agriculture, Center for Nutrition Policy and Promotion: *The Food Environment, Eating Out, and Body Weight: A Review of the Evidence, Nutrition Insight 49*, Alexandria, Va., 2012, U.S. Government Printing Office. from: <http://www.cnpp.usda.gov/Publications/NutritionInsights/Insight49.pdf>. Retrieved on August 19, 2013.

[This review cites evidence from the Nutrition Evidence Library (NEL) linking frequency of meals away from home and risk of overweight, and helps us understand why this occurs.]

Wellman NS, Borra ST, Schleman JC, et al: Trends in news media reporting of food and health issues. *Nutr Today* 46(3):123, 2011. May-June.

[These authors help us understand how and why nutrition and health misinformation gets publicized and how we as health professionals can address this.]

Websites of Interest

- U.S. Department of Agriculture: Nutrition Evidence Library, 2013. This website provided the scientific evidence reviewed by the 2010 Dietary Guidelines Advisory Committee in preparation of their report. http://www.cnpp.usda.gov/NEL.htm.
- U.S. Department of Health and Human Services, 2008. *Physical Activity Guidelines for Americans*. This Web site presents science-based physical activity guidelines for both youth and adults along with educational materials for health professionals and consumers. http://www.health.gov/paguidelines/guidelines/default.aspx.
- U.S. Department of Agriculture, Food Surveys Research Group: *What We Eat in America: Data from the National Health and Nutrition Examination Survey*. This site describes the food and nutrient intakes of Americans according to age, sex, race, ethnicity, and economic status. www.ars.usda.gov/Services/docs.htm?docid=15044.
- U.S. Department of Health and Human Services, National Heart, Lung and Blood Institute: *Keep an Eye on Portion Distortion*. This site describes portion sizes and how they have changed over the years. http://hp2010.nhlbihin.net/portion/keep.htm.
- U.S. Department of Agriculture, Center for Nutrition Policy and Promotion. The MyPlate (ChooseMyPlate.gov) website offers materials for health professionals and practical tips for consumers to use in meal planning; www.ChooseMyPlate.gov.

CHAPTER

2

Digestion, Absorption, and Metabolism

Eleanor D. Schlenker

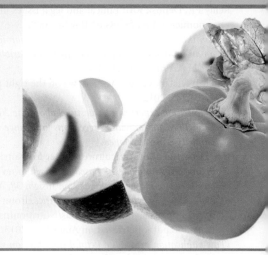

ⓔ EVOLVE WEBSITE

http://evolve.elsevier.com/Williams/essentials/

OUTLINE

HUMAN BODY: THE ROLE OF NUTRITION
Food: Change and Transformation
Importance for Health and Nutrition
The Gastrointestinal Tract
Principles of Digestion
MOVEMENT OF FOOD THROUGH THE DIGESTIVE TRACT
Mouth and Esophagus: Preparation and Delivery
Stomach: Storage and Initial Digestion

Small Intestine: Major Digestion, Absorption, and Transport
Colon (Large Intestine): Final Absorption and Waste Elimination
Gastrointestinal Function and Clinical Applications
Health Promotion
Metabolism

We continue our study of nutrition by looking at what happens to food as it follows its path through the digestive system and is broken down into forms the body can use. We review what must occur to convert the tuna sandwich we had for lunch into the energy-yielding nutrients—glucose, amino acids, and fatty acids—that perform body work. These steps are accomplished through an integrated system that receives the food we take in and transforms it for our use.

The physiologic and biochemical process that turns the food we eat into energy and body tissue has three parts: digestion, absorption, and metabolism. We begin with a review of the gastrointestinal tract and then follow the path of the nutrients to the cells where they nourish and protect us. We will see how all parts must work together to accomplish this task.

HUMAN BODY: THE ROLE OF NUTRITION

FOOD: CHANGE AND TRANSFORMATION

The food we eat contains the nutrients necessary for our survival, but these materials must first be released from other food components and transformed into units the body can use. Through a successive and interrelated system, foods are

broken down into increasingly simple substances that can enter the metabolic pathways in cells. Each section of the gastrointestinal tract has a unique function, but together they form a continuous *whole*. A problem in one section has clinical consequences for the entire system.

IMPORTANCE FOR HEALTH AND NUTRITION

Gastrointestinal function is a partner in nutritional well-being.[1] Food, as it occurs in nature and as we eat it, is not a single substance but a mixture of nutrients and other chemical matter. These substances must be separated so the body can handle each one as an individual unit. Nutrients released from food remain unavailable to the body until they cross the intestinal wall and enter the circulatory system for transport to tissues. Diseases affecting the organs of the gastrointestinal tract or the absorbing surface of the intestinal wall have adverse effects on nutritional status because nutrients are not taken into the body in the amounts needed. At the same time, moderate to severe malnutrition lowers secretion of digestive enzymes and blunts the absorbing structures, further limiting digestion and nutrient passage. This vicious cycle results in rapid and progressive deterioration of nutritional well-being.[1]

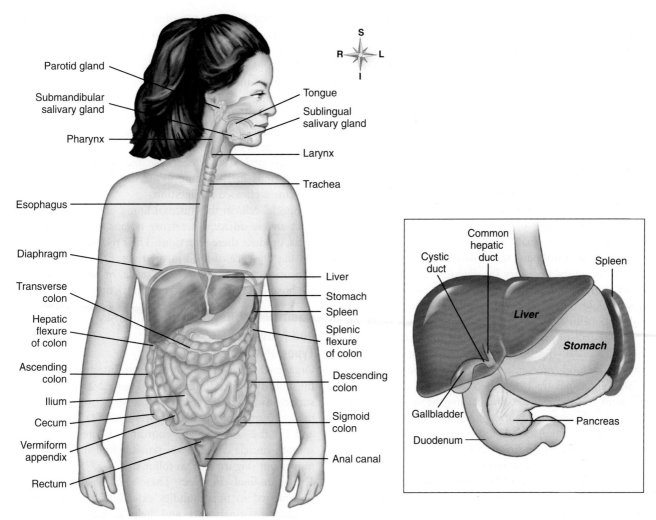

FIGURE 2-1 The gastrointestinal system. The successive parts of the gastrointestinal system carry out multiple activities of digestion that liberate and reform food nutrients for our use. (From Thibodeau GA, Patton KT: *Anatomy and physiology,* ed 7, St. Louis, Mo., 2010, Mosby.)

The output of the gastrointestinal tract is essential to the chemical work that occurs in tissues and cells. This integrated physiochemical system is fundamental to human nutrition in both health and disease. The internal control responsible for maintaining a constant chemical environment and keeping the many functional systems operating in harmony with one another is called **homeostasis**.[2]

THE GASTROINTESTINAL TRACT

Component Parts

The gastrointestinal tract, also called the *alimentary canal,* is a long hollow tube that begins at the mouth and ends at the anus. The specific parts that make up the tract are the mouth, esophagus, stomach, small intestine, large intestine or colon, and rectum. Other organs that lie outside the tract but support its work by secretion of important enzymes and digestive fluids are the pancreas, gallbladder, and liver. Figure 2-1 shows the respective components of the gastrointestinal tract and their relative position to one another. These organs, working as a team, can break down and/or absorb several

kilograms of carbohydrate, one-half kilogram of fat, one-half kilogram of protein, and 20 or more liters of water daily.[2] We will follow these food components as they travel together through the successive parts of the tract.

General Functions

The gastrointestinal tract has the following four major functions:
1. *Receives food:* The mouth is the entrance to the gastrointestinal tract. From here the food moves to the stomach and other organs for digestion and absorption.
2. *Releases nutrients from food:* Digestion and the separation of nutrients from other food components take place in the stomach and small intestine.

KEY TERM

homeostasis State of dynamic equilibrium within the body's internal environment; a balance is achieved through the operation of many interrelated physiologic mechanisms.

3. *Delivers nutrients into the blood:* Absorbing structures called *microvilli* located in the small intestine transfer the nutrients into the portal blood (glucose and amino acids) or lymph (fatty acids). Water is absorbed later in the colon.
4. *Excretes nondigestible waste:* The fecal mass moves from the colon into the rectum where it is stored until excreted. Physical and chemical actions accomplish these tasks.

Sensory Stimulation and Gastrointestinal Function

Both physiologic and psychologic stimuli influence the gastrointestinal tract. The physical presence of food in the mouth, stomach, or small intestine initiates a variety of responses that coordinate the muscular movements and chemical secretions necessary for digestion and absorption. Sensory stimuli, such as seeing, smelling, or being close to food, cause the secretion of digestive juices and muscle motility.[2] Smelling cookies baking, hearing foods sizzle on an outdoor grill, or picking a fresh berry can evoke the physiologic process of digestion. Seeing a sign that advertises your favorite food (or even thinking about food) stimulates the gastrointestinal tract. On the other hand, dreading an unpleasant-tasting medication or recalling the nausea brought on by chemotherapy can repress the desire for food.

The neural responses resulting from the presence or thoughts of food have an important role in food intake and the digestive process. Neural responses prepare the gastrointestinal tract to receive food by initiating the secretion of enzymes and digestive fluids and promoting gastrointestinal motility. They also control the secretion of hormones that influence appetite, food intake, and satiety.[3] Inappropriate changes in neural regulation contribute to poor food intake in some older adults. Feelings of satiety that occur early in the meal limit food intake, resulting in weight loss and frailty.[4] Maintaining positive associations with food and mealtime support efficient digestion and absorption of nutrients.

PRINCIPLES OF DIGESTION

Digestion, the complicated process by which food is broken down and nutrients released, prepares food for body use. Digestion involves two types of actions:
- Chemical breakdown of food into its constituent parts through the action of enzymes and other specialized fluids. Each chemical agent acts on a particular macronutrient in a specific region of the gastrointestinal tract.
- Muscular action including mechanical mixing and propulsive movements controlled by neuromuscular, self-regulating systems. These motions work together to move the food mass along the alimentary canal at the best rate for digestion and absorption.

Gastrointestinal Secretions

Food is digested chemically through the combined action of various secretions of the following four types.

1. *Enzymes:* Certain enzymes attack designated chemical bonds within the structure of nutrient compounds, freeing their component parts.
2. *Hydrochloric acid and buffer ions:* These secretions produce the pH necessary for the activity of certain enzymes.
3. *Mucus:* This sticky, slippery fluid lubricates and protects the inner lining of the gastrointestinal tract and eases the passage of the food mass.
4. *Water and electrolytes:* These agents provide appropriate solutions in the amounts needed to circulate the substances released in digestion.

Special cells in the mucosal lining of the gastrointestinal tract and in adjacent accessory organs, especially the pancreas, produce these secretions. Their release is stimulated by (1) the presence of food in the tract; (2) the sensory nerve network activated by the sight, taste, or smell of food; and (3) hormones specific to certain nutrients.

Gastrointestinal Motility: Muscles and Movement
Types of Muscles
Organized muscle layers in the gastrointestinal wall provide the motility needed for digestion (Figure 2-2). From the outer surface inward, the layers are (1) the **serosa**, (2) a longitudinal muscle layer, (3) a circular muscle layer, (4) the submucosa, and (5) the **mucosa**. The coordinated interaction of four smooth-muscle layers makes possible four different types of movement (Figure 2-3), as follows:

1. *Longitudinal muscles:* These long, smooth muscles arranged in fiber bundles extend lengthwise along the gastrointestinal tract and help propel the food mass forward.
2. *Circular contractile muscles:* The circular smooth-muscle fibers extend around the hollow tube forming the alimentary canal. These contractile rings initiate rhythmic sweeping waves along the tract, pushing the food mass forward. These regularly occurring propulsive movements are called **peristalsis**.
3. *Sphincter muscles:* At strategic points muscle sphincters act as valves—pyloric, ileocecal, and anal—to prevent reflux or backflow and keep the food mass moving in a forward direction.
4. *Mucosal muscles:* This thin embedded layer of smooth muscle produces local constrictive contractions every few centimeters. These contractions mix and chop the food mass, effectively churning and mixing it with secretions to form a semiliquid called **chyme** that is ready for absorption. In summary, the muscles lining the gastrointestinal tract produce the following two types of action:
   - **Tonic** contractions that ensure continuous passage of the food mass and valve control
   - Periodic rhythmic contractions that mix and propel the food mass forward

The alternating contraction and relaxation of these muscles along the tract facilitate digestion and absorption.

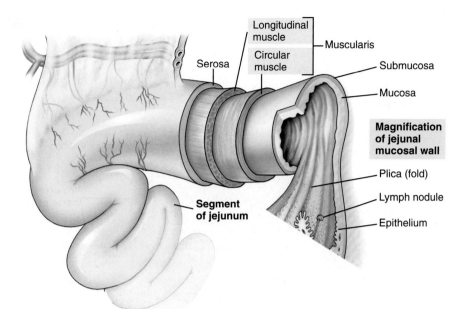

FIGURE 2-2 Muscle layers of the intestinal wall. Notice the five layers of muscle that produce the movements necessary for digestion and moving the food mass forward. (Modified from Thibodeau GA, Patton KT: *Anatomy and physiology*, ed 7, St. Louis, Mo., 2010, Mosby.)

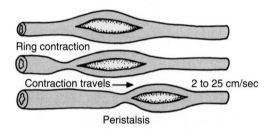

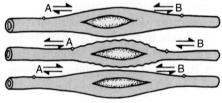

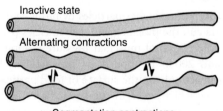

FIGURE 2-3 Types of movement produced by muscles of the intestine: peristaltic waves from contraction of deep circular muscle, pendular movements from small local muscles, and segmentation rings formed by alternate contraction and relaxation of circular muscle.

Nervous System Control

Throughout the gastrointestinal tract, specific nerves regulate muscle action. An interrelated network of nerves within the gastrointestinal wall called the intramural nerve plexus (Figure 2-4) extends from the esophagus to the anus. This network of approximately 100-million nerve fibers regulates the rate and intensity of muscle contractions, controls the speed at which the food mass moves along the tract, and coordinates the digestive process, including the secretion of enzymes and digestive juices.[5]

MOVEMENT OF FOOD THROUGH THE DIGESTIVE TRACT

We have reviewed the integrated muscular and secretory functions that govern the overall operation of the

KEY TERMS

digestion   The process of breaking down food to release its nutrients for absorption and transport to the cells for use in body functions.

serosa   Outer surface layer of the intestines interfacing with the blood vessels of the portal system that goes to the liver.

mucosa   The mucous membrane forming the inner surface of the gastrointestinal tract with extensive nutrient absorption and transport functions.

peristalsis   A wavelike progression of alternating contraction and relaxation of the muscle fibers of the gastrointestinal tract that keeps the food mass moving forward.

chyme   Semifluid food mass resulting from gastric digestion.

tonic   Ongoing low level muscle contraction and relaxation

intramural nerve plexus   Network of nerves in the walls of the intestine that control muscle action and secretions for digestion and absorption.

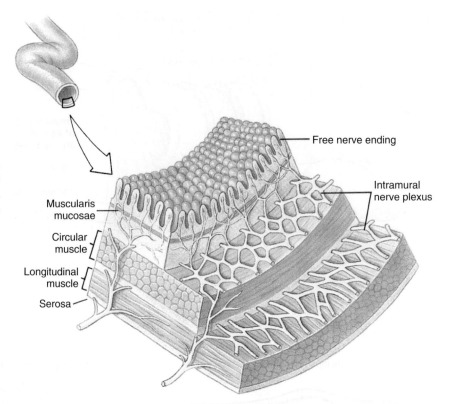

FIGURE 2-4 Innervation of the intestine by the intramural nerve plexus. A network of nerves controls and coordinates the movements of the intestinal muscles. (Courtesy Medical and Scientific Illustration.)

Free nerve ending

Intramural nerve plexus

Muscularis mucosae

Circular muscle

Longitudinal muscle

Serosa

gastrointestinal tract; now we begin to follow this process through its successive stages to see what happens to the food we eat.

MOUTH AND ESOPHAGUS: PREPARATION AND DELIVERY

Eating begins the process by which food is broken down into individual nutrients. The first steps in digestion occur in the mouth, where salivary enzymes act on carbohydrate and all foods are broken down into smaller particles to facilitate the later action of digestive juices. The esophagus delivers the food mass to the stomach.

Taste and Smell

Much of our enjoyment of food comes from its unique flavors and aromas. Taste buds located on the tongue, roof of the mouth, and throat contain chemical receptors that produce the four sensations of taste: salty, sweet, sour, and bitter. Recently, a fifth taste has been identified called *umami,* the taste of amino acids and proteins. Some individuals have a stronger perception of one taste over another, and certain medications produce a bitter taste or loss of taste. Genetically related differences in taste affect our preferences for certain foods. Individuals with enhanced sensitivity to bitter taste are more likely to avoid certain fruits and vegetables and prefer sweet or high-fat foods.[6] Such taste preferences that influence what we eat also affect our risk for obesity or developing

particular chronic diseases or conditions.[7] Patients on chemotherapy often have distorted taste (dysgeusia). Zinc deficiency causes a loss of taste (hypogeusia).

Foods contain volatile components that move from the back of the mouth up into the nasal cavity, where they act on olfactory receptors to produce the pleasant odors we associate with particular foods. In fact, much of what we perceive as a food's taste may actually be its odor. Radiation therapy of the head or neck, Parkinson's disease, and senile dementia of the Alzheimer type often lead to olfactory losses and less interest in eating.

Mastication

Food is broken into smaller particles by biting and chewing. The incisors cut; the molars grind. Jaw muscles provide tremendous force: 55 lb of muscular pressure is applied by the incisors, and 200 lb is applied by the molars.[2] Digestive enzymes can act only on the surface of food particles; therefore chewing, which enlarges the surface area available for enzyme action, is an important step in preparing food for digestion. Chewing also produces finer particles, easing the passage of the food mass down the esophagus and into the stomach. Chewing is necessary to prepare fiber-containing foods such as fruits, vegetables, and whole grains for digestion. Decayed teeth, missing teeth, or poorly fitting dentures make eating difficult. Gingivitis and other diseases of the gums and supporting structures of the teeth may result in mouth pain, infection, or further loss of teeth, thereby restricting food intake and contributing to malnutrition.

TABLE 2-1	COMPARATIVE pH VALUES AND APPROXIMATE DAILY VOLUMES OF GASTROINTESTINAL SECRETIONS	
SECRETION	pH	DAILY VOLUME (mL)
Salivary	6.0-7.4	1000
Gastric	1.0-3.5	1500
Pancreatic	8.0-8.3	1000
Small intestinal	7.5-8.0	1800
Brunner's gland (bicarbonate)	8.0-8.9	200
Bile	7.5-7.8	1000
Large intestinal	7.5-8.0	200
Total		6700

Modified from Guyton AC, Hall JE: *Textbook of medical physiology,* ed 10, Philadelphia, 2000, WB Saunders.

Chemical Digestion

In the mouth, three pairs of salivary glands—parotid, submaxillary, and sublingual—produce a watery fluid containing salivary amylase. This enzyme is specific for starch. The salivary glands also secrete mucus to lubricate and bind the food particles together. Sensory stimuli and even thoughts of favorite or disliked foods influence these secretions. Large amounts of digestive fluids are secreted throughout the gastrointestinal tract (Table 2-1). Saliva secretion alone ranges from 800 mL to 1500 mL a day. Food remains in the mouth for only a short time; thus starch digestion here is brief. However, when salivary amylase binds to starch molecules, it becomes resistant to inactivation by gastric acid, thereby allowing the breakdown of starch to continue in the stomach.[5] A second digestive enzyme released in saliva is lingual lipase, which begins the digestion of fat. Cigarette smoke alters the composition of saliva even in passive smokers,[8] and this effect may contribute to the loss of taste and changes in appetite associated with smoking.[9]

Salivary secretions have other important functions in addition to initiating digestion. They moisten the food particles so they bind together to form a bolus that moves easily down the esophagus, and they lubricate and cleanse the teeth and tissues of the mouth, destroying harmful bacteria and neutralizing any toxic substances entering the mouth. Inadequate secretion leads to the condition known as *dry mouth*. Everyone experiences occasional dry mouth when nervous, upset, or under stress. However, when production of saliva is drastically reduced and prolonged, it leads to swallowing problems as individual particles of food get separated in the esophagus. Infections and ulcers in the mouth, along with tooth decay, are other outcomes of extreme dry mouth, usually referred to as *xerostomia*. Radiation therapy that causes damage to the salivary glands and conditions such as diabetes, Parkinson's disease, and autoimmune deficiency diseases can lead to xerostomia. Various medications for management of cardiac failure, hypertension, depression, or chronic pain contribute to dry mouth in older adults.[10]

Swallowing

Swallowing involves both the mouth and the pharynx. It is intricately controlled by the swallowing center in the brainstem,[2] and damage to these nerves through radiation therapy, age-related changes, or disease makes swallowing difficult. As illustrated in Figure 2-5, the tongue initiates a swallow by pressing the food upward and backward against the palate. From this point on, swallowing goes forward as an involuntary reflex and once begun, cannot be interrupted. Swallowing occurs rapidly, taking less than 1 second, but in that time the larynx must close to prevent food from entering the trachea and moving into the lungs, and the soft palate must rise to prevent food from entering the nasal cavity. Patients must never be fed in a supine position because it increases the risk of food aspiration into the lungs.

Esophagus

The esophagus is a muscular tube that connects the mouth and throat with the stomach and serves as a channel to carry the food mass into the body. Functionally, it has the following three parts[2]:

1. *Upper esophageal sphincter (UES):* The UES controls the entry of the food bolus into the esophagus. Between swallows the UES muscle is closed. Within 0.2 to 0.3 seconds after a swallow, nerve stimuli open the sphincter to receive the food mass.

2. *Esophageal body:* The mixed bolus of food immediately passes down the esophagus, moved along by peristaltic waves controlled by nerve reflexes. Degenerative changes in the muscles or nerves lower the intensity and frequency of the peristaltic waves, slowing passage down the channel. Diabetic neuropathy is one cause of such problems.[11] Pain and discomfort associated with these changes can add to anorexia and weight loss. Gravity aids the passage of food down the esophagus when the person eats in an upright position.

3. *Lower esophageal sphincter (LES):* The LES controls the movement of the food bolus into the stomach. When the LES muscles maintain excessively high muscle tone, they fail to open after a swallow, preventing the passage of food into the stomach. This condition is called *achalasia*, meaning "unrelaxed muscle." (See Chapter 20 for a discussion of this condition.)

Entry Into the Stomach

At the point of entry into the stomach, the gastroesophageal constrictor muscle relaxes to allow the food to pass and then contracts quickly to prevent regurgitation or reflux of the

---

KEY TERMS

gingivitis Red, swollen, bleeding gums, often caused by accumulation of bacterial plaque on the teeth.

pharynx Throat.

bolus Rounded mass of food formed in the mouth and ready to be swallowed.

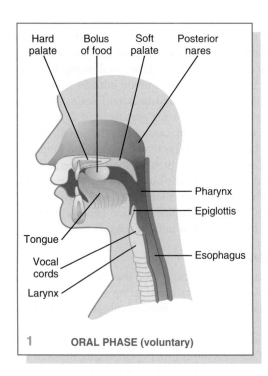

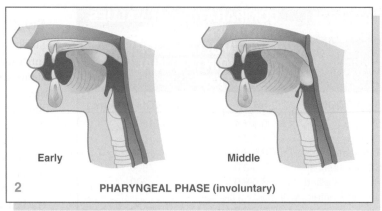

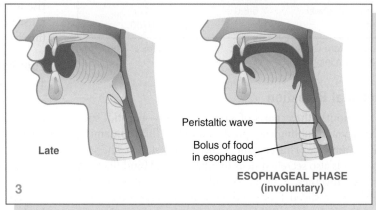

FIGURE 2-5 Swallowing is a highly coordinated task directed by a special nerve center in the hypothalamus. (From Mahan KL, Escott-Stump S, editors: *Krause's food, nutrition, and diet therapy,* ed 12, Philadelphia, 2008, Saunders.)

acidic stomach contents back into the esophagus. When this mechanism fails and regurgitation occurs, one feels what is called *heartburn.* The medical name for this condition is gastroesophageal reflux disease (GERD), and an estimated 10% to 20% of the general population experience GERD on an occasional or chronic basis.[12] GERD damages the tissues of the esophagus, which are unprotected from the destructive effects of gastric acid. Mucus secreted by cells in the stomach wall protects those tissues against the harsh effects of this acid. Obesity, overeating, physical inactivity, smoking, and certain medications contribute to GERD. According to national data, GERD is the leading diagnosis among outpatients who have gastrointestinal disease, and it affects nearly 9 million Americans.[13] The increasing prevalence of obesity contributes to these statistics.[12]

STOMACH: STORAGE AND INITIAL DIGESTION

Motility

The major parts of the stomach are described in Figure 2-6. Muscles in the stomach wall have three motor functions: (1) storage, (2) mixing, and (3) controlled emptying. As the food mass enters the stomach it rests against the stomach walls, which stretch to store as much as 1 L of food and fluid. Local tonic muscle waves increase their kneading and mixing

actions to move the mass of food and secretions toward the pyloric valve at the **distal** end of the stomach. Over time, waves of peristaltic contractions reduce the food mass to the semifluid chyme. Finally, with each wave, small amounts of chyme pass through the pyloric valve into the **duodenum.** The pyloric sphincter periodically constricts and relaxes to control the rate of emptying. The highly acid chyme must be released slowly enough to allow it to be buffered by the alkaline secretions of the small intestine. The caloric density of a meal, along with its volume and composition, influences the rate of stomach emptying. The speed at which food moves from the gastroesophageal sphincter to the distal end of the stomach and into the small intestine influences food intake, as messages to the brain signaling the arrival of food in the small intestine bring about the release of gastrointestinal hormones that induce feelings of satiety.

Chemical Digestion
Types of Secretions
Secretions produced in the stomach include acid, mucus, and enzymes, as follows:
- *Acid:* Hydrochloric acid creates the acidic environment necessary for certain digestive enzymes to work. For example, a pH of 1.8 to 3.5 is needed for the enzyme pepsin to act on protein; at a pH of 5.0 or above, there is little or no pepsin activity.

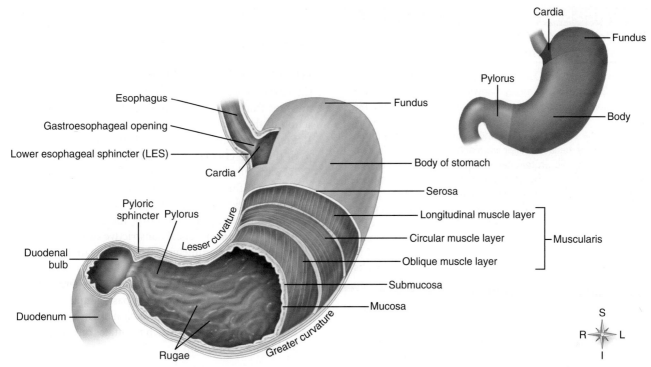

FIGURE 2-6 Stomach. The pyloric sphincter controls passage of the food mass from the stomach into the duodenum, the upper section of the small intestine. See also the five layers of muscle found in the stomach wall. (From Thibodeau GA, Patton KT: *Anatomy & physiology,* ed 7, St. Louis, Mo., 2010, Mosby.)

- *Mucus:* This **viscous** secretion protects the stomach lining from the eroding effect of the acid. Mucus also binds and mixes the food mass and helps move it along.
- *Enzymes:* The major enzyme in the stomach is pepsin, which begins the breakdown of protein. Pepsin is secreted in the form of pepsinogen and activated by hydrochloric acid. The stomach also produces a small amount of gastric lipase (tributyrinase) that acts only on butterfat and has a relatively minor role in overall digestion. Children have a gastric enzyme called *rennin* (not to be confused with the renal enzyme renin) that aids in the coagulation of milk. Coagulation of milk proteins, changing them from a liquid to a semisolid (as occurs when egg white is heated), slows the rate of stomach emptying, ensuring gradual passage of material to the small intestine. Rennin is absent in adults.

Control of Secretions

Stimuli for the release of gastric secretions come from two sources:

1. *Nerve stimuli* are produced in response to the visual and chemical senses, the presence of food in the gastrointestinal tract, and emotional distress. Anger and hostility increase gastric secretions; fear and depression lower secretions and inhibit blood flow to the region and gastric motility.
2. *Hormonal stimuli* are produced when food enters the stomach. Certain food components, especially caffeine,

alcohol, and meat extracts, cause the mucosal cells of the **antrum** to release the local gastrointestinal hormone **gastrin**. Gastrin, in turn, stimulates the secretion of hydrochloric acid. When the pH falls below 3, a feedback mechanism halts the release of gastrin, preventing accumulation of excess acid.[5] A second gastrointestinal hormone, **enterogastrone**, produced in the mucosa of the duodenum, also prevents excessive gastric response by inhibiting secretion of hydrochloric acid and pepsin and slowing gastric motility. (See the Evidence-Based Practice box, "Why Are Many Older Adults Deficient in Vitamin B_{12}?" which describes a problem related to inadequate secretion of gastric acid.)

KEY TERMS

distal   Away from the point of origin.

duodenum   The first section of the small intestine entered by food passing through the pyloric valve from the stomach.

viscous   Sticky.

antrum   Lower section of the stomach.

gastrin   Hormone secreted by mucosal cells in the antrum of the stomach that stimulates the parietal cells to produce hydrochloric acid.

enterogastrone   Hormone produced in the mucous membrane of the duodenum that inhibits gastric acid secretion and motility.

Why Do Older Adults Who Consume Animal Foods Become Deficient in Vitamin B₁₂?

Identify the Problem: Over the years clinicians have observed vitamin B_{12} deficiency among many older adults despite their liberal intakes of meat and other animal foods containing this vitamin.

Review the Evidence: Older adults might develop vitamin B_{12} deficiency because their stomachs no longer produce intrinsic factor, the protein carrier required for absorption of this vitamin. To confirm this diagnosis, older adults with a vitamin B_{12} deficiency were given a labeled dose of crystalline vitamin B_{12} with or without intrinsic factor, and absorption was evaluated by the later appearance of labeled vitamin B_{12} in the urine. It was expected that the vitamin administered without intrinsic factor would remain unabsorbed. Much to the surprise of the researchers, many of these older adults absorbed the vitamin-only test dose, so why were they deficient? Further studies revealed it was not a lack of intrinsic factor but rather a lack of gastric acid. Many older adults secrete very low amounts of hydrochloric acid, and a strongly acid environment is required in the stomach to activate pepsinogen to pepsin, the enzyme needed to break down dietary protein. When animal proteins are not broken down completely, their vitamin B_{12} is not released for absorption and is lost in the feces.

Implement the Findings: Crystalline vitamin B_{12} added to fortified breads, cereals, juices, and vitamin supplements is not bound to protein and is not dependent on an acid environment for absorption. Older adults should be encouraged to include a vitamin B_{12}-fortified food in their diet several times a week to ensure an adequate body supply. Also, we have learned that vitamin B_{12} in milk and dairy products is fairly well absorbed, even if gastric acid secretion is low, because they are more easily digested than meat, poultry, and fish. This finding suggests another reason beyond bone health to consume dairy products.

Bibliography

Allen LH: Bioavailability of vitamin B_{12}. *Int J Vitam Nutr Res* 80(4–5):330, 2010.

Allen LH: How common is vitamin B_{12} deficiency. *Am J Clin Nutr* 89(Suppl):693S, 2009.

Carmel R: Subclinical cobalamin deficiency. *Curr Opin Gastroenterol* 28:151, 2012.

Russell RM, Baik H, Kehayias JJ: Older men and women efficiently absorb vitamin B_{12} from milk and fortified bread. *J Nutr* 131:291, 2001.

Stover PJ: Vitamin B_{12} and older adults. *Curr Opin Nutr Metab Care* 13:24, 2010.

SMALL INTESTINE: MAJOR DIGESTION, ABSORPTION, AND TRANSPORT

Motility

Intestinal Muscle Layers

Review the complex structure of the intestinal wall pictured in Figure 2-2. Coordination of intestinal motility is accomplished by three layers of muscle: (1) the thin layer of smooth muscle embedded in the mucosa with fibers extending up into the villi, (2) the circular muscle layer, and (3) the longitudinal muscle lying next to the outer serosa.

Types of Intestinal Muscle Action

Under the control of the intramural nerve plexus, wall-stretch pressure from food or hormonal stimuli produces muscle action of the following two types:

1. *Propulsive movements:* Peristaltic waves from contractions of the deep circular muscles propel the food mass slowly forward. Fiber and other indigestible materials from plant foods aid this process, providing bulk for the action of these muscles. The presence of food or irritants brings about long sweeping waves over the entire intestine.
2. *Mixing movements:* Local constrictive contractions occurring every few centimeters mix and chop the food particles to form the semiliquid chyme. The interaction of the muscles in the small intestine produces general tonic contractions that ensure continuous passage and valve control, and periodic, rhythmic contractions that mix and propel the food mass forward, which facilitates ongoing digestion and future absorption.

Chemical Digestion
Major Role of the Small Intestine

In comparison to other sections of the gastrointestinal tract, the small intestine carries the major burden of chemical digestion. It secretes several enzymes, each specific for carbohydrate, fat, or protein, and is assisted by other enzymes entering from the pancreas. The small intestine acts as a regulatory center sensing the nutrient content, pH, and osmolarity of its contents, and controls enzyme secretion accordingly.[5]

Types of Secretions

The following four types of digestive secretions complete this final stage of chemical action:

1. *Enzymes:* Specific enzymes act on specific macronutrients to bring about their final breakdown to forms the body can absorb and use (Table 2-2).
2. *Mucus:* Glands located at the entrance to the duodenum secrete large amounts of mucus. As in the stomach, mucus protects the intestinal mucosa from irritation and digestion by the highly acidic chyme. Other cells along the length of the inner intestinal wall secrete mucus when touched by the moving food mass, protecting the mucosal tissues from abrasion.
3. *Hormones:* When signaled by the presence of acid in the food mass entering from the stomach, mucosal cells in the upper part of the small intestine produce the local gastrointestinal hormone secretin.[5] Secretin, in turn, stimulates the pancreas to send alkaline pancreatic juices into the duodenum to buffer the acidic chyme. The intestinal mucosa in the upper duodenum could not withstand the high acid of the entering chyme without the neutralizing action of the bicarbonate-containing pancreatic juice.

TABLE 2-2 SUMMARY OF DIGESTIVE PROCESSES

NUTRIENT	MOUTH	STOMACH	SMALL INTESTINE
Carbohydrate	Salivary amylase breaks down starch to dextrins		Pancreatic amylase breaks down starch to disaccharides: lactose, sucrose, and maltose. Disaccharides are broken down to monosaccharides. Lactase breaks down lactose to glucose and galactose. Sucrase breaks down sucrose to glucose and fructose. Maltase breaks down maltose to glucose and glucose.
Protein		Pepsin and HCl break down protein to polypeptides	Trypsin breaks down proteins and polypeptides to dipeptides. Chymotrypsin breaks down proteins and polypeptides to dipeptides. Carboxypeptidase breaks down polypeptides and dipeptides to amino acids. Aminopeptidase breaks down polypeptides and dipeptides to amino acids. Dipeptidase breaks down dipeptides to amino acids.
Fat	Lingual lipase has a minor role in beginning fat digestion	Tributyrinase breaks down tributyrin (butterfat) to glycerol and fatty acids	Bile emulsifies fat. Pancreatic lipase breaks down fat to glycerol, diglycerides, monoglycerides, and fatty acids.

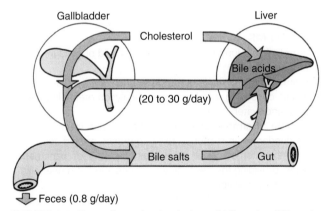

Feces (0.8 g/day)

FIGURE 2-7 Enterohepatic circulation of bile salts. Bile salts are reabsorbed from the small intestine and returned to the liver and gallbladder to be used again and again.

4. *Bile:* Bile emulsifies fat and facilitates its digestion. Bile is produced in the liver as a dilute watery solution and is then concentrated and stored by the gallbladder. When fat enters the duodenum, the local gastrointestinal hormone cholecystokinin (CCK) is secreted by glands in the intestinal mucosa and stimulates the gallbladder to contract and release bile. By means of the *enterohepatic circulation* (Figure 2-7), molecules of bile are reabsorbed and returned to the liver and gallbladder to be used over and over again. CCK also acts on the pancreas to stimulate the release of enzymes that break down fats, proteins, and carbohydrates.[5]

End Products of Digestion

When digestion of the macronutrients is complete, the simplified end products (Table 2-3) are ready for absorption. At

TABLE 2-3 END PRODUCTS OF DIGESTION

MACRONUTRIENT	END PRODUCTS
Carbohydrate	Glucose, fructose, and galactose (monosaccharides)
Fat	Fatty acids, monoglycerides, diglycerides, and glycerol
Protein	Amino acids, dipeptides

times, undigested nutrients remain in the small intestine,[11] causing discomfort or distress. When individuals lack the digestive enzyme lactase, the disaccharide lactose remains in the small intestine and attracts large amounts of fluid, resulting in abdominal pain and diarrhea, nausea, or flatulence.[14] (This condition and its clinical management are discussed later in this chapter.)

Absorption
Surface Structures
Viewed from the outside, the small intestine appears smooth, but the inner surface is quite different. In Figure 2-8 the following three types of convolutions and projections greatly expand the absorbing surface:

1. *Mucosal folds:* Large folds similar to hills and valleys in a mountain range are easily seen with the naked eye.
2. *Villi:* Fingerlike projections on these folds called villi can be seen through a simple compound microscope.
3. *Microvilli:* These extremely small projections on each villus can only be seen with an electron microscope. The array of microvilli covering the edge of each villus is called

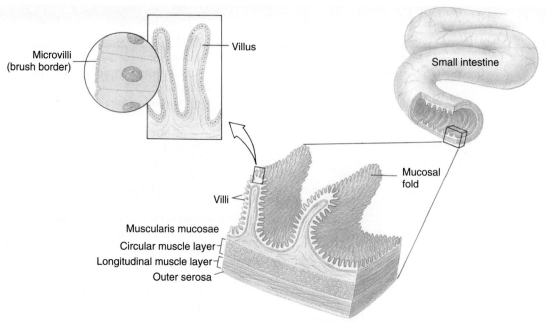

FIGURE 2-8 Absorbing structures of the intestine. Note the structures of the intestinal mucosa that increase the surface area for absorption: mucosal folds, villi, and microvilli. (Courtesy Medical and Scientific Illustration.)

TABLE 2-4	VOLUME OF NUTRIENTS ABSORBED DAILY BY THE GASTROINTESTINAL SYSTEM		
SUBSTANCE	INTAKE (L)	INTESTINAL ABSORPTION (L)	ELIMINATION (L)
Food ingested	1.5		
Gastrointestinal secretions	8.5		
TOTAL	10.0		
Fluid absorbed in small intestine		9.5	
Fluid absorbed in large intestine (colon)		0.4	
TOTAL		9.9	
Feces			0.1

KEY TERMS

osmolarity   Number of millimoles of liquid or solid in a liter of solution.

mucus   Viscous fluid secreted by mucous membranes and glands, consisting mainly of mucin (a glycoprotein), inorganic salts, and water.

secretin   Hormone produced in the mucous membrane of the duodenum in response to the entrance of acid contents from the stomach that stimulates the flow of pancreatic juices, providing the necessary enzymes and the proper alkalinity for their action.

cholecystokinin (CCK)   A peptide hormone secreted by the mucosa of the duodenum in response to the presence of fat that causes the gallbladder to contract and propel bile into the duodenum where it is needed to emulsify the fat.

absorption   Transport of nutrients from the lumen of the intestine across the intestinal wall into the blood (glucose and amino acids) or the lymph (fatty acids).

villi   Fingerlike projections covering the mucosal surface of the small intestine.

microvilli   Minute vascular structures protruding from the villi covering the inner surface of the small intestine that form a "brush border" that facilitates absorption of nutrients.

the *brush border* because it resembles bristles on a brush. Each villus has an ample network of blood capillaries for the absorption of monosaccharides and amino acids, and a central lymph vessel called a *lacteal* for the absorption of fatty acids.

The mucosa, villi, and microvilli together increase the inner surface area of the small intestine approximately 1000 times over that of the outside covering.[2] These specialized structures, plus the contracted length of the small intestine—630 to 660 cm (21 to 22 feet)—produce a tremendously large surface area to capture and absorb nutrients. This absorbing surface, if stretched out flat, would be as large as a tennis or basketball court. The small intestine is one of the most highly developed organs in the body, making possible its tremendous absorptive capacity for food and fluid (Table 2-4).

Mechanisms of Absorption

Absorption of the nutrients dispersed in the water-based solution entering the small intestine involves several transport mechanisms. The particular transport mechanism used depends on the nutrient and the prevailing electrochemical fluid pressure gradient; these are described as follows:

- *Passive diffusion and osmosis:* When there is no opposing fluid pressure, molecules small enough to pass through the capillary membranes diffuse easily into the villi (Figure 2-9). High concentrations of nutrients waiting to move into the capillaries where nutrient concentrations are low create an electrochemical gradient and osmotic pressure that promote absorption.[2]
- *Facilitated diffusion:* Even when the pressure gradient supports absorption, some molecules may be too large to pass easily through the membrane pores and need assistance. Specific proteins located in the membrane facilitate passage by carrying the nutrient across the membrane.
- *Energy-dependent active transport:* Nutrients must cross the intestinal membrane to reach hungry cells even when the flow pressures are against them. Such active work requires extra energy along with a pumping mechanism. A special membrane protein carrier, coupled with the active transport of sodium, assists in the process. The energy-requiring, sodium-coupled transport of glucose is an example of this action. The enzyme sodium/potassium-dependent adenosine triphosphatase (Na^+/K^+-ATPase) in the cell membrane supplies the energy for the pump.
- *Engulfing pinocytosis:* At times, fluid and nutrient molecules are absorbed by pinocytosis. When the nutrient particle touches the absorbing cell membrane, the membrane dips inward around the nutrient, surrounds it to form a vacuole, and then engulfs it. The nutrient is then conveyed through the cell cytoplasm and discharged into the circulation. Smaller whole proteins and fat droplets can be absorbed through pinocytosis (Figure 2-10).

Routes of Absorption

After their absorption, the water-soluble monosaccharides and amino acids enter directly into the portal blood and travel to the liver and other tissues. Fat, which is not water soluble, follows a different route. Fats packaged in a bile complex called a *micelle* (described in more detail in Chapter 4) move into the cells of the intestinal wall, where they are processed into human lipid compounds and joined with a carrier protein. These **lipoproteins**, called *chylomicrons*, flow into the lymph, empty into the cisterna chyli (the central abdominal collecting vessel of the lymphatic system), travel upward into the chest through the thoracic duct, and finally flow into the venous blood at the left subclavian vein. The chylomicrons are rapidly cleared from the blood by a special fat enzyme called *lipoprotein lipase*.

Exceptions to this route of fat absorption are the short-chain fatty acids with 10 or fewer carbons. Because these short-chain fatty acids are water soluble, they can be absorbed directly into the blood along with the carbohydrate and protein breakdown products. However, most dietary fats are made of long-chain fatty acids that are not water soluble and must take the lymphatic route.

COLON (LARGE INTESTINE): FINAL ABSORPTION AND WASTE ELIMINATION

Role in Absorption

Within a 24-hour period, approximately 1500 mL of the remaining food mass leaves the **ileum**, the last section of the

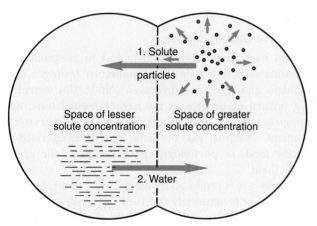

FIGURE 2-9 Movement of molecules, water, and solutes through osmosis and diffusion.

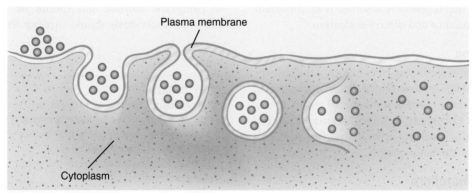

FIGURE 2-10 Pinocytosis, the engulfing of large molecules by the cell. (From Nix S: *Williams' basic nutrition and diet therapy,* ed 13, St. Louis, Mo., 2009, Mosby.)

small intestine, and enters the cecum, the pouch at the entrance to the colon. Passage is controlled by the ileocecal valve. Normally the valve remains closed, but each peristaltic wave relaxes the valve muscle, squirting a small amount of remaining chyme into the cecum. This action holds the food mass in the small intestine long enough to ensure maximal digestion and absorption. Nutrients and other materials, including electrolytes, minerals, vitamins, intestinal bacteria, and nondigestible residue, remain in the chyme delivered to the large intestine.

Water Absorption

The main task remaining for the colon is the absorption of water. The capacity of the colon to absorb water is vast, with a net daily maximum of 5 to 8 L.[2] Normally, from 1.0 to 1.5 L is received from the ileum, and 95% of that is absorbed (see Table 2-4).

Much of the water in the chyme (350 to 400 mL) is absorbed in the first half of the colon. Only 100 to 150 mL remains to form the feces.[2] Absorption of water in the colon is important in the regulation of water balance and the elimination of fecal waste. When the chyme first enters the colon, it is a semiliquid, but water absorption during passage changes it to the semisolid nature of normal feces.

The amount of water absorbed in the colon depends on motility and rate of passage. Poor motility and a slow passage rate, often related to low dietary fiber and low fecal mass, allow greater absorption of water, resulting in hard stools that are difficult to pass, and constipation. Excess motility and too-rapid passage limit the absorption of water and important electrolytes, producing a high volume of loose, watery stool (diarrhea). Diarrhea can result from disease; microbial infection as in foodborne illness; or large amounts of undigested sugar, such as lactose, that exert osmotic pressure and hold vast amounts of fluid. Severe or extended diarrhea leads to dehydration and serious loss of electrolytes.

Mineral Absorption

Sodium and other electrolytes are absorbed from the colon. Intestinal absorption exerts major control on body content of many minerals, and much of our dietary intake is unabsorbed and excreted in the feces. Up to 90% of the calcium and iron in the food we eat is not absorbed. The proportion of a mineral intake that is generally absorbed is an important aspect of nutrient balance and dietary evaluation.

Vitamin Absorption

Conditions in the gastrointestinal tract influence the absorption of vitamins. When gastric acid is lower than normal, vitamin B_{12} is not easily released from animal tissues and is lost in the feces. Conversely, colonic bacteria synthesize vitamin K and biotin, which are actively absorbed and serve as a major source of the body's supply.

Role of Colon Microflora

At birth the colon is sterile, but intestinal bacteria acquired through delivery and infant feeding (human milk or formula)

influence the growth and diversity of particular species. More complex microflora develop after weaning as infants add an increasing number of foods to their diet. The normal diversity of 1000 different species is established by 3 years of age.[15] The gastrointestinal tract contains about 100-trillion microbes—10 times the total number of cells in the human body, and weighing as much as 2 kg.[16] The composition is dynamic in both numbers and species. Dietary intake, genetics, physical environment, use of antibiotics, and immune responses to infection favor one group of bacteria over another. Bacterial populations also differ along the length of the gastrointestinal tract based on differences in structure and pH.[17] Many bacteria ingested with food do not survive the extreme acid environment in the stomach.

Colonic bacteria make up approximately one third of fecal weight,[2] and influence the color and odor of the stool. Colonic bacteria acting on bilirubin produce bile pigments, giving the stool its characteristic brown color; thus, when bile flow is hindered, the feces become clay colored or white. The characteristic odor of the stool comes from amines, especially indole and skatole, formed by the action of bacterial enzymes on amino acids.

Intestinal microflora have many roles. Particular microorganisms produce bothersome gas or increase the risk of gastrointestinal disease. Other species make positive contributions to health. (We discuss these relationships in more detail in the following sections.)

Excessive Gas Production

Colonic bacteria are major contributors to gas production including carbon dioxide (CO_2), molecular hydrogen (H_2), methane, and sometimes hydrogen sulfide. Gas formation is a normal occurrence in the gastrointestinal tract, and, though harmless, is distressing when it causes pain or embarrassment. Intestinal gas, or flatus, can be exaggerated by specific foods or physiologic circumstances in the person eating them.

Usually, gas is produced by the bacterial fermentation of undigested or incompletely absorbed carbohydrate. Humans lack the enzymes necessary to digest the oligosaccharides raffinose and stachyose in legumes that cause the intestinal gas associated with these foods. Certain starches and fibrous materials in whole grains, fruits, and vegetables are resistant to pancreatic amylase and cannot be broken down and absorbed. Individuals should increase their intakes of fiber

---

KEY TERMS

pinocytosis Means of nutrient absorption by which the molecule is engulfed by the cytoplasm of the receiving cell.

lipoproteins Noncovalent complexes of fat with protein that transport lipids in the blood.

ileum The distal section of the small intestine that connects with the colon.

colon The large intestine extending from the cecum to the rectum.

gradually to allow a more comfortable adjustment and prevent gastrointestinal distress.

Excessive gas has social implications. Methane, CO_2, and H_2 are odorless, but hydrogen sulfide carries a striking odor. Hydrogen sulfide most often arises from cruciferous vegetables (cabbage, cauliflower, or broccoli) or large amounts of beer, all high in sulfur. Various over-the-counter products claim to reduce the formation of gas or eliminate gaseous odors, but all have limitations. Individuals should check with their physician before using such preparations.[18] (See the Complementary and Alternative Medicine [CAM] box, "Bismuth and Certain Herbs: A Dangerous Combination," for cautions.)

Waste Elimination

Fully formed and ready for elimination, normal feces are approximately 75% water and 25% solids.[2] Solids include fiber, bacteria, inorganic matter such as minerals, a small amount of fat and its derivatives, some mucus, and sloughed-off mucosal cells.

The mass of food residue now slows its passage. Approximately 4 hours after a meal is eaten, food enters the cecum, having traveled the entire length of the small intestine [630 to 660 cm (21 to 22 feet)]. Approximately 8 hours later, it reaches the sigmoid colon, having traveled an additional 90 cm (3 feet) through the large intestine. In the sigmoid colon, the residue descends still more slowly toward its final destination, the rectum.

The rectum begins at the end of the large intestine immediately past the descending colon and ends at the anus. Feces are usually stored in the descending colon; however, when it becomes full, feces pass into the rectum, resulting in the urge to defecate. Anal sphincters under voluntary control regulate the elimination of feces from the body. As much as 25% of a meal may remain in the rectum for up to 72 hours.

GASTROINTESTINAL FUNCTION AND CLINICAL APPLICATIONS

Chronic Gastrointestinal Distress

Most of the time the gastrointestinal tract is a smoothly working system that allows us to enjoy the food we eat while effectively handling digestion, absorption, and the elimination of waste. However, abdominal pain or bloating, early satiety, postmeal discomfort, nausea, or vomiting are regular occurrences for some individuals, although no disease or structural explanation can be found.[19,20] This situation, referred to as *functional dyspepsia*, adds significantly to health care costs[19] and impacts on vitality and quality of life.[21] Anxiety, emotional stress, depression, various prescription medications, certain foods, and chronic disease all influence gastrointestinal function and may contribute to symptoms in particular individuals.

We need to listen carefully when people tell us about gastrointestinal problems that interfere with eating and their enjoyment of food or that limit their food selections.[22] Health education should point to the dangers of over-the-counter drugs or remedies such as food enzymes claiming to enhance digestion, inappropriate laxatives, or procedures such as colonic irrigation. Chronic digestive problems demand medical assessment and intervention.

(See the Perspectives in Practice box, "Help Your Digestive System Work for You," for practices that support optimal digestive function.)

Lactose Intolerance

Lactose intolerance is a digestive problem related to the inability to digest lactose. Lactose intolerance is estimated to affect as many as 70% of the world's population, including most Asians,[23] although calculations vary if based on self-perception or laboratory testing. In a recent U.S. study, 8% of Caucasian adults, 20% of African-American adults, and 9% of Hispanic adults believed they were lactose intolerant.[24] Individuals with lactose intolerance vary in their ability to digest lactose. They may have symptoms after taking in as little as 6 g or as much as 12 to 18 g of lactose (1 cup of milk contains 12 g of lactose).[14] The problem stems from a deficiency of lactase, the digestive enzyme in the microvilli of the small intestine that breaks lactose into the simple sugars glucose and galactose. When undigested lactose remains in the small intestine and colon, it absorbs large amounts of water and is fermented by resident bacteria, producing diarrhea, bloating, and gas.

Congenital intolerance to lactose is rare; infants usually produce enough lactase to digest the large amounts of lactose in mother's milk. However, loss of lactase activity beyond early childhood is the normal physiologic pattern, with relatively few adults retaining their former capacity for lactose digestion. Before the domestication of cows, lactose was not present in the diet after weaning; therefore this enzyme was

---

 COMPLEMENTARY AND ALTERNATIVE MEDICINE (CAM)

Bismuth and Certain Herbs: A Dangerous Combination

Bismuth-containing medications such as Pepto-Bismol are used to ease gas and bloating. Bismuth also binds with the odor-causing sulfur compounds found in intestinal gas and helps reduce odor and embarrassment. However, when combined with gingko, garlic, ginger, or ginseng, bismuth can have serious side effects. Working together, bismuth and these herbs act as anticoagulants.

Bonci L: *American Dietetic Association guide to better digestion*, Hoboken, NJ, 2003, John Wiley & Sons.

KEY TERMS

bilirubin A reddish bile pigment resulting from the degradation of heme by reticuloendothelial cells in the liver; a high level in the blood produces the yellow skin symptomatic of jaundice.

dyspepsia Gastric distress or indigestion involving nausea, pain, burning sensations, or excessive gas.

PERSPECTIVES IN PRACTICE

Help Your Digestive System Work for You

Our way of eating can either support or stress the normal function of the digestive tract. Positive practices maximize our enjoyment of food and help regulate our food intake.

- Chew your food slowly; allow time for the vapors to enter your sinus cavity and contribute to your sensation of taste.
- Take small bites; eating in a hurry and washing down large mouthfuls with liquid often lead to swallowing an excessive amount of air, causing bloating and belching.
- Wait 15 to 20 minutes before taking second helpings; when food moves from your stomach into your small intestine it triggers feelings of satiety and you may find that you don't need that extra spoonful.
- Try to concentrate on pleasant thoughts or conversation while eating; emotional distress such as fear, anger, or worry can depress the secretion of digestive enzymes and slow peristalsis, leading to gastrointestinal discomfort or upset.
- Focus on your food when eating; try not to combine eating with watching television, completing a homework assignment, or driving to work or class.

- Enjoy the sight, smells, and anticipation of food as you prepare or serve your meal; these responses promote enzyme secretion and digestive function.
- Divide your food across the day; don't consume the majority of your kcalories at one meal; the cells lining the gastrointestinal tract derive most of their energy from the food passing through, and they require a constant supply of nutrients to meet their high metabolic demands.
- Try to eat approximately the same amount of food every day, rather than gorging one day and fasting the next; this supports not only efficient gastrointestinal function but also effective body weight management.

Bibliography

Bonci L: *American Dietetic Association guide to better digestion*, Hoboken, NJ, 2003, John Wiley & Sons.

Harvard Medical School: *The Sensitive Gut, A Harvard Medical School Special Health Report*, Boston, 2012, Harvard Medical School.

Rolls B, Barnett RA: *Volumetrics*, New York, 2000, HarperCollins Publishers.

---

no longer needed. The introduction of a dairy-based culture in particular geographic regions 10,000 years ago likely contributed to the retention of lactase activity among certain European groups. Most populations lose more than 70% of their lactase activity within 3 to 4 years of weaning, although Caucasians often retain high lactase activity through adolescence.[23]

Other conditions can cause or worsen symptoms after eating foods that contain lactose. Irritable bowel syndrome, celiac disease, cystic fibrosis, or other disorders that damage the intestinal mucosa can interfere with the digestion of lactose, and medical diagnosis is often needed to confirm the basis of the malabsorption. Viral infections can cause temporary lactose intolerance. The identification of genes that support the persistence of lactase secretion has enabled the development of genetic testing to confirm true lactose intolerance.[25]

Individuals who appear to have problems digesting lactose may not be lactose intolerant. When adults who believed they were lactose intolerant were given a beverage containing lactose as opposed to a similar beverage that looked and tasted the same but had the lactose removed, their responses were similar, suggesting that lactose itself is not always the major cause of symptoms when consumed in the customary dietary portion of 1 cup of milk.[26] In general, symptoms will not occur with doses of 15 g of lactose or less, especially if consumed with other foods. Symptoms increase when intake rises to 20 g and become acute at levels of 50 g or higher.[27]

Most people who have problems digesting lactose do not need to follow a lactose-free diet, although milk may be limited in favor of other dairy foods. Maldigestion of lactose does not mean that an individual is allergic to milk or dairy foods, although both conditions are sometimes present in the same person. A true milk allergy is caused by the protein in milk, not the lactose.[18]

To increase their intakes of calcium and vitamin D, people with lactose maldigestion might begin to include dairy foods in their diet in the following ways[18]:

- *Add dairy foods gradually:* Begin with a small amount of one dairy food each day, one-quarter cup of milk or one-half ounce of cheese; include only one lactose-containing food per meal. (See Box 2-1 for food lactose content.)
- *Include lactose-containing foods with a meal or snack:* This combination slows the movement of lactose into the intestine and may reduce discomfort.
- *Choose dairy foods low in lactose:* Use lactose-free or lactose-reduced milk. (Acidophilus milk is not lactose-free.) Add lactase enzyme drops (Lactaid or Dairy Ease) to milk to break down some of the lactose. Lactase tablets taken right before eating can reduce discomfort. Aged cheeses such as cheddar or Swiss are lower in lactose than cheese spreads or other processed cheese. Lactose is also found in nondairy foods that have milk as an ingredient. Breads and other baked products, some ready-to-eat breakfast cereals, pancake and cookie mixes, instant potatoes, cream soups, hot dogs, and luncheon meats may contain lactose. Read the Nutrition Facts label, and look for the word *milk* or *whey*. (See Chapter 7 for food sources of calcium for persons who cannot tolerate dairy foods.)

Prebiotics and Probiotics

We sometimes have the perception that all microbes are harmful as we read reports of antibiotic-resistant viruses, outbreaks of foodborne illnesses, or advertisements for antibacterial soap. In contrast, Elie Metchnikoff, a Russian microbiologist who lived in the 19th century, speculated that fermented milk that supplied microbes beneficial to colon

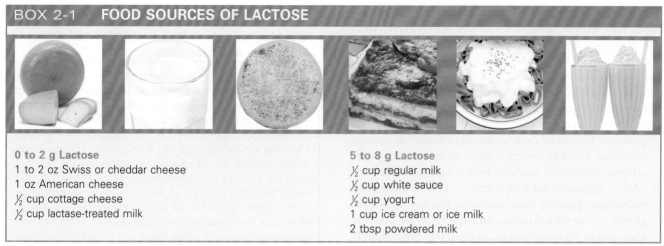

BOX 2-1   FOOD SOURCES OF LACTOSE

0 to 2 g Lactose
1 to 2 oz Swiss or cheddar cheese
1 oz American cheese
½ cup cottage cheese
½ cup lactase-treated milk

5 to 8 g Lactose
½ cup regular milk
½ cup white sauce
½ cup yogurt
1 cup ice cream or ice milk
2 tbsp powdered milk

Data from Bonci L: *American Dietetic Association guide to better digestion,* Hoboken, NJ, 2003, John Wiley & Sons.

BOX 2-2   COLONIC BACTERIA SUPPORT HEALTH IN VARIOUS WAYS

- Produce short-chain fatty acids that nourish the cells of the intestinal mucosa
- Assist in absorbing and activating phytochemicals
- Assist in breaking down binding substances and enabling absorption of minerals
- Prevent harmful bacteria from growing and forming colonies
- Support immune cells that attack harmful body invaders
- Synthesize biotin and vitamin K

---

health contributed to the long life of many peasants in his country. We have since learned that many microbes living in the gastrointestinal tract promote human health; these microbes are new tools for improving gastrointestinal and immune function and treating gastrointestinal disorders (Box 2-2). These microbes and related food components have been termed *prebiotics* and *probiotics* based on their use and intestinal effects. Prebiotics are components found in food that selectively stimulate the growth of one or more species of bacteria in the colon. Probiotics are live microorganisms that result in a health benefit to the host when administered in adequate amounts.[28]

Prebiotics

Prebiotics are indigestible carbohydrates, mostly polysaccharides, that are resistant to the secretions of the stomach and small intestine. They reach the colon generally intact; from there they are fermented and stimulate the growth and activity of healthy bacteria, such as *Lactobacillus* and *Bifidobacterium*.[29,30] Any dietary component that reaches the colon intact is a potential prebiotic. Prebiotics used clinically include oligosaccharides isolated from wheat, onions, bananas, garlic, soybeans, artichokes, and asparagus. Other prebiotics include various fiber derivatives and lactulose, a synthetic disaccharide.[28] Prebiotics found in breast milk support the development of appropriate microflora in the infant's gastrointestinal tract and likely contribute to the immune factors passing to

the breast-fed infant.[29] Prebiotics have been used to treat allergies and eczema in infants and adults.[31]

Prebiotics support increases in health-promoting bacteria and bring about various favorable actions, as follows:

- *Immune function:* Prebiotics exert a profound effect on the immune system by way of their action on microbial populations and the protective cells lining the colon. Prebiotics influence the secretion of antibodies and other agents of the immune system when needed to combat pathogens entering the lower gastrointestinal tract. Prebiotics support the proliferation of health-promoting bacteria that limit the development of harmful bacterial colonies and prevent the binding of pathogens to the intestinal mucosa.[31] Imbalances in gastrointestinal microflora have been implicated in the development of Crohn's disease, inflammatory bowel disease (IBS), and infectious diarrhea.[30]
- *Mineral absorption:* Although most minerals are absorbed in the small intestine, the lower pH of the colon that results from bacterial fermentation stimulates the absorption of calcium, magnesium, zinc, and iron still remaining in the food residue. These bacteria also break down phytate, an indigestible material found in plant foods that binds minerals and prevents their absorption.[31,32] The effect of prebiotics on calcium absorption exerts a positive effect on bone health.
- *Normal laxation:* The fermenting action of bacteria on lactulose relieves constipation and helps avoid dependence on laxatives. Prebiotics added to tube feedings prevent the common problem of diarrhea.[28]
- *Colon cancer:* The fermentation products of health-promoting bacteria may help destroy cancer cells and toxic enzymes produced by harmful bacteria, although further study is needed.[33]

Probiotics

The most commonly used probiotics are lactic-acid bacteria and nonpathogenic yeasts. The benefits of probiotics depend on the particular strain of live bacteria and the active substances it produces. Lactic acid–producing bacteria have been used over the centuries to acidify and preserve foods such as cultured milk and yogurt, cheese, distilled mash, pickled cabbages, and tempeh. Probiotic cultures are available from pharmaceutical companies for clinical use, although quality control regarding the number, activity, and strain of bacteria can be a problem.[28] It is difficult to know how a particular dose of living bacteria will interact with the microflora that already exist in a particular individual. Nevertheless, clinical applications of probiotics now in use include the following:

- *Diarrhea:* Species of *Lactobacillus* are effective in treating infectious diarrhea, which is often rampant in day care centers.[34] Probiotics have also been a successful intervention for antibiotic-induced diarrhea.[35] Loss of the normal microflora resulting from antibiotic therapy allows the growth of harmful bacteria, and the resulting diarrhea adds days to recovery time. In contrast, probiotics seem to have less effect on healthy individuals, as shown when a probiotic drink administered to school-age children, in an effort to reduce infectious disease, did not lower the number of days missed from school.[36]
- *Infant allergies:* Probiotics have the ability to attenuate immune responses and reduce cereal allergies. When given to expectant mothers with a family history of cereal allergy, only half of their infants showed signs of potential allergy.[37]
- *Inflammatory bowel disease:* In patients with ulcerative colitis, treatment with probiotics has supported remission and effectively treated mild to moderate flare-ups. Treatment of Crohn's disease has been less successful.[28,35]
- *Inhibition of* H. pylori: This pathogenic bacterium attaches to the gastric mucosa and has been implicated in the development of peptic ulcer, chronic gastritis, and gastric cancer. Probiotics seem to inhibit its growth and prevent it from burrowing into the stomach lining.[38] (See the Focus on Culture box, "*Helicobacter pylori*: Risk Factor for African Americans and Hispanics," for more information on the prevalence of this condition among various groups.)
- *Gastrointestinal immune response:* Probiotics support the immune cells in the gastrointestinal tract that provide the first line of defense against pathogens entering the body.[28]
- *Lactose intolerance*: Probiotics in the colon help break down lactose, preventing symptoms associated with lactase deficiency.[28]

Although lactic acid–producing bacteria have been used successfully in food and therapeutic preparations, safety is still a concern. Individuals with compromised immune function should not use probiotics without medical supervision, and clinicians have raised concerns about their use with critically ill patients. Contamination of the probiotic with a pathogenic strain or the passage of a probiotic microorganism across the intestinal mucosa and into the blood could lead to sepsis in an adult who lacks normal immune response.[39] Heat-killed probiotic species would provide a safe alternative for individuals at risk, although their potential effectiveness has not been determined.[40] Currently, no legal definitions have been formulated for the terms *prebiotic* or *probiotic*, and as dietary supplements, their product labels are not reviewed for accuracy or efficacy by the U.S. Food and

⊕ FOCUS ON CULTURE

Helicobacter pylori: *Risk Factor for African Americans and Hispanics*

The bacterium *H. pylori* resides in the stomach lining of nearly half of the world's population. In contrast to *Lactobacillus* and *Bifidobacterium*, which carry out many healthful functions in the human colon, *H. pylori* is a known risk factor for dyspepsia, peptic ulcer, chronic gastritis, and gastric cancer. Although a national survey reported that 31% of the U.S. population tested positive for *H. pylori*, prevalence in the African-American and Mexican-American population of the U.S. was nearly twice this number. *H. pylori* infection may contribute to the higher incidence of gastric cancer among African Americans as compared with Caucasians. *H. pylori* infection also affects nutritional status, because it lowers the secretion of gastric acid needed for optimal absorption of various nutrients. Individuals who tested positive for *H. pylori* had lower serum levels of retinol (vitamin A), beta carotene, and folate, despite dietary intakes equivalent to those with higher serum levels who were free of *H. pylori* infection. In another report, low blood levels of ascorbic acid and vitamin B_{12} were restored to normal when the patients' *H. pylori* infection was eradicated. *H. pylori* status is related to socioeconomic variables with higher rates of infection among those with less education, lower income, and poorer living conditions; however, African Americans are still more likely to test positive than Caucasians in a similar situation, suggesting a biologic vulnerability among African Americans.

Bibliography

Epplein M, Cohen SS, Zheng W, et al: Neighborhood socioeconomic characteristics, African ancestry, and *Helicobacter pylori* sero-prevalence. *Cancer Causes Control* 23(6):897, 2012.

Epplein M, Signorello LB, Zheng W, et al: *Helicobacter pylori* prevalence and circulating micronutrient levels in a low-income United States population. *Cancer Prev Res (Phila)* 4(6):871, 2011.

Grad YH, Lipsitch M, Aiello AE: Secular trends in *Helicobacter pylori* seroprevalence in adults in the United States: evidence for sustained race/ethnic disparities. *Am J Epidemiol* 175(1):54, 2012.

Lahner E, Persechino S, Annibale B: Micronutrients (other than iron) and Helicobacter pylori infection: a systematic review. *Helicobacter* 17(1):1, 2012.

Drug Administration.[28] Accurate information relating to the exact strain or species of bacteria, dosage required for effective intervention, safety of a particular product, or product shelf life can be difficult to obtain.[29]

▌HEALTH PROMOTION

Choosing Foods That Contain Prebiotics and Probiotics

Individuals can increase their populations of health-promoting prebiotic and probiotic species by thoughtful food selection. Fruits and vegetables such as bananas, leeks, and asparagus, and whole-grain oatmeal and wheat products are good sources of prebiotics.[41] Yogurt, cheese, and kefir (fermented milk prepared by adding kefir grains to cow's or goat's milk) all contain potentially beneficial live bacteria. Some yogurts currently sold in the U.S. contain not only starter cultures of bacteria, but also added *Lactobacillus* or *Bifidobacterium* to produce a probiotic effect, although label information as to the amount added can be limited. New fermented milk and yogurt products marketed as functional foods and containing known strains of bacteria at probiotic levels are entering the marketplace.[28]

METABOLISM

Following absorption, nutrients are transported to cells to provide energy or produce substances and tissues needed to sustain body functions. Metabolic activities within cells encompass the total spectrum of chemical reactions associated with the final use of the individual macronutrients.

Carbohydrate Metabolism

Glucose is an immediate energy source for all body cells, but it is the preferred energy source for the brain and nervous system. Because glucose is so critical to life, its level in the blood is carefully regulated.

Sources of Blood Glucose

Both carbohydrate and noncarbohydrate molecules are sources of blood glucose, described as follows:
- *Carbohydrate sources:* Three carbohydrate substances can be converted to glucose: (1) dietary starches and sugars, (2) glycogen stored in the liver and muscle, and (3) products of carbohydrate metabolism such as lactic acid and pyruvic acid.
- *Noncarbohydrate sources:* Both protein and fat are indirect sources of glucose. Certain amino acids are called *glucogenic amino acids* because they can form glucose after their amino group (NH_2^+) is removed. About 58% of the protein in a mixed diet is made of glucogenic amino acids. Thus, more than half of dietary protein might ultimately be used for energy if sufficient carbohydrate and fat are not available. After fats are broken down into fatty acids and glycerol, the glycerol portion (about 10% of the fat) can be converted to glycogen in the liver and then to glucose as needed. The formation of glucose from protein, glycerol, and carbohydrate metabolites is called **gluconeogenesis.**

Uses of Blood Glucose

Blood glucose is maintained within a normal range of 70 to 140 mg/dL (3.9-7.8 mmol/L) but is in constant flux as absorbed glucose is transported to cells for immediate use or removed from the circulation and stored as glycogen or fat. Blood glucose is used in three different ways:
- *Energy production:* The primary function of glucose is to supply energy to meet the body's constant demand. An array of metabolic pathways requiring specific and successive enzymes accomplishes this task.

- *Energy storage:* Glucose is stored in two forms: (1) glycogen, which is held in limited amounts in liver and muscle; and (2) fat (adipose tissue), which is the storage form for all excess glucose after energy demands have been met. Only a small supply of glycogen exists at any one time, and it turns over rapidly. In contrast, fat can be stored in unlimited amounts in adipose tissue and provides long-term energy stores.
- *Glucose products:* Small amounts of glucose are used to produce various carbohydrate compounds with important roles in body metabolism. Examples include deoxyribonucleic acid (DNA) and ribonucleic acid (RNA), galactose, and certain amino acids.

These sources and uses of glucose act as checks and balances to maintain normal blood glucose levels, adding or removing glucose as needed.

Hormonal Controls

Several hormones directly and indirectly influence glucose metabolism and regulate blood glucose levels.
- *Blood glucose–lowering hormone:* Only one hormone—insulin—lowers blood glucose. Insulin is produced by the beta cells in the pancreas. These cells are scattered in clusters, forming "islands" in the pancreas, which gives rise to the name *islets of Langerhans* after the German scientist who first discovered them. Insulin lowers blood glucose by the following actions:
  - *Glycogenesis* stimulates the conversion of glucose to glycogen in the liver for energy reserve.
  - *Lipogenesis* stimulates the conversion of glucose to fat for storage in adipose tissue.
  - *Cell permeability* increases, allowing more glucose to enter the cell and be oxidized for energy.
- *Blood glucose–raising hormones:* The following hormones effectively raise blood glucose levels:
  - *Glucagon* produced by the alpha cells in the pancreas acts in opposition to insulin, increasing the breakdown of liver glycogen to glucose and maintaining blood glucose levels during fasting or sleep hours. (The hydrolysis of liver glycogen to yield glucose is called **glycogenolysis.**)
  - *Somatostatin,* produced in the delta cells of the pancreas and in the hypothalamus, suppresses insulin and glucagon and acts as a general modulator of related metabolic activities.
  - *Steroid hormones,* secreted by the adrenal cortex, release glucose-forming carbon units from protein and oppose the actions of insulin.
  - *Epinephrine,* originating from the adrenal medulla, stimulates the breakdown of liver glycogen and quick release of glucose.
  - *Growth hormone (GH)* and *adrenocorticotropic hormone (ACTH),* released from the anterior pituitary gland, oppose the actions of insulin.
  - *Thyroxine,* originating in the thyroid gland, increases the rate of insulin breakdown, increases glucose

absorption from the small intestine, and liberates epinephrine.

Lipid Metabolism
Lipid Synthesis and Breakdown

Two organ tissues—liver and adipose tissue—participate in lipid synthesis and breakdown as partners in lipid metabolism. The fatty acids released from lipids supply body cells with concentrated fuel for energy.

Lipoproteins

Lipid-protein complexes are the transport form of lipids in the blood. An excess of blood lipoproteins produces a clinical condition called *hyperlipoproteinemia*. Lipoproteins are produced (1) in the intestinal wall after the initial absorption of dietary lipids and (2) in the liver for constant recirculation to and from cells. Because lipid and carbohydrate metabolism are interrelated, they involve the same hormones, as follows:

- *GH, ACTH,* and *thyroid-stimulating hormone (TSH),* all coming from the pituitary gland, increase the release of free fatty acids from stored lipids when energy demands are imposed.
- *Cortisol* and *corticosterone* from the adrenal gland cause the release of free fatty acids.
- *Epinephrine* and *norepinephrine* stimulate the breakdown of lipids and release of free fatty acids.
- *Insulin* promotes lipid synthesis and storage, whereas *glucagon* has the opposite effect of breaking down lipid stores to release free fatty acids.
- *Thyroxine* stimulates release of free fatty acids and lowers blood cholesterol levels.

When fatty acids absorbed from the gastrointestinal tract are delivered to the liver and muscle in larger amounts than needed for immediate energy or synthesis of important molecules, the hormone insulin promotes the formation of triglycerides for storage in the adipose tissue. In situations of prolonged physical activity, starvation, physical stress, or other circumstances that require energy beyond what can be supplied by available glycogen, these triglycerides are broken down and their fatty acids released. Free fatty acids are delivered to the liver to be packaged in lipoproteins for transport to cells for meeting energy needs or redeposition in adipose tissue. Muscle cells, including the heart muscle, depend on free fatty acids for their ongoing energy needs.

Protein Metabolism
Anabolism (Tissue Building)

Protein metabolism centers on the critical balance between anabolism (tissue building) and catabolism (tissue breakdown). The process of anabolism builds tissue through the synthesis of new protein. The making of new protein is governed by a definite pattern or "blueprint" provided by DNA in the cell nucleus that calls for specific amino acids. Specific enzymes and coenzymes along with certain hormones—GH, gonadotropins, and thyroxine—control and stimulate the building of tissue protein.

Catabolism (Tissue Breakdown)

Amino acids released by tissue breakdown are reused for making new proteins or, if not needed for protein synthesis, are broken down further and used for other purposes. The breakdown of these amino acids yields two parts: (1) the nitrogen-containing group and (2) the remaining nonnitrogen residue, as follows:

1. *Nitrogen group:* The nitrogen portion is split off first, a process called **deamination**. This nitrogen can be converted to ammonia and excreted in the urine or retained for use in making other nitrogen compounds.
2. *Nonnitrogen residue:* The nonnitrogen residues are called **keto acids**. They can be used to form either carbohydrates or fats, or, with the addition of a nitrogen group, can form a new amino acid. In health, a dynamic equilibrium exists between anabolism and catabolism that sustains growth and maintains sound tissue.

Metabolic Interrelationships

Every chemical reaction occurring in the body is purposeful, and all are interdependent. They have two essential roles: (1) to produce energy, and (2) to support the growth and maintenance of healthy tissue. The controlling agents necessary for these reactions to proceed in an orderly manner are the cell enzymes, their coenzymes (often a vitamin or mineral), and special hormones. Overall, human metabolism is an exciting biochemical process designed to develop, sustain, and protect life.

KEY TERMS

gluconeogenesis   Production of glucose from keto acid carbon skeletons from deaminated amino acids or the glycerol portion of triglycerides.

glycogenolysis   Specific term for the conversion of glycogen into glucose in the liver.

deamination   Removal of an amino group (NH_2) from an amino acid.

keto acid   Amino acid residue after deamination; the glycogenic keto acids can be converted to glucose.

TO SUM UP

Digestion breaks down the food we eat to release and convert nutrients to simple forms that the body can use. Digestion involves two types of activities: mechanical and chemical. Muscle action breaks down food through mixing and churning motions and moves the food mass along the gastrointestinal tract. The chemical activity of gastrointestinal secretions breaks down food into smaller and more simple components for absorption. Monosaccharides (simple sugars) and amino acids are water soluble and pass from the mucosal cells of the small intestine into the portal blood. Long-chain fatty acids must be packaged in lipid-protein complexes that enter the lymph and then pass through the thoracic duct into the general circulation. The enormous population of bacteria found in the colon participates in immune function and the absorption and synthesis of important nutrients. The day-to-day function of the gastrointestinal tract, often taken for granted, represents a highly coordinated and efficient body system. The breakdown products released through digestion—glucose, amino acids, and fatty acids—participate in multiple metabolic pathways under hormonal and enzymatic control, producing energy and the substances and tissues necessary for life and health.

QUESTIONS FOR REVIEW

1. List the muscle types and the motions or movements they provide in each section of the gastrointestinal tract. What are the physiologic or pathologic consequences when (a) movement is absent or too slow and (b) when movement is too rapid?

2. How does the hypothalamus exert control on food intake?

3. You are working with an older adult who suffered a stroke, which resulted in damage to the nerves in his head and throat. What are the implications for his food intake and nutritional well-being?

4. Describe the sources, location of action, and factors that influence the secretion or suppression of digestive enzymes and secretions.

5. It is said that "food doesn't really enter the body until it is absorbed." What does this mean? What mechanisms support the absorption of nutrients against a concentration gradient?

6. You have just eaten a lunch that included a hamburger on a whole-wheat bun, a glass of low-fat milk, and a bunch of grapes. Trace the digestion and final use of each of the macronutrients present in your lunch. What are (a) the enzymes, locations, and breakdown products formed in the complete digestion of these foods; (b) the routes taken by the breakdown products after absorption; and (c) one possible body use?

7. Visit a local supermarket or drug store and examine three over-the-counter medications that claim to (a) reduce stomach acid or (b) alleviate abdominal discomfort or intestinal gas. Make a table that includes each product and list the active ingredients on the product label. Visit the National Library of Medicine/National Institutes of Health MedlinePlus website at http://www.nlm.nih.gov/medlineplus/druginformation.html or consult another drug index to identify the specific actions of each ingredient. What is the mechanism by which each active ingredient is believed to bring about the desired effect? What is the relative safety of this drug based on the possible side effects or contraindications?

8. You are working with a young woman who has indicated that she is lactose intolerant and has deleted all dairy products from her diet: (a) What do you need to know about her symptoms and when they occurred? (b) Develop a daily protocol for gradually adding lactose-containing foods to her diet. (c) Prepare a list of calcium-containing foods that will meet her DRI for calcium if consumption of dairy products is not an option.

9. How might long-term antibiotic use affect the overall function of the gastrointestinal tract? Explain.

10. A patient tells you about an advertisement she saw on the Internet for a probiotic supplement. She frequently experiences stomach discomfort after eating and is wondering if that product will help her. What would you need to know about this product to safely advise her? What would you need to know about her condition and use of other medications?

11. Describe the complementary roles of insulin and glucagon in regulating blood glucose levels. What are the effects of these hormones over the course of a day for an individual who eats breakfast at 7:00 a.m., lunch at 12:00 p.m., and dinner at 6:00 p.m., with no snacks?

REFERENCES

1. Mason JB: Nutrition and gastroenterology: a mutually supportive partnership. *Nutr Clin Care* 7(3):91, 2004.
2. Guyton AC, Hall JE: *Textbook of medical physiology*, ed 10, Philadelphia, 2000, Saunders.
3. Smeets PAM, Erkner A, de Graaf C: Cephalic phase responses and appetite. *Nutr Rev* 68(11):643, 2010.
4. Serra-Prat M, Palomera E, Clave P, et al: Effect of age and frailty on ghrelin and cholecystokinin responses to a meal test. *Am J Clin Nutr* 89:1410, 2009.
5. Klein S, Cohn SM, Alpers DH: The alimentary tract in nutrition. In Shils MA, Olson JA, Shike M, editors: *Modern nutrition in health and disease,* ed 10, Baltimore, Md., 2006, Lippincott Williams & Wilkins.
6. Grimm ER, Steinle NI: Genetics of eating behavior. *Nutr Rev* 69(1):52, 2010.
7. Duffy VB: Variation in oral sensation: implications for diet and health. *Curr Opin Gastroenterol* 23:171, 2007.
8. Avsar A, Darka Ö, Bodrumlu E, et al: Evaluation of the relationship between passive smoking and salivary electrolytes, protein, secretory IgA, sialic acid, and amylase in young children. *Arch Oral Biol* 54:457, 2009.
9. Cena H, Fonte ML, Turconi G: Relationship between smoking and metabolic syndrome. *Nutr Rev* 69:745, 2011.

10. Gonsalves WC, Wrightson AS, Henry RG: Common oral conditions in older persons. *Am Fam Phys* 78:845, 2008.

11. Avunduk C: *Manual of gastroenterology: diagnosis and therapy*, ed 4, Philadelphia, 2008, Lippincott Williams & Wilkins.

12. Singh M, Lee J, Gupta N, et al: 2012. Weight loss can lead to resolution of gastroesophageal reflux disease symptoms. A prospective intervention trial. *Obesity (Silver Spring)* 21(2): 284, 2013.

13. Peery AF, Dellon ES, Lund J, et al: Burden of gastrointestinal disease in the United States: 2012 update. *Gastroenterology* 143(5):1179, 2012.

14. Harrington LK, Mayberry JF: A re-appraisal of lactose intolerance. *Int J Clin Pract* 62:1541, 2008.

15. Wallace TC, Guarner F, Madsen K, et al: Human gut microbiota and its relationship to health and disease. *Nutr Rev* 69(7):392, 2011.

16. Flint HJ: The impact of nutrition on the human microbiome. *Nutr Rev* 70(Suppl 1):S10, 2012.

17. Turner NJ, Thomson BM, Shaw IC: Bioactive isoflavones in functional foods: the importance of gut microflora on bioavailability. *Nutr Rev* 61:204, 2003.

18. Bonci L: *American Dietetic Association guide to better digestion*, Hoboken, NJ, 2003, John Wiley & Sons.

19. Lacy BE, Talley NJ, Locke GR, et al: Review article: current treatment options and management of functional dyspepsia. *Aliment Pharmacol Ther* 36:3, 2012.

20. Oustamanolakis P, Tack J: Dyspepsia: organic versus functional. *J Clin Gastroenterol* 46(3):175, 2012.

21. Aro P, Talley NJ, Agreus L, et al: Functional dyspepsia impairs quality of life in the adult population. *Aliment Pharmacol Ther* 33(11):1215, 2011.

22. Beyer PL: Gastrointestinal disorders: roles of nutrition and the dietetics practitioner. *J Am Diet Assoc* 98:272, 1998.

23. Lomer MCE, Parkes GC, Sanderson JD: Review article: lactose intolerance in clinical practice—myths and realities. *Aliment Pharmacol Ther* 27:93, 2008.

24. Nicklas TA, Qu H, Hughes SO, et al: Self-perceived lactose intolerance results in lower intakes of calcium and dairy foods and is associated with hypertension and diabetes in adults. *Am J Clin Nutr* 94:191, 2011.

25. Mattar R, Ferraz de Campos Mazo DF, Carrilho FJ: Lactose intolerance: diagnosis, genetic, and clinical factors. *Clin Exp Gastroenterol* 5:113, 2012.

26. Savaiano DA, Boushey CJ, McCabe GP: Lactose intolerance symptoms assessed by meta-analysis: a grain of truth that leads to exaggeration. *J Nutr* 136:1107, 2006.

27. Shaukat A, Levitt MD, Taylor BC, et al: Systematic review: effective management strategies for lactose intolerance. *Ann Intern Med* 152(12):797, 2010.

28. Douglas LC, Sanders ME: Probiotics and prebiotics in dietetic practice. *J Am Diet Assoc* 108:510, 2008.

29. Walker WA, Heintz K: Protective nutrients: are they here to stay? *Nutr Today* 47(3):110, 2012.

30. deVos WM, deVos EAJ: Role of the intestinal microbiome in health and disease: from correlation to causation. *Nutr Rev* 70(Suppl 1):545, 2012.

31. Dubert-Ferrandon A, Newburg DS, Walker WA: Part 2: Prebiotics. New medicines for the colon, health benefits. *Nutr Today* 44(2):85, 2009.

32. Roberfroid M, Gibson GR, Hoyles L, et al: Prebiotic effects: metabolic and health benefits. *Br J Nutr* 104(Suppl 2):S1, 2010.

33. Clark MJ, Robien K, Slavin JL: Effects of prebiotics on biomarkers of colorectal cancer in humans: a systematic review. *Nutr Rev* 70(8):436, 2012.

34. Roman BA: Use of probiotics in the management of diarrhea in pediatric patients. *Clin Nutr Insight* 35(10):1, 2009.

35. Quigley EMM: Prebiotics and probiotics: their role in the management of gastrointestinal disorders in adults. *Nutr Clin Prac* 27(2):195, 2012.

36. Lomangino K: Can probiotics prevent infections in healthy children? *Clin Nutr Insight* 36(8):1, 2010.

37. Sanz Y: Gut microbiota and probiotics in maternal and infant health. *Am J Clin Nutr* 94(Suppl):2000S, 2011.

38. Brown AC, Valiere A: Probiotics and medical nutrition therapy. *Nutr Clin Care* 7(2):56, 2004.

39. Whelan K, Myers CE: Safety of probiotics in patients receiving nutritional support: a systematic review of case reports, randomized controlled trials, and nonrandomized trials. *Am J Clin Nutr* 91:687, 2010.

40. Kataria J, Li N, Wynn JL, et al: Probiotic microbes: do they need to be alive to be beneficial? *Nutr Rev* 67(9):546, 2009.

41. Connolly ML, Tuohy KM, Lovegrove JA: Wholegrain oat-based cereals have prebiotic potential and low glycaemic index. *Br J Nutr* 24:1, 2012.

FURTHER READINGS AND RESOURCES

Readings

Andrade AM, Greene GW, Melanson KL: Eating slowly led to decreases in energy intake within meals in healthy women. *J Am Diet Assoc* 108:1186, 2008.

[This research indicates that eating slowly influences appetite regulation and reduces energy intake.]

Bonci L: *American Dietetic Association guide to better digestion*, Hoboken, NJ, 2003, John Wiley & Sons.

[This book is a general reference on dietary interventions for digestive disorders.]

Cao Q, Kolasa KM: Gut check: finding the effective dietary approach. *Nutr Today* 46(4):171, 2011.

[These authors provide insight to dietary approaches for treating common digestive disorders.]

Dubert-Ferrandon A, Newburg DS, Walker WA: Part 2: Prebiotics. New medicines for the colon, health benefits. *Nutr Today* 44(2):85, 2009.

[This publication discusses new uses of prebiotics in patient care.]

Websites of Interest

- National Institutes of Health, National Center for Alternative and Complementary Medicine: This site offers information on herbs sometimes recommended for digestive disorders such as chamomile, ginger, peppermint oil, and turmeric, noting usefulness and risk, if any; http://nccam.nih.gov/health/herbsataglance.htm

- National Institutes of Health, National Digestive Diseases Information Clearing House; Lactose Intolerance: This site describes causes, diagnosis, and useful interventions for lactose maldigesters; http://digestive.niddk.nih.gov/ddiseases/pubs/lactoseintolerance/index.aspx

Carbohydrates

Eleanor D. Schlenker

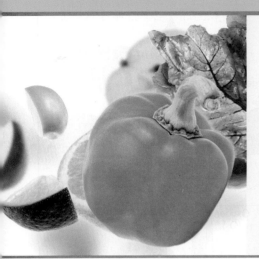

With this chapter we begin our study of the macronutrients—carbohydrates, fats, and proteins. These three nutrients share a unique characteristic: the ability to supply energy.

Carbohydrates are of prime importance in the human diet. Over the ages they have nurtured cultures throughout the world as the major source of energy for work and growth. In recent years researchers have focused attention on digestible and indigestible carbohydrates and their various effects on health. Indigestible carbohydrates, usually referred to as fiber, have specific functions in maintaining gastrointestinal health. Plant foods identified as functional foods have distinct characteristics that positively influence health. Unfortunately, added sugars, which contribute kcalories but little else, are making up a greater proportion of the typical American diet at the expense of complex carbohydrates and fiber.

We will first review the different types of carbohydrate and then examine their functions.

THE NATURE OF CARBOHYDRATE

Basic Fuels: Sugars and Starch

Two forms of digestible carbohydrate occur naturally in plant foods: (1) sugars and (2) starch. Energy on planet Earth comes ultimately from the sun and its action on plants. Using their internal process of photosynthesis, plants transform the sun's energy into the stored fuel of carbohydrate (Figure 3-1). Plants use carbon dioxide (CO_2) from the air and water from the soil—with the plant pigment chlorophyll as a chemical catalyst—to manufacture sugars and starch. The carbohydrates that plants store for their own energy needs become a source of fuel for humans who eat those plants. Because our bodies can rapidly break down starch and sugars, carbohydrates are often referred to as *quick energy foods*. They are our primary source of energy.

Dietary Importance

Carbohydrates make up a major portion of the food of people all over the world. Fruits, vegetables, cereals, grains, and dairy foods supply carbohydrate; in some countries fruits, vegetables, and grains make up 85% of the diet.[1] Rice is one of the world's most important sources of carbohydrate, feeding 3 billion people in the developing world.[2] In the typical American diet, about one half of total kilocalories (kcalories or kcal) come from carbohydrates.[3] Carbohydrate foods are readily available, relatively low in cost, and easily stored. Compared with food items that require refrigeration or have a short shelf life, many carbohydrate foods can be held in dry storage for fairly long periods without spoiling. Modern processing and packaging methods have extended the shelf life of carbohydrate products almost indefinitely.

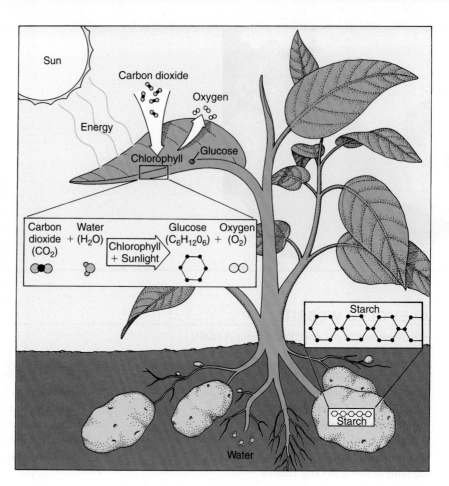

FIGURE 3-1 Photosynthesis. In the presence of sunlight and the green leaf pigment chlorophyll, plants use water and carbon dioxide (CO_2) to produce glucose and starch by capturing the sun's energy and transforming it into chemical energy in the food products stored in their roots, stems, and leaves; through this process oxygen is returned to the atmosphere. (Courtesy Medical and Scientific Illustration.)

CLASSIFICATION OF CARBOHYDRATES

The term *carbohydrate* comes from its chemical nature. Carbohydrates contain the elements carbon, hydrogen, and oxygen, with the hydrogen/oxygen ratio usually that of water (CH_2O). Carbohydrates are classified according to the number of basic sugar or saccharide units that make up their structure. The monosaccharides and disaccharides are referred to as *simple carbohydrates* because of their relatively small size and structure. The polysaccharides, including starch and certain fibers, are called *complex carbohydrates* based on their larger size and more complicated structure.

Monosaccharides

The simplest form of carbohydrate is the monosaccharide, or single sugar. The three monosaccharides important in human nutrition are (1) glucose, (2) fructose, and (3) galactose.

Glucose

Glucose is a moderately sweet sugar found naturally in only a few foods, one being corn syrup. Glucose is the common body fuel oxidized by cells. It is supplied to the body directly from the digestion of starch but is also obtained through conversion of other simple sugars. Glucose (referred to by its older name *dextrose* in hospital intravenous solutions) is the form in which carbohydrates circulate in the blood.

Fructose

Fructose, the sweetest of the simple sugars, is found naturally in fruits and honey. Fructose intake has escalated dramatically since high-fructose corn syrup (HFCS) was introduced for use in processed food. HFCS is the sweetener in many soft drinks, fruit drinks, commercial baked products, and dessert mixes. About 9% of the total energy intake of Americans 2 years of age and older comes from fructose.[4] In humans, fructose is converted to glucose and burned for energy. Fructose is absorbed less efficiently than glucose, and amounts of 25 g to 50 g or more can cause gastrointestinal distress.[5] (An

---

KEY TERMS

carbohydrate Compound made up of carbon, hydrogen, and oxygen; includes starches, sugars, and dietary fiber made and stored in plants; digestible carbohydrates yield 4 kcal/g.

photosynthesis Process by which plants containing chlorophyll are able to manufacture carbohydrate by combining CO_2 from the air and water from the soil with sunlight providing energy and chlorophyll as a catalyst.

monosaccharide Simple sugar; a carbohydrate containing a single saccharide (sugar) unit. The most common monosaccharides are glucose, galactose, and fructose.

TABLE 3-1 PHYSIOLOGIC AND NUTRITIONAL SIGNIFICANCE OF MONOSACCHARIDES

MONOSACCHARIDE	SOURCE	SIGNIFICANCE
D-Glucose*	Fruit juices; hydrolysis of starch, cane sugar, maltose, and lactose	Form of sugar used by the body for fuel; found in blood and tissue fluids
D-Fructose	Fruit and fruit juices; honey; hydrolysis of sucrose from cane sugar	Converted to glucose in the liver and intestine to serve as body fuel
D-Galactose	Hydrolysis of lactose (milk sugar)	Converted to glucose in the liver to be used as body fuel; synthesized in the mammary gland to form lactose for milk; constituent of glycolipids and glycoproteins

*Monosaccharides can exist in D or L forms depending on the position of the hydroxyl group on the right (D) or left (L) side of a specific carbon. Digestive enzymes are stereospecific and act only on D sugars.

TABLE 3-2 PHYSIOLOGIC AND NUTRITIONAL SIGNIFICANCE OF DISACCHARIDES

DISACCHARIDE	SOURCE	SIGNIFICANCE
Sucrose	Cane and beet sugar, sorghum cane, carrots, pineapple	Hydrolyzed to glucose and fructose; fuel for cells
Lactose	Milk	Hydrolyzed to glucose and galactose; fuel for cells; milk production in lactation
Maltose	Starch digestion by amylase or commercial hydrolysis; malt and germinating cereals	Hydrolyzed to yield two molecules of glucose; fuel for cells; can be fermented

FOCUS ON FOOD SAFETY

Honey

Honey is a natural sweetener but in fact contains no vitamins or minerals and has about the same number of kcalories as table syrups. Honey should never be given to infants younger than 1 year because it may contain small amounts of the bacteria spores that produce botulism, a form of food poisoning that is often fatal.

8-oz container of apple juice may contain 16 g of fructose, whereas a 12-oz can of a sweetened soft drink may supply 22 g or more.[5]) (See the Focus on Food Safety box, "Honey," for cautions relating to infant feeding.)

Galactose

The simple sugar galactose is never found free in foods but is released in the digestion of lactose (milk sugar) and then converted to glucose in the liver. This reaction is reversible; in lactation, glucose is reconverted to galactose for use in milk production.

The physiologic and nutritional roles of the monosaccharides (sometimes referred to as *hexoses* because of their six-carbon structure) are summarized in Table 3-1.

Disaccharides

The disaccharides are double sugars made up of two monosaccharides linked together. The three disaccharides of physiologic importance are sucrose, lactose, and maltose. Their monosaccharide components are as follows:

Sucrose = one glucose + one fructose
Lactose = one glucose + one galactose
Maltose = one glucose + one glucose

Notice that glucose is found in each of the disaccharides.

Sucrose

Sucrose is common "table sugar" and is made commercially from sugar cane and sugar beets. It is found naturally in molasses and certain fruits and vegetables (e.g., peaches and carrots) and is added to many processed foods.

Lactose

Lactose is the sugar found in milk and is the least sweet of the disaccharides, only about one sixth as sweet as sucrose. Although milk is relatively high in lactose, cheese, one of milk's products, may contain little or no lactose depending on how the cheese is made. When milk sours in the initial stage of cheese making, the liquid whey separates from the solid curd. The lactose from the milk dissolves into the whey, which is drained away and discarded. The remaining curd is processed into cheese, making it possible for many lactose intolerant individuals to digest cheese, although particular cheeses vary in lactose content.[6] (See Chapter 2 for a review of lactose intolerance.)

Maltose

Maltose occurs naturally in relatively few foods but is formed in the body as an intermediate product in starch digestion. It is found in commercial malt products and germinating cereal grains. The physiologic and nutritional significance of disaccharides is summarized in Table 3-2.

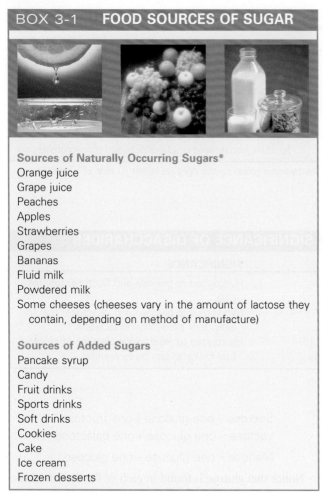

BOX 3-1   FOOD SOURCES OF SUGAR

Sources of Naturally Occurring Sugars*
Orange juice
Grape juice
Peaches
Apples
Strawberries
Grapes
Bananas
Fluid milk
Powdered milk
Some cheeses (cheeses vary in the amount of lactose they
    contain, depending on method of manufacture)

Sources of Added Sugars
Pancake syrup
Candy
Fruit drinks
Sports drinks
Soft drinks
Cookies
Cake
Ice cream
Frozen desserts

Images copyright 2006 JupiterImages Corporation.
*Fruit, fruit juices, and milk containing naturally-occurring sugars
also supply other important nutrients; added sugars supply
kcalories only.

Although sugars occur naturally in fruit and milk, the major portion of sugar in the U.S. diet is added in food preparation or processing.[7] We add sugar when we pour syrup on pancakes or use table sugar to sweeten coffee, tea, or cereal. Various forms of sugar are added to pies, cakes, cookies, candy, soft drinks, fruit drinks, and breakfast cereals. The average daily intake of added sugars in the United States is about 18 tsp (77 g), nearly 15% of total energy intake. Soda is the highest contributor to the added sugar intakes of most adults, whereas fruit drinks contribute most to the added sugar intakes of children ages 2 to 5.[8] Although the consumption of added sugar fell by nearly 25% over the past decade, it still remains above the 2010 *Dietary Guidelines for Americans* recommendation of 8 tsp or less on a 2000 kcal diet.[9] (See Box 3-1 for examples of foods that contain added or naturally occurring sugars.)

Sugar Alcohols

Sugar alcohols (sometimes referred to as *polyols*) are other forms of carbohydrate with sweetening power. Sugar alcohols, such as sorbitol, mannitol, and xylitol, are found in nature but are also used in food processing. Under current labeling laws, processed foods in which sugar alcohols replace

sugar can be labeled as *sugar free*. Sugar alcohols are poorly absorbed in the small intestine and, if absorbed, are poorly metabolized. Sugar alcohols commonly used as sugar replacers add only 0.2 to 3.0 kcal/g when compared with other sugars, which add 4 kcal/g.[10,11] These sweeteners are used in candy, ice cream and other frozen desserts, and baked goods advertised as being artificially sweetened and lower in kcalories. They often replace sugar in products developed to meet the demand for low-carbohydrate foods by those adopting such diets. Sugar alcohols are also attractive to consumers because the bacteria in the mouth that initiate dental caries do not attack them. These sweeteners offer an alternative for those with diabetes, because they do not require insulin for their **metabolism**; however, they do add kcalories. At high intakes, sugar alcohols can cause abdominal distress or exert a laxative effect; hence foods with these sweeteners are best used in moderation.[11]

Polysaccharides

Complex carbohydrates are called *polysaccharides* because they are made up of many (*poly*) single glucose (saccharide) units. Starch is the most important digestible polysaccharide; others are **glycogen** and **dextrin**. Nondigestible polysaccharides, such as cellulose, add important bulk to the diet and are categorized as **dietary fiber**. Box 3-2 displays some common food sources of polysaccharides.

Starch

Starch consists of many coiled and branching chains of single glucose units and yields only glucose on complete digestion. Cooking not only improves the flavor of starch but also softens and ruptures the starch cells, making digestion easier. Starch mixtures thicken when cooked because the substance encasing the starch granules has a gel-like quality that thickens mixtures in the same way as pectin causes jelly to set.

KEY TERMS
disaccharides   Class of sugars composed of two molecules of monosaccharide. The three most common disaccharides are sucrose, lactose, and maltose.
sugar alcohols   Alcohol formed from a simple sugar; sugar alcohols do not react with bacteria in the mouth to form dental caries; most sugar alcohols are poorly digested and absorbed, and yield less than 4 kcal/g.
metabolism   Sum of all the various biochemical and physiologic processes by which the body grows and maintains itself (anabolism), breaks down and reshapes tissue (catabolism), and transforms energy to do its work. Products of these various reactions are called *metabolites*.
glycogen   A polysaccharide made up of many saccharide (glucose) units. Glycogen is the body storage form of carbohydrate (glucose) found mostly in the liver, with lesser amounts in the muscle.
dextrin   Intermediate breakdown product in the digestion of starch.
dietary fiber   Nondigestible carbohydrates and lignin found in plants; dietary fiber is eaten as an intact part of the plant in which it is found.

BOX 3-2   FOOD SOURCES OF COMPLEX CARBOHYDRATES

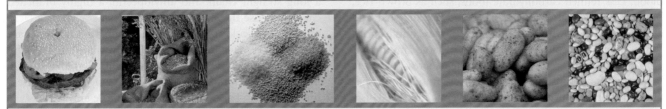

Hamburger buns
Whole-wheat bread
Corn flakes
Baked potato with skin
Sweet potatoes
Corn
Peas
Oatmeal

Rice
Beans
- Grain foods include bread, cereal, rice, and pasta; legumes; and certain vegetables such as potatoes contain large amounts of starch.
- Whole-grain breads and cereals, legumes, vegetables, and whole fruits supply digestible carbohydrates and fiber.

Images copyright 2006 JupiterImages Corporation.

Resistant Starch

At one time it was thought that starch was completely digested and absorbed in the small intestine. Now we know that some starch in particular foods, such as whole grains, potatoes, bananas, and legumes, escapes digestion and enters the colon generally intact.[12,13] This starch, called *resistant starch,* can make up as much as 8% by weight of a food high in starch.[13]

Undigested starch that moves into the colon has an important role in health. Microbial fermentation of resistant starch produces short-chain fatty acids, such as butyric acid, the preferred energy source of cells lining the colon. Available butyric acid helps protect against colonic diseases, such as ulcerative colitis and colon cancer.[14] Resistant starch has many health benefits similar to those of dietary fiber. Based on its health-related properties, food researchers are looking for new ways of processing grains to maximize their content of resistant starch.

Glycogen

Glycogen is the storage form of carbohydrate in animals, whereas starch is the storage form of carbohydrate in plants. Glycogen is synthesized in liver cells and stored in small amounts in liver and muscle. Liver glycogen helps sustain normal blood glucose levels during fasting periods such as sleep hours, and muscle glycogen provides immediate fuel for muscle action. Athletes sometimes practice pregame "glycogen loading" to add fuel stores for athletic competition (see Chapter 14). Dietary carbohydrate is required to maintain normal glycogen stores and prevent the stress symptoms of low-carbohydrate intake—fatigue, dehydration, weakness, and light-headedness. When carbohydrate is not available in sufficient amounts, the body breaks down protein and converts the released amino acids to an energy form. A severe lack of carbohydrate leads to undesirable metabolic effects, such as ketoacidosis, a complication of diabetes (see Chapter 22).

BOX 3-3   BREAKDOWN OF STARCH IN DIGESTION

Starch + Water ⇒ Soluble starch ⇒ Dextrins ⇒ Maltose ⇒ Glucose

Dextrins

Dextrins are polysaccharide compounds formed as intermediate products in the breakdown of starch (Box 3-3).

Oligosaccharides

Oligosaccharides are small fragments of partially digested starch ranging in size from 3 to 10 glucose units. They are formed in digestion and produced commercially by acid hydrolysis. These small starch molecules are used in special formulas for infants and others with gastrointestinal problems because they are easy to digest. Oligosaccharides are also common in sports drinks in which they often contribute almost half of the total glucose.

Some naturally occurring oligosaccharides are formed with bonds that cannot be broken by human enzymes and therefore remain undigested. Two of these—stachyose and raffinose—are found in legumes such as beans, peas, and soybeans, and provide a feast for bacteria in the colon, producing large amounts of gas that result in discomfort and embarrassment.

Glycemic Index

Carbohydrate foods are digested and absorbed at different rates. Refined carbohydrates, such as white bread or corn

KEY TERM
oligosaccharides Intermediate products of polysaccharide digestion that contain from 3 to 10 glucose units.

flakes, are broken down quickly and rapidly absorbed into the blood. Less refined carbohydrate foods, such as brown rice, beans, or apples, also contain fiber and are digested and absorbed more slowly. These differences have implications for blood glucose control. Rapid entry of large amounts of glucose puts stress on the beta cells of the pancreas to secrete larger amounts of insulin to move glucose into body tissues and lower blood glucose levels. The glycemic index (GI) is a relative measure of the effect of different carbohydrate-containing foods on blood glucose levels. A food with a high GI will raise blood glucose to a greater extent than a food with a low GI. The effect of particular foods is compared with the effect of a glucose solution on blood glucose. In clinical practice, GI was measured by studying blood glucose levels over a 2-hour period following ingestion of 50 g of glucose and after consuming a 50-g carbohydrate portion of the test food. Based on its major effect on blood glucose, the glucose dose was assigned the rating of 100, and individual foods were rated accordingly. (See Table 3-3 comparing the GI of various foods.) Although the GI was first introduced as a tool for the management of diabetes, control of blood glucose levels also influences the development of cardiovascular disease, macular degeneration, and inflammation, and affects beta cell function.[15, 16]

Many factors, including the type of digestible carbohydrate, prior cooking, particle size, and presence of fiber, influence the GI of a given food.[17] For example, fruits increase in sugar and decrease in starch as they ripen; as a result, ripe bananas have a higher GI than green bananas. Starches also differ in rate of digestion. Starch exists in two forms: amylose, a long straight chain, and amylopectin, a highly branched chain. Because the starch-digesting enzyme amylase attacks only the molecule at the end of the chain, the straight chain amylose is broken down more slowly than amylopectin, which has many available branch chains. For this reason, potato and wheat, which contain more amylopectin, have a higher GI than barley, which contains more amylose.[17]

Milling, particle size, and indigestible fiber influence the speed of digestion and absorption. Finely milled particles have a higher GI than larger particles because of the greater surface area available to enzyme action. Removal of the bran and fiber from whole grains raises the GI. Hard, compact kernels, such as nuts and legumes, resist penetration of digestive enzymes and are slow to be broken down when compared with porous white bread or high-carbohydrate liquids.

Other macronutrients or foods in the meal influence the GI of the total meal, although not the GI of individual foods.[16] Fat slows gastric emptying and interferes with the action of digestive enzymes so that high-fat items such as ice cream have a low GI, despite their high sugar content. Protein stimulates the secretion of insulin and hastens removal of glucose from the blood, effectively lowering the GI of the meal. Fiber, particularly viscous fiber, thickens the food mass, slowing the digestive process.[17]

Many nutrient-dense foods such as fruits, vegetables, and dairy have relatively low GIs, and whole-grain breads and cereals have moderate GIs when compared with white bread, soda, and fruit drinks. Diets relatively low in overall GI are more likely to meet nutrient requirements.[15]

IMPORTANCE OF CARBOHYDRATES

The complex carbohydrate found in vegetables, legumes, and grains should be the major dietary source of energy. On digestion, starch yields glucose, the favorite energy source of body cells. Fruit and dairy products supply carbohydrate in the form of naturally occurring sugars (fruit contains fructose, and milk contains lactose). Vegetables, legumes, fruits, and grains (especially whole grains) supply other important nutrients, including vitamins, minerals, and fiber. Dairy products are good sources of calcium, magnesium, and protein. Currently, major food sources of starch in the American diet are refined grains, such as white bread and ready-to-eat cereals, white potatoes, pasta, and rice, which are often highly processed and limited in micronutrients. Whole grains include the bran covering of the grain kernel when compared with refined grains from which the bran has been removed. Refined grains are enriched with several B vitamins, iron, and folate but provide less fiber and other trace minerals. Carbohydrate foods high in added sugar supply kcalories but little else. Based on the connection between added sugar and cardiovascular risk factors, including obesity, the American Heart Association recommends a prudent intake not to exceed 100 kcal per day for women and 150 kcal for men.[18] The Perspectives in Practice box, "Cutting Down on Sugar," offers suggestions on how to lower added sugar intake.

TABLE 3-3	GLYCEMIC INDEX OF COMMON CARBOHYDRATE FOODS*
FOOD	GLYCEMIC INDEX
Glucose test dose (50 g)	100
Baked potato (without skin)	98
Corn flakes	80
Jelly beans	80
Bread, white	77
Cupcake, frosted	73
Spaghetti	65
Banana	62
Bread, whole wheat	59
Orange juice	54
Green peas	51
Apple	39
White rice, long grain	38
All-bran cereal	38
Milk, nonfat	37
Kidney beans, canned	36
Fructose	15

Data from Atkinson FS, Foster-Powell K, Brand-Miller JC: International Tables of Glycemic Index and Glycemic Load Values. *Diab Care* 31(12):2281, 2008. (Supplementary Table A1; available online.)

*The test dose of 50 g glucose is assigned the value of 100 and serves as the standard to evaluate other foods.

PERSPECTIVES IN PRACTICE

Cutting Down on Sugar

The MyPlate (ChooseMyPlate.gov) food pattern recommends that empty calories including added sugar should not exceed 260 kcal on a 2000-kcal diet. Consider the following substitutions in your meal plans to lower your intake of added sugar:

- Use fresh fruit, such as berries or sliced bananas or no-sugar-added applesauce, in place of syrup to sweeten pancakes or waffles.
- Drink water, low-fat or nonfat milk, or fruit juice in place of soft drinks, fruit drinks, or sports drinks with added sugar.
- Choose fruit canned in water or juice in place of fruit canned in heavy syrup.
- Select flavored yogurt, lower in added sugar, or yogurt sweetened with nonnutritive sweeteners in place of yogurt with fruit preserves. Purchase unflavored yogurt and add fruit or no-sugar-added applesauce for flavor.
- Look for cake and cookie recipes that use fruit purees as sweeteners in place of sugar.
- Read the food labels on salad dressings, catsup, and other condiments and avoid those with added sugar.

TABLE 3-4	CARBOHYDRATE STORAGE IN AN ADULT MAN (70 kg [154 lb])	
	GLYCOGEN (g)	GLUCOSE (g)
Liver	72	
Muscles	245	
Extracellular fluids		10
Component totals	317	10
TOTAL STORAGE	327	

FUNCTIONS OF CARBOHYDRATES

Energy

The primary function of starch and sugars is to supply energy to cells, especially brain cells that depend on glucose. When carbohydrate is lacking, fats can be used as an energy source by most organ systems; however, body tissues require a constant supply of glucose to function most efficiently.

Body stores of carbohydrate are relatively small but still serve as an important energy reserve. An adult man has about 300 to 350 g of carbohydrate stored in his liver and muscle in the form of glycogen, and another 10 g of glucose circulates in his blood (Table 3-4). Together, this glycogen and glucose will supply the energy for only a half day of moderate activity. To meet the body's constant demand, carbohydrate foods must be eaten regularly and at reasonably frequent intervals.

Special Functions

Carbohydrates have other specialized roles in overall body metabolism.

Glycogen–Carbohydrate Storage

Liver and muscle glycogen are in constant interchange with the body's overall energy system. These energy reserves protect cells, especially brain cells, from depressed metabolic function and injury and support urgent muscle responses.

Protein-Sparing Action

Carbohydrates help regulate protein metabolism. An adequate supply of carbohydrate to satisfy ongoing energy demands prevents the channeling of protein for energy. This protein-sparing action of carbohydrate allows protein to be reserved for tissue building and repair.

Antiketogenic Effect

Carbohydrates influence fat metabolism. The supply of carbohydrate determines how much fat must be broken down to meet energy needs, thereby controlling the formation of *ketones*. Ketones are intermediate products of fat metabolism that normally are produced in very small amounts. However, when carbohydrate is inadequate to meet cell energy needs, as in starvation or uncontrolled diabetes or very low-carbohydrate diets, fat is oxidized at extreme rates. Sufficient amounts of dietary carbohydrates prevent any damaging excess of ketones.

Heart Action

Heart action is a life-sustaining muscle activity. Although fatty acids are the preferred fuel for the heart, the glycogen stored in cardiac muscle is an important emergency source of contractile energy.

Central Nervous System

The brain and central nervous system (CNS) depend on carbohydrate for energy but have very low carbohydrate reserves—enough to last only 10 to 15 minutes. This makes them especially dependent on a minute-to-minute supply of glucose from the blood. Sustained *hypoglycemic* shock causes irreversible brain damage. Providing an adequate morning supply of glucose for brain function may help to explain why individuals who eat breakfast do better in school than those who skip breakfast.[19] Glucose increases the synthesis of acetylcholine, a neurotransmitter that acts on areas of the brain responsible for memory and cognitive function.[20]

RECOMMENDED INTAKE OF CARBOHYDRATE

Dietary Reference Intakes

The Recommended Dietary Allowance (RDA) for carbohydrate is the same for all persons older than 1 year. Children, adolescents, and adults need a minimum of 130 g/day,[21] the amount required to supply the energy demands of the CNS for 1 day. Most people consume more than this minimum amount to meet their overall energy requirement and keep fat and protein intakes at acceptable levels.

Acceptable Macronutrient Distribution Range

A diet rich in plant-based foods supplies important nutrients and fiber, but it is unwise to take in excessive amounts of carbohydrate, just as it is not prudent to severely limit carbohydrate. To provide guidance for developing dietary patterns, nutrition experts established the Acceptable Macronutrient Distribution Ranges (AMDRs) (Box 3-4) for allocating macronutrient intakes in proportion to total kcalories. The adult AMDR for carbohydrate is 45% to 65% of total energy intake.[21] The AMDRs enable us to individualize diets to meet specific health situations and personal food preferences yet encourage sound nutrition habits.

Nonnutritive Sweeteners

Most of us have an inborn desire for foods that are sweet; however, we are faced with the dilemma of moderating our energy intakes to maintain a healthy weight. Nonnutritive sweeteners (NNSs) allow us to indulge our taste for sweets while limiting kcalorie intake. Sweeteners are grouped as *nutritive* or *nonnutritive* depending on the kcalories they add to a food. Sucrose (table sugar) and other natural sugars yield 4 kcal/g. In contrast, NNSs, sometimes referred to as *noncaloric sweeteners,* contribute no kcalories or an insignificant number of kcalories. This is because NNSs have a higher intensity of sweetness when compared with nutritive sweeteners, such as corn syrup or sucrose; thus very small amounts are needed to produce the desired level of sweetness.[10,22]

The Food and Drug Administration (FDA) has approved seven NNSs for use in the United States. They sweeten beverages, baked products, soft drinks, fruit drinks, and candy marketed as low or reduced calorie, and some are available for home preparation or baking. The NNS aspartame contains the amino acid phenylalanine, and aspartame-containing products must carry a label indicating that phenylalanine is present.[10] This protects individuals with phenylketonuria, who lack the enzyme needed to metabolize phenylalanine and so must eliminate it from their diets. The two NNSs most recently approved by the FDA are lo han guo, derived from the plant commonly known as monk fruit, and a purified derivative extracted from the leaves of the stevia plant, common to South America.[10] An example of the intense sweetening power of NNSs is the fact that a 12-oz can of soda may be sweetened with 17 mg of the stevia derivative when

compared with 35 g of sugar (140 kcal). Table 3-5 compares the properties of FDA-approved NNSs. (Note: Although the FDA has approved the stevia derivative for use in food and beverages, the actual stevia leaf has not received FDA-approval for use in foods at this time. It is sold as a dietary supplement, which is not regulated by FDA rules. We will discuss the current legislation relating to dietary supplements in Chapter 9.)[10]

Over the past decade, use of NNS-sweetened beverages increased from 18% to 24% of adults and doubled from 6% to 12% of children,[23] likely fueled by increased concerns about body weight. Of the 85,451 different food products available in 2009, 73% contained caloric sweeteners and 15% contained NNSs, although trends suggest that more consumers are seeking out lower calorie items.[24] Evidence-based evaluations conducted by the Academy of Nutrition and Dietetics concluded that both nutritive sweeteners and NNSs can be used within the context of a balanced diet following the 2010 *Dietary Guidelines for Americans and Dietary Reference Intakes;* however, current evidence is only fair to good that use of NNSs will bring about a loss in body weight.[10] (See the Evidence-Based Practice box, "Do Nonnutritive Sweeteners Help You Lose Weight?" for more discussion.)

CARBOHYDRATES AND ORAL HEALTH

Nutrient intake and oral health have a synergistic relationship that works in both directions. Malnutrition and nutrition-related diseases lead to deterioration of the teeth and supporting tissues of the mouth and gums such that eating becomes difficult and nutrient intake is further compromised. Conversely, infectious diseases of the mouth, such as untreated and progressive periodontal disease, result in systemic infections, worsen glucose control in diabetes, and increase inflammatory responses and cardiovascular risk.[25]

Dental caries is one of the most frequently occurring and preventable infectious diseases of the oral cavity and a major cause of tooth loss.[26] Oral hygiene, diet, and specific nutrients have been related to dental caries. Lack of exposure to fluoride in the form of fluoridated water or fluoride treatments results in tooth enamel that is less resistant to bacterial action and decay. Individuals living in areas where water is fluoridated have an 18% lower rate of dental caries than those who have no exposure to fluoridation.[27]

The amounts and types of dietary carbohydrate and the conditions under which they are eaten influence dental caries. Bacteria in the dental plaque ferment both naturally occurring and added sugars and short-chain starch molecules to form acid. The resulting drop in pH favors the action of the

---

BOX 3-4	ACCEPTABLE MACRONUTRIENT DISTRIBUTION RANGES

Carbohydrate: 45% to 65% of total kcalories
Fat: 20% to 35% of total kcalories
Protein: 10% to 35% of total kcalories

Data from Institute of Medicine, National Academy of Sciences: *Dietary (DRI) reference intakes. The essential guide to nutrient requirements,* Washington, D.C., 2006, National Academies Press.

KEY TERM
nonnutritive sweeteners Substances with sweetening power that are not efficiently absorbed or cannot be metabolized to provide energy or can be used in very minute amounts based on their intense sweetness.

EVIDENCE-BASED PRACTICE

Do Nonnutritive Sweeteners Help You Lose Weight?

Identify the Problem: In an effort to avoid or lose unwanted weight gain, consumers have looked for ways to decrease their kcalorie intake while continuing to enjoy their favorite foods, especially sweet foods. Nonnutritive sweeteners (NNSs) that satisfy the palate and add few if any kcalories would appear to be a welcome alternative, and their use in commercial food processing and home food preparation continues to rise.

Review the Evidence: Although it might be expected that use of NNSs would promote weight loss or at least arrest weight gain, research evidence has not supported this conclusion. Taste experts quoting animal studies suggest that intense sweeteners, such as aspartame or sucralose, create neural responses that increase appetite and food intake;[1] however, evidence from human studies reviewed by the Academy of Nutrition and Dietetics indicated that none of the NNSs used in the United States have this effect in adults.[2] Findings among children are uncertain. The 2010 Dietary Guidelines Advisory Committee evaluated existing evidence as to the effect of NNSs on body weight. Although those who gain weight or have a higher body mass index are more likely to use NNSs, this does not mean that these sweeteners led to their weight gain. Overweight persons often choose NNSs in an effort to address their weight problem. NNSs will influence energy intake and assist in weight loss or weight management *only* if they replace higher-kcalorie foods and beverages.[3]

Implement the Findings: If an individual consumes two 12-oz cans of sugar-sweetened soda each day at a cost of 300 kcal (150 kcal/can), substitution of a calorie-free beverage could over time lead to a modest loss of body weight. However, kcalories "saved" by use of reduced-calorie or calorie-free items cannot be used to add other foods to the diet or enjoy larger portions. Overcompensation for kcalories eliminated with use of NNSs can bring about additional weight gain.[4] Use food labels to evaluate the content of added sugars, naturally occurring sugars, and NNSs in foods and beverages.

References

1. Mattes RD, Popkin BM: Nonnutritive sweetener consumption in humans: effects on appetite and food intake and their putative mechanisms. Am J Clin Nutr 89:1, 2009.
2. Academy of Nutrition and Dietetics: Position of the Academy of Nutrition and Dietetics: use of nutritive and nonnutritive sweeteners. J Acad Nutr Diet 112:739, 2012.
3. U.S. Department of Health and Human Services, U.S. Department of Agriculture: *Report of the Dietary Guidelines Advisory Committee on the Dietary Guidelines for Americans 2010*, Washington, D.C., 2010, Center for Nutrition Policy and Promotion, U.S. Department of Agriculture. from: <http://www.cnpp.usda.gov/DGAs2010-DGACReport.htm>. Retrieved on November 12, 2012.
4. Bellisle F, Drewnowski A: Intense sweeteners, energy intake and the control of body weight. Eur J Clin Nutr 61:691, 2007.

streptococci strain of bacteria that initiates dental caries (Figure 3-2). Children and adolescents who consume higher amounts of added sugar have an increased incidence of dental caries. Although naturally occurring sugars also can lead to tooth decay, citrus fruits with a high proportion of water and all fruits containing citric acid, which stimulates salivary secretion, rinse the teeth and help remove sugars from the enamel's surface. The period of exposure to a sweet solution affects its cariogenic potential. Continuous sipping of a sugar-sweetened beverage throughout the day increases risk of tooth decay.

Prevention of dental caries may be yet another reason to choose whole-grain breads and cereals over highly processed grains and grain foods with added sugar. Unprocessed starch as a large molecule cannot pass through the dental plaque to attack the enamel, whereas shorter-chain oligosaccharides are easily broken down by salivary amylase to yield maltose, a choice substrate for plaque bacteria. Grain-sugar mixtures, such as ready-to-eat breakfast cereals or cakes, are especially cariogenic.[26]

Chronic disease increases an individual's vulnerability to dental caries and tooth loss. Age-related loss of calcium from the bones (or the drastic bone loss occurring in osteoporosis) affects the alveolar bone, resulting in tooth loss. Reduced salivary secretion (dry mouth) associated with diabetes and particular medications accelerates both tooth decay and damage to oral tissues.

IMBALANCES IN CARBOHYDRATE INTAKE

High-Carbohydrate Diets

Although the AMDR recommends that carbohydrate provide 45% to 65% of total energy,[21] individuals have increased their intakes to 75% carbohydrate with intentions of lowering their intakes of fat and kcalories or normalizing blood lipoproteins. When carbohydrate intake exceeds 65% of total kcalories, fat intake may be disproportionately low, jeopardizing the supply of essential fatty acids and vitamins and minerals found in higher-fat foods. Such an increase in dietary carbohydrate can trigger a rise in plasma triglycerides and low-density lipoprotein (LDL) cholesterol, and a drop in high-density lipoprotein (HDL) cholesterol, increasing cardiovascular risk.[21] Excessive carbohydrate intake, with a high

KEY TERMS

cariogenic Promotes the development of dental caries or tooth decay.

low-density lipoprotein (LDL) cholesterol A lipoprotein produced in the liver that transports fatty acids and cholesterol to the cells and tissues; this lipoprotein contains a high proportion of cholesterol.

high-density lipoprotein (HDL) cholesterol A lipoprotein produced in the liver that carries cholesterol from the tissues back to the liver for degradation and elimination.

TABLE 3-5   PROPERTIES AND APPLICATIONS OF COMMON NONNUTRITIVE SWEETENERS

NAME	SWEETENING POWER (COMPARED WITH SUCROSE)	EFFECT OF HEAT	TRADE NAMES	APPLICATIONS
Aspartame	160-220 times sweeter	Degrades during heating and loses sweetening power	NutraSweet, Equal, Sugar Twin (blue box)	Beverages, table sweetener, gelatin, pudding, chewing gum, cold breakfast cereal
Acesulfame-K	200 times sweeter	Stable at baking temperatures	Sweet One, Sweet & Safe	Beverages, table sweetener, baked goods, all-purpose sweetener; excluded for use in meat and poultry
Saccharin*	300 times sweeter	Not affected by heat	Sweet and Low, Sweet Twin, Necta Sweet, Sweet 'N Low Brown	Beverages, table sweetener, chewing gum, baked goods, pudding
Sucralose	600 times sweeter	Not affected by heat in cooking and baking	Splenda	Beverages, desserts, baked goods, candy, table sweetener, all-purpose sweetener
Neotame	7000-13,000 times sweeter	Not affected by heat	Little used in food processing	Approved for general use except for meat and poultry
Stevia (steviol glycosides-rebaudioside A extracted from stevia plant leaves)	250 times sweeter	Shelf-stable in dry forms or liquids	Truvia, Rebiana, PureVia, SweetLeaf	Beverages, cereals, energy bars, table sweetener
Luo Han Guo extract	150-300 times sweeter	May have an aftertaste at high levels	Not commonly used	Table top sweetener, general food ingredient, use with other sweetener blends

Data from Academy of Nutrition and Dietetics: Position of the Academy of Nutrition and Dietetics: use of nutritive and nonnutritive sweeteners. *J Acad Nutr Diet* 117:739, 2012; and Gardner C, Wylie-Rosett J, Gidding SS, et al, on behalf of the American Heart Association Nutrition Committee: Nonnutritive sweeteners: current use and health perspectives. A scientific statement from the American Heart Association and the American Diabetes Association. *Diabetes Care* 35:1798, 2012.
*Limited to <12 mg/fl oz in beverages; 20 mg/serving in individual packages; or 30 mg/serving in processed foods.

proportion of simple carbohydrates or added sugars, brings about rapid elevations in blood glucose, which puts heavy demands on the pancreas for insulin production and release. Whole-grain foods, legumes, or fruits and vegetables high in fiber and other complex carbohydrates are better choices when increasing carbohydrate intake.[28]

Low-Carbohydrate Diets

Diets very low in carbohydrate have been popularized as efficient ways to lose weight. Such diets may restrict carbohydrate intake to 130 g or less,[29] often equaling 10% or less[30] of total kcalories. These regimens bring about weight loss over the short term *if* energy intake is also reduced, and have a favorable effect on metabolic parameters including blood LDL cholesterol, HDL cholesterol, and triglycerides.[31] Nevertheless, questions remain as to their appropriateness when followed for weeks or months.[31,32] It is important that all dietary patterns include the minimum daily servings of fruits, vegetables, and whole grains recommended in the 2010 *Dietary Guidelines for Americans*.[9] These plant-based carbohydrate foods supply health-promoting nutrients and fiber and assist in controlling blood pressure.[33] Low-carbohydrate diets that replace carbohydrate foods with items high in saturated fat add to cardiovascular risk. Low-carbohydrate diets that replace carbohydrate with protein exceeding AMDR

levels increase the burden on the kidneys. A better approach to reducing carbohydrate is eliminating foods high in sugar, such as sugar-sweetened beverages and baked items, and reserving your carbohydrate for fruits, vegetables, dairy foods, and whole grains.

A low-carbohydrate diet changes the energy currency of cells from glucose to fatty acids, although cells of the CNS remain dependent on glucose. This change in body metabolism has proven useful in the treatment of several chronic conditions.[30] Low-carbohydrate diets have been effective in lowering blood glucose levels in some people with diabetes,[29] although severe carbohydrate restriction (below 45% of total kcalories) is not generally recommended. The accelerated breakdown of fat for energy, producing ketones, has an anticonvulsant effect and has been used to treat pediatric epilepsy.[30] The ketosis resulting from low-carbohydrate diets can assist in the management of nonalcoholic fatty liver disease, certain cancers, and neurodegenerative conditions, such as Alzheimer's and Parkinson's diseases.[30] (Note that ketosis as discussed here differs significantly from ketoacidosis, a potentially fatal condition arising in uncontrolled diabetes.) However, even moderate ketosis increases water loss, necessitating attention to water intake. When glucose is in short supply, amino acids are broken down to provide carbon skeletons for glucose synthesis, yielding amino groups that must

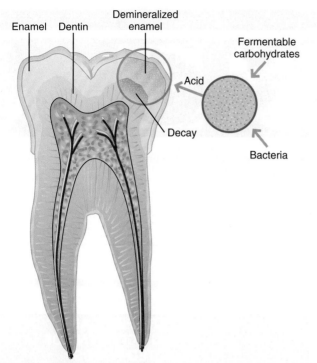

FIGURE 3-2 Dental caries can result from poor dental hygiene and continuous snacking and drinking of items high in added sugar or other refined carbohydrates. (From Mahan LK, Escott-Stump S: *Krause's food and nutrition therapy,* ed 12, St Louis, Mo., 2008, Saunders.)

be disposed of via the urine. Calcium and potassium are also lost in this process, so adequate intakes are critical.[30]

Weight loss patterns among individuals following either low-carbohydrate or high-carbohydrate diets for at least 1 year have not been consistent. Although some individuals following low-carbohydrate regimens lost more weight (5.5 kg as compared with 4.7 kg among those following the high-carbohydrate diets),[34,35] other researchers reported no differences in weight loss between those eating more or less carbohydrate, as long as kcalorie intake was reduced.[36] A 2-year follow-up found that higher intakes of protein coupled with an emphasis on high-fiber complex carbohydrates supported successful weight maintenance.[37] Consuming more protein may help lower energy intakes as protein promotes satiety.

The apparent safety and effectiveness of low-carbohydrate diets with appropriate medical supervision supports the need for more than one dietary approach to weight control, adapted to individual preferences and metabolic needs.[29,35] Regardless, establishing a kcalorie deficit between energy intake and energy expenditure using a combination of foods that support nutritional well-being is the cornerstone of long-term weight management and health.

FIBER: THE NONDIGESTIBLE CARBOHYDRATE

Fiber is the nondigestible material found in whole-grain cereals, fruits, vegetables, and legumes that our grandmothers

referred to as *roughage.* Because humans lack the enzymes necessary to break down these complex carbohydrates into forms that can be absorbed, they travel the length of the gastrointestinal tract and are eliminated in the feces. Fiber's ability to promote regular bowel function has been recognized for generations. All types of fiber are beneficial to health, but different fibers have different physiologic effects; therefore, we need a variety of foods that supply various types. Although most foods contain more than one type of fiber, they likely have more of one than another.

Types of Fiber

In the past, fibers were classified as soluble or insoluble, based on their chemical properties in the laboratory. It was believed that these properties influenced their actions in the body as well. We have since learned that health benefits of fiber are dependent on two characteristics: viscosity and fermentability. Viscous fibers, formerly referred to as *soluble* fibers, influence blood glucose levels and lower LDL-cholesterol levels. Fibers that are fermented by the microflora in the gastrointestinal tract and provide bulk to the stool were referred to as *insoluble* fibers; however, not all viscous fibers are soluble, and not all fibers that influence laxation are insoluble, so these terms are no longer used to describe health benefits, although food labels still use them.[21,38]

For our purposes, fiber is divided into two categories: dietary fiber and functional fiber.[21]

Dietary Fiber

Dietary fiber includes the nondigestible carbohydrates and lignin found intact in plant foods. Several dietary fibers important in human nutrition are described below:
- *Cellulose:* Cellulose is the material in plant cell walls that provides structure. We find it in the stems and leaves of vegetables, in the coverings of seeds and grains, and in skins and hulls. Because humans are unable to break down cellulose, it remains in the digestive tract and contributes bulk to the food mass.
- *Hemicellulose:* This polysaccharide is found in plant cell walls and often surrounds cellulose. Some hemicelluloses help regulate colon pressure by providing bulk for normal muscle action, whereas others are fermented by colonic bacteria.
- *Lignin:* Lignin is the only dietary fiber that is not a carbohydrate. It is a large molecule that forms the woody part of plants and in the intestine combines with bile acids and prevents their reabsorption. Lignin contributes the sandy texture to pears and lima beans.
- *Pectin:* This fiber is found in plant cell walls. It forms a viscous, sticky gel that binds cholesterol and prevents its absorption. Pectin also helps to slow gastric emptying and extend feelings of satiety.
- *Gums:* Plants secrete gums in response to plant injury. In the intestine gums bind cholesterol and prevent its absorption. Bacteria in the colon ferment gums to form short-chain fatty acids that nourish colonic cells (this action is also true of resistant starch).

BOX 3-5 SOURCES OF DIETARY FIBER

Pectin, β-Glucans, Gums
Oatmeal
Oranges
Kidney beans
Carrots
Apples

Cellulose, Hemicellulose, Lignin
Whole-wheat bread
Popcorn
Baked beans
Bananas
Pears

Images copyright 2006 JupiterImages Corporation.

• *β-Glucans:* These water-soluble fibers are found in oats and oat bran, foods that carry a health claim on the label indicating they can reduce the risk of heart disease. (β-glucans interfere with the absorption of cholesterol.)

Box 3-5 gives examples of foods that provide specific varieties of fiber.

Functional Fiber

Functional fibers are nondigestible polysaccharides that have been added to a food to increase its fiber content.[21] The term *functional fiber* is used to distinguish those fibers that are added to foods from those that are intact in plants and eaten in that form. Functional fibers can be isolated from plant foods or manufactured, and they are used as dietary supplements or added to processed foods. A particular fiber can be either a dietary fiber or a functional fiber depending on how it is eaten or used. The pectin in the apple you ate at lunch is considered a dietary fiber. On the other hand, pectin that was isolated from fruit sources and added to homemade or commercial jellies or used as a fiber ingredient in patient tube feedings is classified as a functional fiber. Functional fibers added in food processing must be listed on the food label. Flaxseed and psyllium are two common functional fibers. Flaxseed is a common ingredient in breads and cereals marketed as high fiber. Psyllium, an ingredient in bulk laxatives, is also available as a dietary supplement.

A person's total fiber intake includes both dietary and functional fiber. Selected food sources of dietary fiber and their energy content are listed in Table 3-6. Note that foods high in fiber tend to be low to moderate in kcalories.

KEY TERMS
functional fiber Nondigestible carbohydrates isolated from plant foods or synthesized and added to foods to increase their fiber content.
total fiber Dietary fiber plus functional fiber; the total amount of fiber in an individual's diet from all sources.

TABLE 3-6 DIETARY FIBER AND ENERGY CONTENT OF SELECTED FOODS

FOOD GROUP	SERVING SIZE	DIETARY FIBER (g)	ENERGY (kcal)
Grains Group			
All Bran (wheat flakes)	¾ cup	5.0	95
Wheaties	¾ cup	2.7	95
Shredded wheat (plain)	2 biscuits	5.5	155
Instant oatmeal, cooked	1 package	4.0	150
Cheerios	1 cup	2.6	106
Air-popped popcorn	1 cup	1.2	31
Whole-wheat bread	1 slice	1.9	81
Vegetable Group			
Kidney beans, canned	½ cup	4.4	99
Green peas, frozen, cooked	½ cup	4.4	62
Corn, frozen, cooked	½ cup	2.0	66
Potato, baked, with skin	1 medium	3.8	161
Carrots, raw	1 medium	1.7	25
Broccoli, chopped, frozen, cooked	½ cup	2.8	26
Spinach, frozen, cooked	1 cup	7.0	65
Fruit Group			
Apple, with skin	1 small	3.6	77
Strawberries, sliced	1 cup	3.3	53
Orange	1 medium	3.1	62
Banana	1 medium	3.1	105

Data from U.S. Department of Agriculture, Agricultural Research Service. 2013. USDA National Nutrient Database for Standard Reference, Release 26. Nutrient Data Laboratory Home Page, http://www.ars.usda.gov/ba/bhnrc/ndl.

HEALTH PROMOTION

Health Benefits of Fiber

Dietary fiber influences the food mix in the gastrointestinal tract and gastrointestinal function. Individuals who follow dietary patterns that include higher amounts of dietary fiber are less likely to develop chronic conditions such as type 2 diabetes, cardiovascular disease, or metabolic syndrome,[38,39] and they have lower mortality rates.[40, 41] We outline below the effect of fiber on specific risk factors associated with chronic conditions.

- *Increases fecal mass and promotes laxation:* The capacity of dietary fiber to hold water and bacteria creates its bulk-forming and laxative effects. The added mass helps the food bolus move more rapidly through the small intestine, promoting normal bowel action and preventing or alleviating constipation. A larger food mass in the colon averts the development of diverticula, small pouches that protrude outward through the lining of the colon. When the food residue entering the colon is low in bulk, the muscles must contract more forcefully to move it forward, which over time contributes to the formation of diverticula with risk of inflammation and infection. Dietary fiber has been effective in treating diarrhea and may be useful in treating other gastrointestinal conditions.[38]
- *Promotes growth of beneficial colonic microflora:* Bacteria living in the colon ferment dietary fiber along with resistant starch. This action produces short-chain fatty acids that nourish the cells lining the colon and stimulate their growth.[18] Fiber encourages the proliferation of health-promoting bacteria in the colon and has been used to treat irritable bowel syndrome (see discussion of prebiotic agents in Chapter 2).[38]
- *Binds bile acids and cholesterol:* Fiber binds cholesterol and bile acids in the lower section of the small intestine and prevents their absorption. Bound to fiber, cholesterol and bile acids are eliminated in the feces.[38] When bile acids are lost, cholesterol must be removed from circulating blood lipoproteins to synthesize their replacements, with a resulting decrease in blood cholesterol. Ready-to-eat whole-grain oat cereal has been used to reduce LDL-cholesterol levels.[42]
- *Slows rise in blood glucose and insulin levels:* Foods rich in fiber have a low GI, with their glucose content released slowly into the blood. This slow release prevents a rapid spike in blood glucose after eating. The blunting of blood glucose levels lessens the amount of insulin needed to move glucose into muscle and fat cells, thereby reducing the work of the pancreas. Fiber intake at recommended levels may assist in the prevention and management of diabetes.[38]
- *Assists in weight management:* Fiber lowers the **energy density** of the diet by displacing carbohydrate, fat, or protein in a food, thereby reducing its energy content. A diet containing recommended levels of fiber requires more chewing and promotes satiety, helping to lower food intake. The 2010 Dietary Guidelines Advisory Committee

quoted strong and consistent evidence that in adults, diets lower in energy density support weight loss and weight maintenance.[9,43] Diets lower in energy density include more fruits, vegetables, whole grains, and legumes, and fewer kcalories from fat, baked desserts, and fried foods.[44] Water also lowers the energy density of meals and particular foods, such as soups. In a national survey, individuals who consumed more fiber in the form of beans had lower body weights and lower waist circumferences.[45]

Although dietary fiber performs many actions that support health, much remains to be learned as to its effect on specific chronic conditions.[46] Total fiber intake does not seem to defend against colorectal cancer, although greater use of whole-grain cereals is associated with lower risk.[47] It may be that other dietary components associated with fiber—particular nutrients or phytochemicals—rather than the fiber itself confer resistance to chronic disease (see our later discussion in the section "Functional Foods").

Recommended Fiber Intake

The Adequate Intake (AI) for total fiber is based on the amount expected to lower the risk of coronary heart disease and type 2 diabetes. Men age 50 and younger should consume 38 g/day; those age 51 and older need 30 g/day. The AIs for younger and older women are 25 g/day and 21 g/day, respectively.[21] Unfortunately, consumer directives are inconsistent, as the current nutrition label recommends a fiber intake of 25 g in a 2000-kcal diet, considerably lower than the AI for men.

Fiber intake in the United States is barely half the AI. Mean daily intake is 18.7 g/day for men and 15.5 g/day for women.[48] Women consume more fiber than men based on kcalories (8.1 g/1000 kcal versus 7.0 g/1000 kcal). Whole grains account for nearly half of fiber intake (44%) among U.S. adults, followed by vegetables (21%), fruit (13%), and legumes (10%).[49] The MyPlate (ChooseMyPlate.gov) goal of $4\frac{1}{2}$ cups of fruits and vegetables and three whole-grain servings per day within a 2000-kcal diet provides about 30 g of fiber.[9] (See the Focus on Culture box "Who Eats More Fiber?" to compare intakes among various racial and ethnic groups.)

FUNCTIONAL FOODS: SPECIAL CARBOHYDRATE FOODS

Functional foods, which are foods believed to improve overall health and well-being or reduce the risk of specific diseases or conditions, have attracted the attention of consumers and food processors. All foods are functional at some physiologic level, providing nutrients that furnish energy, build or repair tissues, or support metabolic processes. But functional foods move beyond these necessary roles to provide additional health benefits.[50] Although there is no regulatory definition for functional foods, this market represents about 6% of foods and beverages sold in the United States, with an annual value of $37 billion.[51]

The first foods designated as functional foods were carbohydrate foods. Fruits, vegetables, legumes, and grains contain

Who Eats More Fiber?

The food we choose influences our intake of fiber; thus we see differences in dietary fiber intake across various racial and ethnic groups. Mexican Americans have the highest daily intakes of fiber (20 g) influenced by the fiber-rich beans in their usual meal pattern; intakes among all Hispanics is somewhat lower (18.4 g). Caucasians average 17.3 g, whereas African Americans take in only 13.6 g of fiber each day.[1] Family income also influences fiber intake.[2] Among mothers and children with incomes below 185% of the poverty level and eligible to participate in the Special Supplemental Nutrition Program for Women, Infants and Children (WIC), only 15% of Hispanic mothers and 5.5% of African-American mothers met or exceeded the recommended intake of fiber. The children in these families were even less likely to meet their fiber recommendations (4.4% of Hispanic children and 2% of African-American children had the suggested intake).[2] Weight status is associated with fiber intake, as obese adults tend to have lower intakes of dietary fiber than overweight or normal weight adults.[3]

Higher intakes of dietary fiber, especially fiber derived from whole grains, appear to lower risk of type 2 diabetes and cardiovascular disease, and may help prevent unwanted weight gain.[4] African Americans and Hispanics are especially vulnerable to these chronic conditions. Nutrition education focusing on appropriate fiber-rich foods that fit into customary meal patterns could lower health risk in these groups.

NOTE: See Appendix E for more information on WIC.

References

1. U.S. Department of Agriculture, Agricultural Research Service: Nutrient Intakes from Food: Mean amounts consumed per individual by race-ethnicity and age in the United States. In *What We Eat in America*, NHANES 2009-2010, Bethesda, Md., 2012. at: <www.ars.usda.gov/ba/bhnrc/fsrg>. Retrieved on November 12, 2012.
2. Kong A, Odoms-Young AM, Schiffer LA, et al: Racial-ethnic differences in dietary intake among WIC families prior to food package revisions. *J Nutr Educ Behav* 45(1):39, 2013.
3. King DE, Mainous AG, Lambourne CA: Trends in dietary fiber intake in the United States, 1999-2008. *J Acad Nutr Diet* 112:642, 2012.
4. Ye EQ, Chacko SA, Chou EL, et al: Greater whole-grain intake is associated with lower risk of type 2 diabetes, cardiovascular disease, and weight gain. *J Nutr* 142:1304, 2012.

TABLE 3-7   SELECTED FUNCTIONAL FOODS AND THEIR PROPOSED HEALTH BENEFITS

FUNCTIONAL FOOD	ACTIVE COMPONENT OR INGREDIENT	PROPOSED HEALTH BENEFIT
Whole-grain oats	β-glucans	Reduce risk of heart disease*
Green tea	Catechins	Lower risk of certain cancers
Tomatoes	Lycopene	Lower risk of certain cancers
Fortified margarine	Plant sterols (added ingredient)	Reduce risk of heart disease*
Tree nuts	Monounsaturated fatty acids/ Vitamin E	Reduce risk of heart disease*
Psyllium	Soluble fiber	Reduce risk of heart disease*
Soy	Protein	Reduce risk of heart disease*

Adapted from American Dietetic Association: Position of the American Dietetic Association: functional foods. *J Am Diet Assoc* 109:735, 2009.
*When part of a diet low in saturated fat and cholesterol.

well-known roles in maintaining skin integrity and providing energy.

In our study of nutrition we will look at three categories of functional foods.[50]
1. Conventional or intact foods such as tomatoes, nuts, or whole grains.
2. Modified foods to which a nutrient or active substance has been added. Examples include vitamin D-fortified orange juice, folate-enriched grains, and snack bars or yogurt enhanced with herbs or fish oils or probiotics.
3. Foods for medical or special dietary use intended for individuals with particular conditions or needs. Gluten-free foods for persons with gluten-sensitive enteropathy or foods designed to support weight loss fall in this category.

See Table 3-7 for some examples of functional foods and their bioactive component.

Based on public interest in nonnutrient plant substances known to influence health, many are marketed as dietary supplements, apart from their original food source. Functional components—like nutrients—work best in combination with one another, so eating foods that contain a mixture of these substances offers the best protection against chronic disease.[53] In addition, phytochemicals are found in foods in minute amounts, and not much is known about the safety of using concentrated amounts as found in supplements. Phytochemicals and plant fibers are lost in food processing, so try to choose whole-grain breads and cereals, and eat fruits and vegetables with their skins or peel. For nutrients

tens of thousands of phytochemicals (from the Greek word *phyton* meaning plant). Plants produce phytochemicals to protect themselves against bacteria and viruses, and when the plants are eaten, these substances are absorbed and act as protective factors for humans. Tomatoes were identified early on as a functional food because the lycopene they contain has been associated with reduced risk of prostate cancer.[52] (Lycopene is a carotenoid, which we will discuss in Chapter 6.) The concept of functional foods or ingredients also includes new roles for familiar nutrients. Certain unsaturated fatty acids appear to reduce cardiovascular risk in addition to their such as calcium or vitamin D, which may be difficult to obtain from conventional foods (depending on individual food patterns), the use of available fortified foods can help to meet body needs.

DIGESTION-ABSORPTION-METABOLISM REVIEW

The digestion, absorption, and metabolism of carbohydrates were discussed in Chapter 2. The outline below provides a brief review.

Digestion

The conversion of starch and sugars to glucose begins in the mouth where salivary amylase (ptyalin) from the parotid gland acts on starch to begin its breakdown into dextrins and maltose. No specific enzyme in the stomach acts on carbohydrate; however, by the time the food mass is completely mixed with gastric acid, as much as 20% to 30% of the starch has been broken down to maltose. Enzymes that complete the chemical digestion of carbohydrate come from two sources: the pancreas and the small intestine, as follows:

- *Pancreatic secretions:* Pancreatic amylase entering the duodenum through the common bile duct completes the breakdown of starch to maltose.
- *Intestinal secretions:* Cells within the brush border of the small intestine secrete three disaccharidases, sucrase, lactase, and maltase, which act on their respective disaccharides to release the monosaccharides, glucose, galactose, and fructose (see Table 2-2).

Absorption and Metabolism

Glucose is absorbed by an active pumping system using sodium as a carrier. Of the total carbohydrate absorbed, 80% is in the form of glucose, and the remaining 20% is galactose and fructose.[54] Via the capillaries in the villi, the products of carbohydrate digestion enter the portal blood circulation en route to the liver. Here, fructose and galactose are converted to glucose. Glucose not needed for immediate energy is converted to glycogen or adipose tissue for storage.

KEY TERMS

energy density The relative number of kcalories per unit weight of food; foods high in fat and added sugar have high energy density; vegetables that contain large amounts of water and fiber have low energy density.

amylase A digestive enzyme that breaks down starch; salivary amylase begins the digestion of starch in the mouth; pancreatic amylase enters the small intestine as part of the pancreatic secretions to continue starch breakdown in the duodenum.

sucrase Enzyme that splits the disaccharide sucrose, releasing the monosaccharides glucose and fructose.

lactase Enzyme that splits the disaccharide lactose, releasing the monosaccharides glucose and galactose.

maltase Enzyme that splits the disaccharide maltose, releasing two units of the monosaccharide glucose.

portal An entryway, usually referring to the portal circulation of blood that delivers nutrients absorbed from the small intestine to the liver.

TO SUM UP

Carbohydrates produced by plant photosynthesis supply most of the world's population with its primary source of energy. Fruits, vegetables, grains, legumes, and most milk products provide dietary carbohydrate. Simple carbohydrates—monosaccharides and disaccharides—are easily digested and provide quick energy. Starch, a digestible complex carbohydrate, requires increased breakdown to become available for use, but the final product in the digestion and conversion of both starches and sugars is glucose. Carbohydrates serve special functions through their ability to spare protein, prevent the buildup of ketones, and supply energy for the CNS. Fiber, the nondigestible carbohydrate found in the structural walls, hulls, seeds, leaves, and skins of fruits, vegetables, and whole grains, affects the digestion and absorption of food in ways that are beneficial to health. Carbohydrates should provide 45% to 65% of total kcalories. A healthy diet should emphasize foods containing complex carbohydrates and fiber, with a minimum of added sugar. Plant foods rich in phytochemicals are often referred to as *functional foods* because they contribute to health in ways beyond the actions of the known nutrients they contain.

QUESTIONS FOR REVIEW

1. List the similarities and differences among monosaccharides, disaccharides, and polysaccharides as related to energy value, process of digestion, and applications to weight control. List two food sources of each.
2. What is resistant starch and why is it called resistant? What are its health benefits?
3. For breakfast you had a piece of whole-grain bread with jelly, a banana, and a glass of low-fat milk. List both the digestible and the nondigestible forms of carbohydrate in this meal.
4. A mother tells you that her toddler seems to have chronic diarrhea. The mother has been giving her apple juice as

an afternoon snack rather than milk. What might be contributing to the gastrointestinal upset? What might be a better snack choice?

5. Using the materials on the MyPlate website (www .choosemyplate.gov) and the Nutritrac software found on the Evolve website, determine the daily energy need of a 25-year-old woman who is 5 feet 6 inches tall, weighs 125 lb, and is relatively sedentary. How many grams of carbohydrate should be included in her diet, and how many kcalories should it supply? What is her upper limit for grams of added sugar? How much fiber does she need? Develop a 3-day menu that provides the appropriate amounts of carbohydrate and dietary fiber and does not exceed the limit for sugar.

6. Describe the clinical effects of fiber that may be useful in treating the following conditions: diverticular disease, hyperlipidemia, and type 2 diabetes.

7. Your client Mr. B wants to lose 20 lb before his high school reunion next month. He has decided to eat only meat and other fried foods for the next 4 weeks because he believes a very low-carbohydrate diet will help him lose weight. How would you respond, considering both the pros and the cons of this diet? How would you explain why he needs some carbohydrate? What should be his minimum intake of carbohydrate in grams, and what foods would he need to eat every day to reach this minimum.

8. Why would a glass of orange juice raise an individual's blood glucose more rapidly than a whole orange?

9. Based on the special functions of carbohydrate in the body, explain the mechanisms of the physiologic and metabolic aberrations that result when the body is deprived of carbohydrate.

10. Visit your local grocery store and find two fruit juices, two fruit drinks, and two sports drinks available in single-serving, easy-to-carry containers. Use the nutrition label to construct a table indicating the kcalories, total carbohydrate (g), sugar (g), vitamins, and minerals per 8-oz serving. Check the list of ingredients and indicate which products have added sugar. Do any of these items contain added ingredients to qualify as functional foods? Which are most appropriate for daily use? Which should be limited? Why?

11. Define functional food. Research one of the functional foods listed at the end of this question and determine the following: (a) What are the important phytochemicals or functional components? (b) What effects do these components have on the body? (c) What is an appropriate portion size? Choose one: spinach, blueberries, apples, rolled oats.

12. A client tells you she now uses all nonnutritive sweetened foods and beverages in an effort to lose weight. She drinks on average three 12-oz soft drinks a day and takes a nonnutritive sweetened pudding cup every day in her lunch. Based on the upper limit for intake of aspartame (see Ref. 22), is she exceeding the recommended level?

REFERENCES

1. Englyst HN, Hudson GJ: Carbohydrates. In Garrow JS, James WPT, Ralph A, editors: *Human nutrition and dietetics,* ed 10, Edinburgh, 2000, Churchill Livingstone.

2. Mackey M, Montgomery J: Plant biotechnology can enhance food security and nutrition in the developing world. Part 1. *Nutr Today* 39(2):52, 2004.

3. U.S. Department of Agriculture, Agricultural Research Service: Energy Intakes: Percentages of Energy from Protein, Carbohydrate, Fat, and Alcohol, by Gender and Age. In *What We Eat in America,* NHANES 2009-2010, 2012. from: <www.ars.usda.gov/ba/bhnrc/fsrg>. Retrieved on November 12, 2012.

4. Marriott BP, Cole N, Lee E: National estimates of dietary fructose intake increased from 1977 to 2004 in the United States. *J Nutr* 139:1228S, 2009.

5. Latulippe ME, Skoog SM: Fructose malabsorption and intolerance: effects of fructose with and without simultaneous glucose ingestion. *Crit Rev Food Sci Nutr* 51(7):583, 2011.

6. Lomer MCE, Parkes GC, Sanderson JD: Review article: lactose intolerance in clinical practice—myths and realities. *Aliment Pharmacol Ther* 27:93, 2008.

7. Duffey KJ, Popkin BM: High-fructose corn syrup: is this what's for dinner? *Am J Clin Nutr* 88(6):1722S, 2008.

8. Welsh JA, Sharma AJ, Grellinger L, et al: Consumption of added sugar is decreasing in the United States. *Am J Clin Nutr* 94:726, 2011.

9. U.S. Department of Health and Human Services, U.S. Department of Agriculture: *Report of the Dietary Guidelines Advisory Committee on the Dietary Guidelines for Americans 2010,* Washington, D.C., 2010, Center for Nutrition Policy and Promotion, U.S. Department of Agriculture. from: <http://www.cnpp.usda.gov/DGAs2010-DGACReport.htm>. Retrieved November 12, 2012.

10. Academy of Nutrition and Dietetics: Position of the Academy of Nutrition and Dietetics: use of nutritive and nonnutritive sweeteners. *J Acad Nutr Diet* 117:739, 2012.

11. International Food Information Council: *Sugar alcohols fact sheet,* Washington, D.C., 2009, IFIC Foundation. from: <http://www.foodinsight.org/Resources/ Detail.aspx?topic=Sugar_Alcohols_Fact_Sheet>. Retrieved November 12, 2012.

12. Grabitske HA, Slavin JL: Gastrointestinal effects of low-digestible carbohydrates. *Crit Rev Food Sci Nutr* 49:327, 2009.

13. Murphy MM, Douglass JS, Birkett A: Resistant starch intakes in the United States. *J Am Diet Assoc* 108:67, 2008.

14. Brownawell AM, Caers W, Gibson GR, et al: Prebiotics and the health benefits of fiber: current regulatory status, future research, and goals. *J Nutr* 142:962, 2012.

15. Chiu C-J, Liu S, Willett WC, et al: Informing food choices and health outcomes by use of the dietary glycemic index. *Nutr Rev* 69(4):231, 2011.

16. Wolever TMS: Glycemic index. The measure and its variability—the true state of the science. *Nutr Today* 47(5):214, 2012.

17. Jones JM: Glycemic index. The state of the science, Part 1—The measure and its variability. *Nutr Today* 47(5):207, 2012.

18. Johnson RK, Appel LJ, Brands M, et al, on behalf of the American Heart Association Nutrition Committee: Dietary sugars intake and cardiovascular health. A scientific statement from the American Heart Association. *Circulation* 120:1011, 2009.

19. Pivik RT, Tennal KB, Chapman SD, et al: Eating breakfast enhances the efficiency of neural networks engaged during mental arithmetic in school-aged children. *Physiol Behav* 106:548, 2012.

20. Benton D, Nabb S: Carbohydrate, memory, and mood. *Nutr Rev* 61(5 Pt 2):S61, 2003.

21. Food and Nutrition Board, Institute of Medicine: *Dietary Reference Intakes for energy, carbohydrate, fiber, fat, fatty acids, cholesterol, protein, and amino acids, (macronutrients)*, Washington, D.C., 2002, National Academies Press.

22. Gardner C, Wylie-Rosett J, Gidding SS, et al, on behalf of the American Heart Association Nutrition Committee: Nonnutritive sweeteners: current use and health perspectives. A scientific statement from the American Heart Association and the American Diabetes Association. *Diabetes Care* 35:1798, 2012.

23. Sylvetsky AC, Welsh JA, Brown RJ, et al: Low-calorie sweetener consumption is increasing in the United States. *Am J Clin Nutr* 96:640, 2012.

24. Ng SW, Slining MM, Popkin BM: Use of caloric and noncaloric sweeteners in US consumer packaged foods, 2005-2009. *J Acad Nutr Diet* 112:1828, 2012.

25. American Dietetic Association: Position of the American Dietetic Association: oral health and nutrition. *J Am Diet Assoc* 107:1418, 2007.

26. DePaola DP, Faine MP, Palmer CA: Nutrition and dental medicine. In Shils MA, Olsen JA, Shike M, editors: *Modern nutrition in health and disease*, ed 10, Baltimore, Md., 2006, Lippincott Williams & Wilkins.

27. Food and Nutrition Board, Institute of Medicine: *Dietary Reference Intakes: the essential guide to nutrient requirements*, Washington, D.C., 2006, National Academies Press.

28. Louie JCY, Buyken AE, Brand-Miller JC, et al: The link between dietary glycemic index and nutrient adequacy. *Am J Clin Nutr* 95:694, 2012.

29. Hite AH, Goldstein Berkowitz V, Berkowitz K: Low-carbohydrate diet review: shifting the paradigm. *Nutr Clin Pract* 26:300, 2011.

30. Frigolet ME, Ramos Barragan VE, Tamez Gonzalez M: Low-carbohydrate diets: a matter of love or hate. *Ann Nutr Metab* 58:320, 2011.

31. Abete I, Astrup A, Martinez JA, et al: Obesity and the metabolic syndrome: role of different dietary macronutrient distribution patterns and specific nutritional components on weight loss and maintenance. *Nutr Rev* 68(4):214, 2010.

32. Astrup A, Larsen TM, Harper A: Atkins and other low-carbohydrate diets: hoax or an effective tool for weight loss? *Lancet* 364:897, 2004.

33. Epstein DE, Sherwood A, Smith PJ, et al: Determinants and consequences of adherence to the Dietary Approaches to Stop Hypertension diet in African-American and white adults with high blood pressure: results from the ENCORE trial. *J Acad Nutr Diet* 112:1763, 2012.

34. Sacks FM, Bray GA, Carey VJ, et al: Comparison of weight-loss diets with different compositions of fat, protein, and carbohydrate. *N Engl J Med* 360:859, 2009.

35. Shai I, Schwarzfuchs D, Henkin DY, et al: Weight loss with a low-carbohydrate, Mediterranean, or low-fat diet. *N Engl J Med* 359:229, 2008.

36. de Souza RJ, Bray GA, Carey VJ, et al: Effects of 4 weight-loss diets differing in fat, protein, and carbohydrate on fat mass, lean mass, visceral adipose tissue, and hepatic fat: results from the POUNDS LOST trial. *Am J Clin Nutr* 95:614, 2012.

37. Larsen TM, Dalskov SM, van Baak M, et al: Diet, obesity, and genes (Diogenes Project): diets with high or low protein content and glycemic index for weight-loss maintenance. *N Engl J Med* 363(22):2102, 2010.

38. American Dietetic Association: Position of the American Dietetic Association: health implications of dietary fiber. *J Am Diet Assoc* 108:1716, 2008.

39. Merriam PA, Persuitte G, Olendzki BC, et al: Dietary intervention targeting increased fiber consumption for metabolic syndrome. *J Acad Nutr Diet* 112(5):621, 2012.

40. Streppel MT, Ocké MC, Boshuizen HC, et al: Dietary fiber intake in relation to coronary heart disease and all-cause mortality over 40 y: the Zutphen Study. *Am J Clin Nutr* 88:1119, 2008.

41. Park Y, Subar AF, Hollenbeck A, et al: Dietary fiber intake and mortality in the NIH-AARP Diet and Health Study. *Arch Intern Med* 171(12):1061, 2011.

42. Maki KC, Beiseigel JM, Jonnalagadda SS, et al: Whole-grain ready-to-eat oat cereal, as part of a dietary program for weight loss, reduces low-density lipoprotein cholesterol in adults with overweight and obesity more than a dietary program including low-fiber control foods. *J Am Diet Assoc* 110:205, 2010.

43. Perez-Escamilla R, Obbagy JE, Altman JM, et al: Dietary energy density and body weight in adults and children: a systematic review. *J Acad Nutr Diet* 112:671, 2012.

44. Raynor HA, Looney SM, Steeves EA, et al: The effects of an energy density prescription on diet quality and weight loss: a pilot randomized controlled trial. *J Acad Nutr Diet* 112:1397, 2012.

45. Papanikolaou Y, Fulgoni VL: Bean consumption is associated with greater nutrient intake, reduced systolic blood pressure, lower body weight, and a smaller waist circumference in adults: results from the National Health and Nutrition Examination Survey 1999-2002. *J Am Coll Nutr* 27:569, 2008.

46. Theuwissen E, Mensink RP: Water-soluble dietary fibers and cardiovascular disease. *Physiol Behav* 94:285, 2008.

47. Schatzkin A, Mouw T, Park Y, et al: Dietary fiber and whole-grain consumption in relation to colorectal cancer in the NIH-AARP Diet and Health Study. *Am J Clin Nutr* 85:1353, 2007.

48. U.S. Department of Agriculture, Agricultural Research Service: Table 1. Nutrient Intakes from Food: Mean Amounts Consumed per Individual, by Gender and Age, in the United States, 2009-2010. In *What We Eat in America,* 2009-2010, 2012. from: <http://www.ars.usda.gov/SP2UserFiles/Place/12355000/pdf/0910/Table_1_NIN_GEN_09.pdf>. Retrieved on November 28, 2012.

49. King DE, Mainous AG, Lambourne CA: Trends in dietary fiber intake in the United States, 1999-2008. *J Acad Nutr Diet* 112:642, 2012.

50. American Dietetic Association: Position of the American Dietetic Association: functional foods. *J Am Diet Assoc* 109:735, 2009.

51. Kapsak WR, Rahavi EB, Childs NM, et al: Functional foods: consumer attitudes, perceptions, and behaviors in a growing market. *J Am Diet Assoc* 111:804, 2011.

52. Dwyer JT: Do functional components in foods have a role in helping to solve current health issues? *J Nutr* 137:2489S, 2007.

53. Lila MA: From beans to berries and beyond: teamwork between plant chemicals for protection of optimal human health. *Ann N Y Acad Sci* 1114:372, 2007.

54. Marsh MN, Riley SA: Digestion and absorption of nutrients and vitamins. In Feldman M, Scharschmidt BF, Sleisenger MH, editors: *Gastrointestinal and liver disease*, vol 2, ed 6, Philadelphia, 1998, Saunders.

FURTHER READINGS AND RESOURCES

Readings

Academy of Nutrition and Dietetics: Position of the Academy of Nutrition and Dietetics: oral health and nutrition. *J Acad Nutr Diet* 113:693, 2013.

Gardner C, Wylie-Rosett J, Gidding SS, et al, on behalf of the American Heart Association Nutrition Committee: Nonnutritive sweeteners: current use and health perspectives. A scientific statement from the American Heart Association and the American Diabetes Association. *Diabetes Care* 35:1798, 2012.

Johnson RK, Yon BA: Weighing in on added sugars and health. *J Am Diet Assoc* 110:1296, 2010.

Sylvetsky AC, Welsh JA, Brown RJ, et al: Low-calorie sweetener consumption is increasing in the United States. *Am J Clin Nutr* 96:640, 2012.

[These papers address the physical and dental issues related to excessive sugar consumption and how persons are trying to decrease their sugar intakes.]

Grabitske HA, Slavin JL: Low-digestible carbohydrates in practice. *J Am Diet Assoc* 108:1677, 2008.

[These authors help us identify food sources of low-digestible carbohydrates for use in nutrition counseling.]

Keast DR, Rosen RA, Arndt EA, et al: Dietary modeling shows that substitution of whole-grain for refined-grain ingredients of foods commonly consumed by U.S. children and teens can increase intake of whole grains. *J Am Diet Assoc* 111:1322, 2011.

[This article provides an overview of the effect of whole grains on physical well-being and how to increase intake of whole and refined grain.]

Websites of Interest

• Centers for Disease Control and Prevention, *Nutrition for Everyone—Carbohydrates*: This site describes the different types of carbohydrates, including food sources, suggested intakes, lesser-known whole grains, and label terms for added sugars. www.cdc.gov/nutrition/everyone/basics/carbs.html

• International Food Information Council Foundation: This site contains fact sheets and brochures for both consumers and health professionals describing functional foods and various carbohydrates occurring naturally and used in food processing. www.ific.org/

• Produce for Better Health Foundation: This website promoting the Fruits & Veggies More Matters campaign offers games for children, recipes, and information on portion size, selection, safe handling, and cooking of fruits and vegetables. www.fruitsandveggiesmorematters.org/

• U.S. Department of Agriculture, Center for Nutrition Policy and Promotion; MyPlate (ChooseMyPlate.gov): This site offers information on meal planning, nutritional needs, and menus for different ages, sexes, and activity levels that will supply the recommended amounts of fruits, vegetables, and whole grains. www.choosemyplate.gov/

• U.S. Department of Agriculture, Food and Nutrition Information Center: This site provides a bibliography of cultural and ethnic food and nutrition materials. www.nal.usda.gov/fnic/pubs/bibs/gen/ethnic.html#6

• U.S. Department of Health and Human Services, U.S. Department of Agriculture; *Dietary Guidelines for Americans 2010*: The *Dietary Guidelines* give guidance on increasing intakes of complex carbohydrates and decreasing intakes of sugar. http://www.cnpp.usda.gov/dietaryguidelines.htm

• U.S. National Library of Medicine, U.S. National Institutes of Health: Medline Plus, *Trusted Health Information for You—Carbohydrates*: This website offers materials and information for health professionals and the general public on research news, facts about naturally occurring carbohydrates and artificial sweeteners, and choosing carbohydrate foods. www.nlm.nih.gov/medlineplus/carbohydrates.html

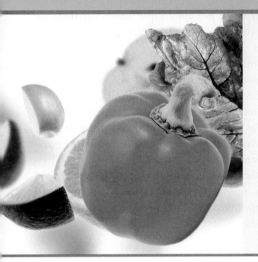

CHAPTER

4

Lipids

Eleanor D. Schlenker

EVOLVE WEBSITE

http://evolve.elsevier.com/Williams/essentials/

OUTLINE

Lipids in Nutrition and Health
Physical and Chemical Nature of Lipids
Fatty Acids and Triglycerides
Food Lipids and Health

Lipid-Related Compounds
Health Promotion
Digestion-Absorption-Metabolism Review

Lipids or fats, as they are commonly called, are the second of the energy-yielding macronutrients and carry mixed messages for consumers. Although we hear that a high-fat diet promotes chronic disease, we also read about the health benefits of the Mediterranean diet, which is moderately high in fat. When consumers were asked why they craved fast-food hamburgers, they gave such answers as, "Has a taste you can't duplicate," "Is warm and inviting," and "Fills that empty spot."[1] In large part, these attributes come from fat. Fats add taste and a pleasant mouth feel to our food and contribute to our "feeling full." Fat itself is an essential nutrient for the fatty acids it contains and has an important role in absorption of the fat-soluble vitamins.

In past years, fat held a prominent place in the American diet, providing the needed kilocalories (kcalories or kcal), for strenuous physical labor. Today we must assess not only how much fat we consume but also what type, because different fats have different effects on our health. Fat is an important component of the total diet,[7] and a low-fat diet is not necessarily a nutritionally adequate diet. In our study of lipids we will learn why we need fat and how to include it in meal planning.

LIPIDS IN NUTRITION AND HEALTH

Health Issues and Lipids

Lipids perform many essential functions in the body, but uncertainties exist as to the types and the amount of fat that we should eat.[3-5] You need what you need, but more is not

better. Health concerns related to dietary fat focus on two issues: (1) the high energy content of fat, and (2) the negative health effects of certain fatty acids. In general, polyunsaturated and monounsaturated fatty acids have positive effects on body function, whereas certain saturated fats and trans fats add to health risk.

Amount of Fat

Fat is energy dense, containing over twice as many kcalories per gram as protein or carbohydrate. Too much fat in the diet supplies more kcalories than may be required for immediate use, with the excess stored as adipose tissue. Over time such increases in body weight—or more precisely body fat—increase risk of type 2 diabetes, hypertension, and heart disease.[6-8] (Increases in body fat and related health problems will be discussed in later chapters.)

KEY TERMS

lipids Chemical group name for fats and fat-related compounds such as cholesterol, lipoproteins, and phospholipids.
fatty acids The building blocks or structural components of fats.
saturated Term used for a substance that is united with the greatest possible number of other atoms or chemical groups. A fatty acid is saturated if all available chemical bonds on its carbon chain are filled with hydrogen. A fat is saturated if the majority of fatty acids making up its structure are saturated.
adipose Cells and tissues that store fat.

65

Type of Fat

Excessive amounts of saturated fats raise blood low-density lipoprotein (LDL) cholesterol levels and promote atherosclerosis, the buildup of fatty deposits on the interior walls of the major arteries that adds to risk of heart attack or stroke. Saturated fat is found primarily in animal sources, although some appear in plant oil. Unsaturated fats, contained mostly in vegetable oils and fatty fish, can modify blood lipids to lower the risk of cardiovascular disease.[6,9] Trans fats produced in the commercial processing of lipids are injurious to health and best eliminated from the diet. It is important to help consumers recognize the different sources and types of fat as these relate to their health.[10]

Functions of Lipids
Food Lipids

Dietary lipids not only support nutrition and health but also add to the joy of eating. Following are descriptions of these important characteristics:

- *Provide energy:* Lipids are a concentrated source of fuel to store and use as needed. Food lipids yield 9 kcal/g when oxidized by the body as compared with carbohydrates and protein, which yield only 4 kcal/g.
- *Supply essential fatty acids:* The essential fatty acids linoleic acid and α-linolenic acid must be obtained in food because they cannot be made by the body or made in the amounts needed.
- *Support absorption of the fat-soluble vitamins:* Lipid must be present in the food mix in the small intestine to provide a vehicle for absorption of the fat-soluble vitamins.
- *Add to food palatability:* Lipids add flavor and a pleasant mouth feel to food. Our food choices are strongly influenced by taste,[10] and textures from lipids enhance our sensory response.
- *Promote satiety:* A meal containing lipids satisfies the appetite for a longer period than a meal containing only carbohydrate and protein. Particular brain cells respond to the mouth feel of fat and influence the region of the brain controlling satiety.[11] Fat contributes texture and body to food mixtures that slow its movement out of the stomach and helps prolong the feeling of fullness.[12]

Body Lipids

Lipids are stored in the body as adipose tissue. This tissue performs many essential tasks, as follows:

- *Storage source of energy:* Lipids are an efficient fuel for all tissues except the brain and central nervous system (CNS). In fact, fatty acids are the preferred fuel of the heart muscle.
- *Thermal insulation:* The layer of lipid deposited directly beneath the skin helps maintain body temperature.
- *Protection of vital organs:* A weblike padding of adipose tissue surrounds vital organs such as the kidneys, protecting them from mechanical shock and providing structural support.

- *Transmission of nerve impulses:* Lipid layers surrounding nerve fibers provide electrical insulation and transmit nerve impulses.
- *Formation of membranes:* Lipids are structural components of cell membranes and help transport nutrients, metabolites, and waste products in and out of cells.
- *Carrier of fat-soluble materials:* Lipids transport the fat-soluble vitamins A, D, E, and K to the cells for metabolic use. Lipoproteins carry lipids to and from the liver and on to body tissues.
- *Precursors of other substances:* Lipids supply fatty acids and cholesterol for the synthesis of various structural and metabolic compounds; brain tissue and the retina contain many fatty acids.

PHYSICAL AND CHEMICAL NATURE OF LIPIDS

Physical Characteristics

The chemical term *lipid* includes fats, oils, and related compounds that are insoluble in water and greasy to the touch. Some food lipids—butter, margarine, or cooking oil—are easily recognized as fats. Other foods that appear to be carbohydrates, such as bakery items or potato chips, often contain significant amounts of fat.[2]

Chemical Characteristics

Lipids are organic compounds consisting of a carbon chain with hydrogen and oxygen atoms attached. Particular lipids may have other radicals or groups of elements attached. Fatty acids and their related compounds are the lipids important in human nutrition. Lipids have something in common with carbohydrates: the same chemical elements that make up carbohydrates—carbon, hydrogen, and oxygen—also make up fatty acids. However, carbohydrates and lipids have two important structural differences:

1. Lipids are more complex, with more carbon (C) and hydrogen (H) atoms and fewer oxygen (O) atoms.
2. The common structural units of lipids are fatty acids, whereas the common structural units of carbohydrates are simple sugars.

We will look first at the unique characteristics of fatty acids—their saturation, chain length, and essentiality—and then focus on the triglycerides built from fatty acids.

FATTY ACIDS AND TRIGLYCERIDES

Characteristics of Fatty Acids: Chain Length

A characteristic of fatty acids important in human nutrition is the length of their carbon chain. Fatty acids in foods range from 4 to 22 carbons (Box 4-1). Chain length affects intestinal absorption. Long-chain fatty acids are more difficult to absorb and require a helping carrier to enter the lymph and then the blood. Short- and medium-chain fatty acids are soluble in water and absorbed directly into the blood. When intestinal diseases injure the absorbing

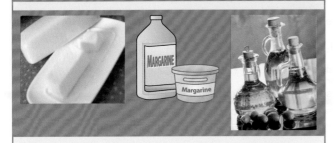
surface of the small intestine, a commercial product called *medium-chain triglyceride* (MCT) oil (made of short- and medium-chain fatty acids) can replace ordinary vegetable oil in food preparation.

Characteristics of Fatty Acids: Saturation

The saturation or unsaturation of a lipid governs its physical characteristics. Saturated fats are hard, less-saturated fats are soft, and unsaturated fats are liquid at room temperature (Box 4-2). These physical differences are based on the ratio of hydrogen atoms to carbon atoms in the fatty acids making up the lipid. If a fatty acid has a hydrogen atom attached at every available space, then it is completely saturated. If the fatty acid has some hydrogen spaces unfilled, then it is unsaturated. The following three terms are used to describe saturation in fats.

1. *Saturated:* Lipids composed mostly of saturated fatty acids are called *saturated fats*. Although saturated fatty acids are usually found in animal foods, the most saturated food fats are two oils from plants: (1) coconut oil, which is 88% saturated, and (2) palm kernel oil, which is 80% saturated.[13] All other saturated fats are of animal origin as found in meat; butter; whole, reduced-fat, and low-fat milk; and other dairy products.

2. *Monounsaturated:* Food lipids that have a high proportion of fatty acids with a pair of hydrogen atoms missing, creating one double bond, are called *monounsaturated fats.* These lipids are generally from plant sources. Canola oil (isolated from rapeseed) and olive oil are primarily monounsaturated fats.

3. *Polyunsaturated:* When fatty acids have four or more spaces unfilled with hydrogen atoms, creating two or more double bonds, they are *polyunsaturated fats.* Many of these fats are from plant sources and include commonly used cooking oils such as corn oil and safflower oil. Polyunsaturated fatty acids with two or more double bonds are also classified according to the position in the carbon chain where the first double bond appears. When the first double bond follows the third carbon atom, counting from the methyl end of the fatty acid, it is referred to as an omega (ω) 3 or *n-3* fatty acid. When the first double bond follows the sixth carbon atom in the chain it is called an omega (ω) 6 or *n-6* fatty acid. Two important fatty acids in human metabolism are linoleic acid, an n-6 fatty acid, and α-linolenic acid, an n-3 fatty acid. These are referred to as essential fatty acids because the body cannot synthesize an n-3 or n-6 fatty acid. The n-3 fatty acids found in fatty fish have a role in cardiovascular health.[3,9]

Essential Fatty Acids

Two different fatty acids—linoleic acid (an n-6 fatty acid) and α-linolenic acid (an n-3 fatty acid) are essential fatty acids for humans. Arachidonic acid, another fatty acid important in human nutrition, can be made from linoleic acid. Two n-3 fatty acids associated with cardiovascular health—(1) eicosapentaenoic acid (EPA) and (2) docosahexaenoic acid (DHA)—can be made from α-linolenic acid

KEY TERMS

lipoproteins Noncovalent complexes of fat with protein. The lipoproteins carry lipids in the plasma; this combination of fat surrounded by protein makes possible the transport of fatty substances in a water-based solution such as plasma.

organic Carbon compounds found in plants or animals.

triglycerides Chemical name for fats that indicates the structure of three fatty acids attached to a glycerol base. Triglycerides are synthesized from excess dietary carbohydrate and fat and stored in adipose tissue; they release free fatty acids into the blood when needed for energy.

linoleic acid An essential fatty acid for humans; an n-6 polyunsaturated fatty acid.

α-linolenic acid An essential fatty acid for humans; an n-3 polyunsaturated fatty acid.

essential fatty acids Fatty acids that must be supplied in the diet because the body cannot make them.

eicosapentaenoic acid (EPA) An n-3 polyunsaturated fatty acid found in fish oil; it helps lower the risk of heart attack or stroke.

docosahexaenoic acid (DHA) An n-3 polyunsaturated fatty acid found in fish oil; it is necessary for brain and neural development in infants and helps lower the risk of heart attack or stroke in adults.

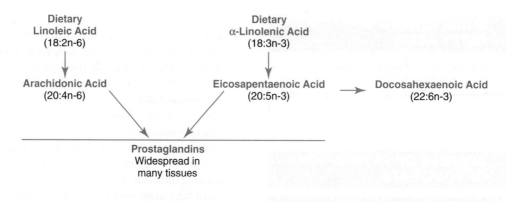

FIGURE 4-1 Linoleic acid and α-linolenic acid (the essential fatty acids) are the starting points for synthesis of various other fatty acids and prostaglandins. Prostaglandins, a type of eicosanoid, help regulate many important body functions.

(Figure 4-1), but these conversion rates are extremely slow,[13,14] and influenced by age, sex, genetics, and overall dietary intake.[15] Therefore, individuals need to obtain these acids from regular servings of fish.

Linoleic acid and α-linolenic acid have the following roles:

- *Skin integrity:* The essential fatty acids strengthen cell membranes and prevent a harmful increase in skin permeability. Essential fatty acid deficiency causes breakdown in skin tissue, with characteristic eczema and skin lesions.[16] Essential fatty acid deficiency seldom occurs with the exception of a patient receiving a parenteral nutrition formula that does not include the essential fatty acids.
- *Regulation of lipid metabolism:* Polyunsaturated fatty acids can reduce blood lipid levels, particularly if they are replacing saturated fat in the diet.[2,15]
- *Growth:* Normal growth requires an adequate supply of the essential fatty acids, and growth is impaired in essential fatty acid deficiency; α-linolenic acid is especially important for the development of brain tissue before and after birth.[16]
- *Gene expression:* The essential fatty acids regulate the production of enzymes needed for synthesis of nonessential fatty acids.[17]
- *Immune function:* Persons with essential fatty acid deficiency have an increased rate of infection.[17]
- *Aggregation of blood platelets:* EPA and DHA prevent unwanted aggregation of blood platelets that blocks the flow of blood in major arteries, causing heart attack or stroke.[18]
- *Synthesis of hormonelike agents:* Essential fatty acids are metabolic precursors of a group of physiologically and pharmacologically active compounds known as *eicosanoids* (see Figure 4-1). **Prostaglandins**, a type of eicosanoid, were first identified in human semen and thought to originate in the prostate gland. Prostaglandins exist in virtually

all body tissues and act as local hormones to direct and coordinate biologic functions. They influence blood pressure, blood clotting, and cardiovascular function.[17]

Dietary Reference Intakes

Adequate Intakes (AIs) have been established for both linoleic and α-linolenic acids. (See Chapter 1 to review the various categories of the Dietary Reference Intakes [DRIs].) Between the ages of 19 and 50, the AI for linoleic acid (an n-6 fatty acid) is 17 g/day for men and 12 g/day for women; past the age of 50, these reference intakes decrease to 14 g/day for men and 11 g/day for women. The AI for α-linolenic acid (an n-3 fatty acid) is 1.6 g/day for all adult men and 1.1 g/day for all adult women.[16] Current surveys indicate that U.S. adults are meeting their requirements for linoleic and α-linolenic fatty acids.[19] Currently there are no specific DRI recommendations for EPA and DHA.

Increased intakes of polyunsaturated fatty acids with multiple double bonds also increase the need for antioxidants to prevent oxidation at double bond sites. We will learn more about the role of vitamin E in preventing unwanted oxidation in Chapter 6.

Special Needs of Infants

Arachidonic acid and DHA play a critical role in the brain and neural development of infants; both are found in breast milk in liberal amounts. Commercial infant formula sold in the United States is fortified with arachidonic acid and DHA to the levels found in human milk.[20] Based on the important role of DHA in both prenatal and postnatal development, some nutrition experts have proposed that both pregnant[21] and lactating women[20] be encouraged to eat one to two portions of oily sea fish per week selected from fish low in mercury and other contaminants. Clinical studies are continuing to evaluate the association between dietary intake

BOX 4-3   FOOD SOURCES OF FATTY ACIDS IMPORTANT TO HEALTH

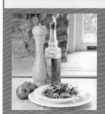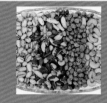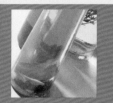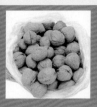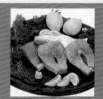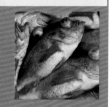

Linoleic Acid: n-6 Fatty Acid (essential)
Safflower oil
Corn oil
Cottonseed oil
Soybean oil
Nuts
Wheat germ

α-Linolenic Acid: n-3 Fatty Acid (essential)
Soybean oil
Flaxseed oil

Canola oil
Walnuts
Wheat germ

Fatty Acids from Fish: n-3 Fatty Acids*
Eicosapentaenoic acid and docosahexaenoic acid
- Herring
- Mackerel
- Halibut
- Salmon
- Canned tuna

Images copyright 2006 JupiterImages Corporation.
*These fatty acids can be synthesized in extremely limited amounts so regular servings of fish are recommended.

of DHA from fish or supplements during pregnancy, the DHA content of breast milk, and infant health outcomes such as visual acuity and cognitive development.[2,22] (More information on selecting low-mercury fish can be found in Chapter 9.)

Food Sources of Essential Fatty Acids

The best sources of the two essential fatty acids are vegetable oils. Corn oil, safflower oil, soybean oil, cottonseed oil, sunflower oil, and peanut oil are rich in linoleic acid (an n-6 acid), and α-linolenic acid (an n-3 acid) is found in flaxseed, soybean oil, and rapeseed oil (canola oil).[14] The *Dietary Guidelines for Americans* recommends that both children and adults consume two servings of fish per week to ensure an adequate supply of EPA and DHA.[2] (Box 4-3 lists food sources of important fatty acids.)

Use of Fish Oil Supplements

Fish oil supplements, which have received increasing attention in the popular press as an alternative to eating fish, should be used only with the supervision of a health care professional. Because EPA and DHA can excessively prolong bleeding time, persons taking anticoagulants including warfarin and aspirin should use such supplements with caution.[14,23]

Structure of Triglycerides

The body stores fatty acids in the form of triglycerides made from three fatty acids attached to a **glycerol** base. When glycerol is combined with one fatty acid, it is called a *monoglyceride;* with two fatty acids, it is a *diglyceride;* and with three fatty acids it is termed a *triglyceride.* **Glycerides** are found in food and also formed in the body. Most natural lipids from animal or plant sources are triglycerides. Triglycerides serve

multiple functions throughout the body. They appear in body cells as oily droplets and circulate in the water-based blood plasma encased in a covering of water-soluble protein. These lipid-protein molecules are called *lipoproteins.*

FOOD LIPIDS AND HEALTH

Degree of Saturation

Food lipids contain a mixture of both saturated and unsaturated fats. Animal sources—meat, milk, and eggs—contain more saturated fats, whereas plant sources, primarily vegetable oils, are more unsaturated. The spectrum of food fats (from saturated to unsaturated) is illustrated in Figure 4-2. In general, saturated fats are solid at room temperature, and the unsaturated plant lipids are free-flowing oils even at low temperatures; however, the exceptions to this usual pattern are important to human health. Coconut oil and palm kernel oil, highly saturated vegetable fats, are used extensively in

---

KEY TERMS

prostaglandins One of a group of naturally occurring substances called eicosanoids derived from long-chain fatty acids; they have multiple local hormone-like actions including regulation of gastric acid secretion, blood platelet aggregation, body temperature, and tissue inflammation.

glycerol An alcohol that is esterified with fatty acids to produce triglycerides and released when fats are hydrolyzed.

glycerides Group name for fats formed from glycerol by the replacement of one, two, or three hydroxyl (OH) groups with a fatty acid. Monoglycerides contain one fatty acid, diglycerides contain two fatty acids, and triglycerides contain three fatty acids. Glycerides are found in animal and plant fats and oils and stored in the adipose tissue.

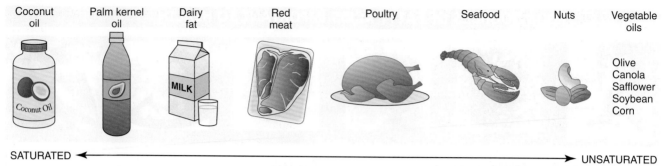

FIGURE 4-2 Spectrum of food fats according to degree of saturation. Note that the two food fats with the highest degree of saturation are plant fats, followed by various animal fats in decreasing order of saturation. In general, plant fats are less saturated.

TABLE 4-1	EFFECTS OF FATTY ACID SATURATION ON BLOOD LIPIDS	
DEGREE OF SATURATION	**NUMBER OF DOUBLE BONDS**	**PHYSIOLOGIC EFFECTS**
Saturated fats	None	Raises blood levels of total cholesterol and low-density lipoprotein (LDL) cholesterol
Monounsaturated fats	One	Decreases blood levels of total cholesterol and LDL cholesterol when substituted for saturated fat
Polyunsaturated fats (includes the essential fatty acids and fish oils)	Two or more	Decreases blood levels of total cholesterol and LDL cholesterol Discourages blood platelet aggregation decreasing risk of unwanted clots
Trans fats	One	Raises blood levels of total cholesterol and LDL cholesterol Decreases blood levels of high-density lipoprotein (HDL) cholesterol

Data from Holligan SD, Berryman CE, Wang L, et al: Atherosclerotic cardiovascular disease. In Erdman JW Jr, Macdonald IA, Zeisel SH, editors: *Present knowledge in nutrition,* ed 10, Ames, Iowa, 2012, International Life Sciences Institute/Wiley-Blackwell.

nondairy creamers and baked goods because they are relatively inexpensive.

The number of double bonds in a fatty acid influences its actions in the body. Certain saturated fats increase cardiovascular risk if eaten in large amounts, although fats with one double bond or more have the opposite effect (Table 4-1). Monounsaturated fatty acids are associated with the health-promoting effects of the Mediterranean diet, a plant-based eating pattern rich in legumes, grains, seeds, and olive oil. Polyunsaturated fats with two or more double bonds include the essential fatty acids and fish oils. Despite the positive effects of unsaturated fats, moderation should be the key.[4,6,9,17,18]

Cis versus Trans Fats

To meet the demand for solid fats for use as table fats or food ingredients the process of hydrogenation was developed. When unsaturated oils are surrounded with hydrogen gas, hydrogen ions attach at available sites, producing a more saturated (or solid) fat. This process turns unsaturated vegetable oils into margarine or vegetable shortenings; however, a particular type of unsaturated fatty acid that is formed in this process, a *trans* fatty acid, is extremely detrimental to health.

In Figure 4-3 we compare the two possible structures of an unsaturated fatty acid. When double bonds occur in nature, the fatty acid chain bends in such a way that both parts are on the same side of the bond. In this case, the fatty

acid is called a *cis* fatty acid, meaning same side. Fatty acids in vegetable oils are in the *cis* form. However, when oils are partially hydrogenated, the normal bend can change with the two structural parts on opposite sides of the bend. This form is called a *trans* fatty acid, meaning opposite side. Commercially hydrogenated lipids used in soft margarine and other food products often contain *trans* fatty acids.

Trans fatty acids have been implicated in the development of coronary artery disease.[24] In addition, they elevate the risk of type 2 diabetes[25] and disrupt essential fatty acid functions in cells[14] (see Table 4-1). In 2006 it became mandatory to add trans fatty acid content to nutrition labels, and since then both the food industry and government agencies have worked to reduce the trans fat content in processed food. Prior to the 2006 mandate even young children were consuming significant amounts of trans fats (the goal is 0 g per day). Mean intake in children ages 3 to 5 was 5 g per day, and teenage boys consumed almost 8 g. Men took in 7 g and women about 5 g. Items contributing the greatest proportions of trans fats were cakes, cookies, and pastries, followed by yeast breads, French fries, ethnic dishes, and tortilla chips.[26] In

> **KEY TERM**
>
> **hydrogenation** Process used to produce margarine and shortening from liquid vegetable oils; when polyunsaturated vegetable oils are exposed to hydrogen gas, hydrogen atoms are added at many of the double bonds, forming a solid fat.

recent years average intake has dropped to 1.3 g per day, although many individuals exceed this level.[27] Based on efforts of public health departments and health professionals, many fast-food restaurants and food manufacturers have voluntarily reduced their use of fats containing trans fatty acids. Several state and city governments including New York City have passed ordinances restricting use of trans fats in local restaurants.[28]

The nutrition label can guide a consumer's intake of fat. Information given includes the grams per serving of total fat, saturated fat, unsaturated fat, and trans fat; however, confusion about portion size can add to intake. Packages assumed to contain one serving are often labeled as containing two servings or more, with the result that actual fat intake is two

or more times what was expected. As for trans fats, it is important for consumers to recognize the difference between none or zero trans fats. None means there are no trans fats present. Conversely, a label can list content as zero *if* the amount of trans fat per serving is 0.5 g or less. Eating several servings of such items adds significant amounts of trans fat to the diet. Fats such as coconut oil and palm kernel oil can be found in the list of ingredients on the food label and be identified as sources of saturated fat. Although we should encourage avoidance of trans fat, it is also important for consumers to understand that a food is not necessarily healthy just because it contains no trans fat.[29] Such a food may be high in total fat or saturated fat and still best eaten in limited amounts. The use of saturated fat in processed food may increase if food manufacturers replace trans fat with forms of saturated fat.[26]

Visible and Hidden Fat

Fat enters the diet in many different forms and foods. Fats are quite visible in butter, margarine, vegetable oil, salad dressing, bacon, and similar added fats; however, less obvious are the fats in milk (unless it is nonfat), egg yolk, cheese, nuts, seeds, and olives, often referred to as *hidden fats*. Other major sources of hidden fats are bakery items, including cake, cookies, crackers, and muffins, or frozen entrees such as baked lasagna (Box 4-4). Meat and poultry have both visible and hidden fat. Even when visible fat has been trimmed away or the skin removed, the remaining portion still contains some fat. Red meat, especially beef, is marbled with tiny fat deposits within the muscle tissue. When evaluating the nutrient intake of a cultural or ethnic group different from your own, it is important to consider potential sources of hidden fat in recipes or added in food preparation (see the Focus on Culture box, "Developing Food Frequency Questionnaires for Culturally Diverse Groups").

Acceptable Macronutrient Distribution Range

The Acceptable Macronutrient Distribution Range (AMDR) for fat is 20% to 35% of total kcalories.[16] This range allows appropriate intake of the essential fatty acids and

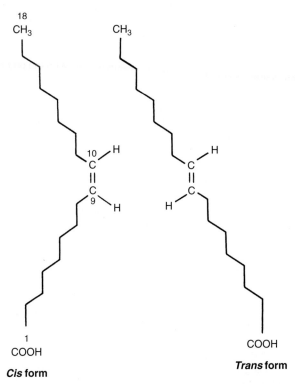

FIGURE 4-3 The *cis* and *trans* forms of a fatty acid.

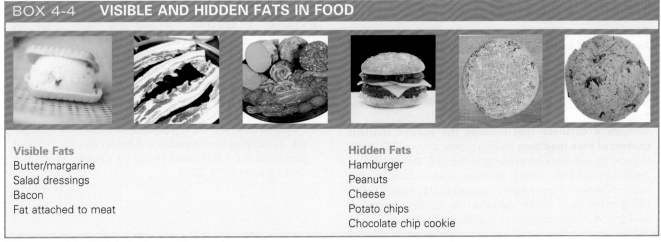

BOX 4-4   VISIBLE AND HIDDEN FATS IN FOOD

Visible Fats
Butter/margarine
Salad dressings
Bacon
Fat attached to meat

Hidden Fats
Hamburger
Peanuts
Cheese
Potato chips
Chocolate chip cookie

Images copyright 2006 JupiterImages Corporation.

FOCUS ON CULTURE

Developing Food Frequency Questionnaires for Culturally Diverse Groups

Food frequency questionnaires (FFQs) are one way of learning what people eat; they provide a tool for evaluating an individual's diet and developing an intervention plan. An FFQ contains a list of common foods from all major food groups, and persons are asked how often they eat each food and the portion size usually eaten. The FFQ can be completed in writing, administered by interview, or entered using a computer-assisted module. Photographs can be especially helpful in defining portion size. When collecting dietary information from individuals who do not speak or read English, it is necessary to translate the FFQ or hire an interviewer who is fluent in their language and familiar with their dietary patterns. Be sure to review your materials with representatives of the target group to be sure that both your words and pictures are clearly understood.[1,2]

Creating a Food Frequency Questionnaire

To obtain an accurate response describing food intake, you must provide a comprehensive list of foods commonly eaten. The list of typical foods eaten by an East Indian or Chinese or Latino family who recently emigrated to the United States will be very different from a list of foods used by those who have come to adopt more typical American patterns. Even among lifelong residents, racial and ethnic differences may exist as to favorite foods such as fruit or vegetable choices.[3] Below is a framework for developing an FFQ for a particular target group.[4]

Step 1

Talk with those who do the cooking about the types of food they prepare for their families. Collect recipes for specific dishes to be sure that you understand what grains, fruits, vegetables, meats, and fats are included in each dish. Certain vegetables may be eaten only as components of mixed dishes and not eaten separately.[5] Check to see what ingredients are available in local shops and what substitutions homemakers need to make when preparing their native dishes. Be sure to talk with both younger and older homemakers. Older families are more likely to retain traditional food patterns, whereas younger homemakers are more likely to adopt store-bought items used by those around them.[6]

Step 2

Group foods according to their nutrient content; put grain foods, protein foods, or calcium-rich foods together.

Step 3

Assign a food name that is familiar to your target group. For example, families from Southeast Asia may recognize broccoli by the name given to Chinese broccoli, kai-lan, or gai-lan.[4]

Step 4

Compile a database that includes the specific nutrient content of each food item that will appear on your FFQ. Many ingredients will likely be available in the U.S. Department of Agriculture (USDA) nutrient database used to calculate the nutrient content of diet records obtained in U.S. food surveys. Using these food values, calculate the nutrient content of mixed food dishes common to your target group.

Special Problems with Fats

Based on the high energy density of fat and its association with chronic disease, we need to obtain good estimates of the types and amounts of fat eaten regularly. Food preparation methods strongly influence fat intake and require particular attention. FFQs developed for use with Native Americans and native Alaskans asked about use of meat, chicken, fish, game meats, and wild birds, if the skin from poultry and birds was eaten, and if these protein foods were fried or otherwise prepared with added fat.[1] Southeast Asian families were found to obtain about 40% of their kcalories from fat, with much of it coming from oil-based curry sauces, whereas Chinese families took in only 34% of their kcalories as fat, yet both added about the same amounts of oil to their stir-fry mixtures.[4] When the researchers looked at the actual foods being prepared, they found their answer. With the stir-fried foods, much of the fat remained in the pan when the food was served; with the thick curry sauces, most of the sauce was eaten along with the other ingredients. It may be helpful to visit a family at mealtime to fully appreciate their food habits.

As groups become more health conscious, it is pertinent to include on FFQs items that are being marketed for their specific nutrient content. For example, when developing an FFQ for individuals trying to lower their fat intake, you might include not only traditional foods but also any highly advertised low-fat or modified-fat foods directed toward your particular audience.

Think about your own ethnic or cultural group. If you were to develop an FFQ for them, then what foods would you include?

References

1. Slattery ML, Murtaugh MA, Schumacher MC, et al: Development, implementation, and evaluation of a computerized self-administered diet history questionnaire for use in studies of American Indian and Alaskan native people. *J Am Diet Assoc* 108:101, 2008.
2. Banna JC, Vera Becerra LE, Kaiser LL, et al: Using qualitative methods to improve questionnaires for Spanish speakers: assessing face validity of a food behavior checklist. *J Am Diet Assoc* 110:80, 2010.
3. Arab L, Cambou MC, Craft N, et al: Racial differences in correlations between reported dietary intakes of carotenoids and their concentration biomarkers. *Am J Clin Nutr* 93:1102, 2011.
4. Kelemen LE, Anand SS, Vuksan V, et al: Development and evaluation of cultural food frequency questionnaires for South Asians, Chinese, and Europeans in North America. *J Am Diet Assoc* 103:1178, 2003.
5. Tseng M, Hernandez T: Comparison of intakes of U.S. Chinese women based on food frequency and 24-hour recall data. *J Am Diet Assoc* 105:1145, 2005.
6. Pakseresht M, Sharma S: Validation of a culturally appropriate quantitative food frequency questionnaire for Inuvialuit population in the Northwest Territories, Canada. *J Hum Nutr Diet* 23(Suppl 1):75, 2010.

fat-containing foods that are rich sources of other important nutrients, yet controls kcalories. The lower end of the range helps with weight management or weight loss, whereas the upper level will promote weight gain in underweight individuals or ensure sufficient kcalories for an active lifestyle or growth. Fat intakes falling below 10% of total kcalories may not supply needed amounts of essential fatty acids.[16]

Appropriate Intakes of Fat and Carbohydrate

The AMDRs for fat (20% to 35% of total kcalories) and carbohydrate (45% to 65% of total kcalories) set a balance between these two energy sources.[16] Popular weight loss regimens often replace carbohydrate with fat and protein to the extent that fat supplies as much as 55% of total kcalories.[30] Patients with type 2 diabetes were found to be consuming diets made up of 45% fat in an effort to lower their intakes of carbohydrates,[31] pointing to the need for nutrition education for this group. At the other extreme, when fat falls below 20% of total kcalories, carbohydrate and protein levels rise disproportionately. (The AMDR for protein is discussed in Chapter 5.)

LIPID-RELATED COMPOUNDS

Cholesterol

Structure

Although cholesterol is not a fat or a triglyceride, it is often discussed in connection with dietary lipids. Cholesterol belongs to a family of substances called steroids and travels in the blood attached to long-chain fatty acids. People sometimes confuse cholesterol with saturated fat because both substances are believed to promote atherosclerosis.

Functions

Cholesterol is required for normal body function and synthesized in the liver. If a person obtained no cholesterol whatsoever from food, the body would still have an adequate supply. Cholesterol has broad roles as follows:

- *Precursor to steroid hormones:* A cholesterol compound in the skin, 7-dehydrocholesterol, is converted to vitamin D when the ultraviolet rays of the sun pass into the skin; cholesterol is also a precursor of estrogen and testosterone.
- *Formation of bile acids:* Cholesterol is used to form bile acids, which emulsify fats and facilitate their digestion; bile acids serve as carriers in fat absorption.
- *Component of brain and nerve tissue:* The brain and nerves include cholesterol in their structure.
- *Component of cell membranes:* Cell membranes contain cholesterol.

Food Sources

Cholesterol is found in animal foods but not plant foods. Egg yolk; meat; whole, reduced-fat, and low-fat milk; cheese; and organ meats supply cholesterol. Animal fats (but *not* plant fats) are rich sources.

Suggested Cholesterol Intake

Because the body can synthesize cholesterol as needed, no DRI is necessary.[16] People are encouraged to limit their intake, keeping in mind that eliminating cholesterol entirely would also eliminate meat, eggs, and some dairy products that provide vitamins and minerals important to health. The American Heart Association recommends that dietary cholesterol be held to 300 mg/day or less, an intake associated with appropriate blood cholesterol levels.[6] In recent years genetic selection has successfully lowered the cholesterol content of eggs and meat; nevertheless, daily intake averages about 333 mg in men and 224 mg in women.[19] Eggs and egg dishes contribute about 25% of cholesterol intake followed by chicken and chicken dishes, beef and beef dishes, burgers, and regular cheese.[2] Upon review of available evidence the 2010 Dietary Guidelines Advisory Committee concluded that one egg a day was acceptable for most individuals; an exception is those with diabetes—these individuals appear to be more vulnerable to the blood-cholesterol raising effect of dietary cholesterol.[2] Certain plant sterols interfere with the absorption of cholesterol and help lower blood cholesterol levels. (See the Evidence-Based Practice box, "Plant Sterols: Weapon for Lowering Blood Cholesterol Levels.")

Lipoproteins

Function

The liver is the body clearinghouse for fatty acids and cholesterol, whether supplied in food or produced in body tissues. When received by the liver, fatty acids and cholesterol are packaged into lipoproteins and released into the circulation for transport to cells.

Lipid Transport

Lipids are insoluble in water, which poses a problem when they need to be carried in a water-based circulatory system. The body solves this problem by producing lipoproteins, a complex of lipids and lipidlike substances surrounded by water-soluble protein. Special compounds called phospholipids are important in the structure of lipoproteins. Phospholipids are molecules in which one of the three fatty acids attached to a glycerol base is replaced with a phosphate (PO_4^{-3}) group that is water soluble and assists in the transport of lipoproteins. Phospholipids in cell membranes help lipid molecules move from the circulatory system into the cell.

Lipoproteins contain fatty acids, triglycerides, cholesterol, phospholipids, and traces of fat-soluble vitamins and steroid hormones. They serve as the major vehicle for lipid transport in the blood.

Classes of Lipoproteins

Lipoproteins are classified according to their density, as determined by their relative content of lipid and protein. The more protein present, the greater the density. The amount of each lipoprotein in the blood is influenced by the time since the last meal and the quantity and type of fat that a person

EVIDENCE-BASED PRACTICE

Plant Sterols: Weapon for Lowering Blood Cholesterol Levels

Identify the Problem: Plant sterols, also known as *phytosterols* or *phytostanols,* are found in small amounts in vegetable oils and grains such as corn, rye, and wheat. The chemical structure of plant sterols is much like that of cholesterol; based on this similarity, plant sterols compete with cholesterol for absorption in the small intestine. Nutrition researchers speculated that plant sterols in the digestive food mix would lower the amount of cholesterol absorbed and delivered to the liver. When less cholesterol is available, the liver produces fewer lipoproteins and blood levels of total cholesterol and LDL cholesterol decline.[1] Unfortunately, plant sterols occur naturally in food in very small amounts, too small to make a difference in cholesterol absorption. Food technologists have since found ways to incorporate plant sterols into food products to increase dietary intake. Table fats, yogurt, orange juice, grain foods, and cereal bars with added plant sterols are examples of new functional foods.[2]

Review the Evidence: Clinical trials with patients having elevated blood cholesterol levels have demonstrated the benefits of plant sterols in the prevention and treatment of cardiovascular disease. A daily intake of 1.5 to 3 g of plant sterols consumed as part of a fortified food or as a dietary supplement lowered LDL cholesterol levels by 5% to 15%,[3,4] and reduced the tendency of blood platelets to form unwanted blood clots.[5] Based on this evidence the U.S. Food and Drug Administration (FDA) approved a health claim to appear on the food label of sterol-containing foods that regular use along with a diet low in saturated fat and cholesterol may reduce the risk of heart disease.[6]

Implement the Findings: We know that plant sterols can help to reduce blood LDL cholesterol levels; however, it is important for patients to realize that individuals who have a higher LDL cholesterol level at baseline are likely to experience greater effects than those with lower baseline levels. The meal at which the sterol-fortified food is consumed also influences its effectiveness. It is best to divide the daily intake of sterol-fortified foods or supplements across two to three meals, or concentrate intake at the noon or evening meal. Sterol-fortified foods are less effective if eaten at breakfast, and this may relate to the diurnal rhythm of body cholesterol synthesis. Sterols consumed in fortified margarine or other fat spreads, salad dressings, or yogurt lead to greater reductions in LDL cholesterol levels than if obtained from fortified grain products or orange juice. More research is needed to determine the effects of particular sterols added to specific foods.[4]

To control kcalorie intake, foods with added sterols must replace, not be used in addition to, the conventional item in the daily meal pattern. An 8-oz serving of orange juice containing 1 g of plant sterols provides 110 kcal but meets the MyPlate (ChooseYourPlate.gov) equivalent of one serving of fruit. Additional fruit servings, however, are best selected from whole fruits that also supply fiber. Table spreads containing about 0.7 g of plant sterols per tablespoon (1 tbsp being the recommended serving size) add 70 kcal and 8 g of fat per serving. Sterol-containing products advertised as "light" spreads usually contain about 50 kcal/tbsp and 5 g of fat. Two tablespoons per day are needed to reach the minimum suggested intake of plant sterols.

Sterol-containing foods appear to be safe for use over long periods of time, although they may adversely affect the absorption of carotenoids and lower blood carotenoid levels. Individuals using sterol-fortified foods should be encouraged to include generous servings of carotenoid-rich foods in their daily diet.[7] (Dark-green, orange, and red vegetables and fruits are good sources of carotenoids. We will learn more about these compounds in Chapter 6.)

References

1. Amiot MJ, Knol D, Cardinault N, et al: Comparable reduction in cholesterol absorption after two different ways of phytosterol administration in humans. *Eur J Nutr* 52(3):1215, 2013.
2. Castro IA, Barroso LP, Sinnecker P: Functional foods for coronary heart disease risk reduction: a meta-analysis using a multivariate approach. *Am J Clin Nutr* 82:32, 2005.
3. Maki KC, Lawless AL, Reeves MS, et al: Lipid-altering effects of a dietary supplement tablet containing free plant sterols and stanols in men and women with primary hypercholesterolaemia: a randomized, placebo-controlled crossover trial. *Int J Food Sci Nutr* 63(4):476, 2012.
4. Abumweis SS, Barake R, Jones PJH: Plant sterols/stanols as cholesterol lowering agents: a meta-analysis of randomized controlled trials. *Food Nutr Res* 52, 2008.
5. Kozlowska-Wojciechowska M, Jastrzebska M, Naruszewicz M, et al: Impact of margarine enriched with plant sterols on blood lipids, platelet function, and fibrinogen level in young men. *Metabolism* 52:1378, 2003.
6. U.S. Food and Drug Administration: Guidance for Industry: A Food Labeling Guide Appendix C: Health Claims, Rockville, Md., U.S. Department of Health and Human Services. from: <www.fda.gov/downloads/Food/GuidanceRegulation/UCM265446.pdf>. Revised October 2009. Retrieved July 13, 2013.
7. Van Horn L, McCoin M, Kris-Etherton PM, et al: The evidence for dietary prevention and treatment of cardiovascular disease. *J Am Diet Assoc* 108:287, 2008.

consumes on a regular basis. The five lipoprotein classes are as follows:

1. *Chylomicrons:* These relatively large particles are formed in the intestinal wall after a meal and carry the digested and absorbed fat to the liver for conversion to other lipoproteins.

2. *Very low-density lipoproteins (VLDLs):* The VLDLs are formed in the liver during the fasting interval between meals. When there is no food in the digestive tract and chylomicrons are not entering the circulatory system, VLDLs transport **endogenous** triglycerides from the liver to tissue cells.

3. *Intermediate-density lipoproteins (IDLs):* IDLs are formed from VLDLs and continue the delivery of endogenous triglycerides to the cells.
4. *Low-density lipoproteins (LDLs):* LDLs are formed from VLDLs and IDLs and carry mainly cholesterol, as most of the triglyceride has already been moved into cells.
5. *High-density lipoproteins (HDLs):* HDLs return cholesterol from the cells to the liver for breakdown and excretion.

Cholesterol, Lipoproteins, and Cardiovascular Risk

The two classes of lipoproteins receiving the most attention in clinical practice are the LDLs and HDLs. Both are primary carriers of cholesterol; thus their levels in the blood have important implications for health. The LDLs transport cholesterol from the liver to the tissues; in fact, about half of the cholesterol circulating in the blood is contained in the LDLs.[32] Conversely, the HDLs return cholesterol from the cells to the liver for excretion. Elevated blood cholesterol in the form of LDL cholesterol promotes atherosclerosis, the underlying pathologic condition in coronary heart disease. High LDL cholesterol levels cause a buildup of fatty plaque on the inner walls of the vessels that supply blood to the heart muscle. Over time, these plaques narrow the lumen of the coronary arteries, decreasing delivery of both oxygen and other nutrients. Interruption of blood to the heart, as a result of a blood clot or built-up plaque, causes a heart attack; a similar occurrence in an artery in the brain results in a stroke (cerebral hemorrhage). In contrast to LDLs, high HDLs slow or prevent the progression of atherosclerosis, lowering cardiovascular risk.

Although both the types and amounts of dietary fat affect LDL and HDL cholesterol levels, it is not that simple. Some people absorb cholesterol more efficiently or synthesize increased amounts regardless of dietary intake. Dietary fat rather than dietary cholesterol may play a role in cholesterol synthesis.[32] Genetic factors affect the production of HDLs and the rate at which cholesterol is eliminated from the body. In Chapter 21 we will learn about dietary and lifestyle interventions and medications to help control blood lipoprotein levels.

HEALTH PROMOTION

Lowering Fat Intake

Despite public health campaigns directed toward lowering dietary fat, fat intake as a proportion of total energy has remained at 33% to 34% over the past decade,[2,33] although total fat intake dropped from 81 g to 77 g.[19] Even with this slight decrease in dietary fat, energy intake actually increased as Americans consumed more kcalories from carbohydrate.[2] Fat intake differs according to sex: on average, men consume 93 g and women consume 66 g each day, based on differences in total kcalorie intake.[19] Fat intake also differs by race and ethnicity. Mexican Americans take in about 30% of their kcalories from fat as compared to Caucasians and African

Americans, who consume 33% of their energy from fat[34]; overall, Mexican Americans consume less total daily fat.[35]

Fast-food adds to intakes of both fat and kcalories. On days when all meals were eaten at home or somewhere other than a fast-food restaurant, men took in 33.6% of their kcalories as fat. On days including a fast-food meal, energy intake rose by 500 kcal and fat intake reached 34.9% of total kcalories.[36] Women increased their energy intake by 220 kcal and their proportion of fat kcalories from 32.7% to 34.6% on days that included a fast-food meal. Carbohydrate intake also increased when eating at a fast-food restaurant.

Dietary fat can be lowered in various ways. Attempting to eliminate all foods high in fat not only lessens intakes of many important nutrients, such as iron, zinc, vitamin E, and essential fatty acids, but also is unlikely to be sustained over time.[30] Alternatively, eating a mix of higher-fat and modified-fat foods effectively lowers dietary fat,[37-39] while maintaining appropriate levels of nutrients contained in higher-fat foods. Including a higher-fat food at mealtime adds to satiety and helps curb the urge to overeat between meals. Limiting portion size is another effective way to reduce both fat and kcalories. A balance of both higher-fat and lower-fat foods is the best strategy for overall good health. (See the Perspectives in Practice box, "Lowering Your Fat Intake," for more ideas on moderating your intake of fats.)

Fat Replacers

Fats serve many functions in food recipes and food preparation. In cooking and baking, fats absorb flavors from various ingredients and help to blend them throughout the food; assist in the heat transfer necessary for browning or crispiness; create a velvety mouth feel in foods such as ice cream, pudding, and cheese; and play a critical role in frying.[40] Fat replacers are ingredients that fulfill these functions but are lower in kcalories. Fruit purees made from apples or prunes

KEY TERMS

cholesterol A fat-related compound; a sterol that is normally found in bile and is a principal constituent of gallstones. Cholesterol is synthesized by the liver and is a precursor of various steroid hormones, such as estrogen and testosterone, and of the vitamin D molecule produced by the action of ultraviolet light on the skin. It is found in animal tissues such as meat, egg yolk, and milk fat.

bile A fluid secreted by the liver and transported to the gallbladder for concentration and storage. It is released into the duodenum on entry of fat and acts as an emulsifier to facilitate enzymatic fat digestion.

complex A chemical compound consisting of several atoms or molecules loosely connected and easily separated. The micelles formed in the lumen of the intestine, which carry fats into the intestinal wall, are bile-lipid complexes.

phospholipids A class of fat-related substances that contain a phosphate group and fatty acids. The phospholipids are important components of cell membranes, nerve tissues, and lipoproteins.

PERSPECTIVES IN PRACTICE

Lowering Your Fat Intake

Consumers need practical suggestions on how to lower their intake of fats, especially unhealthy fats. Encourage small changes that once begun will be continued. Even one change at a time can add up to measurable differences over weeks and months.

Following are some ways to get started:
1. Reduce the fat you add to other foods.
   * Use less butter or margarine on your toast.
   * Be stingy when adding salad dressing.
2. Reduce portion size.
   * Order the small rather than the "supersize" portion of French fries.
3. Eat a favorite high-fat food less often.
   * Have ice cream as a snack or dessert on fewer days of the week; choose fresh fruit on other days.
4. Choose a lower-fat version of a food you eat regularly.
   * Use reduced-fat, low-fat, or fat-free milk in place of whole milk. (Gradually reduce the amount of fat until you reach low-fat or fat-free.)
   * Choose a grilled chicken breast without skin rather than a fried chicken breast with skin.
   * Trim all visible fat from meats.
5. Substitute modified foods lower in fat.
   * Look for reduced-fat mayonnaise and salad dressings. (Be sure to check the kcalorie content.)
6. Eliminate fat when preparing foods.
   * Eat raw carrots without added salad dressing or broccoli without added butter or margarine.
   * Season cooked vegetables with lemon juice, orange juice, or low-sodium chicken broth rather than margarine or butter.

are often used in home baking as fat replacers in cookies and moist cakes. Other fat replacers used as thickeners and emulsifiers have been developed for use in processed foods.

Most fat replacers are carbohydrates—plant polysaccharides, celluloses, or gums—although protein and fat may help provide structure. Several fat replacers have been approved by the FDA for use in the United States.[40] Fat replacers can contribute between 0 and 9 kcal/g, but can be used in smaller amounts than food fats that contain 9 kcal/g. Also, fat replacers are often poorly digested or absorbed, lowering available kcalories. Olestra, a common fat replacer in snack foods, interferes with the absorption of fat-soluble vitamins, so products that contain olestra have added amounts of vitamins A, D, E, and K to compensate for this loss. Blood levels of the fat-soluble vitamins appear to be unchanged in users of olestra-containing foods.[41] Fat replacers that are not digested and remain in the stomach longer might add to satiety and assist in appetite control and weight management; however, it appears that individuals who use foods that contain olestra often compensate for the lower kcalories by consuming a larger amount.[42]

Unfortunately, the general public often assumes that baked goods, frozen desserts, and salad dressings made with fat

replacers are lower in kcalories; this is not always true. In fact, a food containing a fat replacer may contain the same number of kcalories or even more kcalories than its higher-fat counterpart if more sugar has been added to maintain flavor and mouth feel. People who presume they can eat a larger portion of an item made with a fat replacer may be taking in even more kcalories than they would with a smaller portion of the higher-fat item. Better to select snacks from fruit, whole grains, or reduced fat or fat-free dairy foods, which are not only lower in fat but also rich in nutrients.

DIGESTION-ABSORPTION-METABOLISM REVIEW

An overall discussion of digestion is found in Chapter 2. A summary of chemical digestion and the absorption process specific to lipids is provided here for review.

Digestion
Triglycerides in animal and plant foods must be broken down into individual fatty acids for absorption and body use.

Mouth
Lingual **lipase** in the salivary secretions begins the process of lipid digestion.

Stomach
The gastric enzyme specific to lipids is gastric lipase (tributyrinase), which acts on emulsified butterfat. As gastric secretions act on carbohydrates and proteins in the food mix, the lipids begin to separate out, making them more accessible to their own enzymes in the small intestine.

Small Intestine
The major breakdown of lipids begins here. Digestive secretions come from three sources: (1) the biliary tract, (2) the pancreas, and (3) the small intestine, as follows:
1. *Bile from the liver and gallbladder:* The presence of fat in the upper duodenum triggers the release of cholecystokinin (CCK) from the intestinal mucosa, which in turn causes the gallbladder to contract, releasing a flow of bile. Bile acts as an **emulsifier**, preparing lipids for further digestion by (1) breaking them into smaller particles, increasing the surface area accessible to enzyme action, and (2) lowering the surface tension of the finely dispersed globules, enabling enzymes to penetrate more easily. Bile also provides the alkaline medium needed for the action of pancreatic lipase. If bile secretion is hindered, as much as 40% of dietary fat is lost in the feces.
2. *Enzymes from the pancreas:* Pancreatic lipase breaks off one fatty acid at a time from the glycerol base of triglycerides. The initial action yields one fatty acid plus a diglyceride, and continuing action yields another fatty acid plus a monoglyceride. Each successive step becomes more difficult, with the result that less than one third of the fat in the food mass is broken down completely. The final

TABLE 4-2	SUMMARY OF LIPID DIGESTION	
LOCATION	ENZYME	ACTIVITY
Mouth	Lingual lipase (very limited)	Mechanical, mastication
Stomach	No major enzyme	Mechanical separation of fats as protein and starch are digested and go into solution
	Small amount of gastric lipase (tributyrinase)	Butterfat (tributyrin) to fatty acids and glycerol
Small intestine	Bile salts from gallbladder	Emulsifies fats
	Pancreatic lipase	Triglycerides to diglycerides and monoglycerides in turn; then fatty acids and glycerol

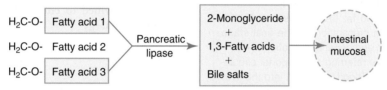

FIGURE 4-4 A micelle complex of fats and bile salts for transport into the intestinal wall. The fatty acid in the *2* position of the triglyceride is the most difficult to remove, and some fat is absorbed in this monoglyceride form.

products of lipid digestion ready to be absorbed are fatty acids, diglycerides, monoglycerides, and glycerol.
3. *Enzyme from the small intestine:* Lecithinase acts on lecithin, a phospholipid, to prepare it for absorption. Table 4-2 summarizes lipid digestion.

Absorption

The task of transporting lipids from the small intestine into the bloodstream takes place in three stages.

Stage I: Initial Lipid Absorption

In the small intestine, bile salts combine with the products of lipid digestion to form **micelles**, a bile-lipid complex. This carrier system (described in Figure 4-4) moves the lipid molecules from the lumen of the intestine into the intestinal wall.

Stage II: Absorption Within the Intestinal Wall

Once inside the wall of the small intestine the bile salts separate from the lipid complex. They are absorbed into the blood and return to the liver via the enterohepatic circulation, ready to carry out their task again. When the lipid products are released from the micellar complex, the following actions take place (Figure 4-5):
1. *Direct absorption of short- and medium-chain fatty acids:* Fatty acids with a chain length of 12 or fewer carbon atoms are absorbed directly into the **portal** blood. As noted earlier, MCT mixtures are helpful with persons who have problems with fat digestion and absorption.
2. *Enteric lipase digestion:* A lipase within the intestinal wall completes the digestion of the remaining diglycerides and monoglycerides, releasing fatty acids and glycerol.
3. *Triglyceride synthesis:* All longer chain fatty acids and glycerol form new human triglycerides, ready for absorption and transport via the lymph.

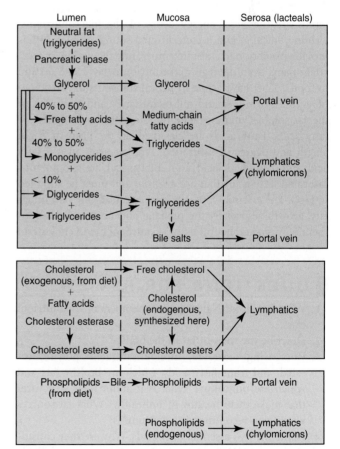

FIGURE 4-5 Absorption of fat, cholesterol, and phospholipids. Note that a large proportion of dietary triglycerides are not completely broken down to fatty acids and glycerol before they combine with bile salts to form the micelle; digestion is completed by the lipase enzyme in the lining of the intestine.

KEY TERMS

chylomicrons   Lipoproteins formed in the intestinal wall after a meal that carry food fats into the lymph and then the general circulation for transport to the liver.

endogenous   Originating from within the body; an example is endogenous cholesterol, which is produced by cells in the liver.

lipase   Group of digestive enzymes that break down triglycerides to fatty acids and glycerol.

emulsifier   An agent that breaks down large fat globules to smaller, uniformly distributed particles increasing the surface area available to digestive enzymes and reducing the surface tension. This is the role of bile in the intestine.

micelles   Complex of bile and fat that carries fat into the wall of the small intestine in preparation for the final stage of absorption into the lymph and general circulation.

portal   An entryway, usually referring to the portal circulation of blood through the liver. Blood is brought into the liver via the portal vein and moves out via the hepatic vein.

enteric   Relating to the intestine.

Stage III: Final Absorption and Transport

The newly formed human triglycerides, along with any other lipid materials present, receive a protein covering to form the lipoproteins called *chylomicrons*. These lipid packages cross the cell membrane to enter the lymphatic system and drain into the portal blood. In the liver the lipids are converted into new lipoproteins for transport to body cells. Review Figure 4-5 to follow lipid absorption through its three stages.

Metabolism

The metabolism of carbohydrates, proteins, and lipids are closely intertwined to effectively meet the body's constant demand for energy.

▊ TO SUM UP

Lipids are the most energy dense of the macronutrients, yielding 9 kcal/g, and a concentrated source of fuel. Lipids provide insulation to assist in temperature regulation, protect vital organs from damage, and contribute flavor and texture to foods. They have a role in neural transmission, structure of steroid hormones and cell membranes, and transport of the fat-soluble vitamins. The building blocks of lipids are fatty acids. Fatty acids are classified on the basis of chain length and degree of saturation. Linoleic acid, an n-6 fatty acid, and α-linolenic acid, an n-3 fatty acid, are two polyunsaturated fatty acids that are *essential* and must be supplied in food. The essential fatty acids are necessary for skin integrity, growth (especially the prenatal and postnatal development of brain and neural tissue), control of blood cholesterol levels, and immune function. Several n-3 fatty acids in fish discourage platelet aggregation and lower the risk of heart attack and stroke. Both the type and amount of dietary lipids affect health. Inappropriately high intakes of fat, especially saturated fats and trans fats, increase cardiovascular risk. The AMDR for fat is 20% to 35% of total kcalories. When lipids provide less than 10% of total kcalories, supplies of the essential fatty acids may be inadequate. Consumers should consult the nutrition label and list of ingredients on processed foods to control their intakes of total fat, trans fat, and saturated fat. Nutrition education should reinforce wise selection of fat-containing and fat-modified foods to maintain a prudent intake of healthy fats, control energy intake, and maximize intakes of vitamins and minerals.

▊ QUESTIONS FOR REVIEW

1. What is a lipid? Name several members of this nutrient class.

2. Describe the roles of fat in the body.

3. Comparing saturated, monounsaturated, polyunsaturated, and trans fatty acids, which are healthy fats and which are unhealthy? What is it about their structures that make them healthy or unhealthy? What fat sources would you recommend to consumers?

4. Name the two essential fatty acids. Why are they considered essential? What happens when they are not available in the amounts needed?

5. You are counseling a patient who has been told that he should lose 10 to 15 lb. His usual fat intake is about 35% of his total energy intake. He has agreed to lower his intake of fat to 30% in an effort to reduce his daily kcalories. What are some strategies that might help him accomplish this? He and his coworkers eat their lunch at fast-food restaurants. Develop two fast-food lunch menus that limit fat and kcalories.

6. Two persons with strong family histories of cardiovascular disease are concerned about their heart health. Both have lowered their cholesterol intake and avoid eating butter. One person started to use a stick margarine made from corn oil and the other a soft tub corn oil margarine. Which person made the better choice? Why?

7. A woman runner has decided to remove all fat from her diet. If she is successful in doing this, then what health problems might she encounter?

8. A consumer tells you that she has begun to read food labels and buys only those items that are made with plant fats rather than animal fats, as she heard that plant fats were healthier. Is this always true? What does she need to

look for on the food label to be sure that she is avoiding unhealthy fats?

9. Go to the grocery store and identify three types of crackers, cookies, or salad dressings that offer both a regular and a reduced-fat or fat-free version. Using the nutrition label, make a chart indicating (a) the serving size, (b) total kcalories per serving, (c) grams of total fat per serving, (d) grams of saturated fat per serving, (e) grams of unsaturated fat per serving, (f) grams of trans fat per serving, (g) grams of sugar per serving, and (h) cost per serving. What nutritional differences did you observe between the regular and reduced-fat or fat-free versions? Was there a cost difference? If so, was the reduced-fat or fat-free version worth the difference in price? How do the regular and reduced-fat or fat-free versions compare in serving size, kcalories, total fat, and sugar?

10. You are asked to provide a 10-minute update on trans fats to a consumer group that is concerned about public health. Develop an outline for your presentation including (a) examples of both processed and restaurant foods that contain trans fats and (b) use of the nutrition label to identify trans fats.

11. You are working with an individual who has been told to reduce his dietary cholesterol. His list of foods indicates that he may have fat-free milk but not reduced-fat or low-fat milk and he doesn't understand why. What would you tell him?

12. Develop a handout of ways that persons can reduce their fat intake.

REFERENCES

1. Moskowitz H, Beckley J, Adams J: What makes people crave fast foods? *Nutr Today* 37:237, 2002.
2. U.S. Department of Health and Human Services, U.S. Department of Agriculture: *Report of the Dietary Guidelines Advisory Committee on the Dietary Guidelines for Americans 2010,* Center for Nutrition Policy and Promotion, Washington, D.C., 2010, U.S. Department of Agriculture. from: <http://www.cnpp.usda.gov/DGAs2010-DGACReport.htm>. Retrieved November 12, 2012.
3. Kris-Etherton P, Fleming J, Harris WS: The debate about n-6 polyunsaturated fatty acid recommendations for cardiovascular health. *J Am Diet Assoc* 110:201, 2010.
4. Astrup A, Dyerberg J, Elwood P, et al: The role of reducing intakes of saturated fat in the prevention of cardiovascular disease: where does the evidence stand in 2010? *Am J Clin Nutr* 93:684, 2011.
5. Bray GA: Is dietary fat important? *Am J Clin Nutr* 93:481, 2011.
6. Van Horn L, McCoin M, Kris-Etherton PM, et al: The evidence for dietary prevention and treatment of cardiovascular disease. *J Am Diet Assoc* 108:287, 2008.
7. Sharabi Y: Management of the unholy trinity: diabetes-obesity-hypertension (diabesotension). *Diabetes Metab Res Rev* 2012.
8. Bray GA, Wilson JF: In the clinic. Obesity. *Ann Intern Med* 149(7):ITC4–1-15, 2008.
9. Baum SJ, Kris-Etherton PM, Willett WC, et al: Fatty acids in cardiovascular health and disease. *J Clin Lipidology* 6:216, 2012.
10. International Food Information Council Foundation: *2012 Food & Health Survey: Consumer Attitudes toward Food Safety, Nutrition and Health,* May 23, 2012, International Food Information Council. at: <http://www.foodinsight.org/Content/5519/IFICF_2012_FoodHealthSurvey.pdf>. Accessed on December 6, 2012.
11. Rolls ET: Sensory processing in the brain related to the control of food intake. *Proc Nutr Soc* 66:96, 2007.
12. Samra RA: Fats and Satiety. In Montmayeur JP, le Coutre J, editors: *Fat detection: taste, texture, and post ingestive effects,* Boca Raton, Fla., 2010, CRC Press.
13. Jones PJH: Papamandjaris AA: Lipids: cellular metabolism. In Erdman JW Jr, Macdonald IA, Zeisel SH, editors: *Present knowledge in nutrition,* ed 10, Ames, Iowa, 2012, International Life Sciences Institute/Wiley-Blackwell.
14. Institute of Medicine, Otten JJ, Hellwig JP, Meyers LD, editors: *Dietary reference intakes: the essential guide to nutrient requirements,* Washington, D.C., 2006, National Academies Press.
15. Holligan SD, Berryman CE, Wang L, et al: Atherosclerotic cardiovascular disease. In Erdman JW Jr, Macdonald IA, Zeisel SH, editors: *Present knowledge in nutrition,* ed 10, Ames, Iowa, 2012, International Life Sciences Institute/Wiley-Blackwell.
16. Food and Nutrition Board, Institute of Medicine: *Dietary Reference Intakes for energy, carbohydrate, fiber, fat, fatty acids, cholesterol, protein, and amino acids (macronutrients),* Washington, D.C., 2002, National Academies Press.
17. Riediger ND, Othman RA, Suh M, et al: A systematic review of the roles of n-3 fatty acids in health and disease. *J Am Diet Assoc* 109:668, 2009.
18. Mozaffarian D, Wu JHY: (n-3) Fatty acids and cardiovascular health: are effects of EPA and DHA shared or complementary? *J Nutr* 142:614S, 2012.
19. U.S. Department of Agriculture, Agricultural Research Service: Nutrient Intakes from Food: Mean Amounts Consumed per Individual by Gender and Age in the United States, 2009-2010. In *What We Eat in America,* NHANES 2009-2010. 2012. at: <http://www.ars.usda.gov/SP2UserFiles/Place/12355000/pdf/0910/Table_1_NIN_GEN_09.pdf>. Accessed on November 15, 2012.
20. Makrides M: Outcomes for mothers and their babies: do n-3 long-chain polyunsaturated fatty acids and seafoods make a difference? *J Am Diet Assoc* 108:1622, 2008.
21. Carlson SE: Docosahexaenoic acid supplementation in pregnancy and lactation. *Am J Clin Nutr* 89(Suppl):678S, 2009.
22. Makrides M, Gibson RA, McPhee AJ, et al: Effect of DHA supplementation during pregnancy on maternal depression and neurodevelopment of young children: a randomized trial. *JAMA* 304:1675, 2010.
23. Kris-Etherton PM, Hill AM: n-3 Fatty acids: food or supplements. *J Am Diet Assoc* 108:1125, 2008.

24. Trumbo PR, Shimakawa T: Tolerable upper intake levels for trans fat, saturated fat, and cholesterol. *Nutr Rev* 69(5):270, 2011.
25. Riserus U, Willett WC, Hu FB, et al: Dietary fats and prevention of type 2 diabetes. *Prog Lipid Res* 48:44, 2009.
26. Kris-Etherton PM, Lefevre M, Mensink RP, et al: Trans fatty acid intakes and food sources in the U.S. population: NHANES 1999-2002. *Lipids* 47:931, 2012.
27. Doell D, Folmer D, Lee H, et al: Updated estimate of *trans* fat intake by the US population. *Food Addit Contam Part A* 29(6):861, 2012.
28. Remig V, Franklin B, Margolis S, et al: Trans fats in America: a review of their use, consumption, health implications and regulation. *J Am Diet Assoc* 110:585, 2010.
29. Eckel RH, Kris-Etherton P, Lichtenstein AH, et al: Americans' awareness, knowledge, and behaviors regarding fats: 2006-2007. *J Am Diet Assoc* 109:288, 2009.
30. Gardner CD, Kim S, Bersamin A, et al: Micronutrient quality of weight-loss diets that focus on macronutrients: results from the A TO Z study. *Am J Clin Nutr* 92:304, 2010.
31. Ma Y, Olendzki BC, Hafner AR, et al: Low-carbohydrate and high-fat intake among adult patients with poorly controlled type 2 diabetes mellitus. *Nutrition* 22(11–12):1129, 2006.
32. Grundy SM: Nutrition in the management of disorders of serum lipids and lipoproteins. In Shils ME, Shike M, Olson J, editors: *Modern nutrition in health and disease*, ed 10, Baltimore, Md., 2006, Lippincott Williams & Wilkins.
33. U.S. Department of Agriculture, Agricultural Research Service: Energy Intakes: Percentages of Energy from Protein, Carbohydrate, Fat, and Alcohol, by Gender and Age. In *What We Eat in America*, NHANES 2009-2010, 2012. at: <http://www.ars.usda.gov/SP2UserFiles/Place/12355000/pdf/0910/Table_5_EIN_GEN_09.pdf>. Accessed on November 12, 2012.
34. U.S. Department of Agriculture, Agricultural Research Service: Energy Intakes: Percentages of Energy from Protein, Carbohydrate, Fat, and Alcohol, by Race/Ethnicity and Age. In *What We Eat in America*, NHANES 2009-2010. What We Eat in America, NHANES 2009-2010, 2012. at: <http://www.ars.usda.gov/SP2UserFiles/Place/12355000/pdf/0910/Table_6_EIN_RAC_09.pdf>. Accessed on November 12, 2012.
35. U.S. Department of Agriculture, Agricultural Research Service: Nutrient Intakes from Food: Mean Amounts Consumed per Individual by Race/Ethnicity and Age in the United States, 2009-2010. In *What We Eat in America*, NHANES 2009-2010, 2012. at: <http://www.ars.usda.gov/SP2UserFiles/Place/12355000/pdf/0910/Table_2_NIN_RAC_09.pdf>. Accessed on November 15, 2012.
36. Bowman SA, Vinyard BT: Fast food consumption of U.S. adults: impact on energy and nutrient intakes and overweight status. *J Am Coll Nutr* 23:163, 2004.
37. Ledikwe JH, Blanck HM, Khan LK, et al: Low-energy-density diets are associated with high quality in adults in the United States. *J Am Diet Assoc* 106:1172, 2006.
38. Raynor HA, Looney SM, Steeves EA, et al: The effects of an energy density prescription on diet quality and weight loss: a pilot randomized controlled trial. *J Acad Nutr Diet* 112:1397, 2012.
39. Phelan S, Lang W, Jordan D, et al: Use of artificial sweeteners and fat-modified foods in weight loss maintainers and always-normal weight individuals. *Int J Obesity* 33:1183, 2009.
40. American Dietetic Association: Position of the American Dietetic Association: fat replacers. *J Am Diet Assoc* 105:266, 2005.
41. Neuhouser ML, Rock CL, Kristal AR, et al: Olestra is associated with slight reductions in serum carotenoids but does not markedly influence serum fat-soluble vitamin concentrations. *Am J Clin Nutr* 83:624, 2006.
42. Jandacek RJ: Review of the effects of dilution of dietary energy with olestra on energy intake. *Physiol Behav* 105:1124, 2012.

FURTHER READINGS AND RESOURCES

Readings
Flores G, Maldonado J, Duran P: Making tortillas without lard: Latino parents' perspectives on healthy eating, physical activity, and weight-management strategies for overweight Latino children. *J Acad Nutr Diet* 112:81, 2012.
[Dr. Flores and his collaborators help us understand the cultural issues in helping families choose healthier foods and ingredients.]
Martin CK, Thomson JL, LeBlanc MM, et al: Children in school cafeterias select foods containing more saturated fat and energy than the Institute of Medicine recommendations. *J Nutr* 140:1653, 2010.
Whitfield Jacobsen PA, Prawitz AD, Lukaszuk JM: Long-haul truck drivers want healthful meal options at truck-stop restaurants. *J Am Diet Assoc* 107:2125, 2007.
[These articles present ideas for nutrition intervention among particular age and lifestyle groups.]
Kris-Etherton P, Fleming J, Harris WS: The debate about n-6 polyunsaturated fatty acid recommendations for cardiovascular health. *J Am Diet Assoc* 110:201, 2010.
[This article describes the differences of opinion that exist among health professionals regarding appropriate intakes of dietary fat.]
Remig V, Franklin B, Margolis S, et al: Trans fats in America: a review of their use, consumption, health implications and regulation. *J Am Diet Assoc* 110:585, 2010.
[This article provides insight as to local and state efforts to reduce the amounts of trans fat in processed foods and fast-food restaurants, and what success has been achieved.]

Websites of Interest
- International Food Information Council Foundation: This site contains fact sheets and brochures for both consumers and health professionals on food fats and fat replacers. http://www.foodinsight.org/Default.aspx?tabid=85&xsq=fats
- National Heart, Lung and Blood Institute, National Institutes of Health: Information for the Public: This government agency provides tutorials on various aspects of heart disease, recipe books for good eating that include cultural and ethnic food patterns, and health assessment tools, including a menu planner to help monitor fat intake. www.nhlbi.nih.gov/health/index.htm

Proteins

Eleanor D. Schlenker

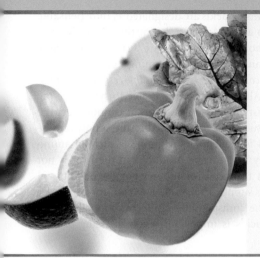

ⒺEVOLVE WEBSITE

http://evolve.elsevier.com/Williams/essentials/

This chapter describing protein completes our sequence of the macronutrients. Protein is quite different from carbohydrate or fat. First, it is the body's major source of nitrogen, the essential element of all living things. Second, its main task is forming body tissue using its individual building units, the amino acids. Protein is critical to growth and health, and protein deficiency associated with crop failure, poverty, or other food shortages causes widespread malnutrition and death among infants, children, and adults in the developing world. In affluent societies intakes of protein—especially animal protein—have escalated and in some individuals may be inappropriately high. Protein is critical to the rehabilitation of patients recovering from surgery, trauma, or serious illness. Our growing understanding of the health benefits of plant proteins encourages their use in menu planning for all age groups.

PHYSICAL AND CHEMICAL NATURE OF PROTEINS

General Definition

In 1838 when Dutch chemist Johann Mulder first identified protein as a substance in all living things, it is unlikely he realized the importance of his discovery. Proteins shape our lives. Protein enzymes break down our food into nutrients the cells can use. As antibodies they shield us from disease.

Peptide hormones carry messages that coordinate continuous body activity. They guide our growth in childhood and maintain our bodies thereafter; they make us each unique.

Chemical Nature

The structural units of proteins—the **amino acids**—are the working currency of protein in body cells. Amino acids contain carbon, hydrogen, and oxygen—the same three elements that make up carbohydrates and fats; however, amino acids and their proteins have the additional element nitrogen. Protein is about 16% nitrogen. Several amino acids also contain sulfur.

The term *amino acid* tells us they have a dual nature. The word *amino* refers to a base or alkaline substance, so at once we have a contradiction. How can a chemical substance be both a base and an acid, and why is this important? Consider the significance of this fact as we learn more about amino acids and their roles in the body.

General Pattern and Structure

A common structural pattern holds for all amino acids. This pattern is built around a central α-carbon, with several attached chemical groups (Figure 5-1) as follows:
- *Amino (base, NH_2) group:* The **amino group** contains the essential element nitrogen and in solution carries a positive charge.

- *Carboxyl (acid, COOH) group:* The **carboxyl group** is found in all acids, and in solution carries a negative charge.
- *An attached radical (R) group:* The *R* stands for *radical*, a general term referring to a group of elements attached to a chemical compound. In this case it refers to the attached side chains on amino acids; each one is different. The distinctive side chain on an amino acid gives it a unique size, shape, and set of properties.[1,2] Compare the structure of the two simplest amino acids—glycine and alanine (Figure 5-2)—with the larger and more complex amino acid arginine (Figure 5-3), with its extended carbon chain (R) and three additional amino groups.

Twenty different amino acids are used to build body proteins.[3] Each has the same core pattern but a specific and different side group. The dual chemical structure of amino acids, including both acid and base groups, gives them a unique **amphoteric** nature, meaning that an amino acid can behave as either an acid or a base, depending on the **pH** of the solution in which it is found. This makes it possible for amino acids to act as **buffers**, important in clinical care.

Essential Amino Acids

Of the 20 amino acids used to build body proteins, nine cannot be synthesized by the body and must be supplied in food. These nine amino acids are designated as **indispensable (essential) amino acids.** Another five of the 20 can be synthesized in the amounts needed and are termed **dispensable (nonessential) amino acids.** The remaining six fall in between and are known as *conditionally indispensable (essential) amino acids* (Box 5-1).[3] Although the body is able to synthesize the conditionally indispensable amino acids, it cannot meet the demand when tissue needs are elevated or the supply of necessary **precursors** is inadequate. Arginine is such an amino acid. The quantity that can be produced in the liver is not sufficient to meet the needs of the newborn, so additional amounts must be supplied in food. The concept of *dietary* essentiality for the indispensable and conditionally indispensable amino acids is important when assessing protein quality.

THE BUILDING OF PROTEINS

Protein Structure

Peptide Bond

The dual chemical nature of amino acids, with a base group on one end and an acid group on the other, enables them to form the unique chain structure found in all proteins. The

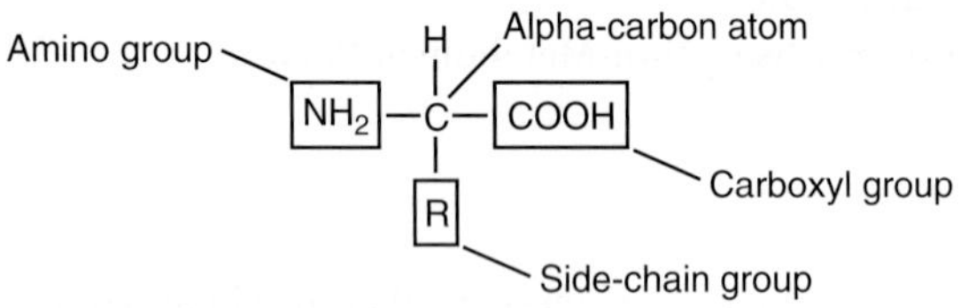

FIGURE 5-1 Basic structure of an amino acid.

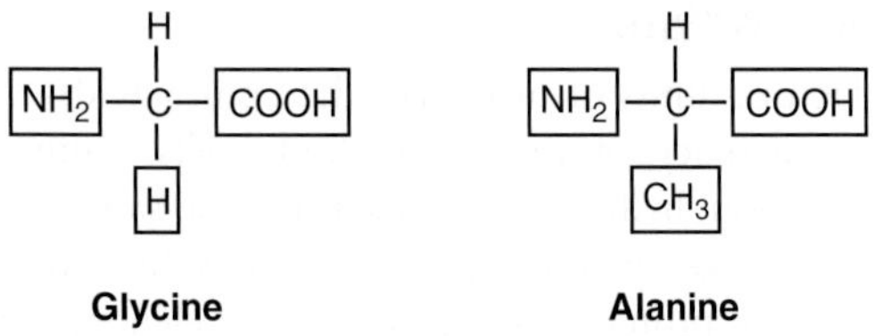

FIGURE 5-2 Structure of the amino acids glycine and alanine.

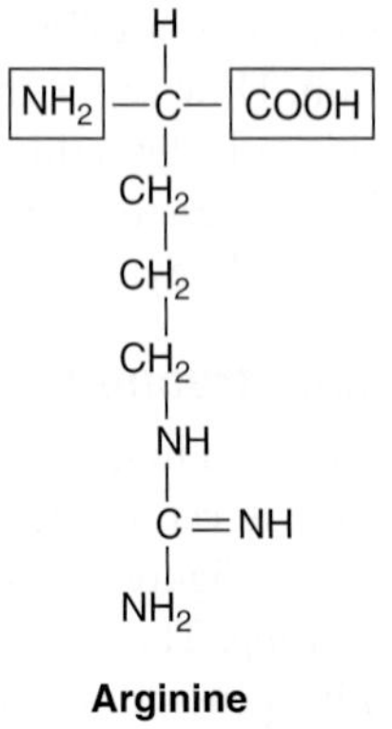

FIGURE 5-3 Structure of the amino acid arginine.

BOX 5-1   CATEGORIES OF AMINO ACIDS

Indispensable (Essential)
- Histidine
- Isoleucine
- Leucine
- Lysine
- Methionine
- Phenylalanine
- Threonine
- Tryptophan
- Valine

Dispensable (Nonessential)
- Alanine
- Aspartic acid
- Asparagine
- Glutamic acid
- Serine

Conditionally Indispensable (Conditionally Essential)
- Arginine
- Cysteine
- Glutamine
- Glycine
- Proline
- Tyrosine

Data from Food and Nutrition Board, Institute of Medicine: *Dietary Reference Intakes for energy, carbohydrate, fiber, fat, fatty acids, cholesterol, protein, and amino acids (macronutrients)*, Washington, D.C., 2002, National Academies Press.

KEY TERMS

amino acids   Acids containing the essential element nitrogen within an amino group—NH_2. Amino acids are the structural units of protein.

amino group   The monovalent radical, NH_2, an essential component of all amino acids.

end amino group of one amino acid joins with the end carboxyl group of the amino acid next to it. This joining of amino acids is called a *peptide bond*. Specific amino acids are joined in a particular sequence to form long chains called *polypeptides,* and specific polypeptides come together to form proteins. Polypeptides vary in length from relatively short chains of 3 to 15 amino acids called *oligopeptides* to medium-sized polypeptides with chains of 21 to 30 amino acids such as insulin. Larger still are complex proteins made up of several hundred amino acids.

To build a compact structure, long polypeptide chains coil or fold back in a spiral shape called a **helix**. Other proteins form a pleated sheet held together by strengthening cross-links of sulfur and hydrogen bonds. Learning more about the structure of body proteins helps medical researchers develop effective medications and understand how genes influence disease risk.

Types of Proteins

Proteins are a widely diverse group of compounds. They have important roles in body structure and metabolism made possible by their specific content and placement of amino acids. Consider the following examples.

Myosin

This fibrous protein found in muscle (Figure 5-4) is built from chains of 153 amino acids that coil and unfold as needed. Shaped into long rods, these fibers end in two-headed bundles so that they can change shape and bend, making it possible to tighten and contract muscles and then relax them.

Collagen

This structural protein contains three separate polypeptide chains that wind around each other to produce a triple helix (Figure 5-5). Thus reinforced, collagen is shaped into long rods and bundled into stiff fibers to do its job of strengthening bone, cartilage, and skin to maintain body form.

Hemoglobin

This globular protein (Figure 5-6) includes four globin polypeptide chains per molecule of hemoglobin. Each chain has several hundred amino acids conjugated with a nonprotein, the iron-containing pigment called *heme*. The globin wraps around the heme and forms protective pockets to secure the iron. The iron in heme has a special ability to bind oxygen, and as part of the red blood cell delivers oxygen to the tissues and returns carbon dioxide for excretion via the lungs.

Albumin

Albumin is the major plasma protein and has a compact globular shape. It consists of a single polypeptide chain of 584 amino acids, twisted and coiled into helix structures held together by disulfide bridges.[4] Albumin serves as a carrier

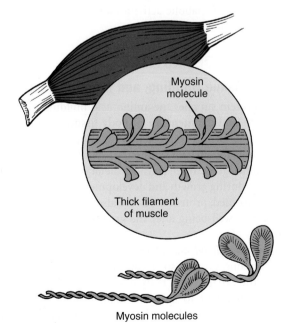

FIGURE 5-4 Myosin molecule

Thick filament of muscle

Myosin molecules

FIGURE 5-4 Myosin is a globular protein in muscle that combines with actin to form actomyosin, the fundamental contractile unit of muscle.

KEY TERMS

carboxyl group The monovalent radical, COOH, found in organic acids.

amphoteric Having opposite characteristics; capable of acting either as an acid or a base or combining with an acid or a base.

pH A scale ranging from 1 to 14 that describes the hydrogen ion concentration of a solution and its relative acidity or alkalinity; 7 is neutral, with lower numbers becoming progressively more acidic and higher numbers becoming progressively more alkaline.

buffers Mixtures of acid and alkaline components that as part of a solution protect against large changes in pH even if strong acids and bases are added. If an acid is added, then the alkaline partner reacts to counteract the acidic effect. If a base is added, then the acid partner reacts to counteract the alkalizing effect. This process keeps body fluids at the pH levels required for life.

indispensable (essential) amino acids Amino acids that the body cannot synthesize or cannot synthesize in sufficient amounts to meet body needs so must be supplied in the diet.

dispensable (nonessential) amino acids Amino acids that can be synthesized by the body from available precursors.

precursor A substance from which another substance is derived.

peptide bond The characteristic joining of amino acids to form proteins. Such a chain of amino acids is termed a *peptide*.

helix A coiled structure found in protein. Some are simple chain coils; others are made of several coils, as the triple helix.

synthesis The making of a substance or compound by the body.

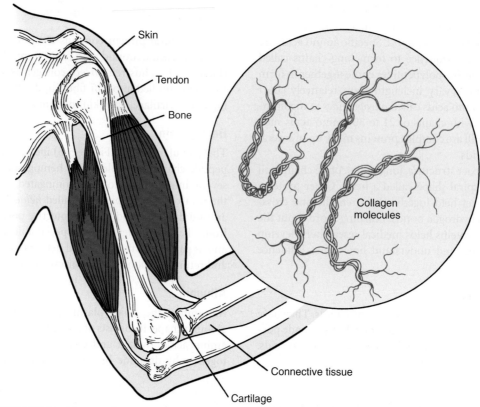

FIGURE 5-5 Tissues that contain collagen, a structural protein forming connective tissue.

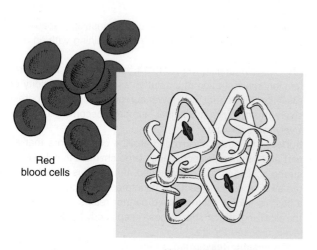

FIGURE 5-6 Hemoglobin is the iron-containing protein in red blood cells that carries oxygen to body cells and tissues and returns carbon dioxide to the lungs for excretion.

protein for drugs, hormones, enzymes, and trace elements. It helps maintain fluid balance by exerting colloidal pressure in the capillaries that forces the flow of nutrients and fluids into the cells and the return of fluid and waste products out of the cells. (The role of albumin in maintaining fluid balance is described in detail in Chapter 7.) In serious illness, albumin is broken down to supply amino acids for the synthesis of new proteins to meet the body emergency.

Proteins with Special Roles

Other proteins with special structural or metabolic roles include the antibodies of the immune system and the blood protein fibrinogen, important in blood clotting. Hormones such as insulin and thyroxin and the enzymes that regulate our day-to-day metabolic activities and produce energy for work are proteins.[2]

FUNCTIONS OF PROTEIN

Growth, Tissue Building, and Maintenance

Dietary protein supplies the amino acid building blocks for the growth and maintenance of body tissues across the life cycle. It must furnish amino acids in the appropriate patterns and amounts for efficient synthesis of specific structural molecules. Although we often consider dietary protein to be most important during growth and development when new tissues are being formed, protein needs are also important for maintenance and well-being after the growth potential has been realized.

Infancy, childhood, and adolescence: Every cell in the human body contains protein so a constant supply is needed to support the expansion of body tissue as an individual grows from a 7-lb infant to a 160-lb man. Protein is especially important to support the rapid growth occurring in the first years of life when protein deficits can have lifelong effects. Protein needs escalate approaching the adolescent growth spurt as bone matrix and muscle tissues expand rapidly.

Good quality protein is needed to support fetal growth and the production of milk.

Adult maintenance: Following the attainment of full growth and maturity, protein requirements reach a steady state based on replacing lost cells and worn-out protein molecules. Loss of cells from the skin and gastrointestinal tract; new cells formed in growth of hair and nails; and formation of enzymes, hormones, and other control proteins constitute daily protein needs. Individuals who participate in strength training and muscle growth require additional protein. Protein requirements demand special attention following recovery from serious illness when depleted protein stores must be replenished.

Specific Physiologic Roles

All amino acids participate in tissue growth and maintenance. Some, however, have important metabolic roles of their own, as follows:

- *Form neurotransmitters for brain and nerve function*[5]: Methionine assists in the formation of choline, a precursor of acetylcholine, and tyrosine is used to synthesize the neurotransmitters dopamine and epinephrine; tryptophan is the precursor of the neurotransmitter serotonin. Age-related decreases in the neurotransmitter dopamine are associated with Parkinson's disease, with muscle tremors and rigidity.[6]
- *Form other amino acids:* Methionine is the precursor of the conditionally indispensable amino acid cysteine, as well as carnitine and taurine; carnitine transports long-chain fatty acids into the mitochondria for energy production, and taurine, found in bile salts, also regulates fluid pressure in the eyes.
- *Form hormones:* Phenylalanine is the precursor of the conditionally indispensable amino acid tyrosine needed to make thyroxin and epinephrine.
- *Support immune function:* Protein is needed to make antibodies for the immune system. Protein molecules referred to as cytokines participate in the acute phase response that brings about alterations in body metabolism needed to handle the demands resulting from critical illness, burns, or trauma.
- *Maintain fluid balance:* Plasma proteins control the flow of fluids, nutrients, and waste products back and forth between the capillaries and the cells. When protein is lacking in quantity or quality and serum proteins such as albumin are not produced in the amounts needed, body fluids accumulate in the tissues and abdomen, resulting in the edema associated with the protein-deficiency disease, kwashiorkor. Low serum albumin complicated by liver disease can lead to ascites.
- *Formation of lipoproteins:* Amino acids supply nitrogen for synthesis of the nitrogen-containing lipoproteins that transport fatty acids and triglycerides from the liver to body cells.
- *Formation of genetic materials:* The synthesis of DNA (deoxyribonucleic acid) and RNA (ribonucleic acid) requires various amino acids.
- *Formation of enzymes and control molecules:* All body enzymes are proteins; examples are the digestive enzymes that break down our food to a form that the body can use for energy and tissue building.

Role in Critical Care

Particular amino acids are beneficial in treating catabolic illness when breakdown and loss of skeletal muscle become critical. Branched chain amino acids—leucine, isoleucine, and valine—have positive effects on protein metabolism in cancer patients for whom malnutrition and body wasting are life threatening.[7,8] Leucine reverses the muscle wasting associated with bed rest by stimulating protein synthesis while decreasing protein breakdown. Although increased amounts of certain amino acids can improve patient status, this should not give license to self-medication with over-the-counter amino acid supplements.

Role as Energy Source

Protein contributes to overall energy metabolism as needed. Protein is seldom used for energy in the fed state when glucose is readily available; however, it may be called upon in the fasting state. In strenuous aerobic exercise protein may be used as an additional source of energy.[11] Before amino acids can be burned for energy the nitrogen-containing amino group must be removed, and then the remaining carbon skeleton is converted to either glucose or fat. In adults about 17 to 25 g of every 100 g of dietary protein is not needed for tissue building or repair and is oxidized for energy.[3] This breakdown of amino acids to a form that can be burned for energy in itself requires energy, leading to the popularization of high-protein diets for weight reduction.[12] Adequate carbohydrate spares protein for its primary purpose of tissue growth and repair.

PROTEIN AND NITROGEN BALANCE

Concept of Balance

Interdependent checks and balances keep the body in working order. This is true for protein ebb and flow, with tissues being built and broken down, and body materials being stored and released. These coordinated activities enable the body to respond to any situation disturbing its normal cycles.

Protein Reserves

The average man contains about 11 kg of protein.[3] Forty percent is in the skeletal muscle with the remainder in skin, blood, kidney, liver, brain, and other organs. Body distribution of protein changes with growth and development. The newborn has relatively little skeletal muscle, with proportionately more protein in the brain and visceral organs.

In contrast to the substantial fat reserves held by most people, body protein reserves are quite limited. What we call the *labile protein reserves,* meaning they are easily broken down to meet immediate needs, make up only about 1% of total body protein; like glycogen, these reserves are sufficient to maintain body functions for only a short period of time.[3]

The labile protein reserves are intended to provide amino acids for an emergency; if the condition continues, as in chronic illness or body wasting, then these reserves are rapidly depleted and skeletal muscle is broken down to furnish amino acids as needed. Muscle has an important role in overall body metabolism, and extreme loss of muscle mass is a predictor of mortality.[13]

Protein Balance

The concept of balance as applied to **protein balance** refers to the steady state between protein synthesis (**anabolism**) and protein breakdown (**catabolism**). In periods of growth, such as infancy or childhood, or the enlargement of muscle as a result of strength training, protein synthesis exceeds breakdown, with a net gain of new tissue (Box 5-2). When food intake is drastically reduced, as in famine or extreme voluntary food restriction, tissue breakdown exceeds synthesis as body protein is broken down to yield energy, with a net loss of body protein. Protein catabolism is accelerated during periods of critical illness as amino acids are needed for the synthesis of new proteins to fight infection, and other body responses to metabolic stress cause protein breakdown and loss of nitrogen in the urine. Serious injury, such as extensive burns, or surgery, or infection are accompanied by catabolic protein losses that continue despite a high protein intake. When healing has begun or the illness has subsided, rehabilitation can bring about increased protein anabolism and gains in body tissue.

Finely tuned mechanisms regulate protein synthesis and breakdown across all body tissues. When less protein is supplied in the diet, protein is conserved and protein losses are minimized. When fighting infection the body uses available protein reserves to obtain amino acids for making immune cells or other proteins necessary to preserve life. When more protein is available than is needed for body growth or repair and protein reserves are at the optimal level, amino acids are broken down and used for energy or stored as fat. In healthy individuals adjustments in protein balance on a day-to-day basis manage the daily variations in protein intake or short-term emergencies.

Various processes and protein compartments participate in control of protein metabolism, as follows:

- *Protein turnover:* Protein turnover is the process by which body proteins are continuously broken down and the released amino acids made into new proteins.[3] New proteins replace worn-out proteins, and different proteins are formed to meet changing needs. When an amino acid labeled with a radioactive carbon atom is incorporated into a protein food and eaten, it can be traced; that is, we can follow its journey through the body. By these studies we learned that amino acids are rapidly incorporated into body proteins. Then, when these proteins are broken down, they are reused to form new proteins. Protein turnover varies among tissues. Turnover rates are higher in the intestinal mucosa, liver, pancreas, kidney, and plasma, tissues that are more metabolically active, and lower in muscle, brain, and skin. Protein turnover is very slow in structural tissues such as collagen. Total body protein turnover is higher in infants and children who are growing rapidly and lower in older adults.

- *Protein compartments:* Body protein is divided between two compartments: (1) tissue protein and (2) plasma protein. Protein from one compartment may be drawn to supply a need in the other. Muscle tissue becomes an important source of amino acids in periods of stress or low-protein intake. Plasma proteins such as prealbumin have rapid turnover and are early indicators of protein catabolism brought on by inflammation, surgery, cancer, or other serious illness. Levels of plasma prealbumin can identify patients at risk of nutritional deficiency or in need of nutrition intervention.[14,15] Low plasma albumin is characteristic of children with kwashiorkor, the protein deficiency disease seen in countries with food shortages.

BOX 5-2   CONDITIONS OF PROTEIN GAIN AND LOSS

Anabolism (net gain in body protein)
- Infant growth
- Muscle building (strength training)
- Pregnancy (building of maternal and fetal tissues)
- Production of milk in lactation
- Rehabilitation of a malnourished patient

Catabolism (net loss in body protein)
- Cancer cachexia
- Sepsis
- Acquired immune-deficiency syndrome (AIDS) wasting
- Pressure ulcers
- Burns or trauma

KEY TERMS

carnitine A naturally occurring amino acid ($C_{17}H_{15}NO_3$) formed from methionine and lysine that transports long-chain fatty acids into the mitochondria where they are oxidized for energy.

taurine A sulfur-containing amino acid, $NH_2(CH_2)_2 \bullet SO_2OH$, formed from the indispensable (essential) amino acid methionine. It is found in lung and muscle tissues and in bile and breast milk.

ascites Accumulation of fluid in the abdomen occurring when blood albumin levels fall below normal and fluid exchange between the cells and the blood is disrupted; may be a complication of liver disease, cancer, or congestive heart failure.

labile Easily changed or modified; unstable.

protein balance The balance between the building up (anabolism) and the breaking down (catabolism) of body tissues as necessary to maintain positive growth and maintenance.

anabolism The building of body tissue.

catabolism The breaking down of body tissue; the opposite of anabolism.

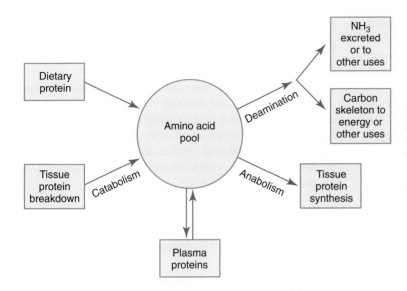

FIGURE 5-7 Flow between protein compartments and the amino acid pool. Amino acids are constantly entering and leaving the body's amino acid pool to form new proteins or other nitrogen-containing compounds, to be converted to carbohydrate and used for energy, or to be converted to fat for storage.

Although albumin is not a specific marker of protein deficiency, it alerts the clinician to the need for comprehensive nutrition assessment.[16] Plasma protein levels are restored to normal when the disease or catabolic stress has abated and protein and kilocalories (kcalories or kcal) become available.[14]

• *Metabolic amino acid pool:* Amino acids derived from tissue breakdown or supplied by dietary protein contribute to a common metabolic "pool." Amino acids from this pool are used to synthesize body proteins as needed. Figure 5-7 summarizes the many aspects of protein metabolism.

Nitrogen Balance

Protein balance is sometimes described as **nitrogen balance**. Nitrogen balance involves all of the nitrogen in the body— protein nitrogen as well as nonprotein nitrogen in such compounds as urea, uric acid, and ammonia. Nitrogen balance is the net result of nitrogen gain and loss across all body tissues. **Negative nitrogen balance** occurs when body nitrogen loss exceeds the nitrogen taken in from food as occurs in long-term illness, hypermetabolic wasting disease, and inadequate protein intake. **Positive nitrogen balance** occurs during growth or pregnancy or strength training as more nitrogen is retained. Healthy persons with an adequate protein intake are in **nitrogen equilibrium** with nitrogen intake and loss about equal on a daily basis.

PROTEIN QUALITY

Evaluating Food Proteins

The nutritional quality of a protein relates to its ability to sustain the growth and repair of body tissues and is based on the following two characteristics[17]:

1. *Protein digestibility:* To be of use to the body, amino acids must be released from other food components and made available for absorption. If nondigestible components in the food prevent this breakdown, then the amino acids are lost in the feces.

2. *Amino acid composition:* All 20 amino acids needed to make body proteins must be available at the same time for new tissues to be formed; therefore food proteins should supply each of the indispensable amino acids in the amount required. Other sources of amino (NH_2) groups in a food protein can be used to synthesize any dispensable amino acids needed.

Comparing Food Proteins

The nutritive value of a food protein is often expressed as its amino acid score, a value based on both its digestibility and amino acid composition. The amino acid reference pattern used to evaluate proteins is quite similar to the pattern of egg white, the reference protein often used in nutrition studies. When evaluating an amino acid score, it is important to identify the **limiting amino acid** (or acids). A limiting amino acid is any indispensable amino acid falling below the amount recommended in the amino acid reference pattern. For protein synthesis to take place, all indispensable amino acids must be available in the required amount. Thus the limiting amino acid "limits" or hinders the body from effectively using the other amino acids in that protein regardless of their adequacy. When one or two limiting amino acids are identified in a food protein having optimal levels of the other indispensable amino acids, that protein can be combined with another food protein that will supply the amino acid or acids needed. A comparison of the amino acid scores and digestibility of various protein foods is found in Table 5-1. In general, proteins from animal sources have higher scores than those from plant sources.

Amino Acid Content of Plant and Animal Foods

Plant and animal foods differ in their content of indispensable amino acids. Animal foods contain all of the indispensable amino acids in the amounts and ratio needed to support protein synthesis and are referred to as **complete proteins**. These foods include eggs, milk, cheese, meat, poultry, and fish (Box 5-3). Plant proteins vary in quality but are **incomplete proteins**; either they supply less than the required amount of one or more indispensable amino acids, or they are missing an indispensable amino acid (Box 5-4). However, several plant proteins eaten together or combined with a small amount of animal protein can supply the amino acids required to support tissue growth and repair.[3,18] This concept of complementary proteins, by which one protein helps meet the amino acid shortage in another, has been at work in the traditional food patterns of families worldwide. See Figure 5-8 for examples of complementary vegetable proteins. Soy protein, although lower in methionine than animal protein, meets the amino acid needs of adults. (See the Focus on Culture box, "Soy: A Protein Source Since Ancient Times," to learn more about soy foods.)

TABLE 5-1	COMPARATIVE QUALITY OF SELECTED FOODS ACCORDING TO AMINO ACID SCORE AND DIGESTIBILITY	
FOOD	**AMINO ACID SCORE**	**DIGESTIBILITY**
Egg	100	100
Cow's milk	95	95
Beef	89	95
Soy flour	47	86
Peanuts	65	94
Polished rice	57	89
Whole wheat	53	87
Sesame seeds	42	90
Peas	37	88

Data from Committee on Amino Acids, Food and Nutrition Board: *Improvement of protein nutriture,* Washington, D.C., 1974, National Academy of Sciences; and Hopkins, DT: Effects of variation in protein digestibility. In Bodwell CE, Adkins JS, Hopkins DT, editors: *Protein quality in humans: assessment and in vitro estimation,* Westport, Conn., 1981, Avi Publishing Company.

PROTEIN REQUIREMENTS

Factors Influencing Protein Requirements

Protein Quality

The quality of dietary protein and its amino acid composition influence the type and amount needed. Individuals who consume some animal protein along with plant protein will have an adequate supply of all amino acids. Those who eat no animal protein should emphasize a wide variety of complementary plant proteins to ensure appropriate amounts of the indispensable amino acids.

Protein Digestibility

Food processing and food preparation affect amino acid availability. Heat applied in drying or baking causes chemical

> **KEY TERMS**
> **nitrogen balance**   The metabolic balance between nitrogen intake from dietary protein and nitrogen losses in urine, feces, sweat, and cells; dietary protein is 16% nitrogen (6.25 g dietary protein contains 1 g of nitrogen).
> **negative nitrogen balance**   The situation when nitrogen intake from dietary protein does not equal nitrogen losses through urine, feces, sweat, and cells lost from the skin and gastrointestinal tract; negative nitrogen balance results in a net loss of nitrogen from the body.
> **positive nitrogen balance**   The situation when nitrogen intake from dietary protein exceeds nitrogen losses through the urine, feces, sweat, and cells lost from the skin or gastrointestinal tract; positive nitrogen balance results in a net increase in body nitrogen.
> **nitrogen equilibrium**   The situation that occurs when nitrogen intake from dietary protein equals total nitrogen losses.
> **limiting amino acid**   The indispensable amino acid present in a food in the lowest amount as compared with the reference amino acid pattern.
> **complete protein**   A protein that contains all indispensable amino acids in the amounts needed according to the reference amino acid pattern.
> **incomplete protein**   A protein with a lower amount of one or more of the indispensable amino acids as compared with the reference amino acid pattern or missing an indispensable amino acid needed to form body proteins.

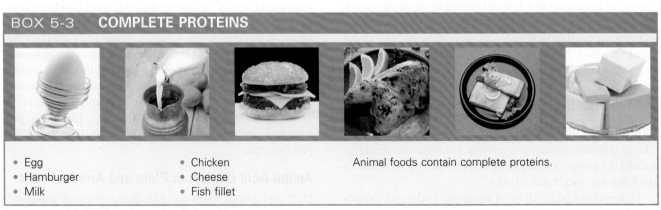

BOX 5-3   COMPLETE PROTEINS

- Egg
- Hamburger
- Milk
- Chicken
- Cheese
- Fish fillet

Animal foods contain complete proteins.

Images copyright 2006 JupiterImages Corporation.

🌐 FOCUS ON CULTURE

Soy: A Protein Source Since Ancient Times

Families throughout Asia have used soybeans for centuries. In China, Japan, Vietnam, Indonesia, the Philippines, Cambodia, and Laos, soybeans in various forms are a dietary staple and a major source of protein. Traditional soy foods such as tofu, tempeh, and soy milk were introduced by newcomers to the United States and have gained broad acceptance. Vegetarians, those who are lactose intolerant, and others looking to expand their food horizons have adopted soy foods. A growing interest in Asian cooking and the increasing popularity of ethnic restaurants have encouraged more people to try these foods.

The most important soy-based protein foods are tofu and tempeh, described as follows:

- *Tofu:* In Chinese, *fu* means "riches," so tofu is usually served at New Year's celebrations to bring good luck. Tofu is made by a process similar to cheese making. A coagulating agent such as calcium sulfate, vinegar, or lemon juice is added to pureed soybeans. After the curd has formed, it is placed in molds to form cakes and the liquid whey is discarded. Tofu made with calcium sulfate has higher calcium content. Some types of tofu look much like farmer cheese, but they are very different in flavor. While most cheeses have strong flavors, tofu is very bland and absorbs flavors from other foods. This makes it an excellent addition to cooked mixed dishes with a variety of seasonings or highly spiced ingredients. Tofu is available in two forms: (1) soft and (2) firm. Soft tofu can be mashed and used in recipes in place of ground beef or ricotta cheese; firm tofu can be grilled or stir-fried. Tofu has a limited shelf life, so consumers should check the expiration date on the package and be sure to keep it refrigerated.
- *Tempeh:* This soy food originated in Indonesia and is a mixture of soy and grain. When fermented, it becomes a firm mass that can be sliced or made into patties. Tempeh has more flavor than tofu and is a rich source of protein.

Soybeans are mixed with other ingredients to make sauces and seasonings used in Asian cooking.

Several of these mixtures are described below:

- *Hoisin sauce:* Used in Chinese cooking, hoisin sauce is a combination of fermented soybeans, water, flour, sugar, and garlic.
- *Miso:* Miso originated in Japan and is a fermented mixture of soybeans and rice or barley. It is a pungent, salty paste used as a seasoning or soup base. Miso is very high in sodium, containing 900 mg of sodium or more per tablespoon.
- *Soy sauce:* This seasoning is a combination of steamed rice, roasted soybeans, and salt that is fermented. Based on its high sodium content, it should be used in moderation.

Tofu and tempeh are available in supermarkets and Asian food stores and add variety and nutrition to the meal pattern. If you have not tasted these foods, look for an Asian cookbook in your local library or ask a classmate to share a family recipe.

Bibliography

Diabetes Care and Education Practice Group of the American Dietetic Association, Goody CM, Drago L, editors: *Cultural food practices*, Chicago, 2010, American Dietetic Association.

Kittler PG, Sucher KP: *Cultural foods: traditions and trends*, Belmont, Calif, 2000, Wadsworth/Thompson Learning.

Margen S, editor: *The wellness encyclopedia of food and nutrition*, New York, 1992, Health Letter Associates.

BOX 5-4 INCOMPLETE PROTEINS

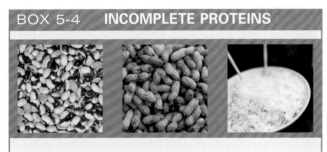

- Soy meat analog
- Beans
- Peanuts
- Rice
- Tofu
- Sesame seeds

Plant foods are incomplete proteins, but two or more can be combined to form a complete protein.

Images copyright 2006 JupiterImages Corporation.

bonding between some sugars and amino acids, forming compounds that cannot be digested. Lysine, methionine, and cysteine can be lost in this way.[19] Protein digestion and amino acid absorption are influenced by the time interval between meals, with longer intervals lowering the competition for available enzymes and absorption sites.

Tissue Growth

Protein requirements reflect the growth patterns of infancy, childhood, and adolescence. Pregnancy and lactation increase protein needs.

Energy Content of the Diet

When carbohydrate intake is sufficient to meet energy needs, dietary protein can be used exclusively for tissue building. This is often referred to as the protein-sparing action of carbohydrate. Dietary carbohydrates also support protein synthesis by stimulating the release of insulin, which promotes the use of amino acids for protein synthesis.

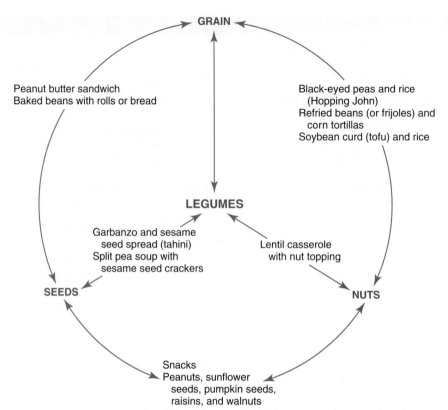

FIGURE 5-8 Complementary vegetable proteins. Examples of common plant foods that when eaten together supply the amounts of essential amino acids required for protein synthesis. (Redrawn from Stanfield PS, Hui YH: *Nutrition and diet therapy: self-instructional modules,* ed 4, Sudbury, Mass., 2003, Jones & Bartlett, with permission.)

Health Status

Conditions and diseases that increase the rate of protein turnover and tissue breakdown raise the protein requirement. After trauma or surgery, amino acids are needed for wound healing and formation of new tissue, as well as the production of infection-fighting immune factors. Serious burns with extensive tissue destruction substantially increase protein needs. In critically ill patients protein requirements may reach 1.5 to 2.0 g/kg of body weight or 2 to 2½ times the usual recommendation.[20-22] Amino acid supplementation helps limit the loss of muscle protein that occurs with immobilization.[23]

Muscle protein synthesis is influenced not only by the amount of protein available but also by the time frame in which the protein is consumed. Individuals undergoing resistance training can benefit from eating some high-quality protein during or immediately following the activity.[24,25]

Dietary Reference Intakes
Protein

The Recommended Dietary Allowance (RDA) for protein is 0.8 g/kg body weight or 56 g/day for men and 46 g/day for women.[3] This intake should maintain body tissues and replace daily nitrogen losses via the urine, feces, and sweat. An additional 25 g/day is needed for pregnancy and lactation. Protein requirements of infants and children vary according to age and stage of growth.

A Tolerable Upper Intake Level (UL) has not been established for protein; however, the safety of protein intakes well in excess of the RDA is a concern. Protein waste products are excreted via the urine, and high protein intakes lead to dehydration if fluid intake is not adjusted accordingly. It is recommended that protein intake, under normal conditions, not exceed two times the RDA.[3]

Amino Acids

Individuals meeting the RDA who eat both animal and plant proteins will have an adequate supply of the indispensable amino acids. If no animal foods are consumed, then an intake of mixed plant proteins obtained from legumes (including soy), grains, nuts, seeds, and vegetables can supply amino acids in the pattern needed, although it is important to select a wide variety of plant proteins.[18] The specific amino acid requirements of particular age groups are described in Ref. 3, accessible on the website of the National Academy of Sciences (see the Evolve website accompanying this text).

ULs have not been set for individual amino acids because imbalances and toxicity are not usually a hazard when amino acids are supplied in food. However, supplements that exaggerate the intake of one or more amino acids interfere with protein synthesis and can lead to toxicity.[3] Leucine has become popular among both amateur and professional athletes based on its ability to promote protein synthesis, and at high levels presents a risk to health.[26] Methionine, cysteine, and histidine supplements have adverse effects if taken over long periods.[27]

Acceptable Macronutrient Distribution Range

The Acceptable Macronutrient Distribution Range (AMDR) for protein is 10% to 35% of total kcalories.[3] Protein needs are generally met if protein makes up 10% of energy intake; however, if total energy intake is low, then it may be necessary to obtain more kcalories from protein to meet the RDA. The suggested kcalorie range for protein provides flexibility with the suggested proportions of fat and carbohydrate to achieve a healthy diet pattern. Diets ranging from 15% to 27% protein that emphasized healthy fats, vegetables, moderate amounts of fruits and grains, and limited sweets had a positive effect, lowering risk factors for coronary heart disease.[28]

PROTEIN INTAKE

Protein-Energy Malnutrition

Protein intake differs widely across population groups, with some getting far more and others far less than they need. Protein-energy malnutrition (PEM) is a major health problem in many developing countries where protein intakes are low in both quantity and quality. More than 6 million children die each year from protein-related deficiencies.[3] PEM also contributes to the morbidity and mortality associated with infectious diseases such as malaria, respiratory tract infections, and gastroenteritis. Based on more than 13,000 hospital admissions over a period of 5 years in rural Africa, malnutrition was estimated to be the underlying cause of half of the inpatient illness and deaths of young children.[29]

Two forms of extreme malnutrition occurring across all age groups when food supplies are insufficient are kwashiorkor and marasmus (Figure 5-9). Marasmus represents extreme starvation with deficits of energy, protein, and micronutrients. These patients have little or no body fat and exhibit extreme wasting. Rehabilitation must be implemented on a gradual basis to avoid refeeding syndrome, with severe complications or death. Kwashiorkor occurs in children and adults when diets are deficient in protein and likely limiting in energy and micronutrients as well. The word *kwashiorkor* comes from a Ghanaian word meaning "illness striking a child when the second child is born," as it frequently befell a child when a new baby replaced him at the breast, and weaning foods were inadequate to meet his nutritional needs. This form of PEM results in a characteristic edema, hypoalbuminemia, skin lesions, and fatty liver. The primary cause of PEM is most often a lack of food supplying appropriate levels of nutrients; however, impaired digestion or absorption, infection, chronic or acute vomiting, or diarrhea are secondary causes or contributors to this condition.

Amounts and Types of Protein

Plant researchers are working to improve the amino acid patterns of grains such as rice[30] and maize[31] that are dietary staples for millions of people around the world who take in

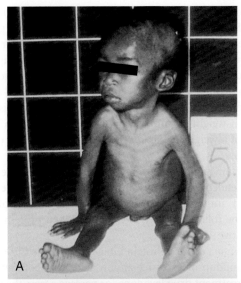

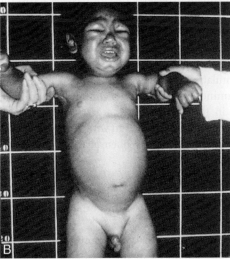

FIGURE 5-9 Protein-energy malnutrition (PEM). **A,** Marasmus results from starvation, a diet lacking in both kcalories and protein. **B,** Kwashiorkor results from a diet that may be sufficient in kcalories but is deficient in protein. Note the abdominal bloating typical of kwashiorkor. (From Thibodeau GA, Patton KT: *The human body in health & disease,* ed 5, St Louis, Mo., 2010, Mosby.)

little or no animal protein. At the other extreme, most people in the United States meet or exceed their RDA for protein, with much coming from animal sources.[32] Average protein intakes of adults are more than 1 and ½ times their Dietary Reference Intake (DRI).[33,34] Protein intakes are also high among U.S. children. One half of the fast-food meals marketed to children contain 16 g or more of protein; this equals 123% of the daily protein allowance for 3-year-olds and 84% of the day's needs for those ages 4 to 8.[35]

Clinical Applications: Protein Intake
Low-Protein Diets

We often associate low-protein diets with the severe PEM evident in famine-ravaged countries; however, degrees of malnutrition exist in all areas of the world, including the United States. Children with chronic PEM have poor growth (low weight for height) and stunting (low height for age).[3] When protein status is marginal immune function is impaired, contributing to the chronic respiratory infections and diarrhea that trouble many poorly nourished children and adults. Low protein intake during pregnancy increases the risk of a low-birth-weight infant. Inappropriately low protein intake as part of a weight reduction regimen, promotes loss of lean body mass.

In certain clinical situations, however, protein intake below recommended levels is warranted. In that case it becomes especially important to choose protein high in biological value. The following serve as examples when protein intake may be low:

- *Parkinson's disease:* Protein intake is controlled to prevent the buildup of excessive amino acids that compete with the treatment drug levodopa for passage across the blood-brain barrier.[6]
- *Phenylketonuria (PKU):* Individuals with this inborn error of metabolism lack the enzyme required to metabolize the indispensable amino acid phenylalanine, and accumulation of inappropriately high blood levels of this amino acid results in mental retardation. All infants born in the United States are tested for PKU at birth, and immediate intervention with a protein-restricted diet limiting the intake of phenylalanine prevents harmful changes.
- *Chronic kidney disease (CKD):* When kidney function declines, protein intake is reduced to minimize the burden of excreting urea and other nitrogen-containing waste.[36]
- *Vegan diets:* Individuals who consume no animal foods and must obtain all of their protein from plant sources may have marginal protein intakes based on the added bulk of plant protein foods. Protein may provide only 10% of total kcalories, the minimum AMDR.[3,18]

High-Protein Diets

High-protein diets moved into the spotlight when media attention focused on weight-loss regimens that restricted carbohydrate in preference to protein and fat. Protein intakes up to 25% or more of total kcalories (about 1.2 g protein/kg) support weight loss and effective energy regulation.[37-39] A major benefit of a weight-loss diet high in protein is its positive effect on satiety, which continues even as energy intake declines, and promotes adherence to the dietary regimen.[39] Protein also increases energy expenditure as compared with carbohydrate and fat, based on the extra kcalories needed to remove the amino group from amino acids and enable their use as a fuel.[39] Liberal protein intakes protect muscle mass during long-term weight reduction and help prevent sarcopenia, the age-related loss of muscle that contributes to frailty.[40] Retention of muscle mass promotes weight management as these tissues add to basal energy needs and contribute to the overall energy requirement.[39] Nevertheless, a reduction in kcalorie intake and/or increase in energy expenditure are still key to weight loss, regardless of the proportion of specific macronutrients. Personal preferences, cultural food patterns, and metabolic considerations should form the basis for individual interventions, while keeping protein intake within the AMDR upper limit of 35%.

Although high-protein diets have some advantages, their long-term effects on calcium balance[3,41] and renal function[42,43] remain under discussion. High intakes of protein, particularly animal protein, can increase urinary calcium; however, protein also stimulates the release of stomach acid and promotes calcium absorption.[3] Attention to water needs should be a part of a dietary protein prescription.[44]

HEALTH PROMOTION

Health Benefits of Plant Proteins

Soy foods and other legumes supply good-quality protein along with an array of important nutrients and phytochemicals with roles in preventing chronic disease.[18,45-48] Soy foods contain phytochemicals thought to have estrogen-like activity that may help prevent bone loss in older women.[46] Higher intakes of flavonoids, a class of phytochemicals found in soy, peanuts, and many fruits and vegetables, were associated with lower risk of stroke and mortality in older adults followed for 7 years.[47] Persons eating legumes at least four times a week had a lower risk of cardiovascular disease than those eating these foods less than once a week,[49] and regular use of legumes improved glucose control among patients with type 2 diabetes.[50] Vegetable protein foods also contain healthy fats. One cup of tofu or soybean curd supplies nearly 25%, and one cup of chickpeas supplies 12% of the RDA for linoleic acid in men.[3,51] Tree nuts and peanuts, often considered snack items rather than alternate sources of protein, are rich in antioxidants, trace minerals, and essential fatty acids,[52] and add rich protein to sandwiches and stews. Beans and nuts are important foods in the Mediterranean diet and likely contribute to the healthful benefits attributed to that diet.[53] (See the Evidence-Based Practice box, "Effect of Soy on Cardiovascular Risk," to learn more about these relationships.)

Nutritional Contributions of Animal Proteins

Proteins from animal sources—meat, fish, poultry, eggs, and milk—provide all of the indispensable amino acids in the appropriate amounts. Used alone or in combination with vegetable proteins, animal proteins meet the amino acid needs of children and adults. Animal foods supply trace minerals such as iron and zinc that are difficult to obtain in sufficient amounts from plant foods based on their lower content and interfering substances. Dairy foods are rich in calcium and riboflavin and provide preformed vitamin A. Vitamin B_{12} and vitamin D occur naturally in animal foods only.[54]

VEGETARIAN DIETS

Vegetarian diets existed in ancient times as described in early Greek culture. People choose to follow a plant-based diet and

EVIDENCE-BASED PRACTICE

Effect of Soy on Cardiovascular Risk

Identify the Problem: Soy has received increasing attention not only as a high-quality plant protein but also for its perceived properties in reducing cardiovascular risk. In 1999 the U.S. Food and Drug Administration (FDA) approved the addition of a health claim to the nutrition label of foods that contain soy, indicating that soy was protective against heart disease. This was followed in 2000 by an advisory from the American Heart Association recommending the use of soy protein with a diet low in saturated fat and cholesterol. Based on evidence available at the time, soy foods were believed to exert positive effects on low-density lipoprotein (LDL) cholesterol, high-density lipoprotein (HDL) cholesterol, serum triglycerides, and blood pressure.

Review the Evidence: Since then, researchers have continued to evaluate the impact of soy protein and its phytochemical content on cardiovascular risk. Emerging evidence has led to some debate regarding the effect of soy on various risk factors as described below:

Blood lipoproteins: Critical evaluation of new evidence by the American Heart Association[1] and the Academy of Nutrition and Dietetics (formerly the American Dietetic Association)[2] concluded that soy has no major effect on blood LDL cholesterol in individuals with normal levels. In those with elevated levels, one serving or more of soy protein each day brought about a decrease of 4.0% to 5.5% in blood LDL cholesterol and an increase of about 3% in blood HDL cholesterol.[3]

Blood pressure levels: Increased intakes of vegetable protein including soy protein are associated with lower blood pressures; however, this effect may result from the fiber or other nutrient(s) contained in these foods. The 2010 Advisory Committee on the Dietary Guidelines for Americans concluded that soy protein does not offer any special protection against high blood pressure.[4]

Implement the Findings: So are soy products good foods? Soy is not only a high-quality protein but also a rich source of vitamins, minerals, phytochemicals, antioxidants, and polyunsaturated fats. Replacing animal foods containing saturated fat and cholesterol with soy on an occasional basis provides a healthy balance of vegetable and animal proteins that supports overall health and well-being. Based on the positive health effects of vegetable proteins, nonvegetarians will benefit from meatless meals once or twice a week; however, soy protein in itself is not likely to bring about a significant improvement in blood lipid levels or blood pressure.

This example of new findings regarding soy that call into question previous conclusions about its effect on health reinforces the need for continuous review of the literature in our professional practice. New research alerts us to new roles of particular foods and provides us with more realistic appraisal of their benefit.

References

1. Sacks FM, Lichtenstein A, Van Horn L, et al: Soy protein, isoflavones, and cardiovascular health. An American Heart Association Science Advisory for Professionals from the Nutrition Committee. *Circulation* 113:1034, 2006.
2. Van Horn L, McCoin M, Kris-Etherton PM, et al: The evidence for dietary prevention and treatment of cardiovascular disease. *J Am Diet Assoc* 108:287, 2008.
3. Anderson JW, Bush HM: Soy protein effects on serum lipoproteins: a quality assessment and meta-analysis of randomized, controlled studies. *J Am Coll Nutr* 30(2):79, 2011.
4. U.S. Department of Health and Human Services, U.S. Department of Agriculture: *Report of the Dietary Guidelines Advisory Committee on the Dietary Guidelines for Americans 2010*, Washington, D.C., 2010, Center for Nutrition Policy and Promotion, U.S. Department of Agriculture. from: <http://www.cnpp.usda.gov/DGAs2010-DGACReport.htm>. Retrieved July 17, 2013.

limit or exclude animal foods for many reasons. Several major world religions including Hinduism and Buddhism advocate avoidance of meat for the preservation of animal life. Ethical considerations were the overwhelming motive for selecting a vegetarian or vegan food pattern, followed by concerns for health, among an urban and university group.[55] Sustainability of the food supply and protection of the environment are growing issues in many parts of the world. From the environmental perspective, production of animal protein requires more than 3 times the water, 13 times the fertilizer, and about 1.5 times more pesticides than production of plant protein. The greatest contributor to this need for resources is beef.[56] Land requirements for producing meat protein are about 10 times greater than for producing plant protein.[57] These reports have led some individuals to adopt a plant-based diet to assist in reducing food shortages throughout the world.

Although diet patterns that emphasize plant foods are generally referred to as *vegetarian diets*, they are exceedingly difficult to quantify. Vegetarian diets differ greatly according to the types of animal foods they include or exclude, as follows:

- Ovo-lacto-vegetarian (includes all plant foods, dairy, and eggs)
- Lactovegetarian (includes all plant foods and dairy)
- Pescovegetarians (includes all plant foods, dairy, eggs, and fish)[58]
- Vegan (includes plant foods only)
- Semi-vegetarian (includes predominantly plant foods with eggs, dairy, and fish or chicken on occasion)[55]

About 5 million people, or 2.3% of the population in the United States, describe themselves as vegetarians who never eat meat, fish, or poultry; 1.4% are vegans.[18] Restaurants have responded to new interest in vegetarian diets, with 71% of chefs noting that vegetarian dishes are "perennial favorites." Most fast-food restaurants offer a soy burger or meatless option. The U.S. market for vegetarian foods including meat analogs made with soy, fortified nondairy milk, and vegetarian entrees has grown to over $1.2 billion in annual sales.[18] The availability of these foods in the marketplace assists vegetarians in meal planning and obtaining required nutrients.

Nutritional Implications of Vegetarian Diets

Vegetarian diets, including vegan diets, will support growth and well-being across the life cycle *if* they are well planned. Conversely, vegetarian and vegan diets, as well as diets that include all types of animal foods, will be inadequate if items high in fat and sugar and low in important nutrients are emphasized. In general, the more restrictive the diet, the more planning is required to avoid nutrient deficiencies.

For vegetarians who include eggs or vitamin D–fortified dairy foods in their meal patterns, protein, vitamin D, and vitamin B_{12} are in good supply. Vegans need to include a wide variety of legumes, nuts, and grains to obtain sufficient amounts of indispensable amino acids and must seek out fortified foods to obtain vitamin D and vitamin B_{12}. Soy milk, rice milk, and orange juice are often fortified with vitamin D and calcium to the amounts found in cow's milk, and may have added vitamin B_{12}. Fortified breakfast cereals and vegetarian support formula yeast are other sources of vitamin B_{12} as are certain meat analogs made with soy protein. Vegetarians must read labels carefully to determine sources of important nutrients. Vegans are at risk for inadequate intakes of vitamin D and vitamin B_{12}, and supplements may be necessary.[59-61]

Long-chain n-3 fatty acids can be limited in vegetarian or vegan meal patterns that do not include fish. Eggs contain small amounts of n-3 fatty acids as do flaxseed, canola, and soybean oils.[61] Nuts, especially walnuts, are good sources of α-linolenic acid, the precursor for docosahexaenoic acid (DHA) and eicosapentaenoic acid (EPA), but as noted in Chapter 4, conversion to DHA and EPA is very slow.[18,59] DHA supplements are well absorbed and provide an alternative to fish.[59,62]

Minerals require special attention in the vegetarian or vegan diet.[61] Calcium intakes of lactovegetarians are similar to or even higher than nonvegetarians; however, calcium intakes of vegans fall below both groups.[59] Calcium is well absorbed from broccoli, Chinese cabbage, collards, and bok choy (all vegetables low in oxalate).[63] Spinach and Swiss chard, however, are poor sources of calcium based on their oxalate content, which interferes with calcium absorption. Fortified soy milk, rice milk, fruit juices, and breakfast cereals supply calcium.

Iron and zinc are found naturally in many plant foods; however, phytates interfere with their absorption. Including a vitamin C source at the same meal facilitates iron absorption, and soaking beans before cooking makes the iron more available. Fortified grains and cereals add iron in a form that can be absorbed. Despite lower intakes, iron deficiency anemia is no more prevalent among vegetarians than nonvegetarians, suggesting that vegetarians may compensate with a higher percentage of absorption.[18] Based on their plentiful intakes of legumes, nuts, and unrefined grains, vegans

are likely to reach their DRI for zinc, although absorption of that nutrient also may be impaired by phytates and fiber. Soaking beans, grains, and seeds, and the leavening action in bread improve the availability of zinc.[59] Fruits and vegetables provide many sources of vitamin A and the carotenoids, vitamin K, the B complex vitamins (with the exception of vitamin B_{12}), and potassium.

Generally, plant-based diets contain more fiber, antioxidants, carotenoids, and phytochemicals, and less saturated fat than the average diet, depending on the animal foods included.[18] Vegetarians eat more fruits and dark green vegetables than nonvegetarians and twice the whole grains and legumes.[64]

Planning Vegetarian Diets

Vegetarian diets are planned as any diet is planned, to include needed amounts of essential nutrients and sufficient kcalories for energy. The U.S. Department of Agriculture has developed guidelines listing the food groups and amounts needed to supply the essential nutrients in a nonvegetarian food pattern, a lacto-ovo-vegetarian food pattern, and a vegan food pattern at an energy level of 2000 kcal.[60a] Note that all protein comes from vegetable sources in the vegan food plan with eggs and milk contributing protein in the lacto-ovo-vegetarian plan. A vegetarian food guide from the Academy of Nutrition and Dietetics (formerly the American Dietetic Association) offers guidance and alternative food sources of important nutrients to assist in planning nutritionally sound plant-based diets (Figure 5-10).[61] Portion sizes of equivalent protein foods are described in Box 5-5.

Individuals accustomed to food patterns that include meat may find it difficult to adopt new meal patterns, even if motivated by health or environmental concerns.[65] This hesitation

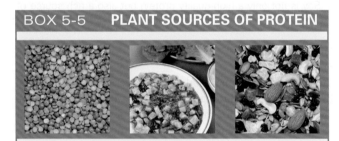

BOX 5-5   PLANT SOURCES OF PROTEIN

Each of the following servings provides at least 4 to 6 g of protein: A plant protein can be combined with a small amount of animal protein to form a complete protein or two or more different plant proteins can be combined to form a complete protein (see Figure 5-8).

- Cooked beans, peas, or lentils: $\frac{1}{2}$ cup
- Tofu or tempeh: $\frac{1}{2}$ cup
- Nut butter: 2 tbsp
- Nuts: $\frac{1}{4}$ cup
- Tahini (sesame seed butter): 2 tbsp
- Meat (soy) analog: 1 oz

Data from Messina V, Melina V, Mangels AR: A new food guide for North American vegetarians. *J Am Diet Assoc* 103:771, 2003. Images copyright 2006 JupiterImages Corporation.

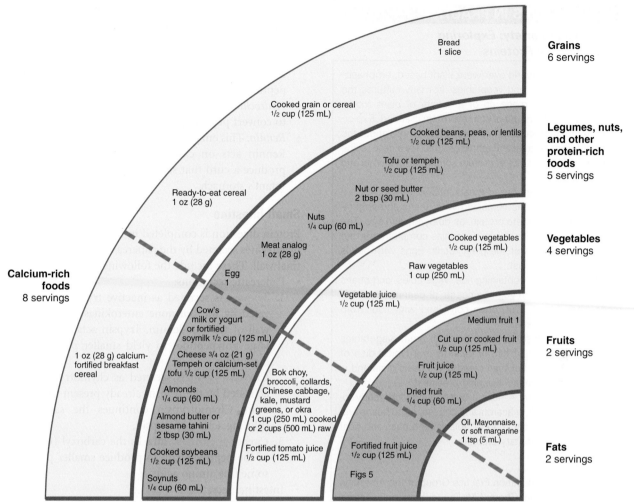

FIGURE 5-10 Vegetarian food guide rainbow. Notice the slice of the rainbow calling attention to the foods in each group that are good sources of calcium. (Redrawn from Messina V, Melina V, Mangels AR: A new food guide for North American vegetarians. *J Am Diet Assoc* 103:771, 2003; reprinted with permission from the Academy of Nutrition and Dietetics, formerly the American Dietetic Association.)

may relate to the familiar meal triangle including a meat, a starch, and a vegetable, and the need to find a substitute for the meat, fish, or poultry. This perception was evaluated by asking people if they preferred meals that combined ingredients, such as pasta with added ground meat, or meals with separate components such as a chicken leg, baked potato, and vegetable. Responses differed by age—older individuals much preferred the food items arranged separately, whereas younger people were more receptive to mixed dishes.[65] Vegetarian food plans are often based on mixtures that combine beans and nuts to achieve a full set of indispensable amino acids. The 7-day sample menu cycle found on the MyPlate website (www.choosemyplate.gov) includes several vegetarian meals and substitution of soy milk or other soy products could adapt other menus to the vegan lifestyle.

Use of complementary proteins to obtain sufficient amounts of the indispensable amino acids is especially important when planning a vegan diet. Review Figure 5-8 and see the Perspectives in Practice box, "Increase Your Variety: Exploring Complementary Proteins," to consider food combinations for the daily plan.

Vegetarian Diets and Chronic Disease

Vegetarian diets represent a wide diversity of dietary practices and are often described by what is omitted rather than by what is included.[59] When a vegetarian diet is well planned, it promotes health and lowers the risk of chronic disease. Vegetarians in comparison to nonvegetarians tend to have diets lower in saturated fat, and higher in fiber, fruits and vegetables, whole grains, and phytochemicals, all of which are associated with the prevention of cardiovascular disease and cancer.[59] Blood levels of LDL cholesterol are lower,[18] HDL cholesterol levels are higher,[66] and body weights are lower[66] among vegetarians as compared with semi-vegetarians or nonvegetarians, and may help explain their resistance to heart disease[18] and metabolic syndrome.[66]

PERSPECTIVES IN PRACTICE

Increase Your Variety: Exploring Complementary Proteins

Traditional diets the world over were plant based, emphasizing cereals, legumes, and vegetables. In many cultures the main dish is a stew made up of a variety of plant foods; sometimes a small amount of animal protein is added. Exploring complementary proteins is a way to learn more about the foods of different cultural and ethnic groups. Try a new recipe and calculate the amounts of protein coming from animal and vegetable sources.

Some traditional plant-based meals follow:

- *Mexican:* Corn tortillas combined with beans and vegetables provide a complete protein, as do beans and rice. The addition of cheese to stews or tortillas complements the incomplete proteins of the grain foods. Eggs with beans are a favorite breakfast.
- *East Indian:* A stew containing rice, vegetables, and beans might be served with yogurt, cheese, or peanuts. Bread is made from wheat flour, often combined with flour from ground peas or beans.
- *Hmong (Vietnamese):* Rice mixed with green vegetables and small amounts of fish or peanuts is a typical dish of this region. Rice rather than bread is the basic grain and is included in every meal, including breakfast.
- *Traditional American:* A peanut butter sandwich, ready-to-eat cereal with milk, macaroni and cheese, pinto beans and corn bread, and "hoppin John" (black-eyed peas and rice) illustrate complementary proteins.

Bibliography

Diabetes Care and Education Practice Group of the American Dietetic Association, Goody CM, Drago L, editors: *Cultural food practices*, Chicago, 2010, American Dietetic Association.

Kittler PG, Sucher KP: *Cultural foods: traditions and trends*, Belmont, Calif, 2000, Wadsworth/Thompson Learning.

DIGESTION-ABSORPTION-METABOLISM REVIEW

Food proteins must be broken down into their building units—the amino acids—to meet body needs. A brief review of this process is outlined in the following section. (See Chapter 2 for a detailed discussion of digestion, absorption, and metabolism.)

Digestion
Mouth

The only digestive action on proteins in the mouth is the mechanical effect of chewing, breaking food into smaller particles for passage into the stomach.

Stomach

The enzymatic breakdown of protein begins in the stomach. Three chemical agents in the gastric secretions initiate this process: (1) **pepsin**, (2) hydrochloric acid, and (3) rennin.

- *Pepsin:* Pepsin is released by the chief cells in the stomach wall as the inactive **proenzyme** pepsinogen and requires hydrochloric acid to be transformed into the active enzyme pepsin. Pepsin splits the peptide linkages between amino acids, breaking large polypeptides into successively smaller peptides.
- *Hydrochloric acid:* This provides the acid medium needed to convert pepsinogen to pepsin.
- *Rennin:* This enzyme exists only in infancy and childhood. Rennin acts on casein, the major protein in milk, to produce a curd that slows the passage of food out of the infant's stomach.

Small Intestine

Protein digestion is completed in the small intestine assisted by enzymes secreted by the pancreas and glands in the intestinal wall. These include the following:
- Pancreatic secretions:
  1. **Trypsin** is secreted as inactive trypsinogen and activated by the hormone enterokinase produced in the wall of the duodenum. Trypsin acts on proteins and large polypeptides to yield smaller polypeptides and dipeptides.
  2. **Chymotrypsin** is secreted as chymotrypsinogen and activated by the trypsin already present in the duodenum. Chymotrypsin continues the same protein-splitting action of trypsin.
  3. **Carboxypeptidase** attacks the carboxyl (COOH) end of the peptide chain to produce smaller peptides and some free amino acids.
- Intestinal secretions:
  1. **Aminopeptidase** releases amino acids one at a time from the amino (NH_2) end of the peptide chain to produce smaller short-chain peptides and free amino acids.

KEY TERMS

pepsin   A gastric enzyme that breaks large protein molecules into shorter-chain polypeptides; gastric hydrochloric acid is required to activate pepsin.

proenzyme   An inactive precursor converted to the active enzyme by the action of an acid or other enzyme.

trypsin   A pancreatic enzyme secreted into the small intestine that acts on proteins and polypeptides to yield smaller peptides and dipeptides.

chymotrypsin   A pancreatic enzyme secreted into the small intestine that breaks peptide linkages forming smaller polypeptides and dipeptides.

carboxypeptidase   A protein-splitting enzyme secreted by the pancreas into the small intestine that splits the peptide bond at the carboxyl (COOH) end of the chain, producing smaller peptide chains and free amino acids.

aminopeptidase   A protein-splitting enzyme secreted by the intestinal mucosa that releases amino acids one at a time from the amino (NH_2) end of the peptide chain to produce smaller short-chain peptides and free amino acids.

2. **Dipeptidase** breaks any remaining dipeptides into two free amino acids.

   A summary of the steps in protein digestion can be reviewed in Table 2-2.

Absorption

Amino acids are absorbed by an energy-requiring, sodium-assisted transport system and enter the portal blood for passage to the liver. A few short-chain peptides and smaller intact proteins escape digestion and are absorbed in that form. Most are broken down as they cross the intestinal wall; however, those protein molecules that pass into the blood intact may play a part in the development of immunity and protein sensitivity. We know that antibodies in the mother's colostrum, the first milk secreted after birth, are passed on to her nursing infant. Inadvertent absorption of intact proteins has been implicated in the development of some food allergies.[73]

Metabolism

The construction sites for building tissue proteins are in the cells. Each cell, depending on its nature and function, requires a unique mix of amino acids to build the specific proteins needed. The metabolic activities of protein are interwoven with those of carbohydrate and fat, which provide the energy to drive ongoing tissue growth and repair.

> **KEY TERM**
>
> **dipeptidase** Final enzyme in the protein-splitting series that cleaves dipeptides to yield two free amino acids.

TO SUM UP

The primary function of dietary protein and its constituent amino acids is to build and repair body tissues and form the regulatory proteins that direct important metabolic tasks. Of the 20 amino acids used to build proteins, 9 cannot be synthesized by the body and are referred to as *indispensable* or *essential amino acids;* another 6 cannot be synthesized in adequate amounts under conditions of stress or accelerated growth and are considered *conditionally indispensable.* The remaining five amino acids can be synthesized by the body and are termed the *dispensable* or *nonessential amino acids.* Both indispensable and conditionally indispensable amino acids must be supplied in the diet. Animal proteins are considered complete proteins because they contain all the indispensable amino acids in the amounts and ratios needed for protein synthesis. Plant proteins or incomplete proteins are missing one or more indispensable amino acids or contain less than the amounts needed to make new proteins. Plant proteins can be mixed with animal proteins or with each other to provide the necessary proportions of all amino acids for body growth and maintenance. Certain amino acids such as leucine and glutamate have therapeutic application in meeting the escalated needs of patients in critical care. Protein requirements are influenced by growth, food protein quality, health status, and the availability of carbohydrate as an energy source. In many countries protein shortages lead to malnutrition with body wasting, stunted growth, chronic infection, and disease. In the United States, overconsumption rather than underconsumption of protein is becoming a problem. Vegetarian food plans emphasizing plant proteins can meet nutrient needs at all stages of the life cycle if well planned. Vegan food plans excluding all animal foods require supplementation or foods fortified with vitamin D and vitamin B_{12} to meet nutritional needs. Well-planned vegetarian diets are appropriate interventions for the treatment of both type 2 diabetes and obesity.

QUESTIONS FOR REVIEW

1. What is the difference between an indispensable, a dispensable, and a conditionally indispensable amino acid? Indicate appropriate food sources of each.
2. What is meant by protein turnover, and how does it relate to nitrogen balance?
3. Distinguish between protein anabolism and protein catabolism. Describe a clinical situation in which protein anabolism exceeds protein catabolism and one in which the opposite is true.
4. Explain the term *protein-sparing effect.* What happens to protein requirements in poorly planned weight-loss diets that are inappropriately low in carbohydrate?
5. Describe the factors that influence dietary protein needs.
6. A pediatrician told a vegan couple that their 2-year-old daughter was falling behind in her growth rate. What dietary factors are likely related to her poor growth? Using the various tools for developing vegetarian food plans presented in this chapter, plan 1 day of meals for this child, indicating food amounts that would meet her protein and energy needs and respect the vegan food pattern. (Protein and energy needs according to age and gender can be found at MyPlate [ChooseMyPlate.gov] accessible at http://www.choosemyplate.gov or on the front inside cover of your textbook.)
7. Protein intakes two to three times the RDA are not uncommon in the United States. Using the food values found on

the Evolve website that accompanies your textbook, calculate the energy value and the number of grams of protein in a fast-food meal that includes one double-patty cheeseburger, a large serving of French fries, and a 12-oz milkshake. Compare the total grams of protein and the total

kcalories with the protein and energy DRIs for a 16-year-old boy. What proportion of his daily protein and energy needs are provided in this meal?

8. How does poor gastric acid secretion influence protein nutrition?

REFERENCES

1. Matthews DE: Proteins and amino acids. In Shils ME, Olsen JA, Shike M, editors: *Modern nutrition in health and disease*, ed 10, Baltimore, Md., 2006, Lippincott Williams & Wilkins.
2. Gropper SS, Smith JL, Groff JL: *Advanced nutrition and human metabolism*, ed 5, Belmont, Calif., 2008, Cengage Learning.
3. Institute of Medicine: *Dietary Reference Intakes for energy, carbohydrate, fiber, fat, fatty acids, cholesterol, protein, and amino acids (macronutrients)*, Washington, D.C., 2002, National Academies Press.
4. Guyton AC, Hall JE: *Textbook of medical physiology*, ed 10, Philadelphia, Pa., 2000, Saunders.
5. Pencharz PR, Young VR: Protein and amino acids. In Bowman BA, Russell RM, editors: *Present knowledge in nutrition*, ed 9, Washington, D.C., 2006, International Life Sciences Institute.
6. Timiras PS: *Physiological basis of aging and geriatrics*, ed 4, New York, 2007, Taylor & Francis.
7. Jonker R, Engelen MPK, Deutz NEP: Role of specific dietary amino acids in clinical conditions. *Br J Nutr* 108(Suppl 2):S139, 2012.
8. Bozzetti F, Bozzetti V: Is the intravenous supplementation of amino acid to cancer patients adequate: a critical appraisal of literature. *Clin Nutr* 32(1):142, 2013.
9. Reference deleted in proofs.
10. Reference deleted in proofs.
11. Williams MH: Sports nutrition. In Shils ME, Olsen JA, Shike M, editors: *Modern nutrition in health and disease*, ed 10, Baltimore, Md., 2006, Lippincott Williams & Wilkins.
12. Bender DA: The metabolism of "surplus" amino acids. *Br J Nutr* 108(Suppl 2):S113, 2012.
13. Wolfe RR: The underappreciated role of muscle in health and disease. *Am J Clin Nutr* 84:475, 2006.
14. Fuhrman MP, Charney P, Mueller CM: Hepatic proteins and nutrition assessment. *J Am Diet Assoc* 104:1258, 2004.
15. Rambod M, Kovesdy CP, Bross R, et al: Association of serum prealbumin and its changes over time with clinical outcomes and survival in patients receiving hemodialysis. *Am J Clin Nutr* 88:1485, 2008.
16. Hoffer LJ: Metabolic consequences of starvation. In Shils ME, Olsen JA, Shike M, editors: *Modern nutrition in health and disease*, ed 10, Baltimore, Md., 2006, Lippincott Williams & Wilkins.
17. Millward DJ, Layman DK, Tomé D, et al: Protein quality assessment: impact of expanding understanding of protein and amino acids for optimal health. *Am J Clin Nutr* 87(Suppl):1576S, 2008.
18. American Dietetic Association: Position of the American Dietetic Association: vegetarian diets. *J Am Diet Assoc* 109:1266, 2009.
19. Rutherfurd SM, Moughan PJ: Available versus digestible dietary amino acids. *Br J Nutr* 108(Suppl 2):S298, 2012.
20. Jeejeebhoy KN: Parenteral nutrition in the intensive care unit. *Nutr Reviews* 70(11):623, 2012.
21. Genton L, Pichard C: Protein catabolism and requirements in severe illness. *Int J Vitam Nutr Res* 81(2–3):143, 2011.
22. McClave SA, Martindale RG, Vanek VW, et al: Guidelines for the provision and assessment of nutrition support therapy in the adult critically ill patient: Society of Critical Care Medicine (SCCM) and the American Society for Parenteral and Enteral Nutrition (ASPEN). *J Parenter Enteral Nutr* 33:277, 2009.
23. Ferrando AA, Paddon-Jones D, Hayes NP, et al: EAA supplementation to increase nitrogen intake improves muscle function during bed rest in the elderly. *Clin Nutr* 29:18, 2010.
24. Beelen M, Koopman R, Gijsen AP, et al: Protein coingestion stimulates muscle protein synthesis during resistance-type exercise. *Am J Physiol Endocrinol Metab* 295:E70, 2008.
25. Brooks N, Cloutier GJ, Cadena SM, et al: Resistance training and timed essential amino acids protect against the loss of muscle mass and strength during 28 days of bed rest and energy deficit. *J Appl Physiol* 105:241, 2008.
26. Pencharz PB, Elango R, Ball RO: Determination of the tolerable upper intake level of leucine in adult men. *J Nutr* 142:2220S, 2012.
27. Garlick PJ: The nature of human hazards associated with excessive intake of amino acids. *J Nutr* 134:1633S, 2004.
28. Swain JF, McCarron PB, Hamilton EF, et al: Characteristics of the diet patterns tested in the optimal macronutrient intake trial to prevent heart disease (OmniHeart): options for a heart-healthy diet. *J Am Diet Assoc* 108:257, 2008.
29. Bejon P, Mohammed S, Mwangi I, et al: Fraction of all hospital admissions and deaths attributable to malnutrition among children in rural Kenya. *Am J Clin Nutr* 88:1626, 2008.
30. Potrykus I: Nutritionally enhanced rice to combat malnutrition disorders of the poor. *Nutr Rev* 61(6, II):S101, 2003.
31. Nuss ET, Tanumihardjo SA: Quality protein maize for Africa: closing the protein inadequacy gap in vulnerable populations. *Adv Nutr* 2:217, 2011.
32. Shay CM, Van Horn L, Stamler J, et al: Food and nutrient intakes and their associations with lower BMI in middle-aged US adults: the International Study of Macro-/Micronutrients and Blood Pressure (INTERMAP). *Am J Clin Nutr* 96:483, 2012.
33. U.S. Department of Agriculture, Agricultural Research Service: Nutrient Intakes from Food: Mean Amounts

Consumed per Individual by Gender and Age in the United States, 2009-2010, *What We Eat in America*, NHANES 2009-2010. 2012. at: <www.ars.usda.gov/SP2UserFiles/Place/12355000/pdf/0910/Table_1_NIN_GEN_09.pdf>. Accessed on July 17, 2013.

34. Fulgoni VL: Current protein intake in America: analysis of the National Health and Nutrition Examination Survey, 2003-2004. *Am J Clin Nutr* 87(Suppl):1554S, 2008.

35. O'Donnell SI, Hoerr SL, Mendoza JA, et al: Nutrient quality of fast food kids meals. *J Am Diet Assoc* 88:1388, 2008.

36. Burrowes JD: New recommendations for the management of diabetic kidney disease. *Nutr Today* 43:65, 2008.

37. Wycherley TP, Moran LJ, Clifton PM, et al: Effects of energy-restricted high-protein, low-fat compared with standard-protein, low-fat diets: a meta-analysis of randomized controlled trials. *Am J Clin Nutr* 96:1281, 2012.

38. Soenen S, Bonomi AG, Lemmens SGT, et al: Relatively high-protein or "low-carb" energy-restricted diets for body weight loss and body weight maintenance. *Physiol Behavior* 107:374, 2012.

39. Westerterp-Plantenga MS, Lemmens SG, Westerterp KR: Dietary protein—its role in satiety, energetics, weight loss and health. *Br J Nutr* 180(Suppl 2):S105, 2012.

40. Paddon-Jones D, Short KR, Campbell WW, et al: Role of dietary protein in the sarcopenia of aging. *Am J Clin Nutr* 87(Suppl):1562S, 2008.

41. Institute of Medicine, Otten JJ, Hellwig JP, et al, editors: *Dietary Reference Intakes: the essential guide to nutrient requirements*, Washington, D.C., 2006, National Academies Press.

42. Juraschek SP, Appel LJ, Anderson CAM, et al: Effect of a high-protein diet on kidney function in healthy adults: results from the OmniHeart Trial. *Am J Kidney Dis* 61(4):547, 2013.

43. Bernstein AM, Treyzon L, Zhaoping LI: Are high-protein, vegetable-based diets safe for kidney function? A review of the literature. *J Am Diet Assoc* 107:644, 2007.

44. Martin WF, Cerundolo LH, Pikosky MA, et al: Effects of dietary protein intake on indexes of hydration. *J Am Diet Assoc* 106:587, 2006.

45. American Dietetic Association: Position of the American Dietetic Association: functional foods. *J Am Diet Assoc* 109:735, 2009.

46. Xiao CW: Health effects of soy protein and isoflavones in humans. *J Nutr* 138:1244S, 2008.

47. McCullough ML, Peterson JJ, Patel R, et al: Flavonoid intake and cardiovascular disease mortality in a prospective cohort of US adults. *Am J Clin Nutr* 95:454, 2012.

48. Egert S, Rimback G: Which sources of flavonoids: complex diets or dietary supplements? *Adv Nutr* 2:8, 2011.

49. Bazzano LA, He J, Ogden LG, et al: Legume consumption and risk of coronary heart disease in U.S. men and women: NHANES I epidemiologic follow-up study. *Arch Intern Med* 161:2573, 2001.

50. Jenkins DJ, Kendall CW, Augustin LS, et al: Effect of legumes as part of a low glycemic index diet on glycemic control and cardiovascular risk factors in type 2 diabetes mellitus: a randomized controlled trial. *Arch Intern Med* 22:1, 2012.

51. U.S. Department of Agriculture, Agricultural Research Service. 2012. USDA National Nutrient Database for Standard Reference, Release 25. Nutrient Data Laboratory Home Page

Accessed on July 17, 2013. at: <http://www.ars.usda.gov/ba/bhnrc/ndl>.

52. King JC, Blumberg J, Ingwersen L, et al: Tree nuts and peanuts as components of a healthy diet. *J Nutr* 138:1736S, 2008.

53. Giugliano D, Esposito K: Mediterranean diet and metabolic diseases. *Curr Opin Lipidol* 19:63, 2008.

54. Murphy SP, Allen LH: Nutritional importance of animal source foods. *J Nutr* 133:3932S, 2003.

55. Timko CA, Hormes JM, Chubski J: Will the real vegetarian please stand up? An investigation of dietary restraint and eating disorder symptoms in vegetarians versus non-vegetarians. *Appetite* 58:982, 2012.

56. Marlow HJ, Hayes WK, Soret S, et al: Diet and the environment: does what you eat matter? *Am J Clin Nutr* 89(Suppl):1699S, 2009.

57. Leitzmann C: Nutrition ecology: the contribution of vegetarian diets. *Am J Clin Nutr* 78(Suppl):657S, 2003.

58. Fraser GE: Vegetarian diets: what do we know of their effects on common chronic diseases? *Am J Clin Nutr* 89(Suppl):1607S, 2009.

59. Craig WJ: Nutrition concerns and health effects of vegetarian diets. *Nutr Clin Pract* 25:613, 2010.

60. Pawlak R, Parrott SJ, Raj S, et al: How prevalent is vitamin B_{12} deficiency among vegetarians? *Nutr Reviews* 71(2):110, 2013.

60a. U.S. Department of Health and Human Services, U.S. Department of Agriculture: *Report of the Dietary Guidelines Advisory Committee on the Dietary Guidelines for Americans 2010*, Washington, D.C., 2010, Center for Nutrition Policy and Promotion, U.S. Department of Agriculture, pp B2-21, 22. from: <http://www.cnpp.usda.gov/DGAs2010-DGACReport.htm>. Retrieved July 18, 2013.

61. Messina M, Melina V, Mangels AR: A new food guide for North American vegetarians. *J Am Diet Assoc* 103:771, 2003.

62. Mangat I: Do vegetarians have to eat fish for optimal cardiovascular protection? *Am J Clin Nutr* 89(Suppl):1597, 2009.

63. American Dietetic Association: Position of the American Dietetic Association and Dietitians of Canada: vegetarian diets. *J Am Diet Assoc* 103:748, 2003.

64. Farmer B, Larson BT, Fulgoni VL, et al: A vegetarian dietary pattern as a nutrient-dense approach to weight management: an analysis of the National Health and Nutrition Examination Survey 1999-2004. *J Am Diet Assoc* 111:819, 2011.

65. Schösler H, de Boer J, Boersema JJ: Can we cut out the meat of the dish? Constructing consumer-oriented pathways towards meat substitution. *Appetite* 58:39, 2012.

66. Rizzo NS, Sabate J, Jaceldo-Siegl K, et al: Vegetarian dietary patterns are associated with a lower risk of metabolic syndrome. The Adventist Health Study 2. *Diabetes Care* 34:1225, 2011.

67. Reference deleted in proofs.

68. Reference deleted in proofs.

69. Reference deleted in proofs.

70. Reference deleted in proofs.

71. Reference deleted in proofs.

72. Reference deleted in proofs.

73. Taylor SL, Hefle SL: Food allergy. In Bowman BA, Russell RM, editors: *Present knowledge in nutrition*, ed 8, Washington, D.C., 2001, International Life Sciences Institute.

FURTHER READINGS AND RESOURCES

Readings

American Dietetic Association: Position of the American Dietetic Association: vegetarian diets. *J Am Diet Assoc* 109:1266, 2009.

Messina V, Melina V, Mangels AR: A new food guide for North American vegetarians. *J Am Diet Assoc* 103:771, 2003.

[These papers provide an overview of a vegetarian food guide that will meet nutritional requirements and describe the adequacy of vegetarian food plans.]

O'Donnell SI, Hoerr SL, Mendoza JA, et al: Nutrient quality of fast food kids meals. *J Am Diet Assoc* 88:1388, 2008.

[Does the average fast-food meal contain more protein than might be needed or appropriate for a young child? These researchers tell us which nutrients are low and which are high in these meals.]

Websites of Interest

- National Institutes of Health, National Library of Medicine: Medline Plus: Trusted Health Information for You. This site provides links to many resources on protein needs throughout the life cycle: http://www.nlm.nih.gov/medlineplus/dietaryproteins.html; and information on vegetarianism including planning healthy diets, dangers of inadequate diets, and sources of problem nutrients: http://www.nlm.nih.gov/medlineplus/vegetariandiet.html; information is provided in English and Spanish.

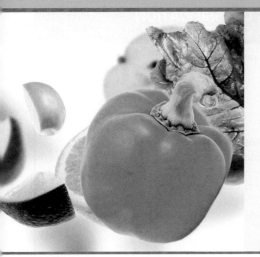

Vitamins

Eleanor D. Schlenker

EVOLVE WEBSITE

http://evolve.elsevier.com/Williams/essentials/

OUTLINE

Here we begin our study of the non–energy-yielding micronutrients: vitamins and minerals. First, we look at the vitamins: why we need them and how we obtain them.

No other group of nutritional elements has so captured the interest of scientists, health professionals, and the general public as the vitamins. Researchers are discovering new roles for vitamins in preventing chronic disease that exceed their known functions as nutrients. Consumers are being bombarded with opinions about vitamin needs that run the gamut from wise and thoughtful use to wild flagrant abuse. Health professionals are trying to learn more about functional foods and the vitamin-like substances they contain, and how these substances interact with known vitamins. In time we may identify new vitamins essential to human health.

VITAMINS: ESSENTIAL NUTRIENTS

General Nature

Most of the vitamins we know about today were discovered between 1900 and 1950. The name *vitamin* was adopted when one of the scientists working with a nitrogen-containing substance called an amine named his discovery *vitamine* ("vital amine"), thinking this was the common nature of all vitamins. At first, a letter designation was given to each new vitamin; however, as the number grew this became confusing, and scientific names based on the structure or function of the vitamin were developed. Letter designations have been retained for the fat-soluble vitamins, because for each of these vitamins a number of closely related compounds have similar metabolic activities and structures.[1]

What Is a Vitamin?

To be classified as a vitamin, a compound has to meet several criteria:

> **KEY TERM**
> **amine** An organic compound containing nitrogen. Amino acids and pyridoxine (vitamin B$_6$) are examples of amines.

- It must be an organic dietary substance that is not energy producing, as are carbohydrate, fat, and protein.
- It is needed in very small quantities to perform a particular metabolic function and prevent an identified deficiency disease.
- It cannot be synthesized by the body, so it must be supplied in food.

These principles form the basis for establishing that a vitamin is essential. However, more must be learned about vitamin requirements, how vitamin needs can be met by the available food supply, and current dietary habits influencing vitamin intake.[2] Other vitamin-like substances in food that appear to promote health and increase resistance to chronic diseases are also being identified. In time, new substances may be added to the list of essential vitamins.

Basic Principles

Over the years we have learned more about individual vitamins and how they interact with each other and other nutrients in carrying out their work. The following principles will guide our study of these nutrients:

- *Individual vitamins are multifunctional:* Most vitamins have multiple roles or actions in the body, sometimes working independently and sometimes working cooperatively with other nutrients. For example, while we associate vitamin A with its major role of helping us see in dim light, this vitamin also maintains the mucous membranes that protect against infection.
- *One vitamin cannot substitute for another vitamin:* All vitamins must be available in sufficient amounts for the body to function normally and for tissues to remain healthy. For example, an abundant supply of vitamin C cannot take the place of folate in preventing a neural tube defect (NTD).
- *Vitamins work together in carrying out body functions:* The formation and maturation of red blood cells require the actions of folate, pyridoxine, vitamin B_{12}, and ascorbic acid, along with several important minerals.
- *Vitamins function best when all are present in the appropriate proportions:* High-potency vitamin A supplements interfere with the action of vitamin D, decreasing calcium absorption and increasing the risk of hip fracture.

These functional truths underscore the importance of eating a variety of foods to obtain essential vitamins and other important substances that contribute to health.

Classification

As the vitamins were discovered, they were grouped according to their solubility in fats or water, and this system has continued (Box 6-1).

Fat-Soluble Vitamins

The fat-soluble vitamins are A, D, E, and K. They are closely associated with body lipids and are easily stored. Their functions are usually related to structural activities with proteins.

BOX 6-1   CLASSIFICATION OF VITAMINS

Fat-Soluble Vitamins
- A
- D
- E
- K

Water-Soluble Vitamins
- Vitamin C (ascorbic acid)
- Thiamin
- Riboflavin
- Niacin
- Pantothenic acid
- Biotin
- Vitamin B_6 (pyridoxine)
- Folate
- Vitamin B_{12} (cobalamin)

Water-Soluble Vitamins

The water-soluble vitamins are vitamin C and the B-complex family. These vitamins are more easily absorbed and transported, but unlike the fat-soluble vitamins, they cannot be stored except in the general sense of tissue saturation. The B vitamins function mainly as **coenzyme** factors in cell metabolism. Vitamin C works with enzymes that support tissue building and maintenance.

Current Knowledge and Key Questions

In our study we will answer the following questions for each vitamin:

- *Chemical and physical nature:* What is the general structure of the vitamin?
- *Absorption, transport, and storage:* How does the body handle this particular vitamin?
- *Function:* What does this vitamin do?
- *Related deficiency symptoms or disease:* What happens when this vitamin is absent or not available in sufficient amounts?
- *Clinical role in health:* Does this vitamin prevent or ameliorate a chronic disease?
- *Recommended intake and possible toxicity:* How much of this vitamin do we need, and how much is too much? What are the consequences of excessive intake? [See Chapter 1 to review the Dietary Reference Intakes (DRIs).]
- *Food sources:* How do we obtain this vitamin?

In the following sections we discuss the four fat-soluble vitamins and the nine water-soluble vitamins.

FAT-SOLUBLE VITAMINS

VITAMIN A

Chemical and Physical Nature

Vitamin A is the generic name for a group of compounds with similar biologic activity: **retinol**, **retinal**, and retinoic acid. The term *retinoids* refers to the natural forms of vitamin A and its synthetic copies. Retinol, an alcohol of high molecular weight ($C_{20}H_{29}OH$), was given its name based on its specific function in the retina of the eye. It is soluble in fat and fat solvents. Because retinol is insoluble in water, it is fairly stable in cooking.

Forms

There are two dietary forms of vitamin A: (1) preformed vitamin A and (2) provitamin A (Box 6-2):

1. *Preformed vitamin A (retinol):* This is the natural form of vitamin A found only in animal foods and usually associated with fat. Vitamin A is stored mostly in the liver but also in small amounts in the kidneys, lungs, and adipose tissue, so organ meats are a rich source. Other dietary sources are the fat portion of dairy foods, egg yolk, and fish.

2. *Provitamin A or β-carotene:* Plants cannot synthesize vitamin A but instead produce a family of compounds called carotenoids. These substances in plants are eaten by animals and then converted to vitamin A. Thus humans can obtain their vitamin A directly by eating animal tissues or by converting carotenoids obtained from plant foods. The carotenoids were so named because β-carotene ($C_{40}H_{56}$) was found in the yellow and orange pigment in carrots and other vegetables and fruits. Examples of other carotenoids found in plant foods include β-cryptoxanthin, lutein, and zeaxanthin, but not all of these can be converted to vitamin A.

The carotenoids have an important role in human nutrition. β-Carotene, converted to vitamin A in the body, provides about 21% of the total vitamin A intake in the United States.[3] Enzymes found in the mucosal cells of the small intestine and in the liver split the carotenoid molecule to yield retinol. The yellow and red carotenoid pigments in many fruits and vegetables and in red palm oil are the major food sources of vitamin A in most developing countries. Unfortunately, the conversion of carotenes to retinol is much less efficient than we thought (Table 6-1), raising concerns as to whether fruits and vegetables can provide an adequate supply of vitamin A in regions of the world where animal foods are scarce.[4]

Absorption, Transport, and Storage
Substances Needed for Absorption

Whether vitamin A enters the body as preformed vitamin A or as the precursor β-carotene, various materials are needed for its absorption, as follows:

- *Bile salts:* Vitamin A joins with fat, other fat-related compounds, and bile salts in the small intestine to form micelles, a bile-lipid complex. Bile salts are necessary for carrying fats and fat-soluble materials into the intestinal wall for further breakdown. Clinical conditions affecting the biliary system such as a bile duct obstruction, infectious hepatitis, or liver cirrhosis that interfere with production or release of bile salts hinder vitamin A absorption.
- *Pancreatic lipase:* This fat-splitting enzyme released into the upper small intestine carries out the hydrolysis of fat emulsions containing vitamin A. Water-based preparations of retinol are used when lipase secretion and absorption of fat is curtailed, as in cystic fibrosis or pancreatitis.[3]

TABLE 6-1	CONVERSION OF CAROTENOIDS TO VITAMIN A	
AMOUNT CONSUMED	**AMOUNT AVAILABLE TO THE BODY**	
1 mcg retinol	1 mcg retinol	
12 mcg β-carotene	1 mcg retinol	
24 mcg α-carotene or β-cryptoxanthin	1 mcg retinol	

NOTE: Although many carotenoids can be converted to retinol (vitamin A) to help meet body needs, greater amounts of the carotenoids are required to produce one molecule of vitamin A.

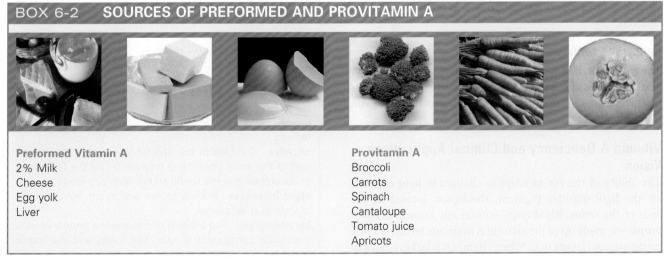

BOX 6-2 SOURCES OF PREFORMED AND PROVITAMIN A

Preformed Vitamin A
2% Milk
Cheese
Egg yolk
Liver

Provitamin A
Broccoli
Carrots
Spinach
Cantaloupe
Tomato juice
Apricots

- *Dietary fat:* Absorption of vitamin A and provitamin A requires the presence of fat to stimulate the release of bile salts and form micelles. At least 3 to 5 g of fat at the same meal is needed to absorb provitamin A.[5]

Age is a factor in absorption. Newborns, especially premature infants, absorb vitamin A poorly. Persons using mineral oil as a laxative reduce their absorption of vitamin A.

Conversion of β-Carotene

β-Carotene can be absorbed and used by the body in its original form or be converted to vitamin A. Although at one time we believed that carotenoids were biologically important only as precursors to vitamin A, we have since learned that as members of that broad category of phytochemicals active in functional foods, they have roles in human health unrelated to the actions of vitamin A. (To learn about the importance of eating a good diet to obtain needed vitamins and phytochemicals rather than depending on supplements, see the Evidence-Based Practice box, "Food or Supplements: Do They Both Produce the Same Results?")

Transport and Storage

The route of absorption of vitamin A and the carotenoids parallels that of fat. In the intestinal mucosa, retinol—whether from preformed animal sources or converted from carotenes—along with intact plant carotenoids are incorporated into the chylomicrons. In this form they enter the bloodstream via the lymphatic system and are carried to the liver for storage or distribution to tissues. Vitamin A is transported to body tissues by special retinol-binding proteins.

The liver is an efficient storage organ for vitamin A, containing up to 80% of the body's total supply. Liver stores are usually sufficient to prevent deficiency for 6 to 12 months and in some individuals for as long as 4 years. The capacity of the liver to store a substantial amount of vitamin A has special significance in parts of the world where vitamin A–containing foods are in short supply, because a prophylactic dose administered every 6 months can prevent mortality and blindness and support normal growth in infants and young children.[6]

Functions of Vitamin A

The role of vitamin A in vision is best known, but vitamin A also influences the integrity of body coverings and linings (epithelial tissues), cell division and differentiation, growth, immunity, and reproductive function.

Vitamin A Deficiency and Clinical Applications
Vision

The ability of the eye to adapt to changes in light depends on the light-sensitive pigment, rhodopsin, located in the rods of the retina. Rhodopsin—commonly known as *visual purple*—is made up of the vitamin A molecule retinal and the protein opsin (Figure 6-1). When vitamin A is lacking, normal rhodopsin cannot be formed and the rods and cones of the

retina become increasingly sensitive to changes in light, causing **night blindness**. This condition is reversed with an injection of vitamin A (retinol), which is readily converted to retinal and then rhodopsin.

Cell Differentiation

This vitamin also controls the differentiation of cells, or in other words, the formation of specialized cells from basic stem cells. Vitamin A is needed to develop and maintain healthy epithelial tissue, which provides our primary barrier to infection. The epithelium includes both the outer skin and the mucous membranes that line many body structures. Without vitamin A the cells formed are dry and flat rather than soft and moist. These dry, flat cells gradually harden to form keratin, a process called **keratinization**. Keratin is a protein that creates dry, scaly tissue, normal for nails and hair but abnormal for skin and mucous membranes. In vitamin

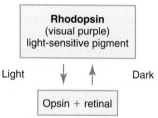

FIGURE 6-1 The vision cycle: light-dark adaptation role of vitamin A.

KEY TERMS

coenzyme A substance that is a necessary partner with a cell enzyme in carrying out a chemical reaction; vitamins are important coenzymes in energy, lipid, and protein metabolism.

retinol Chemical name for vitamin A derived from its function in the retina of the eye producing light-dark adaptation.

retinal The aldehyde form of retinol (vitamin A) derived from the enzymatic splitting of β-carotene in the intestinal wall. In the retina, retinal combines with opsin to form visual pigments.

carotenoids A group of yellow-red-orange pigments widely distributed in plants that act as antioxidants and may have additional health-promoting properties; some carotenoids such as β-carotene can be converted to retinal in the intestinal wall.

precursor A substance from which another substance is derived.

micelles Complex of bile and fat that carries fat into the wall of the small intestine in preparation for the final stage of absorption into the lymph and general circulation.

night blindness Inability to see well in dim light because of vitamin A deficiency.

keratinization The process of creating the protein keratin, a principal component of skin, hair, nails, and the matrix forming tooth enamel.

Food or Supplements: Do They Both Produce the Same Results?

Identify the Problem: The physiologic functions of phytochemicals, the substances associated with the rich yellow, orange, green, blue, and red pigments in fruits and vegetables are distinct from those of the essential vitamins, although we still have much to learn about their specific roles. Because the general public is paying closer attention to nutrition and its relation to lifelong health, sellers of dietary supplements are offering new combinations of both nutrients and non-nutrients to meet this demand. Several of the better known carotenoids such as β-carotene, lycopene, and cryptoxanthin have been isolated from their natural sources and are being marketed in supplement form. However, will we receive the same benefit if we shop in the supplement section and forget about eating fruits and vegetables? What does the research tell us?

Review the evidence: Several long-term follow-up studies have compared supplements that contain antioxidant vitamins and carotenoids with fruit and vegetable intake to determine their effect on chronic disease and mortality. First, individuals who ate more daily servings of fruits and vegetables recorded fewer heart attacks or strokes than those who had fewer daily servings of fruits and vegetables.[1,2] Supplements supplying carotenoids, ascorbic acid, and vitamin E did not offer the same protection against chronic disease as actual fruits and vegetables.[3-5] Over a 20-year follow-up, individuals who ate more blueberries, apples, and pears—all good sources of phytochemicals—were less likely to develop type 2 diabetes.[6]

Implement the findings: Scientists have speculated as to why these dietary components must be eaten in their food form to convey their important benefits. One reason could be that fruits, vegetables, and other plant sources contain a mixture of these chemical substances that work together to bring about important effects on health. To achieve this important **synergy**, they may need to be present in the natural combinations found in food. It may also be that health benefits associated with certain foods come from active substances that we have not yet identified.[7,8] At inappropriately high levels,

known phytochemicals can engage in harmful reactions with various vitamins, trace minerals, and prescription medications,[9] and the concentrated amounts contained in supplements may overestimate body needs.

Supplements such as lutein and cryptoxanthin will not replace plant foods and provide similar health benefits. Fruits and vegetables also add variety and taste to our meals, features that pills cannot deliver. Encourage your patients to head to the fruit and vegetable sections of their local grocery stores, or better yet, start a garden and grow their own.

References
1. Dauchet L, Amouyel P, Hercberg S, et al: Fruit and vegetable consumption and risk of coronary heart disease: a meta-analysis of cohort studies. *J Nutr* 136:2588, 2006.
2. Liu S, Manson JE, Lee I-M, et al: Fruit and vegetable intake and risk of cardiovascular disease: the Women's Health Study. *Am J Clin Nutr* 72:922, 2000.
3. Neuhouser ML, Wassertheil-Smoller S, Thomson C, et al: Multivitamin use and risk of cancer and cardiovascular disease in the Women's Health Initiative cohorts. *Arch Intern Med* 169:294, 2009.
4. Sesso HD, Buring JE, Christen WG, et al: Vitamins E and C in the prevention of cardiovascular disease in men. The Physicians' Health Study II randomized controlled trial. *JAMA* 300:2123, 2008.
5. Voutilainen S, Nurmi T, Mursu J, et al: Carotenoids and cardiovascular health. *Am J Clin Nutr* 83:1265, 2006.
6. Wedick NM, Pan A, Cassidy A, et al: Dietary flavonoid intakes and risk of type 2 diabetes in US men and women. *Am J Clin Nutr* 95:925, 2012.
7. Lila MA: From beans to berries and beyond: teamwork between plant chemicals for protection of optimal human health. *Ann N Y Acad Sci* 1114:372, 2007.
8. Martin C: The interface between plant metabolic engineering and human health. *Curr Opin Biotechnol* 24:1, 2012.
9. Egert S, Rimback G: Which sources of flavonoids: complex diets or dietary supplements? *Adv Nutr* 2:8, 2011.

A deficiency, such abnormal tissue changes occur in many body systems, as follows:
- *Eye:* The cornea dries and hardens, a condition called *xerophthalmia* (Figure 6-2). The tear ducts become dry, robbing the eye of its cleansing and lubricating fluid, and infection follows quickly. In extreme deficiency the keratinization progresses to blindness. Blindness caused by vitamin A deficiency is a world public health problem; each year more than 350,000 preschool children lose their sight and about half die within 1 year of becoming blind.[7]
- *Respiratory tract:* The epithelium lining the nasal passages becomes dry and the cilia are lost, removing a barrier to infectious organisms. Nasal secretions that trap invading particles and remove them from the body are no longer produced.
- *Gastrointestinal tract:* Salivary fluids are no longer secreted, and the mouth becomes dry and cracked, open to invading

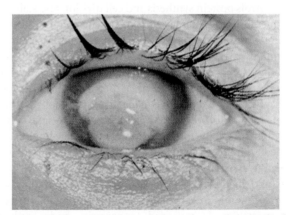

FIGURE 6-2 Xerophthalmia resulting from vitamin A deficiency and a leading cause of blindness in the developing world. (From McLaren DS: *A colour atlas and text of diet-related disorders*, ed 2, London, 1992, Mosby-Year Book Europe Limited.)

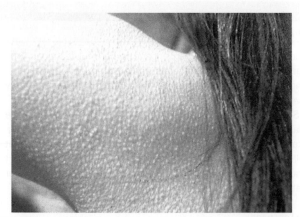

FIGURE 6-3 Follicular hyperkeratosis caused by vitamin A deficiency. (From McLaren DS: *A colour atlas and text of diet-related disorders,* ed 2, London, 1992, Mosby-Year Book Europe Limited.)

bacteria. The esophagus becomes red and inflamed. Mucosal secretions decrease throughout the digestive tract, and tissues dry and slough off, affecting digestion and absorption.

- *Genitourinary tract:* When epithelial tissue begins to break down, problems such as vaginal infections and urinary tract infections ensue.
- *Skin:* As skin becomes dry and scaly, small pustules (hardened, pigmented, papular eruptions) appear around hair follicles, a condition known as *follicular hyperkeratosis* (Figure 6-3).
- *Tooth formation:* Certain epithelial cells surrounding tooth buds in fetal gum tissue that normally become specialized cup-shaped organs called *ameloblasts* do not develop properly. These little organs form the enamel of the developing tooth.

Growth

Vitamin A is essential for the growth of bones and soft tissues as it controls protein synthesis and cell division and stabilizes cell membranes. The growth and maintenance of bone require constant remodeling, reshaping, and expansion. Vitamin A participates in the important job of tunneling out old bone to make way for new bone. Then, the tunnels are filled in to accommodate growth according to the embryonic cartilage model. Although an inadequate supply of vitamin A is detrimental to bone health, so are excessive intakes that cause old bone to be lost more rapidly than new bone can be formed. Among women, intakes of preformed vitamin A exceeding twice the DRI were associated with lower bone mass and increased risk of hip fracture.[8] β-Carotene and other carotenoid precursors of vitamin A supplied in fruits and vegetables do not lead to excessive body levels of vitamin A, nor bone loss. Based on its role in cell growth and differentiation, vitamin A supplements should accompany intervention and treatment of protein-energy malnutrition (PEM).[5]

Reproduction

Vitamin A is needed for normal sexual maturation and function. It participates in gene expression and plays an important role in fetal growth, including development of the central nervous system (CNS).[3] A sufficient intake is required for successful lactation.

Immunity

Poor vitamin A status lowers resistance to infection in two ways: (1) changes in epithelial and mucosal tissues allow disease organisms to enter the body more easily, and (2) vitamin A has a direct effect on immune function. Both cell-mediated and antibody-mediated immunity are impaired when intake is low. Measles is more likely to be fatal in vitamin A–deficient children in developing countries. Immune response returns to normal quite rapidly when vitamin A is restored.[9]

Vitamin A Requirement
Influencing Factors
A number of variables modify the vitamin A needs of a given individual, as follows:
- *Liver stores:* High vitamin A stores can supply body needs for an extended period; those with low body stores depend on day-to-day intakes.
- *Intake of preformed versus provitamin A:* Increased amounts of carotenoids are required to meet the DRI for vitamin A.
- *Illness and infection:* Needs increase to support the production of immune cells and body defenses.
- *Gastrointestinal or hepatic defects:* Gallbladder or liver disease interfering with production of bile salts limits fat absorption and in turn the absorption of vitamin A and carotenoids.

Causes of Vitamin A Deficiency
In the United States the primary cause of vitamin A deficiency is inadequate dietary intake, usually the result of poor food selection rather than unavailability. Fast-food restaurants can influence vitamin A status, as "kids meals" that include a hamburger or chicken sandwich with fries and a sweetened beverage rather than fruit and milk do not meet one third of the DRI for vitamin A.[10] Vitamin A deficiency occurs with poor absorption, inadequate conversion of β-carotene, or liver or intestinal disease. A high intake of alcohol results in loss of vitamin A from the liver even if liver function remains normal.[3] Individuals with fat malabsorption syndromes can develop vitamin A deficiency.

Dietary Reference Intake
The Recommended Dietary Allowance (RDA) for vitamin A is the amount required to maintain optimal liver stores. It is presented in micrograms (mcg) of retinol,[3] and the term **retinol activity equivalent (RAE)** takes into account the ratios for converting carotenoids to vitamin A. Early on, vitamin A was measured in international units (IU), and

some food composition tables still use those units. Many older tables overestimate the amount of vitamin A available from carotenoid-containing foods, such that intakes are calculated to be greater than is true. The RDA for men ages 19 and older is set at 900 mcg, and the RDA for women of this age is 700 mcg. To ensure sufficient vitamin A to support a successful pregnancy and appropriate vitamin A content in breast milk, the RDA increases to 770 mcg in pregnancy and 1300 mcg in lactation.

Vitamin A Toxicity
Hypervitaminosis A

Because the liver can store very large amounts of vitamin A, persons taking high-potency supplements exceeding the Tolerable Upper Intake Level (UL) over months or years can develop toxicity. Impaired vision, gastrointestinal disturbances, and skin abnormalities are evident in both vitamin A deficiency and excess, although expressed in different ways. Daily intakes greater than the UL of 3000 mcg of preformed vitamin A are especially dangerous for pregnant women and can result in congenital malformations,[9] depending on intake. Teens and young adults prescribed acne medications such as isotretinoin (Accutane) and isotretinoin (oral forms), which are nonnutritive sources of vitamin A, need to talk with their doctor when contemplating pregnancy. The increased use of vitamin supplements and fortified foods has created disturbing intakes of preformed vitamin A among some age groups. Supplements often contain as much as two times the RDA and, if combined with highly fortified food items, bring children and adults dangerously close to the UL.[13]

Food Sources of Vitamin A

Animal sources of preformed vitamin A include liver, milk, cheese, butter, egg yolk, and fish. Reduced-fat, lowfat, and fat free milk, as well as certain soy and rice milks, are fortified with vitamin A to the level found naturally in whole milk. Nonanimal products such as margarine, ready-to-eat cereals, and cereal bars are often fortified with vitamin A. Dark-yellow, orange, red, and green vegetables and fruits contain a variety of carotenoids and help meet the vitamin A requirement. Cooked vegetables can be better dietary sources of carotenoids than raw vegetables because cooking helps release these substances from their plant sources, making them more available for absorption. The vitamin A content of selected foods is listed in Box 6-3. (The Focus on Culture box, "Acculturation: How Does It Affect Food Patterns?" points to problems with low intakes of fruits and vegetables among families immigrating to the United States.)

VITAMIN D

Chemical and Physical Nature

When first discovered, vitamin D was classified as a vitamin, although it is now clear that vitamin D is actually a **prohormone**, and in its active form functions as a hormone. Chemically, vitamin D is a sterol and its precursor found in human skin is the lipid molecule 7-dehydrocholesterol. All compounds with vitamin D activity are soluble in fat but not water, and they are heat stable.

Forms

The body uses two forms of vitamin D: (1) ergocalciferol (vitamin D_2) and (2) **cholecalciferol** (vitamin D_3). Vitamin D_2 is formed by irradiating ergosterol found in ergot (a fungus growing on rye and other cereal grains) and yeast. The more important form is vitamin D_3, made by the action of ultraviolet light from the sun on the 7-dehydrocholesterol in the skin and found naturally in fish liver oils. Vitamin D_3 is also the form used in the fortification of milk and other dairy products, cereals, and juice.

Absorption, Transport, and Storage
Absorption

Vitamin D is absorbed in the small intestine as part of the micelles, as are all fat-soluble vitamins. Conditions associated with malabsorption such as celiac disease, cystic fibrosis, Crohn's disease, or pancreatic insufficiency hinder vitamin D absorption.

Active Hormone Synthesis

The active hormone form of vitamin D is 1,25-dihydroxycholecalciferol [$1,25(OH)_2D_3$], with the chemical name **calcitriol**. Calcitriol is produced by the combined action of the skin, liver, and kidneys, an overall process referred to as the *vitamin D endocrine system*.

We will look at each of the following three steps in this process (Figure 6-4):

1. *Skin:* When 7-dehydrocholesterol, the vitamin D precursor in the skin, is exposed to the ultraviolet rays of the sun, it is converted into vitamin D_3. The amount produced depends on the length and intensity of sun exposure and skin pigment. For those living in northern climates, sun exposure is not sufficient to supply all of their vitamin D needs, especially in the winter months.[14] People who are confined indoors and those residing in crowded city areas with high air pollution do not receive adequate ultraviolet exposure to synthesize vitamin D. Dark skin pigment prevents ultraviolet rays from reaching the deep layer in the skin where synthesis of vitamin D_3 occurs. The use of sunscreen with a sun protection factor of 8 lowers vitamin D production by as much as 95%[14]; however, staying in the shade and wearing long sleeves may influence blood vitamin D levels to an even greater extent than use of

---

KEY TERMS

retinol activity equivalent (RAE) Unit of measure for dietary sources of vitamin A, including preformed retinol and the provitamins β-carotene, α-carotene, and β-cryptoxanthin.

prohormone A substance that when converted to its active form acts as a hormone; vitamin D obtained from food or synthesized in the skin is a prohormone, and its active hormonal form is called *calcitriol*.

BOX 6-3   FOOD SOURCES OF VITAMIN A

Food Source	Quantity	Vitamin A (mcg RAE)*
Grains Group		
Fortified ready-to-eat cereals		
Instant oatmeal (plain)	1 packet	230
Special K	1 cup	225
Cheerios	1 cup	277
Wheaties	3/4 cup	150
Vegetable Group		
Sweet potato, baked in skin	1 medium	1096
Pumpkin, canned	½ cup	953
Spinach, leaf, frozen, cooked	½ cup	573
Collard greens, frozen, cooked	½ cup	488
Carrot, raw	1 medium (7½ inches)	601
Chinese cabbage (bok choy), cooked	1 cup	360
Lettuce, dark green	1 cup	205
Peppers, red, sweet, chopped	½ cup	117
Broccoli, raw	6 florets	99
Brussels sprouts, frozen, cooked	1 cup	71
Fruit Group		
Cantaloupe	⅛ melon	117
Apricots, canned in juice	½ cup	104
Watermelon	1 wedge (4 × 8 inches)	80
Meat, Beans, Eggs, and Nuts Group		
Chicken livers, cooked	1	1752
Clams, canned	3 oz	127
Milk Group		
Milk, nonfat, fortified	1 cup	149
Milk, 1% milk fat, fortified	1 cup	142
Milk, whole, 3.5% fat, unfortified	1 cup	112
Soy milk, unfortified	1 cup	00
Cheddar cheese	1 oz	75
Fats, Oils, and Sugar		
Margarine, tub	1 tbsp	116
Butter	1 tbsp	97

Data from U.S. Department of Agriculture, Agricultural Research Service: *USDA National Nutrient Database for Standard Reference, Release 26,* 2013. Nutrient Data Laboratory Home Page: <http://www.ars.usda.gov/ba/bhnrc/ndl>.
Images copyright 2006 JupiterImages Corporation.
Recommended Dietary Allowances for adults: women, 700 mcg RAE; men, 900 mcg RAE.
*1 RAE (retinol activity equivalent) = 1 mcg retinol.

sunscreen.[15] Obesity influences blood vitamin D levels because body vitamin D is sequestered in body fat.[16]

2. *Liver:* Vitamin D, whether produced in the skin or obtained from dietary sources, is transported to the liver where it is converted to **25-hydroxycholecalciferol [25(OH)D₃].**

This intermediate metabolite goes on to the kidneys for final activation.

3. *Kidneys:* In the kidneys a special enzyme completes the last step in forming the physiologically active vitamin D hormone 1,25-dihydroxycholecalciferol [1,25(OH)₂D₃],

FOCUS ON CULTURE

Acculturation: How Does It Affect Food Patterns?

The term *acculturation* refers to the adoption of local customs and practices by families entering a new country, and how such changes influence disease risk. Those who move to a different part of the world begin to develop the chronic diseases of their host country, based on changes in their diet and environment. Families who move to the United States are more likely to become obese than their counterparts who remain in their home country. Latinos taking up residence in the United States increase their intakes of fat, sugars, and sweetened beverages, but decrease their use of fruits and vegetables, including beans. These changes lower their intakes of fiber, provitamin A, and the B-complex vitamins. The longer they reside in the United States, the more their intakes of these foods decrease.[1,2]

The availability of fruits and vegetables in their new neighborhoods as compared with their former neighborhoods may contribute to these changes. Latino homemakers accustomed to purchasing fresh produce at local street markets in Mexico or Puerto Rico must adjust to different marketing environments and likely higher prices. Shoppers mention that fruits and vegetables purchased in the United States taste different from those obtained in their home country, which could relate to degree of ripeness, cultivar, or how one remembers the food "at home."[1] Full-time employment also influences food choices. Honduran women working outside the home noted that they were full-time homemakers in Honduras, allowing more time to prepare food.[2]

The language spoken in the home can predict degree of acculturation and food patterns. When foods eaten by women born in the United States and women born in Mexico were compared on the basis of language spoken at home, those using Spanish had higher intakes of fruits, vegetables, and beans than those speaking English, regardless of birthplace.[3] Mexican-American women born in the United States who spoke predominantly English used fewer fruits, green leafy vegetables, and beans, and the most fried potatoes of any group. They consumed only two thirds as many beans as their counterparts born in the United States who spoke predominantly Spanish, and less than half as many beans as homemakers born in Mexico who still spoke predominantly Spanish.

Relatively few Hispanic adults consume the recommended servings of fruits and vegetables,[4,5] and they fall behind in their intakes of vitamin A and important B-complex vitamins. Only 38% of Hispanic adults have two servings of fruit per day and only 19% have three servings of vegetables per day. Among Puerto Rican adults in Massachusetts, greater use of English and higher socioeconomic status were associated with higher intakes of fruits and nonstarchy vegetables.[6] Income may play an important role in dietary acculturation.

Changes in food patterns may proceed more slowly when language holds ties to a native culture. Health professionals working with populations new to a host country must recognize the role of language and income in the acculturation process.

References
1. Kittler PG, Sucher KP, Nahikian-Nelms M: *Food and culture,* ed 6, Belmont, Calif., 2012, Wadsworth/Cengage Learning.
2. Ayala GX, Baquero B, Klinger S: A systematic review of the relationship between acculturation and diet among Latinos in the United States: implications for future research. *J Am Diet Assoc* 108(8):1330, 2008.
3. Montez JM, Eschbach K: Country of birth and language are uniquely associated with intakes of fat, fiber, and fruits and vegetables among Mexican-American women in the United States. *J Am Diet Assoc* 108:473, 2008.
4. Kirkpatrick SI, Dodd KW, Reedy J, et al: Income and race/ethnicity are associated with adherence to food-based dietary guidance among US adults and children. *J Acad Nutr Diet* 112:624, 2012.
5. Grimm KA, Blanck HM: Survey language preference as a predictor of meeting fruit and vegetable objectives among Hispanic adults in the United States, Behavior Risk Factor Surveillance System, 2009. *Prev Chron Dis* 8(6): A133, 2011. at: <http://www.cdc.gov/pcd/issues/2011/nov/11_0091.htm>. Accessed on December 27, 2012.
6. Van Rompay MI, McKeown N, Castaneda-Sceppa C, et al: Acculturation and sociocultural influences on dietary intake and health status among Puerto-Rican adults in Massachusetts. *J Acad Nutr Diet* 112:64, 2012.

referred to as calcitriol. Individuals with kidney disease are often unable to convert vitamin D to its active form.

Functions of Vitamin D

Vitamin D is associated mostly with calcium and phosphorus absorption and bone formation, although we continue to learn of other functions important to health.

Control of Calcium and Phosphorus Levels in Bone and Blood

The vitamin D endocrine system cooperates with parathyroid hormone and calcitonin to (1) stimulate the active transport of calcium and phosphorus in the small intestine, (2) promote bone mineralization, and (3) maintain blood calcium at normal levels. Each hormone—calcitriol, parathyroid hormone, and calcitonin—has a specific role in controlling bone and blood calcium levels. Vitamin D brings about the synthesis of important proteins that act on the intestine to stimulate calcium and phosphorus absorption and facilitate their deposition in bone tissue. Parathyroid hormone and calcitonin are responsible for keeping blood calcium and phosphorus levels in the normal ranges to support bone deposition.

Vitamin D Deficiency and Clinical Applications
Bone Disease

Without sufficient vitamin D the body cannot build or maintain normal bone. In children the vitamin D deficiency disease is called *rickets* and results in a malformed skeleton (Figure 6-5). Vitamin D–deficient adults develop osteomalacia in which previously deposited bone mineral is mobilized, resulting in bone pain and weak, brittle bones. Osteomalacia occurs in women of childbearing age who have little exposure to sunlight, diets low in calcium and vitamin D, and frequent pregnancies followed by periods of lactation. Older adults who use antacids that contain aluminum are at risk of osteomalacia because aluminum binds phosphorus and causes it to be excreted along with calcium. Osteomalacia sometimes accompanies **osteoporosis**, another bone disease common in older men and women that is treated with vitamin D (see Chapter 7).

The widespread use of vitamin D–fortified milk had nearly eliminated rickets in the United States, but the disease is making a comeback among breast-fed infants who do not receive vitamin D supplements.[22] Breast milk is generally low in vitamin D, and especially so among mothers with poor vitamin D status. It is recommended that infants in northern climates and all African-American infants be given vitamin D supplements. (The vitamin D needs of breast-fed infants will be discussed further in Chapter 12.)

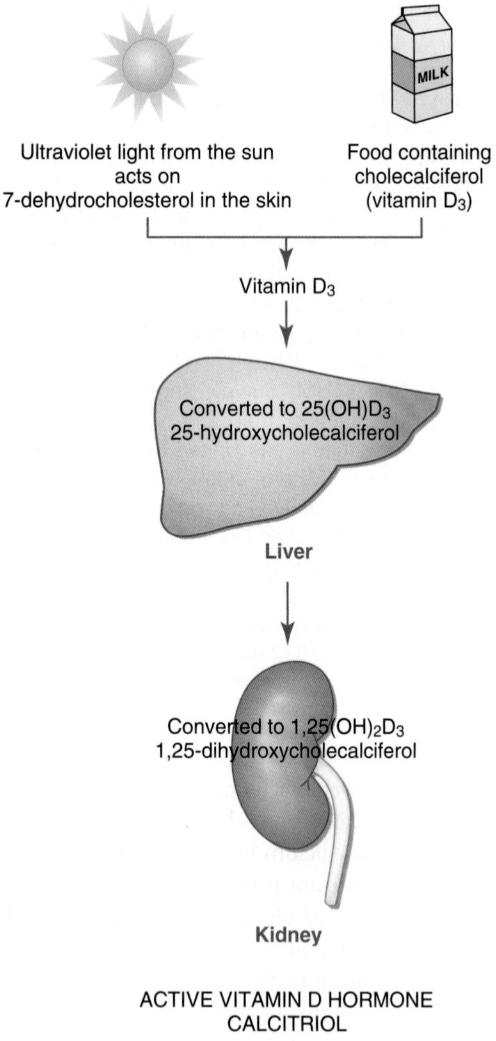

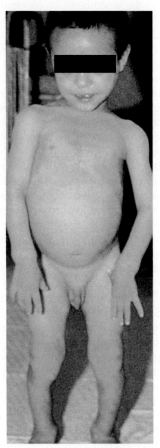

FIGURE 6-5 Bowlegs in rickets resulting from a lack of vitamin D. (From McLaren DS: *A colour atlas and text of diet-related disorders,* ed 2, London, 1992, Mosby-Year Book Europe Limited.)

Ultraviolet light from the sun acts on 7-dehydrocholesterol in the skin

Food containing cholecalciferol (vitamin D₃)

Vitamin D₃

Converted to 25(OH)D₃
25-hydroxycholecalciferol

Liver

Converted to 1,25(OH)₂D₃
1,25-dihydroxycholecalciferol

Kidney

ACTIVE VITAMIN D HORMONE
CALCITRIOL

FIGURE 6-4 Formation of the active vitamin D hormone. Vitamin D undergoes a conversion in the liver and then a second conversion in the kidneys to form the vitamin D hormone calcitriol. Notice that vitamin D is handled the same way whether it was synthesized in the skin or obtained from dietary sources.

KEY TERMS

7-dehydrocholesterol   A precursor cholesterol compound in the skin that when irradiated by sunlight produces cholecalciferol (D₃).

cholecalciferol   Chemical name for vitamin D in its inactive form. When cholecalciferol is consumed in food or synthesized in the skin, its first activation step occurs in the liver; the final activation step is completed in the kidneys to form the active vitamin D hormone calcitriol.

calcitriol   Activated hormone form of vitamin D is 1,25-dihydroxycholecalciferol [1,25(OH)₂D₃].

25-hydroxycholecalciferol   [25(OH)D₃]   Intermediate product formed in the liver in the process of forming the active vitamin D hormone.

calcitonin   A polypeptide hormone secreted by connective tissue cells in the thyroid gland that promotes calcium excretion via the urine when blood calcium levels rise above normal.

Because of its active regulatory role in balancing bone mineral absorption and deposition, vitamin D has been used to treat renal osteodystrophy. This condition is secondary to renal failure and results in defective bone formation.

Vitamin D Requirement
Influencing Factors
Setting dietary recommendations for vitamin D is complicated by differing degrees of sun exposure and skin synthesis. Those individuals who work indoors must obtain more of their vitamin D from dietary sources than people who work outdoors. Individuals who reside in northern latitudes are more vulnerable to vitamin D deficiency. Older adults are less able to synthesize vitamin D regardless of sun exposure because of aging changes in the skin.[23]

Dietary Reference Intake
The current DRI estimates the amount of dietary vitamin D required to sustain appropriate blood levels when sun exposure is minimal. The RDA for ages 1 to 70 is 15 mcg (600 IU). For adults over age 70 it increases to 20 mcg (800 IU)[23] based on body changes that occur as people age. Infants pose special problems. Vitamin D–fortified formula and cereal provide the current Adequate Intake (AI) of 10 mcg or 400 IU; however, breast-fed infants require supplementation.

Vitamin D Toxicity
Vitamin D is stored in the adipose tissue and released slowly, so toxic amounts can accumulate when intake is inappropriately high. Toxicity usually results from inappropriate doses of vitamin D supplements, not fortified foods. Adults exceeding the UL of 100 mcg (4000 IU) may develop hypercalcemia with progressive muscle weakness, bone pain, bone fractures, and falls. Blood levels of vitamin D that exceed established norms are associated with cardiovascular disease, certain cancers including those of the pancreas and prostate, and increased risk of death. African Americans appear to be at greater risk of these complications than other groups.[23] Symptoms of toxicity in young children include failure to thrive and calcium deposits in soft tissues such as the kidneys.

HEALTH PROMOTION
Implications of Vitamin D Deficiency
Leaders in nutrition and public health[11] are calling attention to the broad spectrum of individuals who are vitamin D deficient. Medical advice for reducing skin cancer encourages people to use sunscreen. Frail older people seldom venture outdoors. Youth are more likely to entertain themselves with video games or the Internet than participate in outdoor activities. Dietary surveys conducted by the U.S. Department of Agriculture (USDA) indicate that males and females between the ages of 12 and 19 are taking in 6.7 mcg and 4.7 mcg of vitamin D, respectively[24] (the RDA is 15 mcg). This puts them at risk for poor calcium absorption at a time when bone mineral deposition should be reaching its peak. Low-income, African-American, and Hispanic youth are most likely to have low blood vitamin D levels.[23] The majority of Americans do not obtain sufficient amounts of dietary vitamin D.[11] Although over one third take vitamin D supplements, their combined intake from food and supplements still leaves many deficient.[11] These groups are at risk of poor bone health leading to fractures, falls, and related complications.

Food Sources of Vitamin D
Natural sources of vitamin D are few. Vitamin D_2 is found only in yeast and vitamin D_3 mostly in fish liver oils. Fatty fish such as mackerel or salmon provide significant amounts of vitamin D, and egg yolk contains a small amount. Major dietary sources are fortified foods. Milk was selected as a practical carrier more than 50 years ago because it contained calcium and phosphorus and was commonly used by children. The vitamin D added to milk is standardized at 10 mcg (400 IU)/qt, and other dairy foods such as yogurt have added vitamin D. Fortification of milk was credited with eradicating rickets in the United States in the 1930s; however, less use of milk in preference to soft drinks and fruit drinks has lowered intakes of calcium and vitamin D. Margarine is fortified with 37.5 mcg (1500 IU)/lb to serve as a butter substitute, and various ready-to-eat cereals have added vitamin D. Juices, soy milk, and rice milk fortified with calcium and vitamin D to the level usually found in cow's milk are potential sources for the lactose intolerant. Increasing servings of fish would support intakes of both healthy fats and vitamin D. Food sources of vitamin D are displayed in Box 6-4.

VITAMIN E
Chemical and Physical Nature
Scientists studying reproduction in laboratory animals first discovered vitamin E. Because of its association with birth and its chemical structure as an alcohol, it was named tocopherol from the Greek word *tokos*, meaning childbirth. Vitamin E came to be known as the *antisterility vitamin*, although this has been demonstrated in laboratory animals only, not in humans.

Forms
Vitamin E is the generic name given to a group of eight compounds having to some degree the biologic activity of α-tocopherol. Vitamin E is a pale yellow oil, stable to acids and heat, and insoluble in water. It oxidizes very slowly, which gives it an important role as an antioxidant.[26]

Absorption, Transport, and Storage
Vitamin E is absorbed in the micelles with the aid of bile salts and transported in the chylomicrons. Vitamin E is stored in the liver and adipose tissue where it is held in bulk liquid droplets. Mobilization of α-tocopherol from these storage sites occurs very slowly.

Functions of Vitamin E
Antioxidant Activity
In our study of the vitamins we will continue to hear the term *antioxidant* and the role such nutrients play in destroying molecules called *free radicals*. Free radicals have an unpaired electron and are constantly on the lookout for another molecule with an unpaired electron that they can join with. Free radicals are highly active molecules, and the oxidation reactions they initiate are very damaging to body tissues. Free radicals are formed as by-products of normal cell metabolism but also originate in tobacco smoke, car exhaust fumes, and other air pollutants.

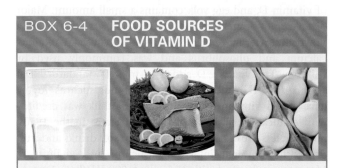

BOX 6-4   FOOD SOURCES OF VITAMIN D

Vitamin D occurs naturally in eggs and fish. Fortified dairy foods, soy milk, juices, and cereals are other good sources for persons with limited exposure to sunlight.

Food Source	Quantity	Vitamin D (mcg)
Grains Group		
Fortified ready-to-eat cereal (e.g., Total)	¾ to 1 cup	1.0-2.5
Fruit Group		
Orange juice, fortified*	1 cup	2.5
Meat, Beans, Eggs, and Nuts Group		
Tuna fish, canned in oil†	3 oz	5.7
Tuna fish, canned in water†	3 oz	1.0
Egg yolk, large	1	0.9
Milk Group		
Milk, fortified* (includes nonfat, 1%, and 2% fat)	1 cup	2.9
Milk, whole (3.5% fat)	1 cup	3.2
Soy milk, fortified*	1 cup	2.9

Data from U.S. Department of Agriculture, Agricultural Research Service: *USDA National Nutrient Database for Standard Reference, Release 26,* 2013. Nutrient Data Laboratory Home Page: <http://www.ars.usda.gov/ba/bhnrc/ndl>.
Images copyright 2006 JupiterImages Corporation.
Recommended Dietary Allowance for adults: ages 19-70, 15 mcg (600 IU); ages ≥71, 20 mcg (800 IU).
*Consumers should check the nutrition label to be sure the product selected is fortified with vitamin D.
†Note the difference in vitamin D content between canned tuna fish packed in oil or water.

Polyunsaturated fatty acids having several double bonds and the tissues where they are found are especially vulnerable to attack. Cell membranes contain a high proportion of polyunsaturated fatty acids, and oxidation by free radicals alters their structure and destroys their ability to recognize harmful substances and prevent them from entering the cell. Brain tissue and nerve fibers are high in unsaturated fatty acids. Deoxyribonucleic acid (DNA) and other proteins in the cell nucleus if modified by unwanted oxidation reactions produce molecules that are ineffective in carrying out body functions. Antioxidants such as vitamin E join with the unpaired electron of free radicals and interrupt the chain of oxidation reactions. Vitamin E is nature's most potent antioxidant.

Partnership with Selenium
In addition to vitamin E, a second line of defense against free radical damage is an enzyme containing selenium, a trace mineral. Selenium can spare vitamin E and reduce the vitamin E requirement. In this partnership role, vitamin E can also reduce the selenium requirement.

Vitamin E Deficiency and Clinical Applications
Premature Infants
Vitamin E deficiency has disastrous effects on red blood cells. When polyunsaturated fatty acids in the lipid membranes of red blood cells are exposed to oxidation, the membranes break, the cell contents are lost, and the cell is destroyed. Continued loss of red blood cells leads to anemia, and this vitamin E–deficiency disease is called hemolytic anemia. Premature infants are especially vulnerable to hemolytic anemia because they miss the last month or two of fetal life when vitamin E stores are normally built up. This condition responds positively to vitamin E therapy[32] and is prevented with vitamin E supplementation at birth. Adequate intake during pregnancy can help ensure optimum vitamin E stores in the full-term infant.

Children and Adults
In older children and adults vitamin E deficiency presents a different set of symptoms associated with the nervous system.[32] Nerves affected are (1) the spinal cord fibers that control physical movement such as walking and (2) the retina

> **KEY TERMS**
> **osteoporosis** Abnormal loss of bone mineral and matrix leading to porous, fragile bone that is prone to fracture or deformity; common disease of aging in older men and women.
> **osteodystrophy** Defective bone formation.
> **tocopherol** Chemical name for vitamin E; it functions as an antioxidant to preserve structural membranes and other tissues with a high content of polyunsaturated fatty acids.
> **antioxidant** A substance that prevents the formation and destructive actions of free radicals.

of the eye. These problems were identified in children with cystic fibrosis and pancreatic insufficiency that had defective absorption of fat and fat-soluble vitamins. Vitamin E deficiency disrupts the making of myelin, the protective lipid covering of the nerve cell axons that helps transmit messages along to muscles. The lack of vitamin E also leads to degeneration of the pigment in the rods and cones of the retina that depend on vitamin E to prevent oxidation damage. Optimum intakes of vitamin E and other antioxidants may be especially important for cystic fibrosis patients who have high tissue oxidation related to their disease.[33] Regular vitamin E replacement therapy is also needed for those with fat malabsorption syndromes.

Vitamin E Requirement
Dietary Reference Intake
The RDA is expressed in milligrams of α-tocopherol, the form of vitamin E with high biologic activity. About 80% of the vitamin E from dietary sources (including fortified foods) is α-tocopherol, and about 20% is other forms. The RDA is 15 mg for both males and females ages 14 and older,[26] but actual intake falls much below this level. In the United States adult men average 8.9 mg/day of α-tocopherol and adult women average 7.1 mg/day[24]; nevertheless, only 5% of adults examined in recent national surveys had blood vitamin E levels categorized as deficient.[11]

Vitamin E Toxicity
No toxicity syndrome has been identified for vitamin E; however, clinicians warn against self-prescribed supplementation. Several recent clinical trials observed increased mortality among those taking in very high levels of vitamin E.[27,28] Over-the-counter supplements often contain as much as 268 mg to 540 mg of α-tocopherol (18 to 36 times the RDA). The UL for vitamin E is 1000 mg.[26] Intakes above recommended levels can interfere with blood platelet aggregation and prevent normal blood clotting. This is particularly important information for persons with low intakes of vitamin K or patients using anticlotting medications.

Food Sources of Vitamin E
Vegetable oils are rich dietary sources of vitamin E. Sunflower, safflower, and canola oils contain the highest amounts, followed by corn oil and olive oil.[34] As might be expected, these oils are also rich sources of polyunsaturated fatty acids which vitamin E protects from oxidation. Other vitamin E sources include peanut butter, nuts, and certain vegetables and fruits, especially tomatoes and spinach. Fortified ready-to-eat cereals contribute significantly to intake, and the vitamin is well absorbed from these foods.[35] Box 6-5 lists major food sources of vitamin E.

VITAMIN K

Chemical and Physical Nature
The studies of Henrik Dam, a biochemist at the University of Copenhagen working on a hemorrhagic disease in chicks, led to the discovery of vitamin K. Because of its blood-clotting function, he called it the *koagulations vitamin,* or vitamin K. For this discovery he received the Nobel Prize in physiology and medicine.

Chemical Nature
The form of vitamin K found in plants is named phylloquinone for its chemical structure. Phylloquinone is the major dietary form and is widely distributed in both animal and plant foods. Menaquinone is synthesized by intestinal bacteria, but either form can be used by the body. A water-soluble analog of vitamin K, menadione, can be absorbed directly into the portal blood,[36] making it an important source for individuals with fat malabsorption.

Absorption, Transport, and Storage
Both phylloquinone and menaquinone require pancreatic lipase and bile salts for absorption. In the liver, vitamin K is stored in small amounts but excreted rapidly after administration of therapeutic doses.

Functional Roles of Vitamin K
Blood Clotting
The major function of vitamin K is to initiate liver synthesis of four proteins necessary for blood clotting.[26] Each clotting factor is in the form of an inactive precursor that depends on vitamin K for activation. This activation step converts the precursor protein prothrombin to thrombin, which in turn acts on the precursor fibrinogen to form fibrin and complete the clotting process. Both calcium ions and vitamin K are needed for normal blood clotting. Vitamin K requires a functioning liver to carry out its tasks. When liver damage is the cause of low prothrombin levels and hemorrhage, vitamin K is ineffective as a therapeutic agent. Vitamin K also controls the liver synthesis of other proteins that regulate the speed and duration of coagulation. These regulatory proteins prevent the development of dangerous, unwanted blood clots or thromboses.[3,36]

Bone Metabolism
Vitamin K has a role in bone health, stimulating the synthesis of osteocalcin and other proteins important to bone.[36,37] Bone is constantly being remodeled, and vitamin K–dependent

---

KEY TERMS

anemia Condition of low blood hemoglobin levels caused by too few red blood cells or red blood cells with a low hemoglobin content.

hemolytic anemia An anemia caused by breakdown of the outer membrane of red blood cells and loss of their hemoglobin; occurs in vitamin E deficiency.

myelin Substance made of fat and protein that forms a fatty sheath around the nerve axons to protect and insulate the nerves and facilitate transmission of neuromuscular impulses.

BOX 6-5   FOOD SOURCES OF VITAMIN E

Food Source	Quantity	Vitamin E (mg)
Grains Group		
Fortified ready-to-eat cereal (e.g., Product 19; Total)	¾ to 1 cup	13.5
Rice Krispies	¼ cup	8.8
Cheerios	1 cup	0.2
Vegetable Group		
Spaghetti sauce, tomato	1 cup	6.3
Spinach, frozen, cooked	½ cup	3.4
Meat, Beans, Eggs, and Nuts Group		
Dry-roasted sunflower seeds	¼ cup	8.3
Peanut butter, smooth	2 tbsp	2.9
Sardines, canned	3 oz	1.7
Red kidney beans, canned	1 cup	0.1
Pinto beans	1 cup	1.3
Fats, Oils, and Sugar		
Corn oil	1 tbsp	2.1
Olive oil	1 tbsp	1.9
Safflower oil	1 tbsp	4.6

Data from U.S. Department of Agriculture, Agricultural Research Service: *USDA National Nutrient Database for Standard Reference, Release 26,* 2013. Nutrient Data Laboratory Home Page: <http://www.ars.usda.gov/ba/bhnrc/ndl>.
Images copyright 2006 JupiterImages Corporation.
Recommended Dietary Allowance for adults: 15 mg.

proteins are necessary for the formation of bone matrix and mineral deposition. Children with higher vitamin K intakes have higher bone mineral; however, we do not know if increasing vitamin K will protect against bone loss later in life.[37]

Vitamin K Deficiency and Clinical Applications
Neonatology

The sterile intestinal tract of the newborn cannot supply vitamin K during the first few days of life until normal bacterial flora develop. To prevent hemorrhage during this immediate postnatal period, a prophylactic dose of vitamin K is usually given soon after birth.

Malabsorption

Any defect in fat absorption impairs vitamin K absorption, resulting in slowed blood clotting; thus, several clinical situations demand supplemental vitamin K. Patients with bile duct obstruction are usually given vitamin K before surgery. Children with cystic fibrosis can become deficient, because

frequent use of antibiotics interferes with bacterial synthesis of this vitamin.[33]

Drug Therapy

Several drug-nutrient interactions involve vitamin K. Anticlotting drugs such as Coumadin (warfarin), Plavix (clopidogrel), or Aggrenox (dipyridamole and aspirin) act as **antimetabolites**, preventing the synthesis of blood-clotting

---

KEY TERMS

phylloquinone   A fat-soluble vitamin of the K group found in green plants or prepared synthetically.

menaquinone   Form of vitamin K synthesized by intestinal bacteria.

menadione   A water-soluble analog of vitamin K.

prothrombin   Blood-clotting factor synthesized in the liver and activated by vitamin K.

antimetabolites   Substances bearing a close structural resemblance to an essential nutrient or metabolite that interfere with its physiologic function or use.

factors in the liver and so inhibit the action of vitamin K. When these drugs are used to prevent unwanted clots in the lungs or blood vessels, dietary intake of vitamin K must be closely monitored. Too much vitamin K will oppose the action of the drug and neutralize its effect; too little vitamin K could lead to serious hemorrhage.[38,39] Dark-green leafy vegetables are rich in naturally occurring vitamin K, but other sources also need to be monitored. Snack foods made with Olestra, a noncaloric fat substitute, are fortified with 80 mcg of vitamin K per 1-oz serving, and vitamin K is added to many multivitamin supplements. With extended use of antibiotics much of the intestinal bacterial flora is lost, eliminating one of the body's main sources of vitamin K, and supplements may be required.

Vitamin K Requirement
Dietary Reference Intake
It is difficult to set a DRI for vitamin K because at least part of the requirement can be met by intestinal bacterial synthesis. Moreover, reliable information as to the vitamin K content of many foods or its bioavailability is lacking. With this in mind the expert committee established an AI rather than an RDA. For men ages 19 and older the AI is 120 mcg/day, and for women it is 90 mcg/day.[3] These values represent the median intakes of nearly 20,000 men and women who participated in national nutrition and health surveys between 1988 and 1994. This intake is adequate to preserve blood clotting, but the amount needed for optimum bone health is not known. Toxicity has not been reported.

Food Sources of Vitamin K
Phylloquinone is found in many vegetables but is highest in dark-green vegetables and liver. Menaquinones occur in milk, meat, and certain cheeses.[36] A list of good food sources can be found in Box 6-6.

Table 6-2 provides a complete summary of the fat-soluble vitamins.

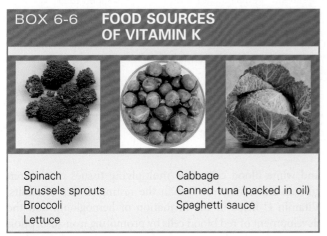

BOX 6-6 FOOD SOURCES OF VITAMIN K

Spinach
Brussels sprouts
Broccoli
Lettuce

Cabbage
Canned tuna (packed in oil)
Spaghetti sauce

Images copyright 2006 JupiterImages Corporation.
Adequate intake for adults: women, 90 mcg; men, 120 mcg.

WATER-SOLUBLE VITAMINS
VITAMIN C (ASCORBIC ACID)
Chemical and Physical Nature
The discovery of vitamin C is associated with the ancient hemorrhagic disease scurvy. Early observations of British sailors led to the detection of an acid in lemon juice that could prevent or cure this disease. Its chemical name *ascorbic acid* is based on its antiscorbutic properties. The structure of vitamin C is similar to glucose, and most animals can convert glucose to ascorbic acid. Humans, however, lack this enzyme. Therefore human scurvy could be called a *disease of distant genetic origin,* an inherited metabolic defect. Vitamin C is an unstable, easily oxidized acid. It is destroyed by oxygen, alkali, and heat.

Absorption, Transport, and Storage
Vitamin C is easily absorbed from the small intestine but requires an acid environment. When gastric hydrochloric acid is lacking, absorption is hindered. In contrast to the fat-soluble vitamins that are stored mostly in the liver, vitamin C is generally distributed throughout the body, maintaining limited tissue saturation. Any excess is excreted in the urine. The total body pool in adults varies from about 2 g to as little as 0.3 g, depending on intake.[26] Optimum tissue saturation can meet day-to-day needs for as long as 3 months when intake is lacking. This explains why generally healthy people in isolated living situations could survive the winter without eating fresh fruits and vegetables.

Breast milk provides sufficient vitamin C for early infancy if the mother is eating a good diet. Cow's milk contains very little vitamin C, as would be expected, because these animals have the enzymes to make their own vitamin C from glucose. Human infant formulas made from cow's milk are supplemented with ascorbic acid.

Functions of Vitamin C
Antioxidant Capacity
Vitamin C, along with vitamin E, is a powerful antioxidant. Vitamin C joins with free oxygen arising from cell metabolism, making it unavailable to fuel the destructive actions of free radicals.

Formation of Intercellular Cement
Vitamin C helps build and maintain many body tissues including bone matrix, cartilage, dentin, and collagen. Collagen is a protein found in the white fibers of connective tissue. When vitamin C is absent, an important ground substance is not formed and collagen fibers are defective and weak.[40] Blood vessels require this cementing substance to form firm capillary walls. In vitamin C deficiency capillaries are fragile and easily ruptured by blood pressure or trauma, and small hemorrhages occur in the skin and other tissues. When vitamin C is restored, the formation of normal collagen follows quickly.[40] Formation of collagen is also important for bone health, providing an appropriate matrix for the

TABLE 6-2   SUMMARY OF FAT-SOLUBLE VITAMINS

VITAMIN	PHYSIOLOGIC FUNCTIONS	RESULTS OF DEFICIENCY	DIETARY REFERENCE INTAKE	FOOD SOURCES
Vitamin A Provitamin: β-carotene Preformed vitamin: retinol	Production of rhodopsin and other light-receptor pigments Formation and maintenance of epithelial tissue Immune function Growth Reproduction Toxic in large amounts	Poor dark adaptation, night blindness, xerosis, xerophthalmia Keratinization of epithelium Growth failure Reproductive failure	Adults Males ages ≥19: 900 mcg RAE* Females ages ≥19: 700 mcg RAE Pregnancy Ages ≤18: 750 mcg RAE Ages ≥19: 770 mcg RAE Lactation Ages ≤18: 1200 mcg RAE Ages ≥19: 1300 mcg RAE	Butter; fortified margarine Whole, fortified low-fat, fortified reduced fat, and fortified nonfat cow's milk Fortified soy milk Dark green, deep yellow, and orange vegetables Yellow and orange fruits
Vitamin D Provitamins: ergosterol (plants); 7-dehydrocholesterol (skin) Vitamins: D₂ (ergocalciferol) and D₃ (cholecalciferol, used in food fortification)	Calcium and phosphorus absorption Calcitriol is major hormone regulator of bone mineral metabolism Possible roles in muscle function and control of cell growth Toxic in large amounts	Faulty bone growth, rickets (in children and youth), osteomalacia (in adults)	Adult males/females Ages 19-70: 15 mcg (600 IU) Ages ≥71: 20 mcg (800 IU) Pregnancy All ages: 15 mcg (600 IU) Lactation All ages: 15 mcg (600 IU)	Fortified cow's milk Fortified soy milk Fortified orange juice Fortified margarine Oily fish (e.g., salmon, tuna) Egg yolk Sunlight on the skin
Vitamin E Tocopherols Most active form is α-tocopherol	Antioxidant Protects cell membranes including red blood cell membranes Partners with selenium in antioxidant function	Anemia in premature infants Increased risk of oxidative damage to body tissues	Adult males/females Ages ≥19: 15 mg Pregnancy All ages: 15 mg Lactation All ages: 19 mg	Vegetable oils Fortified ready-to-eat cereals Nuts Dark green leafy vegetables Tomatoes/spaghetti sauce
Vitamin K K₁ (phylloquinone) K₂ (menaquinone) Analog: K₃ (menadione, water soluble)	Activates blood-clotting factors (e.g., converts prothrombin to thrombin) Participates in bone formation and remodeling (synthesis of osteocalcin) Interferes with anticoagulant therapy	Hemorrhagic disease of the newborn Defective blood clotting Deficiency symptoms produced by anticoagulant and antibiotic therapy	Adults Males ages ≥19: 120 mcg Females ages ≥19: 90 mcg Pregnancy Ages ≤18: 75 mcg Ages ≥19: 90 mcg Lactation Ages ≤18: 75 mcg Ages ≥19: 90 mcg	Green leafy vegetables Canned tuna Spaghetti sauce Synthesized by intestinal bacteria

*Retinol activity equivalent

deposition of bone minerals.[41] Box 6-7 lists common signs of vitamin C deficiency.

Support of General Body Metabolism

Vitamin C is found in greater amounts in metabolically active tissues such as the adrenal and pituitary glands, brain, eyes,

and white blood cells. The multiplying tissues of children contain more vitamin C than the resting tissues of adults. Vitamin C helps in the formation of hemoglobin and the development of red blood cells by promoting iron absorption and assisting in the removal of iron from the protein-iron complex called *ferritin*, in which it is stored.

Vitamin C participates in other functions of metabolic importance, as described below:

- Assists in the synthesis of carnitine, an amino acid that transports long-chain fatty acids into cell mitochondria where they are burned for energy.
- Assists in the synthesis of neurotransmitters such as norepinephrine and receptors for the neurotransmitter acetylcholine.
- Supports the action of the mixed-function oxidase system that metabolizes drugs and breaks down carcinogens and other foreign molecules; this system also sequesters lead and other heavy metals and neutralizes their effects.
- Controls the conversion of phenylalanine, an indispensable amino acid, to tyrosine, a conditionally indispensable amino acid; this is clinically important in children with phenylketonuria.

Clinical Applications

- *Wound healing:* The role of vitamin C in forming the cement for building supporting tissues creates added demands in traumatic injury or surgery when extensive tissue regeneration is required. Formulas for parenteral feeding generally provide 100 mg/day of vitamin C. Protocols for burn patients with elevated needs for tissue growth and defense against infection call for 1000 mg/day.[42]
- *Fever and infection:* The body's response to infection depletes tissue vitamin C stores. Fever adds to losses because it accompanies infection and produces a catabolic effect.
- *Growth:* Additional vitamin C is required during periods of rapid growth in infants and children. An adequate supply is critical in pregnancy to support fetal development and expansion of maternal tissues. Pregnant women who smoke may have elevated needs.[43]
- *Stress and body response:* Body stress arising from injury, illness, debilitating disease, or emotional upset calls on vitamin C stores. The adrenal glands, which have a primary role in stress response, contain large amounts of vitamin C.

Vitamin C Requirement
Dietary Reference Intake
The RDA for vitamin C is set at the level required to maintain tissue saturation and provide antioxidant protection of body cells and membranes. For men the RDA is 90 mg.[26] Based on their smaller body size the RDA for women is 75 mg. Cigarette smokers require an additional 35 mg. Additional vitamin is needed in pregnancy, lactation, and periods of growth.

Vitamin C Toxicity
Vitamin C intakes exceeding the recommended level have been promoted for curing the common cold, protecting against degenerative disease, and delaying the signs of aging. A survey of nearly 3000 breast cancer survivors found that 24% were taking daily supplements of 1000 mg or more.[50] Inappropriate supplement use could cause adverse interactions with ongoing drug therapy. The UL for ascorbic acid is set at 2000 mg; gastrointestinal symptoms and diarrhea have been observed at higher levels.[26]

Food Sources of Vitamin C
The best known sources of vitamin C are citrus fruits and tomatoes. Broccoli, salad greens, strawberries, watermelon, cabbage, and sweet potatoes are other good sources. Vitamin C is easily oxidized when exposed to the air or heated, so storage, preparation, and cooking methods must be chosen carefully to preserve vitamin content (Box 6-8). Vitamin C is quite stable in acid solutions, so citrus and tomato products remain good sources even if heated. Box 6-9 lists the vitamin C content of various foods. A summary of vitamin C functions and requirements is found in Table 6-3. (For tips on the proper handling of fresh fruits and vegetables, see the Focus on Food Safety box, "Did You Wash That Orange?")

FOCUS ON FOOD SAFETY
Did You Wash That Orange?
Oranges, apples, pears, grapes, bananas, and raw carrots are healthy snacks and travel well in a backpack or school bag. But all fresh produce must be washed before you eat or cook it to remove any remaining pesticides, soil particles, and bacteria that accumulated as it was picked, shipped, and handled in the store. Fruits and vegetables to be peeled still need to be washed. When your hands touch the unwashed banana peel, you will transfer those bacteria to the fruit as you peel it. It is also important to wash all "prewashed" vegetables and salad greens to be sure that all soil particles and bacteria have been removed.

BOX 6-7 SIGNS OF VITAMIN C DEFICIENCY
- Easy bruising
- Pinpoint hemorrhages of the skin (petechiae)
- Weak bones that fracture easily
- Poor wound healing
- Bleeding gums (often termed *gingivitis*)
- Anemia

KEY TERMS
scurvy A hemorrhagic disease caused by lack of vitamin C.
collagen Protein substance of the white fibers of skin, tendon, bone, cartilage, and other connective tissue.
parenteral A mode of feeding that does not use the gastrointestinal tract but instead provides nutrition by intravenous delivery of nutrient solutions.

BOX 6-8   FOOD PREPARATION METHODS TO PREVENT VITAMIN LOSS

Vitamins can be destroyed by heat, light, or the action of oxygen from the air. Water-soluble vitamins, especially vitamin C, are particularly vulnerable to such loss. The following storage and preparation practices help retain vitamins in fruits and vegetables:

- Store cut-up fruits and vegetables in the refrigerator in tightly covered containers that protect them from light and oxygen; when preparing fresh fruit or vegetables for salads or cooking, try to minimize the length of time they are exposed to the air.
- Avoid cutting fruits and vegetables into very small pieces; this increases the surface area for nutrient loss.
- Cook vegetables for a *limited* amount of time in a *limited* amount of water in a tightly covered pan to retain nutrients, flavor, color, and texture. (Vegetables should be tender but still retain their shape.)

- Steam vegetables in a steamer basket with the water below to prevent the dissolving of nutrients into the water; vegetables need not be covered with water as the steam in the covered container will soften the food.
- Use the microwave to reduce the time and amount of water needed for cooking, but avoid overcooking. Remember that foods continue to cook for several minutes after being removed from the microwave.
- Stir-fry vegetables using only a small amount of fat to conserve nutrients and food quality.
- Fruits and vegetables add color and variety to meals, along with important nutrients. Include both raw and cooked vegetables to add interest to menus.

BOX 6-9   FOOD SOURCES OF VITAMIN C

Food Source	Amount	Vitamin C (mg)
Vegetable Group		
Tomato soup, canned, water added	1 cup	15
Vegetable juice cocktail	1 cup	72
Pepper, chili, red	1	65
Peppers, sweet, green, chopped	½ cup	60
Peppers, sweet, red, chopped	½ cup	95
Broccoli, cooked	½ cup	50
Cole slaw,	1 cup	28
Sweet potato, canned, vacuumed packed	½ cup	34
Cauliflower, frozen, cooked	½ cup	28
Fruit Group		
Strawberries	1 cup	98
Orange juice, frozen, reconstituted	1 cup	97
Grape juice, fortified	1 cup	63
Orange	1 medium	63
Cantaloupe	⅛ melon	25
Watermelon	1 wedge (4 × 8 inches)	23
Other		
Fruit punch, fortified	1 cup	73

Data from U.S. Department of Agriculture, Agricultural Research Service: *USDA National Nutrient Database for Standard Reference, Release 26,* 2013. Nutrient Data Laboratory Home Page: <http://www.ars.usda.gov/ba/bhnrc/ndl>.
Images copyright 2006 JupiterImages Corporation.
Recommended Dietary Allowances for adults: women, 75 mg; men, 90 mg.

TABLE 6-3 SUMMARY OF VITAMIN C (ASCORBIC ACID)

PHYSIOLOGIC FUNCTIONS	CLINICAL APPLICATIONS	DIETARY REFERENCE INTAKE	FOOD SOURCES
Antioxidant activity	Wound healing	Adults	Citrus fruits and berries
Collagen synthesis	Tissue formation	Males ages ≥19: 90 mg	Vegetables: broccoli, cabbage,
General metabolism	Fevers and infections	Females ages ≥19: 75 mg	chili peppers, potatoes,
Makes iron available for	Stress reactions	Pregnancy	tomatoes
hemoglobin synthesis	Growth	Ages ≤18: 80 mg	
Controls conversion of the	Scurvy (classic deficiency	Ages ≥19: 85 mg	
amino acid phenylalanine	disease)	Lactation	
to tyrosine		Ages ≤18: 115 mg	
		Ages ≥19: 120 mg	

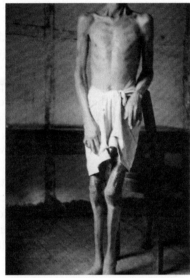

FIGURE 6-6 Beriberi is a thiamin-deficiency disease characterized by extreme weakness, paralysis, and wasting related to the inability to metabolize glucose for energy. (From McLaren DS: *A colour atlas and text of diet-related disorders,* ed 2, London, 1992, Mosby-Year Book Europe Limited.)

THE B VITAMINS

DEFICIENCY DISEASES AND VITAMIN DISCOVERIES

The discovery of the B vitamins is a story of people dying of a puzzling, age-old disease for which no cure existed. Eventually it was learned that common, everyday food held the answer. The paralyzing disease was beriberi, which plagued East Asia for centuries (Figure 6-6). It was named by the native words, *I can't, I can't,* which described its crippling effects. The "vitamine" connection was established when an American chemist, R.R. Williams, used extracts of rice polishings to cure the epidemic infantile beriberi. The food factor that brought the cure was labeled *water-soluble B,* because it was thought to be a single vitamin. Now we know several vitamins exist in the B group, all water-soluble but with unique metabolic functions. Each of the B vitamins has been given a specific chemical name.

COENZYME ROLE

The B vitamins have important metabolic roles as coenzyme partners with cell enzymes that control energy metabolism and build tissue. Eight vitamins are in this group. First we consider the three associated with classic deficiency diseases—thiamin, riboflavin, and niacin; then the more recently discovered coenzyme factors—pantothenic acid, biotin, and pyridoxine (vitamin B_6); and, finally, the important blood-forming factors—folate and vitamin B_{12} (cobalamin).

THIAMIN

The search for the cause of beriberi was successfully concluded with the identification of thiamin. Its nature and metabolic role were clarified in the early 1930s.

Chemical and Physical Nature

Thiamin is a water-soluble and fairly stable vitamin, although it is destroyed in alkaline solutions. Its name comes from its chemical ring-like structure.

Absorption, Transport, and Storage

Thiamin is absorbed most efficiently in the acid environment of the upper small intestine before the food mass is buffered by the alkaline fluids entering from the pancreas. Thiamin is not stored in large amounts, so a continuous dietary supply is needed.[51] Tissue thiamin responds rapidly to increased metabolic demand such as occurs in fever, high muscular activity, pregnancy, and lactation. Tissue stores depend on both thiamin intake and general diet composition. Carbohydrate increases the need for thiamin, whereas fat and protein spare thiamin. When the tissues are saturated, unused thiamin is excreted in the urine.

KEY TERMS

beriberi A disease of the peripheral nerves caused by thiamin deficiency.

pantothenic acid A member of the B vitamin complex widely distributed in nature and throughout body tissues; it functions as a part of coenzyme A (CoA), important in lipid and carbohydrate metabolism.

Function of Thiamin
Coenzyme Role
Thiamin functions as a control agent in energy metabolism. When combined with phosphorus to form thiamin pyrophosphate (TPP), it serves as a coenzyme in reactions involving glucose. About 90% of body thiamin is in the coenzyme form.[51] The symptoms of beriberi can be traced to the loss of energy usually provided by glucose metabolism.

Thiamin Deficiency and Clinical Applications
When thiamin levels are insufficient to support cellular energy metabolism, clinical effects become apparent, as follows:

- *Gastrointestinal system:* Anorexia, constipation, gastric atony, and poor hydrochloric acid secretion progress as the deficiency continues. When the cells of the smooth muscles and the secretory glands do not receive enough energy from glucose, they cannot perform the digestive work needed to supply still more glucose to meet body needs. This vicious cycle accelerates as the deficiency continues.
- *Nervous system:* The CNS depends on glucose to do its work. Without sufficient thiamin to provide this constant fuel, nerve activity is impaired, alertness and reflex responses are diminished, and general apathy and fatigue take over. If the deficiency continues, then lipogenesis is hindered, followed by damage to the myelin sheaths, which is the lipid tissue covering the nerve fibers. This causes increasing nerve irritation, pain, and prickly or deadening sensations. If unchecked, then paralysis will result as in the classic deficiency disease beriberi.
- *Cardiovascular system:* The heart muscle weakens, leading to cardiac failure and edema of the lower extremities.
- *Musculoskeletal system:* Inadequate TPP in muscle tissue results in widespread chronic pain that responds to thiamin therapy.

Thiamin status is evaluated by the activity of a TPP-dependent enzyme transketolase found in red blood cells. This is a common test to determine whether a clinical observation is related to thiamin deficiency or another cause.

Thiamin Requirement
Dietary Reference Intake
The thiamin requirement is based on energy intake with a minimum of 0.3 mg of thiamin/1000 kcal. To provide a margin of safety the RDA is set at 1.2 mg for men and 1.1 mg for women.[51] Additional thiamin is needed during pregnancy and lactation. Because the kidneys excrete excess thiamin, there are no reports of toxicity arising from oral doses up to 50 mg. No UL has been established.

Clinical Applications
Several conditions influence thiamin needs:
- *Alcohol abuse:* Thiamin is important when planning nutritional intervention for patients with alcohol problems.[51] Both a primary deficiency (an inadequate diet) and a conditioned deficiency (the effect of alcohol) contribute to thiamin malnutrition and, over time, serious neurologic disorders. Alcohol interferes with the active absorption of thiamin resulting in rapid depletion of tissue stores.
- *Acute illness or disease:* Fever and infection increase energy requirements and the need for thiamin. Patients on hemodialysis lose thiamin and require supplementation to prevent deficiency.
- *Normal growth and development:* Thiamin needs increase in pregnancy and lactation to meet the demands of rapid fetal growth, the elevated metabolic rate of pregnancy, and milk production. Continuing growth throughout infancy, childhood, and adolescence requires attention to thiamin intake. At any point in the life cycle, the larger the body and its tissue mass, the greater are the cellular energy requirements and need for thiamin.
- *Cardiovascular function:* Various diuretics used to manage hypertension and cardiac failure promote urinary loss of thiamin and increase the thiamin requirement.[21] If thiamin intake is low, then these patients can develop a thiamin deficiency that worsens their cardiac symptoms. The B vitamins might work together in supporting cardiac and circulatory function, as thiamin, riboflavin, and folate intakes were found to be inversely associated with systolic blood pressure.[52]
- *Gastric bypass surgery:* Thiamin supplementation is likely to be necessary after gastric bypass surgery because energy intake is drastically reduced and absorption less efficient. Thiamin deficiency may play a role in the neurologic and CNS complications that sometimes occur following bariatric surgery.[53]

Food Sources of Thiamin
Thiamin is widespread in plant and animal foods, although the amount found in individual foods is usually small. As a result intakes can be low when kilocalories (kcalories or kcal) are markedly curtailed. Major sources in the American diet are whole grain and enriched breads, ready-to-eat cereals, and legumes. Lean pork and beef are also good sources. Thiamin is extremely water soluble and readily lost in cooking water (review Box 6-8). Box 6-10 lists foods containing thiamin.

RIBOFLAVIN

Discovery
In 1897 a London chemist observed in milk whey a water-soluble pigment with a peculiar yellow-green fluorescence. However, it was not until 1932 that researchers in Germany actually discovered riboflavin.[54] This vitamin was given the chemical name *flavin* from the Latin word for yellow. Later,

---

KEY TERM
thiamin pyrophosphate (TPP) Active coenzyme form of thiamin needed for carbohydrate metabolism.

BOX 6-10 FOOD SOURCES OF THIAMIN

Food Source	Amount	Thiamin (mg)
Grains Group		
Ready-to-eat cereals		
Product 19	1 cup	1.50
Total Raisin Bran	1 cup	1.48
Rice Krispies	1¼ cup	0.51
Wheaties	1 cup	0.76
Corn flakes	1 cup	0.38
Instant oatmeal	1 packet	0.46
Rice, white, long grain, cooked, enriched	1 cup	0.34
Pancake, frozen, ready to eat	3 in	0.25
Bagel, enriched	3 in	0.42
Macaroni/spaghetti, enriched	1 cup	0.38
Hamburger roll, enriched	1	0.28
Bread, white, enriched	1 slice	0.13
Vegetable Group		
Green peas, frozen, cooked	½ cup	0.23
Potatoes, mashed, prepared from instant flakes	½ cup	0.10
Tomato juice, canned	1 cup	0.11
Fruit Group		
Orange juice, frozen, reconstituted	1 cup	0.20
Grapes (red or green)	1 cup	0.11
Meat, Beans, Eggs, and Nuts Group		
Pork, roasted, lean	3 oz	0.47
Ham, baked, lean	3 oz	0.58
Kidney beans, cooked	1 cup	0.28
Baked beans, canned, plain or vegetarian	1 cup	0.24
Milk Group		
Milk, 3.5% fat, 2% fat, or nonfat (may vary slightly)	1 cup	0.11

Data from U.S. Department of Agriculture, Agricultural Research Service: *USDA National Nutrient Database for Standard Reference, Release 26,* 2013. Nutrient Data Laboratory Home Page: <http://www.ars.usda.gov/ba/bhnrc/ndl>.
Images copyright 2006 JupiterImages Corporation.
Recommended Dietary Allowances for adults: women, 1.1 mg; men, 1.2 mg.

when it was found to contain a sugar called *ribose*, the name *riboflavin* was officially adopted.

Chemical and Physical Nature

Riboflavin is a yellow-green fluorescent pigment that forms yellowish-brown, needlelike crystals. It is water soluble and relatively heat stable but easily destroyed by light and irradiation.

Absorption, Transport, and Storage

Riboflavin is easily absorbed in the upper small intestine. Bulk fiber supplements such as psyllium, especially when taken with milk or near mealtimes, can hinder riboflavin absorption and contribute to deficiency. Body stores are limited, although small amounts are found in the liver and kidney. Day-to-day tissue needs must be supplied in the diet.

Functions of Riboflavin
Coenzyme Role

Riboflavin is a part of the cell enzymes called *flavoproteins*. These enzymes—flavin mononucleotide (FMN) and flavin adenine dinucleotide (FAD)—are integral to both energy metabolism and deamination. Deamination is the removal of a nitrogen-containing amino group from an existing amino acid so that a new amino acid can be formed. Accordingly, riboflavin is active in both energy production and tissue building.

Riboflavin Deficiency and Clinical Applications

Riboflavin deficiency leads to the condition termed ariboflavinosis. This includes a combination of clinical signs that center on tissue inflammation and breakdown and poor healing of even minor injuries (Box 6-11 and Figure 6-7). Tissues subject to persistent abrasion that require continual replacement, such as the cells in the corners of the mouth, are affected first. Riboflavin deficiency seldom occurs alone but rather develops in combination with other B vitamin deficits. Because riboflavin is light sensitive, infants with elevated blood levels of bilirubin who are treated with phototherapy may require additional riboflavin.

Riboflavin Requirement
Dietary Reference Intake

The RDA for riboflavin is based on the amount needed to sustain optimal levels of the flavoprotein enzymes. Recommended intakes are 1.3 mg/day for adolescent and adult men

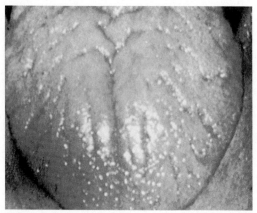

FIGURE 6-7 Glossitis resulting from riboflavin deficiency. (From McLaren DS: *A colour atlas and text of diet-related disorders*, ed 2, London, 1992, Mosby-Year Book Europe Limited.)

and 1.1 mg/day for adolescent and adult women.[51] The higher level for men relates to their higher kcalorie intakes and larger body size. No UL has been set for riboflavin, but supplements exceeding the RDA still carry risk.

Populations at Risk

Certain groups have special needs. Patients on hemodialysis must replace the riboflavin lost in the dialysate fluids.[51] Pregnant and lactating women and infants and children are at risk of riboflavin deficiency based on their rapid tissue growth and high energy and protein metabolism. People who engage in regular physical activity seem to have a greater need for riboflavin, likely related to increased energy expenditure and muscle maintenance and repair.[55] Individuals who are lactose intolerant and avoid milk may be low in riboflavin.

Food Sources of Riboflavin

Major sources of riboflavin are milk and cheese. One quart of cow's milk or fortified soy milk contains 2 mg of riboflavin, more than the daily requirement. Because riboflavin is destroyed by exposure to ultraviolet light, milk is usually packaged in cardboard or opaque plastic containers. Nursing mothers who store breast milk need to be reminded of potential riboflavin losses from glass containers. Other good sources of riboflavin are meat, whole or enriched grains and ready-to-eat cereals, and vegetables. Riboflavin is stable to heat and not easily destroyed with proper cooking. Box 6-12 describes some food sources of riboflavin.

NIACIN

The age-old disease related to niacin is pellagra. It is characterized by a typical dermatitis and eventually leads to fatal effects on the nervous system.[56] Pellagra was first observed in 18th-century Europe and was common in the southern region of the United States in the early 1900s among families whose diet was largely based on corn. The American physician Joseph Goldberger noticed that children who did not have pellagra had higher intakes of meat and milk. His investigation established that pellagra was related to a food factor, not an infectious organism. However, it was not until 1937 that a researcher at the University of Wisconsin associated niacin with pellagra by using it to cure a related disease—black tongue—in dogs.

BOX 6-11   SIGNS OF RIBOFLAVIN DEFICIENCY

- Lips become swollen and cracked with characteristic cracks at the corners of the mouth (**cheilosis**).
- Nasal angles develop cracks and irritation.
- Tongue becomes swollen and reddened (**glossitis**) (see Figure 6-7).
- Extra blood vessels develop in the cornea (corneal vascularization).
- Eyes burn, itch, and tear.
- Skin becomes greasy and scaly, especially in skinfolds (**seborrheic dermatitis**).

KEY TERMS

ariboflavinosis   Group of clinical manifestations of riboflavin deficiency.
cheilosis   Cracks and scaly lesions on the lips and mouth resulting from riboflavin deficiency.
glossitis   Swollen, reddened tongue; symptom of riboflavin deficiency.
seborrheic dermatitis   Greasy scales and crusts that appear on the skin and moist folds of the body in riboflavin deficiency.

BOX 6-12 FOOD SOURCES OF RIBOFLAVIN

Food Source	Amount	Riboflavin (mg)
Grains Group		
Ready-to-eat cereals		
Product 19	1 cup	1.71
Wheaties	¾ cup	0.84
Rice Krispies	1¼ cup	0.43
Corn flakes	1 cup	0.43
Instant oatmeal	1 packet	0.38
Waffle, frozen, ready to eat	1	0.23
Bagel	3½ in	0.18
Rice, white, long grain, enriched, cooked	1 cup	0.03
Bread, white, enriched	1 slice	0.06
Vegetable Group		
Spinach, frozen, cooked	½ cup	0.17
Broccoli, cooked	½ cup	0.10
Meat, Beans, Eggs, and Nuts Group		
Pork, lean, braised	3 oz	0.23
Egg, hard-cooked	1	0.23
Turkey, dark meat, roasted	3 oz	0.32
Kidney beans, canned	1 cup	0.17
Baked beans, canned, plain or vegetarian	1 cup	0.10
Milk Group		
Yogurt, low fat, with fruit	1 cup	0.40
Milk, 2% fat, 1% fat, nonfat	1 cup	0.42
Pudding, instant, chocolate	½ cup	0.22
Cottage cheese, low fat	½ cup	0.22

Data from U.S. Department of Agriculture, Agricultural Research Service: *USDA National Nutrient Database for Standard Reference, Release 26*, 2013. Nutrient Data Laboratory Home Page: <http://www.ars.usda.gov/ba/bhnrc/ndl>.
Images copyright 2006 JupiterImages Corporation.
Recommended Dietary Allowances for adults: women, 1.1 mg; men, 1.3 mg.

Chemical and Physical Nature

Niacin exists in two forms: (1) nicotinic acid and (2) nicotinamide. Nicotinic acid is easily converted to nicotinamide, which is water soluble, stable to acid and heat, and forms a white powder when crystallized.

Niacin also bears a close connection to the essential amino acid tryptophan, as described below:

• *Precursor role of tryptophan:* Curious observations by early researchers raised puzzling questions. Why was pellagra rare in some populations whose diets were low in niacin but common in others whose diets were higher in niacin? Why did milk, which is low in niacin, cure or prevent pellagra? Why was pellagra so common in families subsisting on diets high in corn? Then came the key discovery—tryptophan can be used by the body to make niacin. In

other words, tryptophan is a precursor of niacin. Milk prevents pellagra because it is high in tryptophan. A corn-based diet results in pellagra because it is low in both tryptophan and niacin, but this depends on how the corn is prepared. In the American South, where corn was eaten as a vegetable or made into corn bread or corn meal, the bound niacin present in corn could not be released and absorbed. In Mexican families who soaked corn in lime (alkali) when preparing tortillas, pellagra was rare because the lime treatment released the bound niacin so it was able to be absorbed.[56] Others with diets low in niacin escaped pellagra because they had adequate intakes of animal protein that supplied tryptophan.

• Niacin equivalent (NE): The tryptophan-niacin relation led to the development of the unit of measure called a *niacin equivalent (NE).* In general, 60 mg of tryptophan can produce 1 mg of niacin, the amount designated as the NE. This is the unit used in the DRI for niacin.[51]

Functions of Niacin

Coenzyme Role

Niacin has two coenzyme forms: (1) nicotinamide-adenine dinucleotide (NAD) and (2) nicotinamide-adenine dinucleotide phosphate (NADP). In these forms, niacin partners with riboflavin in the cellular enzyme systems that convert amino acids and glycerol to glucose and then oxidize the glucose to release energy. (Recall that glycerol is obtained from the hydrolysis of triglycerides.)

Use as a Drug

Pharmacologic doses of nicotinic acid have been prescribed for cardiovascular patients in an effort to raise blood high-density lipoprotein (HDL) cholesterol levels and lower low-density lipoprotein (LDL) cholesterol and triglyceride levels. However, at therapeutic levels of 50 to 3000 mg (the RDA is 14 to 16 mg) nicotinic acid acts as a vasodilator, causing skin flushing and itching. Harmful side effects can include gastrointestinal upset, hyperglycemia, and liver damage, so patients treated with these doses require constant medical supervision (see Chapter 21).[56,57]

Niacin Deficiency and Clinical Applications

Niacin deficiency and pellagra result in muscle weakness, anorexia, and indigestion. More specific symptoms involve the skin and nervous system, and skin areas exposed to sunlight develop a dark, scaly dermatitis (Figure 6-8). If the

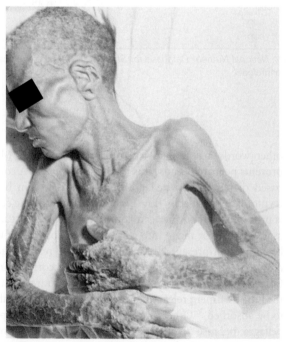

FIGURE 6-8 Pellagra is caused by niacin deficiency. (From McLaren DS: *A colour atlas and text of diet-related disorders,* ed 2, London, 1992, Mosby-Year Book Europe Limited.)

deficiency continues, then deterioration of the CNS leads to confusion, disorientation, neuritis, and finally death.

Niacin Requirement
Dietary Reference Intake

The current RDAs are 16 mg NE/day for adolescent and adult men and 14 mg NE/day for adolescent and adult women.[51] These recommendations allow for gender differences in energy intake and body size, as well as the availability and relative efficiency of converting tryptophan to niacin. Rapid growth, pregnancy, lactation, physical activity, or the need to replace tissues after surgery or trauma increases the need for niacin.

Food Sources of Niacin

Meat and dairy products are major sources of niacin and are also high in tryptophan. Other foods include peanuts, dried beans and peas, and whole-grain or enriched breads and ready-to-eat cereals. Corn and rice are relatively poor sources because they are low in tryptophan. Box 6-13 lists some comparative food sources of niacin.

PANTOTHENIC ACID

Discovery

Pantothenic acid is found in all living things and participates in many body functions.[51] Intestinal bacteria synthesize considerable amounts. This source, along with its occurrence in a wide variety of foods, makes pantothenic acid deficiency unlikely.

Chemical and Physical Nature

Pantothenic acid is a white crystalline compound. It is readily absorbed in the small intestine and combines with phosphorus to make the active molecule acetyl coenzyme A (CoA). In this form, pantothenic acid has broad metabolic presence and use throughout the body. No known toxicity or natural deficiency exists.

Functions of Pantothenic Acid

As an essential constituent of CoA, pantothenic acid controls metabolic reactions involving carbohydrate, fat, and protein.[51]

Pantothenic Acid Requirements

The AI of 5 mg/day for all adults will replace the pantothenic acid lost daily in the urine. No UL exists for this nutrient.[51]

Food Sources of Pantothenic Acid

Pantothenic acid is found in both plant and animal foods. Good sources include egg yolk, milk, and broccoli.

> **KEY TERM**
> **niacin equivalent (NE)** A measure of the total dietary sources of niacin; 1 NE equals 1 mg of niacin or 60 mg of tryptophan.

BOX 6-13 FOOD SOURCES OF NIACIN

Food Source	Amount	Niacin (mg NE)*
Grains Group		
Ready-to-eat cereals		
Product 19	1 cup	20.0
Wheaties	1 cup	10.1
Rice Krispies	1¼ cup	5.9
Corn flakes	1 cup	5.0
Instant oatmeal	1 packet	5.4
Bagel, enriched	3 in	2.8
Spaghetti, enriched	1 cup	2.4
Bread, white, enriched	1 slice	1.2
Vegetable Group		
Spaghetti sauce, no meat	1 cup	10.3
Potato, baked, flesh only	1 medium	2.2
Sweet potato, baked	1 medium	1.7
Meat, Beans, Eggs, and Nuts Group		
Chicken breast, roasted	½	11.8
Tuna, light, canned in water	3 oz	8.6
Haddock, baked	3 oz	3.5
Beef, ground meat patty	3 oz	4.9
Peanuts, dry roasted	1 oz (about 28)	3.8

Data from U.S. Department of Agriculture, Agricultural Research Service: *USDA National Nutrient Database for Standard Reference, Release 26*, 2013. Nutrient Data Laboratory Home Page: <http://www.ars.usda.gov/ba/bhnrc/ndl>.
Images copyright 2006 JupiterImages Corporation.
Recommended Dietary Allowances for adults: women, 14 mg NE; men, 16 mg NE.
*1 mg NE (Niacin Equivalent) = 1 mg niacin or 60 mg tryptophan.

BIOTIN

General Nature of Biotin

Biotin is a sulfur-containing vitamin, and the minute traces in the body perform multiple metabolic tasks. Natural deficiency is unknown; however, induced deficiencies have occurred in patients on long-term parenteral nutrition that omitted biotin. The protein avidin found in raw egg white binds biotin and, if consumed regularly, induces biotin deficiency. Cooking denatures this protein and destroys its ability to combine with biotin. (Raw eggs also carry the risk of food-borne illness that can be fatal to young children, older adults, and those with compromised immune function.) No known toxicity exists for biotin.

Functions of Biotin

Biotin functions as a partner with CoA in reactions that transfer carbon dioxide (CO_2) from one compound to another. Examples of this cofactor at work include (1) the synthesis of fatty acids, (2) the synthesis of amino acids,

and (3) CO_2 fixation to form purines for making genetic material.

Biotin Requirement

Because the amount of biotin needed is so small, the AI for this nutrient is 30 mcg/day for all adults.[51] Intestinal bacterial synthesis adds to the body's supply.

Food Sources of Biotin

Biotin is found in many foods, but its bioavailability varies greatly. The biotin in corn and soy is well absorbed, whereas the biotin in wheat is almost totally unavailable. Excellent food sources include egg yolk, liver, tomatoes, and yeast.

VITAMIN B₆ (PYRIDOXINE)

Chemical and Physical Nature

The chemical structure of vitamin B_6 is a pyridine ring, which accounts for its name. It is water soluble and heat stable but sensitive to light and alkali.

Forms

Vitamin B₆ is the generic term for the three forms of this vitamin found in nature: (1) pyridoxine, (2) pyridoxal, and (3) pyridoxamine. All three forms are equally active as precursors of the coenzyme pyridoxal phosphate (B_6–PO_4), or PLP.[51]

Absorption, Transport, and Storage

Vitamin B_6 is well absorbed in the upper segment of the small intestine. It is stored in muscle but found in tissues throughout the body, evidence of its many metabolic activities involving protein.

Functions of Vitamin B₆
Coenzyme in Protein Metabolism

In its active phosphate form (PLP), vitamin B_6 is a coenzyme in more than 100 amino acid reactions involving the synthesis of important proteins. Examples include the following:

- *Neurotransmitters:* PLP is needed to convert the essential amino acid tryptophan to serotonin, which carries messages across the cells in the brain; it helps to form γ-aminobutyric acid (GABA) found in the gray matter of the brain.
- *Amino group transfer:* PLP transfers nitrogen-containing amino groups from amino acids to form new amino acids and release carbon residues for energy.
- *Niacin:* PLP controls formation of niacin from tryptophan.
- *Hemoglobin:* PLP incorporates amino acids into heme, the nonprotein core of hemoglobin.
- *Immune function:* PLP participates in the production and release of antibodies and immune cells.

Coenzyme in Fat Metabolism

PLP converts the essential fatty acid linoleic acid to arachidonic acid.

Vitamin B₆ Deficiency and Clinical Applications

Vitamin B_6 is key in a number of clinical situations:

- *Anemia:* A lack of vitamin B_6 interrupts heme formation, resulting in a hypochromic anemia. This occurs despite a ready supply of iron and is reversed when vitamin B_6 is restored.
- *CNS abnormalities:* Vitamin B_6 controls brain function through its role in the formation of serotonin and GABA. When a batch of commercial infant formula was mistakenly heated to a very high temperature, destroying the vitamin B_6, babies fed this formula experienced increasing irritability progressing to convulsions. Immediate supplementation with vitamin B_6 restored their normal function. Certain forms of seizures occurring in patients deficient in this vitamin responded to treatment with vitamin B_6.[58] Appropriate vitamin B_6 status supports cognitive function in older adults.[59]
- *Physiologic demands in pregnancy:* Vitamin B_6 deficiency has been identified in mothers with preeclampsia (hypertension with edema and proteinuria) and eclampsia (convulsions).[51] Growth of the fetus along with rising metabolic needs of the mother increase the need for this vitamin.
- *Chronic disease:* Patients in end-stage renal disease undergoing hemodialysis require vitamin B_6 supplements to maintain normal blood levels.[64]
- *Medications:* The drug isoniazid (isonicotinic acid hydrazide [INH]) used to treat tuberculosis is a vitamin B_6 antagonist; vitamin B_6 intakes of 50 to 100 mg/day are needed to overcome this effect. Levodopa, a medication for Parkinson's disease, lowers blood PLP levels.[51] Oral contraceptive users have low PLP levels despite intakes equal to or exceeding the RDA, putting them at risk of poor vitamin status in a future pregnancy.[65]

Vitamin B₆ Requirement
Dietary Reference Intake

The RDA is expected to maintain optimum blood PLP levels in most individuals,[51] although relatively high protein intakes increase the need for vitamin B_6. Men and women ages 19 to 50 should take in 1.3 mg/day. Older adults require higher amounts, and older men need more than older women. For men older than age 50 the RDA is 1.7 mg/day; for women of this age it is 1.5 mg/day. Smokers may require higher amounts than nonsmokers.[66]

Vitamin B₆ Toxicity

Vitamin B_6 is one of the two water-soluble vitamins, along with vitamin C, with a demonstrated and physiologically deleterious toxicity. Vitamin B_6 toxicity was reported in women taking supplements 1000 times the RDA in the belief that such a dose would alleviate premenstrual syndrome. Such intakes interfere with muscle coordination and over time damage the nervous system.[51] Fortunately for these women the symptoms gradually disappeared after the supplements were discontinued. The UL for vitamin B_6 is 100 mg/day.

Food Sources of Vitamin B₆

Vitamin B_6 is widespread among many foods but usually in rather small amounts. Good sources include whole grains, legumes, meat, poultry, bananas, and potatoes. Enriched and fortified breads and cereals are major contributors of vitamin B_6 in the United States.[67] Box 6-14 displays some food sources of this vitamin.

FOLATE

Discovery

Folates were first extracted from dark leafy vegetables and given the name *folic acid* from the Latin word for *leaf.* Studies investigating anemia among poor pregnant Indian women led to the discovery of this vitamin group.[51]

Chemical and Physical Nature

Folic acid, a yellow crystal, has the chemical name of *pteroylmonoglutamic acid* based on its structure. Folic acid is seldom found naturally but is the form used in supplements and fortified foods. Naturally occurring folate or food folate is the compound pteroylpolyglutamate, which contains additional glutamic acid molecules.[51] Both forms are well used by the body.

Absorption, Transport, and Storage

The absorption of folate depends on the source. About 50% of the folate occurring naturally in plant foods (food folate) is absorbed, compared with 85% of the folic acid added to fortified foods. Conversion factors have been developed for calculating folate intake (Box 6-15).[68]

BOX 6-14 FOOD SOURCES OF VITAMIN B₆ (PYRIDOXINE)

Vitamin B_6 (pyridoxine) is found in both plant and animal foods, although the milk group has low amounts. Ready-to-eat cereals, potatoes, and poultry are especially good sources.

Food Source	Amount	Vitamin B_6 (mg)
Grains Group		
Corn flakes	1 cup	0.50
Instant oatmeal	1 packet	0.51
Vegetable Group		
Potato, baked, flesh only	1 medium	0.47
Spaghetti sauce, tomato, no meat	1 cup	0.46
Fruit Group		
Banana	1	0.43
Meat, Beans, Eggs, and Nuts Group		
Chicken breast, roasted	½	0.52
Tuna, light, canned, packed in water	3 oz	0.27
Beef, ground beef patty	3 oz	0.31
Baked beans, canned, plain or vegetarian	1 cup	0.21

Data from U.S. Department of Agriculture, Agricultural Research Service: *USDA National Nutrient Database for Standard Reference, Release 26*, 2013. Nutrient Data Laboratory Home Page: <http://www.ars.usda.gov/ba/bhnrc/ndl>.
Images copyright 2006 JupiterImages Corporation.
Recommended Dietary Allowances for adults: men and women, ages 19-50, 1.3 mg; women, ages ≥51, 1.5 mg; men, ages ≥51, 1.7 mg.

Functions of Folate
Coenzyme Role

Folate is the coenzyme that attaches single carbons to metabolic compounds. Several key molecules provide examples, as follows:

- *Purines:* Nitrogen-containing compounds in genetic material that participate in cell division and the transmission of inherited traits.
- *Thymine:* A component of DNA, the material in the cell nucleus that controls and transmits genetic characteristics.
- *Hemoglobin:* Heme is the iron-containing nonprotein portion of hemoglobin that transports oxygen and CO_2 in the blood.

Folate Deficiency and Clinical Applications
Anemia

A nutritional **megaloblastic anemia** occurs in simple folate deficiency. Because folate needs are high during periods of rapid growth, folate deficiency anemia is most likely to occur in pregnant women, growing infants, and young children. Adolescent girls who severely limit their food intake are also at risk.

Presence of Gastric Acid

An acid environment is required to release food folate from its food source and enable its absorption. Low hydrochloric acid secretion in the stomach, a common problem in older people, or use of medications that raise the pH in the gastrointestinal tract adversely affect folate status.[69]

BOX 6-15 CALCULATING DIETARY FOLATE EQUIVALENTS

- 1 mcg of food folate (occurring naturally in a food) = 1 dietary folate equivalent (DFE).
- 1 mcg folic acid (added in food fortification) = 1.7 mcg DFE (Folic acid added to a food is absorbed more efficiently than naturally occurring food folate.)

To estimate the DFEs in foods such as fortified breakfast cereals in which most or all of the folate is added folic acid, use the percentage daily value listed on the food label:

% Daily value × 400 mcg (the daily value for folic acid) × 1.7 = DFEs per serving

Data from Suitor CW, Bailey LB: Dietary folate equivalents: interpretation and application. *J Am Diet Assoc* 100:88, 2000.

KEY TERMS
antagonist A substance that acts in opposition to another physiologic substance preventing its normal action; vitamin antagonists prevent the usual action of the vitamin.
megaloblastic anemia Anemia characterized by abnormally large immature red blood cells; occurs in vitamin B_{12} or folate deficiency.

Medications

The drug amethopterin (methotrexate) used in cancer treatment is a folate antagonist and prevents the synthesis of DNA and purines, thereby preventing the growth of the cancer. High intakes of folate interfere with the action of the drug phenobarbital used to control seizures.[51]

Folate and Birth Defects

Neural tube defects (NTDs), a worldwide vitamin-related problem, are congenital abnormalities occurring when the spinal cord and its coverings fail to develop normally. If part of the brain fails to develop (anencephaly), then the infant is likely to die shortly after birth. The more common NTD is spina bifida, in which the neural tube fails to close during embryonic development and the spinal cord remains on the outside of the body (Figure 6-9). In less severe cases a child may live a productive life if surgical and medical intervention is effective, but for many a normal life is not achievable.

Folate is essential for the formation and closure of the neural tube in the early weeks of fetal development (between day 21 and day 28 of gestation), before a woman is even aware that she might be pregnant. Therefore it is critical that a mother be in good folate status *before* conception occurs. In 1998, to combat this problem, the U.S. Food and Drug Administration (FDA) instituted a mandatory folate fortification program requiring the addition of 140 mcg of folic acid per 100 g of flour or uncooked grain. In practical terms, one slice of fortified bread and one serving of fortified pasta (½ cup) provide 136 mcg, or about one third of the RDA.[51] Many ready-to-eat cereals provide 400 mcg of folate per serving or 100% of the RDA.

Although folate fortification has been declared a public health success based on the significant decline in NTD-related births, it remains controversial.[70-72] First, excessive folate intake can mask a vitamin B_{12} deficiency (this will be

discussed in more detail in the section on folate toxicity). More recently it was reported that high intakes of folate-fortified foods promoted the growth of existing tumors in the colon.[72] A continuing question is how we achieve optimum folate status in women of child-bearing age while avoiding negative effects on men and older adults who eat numerous servings of grain products and also take folate supplements.

Folate and Chronic Disease

When folate is in short supply, the conversion of methionine (an essential amino acid) to cysteine (a nonessential amino acid) cannot be completed and homocysteine (the intermediate product) accumulates in the blood. Elevated plasma homocysteine levels may contribute to the worsening of various chronic conditions including cardiovascular disease,[73,74] osteoporosis,[41] and age-related cognitive impairment.[59]

Folate Requirement
Dietary Reference Intake

The RDA for adolescents and adults is 400 mcg/day and increases to 600 mcg/day in pregnancy.[51] Women of reproductive age average 155 to 165 mcg of folic acid daily from fortified foods.[78] Folic acid intake from fortification is lowest among African-American women (136 mcg).

Folate Toxicity

The UL for folate is 1000 mcg/day,[51] and supplements exceeding the recommended intake of 400 mcg are best avoided. The basis for concern is the relationship between folate and vitamin B_{12}. If vitamin B_{12} levels are low but folate levels are high, then folate will substitute for vitamin B_{12} in the formation of red blood cells and prevent the development of a megaloblastic anemia. However, vitamin B_{12} also has a critical role in maintaining nerve tissue, and folate cannot meet that

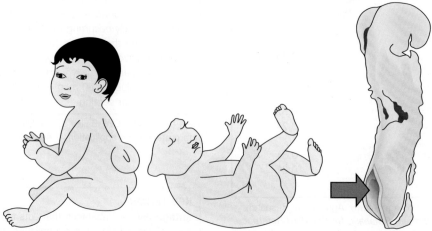

FIGURE 6-9 Neural tube defects (NTDs) include spina bifida and anencephaly. Many NTDs result from a lack of folate needed to close the neural tube that becomes the spinal cord in the developing fetus. (Redrawn from Centers for Disease Control and Prevention: Facts about anencephaly and Facts: spina bifida, Atlanta, 2013. Retrieved from: <http://www.cdc.gov/ncbddd/birthdefects/anencephaly.html> and <http://www.cdc.gov/ncbddd/spinabifida/facts.html>.)

BOX 6-16   FOOD SOURCES OF FOLATE

Food Source	Amount	Folate (mcg DFE)*
Grains Group		
Fortified ready-to-eat cereals		
Product 19	1 cup	676
Wheaties	1 cup	336
Corn flakes	1 cup	163
Instant oatmeal	1 packet	126
Rice, white, long grain, cooked, enriched	1 cup	215
Spaghetti, enriched, cooked	1 cup	167
Hamburger roll, enriched	1	74
Bread, white, enriched	1 slice	43
Vegetable Group		
Spinach, frozen, cooked	½ cup	115
Broccoli, cooked	½ cup	84
Lettuce, dark green (romaine or similar)	1 cup	64
Tomato juice, canned	1 cup	49
Fruit Group		
Orange juice, frozen, reconstituted	1 cup	110
Strawberries	1 cup	40
Meat, Beans, Eggs, and Nuts Group		
Kidney beans, canned	1 cup	67

Data from U.S. Department of Agriculture, Agricultural Research Service: *USDA National Nutrient Database for Standard Reference, Release 26*, 2013. Nutrient Data Laboratory Home Page: <http://www.ars.usda.gov/ba/bhnrc/ndl>.
Images copyright 2006 JupiterImages Corporation.
Recommended Dietary Allowance for adults: 400 mcg.
*1 mcg DFE (Dietary Folate Equivalent) = 1 mcg food folate.

need. The appearance of a megaloblastic anemia is often the first alert to vitamin B_{12} deficiency. If high intakes of folate "mask" this effect, then irreversible damage to the nervous system continues unabated.

Food Sources of Folate

Folate is widely distributed in plant foods. Good sources include dark green leafy vegetables, citrus fruits, tomatoes, cantaloupe, and legumes, as well as fortified grains. Ready-to-eat cereal is a major contributor of folic acid in the U.S. diet.[11] Box 6-16 summarizes food sources of folate.

VITAMIN B₁₂ (COBALAMIN)

Discovery

The discovery of vitamin B_{12} coincided with the search for a cure for **pernicious anemia**.[79] In 1948 workers crystallized a red compound from liver that controlled both the blood-forming defect and the nerve degeneration associated with pernicious anemia. This molecule was numbered *vitamin B₁₂* and later named *cobalamin*, based on the single red atom of the trace element cobalt at its center.

Chemical and Physical Nature

Vitamin B_{12} is a complex red crystal of high molecular weight. It occurs as a protein complex in animal foods only. Vitamin B_{12} is synthesized by bacteria in the intestinal tract of herbivorous animals, although some bacterial synthesis also occurs in the human intestine.

KEY TERM
pernicious anemia A macrocytic anemia caused by the absence of intrinsic factor necessary for absorption of vitamin B_{12}; the condition is treated with intramuscular injections of vitamin B_{12}.

Absorption, Transport, and Storage

Vitamin B_{12} is split from its protein complex by the hydrochloric acid in the stomach and then bound to a specific protein called *intrinsic factor*, secreted by the mucosal cells lining the stomach. This vitamin B_{12}–intrinsic factor complex then moves into the intestine, where special receptors in the wall of the ileum absorb it. The loss of gastric acid or failure of the gastric mucosa to secrete intrinsic factor will impair absorption and result in vitamin B_{12} deficiency.

Approximately 50% of body vitamin B_{12} is stored in the liver, with the remainder distributed among active tissues. The amounts are minute but held tenaciously and only slowly depleted. Vitamin B_{12} deficiency does not become apparent for 3 to 5 years after a gastrectomy and loss of required secretions.

Functions of Vitamin B_{12}
Basic Coenzyme Role

Vitamin B_{12} participates in amino acid metabolism and formation of the heme portion of hemoglobin. It has a role in the synthesis of important lipids and proteins that form the myelin sheath covering the nerves of the brain and spinal cord.

Vitamin B_{12} Deficiency and Clinical Applications

Vitamin B_{12} deficiency disrupts blood formation and affects cognitive function:

- *Pernicious anemia:* The megaloblastic anemia arising from vitamin B_{12} deficiency took on the name *pernicious anemia* because it is fatal if left untreated. When this vitamin is lacking, the production of red blood cells is halted because the heme portion of the hemoglobin molecule cannot be synthesized, and the activated molecule of folate needed to assist in the process cannot be formed. The root cause of pernicious anemia is a lack of intrinsic factor required for vitamin B_{12} absorption; thus another way must be found to supply this vitamin. A monthly intramuscular injection of 1000 mcg controls the blood-forming disorder and prevents the degenerative effects on the nervous system.[80]
- *Cognitive function:* Vitamin B_{12} deficiency causes fatigue, lassitude, and a decline in cognitive and thought processes as damage to the nervous system continues. Even in the absence of overt deficiency, long-term studies indicate that older adults with lower blood vitamin B_{12} levels are more likely to experience cognitive decline[81,82] and depression[82,83] than those with normal levels. Excessively high blood folate levels exacerbated the cognitive losses associated with vitamin B_{12} deficiency.[81] Supplementation with vitamin B_{12} helped to alleviate depressive symptoms.[83]
- *Low gastric acid secretion:* As many as 30% of people above age 50 have low gastric acid levels,[84] putting them at risk of vitamin B_{12} deficiency. Latinos appear to be especially vulnerable based on genetic factors,[85] as their vitamin B_{12} intakes generally exceed the RDA.[24] The form of vitamin B_{12} used in food fortification and vitamin supplements is not bound in a protein complex and does not require gastric acid for effective absorption. Use of vitamin B_{12}–fortified foods several times each week will supply the amount needed. Based on the growing numbers of older adults and increased intakes of folic acid from mandatory fortification, researchers have proposed that vitamin B_{12} fortification of flour also be considered.[86]

Vitamin B_{12} Requirement

The amount of required vitamin B_{12} is minute. The RDA is 2.4 mcg for both younger and older adults.[51]

Food Sources of Vitamin B_{12}

In nature, vitamin B_{12} is found only in animal foods; rich sources include lean meat, fish, poultry, milk, eggs, and cheese. For individuals who consume any animal foods, the recommended intake is easily obtained. Vegans and individuals with low gastric acid levels can meet their requirement from fortified grains, cereals, juices, and soy milk, or vitamin B_{12} supplements. Box 6-17 lists various sources.

A summary of the water-soluble B vitamins is found in Table 6-4.

As we conclude our discussion of this important micronutrient group, consider your own vitamin intake and review the Perspectives in Practice box, "Choosing a Vitamin-Mineral Supplement: Do I Need One?"

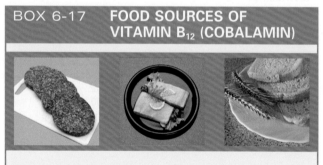

BOX 6-17   FOOD SOURCES OF VITAMIN B_{12} (COBALAMIN)

Vitamin B_{12} (cobalamin) is found naturally in animal foods only, but various grain foods and juices are fortified with this vitamin. Vegans who consume no animal foods and older persons with reduced gastric acid levels should check the nutrition label to identify products with added vitamin B_{12}.

Naturally Occurring Sources of Vitamin B_{12}
Meat patty
Chicken leg
Fish serving
Milk
Cheese

Examples of Nonanimal Foods Sometimes Fortified with Vitamin B_{12}
Ready-to-eat cereal
Bread
Orange juice

Images copyright 2006 JupiterImages Corporation.
Recommended Dietary Allowance for adults: 2.4 mcg.

TABLE 6-4   SUMMARY OF B-COMPLEX VITAMINS

VITAMIN	COENZYME: PHYSIOLOGIC FUNCTIONS	CLINICAL APPLICATIONS	DIETARY REFERENCE INTAKE	FOOD SOURCES
Thiamin	Carbohydrate metabolism Thiamin pyrophosphate (TPP): oxidative decarboxylation	Beriberi (deficiency) Neuropathy Wernicke-Korsakoff syndrome (alcoholism) Depressed muscular and secretory functions	Adults Males ages ≥19: 1.2 mg Females ages ≥19: 1.1 mg Pregnancy All ages: 1.4 mg Lactation All ages: 1.4 mg	Pork, beef, organ meats Whole or enriched grains and cereals Legumes
Riboflavin	General metabolism Flavin mononucleotide (FMN) Flavin adenine dinucleotide (FAD)	Cheilosis, glossitis, seborrheic dermatitis	Adults Males ages ≥19: 1.3 mg Females ages ≥19: 1.1 mg Pregnancy All ages: 1.4 mg Lactation All ages: 1.6 mg	Milk products Organ meats Enriched grains and cereals
Niacin (nicotinic acid, nicotinamide)	General metabolism Nicotinamide adenine dinucleotide (NAD) Nicotinamide adenine dinucleotide phosphate (NADP)	Pellagra (deficiency) Weakness, anorexia Scaly dermatitis Neuritis Death (if untreated)	Adults Males ages ≥19: 16 mg NE* Females ages ≥19: 14 mg NE Pregnancy All ages: 18 mg NE Lactation All ages: 17 mg NE	Meat and dairy foods containing tryptophan Peanuts Enriched grains and cereals
Vitamin B₆ (pyridoxine, pyridoxal, pyridoxamine)	General metabolism Pyridoxal phosphate (PLP): transamination and decarboxylation reactions	Reduced serum levels associated with pregnancy and use of certain oral contraceptives Antagonized by isoniazid, penicillamine, and various other drugs	Adult males Ages 19-50: 1.3 mg Ages ≥51: 1.7 mg Adult females Ages 19-50: 1.3 mg Ages ≥51: 1.5 mg Pregnancy All ages: 1.9 mg Lactation All ages: 2.0 mg	Meat, organ meats Whole grains and cereals Legumes Bananas
Pantothenic acid	General metabolism Coenzyme A (CoA): metabolize carbohydrates, fats, and amino acids	Many roles through acyl transfer reactions (e.g., lipogenesis, amino acid activation, and formation of cholesterol, steroid hormones, and heme)	Adults Males/females ages ≥19: 5 mg Pregnancy All ages: 6 mg Lactation All ages: 7 mg	Egg, milk, liver
Biotin	General metabolism CO_2 transfer reactions	Deficiency induced by avidin (a protein in raw egg white) and by antibiotics	Adults Males/females ages ≥19: 30 mcg Pregnancy All ages: 30 mcg Lactation All ages: 35 mcg	Egg yolk, liver Synthesized by intestinal bacteria
Folate (folic acid)	General metabolism Single carbon transfer reactions (e.g., purine nucleotide, thymine, heme synthesis)	Megaloblastic anemia Elevated blood homocysteine levels Neural tube defect–affected pregnancy	Adults Males/females ages ≥19: 400 mcg Pregnancy All ages: 600 mcg Lactation All ages: 500 mcg	Green leafy vegetables Oranges, orange juice, tomatoes Liver and organ meats Fortified breads and cereals

Continued

TABLE 6-4　SUMMARY OF B-COMPLEX VITAMINS—cont'd

VITAMIN	COENZYME: PHYSIOLOGIC FUNCTIONS	CLINICAL APPLICATIONS	DIETARY REFERENCE INTAKE	FOOD SOURCES
Vitamin B$_{12}$ (cobalamin)	General metabolism Methylation reactions in synthesis of amino acids, heme) Synthesis and maintenance of myelin sheath surrounding nerves	Pernicious anemia induced by lack of intrinsic factor for B$_{12}$ absorption Megaloblastic anemia Peripheral neuropathy Changes in cognitive function Deficiency occurs on a vegan diet with no animal foods and no B$_{12}$ supplements or fortified foods Deficiency can result from low gastric acid secretion hindering B$_{12}$ absorption	Adults Males/females ages ≥19: 2.4 mcg Pregnancy All ages: 2.6 mcg Lactation All ages: 2.8 mcg	Meat, milk, cheese, egg, liver (found in all animal foods) Fortified cereals, juices, and soy milk

*Niacin equivalent

PERSPECTIVES IN PRACTICE

Choosing a Vitamin-Mineral Supplement: Do I Need One?

The general public is constantly bombarded by advertisements urging them to purchase a vitamin or mineral supplement to prevent or cure real or imagined nutrient deficiencies. Sales of dietary supplements now exceed $25.2 billion[1] and continue to grow. The FDA estimates more than 29,000 supplements are currently on the market, including nutritional, herbal, botanical, and sports products.[2]

The best strategy for obtaining appropriate amounts of vitamins and minerals is to eat a variety of nutrient-dense foods.[3] Fortified foods such as breakfast cereals or juices can add vitamins or minerals that are difficult to obtain in sufficient amounts. Certain individuals at particular stages in their life cycle or with elevated needs may require supplements to meet their recommended intakes as follows[3-5]:

- Older adults with low levels of gastric acid who are less able to absorb vitamin B$_{12}$ from animal sources and vegans who eat no animal foods require vitamin B$_{12}$–fortified foods or supplements.
- Women of childbearing age who may become pregnant require 400 mcg of folate daily to prevent neural tube defects; folic acid added to fortified foods and supplements is better absorbed than naturally occurring folate.
- Pregnant women are unlikely to meet their iron requirement of 27 mg from food alone, even including fortified foods, and are usually prescribed a supplement.
- Youth and adults who drink limited amounts of milk or calcium-fortified beverages will need a supplement to reach their calcium goals of 1000 to 1300 mg, depending on age.
- Children and adults who eat or drink limited amounts of vitamin D–containing foods and do not spend time outdoors

in the sun will need a supplement to meet their DRI of 600 IU (15 mcg); individuals over age 70 will need 800 IU (20 mcg).[4,5]

- Older adults with low energy needs and others who eat very limited amounts of food in an effort to lose weight will benefit from a multivitamin-mineral supplement. Daily energy intakes less than 1500 to 1600 kcal are unlikely to meet the required amounts of all nutrients.
- Individuals with disease conditions such as cystic fibrosis that interfere with fat absorption, or who have had bariatric surgery, or who are undergoing hemodialysis will require continuing evaluation of their nutritional status and need for supplements.

Recommendations for the use of vitamin-mineral supplements must be individualized and based on need as determined by a health professional. No one piece of advice fits all. For those individuals who cannot or will not achieve nutritional adequacy with food only, consider the following guidelines when recommending supplements:

Guidelines for Selecting A Vitamin-Mineral Supplement

- Use supplements in addition to, not in place of, real food. A poor diet with added supplements is still a poor diet.
- Avoid multivitamin-mineral supplements or single-nutrient supplements that exceed 100% of the DRI for any nutrient. Individuals using highly fortified foods such as a cereal that supplies 100% of the DRI for most vitamins and minerals must consider whether a supplement is really necessary.

Choosing a Vitamin-Mineral Supplement: Do I Need One?—cont'd

- If using more than one supplement be sure to add the amounts of any nutrient supplied in each. Total intake should not exceed the DRI for any vitamin or mineral.
- Check with a physician or other health professional who can evaluate the relative benefits and risks before beginning a supplement. Inappropriately high amounts of certain vitamins or minerals can interfere with the action of particular prescription or over-the-counter medications or become toxic.[6]
- Be sure to store your vitamin-mineral supplement in a cool, dry place, not the kitchen or bathroom or other area with high heat and humidity. Vitamins such as vitamin C that are easily oxidized will absorb moisture when the bottle is opened and deteriorate rapidly.[7]

References

1. Marcasan W: How can I help my clients sort out the conflicting and confusing information regarding dietary supplements? *J Am Diet Assoc* 110:1408, 2010.
2. American Dietetic Association: Position of the American Dietetic Association: fortification and nutritional supplements. *J Am Diet Assoc* 105:1300, 2005.
3. American Dietetic Association: Position of the American Dietetic Association: nutrient supplementation. *J Am Diet Assoc* 109:2073, 2009.
4. Bailey RL, Fulgoni VL, Keast DR, et al: Examination of vitamin intakes among US adults by dietary supplement use. *J Acad Nutr Diet* 112:657, 2012.
5. Fulgoni VL, Keast DR, Bailey RL, et al: Foods, fortificants, and supplements: where do Americans get their nutrients? *J Nutr* 141:1847, 2011.
6. Sheth A, Khurana R, Khurana V: Potential liver damage associated with over-the-counter vitamin supplements. *J Am Diet Assoc* 108:1536, 2008.
7. Hiatt AN, Taylor LS, Mauer LJ: Influence of simultaneous variations in temperature and relative humidity on chemical stability of two vitamin C forms and implications for shelf life models. *J Agric Food Chem* 58(6):3532, 2010.

TO SUM UP

A vitamin is an organic, non–energy-yielding substance that is (1) required in very small amounts; (2) participates in specific metabolic functions, often as a coenzyme; and (3) must be supplied in the diet. The metabolic tasks of the fat-soluble vitamins A, D, E, and K involve the synthesis of important proteins related to vision, blood clotting, and bone health. Vitamin A influences the differentiation of cells and tissues, and vitamin E, a powerful antioxidant, protects polyunsaturated fatty acids in membranes and neural tissue from harmful free radicals. The fat-soluble vitamins are absorbed and transported with lipids and easily stored; thus excessive intake can lead to toxicity.

The water-soluble vitamins including ascorbic acid and the B-complex vitamins are synthesized by plants and (with the exception of vitamin B_{12} found only in animal sources) are supplied in both plant and animal foods. They function as coenzymes in cell metabolism and protein synthesis and must be consumed regularly as body stores are limited. Excess intake is excreted in the urine. Ascorbic acid functions as an antioxidant and is important for tissue integrity. Folate and vitamins B_6 and B_{12} have important roles in formation of red blood cells and development and function of nerve structures. Vitamin B_6 and ascorbic acid have shown evidence of toxicity with excessive supplement use, and intakes of folate above recommended levels can interfere with the body's use of vitamin B_{12}. Water-soluble vitamins, especially vitamin C and folate, are easily oxidized and appropriate cooking and storage practices are required to prevent losses from food sources.

QUESTIONS FOR REVIEW

1. Explain how the absorption and storage of a vitamin influence the risk of deficiency and toxicity. Provide several examples to illustrate this concept.
2. List and describe three health problems resulting from a vitamin A deficiency. A young man with cystic fibrosis has just been diagnosed with night blindness although he eats a variety of dark green and deep yellow vegetables and fruits. How would you explain this?
3. What organ systems participate in the formation of the vitamin D hormone calcitriol, and what are their roles? How has the use of sunscreen and choice of soft drinks rather than milk increased the vulnerability of youth to vitamin D deficiency? How does renal failure impact vitamin D function?
4. What is an antioxidant, and how does it protect body tissues? A woman tells you that she is taking 1000 mg of vitamin E daily to prevent signs of aging. How would you advise her?
5. A patient tells you that he is taking multiple vitamin supplements including 1000 mg of ascorbic acid, 5 mg of thiamin, 10 mg of riboflavin, and 50 mg of vitamin B_6. How would you evaluate this vitamin regimen? What

advice would you give him and why? Develop menus for 2 days that include good food sources of these vitamins.

6. Name the B vitamins involved in blood formation. Describe their roles and interactions.

7. Is there a need for vitamin B_{12} fortification of grains? Cite evidence to justify your position.

8. Visit a grocery store and from the food label record the folate content per serving of (1) two different breads, (2) two different ready-to-eat cereals, and (3) two rice or pasta dishes. Rice and pasta dishes may be dry mixes or frozen entrees. Using these foods, develop menus for 2 days that include at least six servings from the grains group and provide at least 400 mcg of folate.

REFERENCES

1. Carpenter KJ, Harper AE: Evolution of knowledge of essential nutrients. In Shils ME, Shike M, Olson J, editors: *Modern nutrition in health and disease*, ed 10, Baltimore, Md., 2006, Lippincott Williams & Wilkins.

2. Russell RM: Current framework for DRI development: what are the pros and cons? *Nutr Rev* 66(8):455, 2008.

3. Food and Nutrition Board, Institute of Medicine: *Dietary Reference Intakes for vitamin A, vitamin K, arsenic, boron, chromium, copper, iodine, iron, manganese, molybdenum, nickel, silicon, vanadium, and zinc*, Washington, D.C., 2001, National Academies Press.

4. Tang G, Hu Y, Yin S-A, et al: β-carotene in golden rice is as good as β-carotene in oil at providing vitamin A to children. *Am J Clin Nutr* 96:658, 2012.

5. Solomons NW: Vitamin A. In Erdman JW Jr, Macdonald IA, Zeisel SH, editors: *Present knowledge in nutrition*, ed 10, Ames, Iowa, 2012, International Life Sciences Institute/Wiley-Blackwell.

6. Mayo-Wilson E, Imdad A, Herzer K, et al: Vitamin A supplements for preventing mortality, illness, and blindness in children aged under 5: systematic review and meta-analysis. *BMJ* 25:343:d5094, 2011.

7. Kraemer K, Waelti M, de Pee S, et al: Are low tolerable upper intake levels for vitamin A undermining effective food fortification efforts? *Nutr Reviews* 66:517, 2008.

8. Ahmadieh H, Arabi A: Vitamins and bone health: beyond calcium and vitamin D. *Nutr Reviews* 69(10):584, 2011.

9. Ross AC: Vitamin A and carotenoids. In Shils ME, Shike M, Olson J, editors: *Modern nutrition in health and disease*, ed 10, Baltimore, Md., 2006, Lippincott Williams & Wilkins.

10. O'Donnell SI, Hoerr SL, Mendoza JA, et al: Nutrient quality of fast food kids meals. *Am J Clin Nutr* 88:1388, 2008.

11. U.S. Department of Health and Human Services, U.S. Department of Agriculture: *Report of the Dietary Guidelines Advisory Committee on the Dietary Guidelines for Americans 2010*, Washington, D.C., 2010, Center for Nutrition Policy and Promotion, U.S. Department of Agriculture. from: <http://www.cnpp.usda.gov/DGAs2010-DGACReport.htm>. Retrieved November 12, 2012.

12. Reference deleted in proofs.

13. Penniston KL, Tanumihardjo SA: Vitamin A in dietary supplements and fortified foods: too much of a good thing. *J Am Diet Assoc* 103:1185, 2003.

14. Holick MF, Chen TC, Lu Z, et al: Vitamin D and skin physiology: a D-lightful story. *J Bone Miner Res* 22(Suppl 2):V27, 2007.

15. Linos E, Keiser E, Kanzler M, et al: Sun protective behaviors and vitamin D levels in the US population: NHANES 2003-2006. *Cancer Causes Control* 23:133, 2012.

16. Ganji V, Zhang X, Tangpricha V: Serum 25-hydroxyvitamin D concentrations and prevalence estimates of hypovitaminosis D in the U.S. population based on assay-adjusted data. *J Nutr* 142:498, 2012.

17. Reference deleted in proofs.

18. Reference deleted in proofs.

19. Reference deleted in proofs.

20. Reference deleted in proofs.

21. McKeag NA, McKinley MC, Woodside JV, et al: The role of micronutrients in heart failure. *J Acad Nutr Diet* 112:870, 2012.

22. Taylor SN, Wagner CL, Hollis BW: Vitamin D supplementation during lactation to support infant and mother. *J Am Coll Nutr* 27:690, 2008.

23. Food and Nutrition Board, Institute of Medicine: *DRI, Dietary Reference Intakes: calcium, vitamin D*, Washington, D.C., 2011, National Academies Press.

24. U.S. Department of Agriculture, Agricultural Research Service: Nutrient Intakes from Food: Mean Amounts Consumed per Individual by Gender and Age in the United States, 2009-2010. In *What We Eat in America*, NHANES 2009-2010. 2012. at: <www.ars.usda.gov/ba/bhnrc/fsrg>. Accessed on November 15, 2012.

25. Reference deleted in proofs.

26. Food and Nutrition Board, Institute of Medicine: *Dietary Reference Intakes. The essential guide to nutrient requirements*, Washington, D.C., 2006, National Academies Press.

27. Biesalski HK, Grune T, Tinz J, et al: Reexamination of a meta-analysis of the effect of antioxidant supplementation on mortality and health in randomized trials. *Nutrients* 2:929, 2010.

28. Bjelakovic G, Nikolova D, Gluud LL, et al: Antioxidant supplements for prevention of mortality in healthy participants and patients with various diseases (review). *The Cochrane Library* (3):2012.

29. Reference deleted in proofs.

30. Reference deleted in proofs.

31. Reference deleted in proofs.

32. Traber MG: Vitamin E. In Shils ME, Shike M, Olson ML, editors: *Modern nutrition in health and disease*, ed 10, Baltimore, Md., 2006, Lippincott Williams & Wilkins.

33. Maqbool A, Stallings VA: Update on fat-soluble vitamins in cystic fibrosis. *Curr Opin Pulm Med* 14:574, 2008.

34. U.S. Department of Agriculture, Agricultural Research Service: USDA National Nutrient Database for Standard Reference, Release 25. at: <http://www.ars.usda.gov/ba/bhnrc/ndl>. Accessed on December 14, 2012.

35. Leonard SW, Good CK, Gugger ET, et al: Vitamin E bioavailability from fortified breakfast cereal is greater than that from encapsulated supplements. *Am J Clin Nutr* 79:86, 2004.

36. Suttie JW: Vitamin K. In Shils ME, Shike M, Olson J, editors: *Modern nutrition in health and disease*, ed 10, Baltimore, Md., 2006, Lippincott Williams & Wilkins.

37. Cashman KD, O'Connor E: Does vitamin K_1 intake protect against bone loss in later life? *Nutr Rev* 66:532, 2008.

38. Rohde LE, de Assis MC, Rabelo ER: Dietary vitamin K intake and anticoagulation in elderly patients. *Curr Opin Clin Nutr Metab Care* 10(1):1, 2007.

39. Marcason W: Vitamin K: what are the current dietary recommendations for patients taking Coumadin? *J Am Diet Assoc* 107:2022, 2007.

40. Guyton AC, Hall JE: *Textbook of medical physiology*, ed 10, Philadelphia, Pa., 2000, Saunders.

41. Ahmadieh H, Arabi A: Vitamins and bone health: beyond calcium and vitamin D. *Nutr Reviews* 69(10):584, 2011.

42. Winkler MA, Manchester S: Medical nutrition therapy for metabolic stress, sepsis, trauma, burns, and surgery. In Mahan KL, Escott-Stump S, editors: *Krause's food, nutrition, & diet therapy*, ed 12, Philadelphia, Pa., 2007, Saunders.

43. Cogswell ME, Weisberg P, Spong C: Cigarette smoking, alcohol use and adverse pregnancy outcomes: implications for micronutrient supplementation. *J Nutr* 133:1722S, 2003.

44. Reference deleted in proofs.

45. Reference deleted in proofs.

46. Reference deleted in proofs.

47. Reference deleted in proofs.

48. Reference deleted in proofs.

49. Reference deleted in proofs.

50. Rock CL, Newman VA, Neuhouser ML, et al: Antioxidant supplement use in cancer survivors and the general population. *J Nutr* 134:3194S, 2004.

51. Food and Nutrition Board, Institute of Medicine: *Dietary Reference Intakes for thiamin, riboflavin, niacin, vitamin B_6, folate, vitamin B_{12}, pantothenic acid, biotin, and choline*, Washington, D.C., 1998, National Academies Press.

52. Tzoulaki I, Patel CJ, Okamura T, et al: A nutrient-wide association study on blood pressure. *Circulation* 126:2456, 2012.

53. Frantz DJ: Neurologic complications of bariatric surgery: involvement of central, peripheral, and enteric nervous systems. *Curr Gastroenterol Rep* 14:367, 2012.

54. McCormick DB: Riboflavin. In Shils ME, Shike M, Olson J, editors: *Modern nutrition in health and disease*, ed 10, Baltimore, Md., 2006, Lippincott Williams & Wilkins.

55. Powers HJ: Riboflavin (vitamin B-2) and health. *Am J Clin Nutr* 77:1352, 2003.

56. Bourgeois C, Cervantes-Laurean D, Moss J: Niacin. In Shils ME, Shike M, Olson J, editors: *Modern nutrition in health and disease*, ed 10, Baltimore, Md., 2006, Lippincott Williams & Wilkins.

57. MacKay D, Hathcock J, Guarneri E: Niacin: chemical forms, bioavailability, and health effects. *Nutr Reviews* 70(6):357, 2012.

58. Gerlach AT, Thomas S, Stawicki SP, et al: Vitamin B_6 deficiency: a potential cause of refractory seizures in adults. *JPEN* 35:272, 2011.

59. Selhub J, Troen A, Rosenberg IH: B vitamins and the aging brain. *Nutr Reviews* 68(Suppl 2):S122, 2010.

60. Reference deleted in proofs.

61. Reference deleted in proofs.

62. Reference deleted in proofs.

63. Reference deleted in proofs.

64. Corken M, Porter J: Is vitamin B_6 deficiency an under-recognized risk in patients receiving haemodialysis? A systematic review: 2000-2010. *Nephrology* 16:619, 2011.

65. Wilson SMC, Bivins BN, Russell KA, et al: Oral contraceptive use: impact on folate, vitamin B_6, and vitamin B_{12} status. *Nutr Reviews* 69(10):572, 2011.

66. Morris MS, Picciano MF, Jacques PF, et al: Plasma pyridoxal 5′-phosphate in the US population: the National Health and Nutrition Examination Survey, 2003-2004. *Am J Clin Nutr* 87:1446, 2008.

67. Fulgoni VL, Keast DR, Bailey RI, et al: Foods, fortificants, and supplements: where do Americans get their nutrients? *J Nutr* 141:1847, 2011.

68. Suitor CD, Bailey LB: Dietary folate equivalents: interpretation and application. *J Am Diet Assoc* 100(1):81, 2000.

69. Gregory JF: Case study: folate bioavailability. *J Nutr* 131:1376S, 2001.

70. Crider KS, Bailey LB, Berry RJ: Folic acid food fortification—its history, effect, concerns, and future directions. *Nutrients* 3:370, 2011.

71. Heseker HB, Mason JB, Selhub J, et al: Not all cases of neural-tube defect can be prevented by increasing the intake of folic acid. *Br J Nutr* 102:173, 2009.

72. Solomons NW: Food fortification with folic acid: has the other shoe dropped? *Nutr Rev* 65:512, 2007.

73. Varela-Moreiras G, Murphy MM, Scott JM: Cobalamin, folic acid, and homocysteine. *Nutr Reviews* 67(Suppl 1):S69, 2009.

74. Abraham JM, Cho L: The homocysteine hypothesis: still relevant to the prevention and treatment of cardiovascular disease? *Cleveland Clin J Med* 77(12):911, 2010.

75. Reference deleted in proofs.

76. Reference deleted in proofs.

77. Reference deleted in proofs.

78. Bailey RL, Dodd KW, Gahche JJ, et al: Total folate and folic acid intake from foods and dietary supplements in the United States: 2003-2006. *Am J Clin Nutr* 91:231, 2010.

79. Carmel R: Cobalamin (Vitamin B_{12}). In Shils ME, Shike M, Olson J, editors: *Modern nutrition in health and disease*, ed 10, Baltimore, Md., 2006, Lippincott Williams & Wilkins.

80. Carmel R: How I treat cobalamin (vitamin B_{12}) deficiency. *Blood* 112:2214, 2008.

81. Morris MS, Selhub J, Jacques PF: Vitamin B-12 and folate status in relation to decline in scores on the Mini-Mental State Examination in the Framingham Heart Study. *JAGS* 60:1457, 2012.

82. Moorthy D, Peter I, Scott TM, et al: Status of vitamins B-12 and B-6 but not of folate, homocysteine, and the methylenetetrahydrofolate reductase C677T polymorphism are associated with impaired cognition and depression in adults. *J Nutr* 142:1554, 2012.

83. Skarupski KA, Tangney C, Li H, et al: Longitudinal association of vitamin B-6, folate, and vitamin B-12 with depressive symptoms among older adults over time. *Am J Clin Nutr* 92:330, 2010.

84. Allen LH: How common is vitamin B-12 deficiency? *Am J Clin Nutr* 89:693S, 2009.

85. Campbell AK, Miller JW, Green R, et al: Plasma vitamin B_{12} concentrations in an elderly Latino population are predicted

by serum gastrin concentrations and crystalline vitamin B$_{12}$ intake. *J Nutr* 133:2770, 2003.

86. Green R: Is it time for vitamin B$_{12}$ fortification? What are the questions? *Am J Clin Nutr* 89(Suppl):712S, 2009.

FURTHER READINGS AND RESOURCES

Readings

Flores G, Maldonado J, Duran P: Making tortillas without lard: Latino parents' perspectives on healthy eating, physical activity, and weight-management strategies for overweight Latino children. *J Acad Nutr Diet* 112:81, 2012.

[Dr. Flores and his collaborators help us understand the cultural issues in helping families choose healthier foods and ingredients.]

Martin CK, Thomson JL, LeBlanc MM, et al: Children in school cafeterias select foods containing more saturated fat and energy than the Institute of Medicine recommendations. *J Nutr* 140:1653, 2010.

Whitfield Jacobsen PA, Prawitz AD, Lukaszuk JM: Long-haul truck drivers want healthful meal options at truck-stop restaurants. *J Am Diet Assoc* 107:2125, 2007.

[These articles present ideas for nutrition intervention among various age and lifestyle groups.]

Kris-Etherton P, Fleming J, Harris WS: The debate about n-6 polyunsaturated fatty acid recommendations for cardiovascular health. *J Am Diet Assoc* 110:201, 2010.

[This article describes the differences of opinion that exist among health professionals regarding appropriate intakes of dietary fat.]

Remig V, Franklin B, Margolis S, et al: Trans fats in America: a review of their use, consumption, health implications and regulation. *J Am Diet Assoc* 110:585, 2010.

[This article provides insight as to local and state efforts to reduce the amounts of trans fat in processed foods and fast food restaurants, and what success has been achieved.]

Websites of Interest

- International Food Information Council Foundation: This site contains fact sheets and brochures for both consumers and health professionals on food fats and fat replacers. http://www.foodinsight.org/Default.aspx?tabid=85&xsq=fats
- National Heart, Lung, and Blood Institute, National Institutes of Health: Information for the Public: This government agency provides tutorials on various aspects of heart disease, recipe books for good eating that include cultural and ethnic food patterns, and health assessment tools, including a menu planner to help monitor fat intake. http://www.nhlbi.nih.gov/health/index.htm, http://www.nhlbi.nih.gov/health/index.htm

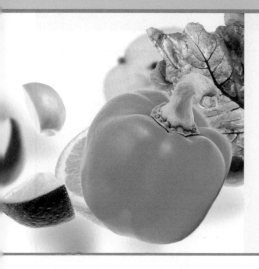

CHAPTER 7

Minerals and Water

Eleanor D. Schlenker

EVOLVE WEBSITE

http://evolve.elsevier.com/Williams/essentials/

OUTLINE

With this chapter we complete our review of the two remaining classes of nutrients: minerals and water. As individual elements, minerals seem simple in comparison to the complex structures of vitamins, but they fulfill equally important roles. New technologies that make it possible to measure extremely small quantities of trace minerals in body tissues have opened new opportunities to study the roles of these nutrients and how they interact with vitamins to maintain body function and prevent disease. In time we may identify additional minerals essential to human health. An equally important but often overlooked nutrient is water. Water is second only to oxygen in that it is vital for survival. Growing interest in sports nutrition and athletic performance has brought new attention to water as a beverage, and bottled water is now the bottled drink with the highest sales volume.

As with the vitamins we will focus on why we need these nutrients and how we obtain them.

MINERALS IN HUMAN NUTRITION

Comparison of Vitamins and Minerals

The two classes of micronutrients, vitamins and minerals, have both similarities and differences (Table 7-1). Vitamins are complex organic molecules that serve primarily as coenzymes or regulators of body metabolism, especially energy metabolism. Minerals, in contrast, are simple elements with important roles in both structure and function. Minerals also serve as cofactors in many important enzyme systems, and, in fact, sometimes partner with vitamins in regulating

TABLE 7-1   COMPARISONS OF VITAMINS AND MINERALS

CHARACTERISTIC	MINERALS	VITAMINS
Similarities		
Essentiality	Must be obtained in food	Must be obtained in food
Unique role	One cannot substitute for another	One cannot substitute for another
Interactions	Interferes with other minerals if present in inappropriate amounts	Interferes with other vitamins if present in inappropriate amounts
Impact on chronic disease	May have a role in prevention of chronic disease	May have a role in prevention of chronic disease
Differences		
Structure	Simple organic elements	Complex organic structures
Absorption	Problems in absorption caused by interfering or binding substances	More easily absorbed
Classification	Based on amount needed by the body (major minerals or trace elements)	Based on solubility in water or lipid
Roles in body	Structural and metabolic	Only metabolic
Relative amount needed	Varies among minerals (more needed for structural roles)	Needed in very minute amounts
Stability	Seldom destroyed in cooking	Easily destroyed in cooking

essential metabolic functions. As was true for vitamins, an excess of one mineral cannot remedy a deficit of another, making it important to eat a wide variety of foods.

Cycle of Minerals

On Earth we live within a vast slow-motion cycle of minerals essential to life. Elements present in water find their way into rocks and soil; through plants they find their way to animals and humans.[1] At one time our access to these elements depended on luck—where we happened to live—because most people obtained all of their food from nearby farms. However, with expanding knowledge of how these elements are incorporated into foods, plus the fact that much of the food we eat is grown outside of our immediate surroundings, people living in all parts of the world have the potential to receive adequate mineral nutrition.

Metabolic Roles
Differing Functions

The roles of minerals in the body are as varied as the elements themselves. They participate in an impressive array of structural and metabolic activities:
- *Structural:* Calcium and phosphorus give strength to bones and body frame. Iron provides the core for the heme in hemoglobin that carries oxygen to the tissues and returns carbon dioxide to the lungs for excretion.
- *Metabolic:* Ionized sodium and potassium exercise control over body water. Iodine is a necessary constituent of the thyroid hormone that sets the rate of metabolism in the cells. Iron is a cofactor in the mitochondrial enzyme system that supplies our body with energy.

Some minerals such as iron contribute to structure and function. Far from being static and inert, minerals are active participants in many systems that support life.

Differing Amounts

Minerals differ from vitamins in the amounts needed. All vitamins are required in very small amounts, but minerals vary depending on their role. A man weighing 150 lb has almost 3 lb of calcium in his body, most of it in the skeleton. This same man contains only about 3 g ($\frac{1}{10}$ oz) of iron, found mainly in the hemoglobin of red blood cells.

Concept of Bioavailability

In general minerals are absorbed less efficiently than vitamins. The amount of mineral in a food as determined by laboratory analysis may not be the amount that can be absorbed. The term bioavailability refers to the proportion of a food nutrient that can be successfully absorbed and made available for body use. Bioavailability is influenced by the food source and the host, as follows[2]:
- *Binding substances:* In some plants, minerals are bound in chemical complexes and not easily released. Oxalates in green leafy vegetables and phytates in whole grains bind minerals and prevent their absorption.
- *Gastric acidity:* Most minerals are better absorbed in an acid environment.
- *Chemical form:* Iron cannot be absorbed in the ferric form; it must first be reduced to ferrous iron for absorption to take place.
- *Other foods in the meal:* Some foods, such as tea, contain substances that interfere with the absorption of certain minerals.

KEY TERMS
hemoglobin   Oxygen-carrying pigment in red blood cells.
bioavailability   Amount of a nutrient in a food that is absorbed and available to the body for metabolic use.

> ### BOX 7-1   ESSENTIAL MAJOR MINERALS AND TRACE ELEMENTS
>
> **Major Minerals (*Required Intake ≥100 mg/day*)**
>
> | | |
> |---|---|
> | Calcium (Ca) | Potassium (K) |
> | Phosphorus (P) | Chloride (Cl) |
> | Magnesium (Mg) | Sulfur (S) |
> | Sodium (Na) | |
>
> **Trace Elements (*Required Intake <100 mg/day*)***
>
> | | |
> |---|---|
> | Iron (Fe) | Chromium (Cr) |
> | Iodine (I) | Selenium (Se) |
> | Zinc (Zn) | Fluoride (F) |
> | Copper (Cu) | Molybdenum (Mo) |
> | Manganese (Mn) | |

*Cobalt is found in the body only as a component of vitamin B_{12}, not as an individual trace element.

- *Body need:* Various minerals such as iron are absorbed at higher rates in periods of active growth, pregnancy, and lactation.

  Bioavailability issues make it difficult to set dietary recommendations for minerals.

Classification

The essential minerals are organized into two groups: (1) major minerals and (2) trace elements. Minerals that are required in amounts of more than 100 mg/day are called *major minerals*, not because they are more important but because there are more of them in the body. Those needed in smaller amounts are called *trace elements*, and a few that are required in only minute amounts are referred to as *ultratrace elements*.

The seven minerals present in the body in large amounts are calcium, phosphorus, magnesium, sodium, potassium, sulfur, and chloride. Nine trace elements that occur in very small amounts are also essential for human health. All essential minerals are listed in Box 7-1. We will review five aspects of each: (1) absorption, (2) physiologic function, (3) clinical applications, (4) daily requirement, and (5) food sources.

MAJOR MINERALS

CALCIUM

Of all the minerals in the body, calcium is present in the largest amount. The adult woman contains about 1000 g (2.2 lb) of calcium, and the adult man contains about 1200 g (2.6 lb). Total body calcium reflects the constant interchange of calcium supplied in food or supplements, calcium stored in the skeleton, and urinary calcium loss. Calcium balance is applied at three levels: (1) the intake-absorption-excretion balance, (2) the bone-blood balance, and (3) the calcium-phosphorus blood serum balance.

Intake-Absorption-Excretion Balance
Calcium Intake

Calcium has been identified as a nutrient of importance to public health in respect to bone health. Except for children ages 1 to 3, the majority of the population is not meeting their RDA (Recommended Dietary Allowance).[3]

Calcium intake in early life can have lifelong implications for bone health. Caucasian women who reported low milk intake as children and adolescents had lower bone mass in later life and were more likely to experience hip fractures.[11]

Calcium Absorption

About 25% of ingested calcium is absorbed, although it can reach 60% in infancy or other periods of high demand. Absorption falls to very low levels in advanced age.[12] Calcium is absorbed in the small intestine, chiefly the duodenum. Here the gastric acidity is still effective, but as the food mass is buffered by pancreatic juices and becomes more alkaline, absorption is reduced.

Factors Increasing Calcium Absorption. The following factors increase calcium absorption:

- *Vitamin D hormone:* Vitamin D is necessary for the active transport of calcium. Calcitriol, the vitamin D hormone, controls the synthesis of a calcium-binding protein that carries the mineral across the mucosal cell and into the blood.[11]
- *Body need:* Physiologic conditions over the life cycle—growth, pregnancy, lactation, and older age—influence the rate of absorption. Absorption is higher in times of greater need, such as pregnancy or the adolescent growth spurt.
- *Amount of calcium in the diet:* Percent absorption increases when intake is limited; at high calcium intakes a smaller proportion is absorbed, although the net amount may be higher.
- *Acidic environment:* Lower pH or a more acidic environment favors the solubility of calcium and enhances absorption.
- *Dietary protein and carbohydrate:* Optimal protein intake supports bone health and increases calcium absorption by promoting gastric acid secretion.[13] Lactose enhances calcium absorption through the action of the intestinal bacterium *Lactobacilli*, which produces lactic acid and lowers intestinal pH.

Factors Decreasing Calcium Absorption. The following factors decrease calcium absorption:

- *Vitamin D deficiency:* A lack of vitamin D or inability to form the active vitamin D hormone calcitriol as a result of liver or kidney disease depresses absorption.
- *Fat malabsorption:* Excessive amounts of fatty acids remaining in the small intestine combine with calcium to form insoluble soaps that cannot be absorbed.
- *Fiber and other binding agents:* Dietary fiber can bind calcium and hinder its absorption. Other binding agents include oxalic acid and phytic acid. Oxalic acid is found in varying amounts in green leafy vegetables, which makes some better sources of calcium than others. The outer

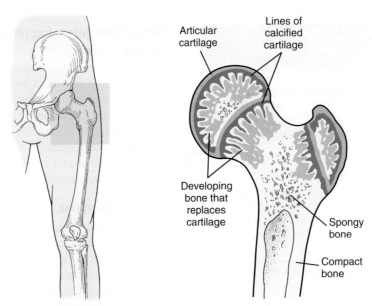

FIGURE 7-1 Bone and cartilage development.

hull of many cereal grains, especially wheat, contains phytates.
• *Alkaline environment:* Calcium is insoluble in an alkaline medium (a high pH) and poorly absorbed. Overuse of antacids will lower calcium absorption.

Calcium Excretion
Calcium balance is controlled primarily at the point of absorption, as is true for many minerals. A large proportion of dietary calcium (50% to 90%) remains unabsorbed and is eliminated in the feces. A small amount of calcium, about 200 mg/day, is excreted in the urine to maintain normal levels in body fluids.

Bone-Blood Balance
Calcium in the Bones
The skeleton is the major site of calcium storage. Bones and teeth contain about 99% of body calcium, but these stores are not static. Bone is constantly being built and reshaped according to period of growth and hormonal influences (Figure 7-1). As much as 700 mg of calcium enters and leaves the bones each day. Under certain conditions withdrawals exceed deposits: immobility from a body cast or the bone disease osteoporosis results in excessive calcium withdrawal and loss.

Calcium in the Blood
The small amount of body calcium that is not in bone—about 1%—circulates in the blood and other body fluids. Blood calcium exists in two forms:
1. *Bound calcium:* About 40% of the calcium in the blood is bound to plasma proteins and not *diffusible,* that is, not able to move into cells or enter into other activities.

2. *Free ionized calcium:* Free calcium carrying an electrical charge moves about unhindered and diffuses through membranes to control body functions. Free calcium accomplishes a great deal of metabolic work because it is in an activated form. Free calcium is critical to ongoing tissue metabolism and so is more closely regulated than bound calcium. When calcium intake is low and blood calcium levels drop, calcium is mobilized from the bones to restore levels to normal.

Calcium-Phosphorus Serum Balance
The final level of calcium balance is the calcium-phosphorus balance in the serum. These two minerals maintain a defined relationship based on their relative solubility. The calcium-phosphorus serum balance is the solubility product of calcium and phosphorus expressed in milligrams per deciliter (mg/dL). Normal calcium serum levels are 10 mg/dL in children and adults. For phosphorus, normal levels are 4 mg/dL in adults and 5 mg/dL in children. Thus the normal serum calcium-phosphorus solubility products are $10 \times 4 = 40$ in adults and $10 \times 5 = 50$ in children. Any situation that increases the serum phosphorus level will decrease the serum calcium level to keep the calcium-phosphorus solubility product constant. A drop in serum calcium interferes with important functions such as muscle contraction, including contraction of the heart muscle.

The three hormones that work together to maintain calcium balance are the parathyroid hormone (PTH), the vitamin D hormone calcitriol, and the hormone calcitonin. The cooperative action of these hormones is an example of the synergism among metabolic control agents:
1. *Parathyroid hormone:* The parathyroid glands lying adjacent to the thyroid glands are particularly sensitive to

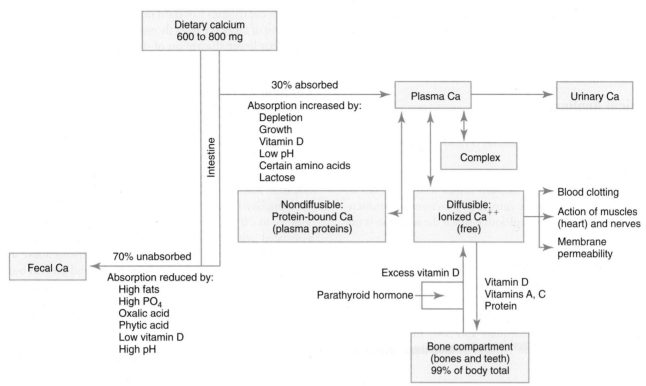

FIGURE 7-2 Calcium metabolism. Note the relative distribution of calcium in body tissues.

changes in the blood level of free ionized calcium. When ionized calcium levels begin to fall, PTH is released and restores the levels to normal by the following actions:

- Stimulates the intestinal mucosa to absorb more calcium
- Rapidly withdraws calcium from bone
- Increases calcium reabsorption and phosphorus excretion by the kidneys

2. *Vitamin D hormone (calcitriol):* Calcitriol cooperates with PTH to control the absorption of calcium in the small intestine and regulate the deposit of calcium and phosphorus in bone. Calcitriol exerts more control on calcium absorption and its deposit in bone, and PTH exerts more control on calcium withdrawal from bone and kidney excretion of phosphorus.

3. *Calcitonin:* Calcitonin is produced by special C cells in the thyroid gland. It prevents an abnormal rise in serum calcium by modulating the release of bone calcium. Thus its action counterbalances that of PTH to keep serum calcium at normal levels. The overall relationship of the factors involved in calcium balance and regulation is illustrated in Figure 7-2.

Physiologic Functions of Calcium
Bone Formation

Calcium along with phosphorus gives strength and rigidity to the skeleton. Building and maintaining bone mass is accomplished through the action of specialized cells that handle the deposit and withdrawal of bone calcium.

Tooth Formation

Special organs in the gums deposit calcium to form teeth, and this mineral exchange continues as in bone. Calcium deposit and withdrawal occur mainly in the dentin and cementum. Very little exchange occurs in the enamel once the tooth is formed.

General Metabolic Functions

The relatively small amount of ionized calcium in blood and body fluids has an amazing number of physiologic roles:

- *Blood clotting:* Serum calcium ions are required for the cross-linking of fibrin, giving stability to the fibrin threads.
- *Nerve transmission:* A current of calcium ions triggers the flow of signals from one nerve cell to another. Calcium ions in cells of the cardiac muscle direct the nerve signals to these fibers.
- *Muscle contraction and relaxation:* Ionized serum calcium initiates the contraction of muscle fibers and controls their return to steady state. Calcium ions released into the cytoplasm of the muscle cell create the attractive forces between actin and myosin that result in the contraction of the muscle fiber. This action of calcium is particularly critical to the constant contraction-relaxation cycle of the heart muscle. Calcium channel blockers slow heart action by preventing this release of calcium.
- *Cell membrane permeability:* Ionized calcium controls the passage of fluids and **solutes** across cell membranes by its effect on the intercellular membrane cement.

- *Enzyme activation:* Calcium ions activate certain cell enzymes, particularly those that release energy for muscle contraction. They have a similar role with protein-splitting enzymes and the lipase enzyme that digests fat.

Clinical Applications

Disruption of the physiologic and metabolic functions of calcium is associated with several clinical problems.

Tetany

A drop in serum ionized calcium causes tetany, marked by severe, intermittent spastic muscle contractions and muscular pain. Seizures and convulsions ensue if the situation is not corrected.

Rickets and Osteomalacia

A deficiency of vitamin D hormone causes rickets in growing children and osteomalacia in adults. When exposure to sunlight is limited and dietary intake of vitamin D is poor, calcium absorption is inadequate and bone mineral is lost. (See Chapter 6 to review vitamin D and these deficiency diseases.)

Resorptive Hypercalciuria and Renal Calculi

Resorption of bone calcium and its excretion in the urine accelerates during prolonged immobilization. A full-body cast, spinal cord injury, or body brace after a back injury decreases the normal muscle tension needed to preserve bone. The subsequent rise in urinary calcium increases the risk of renal stones.

Calcium and Health

Bone Disease

A calcium-related condition increasing in prevalence with the growth of the aging population is osteoporosis, estimated to affect 6 million women and 1 to 2 million men at an annual cost of $14 billion.[13] With advancing age and loss of bone mineral, bones become progressively more fragile, with increasing risk of fractures, physical disability, and mortality.[11] Loss of the steroid hormones estrogen and testosterone bring about alterations in calcium balance such that bone is broken down more rapidly than it can be replaced, with a net loss of bone mass and changes in bone structure (Figure 7-3).[12]

Metabolic Disease

Low calcium intake or limited use of dairy foods has been put forth as a possible contributor to chronic conditions unrelated to bone health, including obesity,[17-19] hypertension,[20,21] and certain types of cancer.[22] Clinical trials evaluating calcium intake and weight management over periods of 2 to 6 years[17,18] found that participants had less weight gain and greater weight loss with higher intakes of dairy foods containing calcium; in fact, increased servings of dairy foods were more important than total calcium intake.

Calcium contributes to weight management by increasing the excretion of fat in the feces through the formation of calcium soaps that lower absorption of dietary fat.[19]

Calcium Requirement
Dietary Reference Intake

Concerns about the amount of calcium required for lifetime maintenance of healthy bones led to the current Dietary Reference Intakes (DRIs).[12] For youths 9 to 18 years of age, the RDA of 1300 mg/day ensures maximum deposition of bone calcium. Men and women ages 19 to 50 should take in 1000 mg/day to maintain positive calcium balance; women ages 51 to 70 require 1200 mg to offset the calcium losses associated with menopause, whereas for men in this age group, the RDA remains at 1000 mg. All persons above age 70 require 1200 mg to support bone health and prevent bone loss. Intakes greater than the Tolerable Upper Intake Level (UL) of 2500 mg/day for adults under age 51 and 2000 mg/day for adults age 51 and older, can interfere with the absorption of other important minerals or lead to complications

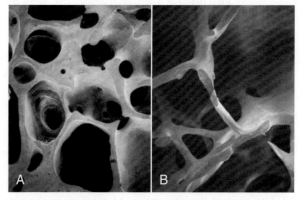

Normal bone   Bone with osteoporosis

FIGURE 7-3 Comparison of normal and osteoporotic spongy bone. Scanning electron micrograph (SEM) of **(A)** normal bone, and **(B)** bone with osteoporosis. Note the loss of bone linkages and enlarged pores in the osteoporotic bone. (From Kumar V, Abbas A, Fausto N: *Robbins basic pathology,* ed 7, Philadelphia, Pa., 2002, Saunders.)

KEY TERMS

osteoporosis The abnormal loss of bone mineral and matrix leading to porous, fragile bone tissue with enlarged spaces that is prone to fracture or deformity; common disease of aging in both men and women.

calcitonin A polypeptide hormone secreted by the C cells in the thyroid gland in response to hypercalcemia, which lowers calcium and phosphorus levels in the blood.

solutes Particles of a substance in solution; a solution consists of a solute and a dissolving medium (solvent), usually a liquid.

such as kidney insufficiency and milk-alkali syndrome. Milk-alkali syndrome got its name from the condition that arose when patients with peptic ulcers were treated with large amounts of antacids (alkaline) such as calcium carbonate over a long period of time. This shifts the body's acid-base balance to alkaline and results in calcium deposits in the kidneys and other soft tissues. Milk-alkali syndrome is seldom seen today unless an individual takes large amounts of a calcium-containing antacid such as Tums to increase their calcium intake. When using antacid products, calcium intake should not exceed 1500 mg a day.

Sources of Calcium

Calcium is highly available from dairy products, making these foods ideal sources. One quart of cow's milk supplies 1200 mg of calcium along with 10 mg (400 IU) of vitamin D. Green leafy vegetables such as bok choy, broccoli, and kale are good sources, but spinach, collard greens, sweet potatoes, and beans are high in oxalic acid, which compromises bioavailability. Whole grains and nuts contain phytic acid, making these foods poor sources. Calcium-fortified soy milk, juices, and cereals meet calcium needs for the lactose intolerant. Aged cheeses such as cheddar or Swiss, good sources of

calcium, are low in lactose. It is important to emphasize low-calorie, reduced-fat, low-fat, or nonfat dairy foods to young women for whom weight gain is a major concern.[23] Box 7-2 suggests additional food sources of calcium.

Calcium Supplements

Many persons cannot or will not consume enough calcium-rich foods to meet their requirement and depend on supplements. Table 7-2 outlines criteria to be considered in selecting and using calcium supplements. To help meet all dietary requirements, it is best to obtain at least half your daily calcium from food that will supply other important nutrients in addition to calcium and will also provide calcium in a highly bioavailable form. (For further reading on calcium and bone health see the Evidence-Based Practice box, "Optimum Calcium Intake: Can We Minimize Bone Loss?")

PHOSPHORUS

Phosphorus is closely associated with body calcium, although it has some unique characteristics and functions of its

TABLE 7-2   CHOOSING A CALCIUM SUPPLEMENT

CHARACTERISTIC	RECOMMENDATION
Amount of elemental calcium present	Calcium compounds contain different amounts of elemental calcium; calcium carbonate is 40% calcium by weight, but calcium citrate is only 21% calcium; you would need twice as much calcium citrate to get the same amount of calcium.
Absorption	Calcium carbonate, calcium citrate, and calcium citrate malate (the form found in fortified juices) are all well absorbed; calcium citrate is better absorbed than calcium carbonate when gastric acid is low.
Purity	Do not use supplements made from bone meal, oyster shell, or dolomite because they may contain lead or other toxic elements; coral calcium may contain lead and mercury; look for a well-known brand of pharmaceuticals or check for the USP (United States Pharmacopeia) symbol or the word "purified."
Dose	Calcium is absorbed best when taken in doses of 500 mg or less; depending on need, take divided doses of 500 mg each rather than one dose of 1000 mg.
When best taken	Calcium carbonate is best absorbed with food; calcium citrate can be taken anytime.
Combination products	Some calcium supplements are combined with other nutrients such as phosphorus, magnesium, or vitamin D; phosphorus is readily available in the U.S. diet and not needed in supplements; unless vitamin D is being provided in another supplement, it could be included here.
Potential interactions	Calcium can decrease the absorption of various medications including phenytoin and tetracycline, and interacts with thiazide and similar diuretics; medications to be taken on an empty stomach should not be taken with a calcium supplement; persons on prescription or over-the-counter medications should check with their physician or pharmacist before adding a calcium supplement.
Form	Calcium supplements are available in tablets, gel capsules, liquids, and chewables; chewables and liquids might be helpful for those with difficulty swallowing.
Ability to dissolve in the stomach	Chewables and liquids are broken down before they enter the stomach; to test a tablet place one in warm water for 30 minutes and stir occasionally; if it has not dissolved in this time it likely will not dissolve in your stomach.

Data from National Institutes of Health: Medline Plus. Trusted Health Information for You. *Calcium supplements,* Bethesda, Md., 2013, U.S. Department of Health and Human Services. Retrieved July 25, 2013 from: <www.nlm.nih.gov/medlineplus/ency/article/007477.htm>; Office of Dietary Supplements: *Dietary supplement fact sheet: calcium,* Bethesda, Md., 2013, National Institutes of Health, U.S. Department of Health and Human Services. Retrieved July 25, 2013 from: <http://ods.od.nih.gov/factsheets/calcium.asp>; Blumberg S: Is coral calcium a safe and effective supplement? *J Am Diet Assoc* 104:1335, 2004.

BOX 7-2   FOOD SOURCES OF CALCIUM

Food Source	Amount	Calcium (mg)
Grains Group		
Fortified ready-to-eat cereals		
Total	¾ cup	1000
All Bran	½ cup	121
Cheerios	1 cup	112
Bread, white, commercially prepared	1 slice	73
Bread, whole wheat, commercially prepared	1 slice	52
Vegetable Group		
Vegetable juice (fortified)	8 fl oz	299
Collard greens (cooked)	1 cup	268
Potato (baked), flesh and skin	1 med	26
Kale (frozen, cooked)	1 cup	179
Broccoli (frozen, cooked)	½ cup	47
Fruit Group		
Orange juice (fortified)	8 fl oz	300
Figs (dried)	2 figs	28
Meat, Beans, Eggs, and Nuts Group		
Soybeans (mature beans, cooked)	1 cup	175
Almonds (roasted)	1 oz (24 nuts)	76
Milk Group		
Yogurt (fruited, low fat)	8 oz container	345
Milk, (nonfat, reduced-fat, whole)	1 cup	299
Soy milk (fortified with calcium)	1 cup	300
Soy milk (unfortified)	1 cup	61
Fats, Oils, and Sugar		
These foods do not supply calcium		

Data from U.S. Department of Agriculture, Agricultural Research Service: *USDA National Nutrient Database for Standard Reference, Release 26.* Nutrient Data Laboratory Home Page, *2013.* <http://www.ars.usda.gov/ba/bhnrc/ndl>.
Images copyright 2006 JupiterImages Corporation.
RDA for adults: men ages 19-70, 1000 mg; women ages 19-50, 1000 mg; men ages >70, 1200 mg; women ages >50, 1200 mg.

own. The adult human body contains about 850 g (1.9 lb) of phosphorus, with 85% in the skeleton, 14% in the soft tissues, and the remaining 1% in extracellular fluids (ECFs) and cell membranes. Phosphorus makes up about 1% of body weight.

Absorption-Excretion Balance
Absorption
Free phosphate is absorbed along the entire length of the small intestine. Absorption is regulated by the vitamin D hormone calcitriol and phosphate carrier proteins.[24] Phos-

phorus exists in food joined with calcium and must be split off as a free mineral to be absorbed. An excess of other minerals such as aluminum or iron or calcium depresses phosphorus absorption. Phytates in whole grains prevent its absorption.

Excretion
Phosphorus is excreted via the kidneys, which help regulate serum phosphorus levels. Usually 85% to 95% of the plasma phosphate filtered by the renal glomeruli is reabsorbed along with calcium under the influence of vitamin D hormone.

EVIDENCE-BASED PRACTICE

Optimum Calcium Intake: Can We Minimize Bone Loss?

Define the Problem: The graying of our population has brought new attention to age-related bone loss and the financial and human cost of osteoporosis and bone fracture. Hip fractures resulting from brittle bones result in loss of independence in 10% to 20% of those affected. Bone health has moved into the forefront as a public health problem, and new drugs have been introduced to treat bone loss. Are there alternatives to these treatments?

Review the Evidence: Although optimal intakes of calcium along with sufficient vitamin D to promote absorption should stem the loss of bone mineral mass, research trials have not always reached the same conclusions. Postmenopausal women given 1000 mg to 1200 mg of calcium daily in the form of a well-absorbed supplement were monitored for 1 to 5 years, and their bone mineral mass compared with those of similar age given a **placebo**. Participants receiving the calcium had an increase in bone mass of 1% to 2% at the wrist, vertebrae, and hip, whereas those given the placebo showed no gain and in most cases lost bone.[1] Any gain in bone mineral mass averts the lower threshold where bone fracture is likely to occur. However, Prince and his co-workers[1] carried their evaluation one step further: They separated the women who consumed at least 80% of their calcium supplements from those who consumed less. Those women who took their supplements regularly had a 33% reduction in risk of hip fracture.

Implement the Findings: Adults can promote their bone health by following the guidelines suggested below:

- Maintain a consistent intake of 1000 to 1200 mg of calcium each day, depending on your age.[2] If you use supplements, then put them in a prominent place and establish a regular schedule for when you take them.
- Maintain a dietary intake of 600 to 800 IU of vitamin D each day[2]; use fortified foods or choose calcium supplements that also supply vitamin D.
- Maintain a healthy lifestyle that includes regular physical activity; weight-bearing exercise and strength training support retention of bone mass.
- Have a bone scan on a regular basis to monitor bone status before a fracture occurs.

For those individuals who have already lost significant bone mass and are at risk of bone fracture, drug intervention may be required. Meeting target intakes of calcium and vitamin D during adulthood minimizes bone loss.

References

1. Prince RL, Devine A, Dhaliwal SS, et al: Effects of calcium supplementation on clinical fracture and bone structure: results of a 5-year, double-blind, placebo-controlled trial in elderly women. *Arch Intern Med* 166:869, 2006.
2. Food and Nutrition Board, Institute of Medicine: *Dietary Reference Intakes for calcium and vitamin D*, Washington, D.C., 2011, National Academies Press.

However, when phosphate must be excreted to preserve the normal serum calcium-phosphorus balance, PTH overrides vitamin D hormone and increases excretion.

Bone-Blood-Cell Balance

Bone

The phosphorus in the skeleton and teeth is combined with calcium. Bone phosphorus is in constant interchange with the phosphorus in blood and other body fluids.

Blood

The normal adult range for serum phosphorus is 3.0 to 4.5 mg/dL; levels below 2.5 mg/dL or above 5.0 mg/dL demand immediate medical attention.[24] High phosphorus intakes leading to elevated serum levels stimulate PTH release and mobilization of bone calcium to restore the normal serum calcium-phosphorus balance. Antacids that contain aluminum bind phosphorus and lower serum levels.

Cells

In its active phosphate form, phosphorus works with proteins, lipids, and carbohydrates to produce energy,

build and repair tissues, and act as a buffer to maintain appropriate pH.

Hormonal Controls

Because calcium and phosphorus work closely together, phosphorus balance is under the control of the vitamin D

KEY TERMS

resorption Breakdown of body tissue; often used to refer to the breakdown of calcified bone tissue, releasing calcium and phosphorus into the blood; parathyroid hormone acts to resorb bone when blood calcium levels fall and calcium is needed to restore normal levels.

placebo An inert and nonharmful substance such as sugar used in clinical studies testing the effects of particular drugs, nutrients, herbs, or other substances on body function. In a controlled clinical trial, one group will receive the active substance being tested, whereas another group will receive the placebo. At the conclusion of the trial, the researcher will review the results from both groups. If changes have occurred in the group receiving the placebo, the researcher will be alerted to a psychologic effect or other unrelated effect that influenced the patient or study outcome.

hormone calcitriol and PTH, two hormones that also control calcium balance. Phosphate depletion results from (1) low intake; (2) poor absorption, usually caused by an interfering substance such as phytate or aluminum; or (3) excessive wasting by the kidney.

Physiologic Functions
Bone and Tooth Formation
Phosphorus helps build bones and teeth. As a component of calcium phosphate, it is constantly deposited and resorbed in the continuing process of bone formation and remodeling.

General Metabolic Activities
Phosphorus is found in every living cell where it participates in overall metabolism. Several specific activities are described below:
- *Absorption of glucose and glycerol:* Phosphorus combines with these molecules to assist their absorption from the intestine. Phosphorus also promotes the reabsorption of glucose in the renal tubules.
- *Transport of fatty acids:* Phospholipids transport fats in the blood.
- *Energy metabolism:* Phosphorus-containing compounds such as adenosine triphosphate (ATP) are high-energy storage molecules that meet instant demands for energy.
- *Buffer system:* The buffer system of phosphoric acid and phosphate helps maintain blood acid-base balance.

Clinical Applications
Changes in the normal serum phosphorus level occur under particular circumstances, as follows:
- *Recovery from diabetic acidosis:* Active carbohydrate absorption and metabolism place a high demand on serum phosphorus, causing temporary hypophosphatemia. Phosphate is combined with glucose to form glycogen.
- *Growth:* Children have higher serum phosphate levels related to their high levels of growth hormone.
- *Hypophosphatemia:* Low serum phosphorus levels occur with intestinal diseases such as sprue and celiac disease that hinder phosphorus absorption. Excessive secretion of PTH (primary hyperparathyroidism) causes inappropriate excretion of phosphorus and hypophosphatemia. Low serum phosphorus may accompany the refeeding syndrome often seen in the first days of nutritional repletion of a severely wasted patient when glycogen stores are being rapidly replenished. One symptom of hypophosphatemia is muscle weakness, because cells are deprived of the phosphorus needed for energy metabolism. If left untreated, then it will lead to metabolic acidosis, heart failure, and sudden death.[25]
- *Hyperphosphatemia:* In renal failure and hypoparathyroidism, excess phosphate accumulates in the serum. This causes the serum calcium level to drop, resulting in tetany.

Highly elevated serum phosphate levels, left untreated, will lead to cardiac paralysis and sudden death.

Phosphorus Requirement
Dietary Reference Intake
The RDA for phosphorus is 1250 mg/day for individuals 9 to 18 years of age and 700 mg/day for all adults over age 18. At one time, the relative intake of calcium to phosphorus was considered important in building and remodeling bone. Phosphorus intakes that were higher than calcium intakes were believed to hinder bone mineral deposition. We have learned since that sufficient amounts of both nutrients are more important than their ratio to each other.[12] Because both minerals are found in many of the same foods, meeting calcium needs will likely provide adequate phosphorus.

Food Sources of Phosphorus
Milk and milk products contain significant amounts of phosphorus. Because phosphorus is important in muscle metabolism, lean meats are a good source. Phosphorus-containing food additives add phosphorus to the typical American diet. Substitution of soft drinks high in phosphorus for milk-based beverages has led to excessive intakes of phosphorus in place of calcium.[12]

SODIUM

Sodium is a plentiful mineral in the body. The average adult contains approximately 100 g (3.5 oz) of sodium. About half circulates in the extracellular fluid (ECF) as free ionized sodium, 40% is found in bone, and 10% resides inside the cell.

Absorption-Excretion Balance
Sodium is easily absorbed in the small intestine; usually no more than 2% remains to be excreted in the feces. The major route of excretion is through the kidneys under the control of **aldosterone**, the sodium-conserving hormone produced in the adrenal cortex. For individuals in temperate climates in a steady state of fluid and sodium balance, urinary sodium excretion is about equal to intake. Sodium is lost in sweat during exercise or in hot environments.

KEY TERM

aldosterone Hormone secreted from the cortex of the adrenal glands that acts on the distal renal tubule to reabsorb sodium in exchange for potassium; the aldosterone mechanism conserves sodium and also water, because water absorption follows sodium reabsorption.

Physiologic Functions of Sodium

Water balance: Ionized sodium is the major guardian of the body water outside the cells. Differences in the sodium concentrations of body fluids largely determine the distribution of water via osmosis from one area to another.

Acid-base balance: In cooperation with chloride and bicarbonate ions, ionized sodium helps regulate acid-base balance.

Cell permeability: The sodium pump located in all cell membranes controls the passage of materials in and out of the cell. Potassium is moved into the cell, and sodium is moved out of the cell. Glucose also moves into the cell via this active transport system.

Muscle action: Sodium ions help transmit electrochemical impulses along nerve and muscle membranes. Potassium and sodium ions work together to balance the response of nerves to stimulation. They control the flow of nerve impulses to muscles and the contraction of muscle fibers.

Sodium Requirement
Dietary Reference Intake

The body can adjust to a wide range of sodium intakes. When intake is low, the body conserves sodium by reducing output in urine and sweat. At high intakes, excretion equals intake. The Adequate Intake (AI) for sodium covers short-term sweat losses from physical activity or exposure to high environmental temperatures. Those with exceptionally high losses, such as endurance runners, will require more sodium.[26] For young adults the AI is 1500 mg of sodium or 3800 mg of table salt. (Sodium chloride or table salt is 40% sodium by weight.) The AI drops to 1300 mg of sodium (about 3300 mg of table salt) for those ages 51 to 70, and to 1200 mg (about 3000 mg of table salt) for those ages 71 and older. These decreases in sodium recommendations as people age are based on their lower energy intakes. The UL is 2300 mg of sodium or 5800 mg of table salt.[26]

Sodium Intake

Current national surveys indicate that 97% of the American public have sodium intakes exceeding the AI.[3] Average intakes for men between the ages of 20 and 69 range from about 3900 mg to 4600 mg, although sodium intake drops to 3200 mg among those ages 70 and over. For women between ages 20 and 69, mean sodium intake falls from about 3200 mg to 2900 mg, with a further drop to 2600 mg beyond age 69.[27] A matter of growing concern for policy makers is the sodium intake of children and teens and its possible role in the development of hypertension in these age groups.[28,29]

▌HEALTH PROMOTION
Sodium and Blood Pressure

The Dietary Guidelines for Americans 2010 Advisory Committee (DGAC) named sodium as one of the dietary components overconsumed in the American diet.[3] Excessive sodium raises blood pressure in African Americans, many middle-aged and older individuals, persons with hypertension, and others who may be salt sensitive, and such groups have been encouraged to lower their sodium intake to 1500 mg.[26] However, the DGAC noted that these segments of the population now comprise over 70% of adults, leading them to recommend a sodium reduction to 1500 mg for the general population.[3] Implementing such a reduction in sodium intake will require time and substantial adjustments in the food supply.[3]

Dietary sodium comes from many sources. Sodium is found naturally in some foods and water, but most (77%) is consumed in the form of salt (sodium chloride) added in food processing. Only 12% of the sodium in the U.S. diet occurs naturally; 6% is added at the table, and 5% is added in cooking (Figure 7-4).[31] Sodium chloride and other sodium-containing compounds are used by food manufacturers for many different purposes (to learn more about dietary intervention for hypertension see the Focus on Culture box, "Low Mineral Intake: Does It Affect Blood Pressure in African Americans?").

Although most persons with liberal intakes of sodium will benefit from lowering their sodium intake, for others, responses in the renin-angiotensin system will increase rather than decrease cardiovascular risk if sodium intake is too low.[37,38] Thus, it is best that all persons consult with a health professional before pursuing a sodium-controlled diet that provides less than the AI (1500 mg) for this nutrient. (Later in this chapter, we will study the role of the renin-angiotensin system.)

Controlling Sodium Intake

Even adults with elevated blood pressure have increased rather than decreased their intakes of sodium in recent years.[39] When individuals are accustomed to liberal use of salt

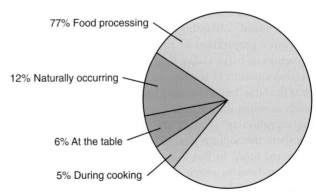

FIGURE 7-4 Sources of dietary sodium. Most of our dietary sodium comes from processed food. (Data from Sebastian RS, Enns CW, Steinfeldt LC, et al: *Discontinuation of data processing step: salt adjustment on designated foods likely to be home prepared, What We Eat in America,* 2012, NHANES, U.S. Department of Agriculture, Agricultural Research Service.)

⊕ FOCUS ON CULTURE

Low Mineral Intake: Does It Affect Blood Pressure in African Americans?

African Americans are at particular risk for elevated blood pressure,[1] with 57% of those ages 18 and over reported to have this condition.[2] Appropriate intakes of calcium, potassium, and magnesium, along with a moderate intake of sodium, influence blood pressure and have been the basis for dietary intervention.[3] The DASH (Dietary Approaches to Stop Hypertension) daily food plan of 7 to 8 grain, 4 to 5 vegetable, 4 to 5 fruit, and 2 to 3 milk servings each day meets or exceeds the DRIs for calcium, potassium, and magnesium and has been successful in helping persons lower their blood pressure and reduce their antihypertensive medication.

According to national surveys African-American adults take in less than half the recommended intakes of potassium, magnesium, and calcium, and fall short of the amounts provided in the DASH diet (see table below).[4] Sodium intake, on the other hand, greatly exceeds the UL of 2300 mg.

Nutrient	Amount in DASH Diet	Intake of African Americans
Potassium	4700 mg	2364 mg
Magnesium	500 mg	261 mg
Calcium	1250 mg	828 mg
Sodium	≤2300 mg	3358 mg

Lowering sodium intake is one step, but equally important is helping African Americans choose more calcium-, potassium-, and magnesium-rich foods. (The DASH food plan can be accessed at: <http://www.cnpp.usda.gov/DGAs2010Policy Document.htm>. *Dietary guidelines for Americans (Policy Document), 2010*, ed 7, Washington, D.C., U.S. Government Printing Office, Appendix 10. DASH will be discussed in detail in Chapter 21.)

References

1. U.S. Department of Health and Human Services: *The seventh report of the Joint National Committee on Prevention, Detection, Evaluation, and Treatment of High Blood Pressure*, Washington, D.C., 2003, U.S. Government Printing Office. NIH Pub No 03-5230.
2. Valderrama AL, Gillespie C, Coleman King S, et al: Vital signs: awareness and treatment of uncontrolled hypertension among adults—United States 2003-2010. *MMWR* 61(35):703, 2012.
3. Epstein DE, Sherwood A, Smith PJ, et al: Determinants and consequences of adherence to the Dietary Approaches to Stop Hypertension diet in African-American and white adults with high blood pressure: results from the ENCORE trial. *J Acad Nutr Diet* 112:1763, 2012.
4. U.S. Department of Agriculture, Agricultural Research Service: Nutrient Intakes from Food: Mean Amounts Consumed per Individual by Race/Ethnicity and Age in the United States, 2009-2010. In *What We Eat in America*, NHANES 2009-2010, 2012. at: <www.ars.usda.gov/ba/bhnrc/fsrg>. Accessed on July 15, 2013.

as a seasoning, adjusting to a reduced level can be difficult. The limited number of reduced-sodium products in the food supply is also a barrier,[3] and foods advertised as "no salt added" or "reduced salt" tend to be higher in cost. Adjusting to a diet within the UL for sodium may be easier if foods naturally lower in sodium are substituted for foods higher in sodium, rather than looking for customary foods with less sodium added.[39] Adapting to a diet lower in sodium is likely to require preparation of more fresh foods seasoned with flavorings or herbs rather than use of heat-and-serve items. Varying amounts of sodium may be added in home cooking or at the table, but it is usually less than is found in processed foods or when dining in restaurants. Most vegetables, with the exception of spinach and celery, are low in sodium. Compare the sodium content of highly processed and less processed foods in Box 7-3. (In Chapter 9 we will use the nutrition label to check the sodium content of processed foods.)

POTASSIUM

Potassium is more than twice as plentiful in the body as sodium. An adult contains about 270 g (9.5 oz) or 4000 mEq (milliequivalents). Most body potassium is inside cells, where it guards intracellular water; however, the relatively small amount of potassium in ECF is important for muscle activity, especially heart muscle activity. Plasma potassium levels are maintained within very narrow limits of 3.5 to 5.0 mEq/L.

Absorption-Excretion Balance

Dietary potassium is readily absorbed in the small intestine and potassium circulating in the gastrointestinal secretions is also reabsorbed. Prolonged vomiting or diarrhea results in serious losses. The principal route of potassium excretion is the urine. Because plasma potassium is critical to heart muscle action, the kidneys guard potassium carefully. At least 70% of the potassium filtered by the kidneys is reabsorbed. Aldosterone, the hormone that acts on the kidneys to conserve sodium, also regulates plasma potassium because potassium is lost in exchange for sodium. Elevated plasma potassium levels stimulate the release of aldosterone. The normal obligatory potassium loss is about 160 mg/day, although certain diuretic drugs lead to greater losses.

Physiologic Functions of Potassium

Water balance: The potassium inside the cells balances with the sodium outside the cells to maintain normal osmotic pressures and water distribution.

BOX 7-3   SODIUM CONTENT OF FOODS*

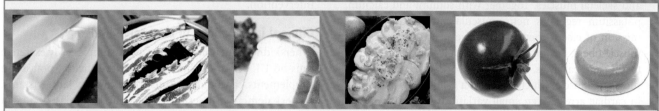

Food Source	Amount	Sodium (mg)
Grains Group		
Ready-to-eat cereals		
Cheerios	1 cup	139
Total	¾ cup	141
All Bran	½ cup	80
Shredded wheat, no salt added	2 biscuits	3
Bread, white, commercially prepared	1 slice	137
Bread whole wheat, commercially prepared	1 slice	146
Vegetable Group		
Potato (baked), flesh and skin	1 medium	17
Potato salad, homemade	1 cup	1323
Tomato, raw	1 medium	6
Stewed tomatoes (canned)	1 cup	564
Broccoli (frozen), cooked, no salt added	½ cup	22
Broccoli (frozen with cheese sauce)	½ cup	402
Meat, Beans, Eggs, and Nuts Group		
Ham (lean)	3 oz	1128
Bacon (broiled/fried)	3 med pieces	326
Ground beef, regular (broiled)	3 oz	64
Tuna, light, canned in water	3 oz	210
Halibut, baked	3 oz	70
Peanuts, dry roasted, without salt	1 oz (28 nuts)	2
Peanut butter, creamy (with salt)	1 tbsp	73
Kidney beans, red, cooked, no salt added	1 cup	4
Baked beans, canned, vegetarian	½ cup	435
Milk Group		
Cottage cheese, creamed, low fat	1 cup	746
Cheddar cheese	1 oz	176
Swiss cheese	1 oz	20
American cheese, processed, pasteurized	1 oz	474
Milk, 1% fat	1 cup	107
Fats, Oils, and Sugar		
Margarine, tub, with salt	1 tbsp	93
Butter (salted)	1 tbsp	91
Butter (unsalted)	1 tbsp	2

Data from U.S. Department of Agriculture, Agricultural Research Service: USDA National Nutrient Database for Standard Reference, Release 26. Nutrient Data Laboratory Home Page, 2013. <http://www.ars.usda.gov/ba/bhnrc/ndl>.
Images copyright 2006 JupiterImages Corporation.
Adequate intake for adults: ages 19-50, 1500 mg; ages 51-70, 1300 mg; ages ≥71, 1200 mg; Tolerable Upper Intake Level for adults: 2300 mg.
*Sodium is added to foods in home food preparation and in food industry processing.

Muscle activity: Potassium is needed for the action of cardiac and skeletal muscles. Together with sodium and calcium, potassium regulates neuromuscular stimulation, transmission of electrochemical impulses, and contraction of muscle fibers. Low plasma potassium leads to muscle irritability and paralysis. This effect is particularly notable for the heart muscle, which develops a gallop rhythm ending in cardiac arrest. Even small variations in plasma potassium are reflected in electrocardiograms (ECGs).

Carbohydrate metabolism: When glucose is converted to glycogen, 0.36 mmol of potassium is stored in each gram of glycogen. When a patient in diabetic acidosis is treated with insulin and glucose, the ensuing rapid production of glycogen draws potassium from the plasma. Serious **hypokalemia** will result if adequate potassium replacement does not accompany treatment. Even moderate potassium deficiency without overt hypokalemia can aggravate existing glucose intolerance.

Protein synthesis: Potassium is required for the storage of nitrogen as muscle protein or other cell protein. When tissue is broken down, potassium is lost along with nitrogen. Amino acid replacement in rehabilitation includes potassium to ensure nitrogen retention.

Control of blood pressure: Potassium helps control blood pressure by offsetting the pressor effect of sodium that raises blood pressure. Persons with higher potassium intakes tend to have lower blood pressures. Potassium also increases the excretion of sodium through the action of aldosterone.

Acid-base balance: Potassium helps protect bone mass and reduces the loss of calcium in the urine. Potassium, along with other bicarbonate-yielding compounds in fruits and vegetables, helps to neutralize sulfur-containing acids produced in the metabolism of meat and other animal protein foods.[40] When potassium and bicarbonate buffers are not available in sufficient amounts, these acids act on bone, releasing bone calcium and lowering bone mass.

Potassium Requirement
Dietary Reference Intake

The AI for potassium is 4700 mg/day for all adults.[26] This intake is expected to lower blood pressure and minimize bone loss, but less than 5% of men and 1% of women reach this goal.[41] Median intakes are 3037 mg for men ages 20 and over and 2279 mg for women of this age; these intakes represent only about two thirds and less than one half, respectively, of the DRI. African-American men and women meet less than half of the AI.[41] Potassium intakes below the DRI are of special concern in light of the elevated intakes of sodium among U.S. adults. Although the *Dietary Guidelines* recommend a sodium-potassium intake ratio of 1500 mg of sodium to 4700 mg of potassium, this is met by less than 2% of the adult population.[42] Based on the age-related increase in blood pressure and loss of bone that occurs in both genders and all race and ethnic groups, increased servings of

high-potassium foods would be a cost-effective public health intervention.

Clinical Implications of Excessive Intake

When kidney function is normal, potassium is easily excreted; thus no UL exists for this nutrient. Nevertheless, potassium supplements can be dangerous, regardless of kidney status. **Hyperkalemia** with serious cardiac arrhythmias occurs in apparently healthy individuals who accidentally or intentionally take potassium supplements. Salt substitutes that contain potassium can be unrecognized sources of potassium. Individuals with diabetes, renal impairment, or heart failure have increased risk of hyperkalemia. Certain medications impair potassium excretion.[26]

Food Sources of Potassium

Potassium as a component of all living cells is found in many foods. Legumes, whole grains, fruits such as oranges and bananas, leafy green vegetables, broccoli, potatoes, meats, and milk supply considerable amounts (Box 7-4). Persons who eat many servings of fruits and vegetables have potassium intakes of about 8 to 11 g/day.[26] In the United States, the top six sources of potassium are reduced-fat and low-fat milk, coffee, chicken and chicken mixed dishes, beef and beef mixed dishes, orange or grapefruit juice, and fried white potatoes.[3] Note that potassium toxicity does not occur from high intakes of potassium-containing foods but rather from potassium supplements.

Based on the amounts found in the body, three additional minerals—magnesium, chloride, and sulfur—are assigned to the major minerals group.

MAGNESIUM

An adult body contains about 25 g of magnesium, a little less than an ounce. Most is combined with calcium and phosphorus in bone, with the remainder distributed in muscle, other tissues, and fluids. Magnesium activates enzymes for energy production and tissue building and has a role in normal muscle action. Magnesium is receiving new attention as an active nutrient related to lowered incidence of atherosclerosis, hypertension, osteoporosis, sudden cardiac death, type 2 diabetes, and metabolic syndrome.[43,44] Older individuals with magnesium intakes that reached at least 80% of the RDA were less likely to develop metabolic syndrome.[45] The relatively high magnesium content in whole grains may contribute to their positive effect in lowering chronic disease risk.[46]

KEY TERM

hyperkalemia   A higher than normal level of potassium in the blood (usually defined as greater than 5.0 mEq/L).

hypokalemia   A lower than normal level of potassium in the blood (usually defined as less than 3.5 mEq/L).

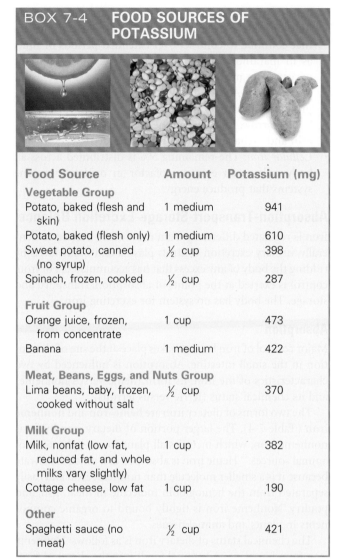

BOX 7-4	FOOD SOURCES OF POTASSIUM		
Food Source		**Amount**	**Potassium (mg)**
Vegetable Group			
Potato, baked (flesh and skin)		1 medium	941
Potato, baked (flesh only)		1 medium	610
Sweet potato, canned (no syrup)		½ cup	398
Spinach, frozen, cooked		½ cup	287
Fruit Group			
Orange juice, frozen, from concentrate		1 cup	473
Banana		1 medium	422
Meat, Beans, Eggs, and Nuts Group			
Lima beans, baby, frozen, cooked without salt		½ cup	370
Milk Group			
Milk, nonfat (low fat, reduced fat, and whole milks vary slightly)		1 cup	382
Cottage cheese, low fat		1 cup	190
Other			
Spaghetti sauce (no meat)		½ cup	421

Data from U.S. Department of Agriculture, Agricultural Research Service: *USDA National Nutrient Database for Standard Reference, Release 26.* Nutrient Data Laboratory Home Page, 2013. <http://www.ars.usda.gov/ba/bhnrc/ndl>.
Images copyright 2006 JupiterImages Corporation.
Adequate intake for adults: 4700 mg.

BOX 7-5	FOOD SOURCES OF MAGNESIUM		
Food Source		**Amount**	**Magnesium (mg)**
Grains Group			
Shredded wheat		2 biscuits	61
Vegetable Group			
Spinach, frozen, cooked		½ cup	78
Meat, Beans, Eggs, and Nuts Group			
Baked beans, canned, vegetarian		1 cup	69
Peanut butter, creamy		2 tbsp	49
Milk Group			
Soy milk		1 cup	61
Milk, reduced fat, low fat, nonfat		1 cup	27

Data from U.S. Department of Agriculture, Agricultural Research Service: *USDA National Nutrient Database for Standard Reference, Release 26.* Nutrient Data Laboratory Home Page, 2013. <http://www.ars.usda.gov/ba/bhnrc/ndl>.
Images copyright 2006 JupiterImages Corporation.
Recommended Dietary Allowance for adults: women ages 19-30, 310 mg; women ages ≥31, 320 mg; men ages 19-30, 400 mg; men ages ≥31, 420 mg.

Magnesium Requirement

The RDA for magnesium is 400 mg for younger men and 310 mg for younger women. To compensate for age-related changes in the kidneys that lead to greater losses, the RDA for persons older than age 30 increases to 420 mg and 320 mg in men and women, respectively.[47]

Food Sources

Magnesium is widespread in nature and unprocessed foods. Whole grains are good sources, but more than 80% of the magnesium is lost when the germ and bran layers of the kernel are removed to produce refined grains. Although milk contains only a modest amount of magnesium, it is a major source in the U.S. diet because it is consumed frequently. Other foods include nuts, soybeans, cocoa, seafood, dried beans and peas, and green vegetables. Except for bananas, fruits are relatively poor sources. Diets rich in vegetables and unrefined grains are higher in magnesium than diets based on highly processed foods and meat. Box 7-5 lists some good sources of magnesium.

CHLORIDE

Chlorine appears in the body as the chloride ion (Cl^-). Chloride accounts for about 3% of body mineral, and most is found in the ECF where it helps control water balance and acid-base balance. Spinal fluid has the highest concentration. A fair amount of ionized chloride is found in the gastrointestinal secretions as a component of gastric hydrochloric acid (HCl). Uncontrolled vomiting and diarrhea with continuing loss of gastric fluids can lead to chloride deficiency with muscle cramps and disturbed acid-base balance.

SULFUR

Sulfur is found in all body cells as a constituent of cell protein. Elemental sulfur forms sulfate compounds with sodium, potassium, and magnesium. Other forms of sulfur include (1) sulfur-containing amino acids such as methionine and cysteine; (2) glycoproteins in cartilage, tendons, and bone matrix; (3) detoxification products formed by intestinal bacteria; (4) organic molecules such as heparin, insulin, coenzyme A (CoA), thiamin, and biotin; and (5) keratin in hair and nails.

The major minerals are summarized in Table 7-3.

ESSENTIAL TRACE ELEMENTS

TRACE ELEMENTS: THE CONCEPT OF ESSENTIALITY

By the simplest definition an essential element is one required to sustain life and, if absent, brings death. For major elements found in relatively large amounts in the body, such a determination is fairly easy based on the quantity available for study. It is more difficult to establish the essentiality of the trace elements because we seem to need so little of them. Trace elements have a required intake of less than 100 mg/day, yet some of them exist in fairly large amounts in our diet and our environment.

Trace elements have two major functions: (1) to catalyze chemical reactions and (2) to serve as structural components of larger molecules. They can be separated into two groups: (1) those that are known to be essential and (2) those for which additional research is needed.

Ten trace elements are considered essential for humans based on defined need and function (see Box 7-1). Several other trace elements are thought to be essential for animals, but researchers have yet to demonstrate a role for them in human health.[47] As we develop better techniques of tissue analysis and functional tests appropriate for human studies, we will learn more about these trace elements and if they are required.

IRON

Of all the micronutrients, iron has the longest history, and the body mechanisms regulating its absorption and use are well understood.

Forms of Iron in the Body

The average adult body contains about 3 to 4 g of iron. This iron is distributed in the following forms, each with a specific metabolic function:
- *Transport iron:* A trace of iron, 0.05 to 0.18 mg/dL, is found in blood plasma bound to the transport carrier protein transferrin.
- *Hemoglobin and myoglobin:* Most body iron, about 70%, resides in the red blood cells as part of the heme portion of the hemoglobin molecule that delivers oxygen to and removes carbon dioxide from body cells. Another 5%

helps form myoglobin, the oxygen-carrying molecule found in the heart and skeletal muscles. Skeletal muscles that continue to contract over extended periods of time, as in marathon runners, require an ongoing supply of oxygen from myoglobin.
- *Storage iron:* About 20% of body iron is stored as the protein-iron compound ferritin in the liver, spleen, and bone marrow. Excess iron is held in the body as hemosiderin and exchanges with ferritin as needed.
- *Cellular iron:* The remaining 5% is distributed across all body cells as an enzyme cofactor in oxidative enzyme systems that produce energy.

Absorption-Transport-Storage-Excretion Balance

Iron is regulated differently from most other nutrients. Generally, urinary excretion controls plasma and tissue levels by ridding the body of any excess that has accumulated. For iron, control is exerted at the points of absorption, transport, and storage. The body has no system for excreting iron.

Absorption

Major control of iron balance takes place at the site of absorption in the small intestine. Absorption is influenced by two characteristics of the iron: its form (heme versus nonheme) and its chemical status (ferric versus ferrous).

The two forms of dietary iron are heme iron and nonheme iron (Table 7-4). The larger portion of dietary iron by far is nonheme iron, which includes all plant sources plus 60% of animal sources.[48] Heme iron is absorbed at a much faster rate because it is a smaller molecule than nonheme iron and easily separated from the hemoglobin molecule in meat, fish, and poultry. Nonheme iron is tightly bound to organic components in plants and animal tissues.

The chemical status of dietary iron is as follows: Nonheme iron found in plant and animal foods is in the chemical form of ferric iron (Fe^{3+}). The gastric acid in the stomach helps separate ferric iron from the organic compounds in which it is bound and reduces it to the more soluble ferrous iron (Fe^{2+}). Ferric iron must be reduced to ferrous iron before it can be absorbed. If not enough gastric acid is available to accomplish this conversion, then the ferric iron is lost in the feces. Approximately 1% to 15% of nonheme iron is absorbed compared with 15% to 45% of heme iron.[49]

Iron distribution and transfer within the absorbing cells of the intestinal mucosa involve several carrier substances. Iron never travels unescorted. First, a protein carrier in the mucosal cell binds the ferrous iron. This protein carrier leaves behind enough iron to serve the needs of the energy-producing mitochondria of the absorbing cell and then delivers specific amounts to waiting carriers that control its destination. These carriers are (1) apoferritin, a protein receptor that combines with iron to form the iron-holding compound ferritin for storage in the cell, and (2) apotransferrin, the protein receptor that combines with iron to form the iron-carrier compound serum transferrin, which circulates in the blood.

TABLE 7-3   SUMMARY OF MAJOR MINERALS

MINERAL	METABOLISM	PHYSIOLOGIC FUNCTIONS	CLINICAL APPLICATIONS	DIETARY REFERENCE INTAKE	FOOD SOURCES
Calcium (Ca)	Absorption according to body need and requiring Ca-binding protein and vitamin D Absorption favored by protein and acidity; Serum levels regulated by vitamin D, parathyroid hormone, and calcitonin Excretion chiefly in feces: 50%-90% of amount ingested Deposition and mobilization in bone tissue is regulated by vitamin D and parathyroid hormone	Constituent of bones and teeth Participates in blood clotting, nerve transmission, muscle action, cell membrane permeability, enzyme activation	Tetany (decrease in serum Ca) Rickets, osteomalacia Osteoporosis Hyperparathyroidism and hypoparathyroidism	Males ages 19-70: 1000 mg Males ages ≥71: 1200 mg Females ages 19-50: 1000 mg Females ages ≥51: 1200 mg Pregnancy Ages ≤18: 1300 mg Ages ≥19: 1000 mg Lactation Ages ≤18: 1300 mg; Ages ≥19: 1000 mg	Milk, cheese, yogurt Green leafy vegetables Whole and fortified grains Legumes, nuts Fortified soy foods Fortified fruit juice
Phosphorus (P)	Absorption with Ca aided by vitamin D and parathyroid hormone and hindered by binding agents Excretion chiefly by kidney according to serum level as regulated by parathyroid hormone Deposition and mobilization in bone compartment is constant	Constituent of bones and teeth Energy metabolism as component of adenosine triphosphate (ATP) Participates in absorption of glucose and glycerol, transport of fatty acids, and buffer system	Growth Recovery from diabetic acidosis Hypophosphatemia: bone disease, malabsorption syndromes, primary hyperparathyroidism Hyperphosphatemia: renal insufficiency, hypoparathyroidism, tetany	Male/female adults Ages ≥19: 700 mg Pregnancy Ages ≤18: 1250 mg Ages ≥19: 700 mg Lactation Ages ≤18: 1250 mg Ages ≥19: 700 mg	Milk, cheese Meat, egg yolk Whole grains Legumes, nuts Soft drinks
Magnesium (Mg)	Absorption according to intake load; hindered by excess fat, phosphate, calcium, protein Excretion (regulated by kidney)	Constituent of bones and teeth Coenzyme in general metabolism, smooth muscle action, neuromuscular irritability Cation in intracellular fluid	Low serum level following gastrointestinal losses Tremor, spasm in deficiency induced by malnutrition, alcoholism	Adults Males ages 19-30: 400 mg Males ages ≥31: 420 mg Females ages 19-30: 310 mg Females ages ≥31: 320 mg Pregnancy Ages ≤18: 400 mg Ages 19-30: 350 mg Ages 31-50: 360 mg Lactation Ages ≤18: 360 mg Ages 19-30: 310 mg Ages 31-50: 320 mg	Milk, cheese Meat, seafood Whole grains Legumes, nuts

Continued

TABLE 7-3   SUMMARY OF MAJOR MINERALS—cont'd

MINERAL	METABOLISM	PHYSIOLOGIC FUNCTIONS	CLINICAL APPLICATIONS	DIETARY REFERENCE INTAKE	FOOD SOURCES
Sodium (Na)	Readily absorbed Excretion chiefly by kidney, controlled by aldosterone	Major cation in extracellular fluid, water balance, acid-base balance Cell membrane permeability Energy-requiring absorption of glucose Normal muscle irritability	Losses in gastrointestinal disorders, diarrhea Fluid-electrolyte and acid-base balance problems Muscle action	Male/female adults Ages 19-50: 1500 mg Ages 51-70: 1300 mg Ages ≥71: 1200 mg UL for all adults: 2300 mg Pregnancy All ages: 1500 mg Lactation All ages: 1500 mg	Salt (NaCl) Sodium compounds used in baking and food processing Milk, cheese, carrots, spinach, beets, celery
Potassium (K)	Readily absorbed Secreted and reabsorbed in gastrointestinal fluids Excretion chiefly by kidney, regulated by aldosterone	Major cation in intracellular fluid, water balance, acid-base balance Normal muscle irritability Glycogen formation Protein synthesis	Losses in gastrointestinal disorders, diarrhea Fluid-electrolyte, acid-base balance problems Muscle action, especially heart muscle Losses in tissue catabolism Treatment of diabetic acidosis: rapid glycogen production reduces serum potassium level Losses with diuretic therapy	Male/female adults All ages: 4700 mg Pregnancy All ages: 4700 mg Lactation All ages: 5100 mg	Fruits Vegetables Legumes, nuts Whole grains Meat
Chloride (Cl)	Readily absorbed Excretion controlled by kidney	Major anion in extracellular fluid, water balance, acid-base balance, chloride-bicarbonate shift Gastric hydrochloric acid—digestion	Losses in gastrointestinal disorders, vomiting, diarrhea, tube drainage Hypochloremic alkalosis	Male/female adults Ages 19-50: 2300 mg Ages 51-70: 2000 mg Ages ≥71: 1800 mg Pregnancy All ages: 2300 mg Lactation All ages: 2300 mg	Salt (NaCl)
Sulfur (S)	Absorbed in elemental form; split from amino acid sources (methionine and cysteine) in digestion and absorbed into portal circulation Excreted by kidney in relation to protein intake and tissue catabolism	Essential component of proteins Detoxification reactions Enzyme activity and energy metabolism through free sulfhydryl group (–SH)	Cystine renal calculi Cystinuria	Adults No specific recommendation: diets adequate in sulfur-containing amino acids are adequate in sulfur	Meat, eggs Milk, cheese Legumes, nuts

TABLE 7-4   CHARACTERISTICS OF HEME AND NONHEME DIETARY IRON

	DIETARY IRON	
	HEME (SMALLER PORTION)	NONHEME (LARGER PORTION)
Food sources	None in plant sources; 40% of iron in animal sources	All plant sources; 60% of iron in animal sources
Absorption	Rapid; transported and absorbed intact	Slow; tightly bound in organic molecules; enhanced by acid and presence of heme iron

The proportion of dietary iron that is absorbed or rejected is determined by the amount of ferritin already present in the intestinal mucosal cells. When all available apoferritin has joined with iron to form ferritin, any additional iron arriving at the binding site is rejected and returned to the lumen of the intestine for excretion in the feces. Most absorption takes place in the upper small intestine.

Three factors favor absorption:

1. *Body need:* In iron deficiency or increased demand as in growth, pregnancy, or weight training, more iron is absorbed.[48] When tissue reserves are ample or saturated, iron is rejected and excreted.
2. *Ascorbic acid (vitamin C) or other acids:* An acidic environment increases iron absorption. Acid reduces ferric iron to ferrous iron, the soluble form that is absorbed. Adding 50 mg of ascorbic acid to a meal by including orange juice or similar acid source can triple the absorption of nonheme iron.[48] Gastric HCl provides the optimal acid medium to prepare iron for absorption.
3. *Animal tissues:* Heme iron improves the absorption of nonheme iron eaten at the same meal. Also, peptides released in digestion of meat, fish, and poultry enhance iron absorption from other food sources.[50]

Five factors hinder iron absorption:

1. *Binding agents:* Phosphates, phytates, and oxalates bind iron and prevent its absorption. Certain vegetable proteins, including soy protein, decrease iron absorption independent of their phytate content. Polyphenols in tea and coffee decrease absorption of nonheme iron.[51]
2. *Low gastric acid:* Partial removal of the stomach reduces the number of acid-secreting cells and decreases absorption of both heme and nonheme iron. Iron supplements are necessary after bariatric surgery.[52] Persons who abuse antacids will have trouble absorbing nonheme iron.[53]
3. *Infection:* Severe infection depresses iron absorption because the body attempts to suppress the supply of iron available to the infectious microorganisms.
4. *Gastrointestinal disease:* Malabsorption syndromes such as celiac disease or steatorrhea hinder iron absorption.
5. *Calcium:* Large amounts of calcium can inhibit the absorption of both heme and nonheme iron consumed at the same meal, and this interaction can influence the iron status of those taking concentrated calcium supplements with meals.[51,54] Adding calcium to meals at the levels normally found in food might be the best approach for optimum absorption of all nutrients.

Transport

After absorption, iron is bound with the protein transferrin for transport to storage sites or body cells. Normally, only 20% to 35% of the iron-binding capacity of transferrin is filled. The remainder serves as a reserve for handling any emergency or variance in iron intake.

Storage

Bound to transferrin, iron is delivered to storage sites in the bone marrow and liver. Here it is recombined with apoferritin to form ferritin, an exchangeable storage form that releases iron as needed. The second less soluble storage form, hemosiderin, provides reserve storage in the liver. From these sites iron is mobilized for hemoglobin synthesis and production of red blood cells or other body cells. Adults use 20 to 25 mg of iron per day for hemoglobin synthesis, but much of this iron was conserved and recycled when old red blood cells were broken down. The average life span of a red blood cell is about 120 days. These interrelationships of body iron absorption-transport-storage are diagrammed in Figure 7-5.

Excretion

Because iron regulation occurs at the point of absorption, only minute amounts are lost through the kidneys. The body also loses iron by the normal sloughing off of skin cells and

---

KEY TERMS

ferritin   Protein-iron compound for storing iron in tissues.

hemosiderin   Insoluble iron oxide-protein compound for storing iron in the liver when the amount of iron in the blood exceeds the storage capacity of ferritin.

heme iron   Form of dietary iron found only in animal sources in the heme portion of hemoglobin. Heme iron is more easily absorbed than nonheme iron.

nonheme iron   The larger portion of dietary iron that includes all plant food sources and 60% of animal food sources. This form of iron is not part of a heme complex and is less easily absorbed.

ferric iron (Fe^{+3})   The oxidized form of iron usually found in food; this form cannot be absorbed and must be reduced to ferrous iron (Fe^{+2}) by the action of gastric acid in order to be absorbed.

ferrous iron (Fe^{+2})   The reduced form of iron that is absorbed in the small intestine.

gastrointestinal cells, as well as through normal gastrointestinal and menstrual blood loss. Heavy menstrual flow, childbirth, surgery, acute and chronic hemorrhage, gastrointestinal disease, or parasitic infestation causes exceptional iron loss and depletes body stores.

Physiologic Functions of Iron

Oxygen transport: Iron is "pocketed" within the heme molecule, the nonprotein portion of hemoglobin in the red blood cell, and carries oxygen to all body cells for respiration and metabolism. Iron has a similar role in myoglobin, which delivers oxygen within muscle cells.

Cellular oxidation: Iron is a component of cell enzyme systems that oxidize glucose and other energy-yielding nutrients.

Immune function: Iron is needed for the production of immune cells and cytokines that attack foreign bacteria invading the body.

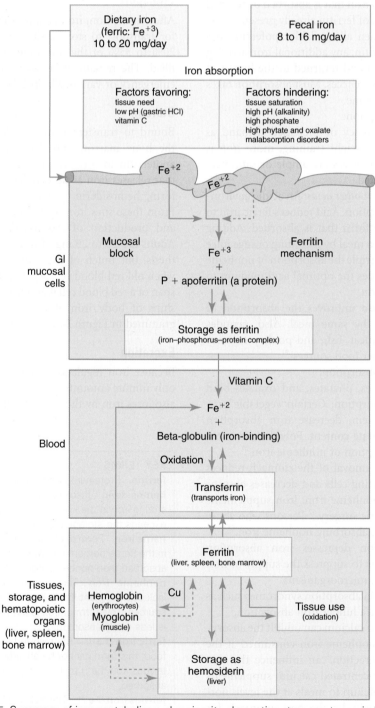

FIGURE 7-5 Summary of iron metabolism, showing its absorption, transport, use in hemoglobin formation, and storage forms (ferritin and hemosiderin).

Growth needs: Positive iron balance is imperative for growth. At birth an infant has a 4- to 6-month supply of iron stored in its liver. Breast-fed infants obtain some iron in breast milk and iron is added to commercial infant formulas. Supplementary iron-rich and iron-fortified foods are introduced to an infant's diet at 4 to 6 months of age to prevent milk anemia.[55] Throughout childhood, iron is needed for continued growth and to build reserves for the physiologic stress of adolescence: muscle development in boys and the onset of menses in girls. Iron needs escalate during pregnancy to produce red blood cells for the mother's expanding blood volume and to build iron reserves in the developing fetal liver. Blood loss in childbirth draws on iron stores.

Brain and cognitive function: Iron is necessary for brain development and the synthesis and breakdown of neurotransmitters. Iron deficiency in the critical periods of gestation and early lactation can have long-lasting negative effects on development of motor skills, social development, and a child's ability to interact with the environment.[56,57] Iron status influenced cognitive function and time to complete mental tasks in young women, with improved performance following treatment for iron deficiency.[58]

Clinical Applications

Clinical abnormalities result from a deficiency or an excess of iron.

Iron Deficiency Anemia

Iron deficiency is a worldwide public health problem and leads to a hypochromic microcytic anemia. Iron deficiency has various causes, described as follows:

- *Low iron intake:* Nutritional anemia develops when iron or other nutrients needed for hemoglobin synthesis and red blood cell production are inadequate. The role of hemoglobin in carrying oxygen to the cells is important in understanding the symptoms of iron deficiency anemia (Box 7-6).
- *Blood loss:* Hemorrhagic anemia results from excessive loss of blood and its associated iron. Aspirin leads to blood loss through the gastrointestinal tract, and its long-term use for pain relief can lower body stores. Severe hemorrhoids cause blood loss.
- *Gastrectomy:* Postgastrectomy anemia develops when gastric acid is insufficient to liberate iron for absorption.
- *Malabsorption:* When the absorbing surface of the small intestine is damaged, iron deficiency anemia follows.

BOX 7-6   SIGNS OF IRON DEFICIENCY

Fatigue
Muscle weakness
Pale color
Decreased resistance to infection
Spoon nails
Angular stomatitis

- *Chronic disease:* Anemia of chronic disease is related to irregularities in the recycling of iron from old red blood cells and the production of new red blood cells, not iron deficiency *per se.* It is associated with infection, inflammatory disorders, heart disease, renal disease, and connective tissue diseases such as osteoarthritis. Found mostly in older adults, this anemia is highly resistant to treatment.
- *Obesity:* Obese youth and adults can experience changes in iron regulation that lower iron absorption and increase risk of iron deficiency, regardless of iron intake.[59]

Worldwide Problem of Iron Deficiency Anemia

Iron deficiency anemia is second only to protein-energy malnutrition as the most prevalent nutritional deficiency worldwide. More than one fourth of the world's population is anemic or iron deficient, with women of childbearing age and children most at risk.[60] Iron deficiency anemia respects neither social class nor geographic location; iron balance in developing countries is precarious based on low intakes of bioavailable iron and iron loss through parasitic infections. For more information on how to identify an iron deficiency anemia see the Perspectives in Practice box, "Nutritional Anemias: How Are They Identified?"

Iron Requirement
Dietary Reference Intake

The RDAs for iron are 18 mg/day for women ages 19 to 50 and 8 mg/day for men ages 19 and older.[48] When the menses cease, the RDA for women is the same as for men—8 mg/day. Pregnancy has a "high iron cost," and the daily allowance rises to 27 mg/day. Iron needs decrease to 9 mg/day during lactation as the menses are usually absent during this period.[48]

Special Considerations for Vegetarians

Individuals who do not eat meat, fish, or poultry need to give special attention to their iron needs. Not only is the bioavailability of iron lower in plant foods, but also heme iron is unavailable to enhance nonheme iron absorption. As a result, overall iron absorption from plant foods is estimated to be about 10% as compared with 18% for the typical American diet. With this in mind it is recommended that vegetarian men take in 14 mg of iron per day and vegetarian premenopausal women take in 33 mg/day. Vegetarian adolescent girls should aim for 26 mg/day.[48] These recommendations are nearly twice those for persons of comparable age and gender who consume a mixed diet, so individual counseling regarding iron sources and supplements is warranted. (See Chapter 5 for a review of plant-based diets.)

Iron Toxicity
Hemochromatosis

Iron toxicity was first identified in a population in Southern Africa who cooked their food in iron vessels and also had a genetic tendency to absorb and store abnormally high amounts of dietary iron. In the United States, accidental iron

PERSPECTIVES IN PRACTICE

Nutritional Anemias: How Are They Identified?

Anemia, a common condition throughout the world, has many different causes. Nutritional anemias occur when a nutrient required to synthesize hemoglobin or red blood cells is lacking. The two most common nutritional anemias are iron deficiency anemia and the megaloblastic anemia related to a lack of dietary vitamin B_{12} or the inability to absorb vitamin B_{12}. These two types of anemia will be the focus of our discussion here.

The cause of a nutritional anemia is evaluated on the basis of various blood parameters, although some characteristics are nonspecific as to the origin of the anemia:

Size of the red blood cell:
- Microcytic cells are small in size relative to normal red blood cells and are characteristic of iron deficiency anemia.
- Macrocytic cells are very large in size relative to normal red blood cells and are often associated with a lack of vitamin B_{12}.

Number of red blood cells:
- The number of red blood cells is decreased in both an iron deficiency and a vitamin B_{12}–related anemia.

Hemoglobin level:
- Women of childbearing age often have lower hemoglobin levels than men due to their monthly blood loss; however, hemoglobin levels are reduced further in both genders in the case of anemia. Low hemoglobin is not a sensitive marker for distinguishing between an iron deficiency and vitamin B_{12}-related anemia.[1]

Specific markers of iron status can help to identify an iron-deficiency anemia.
- Serum iron, which transports iron for metabolic use, falls to low levels as less iron is being absorbed as the iron deficiency worsens.
- Serum ferritin carries iron to storage sites; it falls to low levels as iron becomes less available.
- Transferrin is the protein that binds absorbed iron and delivers it to the bone marrow for production of red blood cells and to body cells for metabolic use; serum transferrin rises as the body attempts to utilize all available iron.
- Serum transferrin saturation indicates the proportion of available transferrin that is bound with iron; normal transferrin saturation is about 20% to 35% but drops to less than 15% in iron deficiency anemia.

A definitive diagnosis of iron deficiency as the cause of a related anemia requires more than one marker of evaluation. Serum ferritin and transferrin saturation are the most sensitive to changes occurring in a true iron deficiency anemia.[2]

References
1. Litchford MD: Assessment: laboratory data. In Mahan LK, Escott-Stump S, editors: *Krause's food and nutrition therapy*, St Louis, Mo., 2008, Saunders.
2. Stopler T: Medical nutrition therapy for anemia. In Mahan LK, Escott-Stump S, editors: *Krause's food and nutrition therapy*, St Louis, Mo., 2008, Saunders.

poisoning occurs in children and adults who overuse iron supplements. However, another cause of iron overload is the genetic disease hemochromatosis, in which iron continues to be absorbed at high rates despite elevated liver stores. It is estimated that 1 in every 385 Americans has this genetic mutation, although not all develop hemochromatosis.[61] Excessive body iron is associated with increased tissue oxidation and production of free radicals and is believed to foster cardiac arrhythmias, liver disease, joint disease, and diabetes.[62] Even moderately elevated iron stores, much lower than those associated with hemochromatosis, appear to increase the risk of type 2 diabetes in otherwise healthy persons.[63,64]

Tolerable Upper Intake Level

Because iron becomes toxic at high levels, iron intake should not exceed 45 mg/day.[48] Although it would seem unlikely that one would reach this level from food alone, current iron fortification policies developed to meet the iron needs of women in the childbearing years add significant amounts of iron to the diet. Individuals who eat more than one serving of a cereal that contains 15 to 18 mg of iron per serving, along with other iron-containing foods, and possibly a multivitamin-mineral supplement with iron, will approach or exceed the UL. Moderately elevated iron stores were found in older

adults who ate large amounts of meat that supplied heme iron and took iron supplements[65] or used alcoholic beverages on a regular basis.[66] (Alcohol increases iron absorption.) Iron supplements should always be approved and supervised by a physician. Acute iron toxicity occurs in children who accidentally consume large amounts of an iron supplement.

Food Sources of Iron

The typical Western diet contains about 5 mg to 7 mg of iron per 1000 kcal. Iron is found in highest amounts in meat, fish, poultry, eggs, dried peas and beans, and whole grain and fortified breads and cereals. Heme iron provides less than 10% of the iron intake of girls and women and less than 12% of the iron intake of boys and men.[48] Fortified grain products such as breakfast bars may contain as much as 24 mg of iron per serving. Box 7-7 lists some comparative food sources of iron.

IODINE

Iodine has worldwide interest, based on the need to identify the cause of goiter and other disorders brought about by iodine deficiency. Iodine is a component of the hormone thyroxine produced in the thyroid gland. The body contains

BOX 7-7   FOOD SOURCES OF IRON

Food Source	Amount	Iron (mg)
Grains Group		
Ready-to-eat cereals		
Total	¾ cup	18.00
Cheerios	1 cup	9.29
All Bran	½ cup	5.46
Rice, white, long-grain enriched, cooked	1 cup	2.86
Rice, brown, long-grain, cooked	1 cup	0.82
Bread, white, commercially prepared	1 slice	1.01
Bread, whole wheat, commercially prepared	1 slice	0.79
Vegetable Group		
Spinach, frozen, cooked	½ cup	1.86
Potato, baked, flesh and skin	1 medium	1.87
Potato, baked, flesh only	1 medium	0.55
Peas, green, canned	½ cup	1.60
Lima beans, frozen, baby, cooked	1 cup	3.53
Broccoli, frozen, cooked	½ cup	0.56
Vegetable juice cocktail, canned	1 cup	0.73
Fruit		
Raisins, seedless	½ cup	1.36
Meat, Beans, Eggs, and Nuts Group		
Ground beef patty, lean	3 oz	2.11
Frankfurter, beef	1	0.59
Ham, canned, lean	3 oz	1.16
Chicken, thigh meat, roasted, without skin	3 oz	1.08
Tuna, light, canned in water	3 oz	1.39
Egg, whole, hard-cooked	1 large	0.60
Soybeans, cooked	½ cup	4.42
Refried beans, canned	½ cup	2.10
Soy patty, vegan	3 oz	2.47
Tofu, firm	3 oz	1.30

Data from U.S. Department of Agriculture, Agricultural Research Service: *USDA National Nutrient Database for Standard Reference, Release 26.* Nutrient Data Laboratory Home Page, 2013. <http://www.ars.usda.gov/ba/bhnrc/ndl>.
Images copyright 2006 JupiterImages Corporation.
Recommended Dietary Allowances for adults: men, 8 mg; women ages 19-50, 18 mg; women ages ≥51, 8 mg.

only 15 to 20 mg of iodine, and 70% to 80% is in the thyroid gland. This gland has a remarkable ability to concentrate iodine.

Absorption-Excretion Balance
Absorption

Iodine is absorbed in the form of iodides. Iodides are then loosely bound to proteins and carried by the blood to the thyroid gland, which takes up as much as it needs for hormone

KEY TERMS
anemia A condition characterized by abnormally low number of red blood cells or hemoglobin content.
hemochromatosis A hereditary disorder causing excessive absorption of iron and its deposition in soft tissues such as joints, heart, and liver; increases risk of diabetes, arthritis, and heart disease.
goiter Enlargement of the thyroid gland caused by lack of available iodine to produce the thyroid hormone thyroxine.

synthesis. About one third of the available iodide is used to produce active thyroid hormone with the remainder used to form hormone precursors for later use.

Excretion

Absorbed iodide not needed by the thyroid gland is excreted in the urine. More than 90% of the iodine taken into the body appears in the urine.

Hormonal Control

Thyroid-stimulating hormone (TSH) from the anterior lobe of the pituitary gland directs the uptake of iodine by thyroid cells in response to plasma thyroid hormone levels. When plasma levels are high, less thyroid hormone is produced. When plasma levels are low, the thyroid cells are stimulated to take up more iodine and produce more hormone. This feedback mechanism maintains a healthy circular balance between supply and demand and is the characteristic pattern of the endocrine glands controlled by the pituitary gland.

Physiologic Function of Iodine
Thyroid Hormone Synthesis

The major function of iodine is in the synthesis of the thyroid hormone, thyroxine. Thyroxine regulates cell oxidation and basal metabolic rate (BMR) by increasing oxygen uptake and the reaction rates of enzyme systems handling glucose. In this role iodine exerts tremendous control over total body metabolism. Thyroid hormone also regulates protein synthesis and myelin formation in the developing brain.[67] Hyperthyroidism and hypothyroidism affect the rate of thyroxine production and the body's overall metabolic rate.

Plasma Thyroxine

Thyroxine is secreted into the bloodstream bound to plasma protein for transport to cells. After completing its work, the hormone is degraded in the liver, and the iodine excreted in the bile.

Clinical Applications
Iodine Deficiency Disorder: Goiter

Endemic goiter, visible as an enlargement of the thyroid gland, is a problem in geographic areas where water and soil, and in turn locally grown foods, contain little iodine. Up to 2 billion people live in iodine-deficient areas, including one third of all school children.[67] Africa, Southeast Asia, the Eastern Mediterranean, and parts of Europe have had widespread iodine deficiency. When iodine is not available in the amounts needed, the thyroid gland cannot produce a normal quantity of thyroxine. Low plasma thyroxine levels signal the pituitary to release TSH, and, without iodine, the thyroid gland responds by making thyroglobulin (a colloid), which accumulates in the thyroid follicles. Over time the gland becomes increasingly engorged and may attain a size of 500 to 700 g (1 to 1½ lb) or more (Figure 7-6).

Salt iodization remains the most cost-effective way to deliver iodine to both humans and livestock and is credited with eradicating iodine deficiency in the United States and Canada. Through the use of iodized salt, the number of countries affected by goiter has dropped from 110 to 32.[68] In remote areas where iodization of salt is not practical, iodized rapeseed oil, monthly doses of potassium iodide to school children, or slow-release iodide added to drinking water has eradicated severe endemic goiter.[69] Goiter also stems from

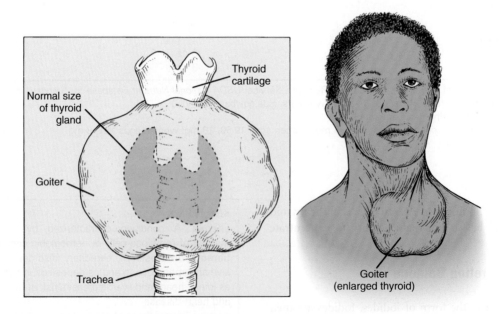

FIGURE 7-6 Goiter. The extreme enlargement shown here reflects an extended duration of iodine deficiency.

eating foods containing substances that inhibit the synthesis of thyroxine. Pearl millet, a cereal grain in the Sudan region of Africa, can cause goiter.

Iodine Deficiency Disorder: Cretinism

Iodine deficiency has been referred to as *the most common cause of preventable brain damage in the world*,[68] and for pregnant and lactating women and their infants, the need is critical. When iodine deficiency is severe during fetal and infant periods of critical brain development, the outcome is **cretinism**, with irreversible mental retardation and disability. Consistent salt-fortification programs provide sufficient iodine to support the elevated needs of pregnancy and the production of breast milk with appropriate iodine content.[68]

Iodine Requirement
Dietary Reference Intake

The RDA for iodine in men and women is 150 mcg/day.[48] To meet the needs of mother and developing fetus, the RDA increases to 220 mcg/day in pregnancy and 290 mcg/day throughout lactation. Because of increased demand for iodine during accelerated growth, the allowance for youth ages 14 to 18 is the same as for adults.

Food Sources of Iodine

Seafood is rich in iodine. Plant foods depend on the iodine content of the soil and the iodine compounds used in food processing. Iodized table salt fortified at the level of 1 mg of iodine per 10 g of salt is a major dietary source in the United States. Calcium and potassium iodates are common additives in commercially produced bread. Avoidance of salt for health reasons likely helps explain the decrease in iodine intakes over the past 30 years.[67]

Common food production and processing methods in the United States add to iodine intake. Dairy farms use iodophors, iodine-containing chemicals, for sanitizing milking machines and milk tanks. Iodine-containing compounds are used as dough conditioners, and iodine supplements are added to animal feeds. For most people iodine intake from food and supplements is unlikely to exceed the UL. Toxicity symptoms usually result from intakes of several grams of iodine.

ZINC

Zinc is a component of over 100 different body enzymes and a factor in growth.[48] Total body zinc ranges from 1.5 g in women to 2.5 g in men. It is present in minute quantities in all body organs, tissues, and fluids. Although zinc is vital throughout life, it is particularly important in periods of growth.[48] Zinc is closely involved with DNA and RNA metabolism and protein synthesis. It is necessary for tissue growth to progress at normal rates.

Absorption-Excretion-Storage

Zinc is absorbed in the midsection of the small intestine, and, as is the case for iron, individuals in poor zinc status absorb a greater proportion of their dietary zinc than individuals in good zinc status. Zinc is excreted primarily via the feces, with very small amounts lost in the urine. Zinc absorption is impaired with long-term alcohol consumption, and greater amounts are lost in the urine, putting these persons at risk of poor zinc status. Zinc is stored primarily in the muscle and bone. A very small amount of body zinc circulates in the plasma but these levels are carefully regulated.

Clinical Applications

Several clinical problems stem from zinc deficiency, as follows:

- *Hypogonadism:* Dwarfism with arrested development and function of the gonads results from pronounced zinc deficiency in childhood and adolescence. Sexual maturation is delayed in male adolescents deprived of zinc.
- *Loss in taste and smell:* Hypogeusia (diminished taste) and hyposmia (diminished smell) are associated with severe zinc deficiency but improve when zinc is restored.
- *Wound healing:* Healing of wounds or tissue injuries from trauma, surgery, or physiologic stress is retarded in those who are zinc deficient. Older adults with pressure sores may benefit from zinc supplementation.
- *Growth, development, and life cycle needs:* Rapid growth in infants, children, and adolescents carries special needs for zinc. When zinc is inadequate, proteins necessary for the linear growth of the long bones are not produced and growth is stunted.[48,70] Poor zinc intake in pregnancy can result in congenital malformations and low infant birth weight. Even subclinical deficiency has adverse effects on brain function in both children and adults.[71]
- *Immune function:* Zinc promotes optimum immune function. Zinc-deficient children are more vulnerable to disability and death from diarrhea.[70] Older individuals with optimum zinc status have greater resistance to infections and less need for antibiotics.[72]
- *Malabsorption:* Malabsorption diseases such as Crohn's disease lead to zinc deficiency. Dietary restrictions imposed in the treatment of these conditions can further limit zinc availability.

Zinc Requirement
Dietary Reference Intake

The RDA for zinc is 11 mg for men and 8 mg for women.[48] Women's needs are lower because of their generally smaller body size. Caregivers need to be reminded of the importance of foods containing zinc for young children. Less than half of the sack lunches preschool children brought to a day care center met one third of the DRI for zinc[73]; the omission of milk in many lunches contributed to the low zinc content.[73]

KEY TERM

cretinism A congenital disease resulting from a lack of iodine and thyroxin secretion, characterized by physical deformity, dwarfism, mental retardation, and often goiters.

Beef is a major zinc source in the United States, accounting for nearly 25% of total intake, followed by ready-to-eat cereals, milk, and poultry.[48] Zinc is better absorbed from diets high in animal protein than diets high in plant protein. Zinc can be a problem for vegetarians because phytates in plant foods bind to zinc and prevent its absorption.[74]

Concentrated zinc supplements can interfere with iron and copper absorption and can lead to poor copper status. Conversely, there is evidence that iron supplements may interfere with zinc absorption if both are taken without food. This raises a concern about the management of supplement use in pregnancy when both nutrients are vital to growth of maternal and fetal tissues.[47] Excessive zinc intake results in gastrointestinal distress, a decrease in blood HDL (high-density lipoprotein) cholesterol, and a suppressed immune system. This is known to occur not as a result of food intake but rather from use of high potency supplements exceeding the UL of 40 mg.[47]

Food Sources of Zinc

Good sources of dietary zinc are seafood (especially oysters), meat, eggs, and milk. Legumes and whole grains contain zinc, but bioavailability is a problem. Box 7-8 lists some foods containing zinc.

COPPER

Copper and iron have many characteristics in common, as listed below:
- Both are components of cell enzymes.
- Both are involved in energy production.
- Both participate in hemoglobin synthesis.

Copper is found in many foods, but deficiency has been reported in patients on total parenteral nutrition (TPN) that excluded copper. Persons using concentrated zinc supplements that interfere with copper absorption can develop copper deficiency. Premature infants fed only cow's milk, which is low in copper, become deficient.[48]

The RDA for copper is 900 mcg/day (0.9 mg/day).[48] Copper, like many trace elements, is lost in food processing. The richest sources are liver, seafood (particularly oysters), nuts, and seeds, with smaller amounts in whole grains and legumes. The Focus on Food Safety box, "Minerals from Cooking Utensils: Safe or Harmful?" describes how copper and other minerals can enter our food in cooking.

MANGANESE

The adult body contains about 20 mg of manganese distributed in the liver, bones, pancreas, and pituitary gland.[48] Manganese is a part of important cell enzymes. Manganese deficiency has been reported in patients with pancreatic insufficiency and protein-energy malnutrition. Although an essential nutrient, manganese is toxic at high levels among miners or other workers with prolonged exposure to manganese dust. Excess manganese accumulates in the liver and central nervous system (CNS), producing psychiatric

BOX 7-8   FOOD SOURCES OF ZINC

Food Source	Amount	Zinc (mg)
Grains Group		
Shredded wheat	2 biscuits	1.38
Oat bran muffin	1 (small)	1.21
Vegetable Group		
Peas, green, canned	1 cup	1.48
Meat, Beans, Eggs, and Nuts Group		
Oysters, breaded, fried	3 oz (6 medium)	74.06
Ground beef patty, lean	3 oz	5.27
Baked beans, canned, vegetarian	1 cup	5.79
Peanut butter, creamy	2 tbsp	0.93
Milk Group		
Milk, nonfat (reduced-fat, low-fat, and whole milk vary slightly)	1 cup	1.03
American cheese, processed, pasteurized	1 oz	0.71

Data from U.S. Department of Agriculture, Agricultural Research Service: *USDA National Nutrient Database for Standard Reference, Release 26.* Nutrient Data Laboratory Home Page, 2013. <http://www.ars.usda.gov/ba/bhnrc/ndl>.
Images copyright 2006 JupiterImages Corporation.
Recommended Dietary Allowance for adults: women, 8 mg; men, 11 mg.

disturbances and neuromuscular symptoms resembling those of Parkinson's disease. Manganese toxicity usually occurs from environmental exposure, not dietary intake.

The AI for manganese is 2.3 mg/day for men and 1.8 mg/day for women.[48] The typical American diet supplies manganese at a level of 1.6 mg/1000 kcal. The best sources are plant foods such as grains, legumes, seeds, nuts, leafy vegetables, tea, and coffee.

CHROMIUM

Chromium is found in minute amounts in liver, soft tissues, and bone, although the precise body total is unknown. Chromium is part of a protein complex that potentiates insulin activity and assists in moving glucose into cells. Through its role with insulin, chromium influences carbohydrate, protein, and fat metabolism. Chromium picolinate is widely advertised as a bodybuilding and weight-loss supplement, despite the fact that no research evidence supports these claims, and, in fact, existing evidence contradicts these claims. (See Chapter 14 for more discussion of chromium picolinate.)

The AI for chromium is 35 mcg/day for men and 25 mcg/day for women ages 19 to 50. Based on the decline in energy intakes, the AIs decrease to 30 mcg and 20 mcg, respectively, after age 50.[48] Information about the chromium content of common foods is sparse. Brewer's yeast is a rich source. Other food sources include liver, cheddar cheese, wheat germ, and whole grains.

SELENIUM

Selenium is deposited in all body tissues except adipose tissue. Concentrations are highest in liver, kidney, heart, and spleen. Selenium is an integral part of an antioxidant enzyme that protects cells and lipid membranes from oxidative damage. Selenium partners with vitamin E, each sparing the other. Highly bioavailable selenium compounds are found in breast milk, suggesting an important role for this element in early life.[75] The RDA for all adults is 55 mcg/day.[76] Plant foods vary in selenium based on the content of the soil in which they were grown. In general, good sources include seafood, legumes, whole grains, lean meats, and dairy products; vegetables have the smallest amounts.

MOLYBDENUM

Molybdenum is an enzyme cofactor in reactions that move hydroxyl (OH^-) groups.[48] The RDA is set at 45 mcg/day for all adults. The amount of molybdenum in foods varies according to the soil content. The richest sources generally include legumes, whole grains, and nuts. Animal products, fruit, and most vegetables are poor sources.

FLUORIDE

Fluoride accumulates in the calcified tissues and protects bones and teeth from mineral loss.[77] If fluoride is present when calcium-phosphorus crystals are being formed, then a fluoride ion (F^-) replaces a hydroxyl ion (OH^-) in the crystal, resulting in a material that is more resistant to resorption. Fluoride-containing crystals are also more resistant to the erosion of bacterial acids formed by microorganisms that feed on fermentable carbohydrates adhering to the teeth and initiate tooth decay.[77]

The AI for fluoride is expected to protect against dental caries. Intake is set at 4 mg/day for men and 3 mg/day for women.[47] Fish, fish products, and teas contain the highest amounts. Fluoridated dental products such as toothpaste and mouthwash contribute to fluoride intake and may approach the amount ingested from food. Adding fluoride to public water supplies in the amount of 1 part per million (ppm) reduces dental caries in those communities. Cooking with fluoridated water increases the level in many foods.

Excessive fluoride intake leads to pitted and discolored teeth, and this condition was first identified in communities where the natural water source was high in fluoride. Enamel fluorosis and skeletal fluorosis are unlikely to occur unless fluoride intake exceeds 10 mg a day for a period of 10 years or more; such intakes are uncommon in the United States. Young children should be monitored to avoid swallowing excessive amounts of dental products that contain fluoride.[47]

The roles of the essential trace elements are summarized in Table 7-5.

OTHER TRACE ELEMENTS

The metabolic functions or need for five other trace elements: arsenic, boron, vanadium, nickel, and silicon are at present undefined. Although they appear to have beneficial roles in various animal species, evidence of their nutritional importance, essentiality, or role in human health is lacking.[47] Insufficient research data are available to set an RDA or AI for these minerals. Based on their potential for toxicity, a UL has been established for boron, nickel, and vanadium.[47]

WATER AND ELECTROLYTES

Water, the last nutrient we will review, is essential to the life of every cell. In our discussions of sodium, potassium, and chloride we noted the roles of these minerals in guarding

TABLE 7-5   SUMMARY OF TRACE ELEMENTS

ELEMENT	METABOLISM	PHYSIOLOGIC FUNCTIONS	CLINICAL APPLICATIONS	DIETARY REFERENCE INTAKE	FOOD SOURCES
Iron (Fe)	Absorption controls body supply; favored by body need, acidity, and reduction agents such as vitamin C; hindered by binding agents, reduced gastric HCl, infection Transported as transferrin, stored as ferritin or hemosiderin Excreted in sloughed cells, bleeding; no body mechanism for excretion	Hemoglobin and myoglobin synthesis, oxygen transport Cell oxidation	Anemia (hypochromic, microcytic) Excess: hemosiderosis, hemochromatosis Growth and pregnancy needs	Adults Males ages ≥19: 8 mg Females ages 19-50: 18 mg Females ages ≥51: 8 mg Pregnancy All ages: 27 mg Lactation Ages ≤18: 10 mg Ages ≥19: 9 mg	Meat, eggs, liver Whole grain and enriched breads and cereals Dark green vegetables Legumes, nuts Acidic foods cooked in iron utensils
Iodine (I)	Absorbed as iodides, taken up by thyroid gland under control of thyroid-stimulating hormone (TSH) Excretion by kidney	Synthesis of thyroxin, which regulates cell metabolism, basal metabolic rate (BMR)	Endemic colloid goiter Cretinism Hypothyroidism and hyperthyroidism	Adults Males/females ages ≥19: 150 mcg Pregnancy All ages: 220 mcg Lactation All ages: 290 mcg	Iodized salt Seafood
Zinc (Zn)	Absorbed in small intestine Stored in many tissues Excretion largely intestinal	Essential coenzyme component; involved with DNA/RNA metabolism and protein synthesis	Growth: hypogonadism Sensory impairment: taste and smell Wound healing, Malabsorption disease	Adults Males ages ≥19: 11 mg Females ages ≥19: 8 mg Pregnancy Ages ≤18: 12 mg Ages ≥19: 11 mg Lactation Ages ≤18: 13 mg Ages ≥19: 12 mg	Beef and other meats, liver Oysters, seafood Milk, cheese, eggs Whole grains Widely distributed in food
Copper (Cu)	Absorbed in small intestine Stored in many tissues	Associated with iron in enzyme systems, hemoglobin synthesis Metalloprotein enzyme component	Hypocupremia: nephrosis and malabsorption Wilson's disease, excess copper storage	Adults Males/females ages ≥19: 900 mcg Pregnancy All ages: 1000 mcg Lactation All ages: 1300 mcg	Meat, liver, seafood Whole grains Legumes, nuts Widely distributed in food

Mineral	Absorption/Excretion	Function	Requirements	Deficiency/Toxicity	Sources
Manganese (Mn)	Absorbed poorly Excretion mainly by intestine	Enzyme component in general metabolism	Adults Males ages ≥19: 2.3 mg Females ages ≥19: 1.8 mg Pregnancy All ages: 2.0 mg Lactation all ages: 2.6 mg	Low serum levels in protein-energy malnutrition Inhalation toxicity	Whole grains and cereals Legumes, soybeans Green leafy vegetables
Chromium (Cr)	Absorbed in association with zinc Excretion mainly by kidney	Associated with glucose metabolism	Adults Males ages 19-50: 35 mcg Males ages ≥51: 30 mcg Females ages 19-50: 25 mcg Females ages ≥51: 20 mcg Pregnancy Ages ≤18: 29 mcg Ages ≥19: 30 mcg Lactation Ages ≤18: 44 mcg Ages ≥19: 45 mcg	Potentiates action of insulin	Whole grains and cereals Brewers' yeast Animal protein foods
Selenium (Se)	Absorption depends on solubility of compound form Excreted mainly by kidney	Component of enzyme glutathione peroxidase Synergistic antioxidant with vitamin E	Adults Males/females Ages ≥19: 55 mcg Pregnancy All ages: 60 mcg Lactation All ages: 70 mcg	Marginal deficiency when soil content is low Deficiency secondary to total parenteral nutrition (TPN) or malnutrition Toxicity observed in livestock	Seafood Legumes Whole grains Vegetables Low-fat meats and dairy foods Varies with soil content
Molybdenum (Mo)	Readily absorbed Excreted rapidly by kidneys Small amount excreted in bile	Component of oxidase enzymes	Adults Males/females ages ≥19: 45 mcg Pregnancy All ages 50 mcg Lactation All ages: 50 mcg	Deficiency unknown in humans	Legumes Whole grains Milk Organ meats Leafy vegetables
Fluoride (F)	Absorbed in small intestine; little known of bioavailability Excreted by kidneys	Accumulates in bones and teeth, increases resistance to resorption	Adults Males ages ≥19: 4 mg Females ages ≥19: 3 mg Pregnancy All ages: 3 mg Lactation All ages: 3 mg	Reduces dental caries Osteoporosis: may reduce bone loss Excess: dental fluorosis	Fish and fish products Tea Drinking water (if fluoridated) Foods cooked in fluoridated water

body water and maintaining its appropriate distribution within and outside of body cells. Now we will see how this is accomplished.

Hydration status is fundamental to health and a vital part of patient care. Three interdependent factors control fluid balance: (1) the water itself (the solvent base for solutions), (2) the various particles in the water (solutes), and (3) the separating membranes that control flow from one compartment to another.

BODY WATER

Body Water Distribution

If you are a woman, your body is about 50% to 55% water; if you are a man, then it is about 55% to 60% water. Men have higher water content because they have proportionately more muscle and less fat. Muscle contains more water than any other tissue except blood. Women have proportionately less muscle and more fat, which is lower in water content.

Functions of Body Water

Body water has many roles (Box 7-9). Much of our body form comes from the turgor water provides for tissues. Cell water furnishes the fluid environment for the vast array of chemical reactions that sustain life. Medications are dissolved in body fluids. The evaporation of water from the skin is an important means of regulating body temperature.

Overall Water Balance: Input and Output

The average adult processes 2.5 to 3 L of water each day. Water enters and leaves the body by various routes (Table 7-6), controlled by the thirst mechanism and regulatory hormones.

Water enters the body in three forms:
- As preformed water taken in as water or in other beverages
- As preformed water in food
- As metabolic water produced by cell oxidation

It is estimated that 81% of fluid intake comes from water and beverages and 19% comes from food.[26] Plain water contributes about a third of the total and other beverages about half.[78] Many common foods contain large amounts of water (Table 7-7). Metabolic water contributes less to total water than do beverages or food. All water, regardless of source, is of equal value in meeting fluid needs.

Water leaves the body via the kidneys, skin, and lungs, as well as through fecal elimination (see Table 7-6). Vomiting and diarrhea bring abnormal fluid losses and serious clinical problems if prolonged. Abnormal loss of body fluid is especially dangerous for infants and children, whose bodies contain a greater proportion of water. More of their body water is outside the cells and more easily lost. Water retention associated with heart failure or electrolyte disturbances requires immediate medical attention. Intake and

TABLE 7-6	APPROXIMATE DAILY ADULT WATER INTAKE AND OUTPUT			
			OUTPUT (LOSS) (mL/day)	
	INTAKE (REPLACEMENT) (mL/day)		OBLIGATORY (INSENSIBLE) (mL/day)	ADDITIONAL (BASED ON NEED) (mL/day)
Preformed in liquids	1200-1500	Lungs	350	
In foods	700-1000	Skin diffusion	350	
Metabolism (oxidation of food)	200-300	Sweat	100	≈250
		Kidneys	900	≈500
		Feces	150	
TOTAL	2100-2800 (≈2600 mL/day)	TOTAL	1850 (≈2600 mL/day)	750

TABLE 7-7	WATER CONTENT OF SELECTED FOODS AND BEVERAGES	
FOOD		PERCENT (%)
Coffee, milk, sports drinks, watermelon, broccoli, lettuce		91-100
Soda, fruit drinks, fruit juice, apples, oranges, grapes		80-90
Peas, frozen desserts, bananas, casseroles		70-79
Meat, fish, poultry		60-69
Bread, pasta		30-40
Cereals, nuts		<5

Data from Campbell S: Dietary Reference Intakes: water, potassium, sodium, chloride, and sulfate. *Nutr MD* 30(6):13, 2004.

BOX 7-9	FUNCTIONS OF BODY WATER

Gives body form and structure
Provides fluid environment for chemical reactions to take place
Dissolves important substances in tissues and cells
Transports nutrients and waste
Controls body temperature
Dissolves medications

KEY TERM

compartment   The collective quantity of material of a given type in the body. The four body compartments are (1) lean body mass (muscle and vital organs), (2) bone, (3) fat, and (4) water.

output must remain in balance to sustain normal hydration levels.

WATER REQUIREMENTS

For years we were told to drink eight glasses of water a day, although it is difficult to find documentation on the origin of this advice.[79,80] References to hydration in the popular press and advertisements for bottled water promote deliberate water consumption. Nutrition experts note that for most individuals fluid needs are met by drinking when thirsty.[26,81]

Dietary Reference Intake

The current AIs for fluid (Table 7-8) are based on the median water intake of participants in recent national surveys[26]; half of the people in each age and gender category drank more than this amount and half drank less. However, questions remain as to the appropriateness of these recommendations. First, quantifying water intake is difficult, and only recently have such questions been added to nutrition surveys.[81,82] Moreover, individuals often consume fluids such as sweetened or alcoholic beverages for reasons other than thirst.[81] Finally, these water guidelines are intended for healthy individuals who are relatively sedentary and live in temperate climates. Older adults with a diminished sense of thirst, athletes engaging in vigorous physical activity of long duration, the critically ill with a high rate of metabolism, persons in very hot environments with high losses of water via sweat, or those doing strenuous physical work require special attention.[26,81]

Fluid intake is related to energy intake. Water, when consumed in place of sugar-sweetened beverages, juice, or milk, is linked with lower energy intake.[81,83] This relationship has application to kcalorie intake and inappropriate weight gain in children and youth.

Clinical Applications

The following clinical situations influence water needs:

- *Uncontrolled diabetes mellitus:* Patients lose excessive amounts of water through the osmotic effect of high urinary glucose and need additional fluid.

- *Cystic fibrosis:* This disease increases fluid needs.
- *High fiber intake:* As dietary fiber increases, so do fluid requirements. Adequate fluid is needed to replace the water absorbed by the fiber in the gastrointestinal tract.
- *High protein intake:* Protein metabolism produces urea and other nitrogenous wastes that must be excreted via the kidneys. Providing an appropriate level of fluid is important for patients given high-protein supplements.
- *Intense physical activity:* Exercise of high intensity or duration such as marathon runs or strenuous physical work requires consistent fluid intake to replace water lost in sweat, thereby enabling this cooling mechanism to continue. A lack of fluid in such situations can lead to heat stroke and death (see Chapter 14).
- *Impaired thirst in older adults:* Some older persons, particularly frail older adults in poor health or who take multiple medications, do not become thirsty when they should, based on aging changes in the thirst center of the hypothalamus.[81] Older adults who suffer from incontinence may voluntarily reduce their fluid intake.
- *Medications:* Diuretics increase fluid output, as do certain analgesics and decongestants.

Water Compartments

Body water is divided into two major compartments: (1) the water outside the cells, known as *extracellular fluid (ECF)* and (2) the water inside the cells, known as *intracellular fluid (ICF)* (Figure 7-7). We describe as follows:

- *ECF:* The water outside the cells makes up about 20% of total body weight. It is divided into four sections: (1) blood plasma, which accounts for about 5% of body weight; (2) interstitial fluid, the water surrounding the cells; (3) secretory fluid, the water circulating in transit; and (4) dense tissue fluid, water in deep connective tissue, cartilage, and bone.
- *ICF:* The water inside the cells makes up about 40% to 45% of total body weight. All of the metabolic activity of organs and tissues takes place within cells, so it could be expected that the amount of water inside the cells would be greater than the amount outside the cells (intracellular water is about double the amount of extracellular water).

FORCES CONTROLLING WATER DISTRIBUTION

Two forces control the distribution of body water: (1) the number of solutes or particles in solution and (2) the membranes that separate water compartments. We will look at the properties of each. (Review Figure 2-9, which illustrates the movement of water across membranes.)

Solutes

A variety of particles are found in body water. Two types control water balance: electrolytes and plasma proteins.

TABLE 7-8	**ADEQUATE INTAKES OF FLUID***	
AGE (YEARS)	MALES	FEMALES
1-3	4 cups	4 cups
4-8	5 cups	5 cups
9-13	8 cups	7 cups
14-18	11 cups	8 cups
≥19	13 cups	9 cups

Data from Food and Nutrition Board, Institute of Medicine: *Dietary Reference Intakes for water, potassium, sodium, chloride, and sulfate*, Washington, D.C., 2004, National Academies Press.
*Expressed as cups of beverages/drinking water with additional fluid to be supplied in food.

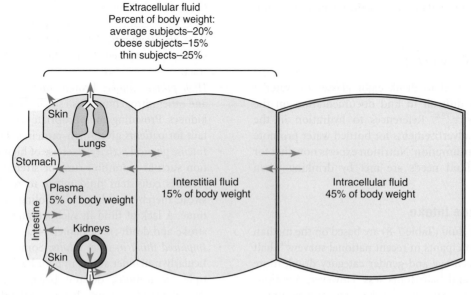

FIGURE 7-7 Body fluid compartments. Note the relative amounts of water in the intracellular (ICF) and extracellular (ECF) compartments. (Data from Gamble JL: *Chemical anatomy, physiology, and pathology of extracellular fluid,* Cambridge, Mass., 1964, Harvard University Press.)

Electrolytes

Several minerals act as major electrolytes in controlling body fluid compartments. In this role they are called *electrolytes* because they are free in solution and carry an electrical charge. Free, charged chemical forms are also called *ions,* a term that refers to atoms, elements, or groups of atoms that in solution carry either a positive or negative electrical charge. An ion carrying a positive charge is called a *cation:* examples are sodium (Na^+), the major cation in extracellular water; potassium (K^+), the major cation in intracellular water; calcium (Ca^{+2}); and magnesium (Mg^{+2}). An ion carrying a negative charge is called an *anion:* examples are chloride (Cl^-), bicarbonate (HCO_3^-), phosphate (HPO_4^{-2}), and sulfate (SO_4^{-2}). By virtue of their small size these ions or electrolytes can diffuse freely across cell membranes and create forces that control the movement of water.

Plasma Proteins

Albumin and globulin, plasma proteins of large molecular size, influence the movement of water in and out of capillaries. In this function these plasma proteins are called *colloids.* Because of their large size, plasma proteins cannot pass through the capillary membrane into the interstitial fluid. Instead they remain in the blood vessels, where they exert **colloidal osmotic pressure (COP)** to maintain vascular blood volume. We will learn more about this process a bit later.

Organic Compounds of Small Molecular Size

Other organic compounds small in size such as glucose, urea, and amino acids diffuse freely in and out of the various fluid compartments but do not influence movement of water unless they are present in abnormally large concentrations. Such a situation occurs in patients with uncontrolled diabetes mellitus, when large amounts of glucose being excreted in the urine cause an abnormal osmotic diuresis or excess water output.

Membranes

Water and solutes move across the separating membranes according to the physiologic mechanisms that handle fluid shifts. These mechanisms include osmosis, diffusion, active transport, and pinocytosis. We learned about these mechanisms in Chapter 2.

KEY TERMS

electrolyte   A chemical element or compound that in solution forms ions carrying a positive (e.g., H^+, Na^+, K^+, Ca^{+2}, and Mg^{+2}) or negative (e.g., Cl^-, HCO_3^-, HPO_4^{-2} and SO_4^{-2}) charge. Electrolytes control fluid concentrations inside and outside the cells.

interstitial fluid   The fluid between cells or in the interspaces of a tissue.

colloidal osmotic pressure (COP)   Osmotic pressure produced by the protein molecules in the plasma. Because proteins are large molecules, they do not pass through the separating membranes of the capillary cells but exert a constant osmotic pull that draws fluid and waste products back into the capillaries for transport to the kidneys for filtration and excretion. Cell proteins exert an osmotic pressure that protects against loss of cell water.

INFLUENCE OF ELECTROLYTES ON WATER BALANCE

Measurement of Electrolytes

The concentration of electrolytes or particles in a given solution determines the chemical activity of that solution. It is the number of particles, not the size of the particles that determines chemical combining power, so electrolytes are measured according to the total number of particles in solution. Each particle contributes chemical combining power according to its valence, not its total weight. The unit of measure commonly used is the *equivalent*. Because we are talking about very small amounts, these measurements are expressed in *milliequivalents (mEq)*, or thousandths of an equivalent. This term refers to the number of ions—cations and anions—in solution in a given volume of body fluid. It is expressed as the number of milliequivalents per liter (mEq/L).

Electrolyte Balance

Electrolytes are distributed in body water compartments in a definite pattern. According to biochemical and electrochemical laws, a stable solution must have equal numbers of positive and negative particles. This means it must be electrically neutral. When shifts or losses occur, compensating shifts and gains must follow to maintain this balance of essential electrochemical neutrality.

Electrolyte Control of Body Hydration

Ionized sodium is the chief cation of ECF, and ionized potassium is the chief cation of ICF. These two electrolytes control the amount of water retained in each compartment. Shifts in water from one compartment to the other reflect changes in the ECF concentration of these electrolytes. The terms *hypertonic* and *hypotonic* refer to the electrolyte concentration of the water outside the cell. When surrounded by a hypertonic solution, water flows out of the cell and the cell becomes dehydrated and shrinks in size. When the cell is surrounded by a hypotonic solution, water flows into the cell, causing it to swell and eventually burst if the situation is not corrected.

INFLUENCE OF PLASMA PROTEINS ON WATER BALANCE

Capillary Fluid Shift Mechanism

Water is constantly circulating through the blood vessels to reach cells; fluid must move out of the vessels to service the tissues and then be drawn back into the vessels to maintain normal transport flow. Two opposing pressures control the movement of water and solute across capillary membranes: (1) the hydrostatic pressure (blood pressure) of the capillary blood flow and (2) the COP from plasma proteins (mainly albumin). The flow of water, nutrients, and waste to and from the cells occurs by the shifting balance of these two pressures. It works as a filtration process driven by the differences in osmotic pressure on either side of the capillary membrane.

When blood first enters the capillary system, the existing blood pressure forces water and small solutes such as glucose out into the tissues to bathe and nourish the cells. The plasma proteins, however, are too large to pass through the pores of the capillary membrane and now exert the greater COP that draws fluid and waste materials back into the capillary circulation. This process is called the capillary fluid shift mechanism. It is one of the most important homeostatic mechanisms in the body for maintaining water balance, without which cells would die. Low serum albumin disrupts this process. Low concentrations of serum albumin lower the COP with the result that less fluid is drawn back into the capillary circulation, leading to fluid retention in the tissues and edema.

Cell Fluid Control

Just as plasma proteins in the capillaries provide COP to maintain the volume of the ECF, cell protein provides the osmotic pressure that maintains the volume of the ICF. Electrolytes also play a role with ionized potassium guarding water within the cell and ionized sodium guarding water outside the cell. This balance supports the sustaining flow of water, nutrients, metabolites, and waste in and out of cells.

INFLUENCE OF HORMONES ON WATER BALANCE

Antidiuretic Hormone

The posterior lobe of the pituitary gland secretes the antidiuretic hormone (ADH), also called *vasopressin*. It controls the reabsorption of water by the kidneys according to body need, acting as a water-conservation mechanism. In times of threatened or actual loss of body water, this hormone is released to retain precious fluid.

ADH is secreted in response to (1) an increase in the concentration of particles in the ECF as measured by receptors in the hypothalamus and (2) decreased blood volume and blood pressure as measured by receptors in the major arteries. Secretion of ADH causes an increase in water reabsorption in the kidney tubule, thereby decreasing the amount of fluid lost via the urine. When ECF concentration and blood volume have returned to normal, ADH secretion is reduced. ADH levels rise in situations when fluid is lost through heavy sweating, fever, or major blood loss.

Aldosterone

Aldosterone is the sodium-conserving hormone associated with the renin-angiotensin-aldosterone system, but it also exerts secondary control over body water. Renin, an enzyme secreted by the kidney in response to reduced blood volume acts on angiotensin, an enzyme in the plasma, which triggers the release of aldosterone from the adrenal cortex. Aldosterone acts on the kidney to reabsorb sodium, but in the process water is also reabsorbed, restoring normal blood volume. The ADH and aldosterone systems work cooperatively to maintain normal hydration and are continuously present at low levels. Both are activated by injury, surgery, or other physiologic stress bringing about losses of body water.

KEY TERMS

valence   The combining power of an element or group of elements.

capillary fluid shift mechanism   Process that controls the movement of water and small molecules (electrolytes, nutrients) between the blood in the capillary and the surrounding interstitial area. Shifts in balance between the intracapillary hydrostatic blood pressure and the colloidal osmotic pressure exerted by the plasma proteins accomplish filtration of water and solutes out of the capillary at the arteriole end and reabsorption at the venule end.

renin-angiotensin-aldosterone system   Three-stage system of sodium conservation and control of water loss; in response to diminished filtration pressure in the kidney nephrons: (1) the kidneys secrete the enzyme renin, which combines with and activates angiotensinogen from the liver; (2) active angiotensin stimulates the adjacent adrenal gland to release the hormone aldosterone; and (3) aldosterone causes reabsorption of sodium in the kidney nephrons and water follows.

TO SUM UP

Minerals are inorganic substances widely distributed in nature. They build body tissues; activate, regulate, and control metabolic processes; and help transmit messages along nerve fibers. Minerals are classified as (1) major minerals and (2) trace elements. Major minerals are required in amounts greater than 100 mg/day, whereas trace elements, measured in units as small as a microgram (mcg), are required in lesser amounts. Seven major minerals and 10 trace elements are known to be essential in human nutrition; others may be essential for humans, but their roles and requirements remain undefined. The major minerals include calcium and phosphorus, with roles in bone health, energy metabolism, and nerve transmission; and magnesium, a participant in many metabolic reactions. Sodium and potassium exert opposing effects on blood pressure, and increased potassium may moderate the pressor effect of sodium. The trace mineral iron (a part of hemoglobin) transports oxygen to the cells and, along with iodine and zinc, regulates growth and body metabolism. Other trace minerals as enzyme partners regulate day-to-day metabolic activities. Sodium, potassium, and chloride particles in body fluids, along with plasma proteins, control the distribution of body water inside (ICF) and outside (ECF) the cells. The capillary fluid shift mechanism makes possible the ongoing delivery of nutrients and removal of waste from body tissues and cells. Maintaining appropriate fluid compartments and hydration status are crucial in clinical care.

QUESTIONS FOR REVIEW

1. List the seven major minerals and describe their (a) physiologic function, (b) problems related to deficiency or excess, and (c) dietary sources.

2. List the 10 trace elements with proven essentiality for humans. Why has it been difficult to establish DRIs for these nutrients?

3. You are working with a teenager who eats no red meat or fish but likes chicken. She is concerned about her weight and limits her food intake to 1600 kcal/day. List the foods with portion sizes that you would select to reach her iron RDA of 18 mg. When making your selections, consider other factors in the diet that will enhance or impede the absorption of the iron provided. (USDA food patterns for various kcalorie levels that conform to the 2010 *Dietary Guidelines for Americans* can be accessed at http://www.cnpp.usda.gov/USDAFoodPatterns.htm.)

4. What causes the edema in protein-energy malnutrition?

5. Why does prolonged diarrhea lead to potassium depletion and what are the consequences?

6. In the early 1900s the Great Lakes and mountainous regions of the United States suffered from endemic iodine deficiency. What was the cause of this? How has it been eliminated?

7. Go to a nearby grocery store or drug store that sells mineral supplements. Check three multi-mineral supplements marketed for children or adults or older adults. Prepare a table that lists each brand and include (a) the percentage of the DRI provided for each mineral and (b) the cost of a 1-day supply of the supplement. Did any of the supplements you examined exceed a UL for the intended age group? If so, then what is the danger of toxicity? Based on cost and content, what specific foods might be better choices as nutrient sources?

8. You are working with a 37-year-old man with gradually increasing blood pressure who has been advised to increase his intakes of potassium and calcium and lower his intake of sodium. When his work takes him on the road he has lunch at a fast-food restaurant; on other days he takes a sandwich from home to eat at his desk. Develop a menu for a fast-food lunch and a packed lunch that will provide 33% of the DRI for potassium and calcium and no more than 33% of the UL for sodium. (He has access to a refrigerator at his worksite for storage of his packed lunch.)

9. You are asked to give a 10-minute talk on water at a meal site for older adults. Prepare an outline of your major points and justify your choice of information to be presented. Develop a handout with suggestions for increasing fluid intake.

REFERENCES

1. Weaver CM, Heaney RP: Calcium. In Shils ME, Shike M, Olson J, editors: *Modern nutrition in health and disease,* ed 10, Baltimore, Md., 2006, Lippincott Williams & Wilkins.

2. Klein S, Cohn SM, Alpers DH: Alimentary tract in nutrition. In Shils ME, Shike M, Olson J, editors: *Modern nutrition in health and disease,* ed 10, Baltimore, Md., 2006, Lippincott Williams & Wilkins.

3. U.S. Department of Health and Human Services, U.S. Department of Agriculture: *Report of the Dietary Guidelines Advisory Committee on the Dietary Guidelines for Americans 2010,* Washington, D.C., 2010, Center for Nutrition Policy and Promotion, U.S. Department of Agriculture. from: <http://www.cnpp.usda.gov/DGAs2010-DGACReport.htm>. Retrieved July 15, 2013.

4. Reference deleted in proofs.

5. Reference deleted in proofs.

6. Reference deleted in proofs.

7. Reference deleted in proofs.

8. Reference deleted in proofs.

9. Reference deleted in proofs.

10. Reference deleted in proofs.

11. Vatanparast H, Whiting SJ: Early milk intake, later bone health: results from using the milk history questionnaire. *Nutr Rev* 62:256, 2004.

12. Food and Nutrition Board, Institute of Medicine: *Dietary Reference Intakes for calcium and vitamin D,* Washington, D.C., 2011, National Academies Press.

13. Heaney RP, Layman DK: Amount and type of protein influences bone health. *Am J Clin Nutr* 87(Suppl):1567S, 2008.

14. Reference deleted in proofs.

15. Reference deleted in proofs.

16. Reference deleted in proofs.

17. Verguand A-C, Peneau S, Chat-Yung S, et al: Dairy consumption and 6-y changes in body weight and waist circumference in middle-aged French adults. *Am J Clin Nutr* 88:1248, 2008.

18. Shahar DR, Schwarzfuchs D, Fraser D, et al: Dairy calcium intake, serum vitamin D, and successful weight loss. *Am J Clin Nutr* 92:1017, 2010.

19. Soares MJ, Murhadi LL, Kurpad AV, et al: Mechanistic roles for calcium and vitamin D in the regulation of body weight. *Obes Rev* 13:592, 2012.

20. Kesteloot H, Tzoulaki I, Brown IJ, et al: Relation of urinary calcium and magnesium excretion to blood pressure. The International Study of Macro- and Micro-Nutrients and Blood Pressure and the International Cooperative Study on Salt, Other Factors, and Blood Pressure. *Am J Epidemiol* 174(1):44, 2011.

21. Kim K, Jung Kang Y, Kim K, et al: Interactions of single nucleotide polymorphisms with dietary calcium intake on the risk of metabolic syndrome. *Am J Clin Nutr* 95:231, 2012.

22. Astrup A: Calcium for prevention of weight gain, cardiovascular disease, and cancer. *Am J Clin Nutr* 94:1159, 2011.

23. Poddar KH, Hosig KW, Nickols-Richardson SM, et al: Low-fat dairy intake and body weight and composition changes in college students. *J Am Diet Assoc* 109:1433, 2009.

24. Knochel JP: Phosphorus. In Shils ME, Shike M, Olson MJ, editors: *Modern nutrition in health and disease,* ed 10, Baltimore, Md., 2006, Lippincott Williams & Wilkins.

25. Marinella MA: Refeeding syndrome in cancer patients. *Int J Clin Pract* 62:460, 2008.

26. Food and Nutrition Board, Institute of Medicine: *Dietary Reference Intakes for water, potassium, sodium, chloride, and sulfate,* Washington, D.C., 2004, National Academies Press.

27. U.S. Department of Agriculture, Agricultural Research Service: Nutrient Intakes from Food: Mean Amounts Consumed per Individual by Gender and Age in the United States, 2009-2010. In *What We Eat in America,* NHANES 2009-2010, 2012. at: <www.ars.usda.gov/ba/bhnrc/fsrg>. Accessed on July 15, 2013.

28. Yang Q, Zhang Z, Kuklina EV, et al: Sodium intake and blood pressure among US children and adolescents. *Pediatrics* 130:611, 2012.

29. Feber J, Ahmed M: Hypertension in children: new trends and challenges. *Clin Sci* 119:151, 2010.

30. Reference deleted in proofs.

31. Sebastian RS, Enns CW, Steinfeldt LC, et al: Discontinuation of Data Processing Step: Salt Adjustment on Designated Foods Likely To Be Home Prepared. In *What We Eat in America,* 2012, NHANES, U.S. Department of Agriculture, Agricultural Research Service. at: <http://www.ars.usda.gov/SP2UserFiles/Place/12355000/pdf/0910/discontinuation%20of%20data%20processig%20step-salt%20adjustment.pdf>. Accessed on January 1, 2013.

32. Reference deleted in proofs.

33. Reference deleted in proofs.

34. Reference deleted in proofs.

35. Reference deleted in proofs.

36. Reference deleted in proofs.

37. Lomangino K: Is salt getting a fair shake? *Clin Nutr Insight* 34(5):1, 2008.

38. Taylor RS, Ashton KE, Moxham T, et al: *Reduced dietary salt for the prevention of cardiovascular disease,* 2011, The Cochrane Collaboration, John Wiley and Sons. at: doi: 10.1002/14651858.CD009217. Accessed on January 1, 2013.

39. Mellen PB, Gao SK, Vitolins MZ, et al: Deteriorating dietary habits among adults with hypertension. DASH dietary accordance, NHANES 1988-1994 and 1999-2004. *Arch Intern Med* 168:308, 2008.

40. Lanham-New SA: The balance of bone health: tipping the scales in favor of potassium-rich, bicarbonate-rich foods. *J Nutr* 138:172S, 2008.

41. Cogswell ME, Zhang Z, Carriquiry AL: Sodium and potassium intakes among US adults: NHANES 2003-2008. *Am J Clin Nutr* 96:647, 2012.

42. Drewnowski A, Maillot M, Rehm C: Reducing the sodium-potassium ratio in the US diet: a challenge for public health. *Am J Clin Nutr* 96:439, 2012.

43. Nielsen FH: Magnesium, inflammation, and obesity in chronic disease. *Nutr Rev* 68(6):333, 2010.

44. Rosanoff A, Weaver CM, Rude RK: Suboptimal magnesium status in the United States: are the health consequences underestimated? *Nutr Rev* 70(3):153, 2011.

45. McKeown NM, Jacques PF, Zhang XL, et al: Dietary magnesium intake is related to metabolic syndrome in older Americans. *Eur J Nutr* 47:210, 2008.

46. Newby PK, Maras J, Bakun P, et al: Intake of whole grains, refined grains, and cereal fiber measured with 7-d diet records and associations with risk factors for chronic disease. *Am J Clin Nutr* 86:1745, 2007.

47. Institute of Medicine, Otten JJ, Hellwig JP, Meyers LD, editors: *Dietary Reference Intakes (DRI). The essential guide to nutrient requirements*, Washington, D.C., 2006, National Academies Press.

48. Food and Nutrition Board, Institute of Medicine: *Dietary Reference Intakes for vitamin A, vitamin K, arsenic, boron, chromium, copper, iodine, iron, manganese, molybdenum, nickel, silicon, vanadium, and zinc*, Washington, D.C., 2001, National Academies Press.

49. Hunt JR, Roughead ZK: Adaptation of iron absorption in men consuming diets with high or low iron availability. *Am J Clin Nutr* 71:94, 2000.

50. Hoppe M, Hulthen L, Hallberg L: The importance of bioavailability of dietary iron in relation to the expected effect from iron fortification. *Eur J Clin Nutr* 62(6):761, 2008.

51. Hurrell R, Egli I: Iron bioavailability and dietary reference values. *Am J Clin Nutr* 91(Suppl):1461S, 2010.

52. Ruz M, Carrasco F, Rojas P, et al: Heme- and nonheme-iron absorption and iron status 12 mo after sleeve gastrectomy and Roux-en-Y gastric bypass in morbidly obese women. *Am J Clin Nutr* 96:810, 2012.

53. Alleyne M, Horne MK, Miller JL: Individualized treatment for iron-deficiency anemia in adults. *Am J Med* 121:943, 2008.

54. Gaitan D, Flores S, Saavedra P, et al: Calcium does not inhibit the absorption of 5 milligrams of nonheme or heme iron at doses less than 800 milligrams in nonpregnant women. *J Nutr* 141:1652, 2011.

55. AAP Committee on Nutrition, Kleinman RE, editors: *Pediatric nutrition handbook*, ed 6, Elk Grove Village, Ill., 2008, American Academy of Pediatrics.

56. Beard JL: Why iron deficiency is important in infant development. *J Nutr* 138:2534, 2008.

57. Black MM, Quigg AM, Hurley KM, et al: Iron deficiency and iron-deficiency anemia in the first two years of life: strategies to prevent loss of developmental potential. *Nutr Rev* 69(Suppl 1):564, 2011.

58. Murray-Kolb LE, Beard JL: Iron treatment normalizes cognitive functioning in young women. *Am J Clin Nutr* 85:778, 2007.

59. Tussing-Humphreys L, Pusatcioglu C, Nemeth E, et al: Rethinking iron regulation and assessment in iron deficiency, anemia of chronic disease, and obesity: introducing hepcidin, *J Acad Nutr Diet* 112:391, 2012.

60. McLean E, Cogswell M, Egli I, et al: Worldwide prevalence of anaemia, WHO vitamin and mineral nutrition information system, 1993-2005. *Public Health Nutr* 12(444):2009.

61. Heath ALM, Fairweather-Tait SJ: Health implications of iron overload: the role of diet and genotype. *Nutr Rev* 61(2):45, 2003.

62. Fleming RE, Ponka P: Mechanisms of disease. Iron overload in human disease. *N Engl J Med* 366:348, 2012.

63. Zhao Z, Li S, Liu G, et al: Body iron stores and heme-iron intake in relation to risk of type 2 diabetes: a systematic review and meta-analysis. *PLoS One* 7(7):e41641, 2012.

64. Rajpathak SN, Wylie-Rosett J, Gunter MJ, et al: Biomarkers of body iron stores and risk of developing type 2 diabetes. *Diabetes Obes Metab* 11:472, 2009.

65. Beard J: Dietary iron intakes and elevated iron stores in the elderly: is it time to abandon the set-point hypothesis of regulation of iron absorption? *Am J Clin Nutr* 76:1189, 2002.

66. Liu JM, Hankinson SE, Stampfer MJ, et al: Body iron stores and their determinants in healthy postmenopausal U.S. women. *Am J Clin Nutr* 78:1160, 2003.

67. Zimmerman MB: Iodine requirements and the risks and benefits of correcting iodine deficiency in populations. *J Trace Elem Med Biol* 22:81, 2008.

68. Zimmerman MB, Andersson M: Assessment of iodine nutrition in populations: past, present, and future. *Nutr Rev* 70(10):553, 2012.

69. Zimmerman MB: Iodine and iodine deficiency disorders. In Shils ME, Shike M, Olson MJ, editors: *Modern nutrition in health and disease*, ed 10, Baltimore, Md., 2006, Lippincott Williams & Wilkins.

70. Fischer Walker CL, Ezzati M, Black RE: Global and regional child mortality and burden of disease attributable to zinc deficiency. *Eur J Clin Nutr* 63:591, 2009.

71. Sandstead HH: Subclinical zinc deficiency impairs human brain function. *J Trace Elem Med Biol* 26(2–3):70, 2012.

72. Barnett JB, Hamer DH, Meydani SN: Low zinc status: a new risk factor for pneumonia in the elderly. *Nutr Rev* 68(1):30, 2009.

73. Sweitzer SJ, Briley ME, Robert-Gray C: Do sack lunches provided by parents meet the nutritional needs of young children who attend child care. *J Am Diet Assoc* 109:141, 2009.

74. Hambidge KM, Miller LV, Westcott JE, et al: Zinc bioavailability and homeostasis. *Am J Clin Nutr* 91(Suppl):1478S, 2010.

75. Burk RF, Levander OA: Selenium. In Shils ME, Shike M, Olson J, editors: *Modern nutrition in health and disease*, ed 10, Baltimore, Md., 2006, Lippincott Williams & Wilkins.

76. Food and Nutrition Board, Institute of Medicine: *Dietary Reference Intakes for vitamin C, vitamin E, selenium, and carotenoids*, Washington, D.C., 2000, National Academies Press.

77. American Dietetic Association: Position of the American Dietetic Association: the impact of fluoride on health. *J Am Diet Assoc* 112:1443, 2012.

78. Kant AK, Graubard BI, Atchison EA: Intakes of plain water, moisture in foods and beverages, and total water in the adult U.S. population—nutritional, meal pattern, and body weight correlates: National Health and Nutrition Examination Surveys 1999-2006. *Am J Clin Nutr* 90:655, 2009.

79. Valtin H: Drink at least eight glasses of water a day. Really? Is there scientific evidence for "8 × 8?" *Am J Physiol Regul Integr Comp Physiol* 283(5):R993, 2002.

80. Grandjean AC, Reimers KJ, Buyckx ME: Hydration: issues for the 21st century. *Nutr Rev* 61(8):261, 2003.

81. Popkin BM, D'Anci KE, Rosenberg IH: Water, hydration, and health. *Nutr Rev* 68(8):439, 2010.

82. Vergne S: Methodological aspects of fluid intake records and surveys. *Nutr Today* 47(4S):S7, 2012.

83. Tate DF, Turner-McGrievy G, Lyons E, et al: Replacing caloric beverages with water or diet beverages for weight loss in adults: main results of the Choose Healthy Options Consciously Everyday (CHOICE) randomized clinical trial. *Am J Clin Nutr* 95:555, 2012.

84. Reference deleted in proofs.

85. Reference deleted in proofs.

86. Reference deleted in proofs.

FURTHER READINGS AND RESOURCES

Readings

Academy of Nutrition and Dietetics: Position of the Academy of Nutrition and Dietetics: the impact of fluoride on health. *J Acad Nutr Diet* 112:1443, 2012.

[Fluoridation of water is one of the top 10 public health initiatives for this century; this article helps us understand the need for fluoride.]

Bailey RL, Fulgoni VL, Keast DR, et al: Dietary supplement use is associated with higher intakes of minerals from food sources. *Am J Clin Nutr* 94:1376, 2011.

[These authors note that individuals with low mineral intakes from food are not taking supplements whereas those who consume adequate minerals in their food are exceeding the UL by their use of supplements.]

Black MM, Quigg AM, Hurley KM, et al: Iron deficiency and iron-deficiency anemia in the first two years of life: strategies to prevent loss of developmental potential. *Nutr Reviews* 69(Suppl 1):S64, 2011.

[These authors help us understand the importance of iron nutrition in early life to prevent loss of cognitive potential.]

Centers for Disease Control and Prevention: Vital signs: food categories contributing the most to sodium consumption—United States, 2007-2008. *MMWR* 61(05):92, 2012. February 10.

Kolasa KM, Sollid K, Edge MS, et al: Blood pressure management: communicating comprehensive lifestyle strategies beyond sodium. *Nutr Today* 47(4):183, 2012.

[Dr. Kolasa and her colleagues provide us with an intervention strategy for high blood pressure that goes beyond sodium intake but note the MMWR report listing the major contributors to sodium intake.]

Fulgoni VL, Keast DR, Auestad N, et al: Nutrients from dairy foods are difficult to replace in diets of Americans: food pattern modeling and an analyses of the National Health and Nutrition Examination Survey 2003-2006. *Nutr Res* 31:759, 2011.

Weaver CM: Back to basics: have milk with meals. *J Am Diet Assoc* 106:1756, 2006.

[These articles point to the difficulty in obtaining important minerals when the diet does not include dairy products; Dr. Weaver shares her experiences in helping her own children meet their calcium requirements.]

Lieberman HR: Hydration and human cognition. *Nutr Today* 45(6S):S33, 2010.

McBurney MI: Drink fluids to maintain hydration and eat to obtain calories. *Nutr Today* 44(1):14, 2009.

Stookey JD: Drinking water and weight management. *Nutr Today* 45(6S):S7, 2010.

[The three preceding articles point to the role of water intake in weight management and overall body regulation].

Websites of Interest

Three government sites provide comprehensive information on dietary supplements, what they are or what they contain, guidelines for their use, and their interactions with prescription and over-the-counter medications:

- National Institutes of Health, National Library of Medicine: Medline Plus, Trusted Health Information for You: *Dietary supplements:* www.nlm.nih.gov/medlineplus/ dietarysupplements.html and National Institutes of Health, Office of Dietary Supplements: www.dietary-supplements.info.nih.gov/.
- U.S. Food and Drug Administration, Center for Food Safety and Applied Nutrition, Office of Nutritional Products, Labeling, and Dietary Supplements: http://www.fda.gov/food/ DietarySupplements/default.htm.
- National Institutes of Health. This site provides information on calcium and bone health: http://www.nlm.nih.gov/medlineplus/ calcium.html.
- National Institutes of Health. This site provides information on sodium and blood pressure: http://www.nlm.nih.gov/ medlineplus/dietarysodium.html.
- U.S. Department of Agriculture. *MyPlate (ChooseMyPlate.gov).* This website describes daily food plans and healthy food choices supplying adequate minerals for all age groups: http://www.ChooseMyPlate.gov.

Energy Balance

Eleanor D. Schlenker

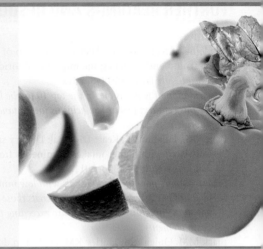

EVOLVE WEBSITE

http://evolve.elsevier.com/Williams/essentials/

OUTLINE

The Human Energy System
Total Energy Requirement
Body Composition: Fatness and Leanness

Health Promotion
Fatness, Thinness, and Health

Thus far we reviewed the three energy-yielding nutrients (carbohydrate, fat, and protein), the micronutrients (vitamins and minerals that catalyze the chemical reactions converting food to energy),and water, which provides the medium in which all of these processes occur. Here we look at the relationship between energy intake and energy expenditure and their combined effect on body composition and body weight.

A sedentary lifestyle, coupled with an abundance of food, puts youth and adults at risk for unwanted weight gain. At the other extreme, an obsession with thinness or food scarcity leads to life-threatening malnutrition.[1] Energy balance is not a simple matter. Energy needs vary under different circumstances and for different body types. Each of us is unique, and our varying body weights and propensity to gain or lose weight reflect this. In this chapter we look at the dynamics of energy metabolism and how these principles apply to a healthy weight.

THE HUMAN ENERGY SYSTEM

Energy Cycles and Energy Transformation

Forms of Human Energy

In the physical world, energy, like matter, is neither created nor destroyed. When we speak of energy being produced, what we really mean is energy being *transformed*. Energy constantly changes form as it moves through various systems. In the human body, metabolic reactions convert the stored chemical energy in food to other forms of energy that carry out body work. The ultimate source of energy is the sun with

its vast reservoir of heat and light (Figure 8-1). By the process of photosynthesis (review Figure 3-1), plants use water and carbon dioxide (CO_2) to transform the sun's energy into carbohydrate, a storage form of chemical energy. In the body, carbohydrate is converted to glucose, which together with fatty acids is metabolized to release energy and support life. The end products of body energy metabolism are water and CO_2. These end products then become available to plants to produce more carbohydrate for human use.

Transformation of Energy

When food with its stored chemical energy is taken into the body, it undergoes many changes that convert it to different storage forms of chemical energy. This chemical energy is then changed further as work is performed. Our bodies use four forms of energy: (1) chemical, (2) electrical, (3) mechanical, and (4) thermal. In the brain, chemical energy is changed to electrical energy for transmitting nerve impulses and carrying out brain activities. Chemical energy is changed to mechanical energy when muscles contract; it is changed to

> **KEY TERM**
>
> **energy** The capacity of a system for doing work; energy is manifest in various forms—motion, position, light, heat, and sound. Energy is interchangeable among these various forms and is constantly being transformed and transferred among them.

thermal energy in the regulation of body temperature. Chemical energy is needed to form new tissues and molecules for growth and metabolism. Throughout all of this work, heat is given off to the surrounding atmosphere and larger biosphere.

In the human body energy is present as either *free energy* or *potential energy*. Free energy is the energy being used at any given moment in the performance of a task. It is unbound and in motion. Potential energy is energy that is stored or bound in a chemical compound and can be converted to free energy when needed. For example, the energy stored in carbohydrate is potential energy. When we eat carbohydrate and it is metabolized, energy is released for body work. As work is completed, this energy, now in the form of heat or thermal energy, is given off into the air. Measurement of the amount of heat produced over time makes it possible for us to express body energy consumption in kilocalories (kcalories or kcal) or units of heat.

Energy Balance: Input and Output

A constant supply of energy is needed to sustain the activities essential to life. Energy is required to support internal needs along with the added expectations of physical activity. Whether the energy used is electrical, mechanical, thermal, or chemical, the supply of free energy and the reservoir of potential energy decrease as the metabolic and physical work of the body continues; therefore, the system must be constantly refueled from an outside source. For the human energy system, this outside fuel source is food.

Energy Control in Human Metabolism

If the energy produced in the body through its many chemical reactions was "exploded" all at once, it would damage tissues and systems, so mechanisms are needed by which energy release can be controlled to support life, not destroy it. Two means of control make this possible: (1) **chemical bonding** and (2) controlled reaction rates.

Chemical Bonding

The primary mechanism controlling energy release in the human system is chemical bonding. The chemical bonds that hold elements together in compounds are energy bonds. As long as the compound stays intact, energy is being exerted to maintain it. When the compound is broken into its parts, this energy is released and becomes available for work.

The following three types of chemical bonds transfer energy:
1. *Covalent bonds:* These bonds are based on the relative combining power of the elements that make up a compound. The carbon atoms in organic compounds such as glucose are held together by covalent bonds.
2. *Hydrogen bonds:* Although weaker than covalent bonds, hydrogen bonds are significant because there are large numbers of them. In addition, the very fact that they are less strong and more easily broken allows them to transfer energy readily from one substance to another. The hydrogen attached to the oxygen molecule in the carboxyl group

(COOH-) of amino acids and fatty acids is an example of this type of bond.
3. *High-energy phosphate bonds:* The high-energy phosphate bonds in the compound **adenosine triphosphate (ATP)** are the major energy source for carrying out body functions. Working like storage batteries for electrical energy, these bonds are the controlling force of energy metabolism in the human cell.

Controlled Reaction Rates

The chemical reactions making up the body's energy system must have controls to manage the speed at which they occur. For example, some reactions that break down protein, if left alone, occur very slowly. If such reactions were not accelerated by **catalysts**, then getting needed energy from the food in a meal could take years. At the same time, chemical reactions must be prevented from occurring too fast, which would release destructive bursts of energy. **Enzymes, coenzymes,** and hormones regulate energy reactions as follows:
- *Enzymes:* Enzymes are proteins produced in the cell under the direction of individual genes. One gene controls the making of one enzyme, and thousands of enzymes exist in every cell. Each enzyme acts on one particular substance, called its **substrate**. The enzyme and its substrate lock together to produce a new reaction product; however, the enzyme itself remains unchanged, ready to do its work over and over again (Figure 8-2). Enzymes often act as catalysts.
- *Coenzymes and cofactors:* Many enzymes require partners to assist in completing their work. These coenzyme

---

KEY TERMS

chemical bonding Process of linking elements or groups of elements in a chemical compound.

adenosine triphosphate (ATP) A high-energy phosphate compound important in energy exchange within the cell. ATP is formed from the nucleotide adenosine with three attached phosphoric acid groups. The splitting off of the terminal phosphate group (PO_4) to produce adenosine diphosphate (ADP) releases bound energy that is transformed to free energy and available for body work. ATP is then re-formed as an energy store for use when needed.

catalyst A chemical or compound that speeds up a chemical reaction but is not changed in the process. In the body, enzymes act as catalysts.

enzymes Complex proteins that act as catalysts to speed the rate of chemical reactions. Enzymes facilitate chemical changes in other substances without themselves being changed in the process. Enzymes are named according to the substance (substrate) on which it acts, with the common suffix "-ase"; for example, sucrase is the enzyme that breaks down sucrose to glucose and fructose.

coenzyme A molecule, usually a vitamin, that partners with an enzyme to bring about a chemical reaction related to energy metabolism or other cell activities.

substrate The specific organic substance on which a particular enzyme acts to produce a new metabolic product.

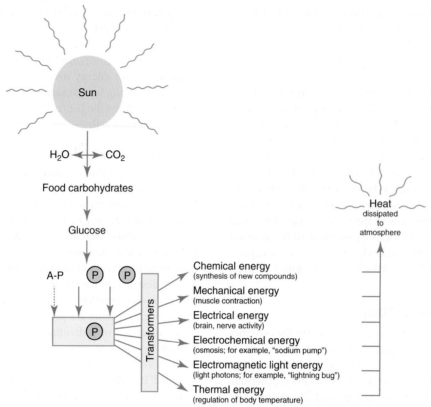

FIGURE 8-1 Transformation of energy from its primary source (the sun) to the forms needed for biologic work.

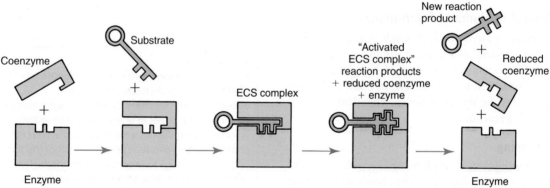

FIGURE 8-2 Lock-and-key concept. An enzyme, coenzyme, and substrate work together to produce a new substance.

partners are often vitamins, especially B-complex vitamins. Various minerals also participate in enzyme reactions and in this role are referred to as *cofactors.* It may be helpful to think of coenzymes and cofactors as another substrate, because in receiving the material being transferred, they are changed or reduced.

- *Hormones:* In energy metabolism hormones act as messengers to trigger or control enzyme action. The rate of oxidation reactions in the tissues—the body's metabolic rate—is controlled by thyroxine (T_4) from the thyroid gland. Another example is the controlling action of insulin on glucose utilization in the cells.

Types of Metabolic Reactions

Two types of reactions occur in the body: (1) anabolic and (2) catabolic. Each requires energy. The process of anabolism synthesizes new and more complex substances as in body growth and repair. The process of catabolism breaks down complex substances to more simple ones, as when worn-out proteins are broken down and their released amino acids used to make new proteins. Both activities release free energy, but the work performed also uses up some free energy. This creates a constant energy deficit that must be met by food.

Sources of Stored Energy

When a person is not taking in food, as in fasting or starvation, the body must draw on its own stores for energy. Sources of stored energy can meet short- or long-term needs, as described below:

- *Glycogen:* Only a 12- to 36-hour reserve of glycogen exists in liver and muscle; it is quickly depleted.
- *Muscle mass:* Energy stores in the form of muscle protein exist in limited amounts but in greater volume than glycogen stores. Although the body tries to limit the breakdown of protein for energy, the need for glucose to fuel the central nervous system (CNS) results in loss of body protein when energy and carbohydrate intakes are inadequate. (Review our discussion in Chapter 5 of deamination of amino acids for glucose production.) Loss of body protein occurs in rapid weight loss and in body wasting or cachexia. It is a cause for concern and requires prompt intervention.
- *Adipose (fat) tissue:* Although fat stores are generally the largest resource of stored energy, the supply varies from person to person.

Measurement of Energy Balance
Kilocalorie

Because the release of energy and work performed by the body produces heat, energy expenditure can be measured in heat equivalents. This measure of heat is the calorie. To avoid having to calculate very large numbers, health professionals use the kilocalorie to describe energy needs. The kilocalorie is equal to 1000 calories; this is the amount of heat required to raise 1 kg of water 1°C. (Materials prepared for the general public use the term *calorie*, although the actual measurement is the kilocalorie.)

Joule

The international (*Système International d'Unités* [SI]) unit of energy measurement is the joule. It equals the amount of energy expended when 1 kg of a substance is moved 1 m by a force of 1 newton (N). The conversion factor for changing kcalories to kilojoules (kJ) is 4.184 (1 kcal = 4.184 kJ). Some nutrition research journals use kilojoules rather than kcalories to describe energy intakes; in clinical practice we use kcalories.

Food Energy Measurement

When helping people develop a food pattern appropriate to their energy needs, it is necessary to know the energy content of individual foods. There are two methods for determining the energy content of foods: (1) direct calorimetry or (2) calculation of approximate composition.

Calorimetry

The kcalorie values of foods given in food tables were determined by the method called *direct calorimetry*.[2] This method uses a metal container called a *bomb calorimeter*, named from its long tubular shape. A weighed amount of food is placed

TABLE 8-1   FUEL FACTORS

ENERGY SOURCE	KCALORIES PER GRAM
Carbohydrate	4
Protein	4
Fat	9
Alcohol	7

inside and the bomb calorimeter is immersed in water. The food is then ignited by an electric spark in the presence of oxygen and burned to ash. The increase in the temperature of the surrounding water indicates the number of kcalories given off by the complete oxidation of the food sample. When you use food tables, remember that these values represent averages from a number of samples of the given food, thus the kcalorie value of a particular serving will vary around that average. Examples of food tables can be found in the Nutritrac program on the Evolve website that accompanies your text.

Approximate Composition

An alternative method of estimating the energy value of a food is by calculating the kcalories contributed by the carbohydrate, fat, and protein content as listed in food tables. These calculations are based on the kcalorie value per gram of each of the energy-yielding macronutrients, values known as their fuel factors (Table 8-1). Note that 1 g of fat contains more than twice the number of kcalories as 1 g of carbohydrate or protein. The fuel factor for alcohol (7 kcal/g) falls midway between fat and that of carbohydrate and protein. Using the method of approximate composition, a food containing 12 g of carbohydrate, 8 g of protein, and 5 g of fat would contain 125 kcal.

Calculation:
Carbohydrate: 12 g × 4 kcal/g = 48 kcal;
Protein: 8 g × 4 kcal/g = 32 kcal;
Fat: 5 g × 9 kcal/g = 45 kcal;
Total: 48 + 32 + 45 kcal = 125 kcal.

Did you recognize this food as a 1-cup serving of reduced-fat (2%) milk?

TOTAL ENERGY REQUIREMENT

The total energy expended by an individual stems from three energy needs: (1) basal metabolism, (2) food intake effect, and (3) physical activity. Physical size and body composition, as well as level of physical activity, influence the energy needs of a given individual.

Basal Metabolic Needs
Basal Metabolic Rate

The basal metabolic rate (BMR) is a measure of the energy required to maintain the body at rest. This is the sum of all chemical activities going on in the body plus the energy needed to fuel the brain, heart, lungs, kidneys, and other organs that must continue to work even when the body rests.[3] Certain small but active tissues such as the brain, liver, gastrointestinal tract, heart, and kidneys make up less than 5% of total body weight but add up to about 60% of basal metabolic activity. The BMR is the largest of the energy needs of most people, accounting for 60% to 70% of the total daily energy expenditure.[4] As described in Box 8-1, the feeding status of the patient and the test environment influence the BMR.[3] Thus, the BMR is seldom measured in clinical practice because of the preparation and details required. Rather, the **resting metabolic rate (RMR)** is more commonly used because it does not require fasting prior to the test. Recognize, however, the RMR may be as much as 10% to 20% higher than the BMR because of energy being expended in the processing of food or the delayed effect of recent physical activity.[3]

Measuring Basal Metabolic Rate

The BMR can be measured by direct or indirect methods of calorimetry, as follows:

- *Direct calorimetry:* Using the direct method, a person is placed in an enclosed chamber that has the capacity to measure body heat production while the person is at rest. This instrument is large and costly and usually found only in research facilities.[2]
- *Indirect calorimetry:* Using the indirect method, a portable instrument called a *respirometer* is brought to the side of the bed or chair. This complete apparatus is often referred to as the *metabolic cart.* As the person breathes through a mouthpiece or ventilated hood, the exchange of gases in respiration, called the *respiratory quotient* (CO_2/O_2), is measured. Because more than 95% of the body's energy comes from oxygen-related reactions,[5] the BMR can be calculated from the amount of oxygen consumed in a given period. The amount of oxygen used equals the amount of heat released. These numbers can be converted to kcalories using standardized equations.
- *Indirect laboratory tests:* The BMR is regulated by the thyroid hormone thyroxine (T_4); thus thyroid function tests can provide indirect measures of BMR and thyroid activity. These tests include measurements of serum thyroid-stimulating hormone (TSH) from the anterior pituitary gland, as well as triiodothyronine (T_3) and T_4. Thyroid hormone levels within the normal range indicate that cell metabolism is occurring at normal rates but cannot be used to calculate BMR.

Factors Influencing Basal Metabolic Rate

Individual characteristics including gender, body size and composition, genetic makeup, and disease state influence the BMR of an individual, explained as follows:

- *Body size and body composition:* Lean body mass (LBM) is the body compartment made up of muscle and vital organs. It is the major factor influencing BMR because of the high metabolic activity of these tissues compared with the less active tissues of fat and bone. Differences in basal energy requirements between men and women of the same height and body weight relate to their differences in body composition. Compared with men, women have less muscle and more fat, resulting in a lower BMR. As humans age, the loss of muscle tissue and to a lesser extent organ tissue, lowers their BMR.[6]

BOX 8-1   REQUIRED CONDITIONS FOR MEASURING BASAL METABOLIC RATE

- Overnight fast (no food for 12 to 14 hours)
- Comfortably resting in a **supine** position
- Relaxed state (no activity up to 1 hour prior)
- Awake but motionless
- Normal body temperature
- Comfortable room temperature (neither hot nor cold)

KEY TERMS

cachexia A wasting condition marked by weakness, extreme weight loss, and malnutrition.

calorie The amount of heat energy needed to raise the temperature of 1 g of water from 14°C to 15°C. Because this is a small unit, nutritionists use the term *kilocalorie*, which equals 1000 small calories. (See also *joule.*)

kilocalorie The *kilocalorie* equals 1000 small calories and is the amount of heat required to raise the temperature of 1 kg of water 1°C; this measure is commonly used to describe the energy content of foods and diets.

joule A unit of energy. The International System of Units uses joules in place of calories to refer to food energy, and many nutrition journals use joules instead of calories (1 kcal = 4.184 kilojoules [kJ], often rounded to 4.2 kJ for ease in calculation).

calorimetry Measurement of amount of heat absorbed or given off. The *direct method* is the measurement of the heat produced by a subject enclosed in a small chamber. The *indirect method* is the measurement of heat produced by a subject based on the amount of oxygen (O_2) taken in and carbon dioxide (CO_2) exhaled.

fuel factors The number of kcalories yielded by 1 g of the macronutrient when completely oxidized. The kilocalorie fuel factor is 4 for carbohydrate and protein, 9 for fat, and 7 for alcohol. Fuel factors are used in computing the energy values of foods and diets (e.g., 10 g of fat yields 90 kcal).

body composition The relative sizes of the four tissue compartments that make up the total body: lean body mass (LBM) (muscles and organs), fat, water, and mineral.

basal metabolic rate (BMR) Amount of energy required to maintain the body at rest after an overnight fast, in a comfortable environmental temperature, with the subject awake. (See also *resting metabolic rate [RMR].*)

resting metabolic rate (RMR) Amount of energy required to maintain the body at rest when in a comfortable environmental temperature and awake. Because of differences in measuring techniques, an individual's RMR and BMR (basal metabolic rate) differ slightly.

supine Lying down.

- *Growth:* The increased anabolic work supported by growth hormone adds to the BMR in childhood, adolescence, pregnancy, and lactation.
- *Fever:* With fever, the BMR increases 7% for each 1°F (0.83°C) rise in body temperature.
- *Disease:* Diseases that increase cell activity such as cancer, cardiac failure, and chronic obstructive pulmonary disease increase BMR and often result in loss of body weight and muscle.[7] Renal disease and sepsis increase the metabolic work of the body and the BMR.[8] The involuntary muscle tremors of Parkinson's disease increase energy needs. Older adults with pressure ulcers have increased basal requirements,[9] and untreated human immunodeficiency virus (HIV) infection can raise resting energy expenditure (REE) by more than 10%.[10] Standard prediction equations based on height and weight underestimate the BMR of children with cystic fibrosis.[11] Conversely, in starvation and protein-energy malnutrition, BMR falls as cell metabolism slows in response to the drop in energy intake and loss of metabolically active tissue.
- *Climate:* BMR rises in response to lower environmental temperatures as the body takes action to increase heat production and minimize heat loss. Opposite reactions that reduce heat production and increase heat loss as environmental temperatures rise also raise the BMR. Unless weather conditions are extreme, these changes in BMR are temporary while the individual adapts to the new environment.
- *Genetics:* Race and ethnicity influence BMR. African Americans have a lower REE per unit of LBM than Caucasians, which may relate to the smaller size of organs with high metabolic rates.[12] Energy prediction equations developed with Caucasian youth do not accurately predict REE in obese Hispanic youth.[13] Studies of the human genome indicate that intrafamily differences in RMR may contribute to higher weight gain and development of metabolic syndrome among particular groups.[14]
- *Age:* Loss of LBM, particularly muscle, results in a drop in REE in frail older adults.[8]

Food Intake Effect (Thermic Effect of Food)

Taking in food stimulates body metabolism as energy is needed to digest, absorb, metabolize, and store nutrients. The kcalories needed to perform these tasks is called the **thermic effect of food (TEF)**. On average, about 10% of the kcalories in a meal or snack are used to process and metabolize that food, although this varies depending on the meal composition. Macronutrients differ in their TEFs. The TEF for fat is 0% to 3%, because fatty acids are easily burned for energy or stored in the form in which they enter the body; therefore, few kcalories are needed for processing or storage. For carbohydrate the TEF is 5% to 10% of its kcalories; for protein the TEF is 20% to 30% of its kcalorie content. The TEF for alcohol is 10% to 30%.[15]

The energy required to metabolize amino acids and synthesize new proteins raises the TEF of this macronutrient, and the TEF effect is especially pronounced with high-quality protein.[15] Removal of the amino group from surplus amino acids to allow their use as an energy source is an energy-intensive process and reduces the kcalories available for future use. These factors contribute to the value of a high-protein diet for weight loss or weight management. The very low TEF of fat, along with its high fuel factor (9 kcal/g), can accelerate weight gain on a high-fat diet.

Physical Activity Needs

Physical activity related to employment, personal care, housekeeping, recreation, organized sports, or fitness training produces wide variations in energy requirements. For sedentary individuals the kcalories expended in physical activity may be only 15% to 20% of their total energy expenditure, as compared with very active persons whose physical activity kcalories may be 50% to 60% of their total.[4] Table 8-2 describes the energy cost of common activities per pound of body weight. For weight-bearing activities, kcalorie expenditure is proportional to body weight; accordingly, such an activity will require more kcalories for an individual with an above-average body weight and fewer kcalories for one whose body weight is below average (Figure 8-3).[3] Obese adolescents can have the same activity energy expenditure as their nonobese counterparts despite less body movement, based on their higher body weight.[16]

The speed at which a person moves also influences the number of kcalories expended. Walking at a speed of 4 mph requires more kcalories than walking at 2 mph, regardless of body weight (see Figure 8-3).[3] Jogging or running at 5 mph requires more than twice the energy than walking at 3.5 mph (see Table 8-2). The energy cost of movement is also influenced by age-related changes in muscle mass and innervation of muscle cells. Older adults had an energy cost 20% higher than younger adults walking a similar distance at the same speed on a level surface.[17] The slower gait observed among older individuals may be a compensatory response to offset the greater energy cost of walking brought about by aging and chronic conditions.[18]

Estimating Energy Requirements

Estimating the total energy requirement for a given individual is difficult. An expert panel defined the estimated energy requirement (EER) as the energy intake that will maintain energy balance in a healthy adult of a certain age, gender, weight, height, and level of physical activity,[3] and developed some numerical equivalents to assist in calculation. Typical ranges for RMR are 0.8 to 1.0 kcal/min for women and 1.1 to 1.3 kcal/min for men (1 kcal/min is about equal to the heat released by a burning candle or 75-watt bulb over the course

> **KEY TERM**
> **thermic effect of food (TEF)** The amount of energy required to digest and absorb food and transport nutrients to the cells. This work accounts for about 10% of the total energy requirement.

TABLE 8-2   ENERGY EXPENDITURE PER POUND PER HOUR FOR VARIOUS ACTIVITIES

ACTIVITY	Kcal/lb/hr*
Daily Activities	
Cleaning	1.36
Cooking	0.91
Driving a car	0.91
Gardening	1.81
Reading, writing while sitting	0.70
Sleeping	0.41
Shoveling snow	2.72
Walking	
Moderate: 3 mph (20 min/mile), level	1.50
Moderate: 3 mph (20 min/mile), uphill	2.73
Brisk: 3.5 mph (17 min/mile), level	1.72
Fast: 4.5 mph (13 min/mile), level	2.86
Running	
5 mph (12 min/mile)	3.63
7 mph (8.5 min/mile)	5.22
9 mph (6.5 min/mile)	6.80
Bicycling	
Light (10-11.9 mph)	2.72
Moderate (12-13.9 mph)	3.63
Fast (14-15.9 mph)	4.54
Sports	
Field hockey	3.63
Golf	2.04
Rollerblading	4.42
Soccer	3.85
Swimming, moderate	3.14
Ultimate Frisbee	3.63
Volleyball	1.81
Weight Training	
Light or moderate	1.36
Heavy or vigorous	2.72

Data from Nieman DC: *Exercise testing and prescription: a health-related approach*, ed 5, New York, 2003, McGraw-Hill; and Nix S: *Williams' basic nutrition and diet therapy*, ed 13, St Louis, Mo, 2009, Mosby-Elsevier.
Energy expenditure also depends on an individual's physical fitness and continuity of exercise.
*Multiply activity factor by weight in pounds by fraction of hour performing activity. Example: a 150-lb person plays soccer for 45 minutes, as follows: 3.18 (factor) × 150 (lb) × 0.75 (hr) = 357.75 calories burned.

TABLE 8-3   FACTORS FOR CALCULATING DAILY ENERGY EXPENDED IN PHYSICAL ACTIVITY

ACTIVITY LEVEL	DEFINITION	PHYSICAL ACTIVITY FACTOR*
Sedentary	Normal activities required for independent living	0.2
Low active	Normal activities required for independent living plus at least 30 to 60 min of moderately intensive activity	0.5
Active	Normal activities required for independent living plus *more* than 60 min of moderately intensive activity or a mix of moderately intensive and vigorous activity	0.7
Very active	Normal activities required for independent living plus 2 hours or more of vigorous activity	1.2

Adapted from Food and Nutrition Board, Institute of Medicine: *Dietary Reference Intakes for energy, carbohydrate, fiber, fat, fatty acids, cholesterol, protein, and amino acids (macronutrients)*, Washington, D.C., 2002, National Academies Press.
*These physical activity factors represent the midpoint of the range for each activity level.

factor that estimates your activity level. Nutrition experts have defined several levels of physical activity and developed factors that estimate the kcalories required (Table 8-3).[3] Consider these definitions and the time span and intensity of activity required. If your only physical activity for the day involves the casual walking and routine tasks we all perform as part of our daily living, then your pattern is sedentary. Additional activity in the form of walking at a brisk pace, running, dancing, sports, or use of fitness equipment is needed for the higher categories of activity. Estimate your personal activity level by keeping a daily record; you may be less active than you think you are (Box 8-2).

Age influences the RMR and EER. As we age, we lose muscle and organ weight, tissues with high metabolic activity, and gain fat, tissue with low metabolic activity. Table 8-4 illustrates the effect of gender, age, and physical activity on the total energy requirement. Within genders individuals have the same body weight, although the older adults will have experienced changes in body composition. Note the significant differences in energy expenditure between sedentary and active adults.

Energy requirements rise during pregnancy, lactation, and other periods of rapid growth and elevated metabolism. (We will estimate energy requirements using specific equations that adjust for height, weight, and age in Chapter 16.)

of a minute).[3] Differences in body dimensions and the proportion of body fat versus muscle influence the RMR and thus the total energy requirement. Individuals with a greater amount of body fat and a lesser proportion of muscle will likely need fewer kcalories.

Because your RMR reflects your body weight, your energy expenditure in physical activity can be calculated using a

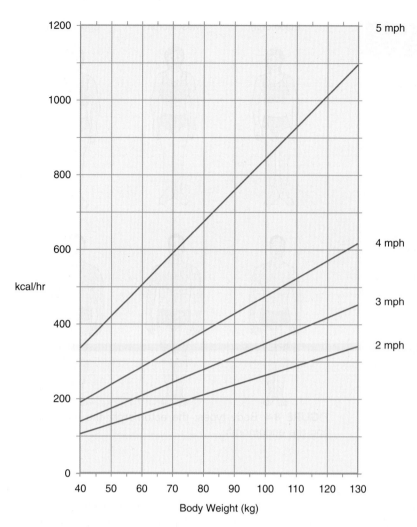

FIGURE 8-3 Effect of body weight on the energy required to walk at different speeds. Both body weight and walking speed influence the kcalories burned. Persons with a higher body weight use more kcalories in weight-bearing activities than persons with a lower body weight; the faster they walk the more kcalories they will use. (Redrawn with permission from Food and Nutrition Board, Institute of Medicine: *Dietary reference intakes for energy, carbohydrate, fiber, fat, fatty acids, cholesterol, protein, and amino acids (macronutrients),* Washington, D.C., 2005, National Academies Press.)

TABLE 8-4	ESTIMATED ENERGY REQUIREMENTS (EERS) BASED ON ACTIVITY LEVEL AND AGE			
	MALE (178 lb, 71 in)* KCALORIES		**FEMALE (132 lb, 61 in)* KCALORIES**	
ACTIVITY LEVEL	**AGE 25**	**AGE 65**	**AGE 25**	**AGE 65**
Sedentary	2685	2285	1869	1589
Low active	2934	2534	2072	1792
Active	3250	2850	2325	2045
Very active	3770	3370	2628	2348

Calculations based on data presented in Food and Nutrition Board, Institute of Medicine: *Dietary Reference Intakes for energy, carbohydrate, fiber, fat, fatty acids, cholesterol, protein, and amino acids (macronutrients),* Washington, D.C., 2002, National Academies Press.
*An individual of this height and weight has a BMI of approximately 25 kg/m², the boundary between normal weight and overweight.

New Research Exploring Total Energy Expenditure

As the prevalence of overweight grows worldwide, medical scientists are exploring physiologic and metabolic factors that might influence energy intake and energy expenditure. New areas of research with potential for future intervention include the following:

- *Action of intestinal microflora:* Particular species of intestinal bacteria may have a role in prevention and treatment of obesity (see the discussion of probiotics in Chapter 2). When the quantities of fatty acids produced by bacterial fermentation exceed the amount needed by the intestinal cells, the excess are absorbed into the body, adding to energy intake.[19] Obese individuals have a different profile of intestinal microflora than the nonobese, and introduction of useful microflora might assist in weight management.[20]
- *Brown fat thermogenesis:* Brown fat is a special adipose tissue capable of high energy metabolism given off as heat. Infants have plentiful amounts of brown fat to assist in their response to cold as they move from the warmth of

BOX 8-2   KEEPING A PHYSICAL ACTIVITY RECORD

To get a true picture of your activity pattern you can keep a physical activity record. Recording your physical activity over a 24-hour period is much like recording your food intake. Prepare a chart that allows you to record the time you start and stop each activity and describe the type of activity. Carry a notebook with you and make entries immediately as changes occur and before you forget. Review the activity expenditure database prior to use, so you are sure to include the appropriate amount of detail when keeping your record. The Evolve website accompanying this text provides a comprehensive listing of day to day activities or refer to Table 8-2. The Center for Disease Control and Prevention also lists the kcalories required for typical activities at http://www.cdc.gov/healthyweight/physical_activity/index.html#calories%20used%20in%20typical%20activities. Using the energy expenditures assigned to your body weight in pounds, calculate your total energy expenditure over a 24-hour period. Keep in mind that databases providing kcalories per activity also account for RMR needs per pound of body weight per unit of time; thus, you need sum only the time-corrected values to estimate your total energy expenditure for the day. If you are trying to increase your physical activity, keeping a log for several days will help you identify times through the day or week when you might add or increase an activity. Keeping a record may also alert you to the fact that you are not as active as you think you are.

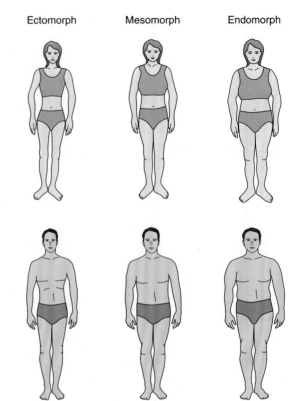

FIGURE 8-4 Body types: the ectomorph, the mesomorph, and the endomorph.

the womb to the ambient temperature surrounding them. Brown fat is lost as individuals move through childhood and adolescence, although adults retain small amounts. Brown fat affects long-term energy balance by raising the BMR.[21] Capsaicin, a compound found in hot peppers, activates brown fat thermogenesis in some individuals.[22]

• *Sleep deprivation:* It is estimated that 30% of Americans get 6 or fewer hours of sleep per night, as life becomes more demanding. Too little sleep influences energy intake and expenditure in several ways: (1) sleep-deprived individuals often experience increases in appetite and crave snack foods high in carbohydrate and fat; (2) lack of sleep reduces one's energy level so that active pursuits are likely avoided; and (3) hormonal changes set up metabolic patterns that contribute to body weight gain.[23] Night shifts and rotating work shifts can disrupt body metabolism and promote unwanted weight gain. Increasing hours of sleep may help bring about weight loss or prevent unwanted weight gain.

BODY COMPOSITION: FATNESS AND LEANNESS

A person's body composition reflects his or her total lifetime nutrient and energy balance.[24] Individuals have different body shapes and sizes depending on their age, gender, genes, body type, and state of health. Ectomorphs have a body type that is generally slender and fragile, mesomorphs have prominent muscle and bone development, and endomorphs have a soft, round physique with some accumulation of body fat (Figure 8-4). Although each body type has a genetic base, dietary intake and physical activity influence how it is expressed. Some body types are associated with better health, whereas others carry increased risk of chronic disease. We need to be sensitive to different body types when developing strategies to improve body composition and health.

Body Weight and Body Fat
Overweight Versus Overfat

Because height and weight are easily measured, they are commonly used to assess health status. It is important to know what these measurements do and do not tell us. The terms *overweight* and *obesity* have different meanings as related to body composition, and these distinctions have implications for health. A football player in peak physical condition can be markedly "overweight" according to standard height-weight charts. That is, the player weighs more than the average person of similar height, but that player's body tissues are likely to be very different. A sedentary man above average weight likely has an excess amount of body fat that is adding to his total body weight; an athlete above average weight is likely to have an exceptionally large amount of muscle. In fact, the overweight athlete may have an even lower proportion of body fat than an individual of average weight. When overweight is the result of excessive body fat rather than enhanced muscle or skeletal tissue, *overfat* or *obese* is the appropriate term. The critical element when evaluating body build and health is body composition. What we really need to know is how much of a person's body weight is fat and how much is fat-free mass (FFM). It is more precise to think in terms of *fatness* and *leanness* rather than body weight or overweight.

Body Compartments

Body compartments are defined on the basis of their comparative size and metabolic activity. The relative amounts of specific body tissues sometimes overlap among compartments. The four-compartment model for evaluating body composition includes lean body mass (LBM), body fat, body water, and mineral mass, as follows:

1. *LBM:* This compartment is made up of active cells from muscle and vital organs and largely determines the BMR and related nutrient needs. In sedentary individuals it accounts for almost the entire energy requirement. LBM includes not only cell protein but also a large amount of water, because muscle cells are about 65% water. This compartment also contains very small amounts of fatty acids found in the membranes of muscle and organ cells. LBM changes in size across the life cycle, with steady growth through childhood and young adulthood and gradual loss in later years. In adults it makes up 30% to 65% of total body weight. Most weight reduction regimens result in a loss of both body fat and LBM. (LBM contains cell protein, cell water, and a very small amount of fat found in membranes, while FFM includes cell protein, all body water both inside and outside of cells, and bone mineral mass—all body tissues except for fat.)

2. *Body fat:* Total body fat reflects both the number and size of the fat cells (**adipocytes**) that form the adipose tissue. Most adipocytes are white fat cells, not the brown fat cells we referred to earlier. In an adult man of normal weight, fat comprises 13% to 21% of body weight. In a woman of normal weight, the range of body fat content is 23% to 31%. These amounts vary with age, body type, exercise, and fitness, and many people have body fat levels markedly greater than or less than these ranges. About one half of all body fat is located in the subcutaneous fat layers under the skin, where it serves as insulation. In children and young adults, the subcutaneous fat provides a useful measure for estimating total body fat. Skinfold thickness measured at various locations on the body such as the triceps, subscapular region, or waist can be applied to existing standards to assess relative leanness or fatness. As individuals grow older, body fat is deposited on the trunk rather than on the extremities; thus waist circumference, waist-to-hip ratio, and waist-to-height ratio become useful tools to evaluate body fatness and health risk.[25-27]

3. *Body water:* Total body water includes both intracellular and extracellular water. Total body water varies with relative leanness or fatness, age, hydration status, and health status. Generally, water makes up about 50% to 65% of body weight. Muscle tissue has high water content, whereas adipose tissue has low water content; thus men have a higher proportion of body water than women because they have more muscle and less fat. Infants have a relatively high proportion of body water, which drops to adult levels by age 2.[9] This makes them especially vulnerable to the dangers of dehydration with continued vomiting or diarrhea.

4. *Mineral mass:* Body minerals found largely in the skeleton account for only 4% to 6% of body weight. Major minerals are calcium and phosphorus located in bone and other body cells and in fluids. Sodium is the major mineral in extracellular fluid (ECF), and potassium is the major mineral in intracellular fluid (ICF).

The following factors influence the relative sizes of body compartments[27]:

- *Gender:* Women have more adipose tissue, and men have more lean tissue, particularly muscle tissue.
- *Age:* Young adults have more LBM and less fat than older adults.
- *Physical activity:* Persons who are physically active have less fat and more LBM than individuals who are sedentary.
- *Race:* African Americans have relatively more bone mineral than Caucasians or Hispanics; Caucasian men tend to have more body fat than African-American men of similar height and weight; Mexican-American women tend to have more body fat than African-American women with similar heights and weights.[28]
- *Climate:* Individuals living in very cold climates develop more subcutaneous fat to insulate against heat loss.

Importance of Body Fat

Although excess body fat is detrimental to health, some body fat is necessary for life. In human starvation, victims die from fat loss, not protein depletion. For mere survival, men require about 3% body fat and women require about 12%; however, for reproductive capacity women require a body fat of about 20%. The initiation of menstruation or **menarche** occurs when the female body attains a certain size or, more precisely, the critical proportion of body fat. Body fat gained during pregnancy serves as an important energy reserve for lactation, and the production of breast milk with its high energy cost usually brings about a gradual loss of these fat stores. Ill-advised dieting during pregnancy in an attempt to avoid normal weight gain interferes with fetal development and can result in a low–birth-weight infant with associated health risks.

KEY TERMS

obesity   Fatness; an excessive accumulation of body fat.
adipocyte   A fat cell.
menarche   The first menstruation with the onset of puberty.

Measuring Body Compartments
Specialized Methods

The classic method for determining body composition is hydrostatic weighing using Archimedes' principle. The individual is first weighed in air and then weighed completely submerged in water. The volume of water displaced is measured, and using standardized equations the relative amounts of LBM and body fat can be calculated. In a new application of this principle, the individual is weighed in air and then introduced to an air-controlled chamber, referred to as a *pod*. The pod can measure the amount of air displaced by the volume of the body (Figure 8-5). Both air and water displacement methods take advantage of the fact that body fat and lean tissue differ in density, and standard calculations can be applied. The air displacement method offers an opportunity for measuring infants, children, older adults, or patients who cannot be weighed under water.[29]

Dual-energy x-ray absorptiometry (DEXA) is an advanced form of radiographic technology that can differentiate among muscle, fat, and bone; this method is used to measure bone mineral density and age-related bone loss. Bioelectrical impedance systems that pass a very small current of electricity through the body can distinguish water, fat, and bone, and are applicable to clinical settings. Body circumferences and skinfold thicknesses are useful and inexpensive methods to estimate body muscle and body fat in the clinical setting. These procedures will be discussed in detail in Chapter 16.

Development of Height-Weight Tables

The Metropolitan Life Insurance Company, using information obtained from their life insurance policyholders, mostly middle-aged Caucasian men, constructed the first height-weight tables in the 1930s. Desirable weights were based on the body weights of the policyholders who lived the longest. Early height-weight tables presented adult reference weights according to age, based on the assumption that weight gain continued throughout adult life. In recent years new concepts have emerged regarding height-weight tables: (1) body weight (and body fat) should not increase as individuals move into middle and older ages, and (2) body build and body fat patterns differ across racial and ethnic groups, so the standard measurements developed using Caucasian populations may not be appropriate for African Americans, Hispanics, or Asians. (See the Focus on Culture box, "Evaluating Body Compartments: One Size Really Doesn't Fit All," to explore this issue further.)

Reference Tables for Clinical Evaluation

Health and nutrition professionals from the Institute of Medicine and the U.S. Department of Health and Human Services have since developed reference standards to define the terms *overweight* and *obesity*.[3,30,31] Appropriate ranges of body weight for adults of a given height can be of use to health professionals in assessing patients and setting goals (see Table 8-5 and Appendix A).[31] Americans are becoming taller and heavier, but body weights have risen at a faster rate than body heights.[32] Since 1960 average body weight in women increased by 24 lb (from 140 to 164 lb), although body height increased less than 1 inch. Men increased in average weight from 166 to 191 lb (a gain of 25 lb), with about an inch increase in height. However, it appears the proportion of U.S. adults who are obese has stabilized, after steady increases in past decades.[33,34] Nearly 74% of men and 64% of women ages 20 and over are either overweight or obese, and these numbers are higher among Hispanic and Mexican-American men, and African-American, Hispanic, and Mexican-American women.

Body Mass Index

In 1871 Quetelet developed the body mass index (BMI), which has replaced body weight as the medical standard to define obesity. Although calculated using body height and weight, BMI provides a better evaluation of appropriate body weight than simple height-weight tables and correlates well with estimates of body fat obtained by underwater weighing. Nevertheless, BMI does not provide a quantitative estimate of body fat and cannot distinguish between excess body fat and increased muscle in persons who weigh more than the standard. Stature influences body composition because taller people have greater bone mass, which adds to their body weight. Thus, individuals with the same BMI may not have the same body composition.[35] Despite these limitations, BMI is a useful tool relating the increase in health risk with excessive body weight, and providing a base line for intervention when more sophisticated equipment is not available.

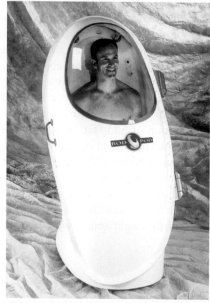

FIGURE 8-5 A pod for measuring body composition. The BOD POD uses air displacement technology to measure body composition. (Courtesy Life Measurement, Inc, Concord, Calif.)

⊕ FOCUS ON CULTURE

Evaluating Body Compartments: One Size Really Doesn't Fit All

Body composition differs among racial and ethnic groups. African Americans have greater bone mineral than Caucasians.[1] Body potassium (a measure of LBM) is higher in African Americans than Caucasians of similar size, and lower in Mexican Americans and Asians.[2]

Total body fat and abdominal fat also vary according to age, gender, and race. All women have a higher percentage of body fat than men, but white men have a higher proportion of abdominal fat than men of other groups.[3] Body mass index (BMI) does not present a true estimate of weight status in certain age and population groups. BMI underestimated the amount of body fat in more than one fourth of older African-American women and in Mexican-American adults of all ages.[4]

Common standards now used to evaluate body fat and health risk are not equally appropriate for all groups. Even slight increases in body fat carry greater health risks for Chinese men and women. Chinese women whose waist-to-hip ratio was above 0.8 had greater mortality risk from coronary heart disease even though their BMI was in the healthy range (less than 25 kg/m^2).[5] Health experts have suggested a cutoff of 23 kg/m^2 rather than 25 kg/m^2 to define overweight, and a level of 25 kg/m^2 rather than 30 kg/m^2 to define obesity in Asians.

New prediction standards are needed to accurately target disease risk and early intervention.

References

1. Katzmarzyk PT, Barreira TV, Harrington DM, et al: Relationship between abdominal fat and bone mineral density in white and African American adults. *Bone* 50:576, 2012.
2. He Q, Heo M, Heshka S, et al: Total body potassium differs by sex and race across the adult age span. *Am J Clin Nutr* 78:72, 2003.
3. Camhi SM, Bray GA, Bouchard C, et al: The relationship of waist circumference and BMI to visceral, subcutaneous, and total body fat: sex and race differences. *Obesity (Silver Spring)* 19(2):402, 2011.
4. Heo M, Faith MS, Pietrobelli A, et al: Percentage of body fat cutoffs by sex, age, and race-ethnicity in the US adult population from NHANES 1999-2004. *Am J Clin Nutr* 95:594, 2012.
5. Zhang X, Shu XO, Yang G, et al: Abdominal adiposity and mortality in Chinese women. *Arch Intern Med* 167:886, 2007.

TABLE 8-5   ADULT BMI CHART

To determine BMI, locate the height of interest in the left-most column and read across the row for that height to the weight of interest. Follow the column of the weight up to the top row that lists the BMI. A BMI of 18.5 to 24.9 is the healthy-weight range, a BMI of 25 to 29.9 is the overweight range, and a BMI of 30 or above is the obese range.

BMI	19	20	21	22	23	24	25	26	27	28	29	30	31	32	33	34	35*
HEIGHT							BODY WEIGHT IN POUNDS										
4 ft 10 in	91	96	100	105	110	115	119	124	129	134	138	143	148	153	158	162	167
4 ft 11 in	94	99	104	109	114	119	124	128	133	138	143	148	153	158	163	168	173
5 ft	97	102	107	112	118	123	128	133	138	143	148	153	158	163	168	174	179
5 ft 1 in	100	106	111	116	122	127	132	137	143	148	153	158	164	169	174	180	185
5 ft 2 in	104	109	115	120	126	131	136	142	147	153	158	164	169	175	180	186	191
5 ft 3 in	107	113	118	124	130	135	141	146	152	158	163	169	175	180	186	191	197
5 ft 4 in	110	116	122	128	134	140	145	151	157	163	169	174	180	186	192	197	204
5 ft 5 in	114	120	126	132	138	144	150	156	162	168	174	180	186	192	198	204	210
5 ft 6 in	118	124	130	136	142	148	155	161	167	173	179	186	192	198	204	210	216
5 ft 7 in	121	127	134	140	146	153	159	166	172	178	185	191	198	204	211	217	223
5 ft 8 in	125	131	138	144	151	158	164	171	177	184	190	197	203	210	216	223	230
5 ft 9 in	128	135	142	149	155	162	169	176	182	189	196	203	209	216	223	230	236
5 ft 10 in	132	139	146	153	160	167	174	181	188	195	202	209	216	222	229	236	243
5 ft 11 in	136	143	150	157	165	172	179	186	193	200	208	215	222	229	236	243	250
6 ft	140	147	154	162	169	177	184	191	199	206	213	221	228	235	242	250	258
6 ft 1 in	144	151	159	166	174	182	189	197	204	212	219	227	235	242	250	257	265
6 ft 2 in	148	155	163	171	179	186	194	202	210	218	225	233	241	249	256	264	272
6 ft 3 in	152	160	168	176	184	192	200	208	216	224	232	240	248	256	264	272	279
6 ft 4 in	156	164	172	180	189	197	205	213	221	230	238	246	254	263	271	279	287
	Healthy Weight						**Overweight**					**Obese**					

Data from National Heart, Lung, and Blood Institute, National Institute of Diabetes and Digestive and Kidney Disease: *Clinical guidelines on the identification, evaluation, and treatment of overweight and obesity in adults. The Evidence Report*, NIH Pub No 98-04083, Bethesda, Md., 1998, National Institutes of Health. Can be accessed at: <http://www.nhlbi.nih.gov/guidelines/obesity/ob_gdlns.pdf>.
*Height and weight equivalents for BMI levels above 35 can be found in Appendix A.

The formula for calculating BMI is as follows:

$$BMI = Weight\ (kg) \div Height\ (m)^2$$

$$Weight: 1\ kg = 2.2\ lb$$

$$Height: 1\ m = 39.37\ inches$$

The desirable BMI range for adults is 18.5 to 24.9 kg/m². Health risks associated with overweight begin at 25 kg/m² and become apparent at 30 kg/m². Values beyond 35 kg/m² indicate severe obesity (Tables 8-5 and 8-6).[3] BMI is often used to evaluate the effects of overweight and obesity on morbidity and mortality. Age and gender become factors when evaluating the mortality risk associated with a rise in BMI, as older adults and women seem to better tolerate overweight or obesity than younger adults or men.[36-38] A recent analysis of 27 studies that followed up on nearly 3 million adults reported that overweight (BMI = 25 to 29.9) was associated with lower all-cause mortality rates, and persons with grade 1 obesity (BMI = 30 to 34.9) had similar mortality rates as those of desirable weight (18.5 to 24.9 kg/m²). BMI measurements of 35 and over carried higher risk of death. These findings have raised questions as to whether all individuals with a BMI of 25 or higher should be approached about weight loss or if identification and intervention for other risk factors is a better approach.[39]

Abdominal Fat/Waist Circumference

Health and disease risk are influenced not only by the amount of body fat but also by where it is positioned. The pear shape, with a smaller waist and larger hip (gynoid shape), is characteristic of younger women and controlled to some extent by the female hormone estrogen. The apple shape, with more fat around the abdomen (android shape), is common in men and postmenopausal women. Because abdominal (visceral) fat raises blood lipid levels and increases the risk of cardiovascular disease, extra weight around one's middle is of greater harm than extra weight on the hips or thighs. An appropriate waist-to-hip ratio (WHR) is 0.9 or less for men and 0.8 or less for women. These ratios indicate a smaller waist and a larger hip measurement.[30] Waist circumference has become a popular tool for evaluating abdominal fat and health status.[38] The threshold for abdominal obesity as defined by waist circumference is greater than or equal to 88 cm (35 inches) in women and greater than or equal to 102 cm (40 inches) in men.[30] (See the Perspectives in Practice box, "Assessing Energy Expenditure and Body Weight," to estimate your energy requirements and evaluate your body weight status.)

HEALTH PROMOTION

Finding a Healthy Weight

For many people a normal body weight cannot be defined.[1] In the traditional sense, overweight and excessive body fat represent an energy imbalance arising from a surplus in energy input (fuel from food) over energy output (total energy expenditure). But it is not that simple. Our genetic makeup influences propensity to weight gain and the amount and position of body fat. Estrogen and testosterone control the differences in body fat between men and women, but other internal mechanisms also lead to differences in fat accretion. Certain individuals have an exceptionally low RMR and a high metabolic efficiency influenced by an inherited obesity gene,[3,14] which adds to their risk of unwanted weight. A genetic link has been identified among certain Native Americans that characterizes their lower energy expenditure and higher BMI and contributes to their elevated risk for type 2 diabetes.[40] Fidgeting and ongoing body movement, sometimes referred to as non-exercise activity thermogenesis (NEAT) increases energy expenditure and helps some people resist weight gain even if overfed.[41,42]

Just as weight gain results from a surplus of kcalories, weight loss should follow a kcalorie deficit. Traditionally it was believed that a shortfall of 3500 kcal would bring about the loss of 1 lb of body weight; however, this can be a false promise, and leading clinicians recommend that it not be used.[43] Body mechanisms designed to preserve body mass can decrease spontaneous activity or lower the RMR, making weight loss more difficult. When weight loss is successful, RMR and energy requirements decrease as body tissue is lost. Adding an exercise component assists in weight management if individuals do not increase their energy intake as a result of the activity.[43] For some individuals the weight loss required to move them into a more appropriate weight range is not possible. Yet, it is critical to interrupt a cycle of continued weight gain. The American Heart Association[44] points to the misperception created by an emphasis on body weight and mortality. Although body weight in the overweight or moderately obese range does not always result in earlier

BMI (kg/m²)	BODY WEIGHT STATUS	BODY FAT (%): MEN	BODY FAT (%): WOMEN
<18.5	Underweight	<13	<23
18.5-24.9	Normal	13-21	23-31
25-29.9	Overweight	21-25	31-37
30-34.9	Obese	25-31	37-42
≥35	Severely obese	>31	>42

TABLE 8-6   BODY MASS INDEX AND PERCENT BODY FAT

From Food and Nutrition Board, Institute of Medicine: *Dietary Reference Intakes for energy, carbohydrate, fiber, fat, fatty acids, cholesterol, protein, and amino acids (macronutrients)*, Washington, D.C., 2005, National Academies Press.

KEY TERM

visceral   Referring to the organs in the abdominal cavity.

PERSPECTIVES IN PRACTICE

Assessing Energy Expenditure and Body Weight

In your professional role you will help clients define their energy needs and assess their body weight and body fat. This exercise provides experience in applying some simple measures.

A. Calculate Your Total Energy Expenditure

Your total energy output per day is the sum of three uses of energy:
1. Resting metabolic rate (RMR).
2. Thermic effect of food (TEF). (The factors we are using to calculate physical activity include the TEF so for this exercise we will not calculate it separately.)
3. Physical activity.

1. Resting Metabolic Rate

Calculate your RMR using one of the following[1]:

Women: 0.9 kcal/kg/hr*

Men: 1.2 kcal/kg/hr

Convert your body weight from pounds (lb) to kilograms (kg): 1 kg = 2.2 lb. Body weight in pounds _____ ÷ 2.2 = _____ kg.

Example: Mr. Frank weighs 176 lb: 176 ÷ 2.2 = 80 kg.

RMR (kcalories) = 0.9 (for women) or 1.2 (for men) × kg body weight × 24 (hours in day) = _____

Example: Mr. Frank weighs 80 kg and the calculation factor for men is 1.2.

RMR (kcalories) = 1.2 × 80 kg × 24 (hours) = 2304 kcal

2. Physical Activity[1]

Calculate your physical activity expenditure:

Calculate the energy cost of your physical activity using your RMR and the activity factor from Table 8-4 that best fits your current activity level.

Physical activity kcalories = RMR × physical activity factor = _____

Example: Mr. Frank's RMR is 2304 kcal, and he is sedentary, so his activity factor is 0.2.

Physical activity kcalories = 2304 × 0.2 = 461 kcal

3. Total Energy Expenditure

To calculate your total energy expenditure (kcalories):

RMR kcalories _____ + physical activity kcalories _____ = _____

Example: Mr. Frank's total energy expenditure: 2304 kcal (RMR) + 461 kcal (physical activity) = 2765 kcal (Total Energy Expenditure)

Refer to the dietary intake record that you completed for the *Perspectives in Practice* box in Chapter 1, and consider the following questions:
a. How does your energy intake compare with your estimated total energy expenditure completed above? Are you taking in more kcalories, fewer kcalories, or about the same number of kcalories as you are using each day?
b. What will be the effect on your body weight if you continue this pattern? What will be the effect on your health status?

B. Evaluate Your Body Weight Using the Body Mass Index[2]

Determine your body mass index (BMI) using Table 8-5 or Appendix A.

BMI = _____

Health risks associated with overweight begin at a BMI of 25, and individuals with a BMI of 30 or greater have increasing levels of risk (see Table 8-6).
a. What is your assessment of your weight status using the BMI? Are you underweight, overweight, or in the healthy range?
b. If you are not in the healthy range, how might you begin to improve your status? (Consider underweight to be as needful of attention as overweight.)

C. Evaluate Your Health Status Using Waist Circumference[2]

Measure your waist circumference (WC) using a nonstretch tape.

WC = _____

If you are a woman, then your waist circumference should not exceed 88 cm (35 inches); if you are a man, it should not exceed 102 cm (40 inches).
a. What is your assessment of your chronic disease risk based on your waist circumference?
b. If you are not in the healthful range, how might you begin to improve your status?

References

1. Food and Nutrition Board, Institute of Medicine: *Dietary Reference Intakes for energy, carbohydrate, fiber, fat, fatty acids, cholesterol, protein, and amino acids (macronutrients)*, Washington, D.C., 2002, National Academies Press.
2. National Heart, Lung, and Blood Institute/National Institute of Diabetes and Digestive and Kidney Diseases: *Clinical guidelines on the identification, evaluation, and treatment of overweight and obesity in adults: the evidence report*, NIH Pub No 98-4083, Bethesda, Md., 1998, National Institutes of Health.

*These factors represent the midpoint of the suggested range for each sex.

death,[36,45] even small increases in body weight can add to risk of chronic conditions that adversely affect quality of life. Conversely, small losses in body weight interrupt or slow such changes. So what should be our approach to a healthy weight?

Developing a Healthy Lifestyle

The goals of weight management go well beyond numbers on a scale, even if a change in weight is one of the objectives.[1] Successful weight management requires a lifelong commitment to positive lifestyle behaviors that emphasize

EVIDENCE-BASED PRACTICE

Is There a Role for Walking in Weight Management?

Identify the Problem: Health educators worldwide are encouraging individuals to increase their physical activity. Walking has many advantages as a form of exercise: It requires no special training, no special equipment other than a good pair of walking shoes, does not cost money, and is considered a safe activity for individuals who are obese or have been sedentary. However, is walking an effective form of physical activity for weight management?

Review the Evidence: Researchers have evaluated walking patterns and weight gain in persons with differing body weights. Levine and colleagues[1] fitted both lean and obese sedentary individuals with locomotion detection devices and found that both had the same number of walking bouts (46 to 47) over the course of the day; however, the lean individuals took more steps with each bout, which added about 3.5 miles to their distance walked. Walking also may be key to slowing the weight gain that occurs between youth and middle age. Among 5000 young adults followed for 15 years, the average weight gain was 2 lb per year, and BMI rose from less than 25 to 29 in women and from less than 25 to 28 in men.[2] Kcalorie intake changed very little over the 15-year span; walking made the difference. Women who walked 4 hours a week gained about 11 lb; those who did not walk gained 19 lb. Among men, weight gain for walkers was 15 lb compared with 24 lb for nonwalkers.

Implement the Findings: Adults are encouraged to perform at least 30 min of moderate-intensity exercise on most days of the week, and walking at a speed of 3 to 4 mph (greater than or equal to 100 steps/min) meets this standard. Although the 30 min of walking can be spread throughout the day, each bout should extend for at least 10 min to meet the expectation for moderate-intensity activity. Daily activities of independent living require about 2500 steps and 30 min of brisk walking will add at least 3000 steps to the daily total.[3] For most people, including older adults or persons with chronic disease, 5500 to 7500 steps per day is an achievable goal.[3] Individuals who stepped in place while television commercials were being aired added 2000 steps to their daily total.[4] Inexpensive pedometers can serve as incentives for individuals starting a walking program.

References

1. Levine JA, McCrady SK, Lanningham-Foster LM, et al: The role of free-living daily walking in human weight gain and obesity. *Diabetes* 57:548, 2008.
2. Gordon-Larsen P, Hou N, Sidney S, et al: Fifteen-year longitudinal trends in walking patterns and their impact on weight change. *Am J Clin Nutr* 89:19, 2009.
3. Tudor-Locke C, Craig CL, Aoyagi Y, et al: How many steps/day are enough? For older adults and special populations. *Int J Behav Nutr Phys Act* 8:80, 2011.
4. Steeves JA, Thompson DL, Bassett DR Jr: Energy cost of stepping in place while watching television commercials. *Med Sci Sports Exerc* 44(2):330, 2012.

sustainable and enjoyable eating habits and daily physical activity.[46,47] A healthy food and activity pattern is a more appropriate goal than weight loss at any cost. A meal plan low to moderate in fat and rich in fruits, vegetables, whole grains, and fiber at an energy level that prevents further weight gain adds to well-being regardless of weight loss. Regular physical activity such as walking lowers the risk of heart attack, even if individuals remain obese.[48] A stable weight, even if above desirable weight, is favored over regular cycles of weight loss followed by even greater weight gain. (Weight loss diets celebrated in the popular press but inappropriate for long-term health and well-being will be discussed in Chapter 15 on obesity.) For more discussion on the benefits of walking, see the Evidence-Based Practice box, "Is There a Role for Walking in Weight Management?")

FATNESS, THINNESS, AND HEALTH

Obesity and Health

Weight-related health problems can be divided into four categories: (1) metabolic, (2) degenerative, (3) neoplastic, and (4) anatomic.

- *Metabolic:* Type 2 diabetes, hypertension, elevated blood lipids, and the constellation of conditions associated with metabolic syndrome often accompany obesity. Regardless of total body fat, abdominal fat increases the risk of metabolic disorders.[49]
- *Degenerative:* Obesity and physical disability are strongly linked.[50] Osteoarthritis and joint problems, atherosclerotic changes, and pulmonary diseases are more serious in obese persons.
- *Neoplastic:* Many forms of cancer including colorectal, breast, prostate, esophageal, and ovarian cancer are more frequent in higher weight categories.
- *Anatomic:* Individuals who exceed a healthy weight have a greater risk of gastroesophageal reflux disease (GERD) and obstructive sleep apnea.

The current prevalence of overweight and obesity will increase health care costs in the years ahead. A 10-year follow-up of Medicare spending among normal weight, overweight, and obese older adults (classifications were based on BMI) indicated growing expenditures related to weight.[51] Spending increased $122 per year among the normal weight beneficiaries, but $230 per year in the overweight group, and $271 per year in the obese group.

Obsession with Thinness

A trend opposite to obesity but equally harmful to health is the model of extreme thinness. Fueled by advertising dollars, an image of thinness drives the marketing of clothes, cosmetics, and food to teenagers and young adults.[52] Social pressures have created an abnormally thin and unrealistic ideal to the point that even fashion models express dissatisfaction with their overall body shapes.[53] Social discrimination against school-age children who are overweight can intensify the fear of weight gain.[54] Boys and girls as young as age 7 perceive their mothers' encouragement to remain thin, and develop restrained eating patterns and dissatisfaction with their bodies.[55] When parents restrict food intake, children may react by overeating when those restricted foods are available outside the home.[56] Guilt feelings after eating certain foods and distorted perceptions of body size often form the basis for serious eating disorders that threaten nutritional and physical health. School programs, voluntary community programs, and sports programs that build self-esteem offer primary prevention for disordered eating.

The ongoing quest for the perfect body has given rise to the chronic dieter who is constantly trying to restrict food intake. Although restrained eating is often seen in women, dieting is also a concern among boys and girls. The family has a role in helping young people develop positive attitudes toward food. Adolescents who reported positive communication and closeness within their families had more frequent meals with family[57] and were less likely to follow inappropriate diets or engage in disordered eating behaviors.[58] Teens participating in weight-related sports are especially vulnerable to unhealthy weight-control practices, and preventive efforts should target parents and coaches.[59]

Eating Disorders: A High Price for Thinness

The number of individuals affected by eating disorders is unknown, as these conditions often exist for some time before clinical detection, and based on their secretive nature, they often go unreported. Prevalence differs according to gender and age. Although female adolescents are especially vulnerable to eating disorders, the incidence among male adolescents is rising. Males often have a history of obesity, which leads them to begin dieting.[60] Anorexia nervosa and bulimia nervosa are more likely to occur among adolescents, whereas binge eating disorder takes place well into adulthood.[61] Older adults are diagnosed with eating disorders. Eating disorders are biologically based mental illnesses that lead to nutritional deficiencies, medical complications, and in the extreme, disability and death. We associate eating disorders with our society's emphasis on thinness, but physicians in Great Britain and France described anorexia nervosa in the 1800s.

Causes of Eating Disorders

Eating disorders have an emotional/behavioral component and a neurophysiologic/genetic component, although genes appear to play a significant role.[62] Alterations in CNS activity directly affect food behavior and the development of eating disorders. Levels of serotonin and other neurotransmitters are altered, and changes in the hypothalamus affect appetite. Personality traits such as perfectionism and obsessive-compulsive behavior are common among individuals with eating disorders. Family dynamics may be part of the environmental stress that adds to the seriousness of these conditions, but families are not the root cause. Eating disorders often coexist with other psychiatric and anxiety-related disorders, and the longer the nutritional deficits and emotional problems continue, the more severe they become. Individuals do not choose to have eating disorders and treatment must address both physiologic and emotional components if restoration is to occur.[62]

For every individual who develops an eating disorder, a particular factor may be more or less important. The growing interest in athletics among children and youth can increase risk of eating disorders or assist in prevention. Those participating in activities in which thinness is expected, such as gymnastics or dance, are at greater risk.[61] Students who take part in school or recreational sports that do not require a thin body are at lower risk. Activities that build self-esteem and help young people feel good about themselves and their accomplishments help protect against eating disorders.

Types of Eating Disorders

The four types of eating disorders recognized by the American Psychiatric Association are (1) anorexia nervosa, (2) bulimia nervosa, (3) binge-eating disorder, and (4) eating disorders not otherwise specified (EDNOS).[61] Each has distinctive diagnostic criteria and symptoms.

Anorexia nervosa means appetite loss from nervous disease. Anorexia nervosa is a form of starvation with excessive weight loss self-imposed at great physical and psychologic cost. Although these patients may have a body weight only 85% of average or a BMI of less than 17.5, they never see themselves as underweight and emaciated but always as fat.[61] This distorted body image often persists during recovery. Low bone mass is a frequent complication because amenorrhea usually accompanies this condition. Sudden death can result from cardiac arrest. Individuals with a higher percentage of body fat at the time of hospital discharge are more likely to have a positive long-term outcome.[63]

Bulimia nervosa, meaning "ox hunger," describes the massive amounts of food consumed by these patients. Because this individual is eating, body weight is usually normal or even above normal. Bulimia nervosa is often associated with depression or difficulty in meeting social or role expectations. Patients are consumed with guilt about their food behavior. Eating episodes are followed by purging through self-induced vomiting, use of laxatives or diuretics, enemas, or excessive exercise, and may occur twice a week or more. Repeated vomiting of the highly acidic stomach contents is harmful to the teeth and tissues of the mouth.[64] This condition is sometimes referred to as the *binge and purge syndrome*.

Binge-eating disorder includes binge-eating episodes but without the purging behavior of bulimia nervosa. Binge eating occurs in response to stress or anxiety, or may soothe or relieve painful feelings. Many of these patients are overweight and have the same medical problems as obese individuals who do not binge eat.[64]

Eating disorders not otherwise specified (EDNOS) may include a combination of the conditions described above or a frequency of symptoms that differ from established diagnostic criteria. Eating problems such as purging syndrome and night-eating syndrome are included here.[64]

Prevention and Treatment

The identification of individuals at risk for eating disorders can prompt early intervention and interrupt the progression of malnutrition. Health professionals and school personnel working with adolescents and athletes should watch for behavioral and clinical signs that indicate those at risk (Box 8-3). Parents need to be alerted to the behavioral and health characteristics of eating disorders and watch for such behaviors in their children. School personnel need to monitor school-based programs intended to combat obesity.[62] Since it is not known which students may be genetically predisposed to an eating disorder, programs promoting weight loss require personal supervision. Individuals with anorexia nervosa will demonstrate characteristic signs of protein-energy malnutrition as the condition worsens; those with bulimia nervosa are less likely to be underweight.

BOX 8-3   SIGNS ASSOCIATED WITH DEVELOPMENT OF EATING DISORDERS IN ADOLESCENTS*

Behavioral Signs
- Obsession with dieting
- Extreme level of exercise
- Dissatisfaction with body size or shape
- Overestimation of kcalorie intake (anorexia nervosa)

Clinical Signs (Anorexia Nervosa)
- Arrested growth and maturation
- Underweight: body mass index (BMI) <17.5
- Dry and yellowish skin
- Growth of fine hair over body (e.g., lanugo)
- Drop in internal body temperature; person feels cold
- Severe constipation
- Low blood pressure, slowed breathing and pulse

Clinical Signs (Bulimia Nervosa)
- Chronically inflamed and sore throat
- Swollen glands in the neck and below the jaw
- Worn tooth enamel and decaying teeth
- Intestinal distress and irritation from laxative abuse
- Severe dehydration from purging of fluids

Data from American Dietetic Association: Position of the American Dietetic Association: nutrition intervention in the treatment of anorexia nervosa, bulimia nervosa, and other eating disorders. *J Am Diet Assoc* 106:2073, 2006; U.S. Department of Health and Human Services, National Institute of Mental Health: *Eating disorders*, NIH Pub No 07-4901, Bethesda, Md., 2007, National Institute of Mental Health.
*Not all of these signs will be observed in all individuals

The treatment of eating disorders requires an experienced team of health professionals including a physician, nurse, dietitian, clinical psychologist or psychiatrist, and dentist. Outpatient services may provide the care needed in less advanced cases, but for life-threatening anorexia nervosa, intense inpatient therapy is essential. The care plan for disordered eating patients should include nutritional, medical, and behavioral intervention. A framework for meals, snacks, and food choices must be implemented on a gradual basis to address the underweight or overweight. Medical complications arising from severe malnutrition, dehydration, habitual vomiting, or excessive use of diuretics and laxatives require immediate attention. The psychologist or psychiatrist on the health care team can address the personal and emotional issues contributing to the condition, and promote healthy behaviors that will sustain the nutritional and medical recovery. Persons with eating disorders can be resistant to treatment, and progress can be slow. An individualized approach to patients and their needs is mandatory for success.

The Problem of Underweight

We have discussed the problem of excessive body weight and body fat, and situations in which individuals deliberately reduce their food intake. Now we consider the causes and effects of underweight caused by lack of food or debilitating illness.

Definition

Extreme underweight is associated with serious health problems in all age groups.[8,65,66] *Underweight,* defined as a BMI of less than 18.5 kg/m², is relatively uncommon in the United States. A national survey identified only 2.2% of adults as underweight,[45] although a regional study found nearly 5% of low-income children between the ages of 2 and 4 to be low weight for height.[67] Low weight for age is associated with more than 2.2 million child deaths in developing countries,[65] and those who do survive often experience long-term growth retardation and disability. Underweight springs from poverty, poor living conditions, long-term illness, or physiologic

KEY TERMS
neoplastic Describing abnormal growth of tissue, usually associated with the formation of tumors.
anorexia nervosa Extreme psychophysiologic aversion to food resulting in life-threatening weight loss. An eating disorder accompanied by a distorted body image considered to reflect fat when the body is actually malnourished and thin from self-starvation.
bulimia nervosa An eating disorder in which cycles of gorging on large quantities of food are followed by self-induced vomiting and use of diuretics or laxatives or extreme levels of exercise to avoid weight gain.
binge-eating disorder An eating disorder in which individuals consume large amounts of food in a short period of time, but without the purging behavior of bulimia nervosa.

- *Poor utilization of available nutrients:* Malabsorption associated with prolonged diarrhea, gastrointestinal disease, or laxative abuse depletes nutrient stores. Cytokines produced by the immune system in response to chronic conditions such as cancer, chronic kidney disease, congestive heart failure, and AIDS accelerate the breakdown of body protein and fat. Cytokines also interfere with the effective utilization of nutritional supplements, making it difficult to reverse the patient's deteriorating condition.[68]

dysfunction. Infants, young children, and older adults are at greatest risk. Resistance to infection is lower, general health is poorer, and physical strength is decreased in seriously underweight individuals.

General Causes

Malnutrition and underweight stem from decreased food intake, increased energy requirements, or poor utilization of ingested nutrients (Box 8-4).

- *Poor food intake:* Lack of sufficient and appropriate food results in failure to thrive in children and older adults. Medications such as digoxin and chemotherapeutic agents contribute to the devastating weight loss known as *cachexia* seen in cardiac failure and cancer. Older people in poverty who live alone and lack transportation to a grocery store risk unwanted weight loss. Skilled nursing facilities are required to monitor body weight, as a patient's inability to self-feed can lead to significant weight loss. Self-imposed food restriction associated with eating disorders can result in life-threatening underweight.
- *Increase in energy requirements:* Long-term **hypermetabolic** conditions such as cancer, acquired immunodeficiency syndrome (AIDS), advanced heart disease, or infection impose energy demands that drain the body's resources. Hyperthyroidism increases caloric requirements. Extensive physical activity without a sufficient increase in energy intake will over time bring about inappropriate weight loss in the normal weight individual.

Nutritional Care

Underweight persons require special nutrition intervention to rebuild body tissues and nutrient stores. Food plans must be adapted to the individual's personal preferences, financial situation, and household concerns, and address any existing disease. The dietary recommendation should be (1) high in kcalories (at least 50% beyond standard needs); (2) high in protein to rebuild tissue; (3) high in carbohydrate to provide a primary energy source in an easily digested form; (4) moderate in unsaturated fats to add kcalories but not exceed recommended limits; and (5) optimum in vitamins and minerals, including supplements when deficiencies require them. A wide variety of food that is well seasoned and attractively presented helps revive a lagging appetite and the desire to eat. Meals and snacks spread throughout the day that include favorite foods increase interest in eating and promote optimal utilization of nutrients. Liquid nutritional supplements add kcalories and key nutrients. In extreme cases, tube feeding or total parenteral nutrition (TPN) may be necessary. (Rehabilitation of undernourished patients will be discussed further in Chapter 19.)

> **KEY TERM**
> **hypermetabolic** Increased rate of body metabolism occurring as a result of infection, trauma, or disease.

TO SUM UP

Food provides the energy that enables the body to continue its physical and metabolic work. Through a series of ongoing metabolic reactions, the chemical energy in food is converted to thermal, electrical, and mechanical energy. The heat produced by body work, expressed in kcalories, serves as a measure of energy taken in and expended. One's total energy requirement is the sum of (1) basal metabolic needs, (2) the food intake effect (TEF), and (3) physical activity. Physical activity is the most variable component, adding relatively few kcalories for sedentary persons but making up one half or more of the total energy requirement of highly active people. Both energy intake and physical activity influence the size of the four major body compartments: (1) lean body mass (LBM), (2) body fat, (3) body water, and (4) mineral mass. Both the amount of body fat and its location on the body influence disease risk, with abdominal fat of greatest concern. Conversely, eating disorders with self-imposed food restriction or purging result in poor health and even death, if prolonged, and treatment prognosis can be poor. Poverty, chronic disease, and medications contribute to underweight through low food intake, poor food utilization, or increased energy requirements. A nutrient- and energy-rich diet combined with ongoing counseling to support the rehabilitation process can in many instances restore a healthy weight.

QUESTIONS FOR REVIEW

1. Define *fuel factor*. Name the fuel factors of the energy-yielding nutrients.

2. List the three components contributing to the total energy requirement. What factors influence the BMR and why? What is the most variable component of the total energy requirement and why?

3. What is the difference between the BMR and the RMR? Which is most often used in clinical practice? Why?

4. Name the four body compartments and describe the tissues found in each. How are they measured?

5. You are performing a nutritional assessment of a man who is 6 feet 2 inches tall and weighs 248 lb. What is his BMI? Is he overweight, overfat, or do you not know? Explain.

6. You are working with a client who wants to lose weight and has found several diets on the Internet. One is a high-fat diet containing 1800 kcal and the other is a high-protein diet, also containing 1800 kcal. Which diet is most likely to produce long-term weight loss? Why?

7. Describe various eating disorders defined by the American Psychiatric Association. What factors contribute to risk of disordered eating?

8. You are working with a single mother and her 3-year-old daughter who are both underweight. They live in a small apartment in a dilapidated building in the inner city. Their electricity was disconnected, thus they have no working equipment for cooking and no refrigeration. They receive a noon and a supper meal at a nearby food program for the homeless. Plan a breakfast and snacks throughout the day that would increase their kcalorie and nutrient intake. (Remember, all foods you suggest must be safely stored at room temperature.)

9. An adolescent girl who weighs 142 lb wants to increase her energy expenditure by 250 kcal a day to encourage weight loss. Develop an activity plan that would mesh with her after-school hours and social time with friends.

10. Visit your local library and review the magazines directed toward young adults. Look for an article that suggests a regimen for weight management for either males or females. Evaluate each protocol in terms of (a) nutritional adequacy as compared with the MyPlate (ChooseMyPlate.gov) recommendations for servings of fruits, vegetables, grains, dairy, protein foods, and oils; (b) development of sustainable food patterns such as bag lunches or eating out; (c) reliance on commercial weight-loss products; and (d) safety for long-term use.

REFERENCES

1. American Dietetic Association: Position of the American Dietetic Association: weight management. *J Am Diet Assoc* 109:330, 2009.

2. Brody T: *Nutritional biochemistry*, ed 2, New York, 1999, Academic Press.

3. Food and Nutrition Board, Institute of Medicine: *Dietary Reference Intakes for energy, carbohydrate, fiber, fat, fatty acids, cholesterol, protein, and amino acids (macronutrients)*, Washington, D.C., 2002, National Academies Press.

4. Das SK, Roberts SB: Energy metabolism in fasting, fed, exercise, and re-feeding states. In Erdman JW, Jr, Macdonald IA, Zeisel SH, editors: *Present knowledge in nutrition*, ed 10, Ames, Iowa, 2012, International Life Sciences Institute & Wiley-Blackwell.

5. Guyton AC, Hall JE: *Textbook of medical physiology*, ed 10, Philadelphia, Pa., 2000, Saunders.

6. Wolfe RR: The role of dietary protein in optimizing muscle mass, function and health outcomes in older individuals. *Br J Nutr* 108(Suppl 2):S88, 2012.

7. Kulstad R, Schoeller DA: The energetics of wasting diseases. *Curr Opin Clin Nutr Metab Care* 10:488, 2007.

8. Evans WJ: Skeletal muscle loss: cachexia, sarcopenia, and inactivity. *Am J Clin Nutr* 91(Suppl):1123S, 2010.

9. Cereda E, Klersy C, Rondanelli M, et al: Energy balance in patients with pressure ulcers: a systematic review and meta-analysis of observational studies. *J Am Diet Assoc* 111:1868, 2011.

10. Kosmiski L: Energy expenditure in HIV infection. *Am J Clin Nutr* 94(Suppl):1677S, 2011.

11. AAP Committee on Nutrition. In Kleinman RE, editor: *Pediatric nutrition handbook*, ed 6, Elk Grove Village, Ill., 2008, American Academy of Pediatrics.

12. Gallagher D, Albu J, He Q, et al: Small organs with a high metabolic rate explained lower resting energy expenditure in African American than in white adults. *Am J Clin Nutr* 83:1062, 2006.

13. Klein CJ, Villavicencio SA, Schweitzer A, et al: Energy prediction equations are inadequate for obese Hispanic youth. *J Am Diet Assoc* 111:1204, 2011.

14. Jacobson P, Rankinen T, Tremblay A, et al: Resting metabolic rate and respiratory quotient: results from a genome-wide scan in the Quebec Family Study. *Am J Clin Nutr* 84:1527, 2006.

15. Westerterp-Plantenga MS, Lemmens SG, Westerterp KR: Dietary protein—its role in satiety, energetics, weight loss and health. *Br J Nutr* 108(Suppl 2):S105, 2012.

16. Westerterp KR: Physical activity as determinant of daily energy expenditure. *Physiol Behav* 93:1039, 2008.

17. Hortobagyi T, Finch A, Solnik S, et al: Association between muscle activation and metabolic cost of walking in young and old adults. *J Gerontol A Biol Sci Med Sci* 66A(5):541, 2011.

18. Schrack JA, Simonsick EM, Chaves PHM, et al: The role of energetic cost in the age-related slowing of gait speed. *J Am Geriatr Soc* 60:1811, 2012.

19. Arora T, Sharma R: Fermentation potential of the gut microbiome: implications for energy homeostasis and weight management. *Nutr Reviews* 69(2):99, 2010.

20. Arora T, Singh S, Sharma RK: Probiotics: interaction with gut microbiome and antiobesity potential. *Nutrition* 29(4):591, 2013.

21. Feng B, Zhang T, Xu H: Human adipose dynamics and metabolic health. *Ann NY Acad Sci* 1281:160, 2013.

22. Yoneshiro T, Aita S, Kawai Y, et al: Nonpungent capsaicin analogs (capsinoids) increase energy expenditure through the activation of brown adipose tissue in humans. *Am J Clin Nutr* 95:845, 2012.

23. Shlisky JD, Hartman TJ, Kris-Etherton PM, et al: Partial sleep deprivation and energy balance in adults: an emerging issue for consideration by dietetic practitioners. *J Acad Nutr Diet* 112:1785, 2012.

24. Heymsfield SB, Baumgartner RN: Body composition and anthropometry. In Shils ME, Shike M, Olson J, editors: *Modern nutrition in health and disease*, ed 10, Baltimore, Md., 2006, Lippincott Williams & Wilkins, pp 751–770.

25. Zhang C, Rexrode KM, van Dam RM, et al: Abdominal obesity and the risk of all-cause, cardiovascular, and cancer mortality. Sixteen years of follow-up in U.S. women. *Circulation* 117:1658, 2008.

26. Ashwell M, Gunn P, Gibson S: Waist-to-height ratio is a better screening tool than waist circumference and BMI for adult cardiometabolic risk factors: systematic review and meta-analysis. *Obes Reviews* 13:275, 2012.

27. Wells JCK: Lessons from body composition analysis. In Bowman BA, Russell RM, editors: *Present knowledge in nutrition*, vol 1, ed 9, Washington, D.C., 2006, International Life Sciences Institute, pp 23–33.

28. Heo M, Faith MS, Pietrobelli A, et al: Percentage of body fat cutoffs by sex, age, and race-ethnicity in the US adult population from NHANES 1999-2004. *Am J Clin Nutr* 95:594, 2012.

29. Baracos V, Caserotti P, Earthman CP, et al: Advances in the science and application of body composition measurement. *J Parenter Enteral Nutr* 36:96, 2012.

30. National Heart, Lung, and Blood Institute/North American Association for the Study of Obesity: *The practical guide: identification, evaluation, and treatment of overweight and obesity in adults*, NIH Pub No 00-4084, Bethesda, Md., 2000, National Institutes of Health. at: <http://www.nhlbi.nih.gov/guidelines/obesity/prctgd_c.pdf>. Accessed on January 25, 2013.

31. National Heart, Lung, and Blood Institute, National Institute of Diabetes and Digestive and Kidney Disease: 1998. *Clinical guidelines on the identification, evaluation, and treatment of overweight and obesity in adults. The Evidence Report*, NIH Pub No 98-04083, National Institutes of Health, Bethesda, Md., 1998, Author. at: <http://www.nhlbi.nih.gov/guidelines/obesity/ob_gdlns.pdf>. Accessed on July 30, 2013.

32. Ogden CL, Fryar CD, Carroll MD, et al: *Mean body weight, height, and body mass index, United States, 1960-2002: advance data, vital and health statistics*, No 347, Washington, D.C., 2004, U.S. Department of Health and Human Services.

33. Ogden CL, Carroll MD, Kit BK, et al: *Prevalence of obesity in the United States*, 2009-2010, NCHS Data Brief, No 82, Atlanta, Ga., 2012, U.S. Centers for Disease Control and Prevention.

34. Flegal KM, Carroll MD, Kit BK, et al: Prevalence of obesity and trends in the distribution of body mass index among US adults, 1999-2010. *JAMA* 307(5):491, 2012.

35. Heymsfield SB, Gallagher D, Mayer L, et al: Scaling of human body composition to stature: new insights into body mass index. *Am J Clin Nutr* 86:82, 2007.

36. de Gonzalez AB, Hartge P, Cerhan JR, et al: Body-mass index and mortality among 1.46 million white adults. *N Engl J Med* 363:2211, 2010.

37. Park V, Hartge P, Moore SC, et al: Body mass index and mortality in non-Hispanic black adults in the NIH-AARP Diet and Health Study. *PLoS ONE* 7(11):e50091, 2012.

38. Jacobs EJ, Newton CC, Wang Y, et al: Waist circumference and all-cause mortality in a large US cohort. *Arch Intern Med* 170(15):1293, 2010.

39. Heymsfield SB, Cefalu WT: Does body mass index adequately convey a patient's mortality risk? *JAMA* 309(1):87, 2013.

40. Traurig MT, Orczewska JI, Ortiz DJ, et al: Evidence for a role of LPGAT1 in influencing BMI and percent body fat in Native Americans. *Obesity (Silver Spring)* 20(12):2426, 2012.

41. Levine JA: Non-exercise activity thermogenesis (NEAT). *Nutr Reviews* 62(7 Pt 2):S82, 2004.

42. Elbelt U, Schuetz T, Hoffmann I, et al: Differences of energy expenditure and physical activity patterns in subjects with various degrees of obesity. *Clin Nutr* 29:766, 2010.

43. Hall KD, Heymsfield SB, Kemnitz JW, et al: Energy balance and its components: implications for body weight regulation. *Am J Clin Nutr* 95:989, 2012.

44. Lewis CE, McTigue KM, Burke LE, et al: Mortality, health outcomes, and body mass index in the overweight range. A science advisory from the American Heart Association. *Circulation* 119:3263, 2009.

45. Flegal KM, Graubard BI, Williamson DF, et al: Excess deaths associated with underweight, overweight, and obesity. *JAMA* 293:1861, 2005.

46. American Dietetic Association: Position of the American Dietetic Association: weight management. *J Am Diet Assoc* 102:1145, 2002.

47. Haskell WL, Lee IM, Pate RR, et al: Physical activity and public health: updated recommendation for adults from the American College of Sports Medicine and the American Heart Association. *Med Sci Sports Exerc* 39:1423, 2007.

48. Wessel TR, Arant CB, Olson MB, et al: Relationship of physical fitness vs body mass index with coronary artery disease and cardiovascular events in women. *JAMA* 292:1179, 2004.

49. Klein S, Allison DB, Heymsfield SB, et al: Waist circumference and cardiometabolic risk: a consensus statement from Shaping America's Health: Association for Weight Management and Obesity Prevention; NAASO, the Obesity Society; the American Society for Nutrition; and the American Diabetes Association. *Am J Clin Nutr* 85:1197, 2007.

50. Reuser M, Bonneux LG, Willekens FJ: Smoking kills, obesity disables: a multistate approach of the U.S. Health and Retirement Survey. *Obesity* 17:783, 2009.

51. Alley D, Lloyd J, Shaffer T, et al: Changes in the association between body mass index and Medicare costs, 1997-2006. *Arch Intern Med* 172(3):277, 2012.

52. Benowitz-Fredericks CA: Body image, eating disorders, and the relationship to adolescent media use. *Pediatr Clin N Am* 59(3):693, 2012.

53. Grivetti L: Psychology and cultural aspects of energy. *Nutr Reviews* 59:S5, 2001.

54. Corsica JA, Hood MM: Eating disorders in an obesogenic environment. *J Am Diet Assoc* 111(7):996, 2011.

55. Anschutz DJ, Kanters LJ, Van Strien T, et al: Maternal behaviors and restrained eating and body dissatisfaction in young children. *Int J Eat Disord* 42:54, 2009.

56. Birch LL, Fisher JO, Davison KK: Learning to overeat: maternal use of restrictive feeding practices promotes girls' eating in the absence of hunger. *Am J Clin Nutr* 78:215, 2003.

57. Berge JM, Wall M, Larson N, et al: Family functioning: associations with weight status, eating behaviors, and physical activity in adolescents. *J Adolesc Health* 52(3):351, 2012.

58. Berge JM, Wall M, Larson N, et al: The unique and additive associations of family functioning and parenting practices with disordered eating behaviors in diverse adolescents. *J Behav Med* 37:205, 2014.

59. Vertalino M, Eisenberg ME, Story M, et al: Participation in weight-related sports is associated with higher use of unhealthful weight-control behaviors and steroid use. *J Am Diet Assoc* 107:434, 2007.

60. Rees L, Clark-Stone S: Can collaboration between education and health professionals improve the identification and referral of young people with eating disorders in schools? A pilot study. *J Adolesc* 29(1):137, 2006.

61. American Dietetic Association: Position of the American Dietetic Association: nutrition intervention in the treatment of eating disorders. *J Am Diet Assoc* 111:1236, 2011.

62. American Dietetic Association: Practice paper of the American Dietetic Association: nutrition intervention in the treatment of eating disorders. 2011. at: <http://www.eatright.org/Members/content.aspx?id=6442464620>. Accessed on July 30, 2013.

63. Mayer LE, Roberto CA, Glasofer DR, et al: Does percent body fat predict outcome in anorexia nervosa? *Am J Psychiatry* 164:970, 2007.

64. Miller CA, Golden NH: An introduction to eating disorders: clinical presentation, epidemiology, and prognosis. *Nutr Clin Prac* 25:110, 2010.

65. Black RE, Allen LH, Bhutta ZA, et al: Maternal and child undernutrition: global and regional exposures and health consequences. *Lancet* 371:243, 2008.

66. Morley JE: Pathophysiology of the anorexia of aging. *Curr Opin Nutr Metab Care* 16:27, 2013.

67. Sherry B, Mei Z, Scanlon KS, et al: Trends in state-specific prevalence of overweight and underweight in 2- through 4-year-old children from low-income families from 1989 through 2000. *Arch Pediatr Adolesc Med* 158:1116, 2004.

68. Morley JE, Thomas DR, Wilson MM: Cachexia: pathophysiology and clinical relevance. *Am J Clin Nutr* 83:735, 2006.

FURTHER READINGS AND RESOURCES

Readings

Corsica JA, Hood MH: Eating disorders in an obesogenic environment. *J Am Diet Assoc* 111(7):996, 2011.

Friend S, Bauer KW, Madden TC, et al: Self-weighing among adolescents: associations with body mass index, body satisfaction, weight control behaviors, and binge eating. *J Acad Nutr Diet* 112(1):99, 2012.

Martin JB: The development of ideal body image perceptions in the United States. *Nutr Today* 45(3):98, 2010.

[These authors explore issues relating to eating and body image and how related disorders can be prevented and treated.]

Farley TA: The role of government in preventing excess calorie consumption. The example of New York City. *JAMA* 308(11):1093, 2012.

Lamont LS, Risica PM: Weight gain and weight management concerns for patients on β-blockers. *Nutr Today* 45(6):250, 2010.

McCrady SK, Levine JA: Sedentariness at work: how much do we really sit. *Obesity (Silver Spring)* 17(11):2103, 2009.

Shlisky JD, Hartman TJ, Kris-Etherton PM, et al: Partial sleep deprivation and energy balance in adults: an emerging issue for consideration by dietetics practitioners. *J Acad Nutr Diet* 112:1785, 2012.

[These articles address issues of energy intake in our society and potential interventions.]

Paddon-Jones D, Westman E, Mattes RD, et al: Protein, weight management, and satiety. *Am J Clin Nutr* 87(Suppl):1558S, 2008.

[Protein may have a role in weight management through its effect on satiety and overall metabolism. These authors provide some examples of its use in weight reduction diets.]

Websites of Interest

- National Heart, Lung, and Blood Institute/North American Association for the Study of Obesity: 2000. *The practical guide: identification, evaluation, and treatment of overweight and obesity in adults.* National Institutes of Health. This book provides a wealth of practical information on meal planning, food selection, and appropriate physical activity for assisting individuals with weight control; Bethesda, Md., NIH Pub No 00-4084: www.nhlbi.nih.gov/guidelines/obesity/prctgd_c.pdf.

- National Institute of Diabetes and Digestive and Kidney Diseases (NIDDK): WIN—Weight-Control Information Network. This site offers up-to-date, science-based information on weight control, obesity, physical activity, and related nutritional issues for health professionals and consumers: http://www.win.niddk.nih.gov/ (materials are available in English and Spanish).

- National Institutes of Health and National Library of Medicine, *Weight control.* This site offers tips on food selection for weight management and links to sites that provide ideas for physical activity: http://www.nlm.nih.gov/medlineplus/weightcontrol.html.

- National Institutes of Health and National Library of Medicine: Medline Plus; *Eating disorders.* This site offers comprehensive information on eating disorders, including causes, symptoms, treatment, and prevention: http://www.nlm.nih.gov/medlineplus/eatingdisorders.html.

- National Institute of Mental Health: *Eating disorders.* This site contains publications with information about eating disorders and how to deal with them: http://www.nimh.nih.gov/health/publications/eating-disorders/complete-index.shtml (materials available in English and Spanish).

- U.S. Department of Health and Human Services, Centers for Disease Control and Prevention: *Physical activity for everyone.* This site offers physical activity programs and information for all age groups, as well as resources for health professionals: http://www.cdc.gov/nccdphp/dnpa/physical/index.htm.

Community Nutrition and the Life Cycle

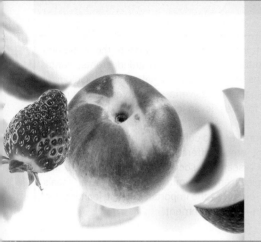

Food Selection and Food Safety

Eleanor D. Schlenker

OUTLINE

We begin a two-chapter section in which we apply our knowledge of nutrition science to the food needs and food safety of individuals and families. We look first at the web of factors that influence our personal food choices, including the ever-changing food environment. Issues such as health and convenience have joined taste and cost as consumer concerns in the marketplace. Although the expanding food supply offers more choices, it has also created a need for increased food regulation. When families produced their own food, they were responsible for its wholesomeness and safety. As our sphere of food access has broadened to include our region, our nation, and the world, food safety has become the responsibility of government and various enforcement agencies. Maintaining a healthy food supply rich in nutrients requires the cooperative efforts of farmers, food processors, and health professionals.

PERSONAL FOOD SELECTION

Food habits, like other human behaviors, do not develop in a vacuum. Rather, they grow out of our cultural, social, and psychologic environment, and the unique experiences that follow each of us throughout our lives.

Cultural Influences
Cultural Identity

Culture can be defined as the accumulation of a group's learned and shared behaviors in everyday life. Culture reveals the knowledge, values, beliefs, attitudes, and practices accepted by members of a group or community that bring a sense of identity and order to their lives.[1] Often the most significant thing about a culture is what is taken for granted. Culture involves not only the obvious aspects of life—language, religion, family structure, and historical heritage—but also daily patterns such as preparing and serving food and caring for children or elders. Culture defines how an individual describes health, perceives illness, and seeks treatment.[1] These facets of daily life are passed from generation to generation and learned as children grow up within the community.

Food in a Culture

Foodways (food customs or traditions) are among the oldest and most deeply rooted aspects of a culture. They determine what is eaten, when and how it is eaten, and who prepares it. An item considered to be a special treat by families in one part of the world can be unacceptable somewhere else. The geography of the land, the agriculture of that locality, experiences related to health and food safety, religious beliefs, and local history and traditions influence what we eat. Throughout history, designated foods or meals have commemorated special events of religious or national significance or rites of passage. Many of these customs remain today.[2] (To learn more about food customs see the Focus on Culture box, "Family Meals: Where Food and Culture Meet.")

⊕ FOCUS ON CULTURE

Family Meals: Where Food and Culture Meet

Over the centuries the family meal has been the setting in which children learn about their culture. Common vocabulary, food-related customs, etiquette, food-related holidays, and intergenerational and gender relationships are learned at the family table. Generally, celebrations such as weddings, birthdays, religious holidays, or secular holidays involve meals more elaborate in preparation and variety than day-to-day fare, and include food items not served at other times. Although Thanksgiving and Christmas mark traditional holiday meals for some groups, Chinese families celebrate New Year with feasting, and Muslims mark the end of Ramadan and the period of fasting with an elaborate meal. In agrarian societies, harvest dinners marked the end of the growing season and the securing of food crops for the coming winter. Sunday dinner has long been a special meal in the Appalachian culture and among African-American families because this was the day of rest when families had time to be together.

Family meals define gender roles and relationships. In East Indian cultures, feeding the family is an important role of the woman of the house. Even if servants or others assist with preparation, the woman of the house delivers the food to the table. Who eats together at mealtime establishes the framework of social standing among family members. In East Asian countries such as China and Japan, and traditional Native American, Arab, and African cultures, men and guests ate first, and then women and children ate. In comparison, African-American,

Latino, and Asian Indian families celebrated the extended family as an important social unit with grandparents, aunts, uncles, and cousins joining in communal meals. Sociologists suggest that the special cohesiveness observed among many African-American families is an outgrowth of the extended family meal.

The blending of families and cultures in the United States has obscured some of these differences in traditional practice. Nevertheless, the research associating better outcomes and healthier food choices among youth who eat regular meals with their families reinforces the importance of the learning and social interaction in this environment.

Bibliography

Barkoukis H: Importance of understanding food consumption patterns. *J Am Diet Assoc* 107:234, 2007.

Goody CM, Drago L, editors: *Cultural food practices*, Chicago, 2010, Diabetes Care and Education Dietetic Practice Group, American Dietetic Association.

Hammons AJ, Fiese BH: Is frequency of shared family meals related to the nutritional health of children and adolescents? *Pediatrics* 127:e1565, 2011.

Kittler PG, Sucher KP, Nahikian-Nelms M: *Food and culture*, ed 6, Belmont, Calif, 2012, Wadsworth/Cengage Learning.

Components of a Cultural Food Pattern

All food patterns share several common characteristics, although they differ in the actual foods they contain. These common dietary components are as follows[2]:

- *Core foods:* core foods, usually complex carbohydrates, are eaten every day and provide the bulk of the energy intake.
- *Complementary foods:* these are items added to improve palatability such as the vegetables or meat added to a rice or pasta meal.
- *Food flavors and preparation:* how foods are prepared and seasoned is distinctive for every group and is as important as the foods themselves.
- *Frequency and timing of meals:* the number of meals or snacks eaten each day, when they are eaten, and the foods they contain, define dietary intake within individuals and cultures.

Maintaining core foods, familiar flavors, and meal sequence serves as a bridge to new meal patterns related to health or other considerations.

Social Influences

Internal Factors

Food has social roles. Food is a symbol of acceptance, warmth, and friendliness. People are more likely to accept food from those they view as friends or supporters. The offering of food is an expected act of hospitality in many cultures. Strong food patterns develop within the primary family unit, and

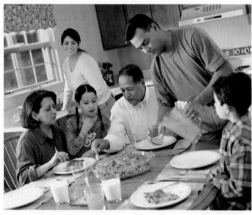

FIGURE 9-1 A family sharing food. Sharing food with visitors to your home is an established custom among many cultural and ethnic groups. (From Food and Nutrition Service, U.S. Department of Agriculture and Food and Nutrition Information Center, National Agricultural Library: *SNAP-Ed Connection: SNAP-Ed photo gallery*, Beltsville, Md., 2005, U.S. Department of Agriculture. Reprinted with permission. from: <http://snap.nal.usda.gov/photo-gallery?mode=mealtime>. Retrieved February 25, 2013.

food practices associated with family celebrations and camaraderie are held tenaciously throughout life (Figure 9-1). Long into adulthood, certain foods trigger a flood of childhood memories and are valued for reasons totally apart from their nutritional contribution. Nevertheless, income, local availability, and market conditions ultimately influence food choices. People eat foods that are readily available and that they have the money to buy.

External Factors

Peer pressure influences food choices. Foods may be viewed as high-prestige foods or associated with low economic status. Those immigrating to the United States may reject their traditional foods in favor of American foods popular among neighbors or classmates. Children plead for a particular snack item if that is what their friends eat. Adolescents are particularly susceptible to the influence of their peers in selecting healthy or unhealthy foods.[3,4]

Psychologic Influences

People who enjoy a bountiful food supply think less about food because it is always available, whereas those with chronic hunger or food cravings think, talk, and dream about food.[5] For most of us, concerns about food are associated with other needs. Maslow's classic hierarchy describes the five levels of human need, each building on the one before[6]:

1. *Basic physiologic needs:* hunger and thirst
2. *Need for safety:* physical comfort, security, and protection
3. *Need to belong:* love, giving and receiving affection
4. *Need for recognition:* self-esteem, sense of self-worth, self-confidence, and capability
5. *Need for self-actualization:* self-fulfillment and creative growth

Although these needs vary with time and circumstance, they help us understand the motivations and actions of others and develop our care plan accordingly. As summarized in Box 9-1, a complex set of physical, social, and psychologic factors influence what a person eats.

THE FOOD ENVIRONMENT

Food in the Marketplace

Family, ethnic, and regional ties are strong influences in our lives, but new technology and mass media put old influences in conflict with new forces, and this is also true for food. New ethnic flavors are displacing traditional recipes, and parents or grandparents who took pride in the dishes they prepared are disheartened if children like the "box" version better. Over 26% of Americans live alone, and they are more likely to cook from scratch or use more sophisticated ready-to-eat items.[7] Traditional families with children under age 18 are being targeted with prepackaged foods that can be prepared in minimal time. These families eat more pasta, macaroni, casseroles, and pizza.[8] With the busy lifestyles of parents and children, more family kitchens are 24-hour commissaries that family members can access at will, heating individual items that accommodate their meal preferences and schedules.[7] Yet, almost half of shoppers report they try to purchase fewer convenience foods to save money.[7] The growing older population will need healthy meals that require limited preparation while also accommodating the changes in taste and smell that accompany aging.[9]

BOX 9-1   FACTORS INFLUENCING FOOD CHOICES

Environmental Factors
- Food availability
- Food technology
- Geography, agriculture, food distribution
- Personal economics, income
- Sanitation, housing
- Season, climate
- Storage and cooking facilities

Social Factors
- Advertising
- Culture
- Education, food and nutrition knowledge
- Political and economic policies
- Religion and social customs
- Social class role, peer pressure
- Social problems, poverty, alcoholism
- Distance from food outlets (e.g., grocery stores, restaurants)

Physiologic Factors
- Allergy, food tolerance or intolerance
- Physical disability
- Health-disease status
- Personal food acceptance
- Energy or nutrient needs
- Medical nutrition therapy

Taste, price, and health, followed by convenience and land sustainability, drive the food purchases of the American public, although consumer age also has an influence. Consumers below age 50 are more driven by price, whereas older groups are more concerned with healthfulness.[10]

Meal Solutions

For those who must respond to the question "What's for dinner?" the meal should be quick and easy.[11] According to a food industry survey, a growing trend is "dining in" with a majority of meals eaten at home (Box 9-2). On average, U.S. families eat dinner at home at least five times each week.[7] Cooking skills that support healthy eating are also getting more attention. Almost 60% of young adults rate their cooking skills as good, compared with only 50% of those above age 45.[7] For those using prepackaged items, multi-portion skillet meals or oven meals are taking precedence over individual heat-and-serve items.[11] Consumer participation, even to a limited extent, brings the food preparation experience closer to that of "cooking from scratch." Parents may feel more positive about dishes to which they add a few fresh ingredients.[11]

Convenience items and fresh items can be combined for a quick and healthy meal. A rotisserie chicken from the supermarket or grilled chicken from a fast-food restaurant served with a frozen vegetable, and fruit or salad in place of French fries, is moderate in kcalories and nutrient dense. A frozen vegetable can be cooked in the microwave in the time it takes to set the table and get the family seated. Packaged salad greens can provide a quick addition to a meal; however, they should not be viewed as "ready to eat" without thorough washing. (Later in this chapter we will discuss recent outbreaks of foodborne illness related to bagged salad greens.) Helping families identify low-fat and nutrient-dense accompaniments to convenience items improves the nutrition of all family members.

Eating Frequency

The number of eating occasions throughout the day, both meals and snacks, influences energy intake. In recent years snacking (defined as any food or beverage other than water taken between meals) has about doubled.[12] Almost 90% of adults have at least one and 40% have three or more snacks each day. Snacks make up 24% of the daily energy intake of adults with alcohol, sugars, and solid fats contributing the highest proportion of kcalories.[12] In some adults, snacks escalated energy intake by as much as 1057 kcal while adding few other nutrients.[13] Among teens, snacks contributed on average 526 kcal per day; those with four or more snacks took in one and one-half times as many kcalories as those who reported no snacks.[14] Many adolescents eating three or more snacks a day also were eating three meals—breakfast, lunch, and dinner.[15]

Smaller meals with snacks (a grazing pattern) rather than one or two very large meals present a healthy eating pattern *if* the energy and nutrient content of all foods eaten are monitored wisely. Individuals who are physically active can benefit from eating more frequently. Older adults who have two or more snacks each day in addition to their regular meals are more likely to meet their energy requirement than those who do not snack.[16] Snacking on fruits, vegetables, low-fat dairy foods, low-fat grain products, or protein foods such as peanut butter or hard-cooked eggs adds important nutrients with low to moderate kcalories. When researchers from the U.S. Department of Agriculture (USDA) evaluated snacking in

relation to overweight and obesity, the number of daily snacks was not related to body mass index (BMI) in either youth[14] or adults.[12] Portion size, energy density of the foods chosen,[17] or lack of physical activity may have a greater role in unwanted weight gain.

Family Meals

Extended working hours for parents and increasing sport and club activities for children can make it difficult to manage family meals. Over the past decade the number of middle and high school students eating five or more meals per week with their families has declined. This is especially true among middle-school youth, girls, Asian families, and limited resource families.[18] Nevertheless, 44% of adolescents still eat at least five meals a week with their parents. Eating together as a family influences nutritional and emotional well-being. The more meals children eat with their parents, the greater their intakes of calcium-rich foods, fruits, and vegetables, and the more likely they are to be of normal weight.[19] Moreover, youth who have dinner regularly with their families have lowered risk of disordered eating, do better in school, and are less likely to use tobacco, alcohol, and drugs.[18]

Family meals also influence the food practices of parents, as mothers and fathers eating more meals with their children ate more fruits and vegetables. Mothers were less likely to indulge in binge eating or inappropriate dietary behaviors.[20] Meal patterns established in youth carry over in succeeding years. Young adults who ate breakfast regularly as adolescents were more likely to eat breakfast regularly when living independently.[21] Men appear to be assuming more responsibility for meal planning and preparation,[22] providing important role models for children and youth. (See the Perspectives in Practice box, "Returning to Hands-On Food," for ideas on how to get started preparing healthy meals.)

Health Concerns

Americans continue to experience frustration regarding the ever-changing nutrition messages flowing from the mass media. In a recent poll consumers noted that choosing what they should or should not eat was more difficult than figuring out their taxes.[10] Still, health ranks among the top three influences on shopping decisions, after taste and price.[10] In one survey 64% of responders reported making recent changes to improve their food choices, and the majority of these changes were directed toward losing weight.[23] Despite the growing prevalence of obesity, the proportion of consumers concerned about their body weight declined from earlier years, suggesting that people are becoming more complacent about their obesity.[23] Parents appear to worry more about the healthfulness of their children's diets than about their own.[10]

Fat, sodium, and kcalories continue to influence food purchases.[10] Two thirds of Americans try to avoid saturated fat, and 75% say they choose foods lower in fat at least some of the time. Kcalorie and sodium content are the most used information on the nutrition label.[23] In contrast, the majority

PERSPECTIVES IN PRACTICE

Returning to Hands-On Food

As the pace of life quickens with growing responsibilities of work, school, and child care, preparing meals at home can seem to be a daunting task. Young adults perceive lack of time as a major barrier to healthful eating.[1,2] Eating on the run can lead to increased intakes of sugar-sweetened beverages, high-calorie fast-food, and saturated fat, and limited intakes of fruits and vegetables. Poor food preparation skills add to the time required to prepare meals at home.

Following are some ways to begin developing skills for quick and healthy meals:

- *Obtain a family cookbook to help you get started:* The Academy of Nutrition and Dietetics, American Heart Association, and American Diabetes Association offer cookbooks with quick and easy recipes that can be prepared in 30 min and support healthy eating for all ages.
- *Supplement take-out foods with healthy items prepared at home:* Add a frozen vegetable or salad and oven-browned French fries (made with frozen potato strips) to the chicken or hamburgers purchased on the way home.
- *Try to make foods in advance to keep in your freezer for quick meals:* Instead of making a meat loaf in a loaf pan, make individual meat loaves in a muffin pan. The muffin meat loaves cook in half the time of a regular meat loaf, and leftovers can be frozen individually to thaw and heat as needed.
- *Use cut-up chicken parts that cook quickly on the cooktop or in the oven:* Look for recipes that use canned low-sodium chicken broth or low-sodium soups as ready-made sauces.
- *Look for skillet meals or casseroles that mix a protein food with pasta or vegetables:* Consider skillet lasagna, tuna noodle casserole, macaroni and cheese, or chicken and broccoli; one-pot cooking also makes for quick cleanup; begin to substitute whole grain pasta for refined pasta.
- *Get familiar with legumes:* Lentils and dried green peas can be added directly to a recipe without soaking; make a pot of lentil soup in the evening or on a weekend afternoon to take care of a dinner the next week.
- *If purchasing frozen entrees, look for those lower in sodium and check the price per ounce:* For a quick dinner, supplement this purchase with a fresh or frozen vegetable or salad.
- *Get friendly with vegetables:* When fresh vegetables are out of season and costly, or when time is short, frozen vegetables that are partially processed are a good option for adding color, texture, and nutrients to your meal; add some cut-up broccoli or carrots to traditional casseroles; avoid frozen vegetables with added sauces high in sodium and fat.

If you have not been cooking, then start by preparing just one or two meals a week. See how fast you develop your cooking skills and perfect some favorite recipes!

References

1. Larson NI, Nelson MC, Neumark-Sztainer D, et al: Making time for meals: meal structure and associations with dietary intake in young adults. *J Am Diet Assoc* 109:72, 2009.
2. Escoto KH, Laska MN, Larson N, et al: Work hours and perceived time barriers to healthful eating among young adults. *Am J Health Behav* 36(6):78, 2012.

of consumers don't pay attention to refined carbohydrates when purchasing food or beverages.[10] Although shoppers are very positive about food items with added benefits for health—for instance, calcium and vitamin D—awareness does not necessarily lead to behavior change. Over 90% of consumers were aware of the association between calcium and bone health, but only 58% were making an effort to consume more calcium.[24]

EXPANDING THE FOOD SUPPLY: BIOTECHNOLOGY AND THE CONSUMER

Throughout human history, new scientific discoveries have created challenges for society. Biotechnology as it relates to agriculture, food processing, and the environment holds the potential to increase the quantity and quality of our food supply. This field of science allows us to alter the deoxyribonucleic acid (DNA) of a plant or animal species by adding or removing a particular gene, likened to cutting a circle of tape, inserting a different piece, and rejoining both ends to the new piece.[25] This was the technique used to develop a new variety of rice with increased β-carotene content,[25] and new microorganisms for use in the making of cheese.[26] However, there are questions about the safety of the food produced using these methods. We will examine some of these issues and the process for biosafety review.

Genetically Modified Plants

Genetically modified (GM) organisms are plants or bacteria in which the natural DNA has been changed in some way to produce a desired trait. Genetic modification can take place through plant breeding methods or through biotechnology in which a gene is transferred from one organism to another. Genetic engineering was first applied in the pharmaceutical industry, and GM bacteria produce human insulin for managing diabetes.

GM food crops were introduced in the 1990s, and their use has grown dramatically. Farmers in at least 25 countries are planting GM species,[26] representing 51% of the soybeans, 31% of the maize, and 5% of the rapeseed (canola oil) produced worldwide.[27] In the United States, the sale and use of GM seeds are regulated by the Food and Drug Administration (FDA), the Environmental Protection Agency (EPA), and the USDA.

Goals for Genetic Modification

Since humans first began to cultivate plants, various practices have been used to improve the yield or desirability of particular species. The use of Mendel's principles of inheritance and the development of hybrid plants led to the green revolution and new varieties of wheat and rice with double the yields. Such advances were credited with reducing food shortages in the developing world.[28]

Genetic modification of food plants has three goals[28]:

1. *Resistance to insects and disease:* Plants carrying a protein that acts as a built-in insecticide enable farmers to reduce their use of pesticides and herbicides.
2. *Increased tolerance to weather conditions:* Varieties able to survive more extreme environmental conditions are less likely to be destroyed by a late frost.
3. *Increased nutritional value:* Genetic modification increased the monounsaturated fatty acid content of soybean oil, and scientists are working on a tomato with increased amounts of lycopene. Grains with increased protein or micronutrients lessen nutrient deficiencies in developing nations.

Corn, soybeans, rapeseed (canola oil), papaya, and squash are among the genetically altered food crops approved for use in the United States.[26]

Safety of Genetically Modified Crops

Both scientists and consumers have voiced concerns about GM foods as follows:

- *Risk of allergic reaction:* Transfer of a known allergen into a new food (e.g., adding a peanut allergen to a corn plant) would make the modified plant unsafe for persons with the allergy.[26]
- *Potential toxicity:* Need to check DNA against a protein database to identify any known harmful protein.[29]
- *Danger to the environment*[26]: Transfer of insect-resistant genes to weeds or invasive plants could be harmful to helpful insects such as butterflies. Farmers are urged to confine GM plants to specific growing areas.

Current labeling regulations do not require the identification of ingredients from GM sources *unless* the modification has increased its allergenicity or reduced its nutrient content.[30] This situation is controversial as many consumers wish to avoid eating GM foods. A requirement that a GM food carry label identification would provide the information needed for making an informed decision.

Biotechnology and Animal Foods
Marker-Assisted Breeding

Conventional breeding methods have produced eggs with less cholesterol and beef with reduced fat. Marker-assisted breeding, which combines the skills of classic breeders with molecular geneticists, offers increased potential for the development of healthy animal foods. When geneticists identify existing DNA patterns that influence traits such as fat composition, breeders can better select for these characteristics.

Bovine Growth Hormone

Growth hormone has an essential role in growth, development, and health. Bovine growth hormone (BGH) extracted from the pituitary glands of cattle has long been used to boost milk production. When it became possible to synthesize bovine somatotropin (bST) using recombinant DNA, farmers petitioned the FDA for permission to use recombinant bovine somatotropin (rbST) in their dairy herds.[31] Following intense review this practice was approved. Evaluation of milk samples from retail stores in 48 states indicated that milk from rbST-treated cows did not differ in bST content from milk obtained from nontreated cows.[32] Nevertheless, many consumers choose to avoid purchasing milk from rbST-treated cows.

When assessing risk, answers are seldom clear-cut; no action or lack of action by either a government agency or an individual is ever completely risk-free. Risk is evaluated according to potential benefits versus potential harm and usually involves numerous and often subtle variables. Available research evidence must form the basis for judgments that serve the public interest.

PROTECTING THE FOOD SUPPLY: REGULATION AND INFORMATION

Government Agencies Responsible for Food Safety
A Shared Regulatory System: USDA and FDA

Regulation of the food supply began more than 100 years ago when Congress charged the USDA with safeguarding the nation's food. Early on, USDA initiated on-site inspection of meatpacking and poultry-processing plants, an enormous job that continues today. The FDA was assigned responsibility for the safety of all foods except meat and poultry. These two agencies work with the EPA to ensure that pesticide residues do not exceed tolerance standards. Interagency cooperation is essential for mounting an effective response to any food-related threat to health. The USDA, FDA, and the Centers for Disease Control and Prevention (CDC) work together to prevent the introduction and spread of such hazards as avian flu or investigate and recall products associated with outbreaks of foodborne illness.

Food and Drug Administration

The FDA enforces all federal regulations intended to keep our food supply safe, pure, and wholesome (Box 9-3).[33] Included in this mandate is the power to seize contaminated and unsafe food, whether grown and processed in the United States or entering from elsewhere. Because it is impossible to inspect all food products before they are sold, the FDA has put in place risk assessment procedures in food manufacturing facilities to prevent contamination. These procedures, referred to as *Hazard Analysis and Critical Control Points* (HACCP), identify potential sources of contamination and help food plant managers set up ways to control them. HACCP requires systematic testing for the presence of dangerous microbes at production points where they might enter the system. The joint efforts of the FDA and USDA to implement HACCP procedures in poultry processing are credited with reducing by half the number of chickens contaminated with *Salmonella*. The FDA also monitors any suspicious behaviors that might be related to intentional food contamination and food bioterrorism.

Food Safety Laws
Approval Process for Drugs

The control of drugs by the FDA began in 1938 with the passage of the Federal Food, Drug, and Cosmetic Act (FFDCA). Any new drug, whether developed in the United States or elsewhere, must undergo intensive testing, often extending over a period of years. The manufacturer must present convincing scientific evidence that the product meets the legal standard of "safe and effective," and formal FDA approval is necessary before the drug can be sold.

Regulation of Food Ingredients and Food Additives

Manufacturers of all foods and food additives are legally obligated to assure the public that their products are safe. For conventional foods the FFDCA requires that the food and all ingredients not be "ordinarily injurious." Ingredients with a long history of use are assumed safe, and such food items may be marketed without prior FDA approval. Cookies made with flour, brown sugar, eggs, butter, and baking soda would meet this standard.

In 1960 the FFDCA was expanded to create two legal classes of food additives as described below:

1. *Generally recognized as safe (GRAS):* The GRAS list includes all food additives and ingredients that were marketed before 1958. The GRAS list includes thousands of additives. One example is the yellow coloring added to margarine that has been in use since the 1930s. Under the law a food is unsafe if an additive "may render injurious" the food product. Food processors are not required to obtain FDA approval to use GRAS list additives; however, the presumed safety of these additives was based on their wide prior use; most were not tested. In 1977 Congress directed the FDA to begin testing the additives on the list, and this is continuing.

2. *Food additives developed since 1958:* For these additives the same legal standard of "may render injurious" applies, but they must undergo rigid testing before approval is obtained. Splenda® (sucralose), a nonnutritive sweetener described in Chapter 3, went through the FDA approval process and is now being sold.

Dietary Supplements

Dietary supplements enjoy a very favorable legal status. In 1994 Congress passed the Dietary Supplement Health and Education Act (DSHEA), which effectively deregulated the dietary supplement industry.[34,35] All substances marketed as supplements prior to 1994 were assumed to be safe, whether or not research evidence existed to support this claim. The dietary supplement industry markets thousands of products containing vitamins, minerals, herbs, botanical compounds, Asian medicinal herbals, and related substances. Under the law these supplements are classified as neither foods nor drugs. No scientific testing that demonstrates either product safety or effectiveness is required. For supplement ingredients developed after 1994, the safety standard is simply that there be no "unreasonable risk." The manufacturer must notify the FDA before marketing such a product, but no prior approval is required.

The DSHEA is a controversial law. Dietary supplements are a major industry, with large advertising budgets and a wide range of products, from single vitamins to complex mixtures. Although a dietary supplement cannot claim to cure a disease, statements about how the human body will respond to the supplement, such as a claim that it will make you burn away unwanted fat, require no substantiating evidence. Supplements containing growth hormone or other potentially dangerous substances said to restore youthful vitality are often marketed to older adults. Steps are urgently needed to ensure consumer safety and honest claims describing appropriate use, expected effects, recommended dose, and potential interactions among drugs, herbs, and nutrients. (See later section on combating food and drug misinformation.)

Agricultural Chemicals

Agricultural chemicals control destructive insects and weeds, improve seed sprouting to increase yield, prevent plant diseases, and improve market quality. However, overuse adds to food pesticide residues and farm workers' exposure to such chemicals. Researchers are helping farmers reduce their use of chemical pesticides through integrated pest management, which uses the natural enemies of insect pests to decrease their population. The FDA has the task of assessing health risks and establishing guidelines for the thousands of agricultural chemicals in development and use.

Organic farming—which bars the use of chemical pesticides and herbicides—is growing in status as consumers become more concerned about the conditions surrounding the production of their food. Over a 10-year period, sales of organic foods grew from $3.6 billion to $21.1 billion.[36] Organic foods are now available in most major supermarkets.

Organic farmers working with soil scientists are developing sustainable systems for growing plant foods and raising beef and poultry. National standards that govern growing procedures and postharvest handling have been established for producers who wish to label their food as "organic." The USDA must certify farmers before they can use the seal of the National Organic Program (Figure 9-2).[37]

Water Contamination

Indiscriminate dumping of waste has raised the concentrations of polychlorinated biphenyls (PCBs), heavy metals such as mercury, and other toxic substances in inland and ocean waters. These pollutants are transferred to fish, shellfish, and other wildlife living in or drinking these waters, and then to the humans who eat them. State and local health departments post advisories to fishermen regarding the safety of fish caught in local waters, and the FDA monitors the mercury content of ocean and farm-raised fish sold in the United States. Although fish is valued for the protein and omega-3 fatty acids it contains, women who are pregnant or nursing or who may become pregnant should monitor their intake and choose fish low in mercury (Box 9-4).[38] This FDA advisory relating to the developing fetus or infant also applies to young children based on the damaging effect of mercury on the developing nervous system.

Government Agencies Responsible for Food Education

Just as several federal agencies share responsibility for food safety, so several groups partner to provide food and health information to the public. The U.S. Department of Health and Human Services (USDHHS) is the major source of health information. The USDA focuses on food and diet

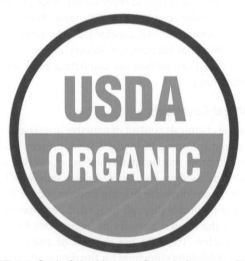

FIGURE 9-2 Seal of the National Organic Program. The U.S. Department of Agriculture (USDA) has developed a certification program to enable organic farmers to label their produce as *organically grown.* (From National Organic Program, Agricultural Marketing Service, U.S. Department of Agriculture: *The organic seal,* Washington, D.C., 2012, U.S. Department of Agriculture. Available at: <www.ams.usda.gov/AMSv1.0/nop>.)

with responsibility for the *Dietary Guidelines for Americans* and MyPlate (choosemyplate.gov). The FDA oversees consumer food and drug education and reviews food labels, food health claims, and false advertising.

Food Labels

To choose food wisely, consumers must know what nutrients they need, the amounts, and where to find them. Over the past 30 years, the FDA, with the advice of experts representing agriculture, foods, nutrition, and health, developed a framework of food labeling to help individuals monitor their nutrient intake.

Early Efforts at Food Labeling

In the mid-1970s, new requirements were set for the food label. All cans and packages had to provide content information including weight, list of ingredients, and the name and address of the manufacturer (Figure 9-3). The goal at that time was to protect consumers from economic risk—giving true information about food weight and ingredients—not health risk. However, surveys indicated that consumers wanted more nutrition information, including amounts of carbohydrate, fat, and protein, total number of kcalories, and key vitamins and minerals.

Original Nutrition Facts Label

The original nutrition facts label became law under the Nutrition Labeling and Education Act of 1990 and has been in use since 1994 (Figure 9-4). This label has been required on all prepared or processed foods such as bread, cereal,

---

BOX 9-4   MERCURY CONTENT OF FISH

Fish Lower in Mercury
- Canned light tuna (albacore or white tuna is higher in mercury than light tuna)
- Pollock
- Salmon
- Catfish
- Shrimp

Fish Higher in Mercury
- Shark
- Swordfish
- King mackerel
- Tilefish

Data from U.S. Food and Drug Administration and U.S. *Environmental Protection Agency: What you need to know about mercury in fish and shellfish: advice for women who might become pregnant, women who are pregnant, nursing mothers, young children,* EPA-823-R-04-005, Washington, D.C., 2004, U.S. Department of Health and Human Services. from: <http://www.fda.gov/Food/FoodborneIllnessContaminants/BuyStoreServeSafeFood/ucm110591.htm>. Retrieved February 26, 2013.
NOTE: Women who are pregnant or nursing or might become pregnant should eat no more than two meals or 12 oz a week of low-mercury fish; these recommendations also apply to young children (but serve smaller portions). Fish sticks and fish sandwiches served at fast-food restaurants are generally made from fish low in mercury.

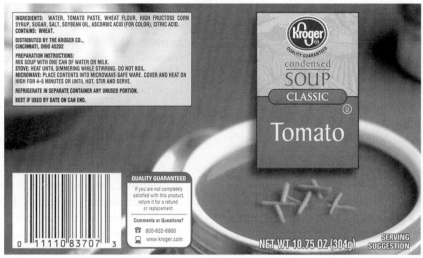

FIGURE 9-3 Example of a food label. Notice that this label also informs the consumer that the product contains wheat—one of eight food allergens that must be clearly stated to protect individuals having this allergy. (Courtesy The Kroger Company, Cincinnati, Ohio.)

Original vs. Proposed

Nutrition Facts	
Serving Size: 1/2 cup (114 g)	
Servings Per Container: 4	
Amount per Serving	
Calories 260	
Calories from Fat 120	
	% Daily Value*
Total Fat 13 g	20%
Saturated Fat 5 g	25%
Trans Fat 0 g	
Cholesterol 30 mg	10%
Sodium 660 mg	28%
Total Carbohydrate 31 g	11%
Dietary Fiber 0 g	0%
Sugars 5 g	
Protein 5 g	
Vitamin A 4% • Vitamin C 1%	
Calcium 15% • Iron 4%	

*Percents (%) of a Daily Value are based on a 2,000 calorie diet. Your Daily Values may vary higher or lower depending on your calorie needs.

Nutrient	2,000 calories	2,500 calories
Total Fat	<65 g	<80 g
Saturated Fat	<20 g	<25 g
Cholesterol	<300 mg	<300 mg
Sodium	<2,400 mg	<2,400 mg
Total Carbohydrate	300 g	375 g
Dietary Fiber	25 g	30 g

1 g Fat = 9 calories
1 g Carbohydrate = 4 calories
1 g Protein = 4 calories

Nutrition Facts	
8 servings per container	
Serving size	2/3 cup (55g)
Amount per 2/3 cup	
Calories	**230**
% Daily Value*	
QUICK FACTS:	
12%	**Total Fat** 8g
12%	**Total Carbs** 37g
	Sugars 1g
	Protein 3g
AVOID TOO MUCH:	
5%	Saturated Fat 1g
	Trans Fat 0g
0%	**Cholesterol** 0mg
7%	**Sodium** 160mg
	Added Sugars 0g
GET ENOUGH:	
14%	Fiber 4g
10%	Vitamin D 2mcg
20%	Calcium 260mg
45%	Iron 8mg
5%	Potassium 235mg

* Footnote on Daily Values (DV) and calorie reference to be inserted here.

FIGURE 9-4 The original Nutrition Facts label as compared with the proposed Nutrition Facts label. The proposed Nutrition Facts label reflects new dietary recommendations and draws attention to calories, portion size, and nutrients lacking in the U.S. diet. (From U.S. Food and Drug Administration [FDA], Silver Spring, Md. Available at: <http://www.fda.gov/Food/GuidanceRegulation/GuidanceDocumentsRegulatoryInformation/LabelingNutrition/ucm385663.htm#images>.)

canned and frozen food, snacks, desserts, and beverages, but it is voluntary for fresh fruits, fresh vegetables, and seafood. The original nutrition facts label describes the serving size and nutrient content as compared with recommended intakes of those nutrients. Health claims on the food label (approved by the FDA) help consumers make choices to lower their risk

of chronic disease. The USDA, rather than the FDA, controls labeling on fresh meat, poultry, and dairy foods.

The nutrition facts label enables consumers to compare the nutritional value of one product with another and make informed choices. The information on the original nutrition facts label is described below[39]:

- *Food amount and energy content:* Food amount is described by weight, serving size, and number of servings in the package or container.
- *Macronutrient content:* Protein, carbohydrate, and fat are listed in grams. Individual amounts of saturated fat, *trans* fat, and cholesterol are also required, and some processors have voluntarily added monounsaturated and polyunsaturated fats. Total carbohydrate is broken down into dietary fiber and sugar. Suggested daily intakes are compared with reference diets of 2000 or 2500 kcal.
- *Vitamin and mineral content:* Sodium and four leader nutrients—vitamin A, vitamin C, calcium, and iron—are required on the original nutrition label. Sodium is listed in milligrams and as a percentage of the suggested upper limit of 2400 mg, the recognized goal at that time. Vitamins and minerals appear as percentages of the Daily Reference Value (DV). The DVs were derived from the1968 edition of the Recommended Dietary Allowances (RDAs), the standards in general use when the original nutrition label was being developed. The DV represented the highest RDA for that nutrient among the various age and gender groups. For example, the DV for iron is 18 mg, the RDA for women of childbearing age. Fortified foods such as cereals also list other vitamins and minerals added in the manufacturing process.

Proposed Changes in the Nutrition Facts Label

Since the original nutrition facts label was introduced in 1994, there have been changes in our knowledge of nutrition science and the food patterns and health of the American people. The prevalence of obesity has escalated across all age groups, and foods high in energy value and added sugars but low in nutrient density constitute a growing proportion of the American diet. Portion sizes have increased such that the reference servings used in the development of the original nutrition label no longer represent what individuals actually eat. The proposed nutrition facts label addresses these issues as described further on. (The original and proposed nutrition facts labels are compared in Figure 9-4).[40]

Label Changes Based on New Nutrition Science

- *Added sugars.* The 2010 Dietary Guidelines for Americans recommended that consumers limit their intakes of added sugars, and the meal plans provided on MyPlate (choosemyplate.gov) include an upper limit to intake of added sugars. The original nutrition label indicates the total amount of sugar in a food but does not indicate what portion is naturally occurring sugar and what portion is added sugars. The proposed label provides consumers with the amount of added sugar and the total sugar (naturally occurring sugar plus added sugar) in the food.
- *Fats.* The proposed food label will continue to note the amounts of total fat, saturated fat, and *trans* fats in a food, but it will not list the total calories coming from fat. Current research suggests that the type of fat in the diet is more important to health than the number of calories obtained from fat.

- *Specific nutrients.* The original nutrition label drew attention to calcium, iron, vitamin A, and vitamin C, problem nutrients at that time. Recent U.S. dietary surveys have revealed that many population groups are deficient in calcium, iron, vitamin D, and potassium, nutrients with important roles in the prevention of chronic disease, and these nutrients will be mandatory on the proposed label. Vitamin A and vitamin C intakes are generally adequate in most U.S. population groups and will no longer be mandatory, although they may be added.
- *Daily Reference Value (DV).* The DV serves two purposes: it establishes a maximum intake for a nutrient such as fat, and it indicates the percentage of the daily requirement of a nutrient, such as calcium, that is provided in a serving. The DVs for several nutrients, including sodium and calcium, are being revised to agree with current Dietary Reference Intakes (DRIs). The maximum intake for sodium will be lowered from 2400 mg to 2300 mg, and the DV for calcium will increase from 1000 mg to 1300 mg.

Label Changes Pertaining to Serving Sizes and Labeling Requirements

- *Reference servings.* The size of food portions consumed by the U.S. population has increased greatly over the past 20 years, and so have the calories and nutrients that go with them (review Figure 1-2). By law reference servings used on nutrition labels must reflect what individuals actually eat, not what dietitians recommend they eat; thus 27 of the 158 reference servings used in labeling will be adjusted to accommodate current eating patterns. Several new reference servings will be developed for use with new foods.
- *Number of servings in a package.* The size and number of servings contained in a package as stated on the original nutrition label were often misunderstood. A food package perceived by the general public to contain a 1-cup single serving that was typically eaten in one sitting could be labeled as containing two, ½ cup servings; consequently the portion actually consumed contained twice the calories expected. The proposed nutrition label will require that packages containing between 150% and 200% of the reference serving, such as a 20-ounce can of soda or a 15-ounce can of soup, must be labeled as containing one serving. Packages containing at least 200% but less than or equal to 400% of the reference serving will require dual labeling, listing information per serving and per package. (See Figure 9-5 describing this concept.)

Refreshed Design

- Information important to health will receive new emphasis. Calorie content and the number of servings per container will be highlighted and printed in bold. The specific amount of a nutrient will be included in addition to the %DV. This could be helpful to individuals requiring lesser amounts of that nutrient, such as men whose iron DRI is only 8 mg, when compared with women of childbearing age, who require 18 mg. The "Amount per Serving" section has been replaced with "Amount per _____," with the blank providing the household measure as, for example, the Amount per Cup. "Total Carbohydrate" has been replaced by "Total Carbs," followed by "Added Sugars." The existing footnote on the original nutrition label that related the %DV to a standard diet containing 2000 or 2500 calories will be replaced with an explanation of the %DV, a concept that is confusing to many consumers.[40] (Compare the original and proposed nutrition facts label in Figure 9-4.)

• The proposed changes to the nutrition facts label were published in the Federal Register, with 90 days allowed for public comment from consumers, food and health professionals, and food manufacturers. When all comments have been read and considered, FDA will release a final rule. Then food manufacturers will have 2 years to implement the required changes.

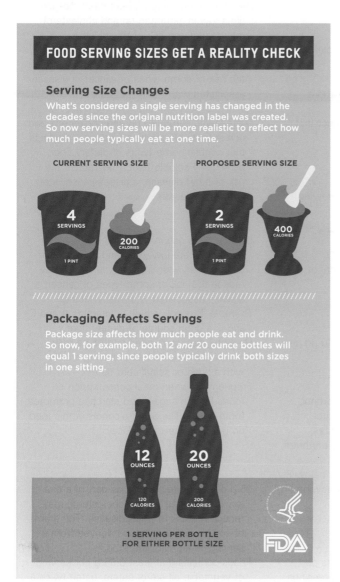

FIGURE 9-5 Serving size changes in the proposed Nutrition Facts label. These changes in serving sizes will more closely reflect the amount of food that people actually eat at one time. (From U.S. Food and Drug Administration [FDA], Silver Spring, Md. Available at: <http://www.fda.gov/Food/Guidance Regulation/GuidanceDocumentsRegulatoryInformation/ LabelingNutrition/ucm385663.htm#images>.)

Nutrition Labeling for Special Conditions

Since the development and implementation of the original nutrition facts label, additional information has been added to the label to assist consumers with special needs or interests, as described below:

• *Health claims:* Health claims are label statements that imply a relationship between the consumption of a nutrient or food substance and a disease or health-related condition; however, there can be no suggestion that the nutrient or substance will cure or mitigate the condition.[39] Based on scientific evidence presented for review, the FDA has approved 15 health claims that address such relationships as calcium, vitamin D, and bone health; soluble fiber and heart health; and folate and neural tube defects (Table 9-1).[41]

• *Labels for special needs:* Some nutrition labels include information for the benefit of certain groups. Animal foods processed under the supervision of a rabbi and meet Jewish dietary standards are labeled as *kosher*.

• *Presence of particular substances*: Foods or beverages containing aspartame must include a warning for the safety of individuals with phenylketonuria who must avoid the amino acid phenylalanine found in this nonnutritive sweetener. The Food Allergen Labeling and Consumer Protection Act requires that foods containing any amount of a major allergen known to cause anaphylactic shock in allergic individuals must be so labeled. These eight allergens are (1) milk (casein), (2) peanuts, (3) tree nuts, (4) fish, (5) shellfish, (6) wheat, (7) eggs, and (8) soybeans.[39] Casein, eggs, wheat flour, and soy are sometimes added in very small amounts to product formulations to provide texture or stability, and would not be apparent to the general consumer if not included on the label. In light of the very minute amounts of these substances that can have lethal consequences in allergic individuals, a label warning must be included. Figure 9-3 provides such an example, as one might not expect to find a wheat ingredient in tomato soup. With sweet baked items it is common to see the notation "this product was produced in a plant that also processes peanuts." It is estimated that 1 in 133 persons in the United States has celiac disease, an immune disorder characterized by a response to

KEY TERMS
anaphylactic shock A serious and sometimes fatal hypersensitivity reaction to a drug, food, toxin, chemical, or other allergen; the patient experiences weakness, sweating, and shortness of breath or such life-threatening responses as loss of blood pressure and shock, respiratory congestion, or cardiac arrest (see *allergens* below).
allergens Substances that cause a hypersensitivity reaction in the body; proteins found in milk, eggs, fish, shellfish, wheat, tree nuts (such as almonds or walnuts), peanuts, and soy can produce serious and sometimes fatal reactions in allergic individuals. The presence of these foods must be indicated on the food label.

TABLE 9-1   HEALTH CLAIMS APPROVED BY THE U.S. FOOD AND DRUG ADMINISTRATION FOR NUTRITION LABELS

CLAIM	FOOD REQUIREMENT	MODEL STATEMENT
Calcium and osteoporosis	High in calcium*	Regular exercise and a healthy diet with enough calcium helps teens and young adult white and Asian women maintain good bone health and may reduce their high risk of osteoporosis later in life.
Sodium and hypertension	Low in sodium	Diets low in sodium may reduce the risk of high blood pressure, a disease associated with many factors.
Dietary fat and cancer	Low fat	Development of cancer depends on many factors. A diet low in total fat may reduce the risk of some cancers.
Dietary saturated fat and cholesterol and risk of coronary heart disease	Low saturated fat Low cholesterol Low fat	Although many factors affect heart disease, diets low in saturated fat and cholesterol may reduce the risk of this disease.
Fiber-containing grain products, fruits, and vegetables, and cancer	A grain product, fruit, or vegetable that contains dietary fiber Low fat Good source of dietary fiber without fortification	Low-fat diets rich in fiber-containing grain products, fruits, and vegetables may reduce the risk of some types of cancer, a disease associated with many factors.
Fruits, vegetables, and grain products that contain fiber, particularly soluble fiber, and risk of coronary heart disease	A fruit, vegetable, or grain product that contains fiber Low saturated fat Low cholesterol Low fat At least 0.6 g soluble fiber per serving (without fortification) Soluble fiber content provided on label	Diets low in saturated fat and cholesterol and rich in fruits, vegetables, and grain products that contain some types of dietary fiber, particularly soluble fiber, may reduce the risk of heart disease, a disease associated with many factors.
Fruits and vegetables and cancer	A fruit or vegetable Low fat Food source (without fortification) of at least one of the following: Vitamin A Vitamin C Dietary fiber	Low-fat diets rich in fruits and vegetables (foods that are low in fat and may contain dietary fiber, vitamin A, or vitamin C) may reduce the risk of some types of cancer, a disease associated with many factors. *Example:* Broccoli is high in vitamins A and C and is a good source of dietary fiber.
Folate and neural tube defects	Good source of folate (at least 40 µg per serving)	Healthful diets with adequate folate may reduce a woman's risk of having a child with a brain or spinal cord defect.
Dietary sugar alcohols and dental caries	Sugar-free Sugar alcohol must be xylitol, sorbitol, mannitol, maltitol, isomalt, lactitol, hydrogenated starch hydrolysates, hydrogenated glucose syrups, erythritol, or a combination Food must not lower plaque pH below 5.7	Frequent between-meal consumption of foods high in sugars and starches promotes tooth decay. The sugar alcohols in this food do not promote tooth decay.
Soy protein and risk of coronary heart disease	At least 6.25 g soy protein per serving Low saturated fat Low cholesterol Low fat	25 g of soy protein a day, as part of a diet low in saturated fat and cholesterol, may reduce the risk of heart disease. The grams of soy protein that can be derived from a serving varies with the food.[†]
Plant sterol/stanol esters and risk of coronary heart disease	At least 0.65 g plant sterol esters per serving of spreads and salad dressings *Or* At least 1.7 g plant stanol esters per serving of spreads or salad dressings Low saturated fat Low cholesterol	Foods containing at least 0.65 g per serving of vegetable oil sterol esters, eaten twice a day with meals for a daily total intake of at least 1.3 g, as part of a diet low in saturated fat and cholesterol, may reduce the risk of heart disease. The grams of vegetable oil sterol esters that can be derived from a serving varies with the food.[†]

TABLE 9-1	HEALTH CLAIMS APPROVED BY THE U.S. FOOD AND DRUG ADMINISTRATION FOR NUTRITION LABELS—cont'd		
CLAIM	**FOOD REQUIREMENT**	**MODEL STATEMENT**	
Monounsaturated fat from olive oil and coronary heart disease	Must contain monounsaturated fat	Eating about 2 tablespoons of olive oil daily may reduce the risk of coronary heart disease due to the monounsaturated fat in olive oil. To achieve this benefit, olive oil should replace a similar amount of saturated fat and not increase the total number of kcalories eaten in a day. The grams of olive oil that can be derived varies with the food.[†]	
Omega-3 (n-3) fatty acids and coronary heart disease	Must contain both EPA and DHA omega-3 (n-3) fatty acids	Eating EPA and DHA omega-3 (n-3) fatty acids may reduce the risk of coronary heart disease. The grams of EPA and DHA fatty acids that can be derived from 1 serving varies with the food.[†]	
Whole grain foods and risk of heart disease and certain cancers	Contains 51% or more whole grain ingredients by weight per serving Good fiber source Low fat	Diets rich in whole grain foods and other plant foods and low in total fat, saturated fat, and cholesterol may reduce the risk of heart disease and some cancers.	
Potassium and the risk of high blood pressure and stroke	Good source of potassium Low sodium Low total fat Low saturated fat Low cholesterol	Diets containing foods that are a good source of potassium and low in sodium may reduce the risk of high blood pressure and stroke.	

Modified from U.S. Food and Drug Administration: *Guidance for industry. A food labeling guide—Appendix C: Health claims*, Rockville, Md., 1994 (rev 1999, 2004, 2008, 2009), Author. Retrieved August 8, 2013 from: <http://www.fda.gov/Food/GuidanceRegulation/GuidanceDocumentsRegulatoryInformation/LabelingNutrition/ucm2006828.htm>.
EPA: Eicosapentaenoic acid; *DHA:* docosahexaenoic acid.
*Food contains, without fortification, at least 10% of the Daily Reference Value for the named vitamin, mineral, or fiber, and less than 13 g fat, 4 g saturated fat, 60 mg cholesterol, and 480 mg sodium per serving.
[†]Label will list the amount found in that particular food serving.

gluten, a protein found in wheat, rye, barley, and sometimes oats. To prevent resulting damage to the lining of the gastrointestinal tract, patients must follow a gluten-free diet. The FDA has defined standards for products carrying the label of "gluten-free" to help patients make informed choices.[42]

Public attention to the energy, fat, sodium, and cholesterol content of foods led to legal definitions for terms such as *low* or *reduced* to protect the public from inappropriate or misleading claims.[40] Nevertheless, confusion about serving sizes and differences between the DVs used on the nutrition label and the Dietary Reference Intakes (DRIs) create misperceptions for users.

Food and Botanicals

New foods and beverages with added herbs or stimulants are blurring the distinction between food and supplements. One product receiving increased scrutiny is "energy drinks" that contain high levels of caffeine and may include added B vitamins, taurine (an amino acid), and the botanicals ginseng, gingko, or milk thistle.[43,44] Energy drinks can be marketed as foods or supplements. Those sold as supplements fall under the 1994 DSHEA,[45] enabling manufacturers to bypass label disclosure of ingredients that appear on the GRAS list, such

as caffeine.[43-45] Energy drinks usually contain about 80 to 140 mg of caffeine per 8-oz serving, the equivalent of 5 oz of coffee or two cans of caffeinated soda[46]; however, some energy drinks contain as much as 500 mg of caffeine per can—the equivalent of about 14 cans of caffeinated soda. A safe intake of caffeine is estimated to be less than 500 mg per day, although individuals with heart disease or liver disease or who take medications that slow the metabolism of caffeine need to consider a lower intake.[43]

Energy drinks and alcohol are a particularly dangerous combination as the high caffeine content of the energy drink reduces the symptoms of intoxication, encouraging even greater alcohol consumption.[46] Excessive energy drink consumption has been related to caffeine-induced seizures,[47] cardiac arrhythmias, and death.[44] Energy drinks often contain as much as 37 g of sugar per 12-oz can; young men participating in a national survey added 477 kcal per week through use of energy drinks.[47]

THE PROBLEM OF MISINFORMATION: FOOD AND HEALTH

For centuries people have been concerned with the safety and wholesomeness of their food. Particular foods were believed to possess healing properties or, conversely, cause illness, and certain religious food laws are likely rooted in food safety. In the absence of formal health care, remedies prepared from local plants and herbs were used to cure ailments as much as possible. In today's world of electronic communication, the Internet, blogs, and other forms of messaging can be used to advertise foods, drugs, herbs, and other plant botanicals as preventives or cures for common conditions. Some unsubstantiated beliefs about food or plant remedies or bogus drugs are harmless, but others carry serious implications for health. False information may be embedded in folklore, built on half-truths, or stem from intentional deception. The FDA supports a vigorous campaign to prevent and prosecute false advertising for particular foods, supplements, or medicines.

False claims usually fall within one of the following categories:

1. The food or product will cure a specific disease or condition.
2. Certain food combinations have special therapeutic effects.
3. Only "natural" foods or plant remedies can meet body needs and prevent disease.

Misleading claims about the healing properties of certain foods or other substances delay appropriate health intervention with a worsening of the illness and possible death. Patients with difficult-to-treat conditions such as cancer, diabetes, or arthritis are especially vulnerable to fraudulent claims for medicines that promise immediate cures and relief from pain. Diagnostic tests sold online are often the products of illegal pharmaceutical operations and result in inaccurate findings that delay treatment or lead to expenditures for unneeded medications from the same online supplier. Products formulated under unsanitary conditions or that contain potentially harmful substances can lead to further illness and critical consequences. Misleading advertising has a high economic cost. As much as $25.2 billion per year is spent on dietary supplements,[48] and many are unnecessary or ineffective.

The FDA Division of Consumer Education conducts an active program of public education through its website. A checklist to assist consumers in separating legitimate products and health advice from those that are harmful and waste money is found in Box 9-5.

FOOD SAFETY AND FOOD PROCESSING

In Chapter 1 we introduced the topic of food safety and the need for vigilance in preparing and handling food. Here we look at the pathogens that cause foodborne illness and ways to prevent contamination on the journey from the farm to the market to the kitchen.

Foodborne Illness
Prevalence and Causes of Foodborne Illness
Many disease-producing microorganisms in our environment have the potential to contaminate our food and water,

| BOX 9-5 | CHECKLIST FOR SPOTTING A HEALTH SCAM |

- Promises a quick or painless cure
- Claims to be made from a special, secret, or ancient formula available from only one source
- Uses testimonials or undocumented case histories from satisfied patients
- Claims to be effective for a wide range of ailments
- Claims to cure a disease such as arthritis or cancer or diabetes that is not fully understood by physicians and medical scientists
- Requires advance payment and claims limited availability of the product

Modified from National Institute on Aging, U.S. Department of Health and Human Services: Age page: *Beware of health scams*, Washington, D.C., 2008, U.S. Department of Health and Human Services.

posing a serious threat to public health. New technologies ranging from refrigerated trucks to freeze-drying to food irradiation have brought major improvements in food handling and food safety, yet Americans are still vulnerable to foodborne pathogens. The distribution of food across continents by large corporations presents opportunities for organisms to enter the food chain and be spread regionally and globally. Fruits and vegetables are often eaten raw or unpeeled, without being washed. Families eat more precooked foods, seafood salads, and deli meats that are vulnerable to spoilage. Meals picked up at food outlets on the way home are kept warm for extended periods, in contrast to cooked meals eaten immediately after preparation. Those who eat at their desks or in their cars while traveling may not take time to wash their hands or use a hand sanitizer.

The CDC is responsible for tracking the incidence of foodborne illness and sharing their findings with other regulatory agencies in an effort to improve food production and handling methods. According to most recent estimates 1 in 6 Americans (or 48 million people) get sick; 128,000 are hospitalized; and 3000 die from foodborne illness each year.[49] A 1999 report estimated morbidity and mortality from foodborne illness as 325,000 hospitalizations and 5000 deaths; however, the more recent lower estimates of hospitalizations and deaths likely reflect differences in data collection procedures rather than actual decreases in incidence.[50,51] Estimating both the true incidence of foodborne illness and the food responsible is difficult. First, many people experiencing illness assume it is the "flu" or other temporary upset and do not seek medical care. Most of us eat various foods at a meal and may not be able to identify the particular cause of any subsequent distress.[49] The food or organism responsible is more likely to be identified if individuals receive medical treatment or if the outbreak involves an entire family or population group who consumed the same food.

Forms of Foodborne Illness
Food infection and food poisoning are two different forms of foodborne illness caused by microorganisms.

- *Bacterial food infection* occurs when individuals eat food contaminated with large colonies of bacteria.
- *Bacterial food poisoning* results from toxins produced by bacteria before the food was eaten.

Bacterial Food Infection. Six common pathogens cause food infection:

1. *Escherichia coli O157:H7:* Most classes of *E. coli* are benign, and some do nutritionally important work such as fermenting resistant starch. However, other strains such as *E. coli* O157:H7 produce toxins that produce severe illness. Found naturally in the intestines of animals and humans, *E. coli* O157:H7 has emerged as a major cause of both individual cases and more extensive outbreaks of inflammatory diarrhea with bloody stool and fever. Serious infections result in renal failure or death. *E. coli* O157:H7 is destroyed by heat, and most outbreaks arise from unpasteurized or undercooked food or contaminated water. Several outbreaks of *E. coli* O157:H7 infection included several deaths that resulted from drinking unpasteurized cider made from apples that had fallen to the ground, been contaminated with animal droppings, and not thoroughly washed. These events led to greater emphasis on the need for pasteurization of juices and beverages. A major outbreak occurred from beef contaminated in processing and then undercooked at a fast-food restaurant.[52] The restaurant incident reminds us that all parties across the food chain—those who process food *and* those who prepare it—are responsible for food safety. Ground beef must be cooked to a temperature of 165°F to safely destroy *E. coli*. *E. coli* is also found in salad greens, which reinforces the need to thoroughly wash these foods.

2. *Salmonella: Salmonella* grow quickly in high-protein foods such as milk, custard, egg dishes, and sandwich fillings. Seafood, especially shellfish such as oysters and clams harvested from polluted waters, are a source of infection. Contamination of eggs with *Salmonella enteritidis* is a worldwide problem. No one should eat raw cookie dough, drink unpasteurized beverages containing milk or egg, or eat undercooked eggs, but these rules are especially important for older adults or others with impaired immune function. Forty percent of deaths from *Salmonella* occur in people over age 65.[53] Symptoms develop slowly, usually 12 to 24 hours after ingestion, with mild to bloody diarrhea with fever.

3. *Campylobacter: Campylobacter* is a cause of acute diarrhea in the United States and around the world. This pathogen is found in raw and undercooked beef, poultry, and seafood; raw milk; and untreated water. It is destroyed by heating food to 160°F or applying appropriate water purification methods. Cross-contamination such as using a cutting board for raw poultry and then using it to chop lettuce without appropriate cleaning is a major cause.[52] *Campylobacter* infection has been associated with Guillain-Barré syndrome and other neuropathies that occur months or years following infection.[54]

4. *Shigella:* First discovered as the cause of a dysentery epidemic in Japan, *Shigella* infection is usually confined to the large intestine and varies from simple cramps and diarrhea to fatal dysentery. Young children are at particular risk of fatal complications, and treatment with antibiotics may be required. *Shigella* are found in the intestinal tract of animals and in contaminated water. They are spread by insects and unsanitary food handling and grow rapidly in moist or protein foods such as milk, beans, tuna, and turkey. Apple cider or raw fruits and vegetables contaminated by animal droppings are sources of *Shigella*. Foods must be washed and cooked thoroughly and chilled quickly to prevent infection.

5. *Listeria:* This microorganism is a major cause of infection after surgery, but only recently was *Listeria monocytogenes* linked with foodborne illness. In older adults, pregnant women, infants, or those with suppressed immune systems, this organism produces diarrhea and flulike fever and headache. Related complications include pneumonia, sepsis, meningitis, endocarditis, and miscarriage. Outbreaks of *Listeria*-related illness have been traced to unpasteurized dairy products, particularly soft Mexican cheeses made with unpasteurized milk. Undercooked poultry and deli foods have been implicated in *Listeria* infections.[55] Pregnant women are advised to heat to steaming all luncheon meats and processed meats to avoid exposure to *Listeria* organisms. Thorough cooking and careful washing of raw fruits and vegetables are preventive measures (see the Focus on Food Safety box, "Do I Really Need to Wash That Melon?").

🎯 FOCUS ON FOOD SAFETY

Do I Really Need to Wash That Melon?

Unwashed or poorly washed vegetables and fruits are common sources of foodborne illness. Produce can become contaminated with *Escherichia coli* O157:H7, *Salmonella,* or *Cyclospora* through contact with animals, fertilizers containing animal waste, contaminated irrigation water, or poor sanitation practices of workers who pick or sort these crops.

Following are safety tips for washing fresh fruits and vegetables:

- *Rinse raw produce under running water,* even if you are not going to eat the skin or rind. Any bacteria on the outer surface will be transferred to your hands or to the knife as you peel or cut and then to the food itself. Rub firm-skinned fruits and vegetables or scrub with a small vegetable brush to remove surface dirt.
- *Remove and discard the outermost leaves* of a head of lettuce or cabbage. Wash each lettuce leaf under running water. Scrub melons thoroughly. Do not dip the entire head of lettuce or melon in a container of water. You may be rinsing in contaminated water.
- *Store fruits and vegetables in the refrigerator within 2 hours of peeling or cutting.* Be especially careful with cut melon. Melons are low in acid as compared with oranges, apples, or pineapple, and this allows more rapid growth of bacteria on cut surfaces when the melon stands at room temperature.

6. *Vibrio:* This family of bacteria includes *V. cholerae,* the pathogen causing cholera. The species generally associated with outbreaks of foodborne illness in the United States is *V. parahaemolyticus,* found in coastal waters. This is a salt-requiring organism and increases in number in warm weather. Persons who eat raw or undercooked fish, oysters, clams, or other shellfish are at high risk. *V. parahaemolyticus* causes a watery diarrhea with abdominal cramps, vomiting, fever, and chills that usually last no more than 3 days. Many incidents go unreported, although it is estimated that at least 1400 cases occur each year.[56] Individuals with compromised immune systems, liver disease, or alcoholism can have serious complications and require medical attention.[56]

Bacterial Food Poisoning. Foodborne illness caused by toxins already present in the food when it is eaten develops rapidly, with symptoms appearing within 1 to 6 hours after eating. The two most common types of bacterial food poisoning are caused by *Staphylococcus* and *Clostridia* species:

1. *Staphylococcal food poisoning: Staphylococcus aureus,* involved in various illnesses such as toxic shock syndrome, is a common cause of food poisoning that affects an estimated 185,000 individuals annually.[57] Symptoms come on suddenly and include severe cramping and abdominal pain with vomiting and diarrhea, along with sweating, headache, and fever. In some cases, shock and **prostration** occur. Recovery is fairly rapid, usually within a day, but depends on the amount of toxin ingested and the general health of the victim.[57] A common source of contamination is an infection on the hand of a food worker, often minor or unnoticed. This bacterium grows rapidly in custard- and cream-filled bakery goods, chicken and ham salads, egg products, and processed meat, cheese, and sauces—all moist foods with a high protein content. There is no change in odor, taste, or appearance of the food, so the consumer has no warning.

2. *Clostridial food poisoning: Clostridium perfringens* spores are in soil, water, dust, and refuse—virtually everywhere. It multiplies in cooked meat and meat dishes and develops its toxin in foods held for extended times after cooking. Outbreaks occur in food service facilities that hold foods for long periods at warming or room temperatures. Prevention rests with thorough cooking, prompt serving after cooking, and immediate refrigeration thereafter.

The toxins produced by another *Clostridium, C. botulinum,* cause more serious and often-fatal food poisoning. Depending on the amount of toxin consumed and the individual response, death ensues within 24 hours. The *botulinum* neurotoxin is the most potent substance known, and consuming only a few milligrams of a food that contains this poison can cause illness and death.[58] Initial complaints are vomiting, weakness, and dizziness. Progressively, the toxin irritates motor nerve cells and blocks transmission of neural impulses, causing gradual paralysis ending in respiratory paralysis. *C. botulinum* spores are found in soils throughout the world and carried on harvested food to the canning process. Like all clostridia, this species is anaerobic (i.e., it

develops in the absence of air). If spores are not completely destroyed in the canning process, this relatively air-free environment provides ideal conditions for toxin production. The commercial canning industry follows processing standards that eliminate the risk of botulism, but cases still result from foods canned at home using inappropriate methods. Boiling for 10 min destroys the toxin (although not the spore), so all home-canned food, no matter how well preserved, should be boiled at least 10 minutes before eating. Native Alaskan food practices involving uncooked or partially cooked meats have resulted in cases of botulism.[58] Table 9-2 summarizes bacterial sources of food contamination.

Viruses. Viruses from the Caliciviridae family, also known as noroviruses, are responsible for over half of all gastroenteritis cases in the United States. There is no vaccine to prevent infection and no drug to cure it.[59] Norovirus infection arises from contaminated fruits and vegetables that are not washed prior to eating, and raw or undercooked shellfish. However, these viruses are also spread via the fecal-oral route. Nursing homes are subject to outbreaks if health care workers disposing of vomitus, feces, or used bed linens or dishes touch food or serving dishes without washing their hands. In food service facilities, illness can spread from worker to worker and on to food. Vomiting and diarrhea resulting from norovirus contamination usually last no more than 1 to 2 days, but this illness and related dehydration can be serious in young children and older adults.

Vulnerability to Foodborne Illness

Foodborne illness has health and economic consequences. Microbial foodborne illness causes acute but self-limiting symptoms, and most people require only general supportive care. However, for young children; older adults; and immune-compromised patients with cancer, recent organ or bone marrow transplants, or autoimmune deficiency diseases, foodborne pathogens can lead to septicemia, acute renal failure, or death. In pregnant women, foodborne illness can result in miscarriage. Medical intervention and lost productivity have an annual cost of $23 billion.[60]

KEY TERMS

dysentery   A number of disorders marked by inflammation of the intestines, especially the colon, and accompanied by abdominal pain and frequent stools containing blood and mucus; it is caused by chemical irritants, bacteria, protozoa, or parasites.

sepsis   Presence of pathogenic microorganisms or their toxins in the blood or other tissues.

meningitis   Inflammation of the meninges, the three membranes that envelop the brain and spinal cord, caused by a bacterial or viral infection and leading to high fever, severe headache, and stiff neck or back muscles.

endocarditis   Inflammation of the endocardium, the serous membrane lining the cavities of the heart.

prostration   Extreme exhaustion.

The increasing use of foods often associated with foodborne illness points to the need for vigilance. In recent years, 46% of reported foodborne illness was attributed to plant foods with major emphasis on leafy vegetables.[61] Bacteria in the soil cling to growing plants and failure to properly wash fruits and vegetables prior to eating or processing transfer these pathogens to humans.[61] Poor sanitation on the part of farm workers or irrigation with polluted water elevates the risk from plant foods. Cheeses made with unpasteurized milk, raw milk as a beverage, or contamination of milk following pasteurization are responsible for 14% of reported foodborne illnesses. Raw or poorly cooked eggs and shellfish are each responsible for 6% of reported outbreaks.[60] Although bacterial contamination of raw poultry has been reduced with vigilance in processing,[62] thorough cooking is necessary. Ground meat, with its expanded surface area for contamination, must be cooked until it is no longer pink. See Figure 9-6 for guidance on appropriate cooking and holding temperatures for various foods. (Using the information you learned about the importance of family meals, the nutrition label, and food safety complete the Case Study box, "Planning the Family Dinner.")

Prevention of Foodborne Illness

Protecting food from bacterial contamination in the home or food service facility begins with appropriate storage. Covered containers or sealable plastic bags for dry, refrigerated, or freezer storage protect food from insects or unwanted contact with other raw foods. Opened packages of dry foods are best kept at the front of the shelf where they are visible and will be used first. Labels on highly perishable foods such as meat, poultry, and fish give directions for preventing spoilage and contamination (Figure 9-7). Raw poultry must be kept separate from other foods and work surfaces. Thorough cooking

TABLE 9-2	**SELECTED EXAMPLES OF BACTERIAL FOODBORNE ILLNESS**		
FOODBORNE ILLNESS	**CAUSATIVE ORGANISMS (GENUS AND SPECIES)**	**COMMON FOOD SOURCE**	**SYMPTOMS AND COURSE**
Bacterial Food Infections			
Salmonellosis	*Salmonella* *S. typhi* *S. paratyphi*	Milk, custards, egg dishes, salad dressings, sandwich fillings, polluted shellfish	Mild to severe diarrhea, cramps, vomiting; appears 12-24 hours after eating; lasts 1-7 days
Shigellosis	*Shigella* *S. dysenteriae*	Milk and milk products, seafood, salads	Mild diarrhea to fatal dysentery (especially in young children); appears 7-36 hours after eating; lasts 3-14 days
Listeriosis	*Listeria* *L. monocytogenes*	Soft cheese made from unpasteurized milk; poultry, seafood, unpasteurized milk, meat products (pâté)	Severe diarrhea, fever, headache, pneumonia, meningitis, endocarditis; can cause miscarriage in pregnant women; symptoms begin after 3-21 days
Vibrio	*Vibrio* *V. parahaemolyticus*	Raw or undercooked oysters, clams, mussels, other shellfish or fin fish;	Watery diarrhea, abdominal cramps, nausea, vomiting, fever, and chills; symptoms occur within 24 hours and usually continue for no more than 3 days; severe complications possible with compromised immune systems, liver disease, or alcoholism
Bacterial Food Poisoning Enterotoxins			
Staphylococcal	*Staphylococcus* *S. aureus*	Custards, cream fillings, processed meats, ham, cheese, ice cream, potato salad, sauces, casseroles	Severe abdominal pain, cramps, vomiting, diarrhea, perspiration, headache, fever, prostration; appears suddenly 1-6 hours after eating; symptoms usually subside within 24 hours
Clostridium perfringens enteritis	*Clostridium* *C. perfringens*	Cooked meats, meat dishes held at warm or room temperature	Mild diarrhea, vomiting; appears 8-24 hours after eating; lasts ≤1 day
Botulism	*Clostridium* *C. botulinum*	Improperly home-canned foods; smoked and salted fish, ham, sausage, shellfish	Severe cases lead to death within 24 hours; initial nausea, vomiting, weakness, dizziness, progressing to motor and sometimes fatal breathing paralysis

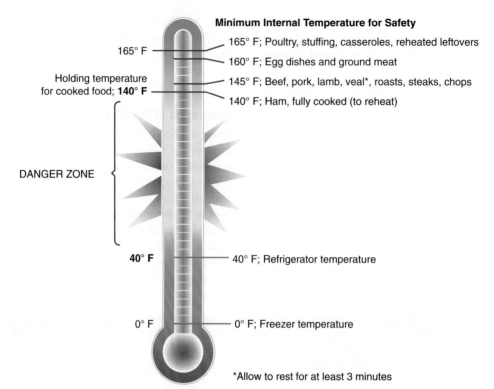

Minimum Internal Temperature for Safety

165° F ———

Holding temperature
for cooked food; **140° F** ———

165° F; Poultry, stuffing, casseroles, reheated leftovers
160° F; Egg dishes and ground meat
145° F; Beef, pork, lamb, veal*, roasts, steaks, chops
140° F; Ham, fully cooked (to reheat)

DANGER ZONE

40° F ———

40° F; Refrigerator temperature

0° F ———

0° F; Freezer temperature

*Allow to rest for at least 3 minutes

FIGURE 9-6 Chart of food temperatures: Danger Zone Stand Time. It is important to keep hot foods hot and cold foods cold. Foods should be held at temperatures below 40°F or above 140°F to prevent microbial growth. Microorganisms grow rapidly between 40°F and 140°F. Meat and poultry products should be cooked to the internal temperature indicated on the chart. (From U.S. Department of Agriculture, Food Safety and Inspection Service: "Danger Zone" 40°F to 140°F. at: <http://www.fsis.usda.gov/wps/portal/fsis/topics/food-safety-education/get-answers/food-safety-fact-sheets/safe-food-handling/danger-zone-40-f-140-f/ct_index>. Accessed on August 29, 2013.)

CASE STUDY

Planning the Family Dinner

Mrs. G is a single parent with two children: a daughter in third grade and a son in ninth grade. Although they ride different buses to school, both children get home about 3:30 p.m. Mrs. G is employed in a real estate office and usually does not get home until about 6:30 p.m. By that time the children have already filled up on snacks and are not really hungry for a meal. Sometimes she calls ahead to tell them that she is stopping at a fast-food restaurant and they should wait to eat with her, but most of the time they get something to eat for themselves. Mrs. G's son has been gaining weight at a faster-than-expected rate and has a body mass index (BMI) of 29. At his most recent physical examination, his blood pressure was higher than normal, and the physician recommended that he moderate his weight gain to improve his long-term health.

Questions for Analysis

1. Is it important that the family eat together when Mrs. G gets home? How would you approach this?

2. What are some appropriate snack foods that the children might have when they get home from school that would hold them over until dinner?

3. What are important facts on the new nutrition label that Mrs. G could use in selecting after-school snacks for her children?

4. USDA food patterns recommend an energy intake of 2400 kcal for a 14-year-old moderately active boy. What should be the upper level of fat and sodium included in his food for the day? If one fourth of his daily energy intake is reserved for snacks, then recommend some food combinations that would not exceed the appropriate amounts of kcalories, sodium, and fat.

5. What might Mrs. G bring home, or what could the children begin to prepare before she arrives home that would provide a quick and healthy meal?

6. Develop five rules for food safety that the children should practice when preparing and eating their after-school snacks.

Safe Handling Instructions

This product was prepared from inspected and passed meat and/ or poultry. Some food products may contain bacteria that could cause illness if the product is mishandled or cooked improperly. For your protection, follow these safe handling instructions.

 Keep refrigerated or frozen.
Thaw in refrigerator or microwave.

 Keep raw meat and poultry separate from other foods. Wash working surfaces (including cutting boards), utensils, and hands after touching raw meat or poultry.

 Cook thoroughly.

 Keep hot foods hot. Refrigerate leftovers immediately or discard.

FIGURE 9-7 The safe handling label provides important information about safe storage and cooking of perishable foods. Labels on fresh and frozen meat, fish, and poultry advise consumers on storing, thawing, and cooking these foods to avoid foodborne illness. (From U.S. Department of Agriculture: *Safe handling label,* Washington, D.C., U.S. Department of Agriculture.)

and time-sensitive storage of protein foods prevents foodborne illness. Fight BAC!, a food safety education program, recommends four simple steps[63]:
- CLEAN: Wash hands and surfaces often.
- SEPARATE: Don't cross-contaminate!
- COOK: Cook to proper temperature.
- CHILL: Refrigerate promptly.

The major personal defense against contracting or spreading foodborne illness is hand washing before touching food and after handling dirty dishes, linens, or trash, or using the bathroom. Thorough hand washing with soap and water is superior to use of waterless hand sanitizer.[59] Use of gloves (following hand washing) is required of food handlers and should be the rule for individuals who serve refreshments or present community food programs. Those with any infectious disease or hand injuries, however slight, must not work with food. Figure 9-8 illustrates proper hand washing.

Food Safety Education

Government agencies, food processors, and health organizations have joined forces to develop food safety education programs and certifications to meet the needs of various groups. The initiative of the Partnership for Food Safety Education called Fight BAC!, described earlier, offers website lessons and publicity materials for consumers and professionals (see http://www.fightbac.org). Fight BAC! presents food safety messages useful to teachers, nutritionists, nurses, or food service managers working with children or adults. The National Restaurant Association Foundation supports a 16-hour national certification program called *ServSafe* for food managers in restaurants, schools, day care centers, hospitals, correctional facilities, and nursing facilities. Most public health departments require all food service managers

THE PROPER WAY TO WASH YOUR HANDS

1 Wet hands.
2 Use soap.
3 Wash hands while counting to 20.
4 Rinse completely.
5 Dry hands with paper towel.
6 Use paper towel to turn off faucet.
7 Put paper towel in trash.

VirginiaTech *Invent the Future*   **Virginia Cooperative Extension**

FIGURE 9-8 Seven-step process for proper hand washing. Failure to wash hands thoroughly before and after food preparation and before eating is a common cause of contamination that leads to foodborne illness. (Courtesy Virginia Cooperative Extension, College of Agriculture and Life Sciences, Virginia Polytechnic Institute and State University, Blacksburg, Va.)

to have the ServSafe certification or equivalent. Training and certification in HAACP is available to food processors through government and university training programs. Healthy People 2020 includes goals for reducing foodborne illness and adopting food safety practices.[64] (To learn more about assessing food safety education needs, see the Evidence-Based Practice box, "Developing Food Safety Education: Assessing Learner Needs.")

Food Preservation and Processing
Preservation Methods

As consumers look for shelf-stable convenience foods to feed their families, food scientists are seeking new ways to maintain freshness and flavor and prohibit microbial growth. Some of the preservation methods used by food processors are the same as those used in the home. Various ways to preserve food are described below:

- *Applying heat:* Cooking increases palatability, softens food for chewing, and prepares food for digestion; however,

heat is also an important means of ensuring food safety. Most bacteria are killed at temperatures of 180°F to 200°F,[65] and heat also inactivates enzymes that cause spoilage. This is why vegetables are first blanched in boiling water to prevent further enzyme activity before being frozen. Pasteurization eliminates pathogens in fluid milk and fruit juices. Factory-canned foods are exposed to temperatures that effectively sterilize the food contents. Foods canned at home using too low a temperature carry the risk of botulism.

- *Keeping food cold:* Microbial activity slows at temperatures below 50°F; thus, refrigeration at 45°F or lower will preserve food for a limited period of time.[65] While freezing prevents microbial growth, bacteria can remain alive, albeit dormant. This is why it is dangerous to refreeze food that has been thawed for some time, as microorganisms have begun to multiply. Cold temperatures will decrease but not eliminate enzyme activity.

- *Removing moisture:* Drying lowers the water activity in a food, and removing available water inhibits the survival

EVIDENCE-BASED PRACTICE

Developing Food Safety Education: Assessing Learner Needs

Identify the Problem: Older adults, cancer patients, organ transplant patients, or those with acquired immune deficiency syndrome are especially vulnerable to critical illness or death from food microbial contamination. Therefore their understanding of home food safety practices is crucial. As health professionals we sometimes believe that we know what our clients need to know. A more effective strategy is to survey your target group or review published studies to determine what *they* see as their information needs and how they would prefer the information be presented.

Review the Evidence: Two groups of investigators[1,2] conducted focus groups* with cancer and organ transplant patients to learn more about the food safety information they were given after being diagnosed, and their preferences on how food safety education should be delivered. Although most participants recognized their vulnerability to foodborne infection, none had made major changes in their food safety behavior. For future food safety education, the patients recommended that special materials be developed for patients according to their particular disease or condition. They also requested that information be science-based, and easy to read and understand. Written materials that they could read at home were preferred over face-to-face classes. Some patients wished they could receive the needed information at their doctors' visits.[1,2] Because patients preferred materials they could read at home, Kosa and co-workers[3] evaluated the effectiveness of web-based versus print delivery to an older group having 12 or fewer years of schooling. While 60% of the web users and 69% of the print readers read all the materials presented to them, the information did not result in behavior change. Follow-up revealed only small improvements in food safety practices regardless of the delivery mode.

Implement the Findings: Determining both information needs and the preferred format for presentation is an important first step in planning a program. Although some individuals enjoy the social setting and interaction with fellow learners, lack of transportation or its cost, or the need to attend to children or other adults in the household can preclude class participation. Providing information at the treatment site should be explored as a model for reaching older patients. Print delivery appeared to be preferred in this older age group, but findings could differ with younger patients who have more web-based experience. Evidence gained from these studies indicates that home-based instruction using either print or online methods can be successful based on review of materials provided; however, the facts presented did not lead to changes in food safety behavior, which was the purpose of the education program. Motivation for learning appears to be more important for successful intervention than how the information is disseminated, and that may be where research on nutrition education must begin.

References

1. Medeiros LC, Chen G, Hillers VN, et al: Discovery and development of educational strategies to encourage safe food handling behaviors in cancer patients. *J Food Prot* 71:1666, 2008.

2. Chen G, Kendall PA, Hillers VN, et al: Qualitative studies of the food safety knowledge and perceptions of transplant patients. *J Food Prot* 73(2):327, 2010.

3. Kosa KM, Cates SC, Godwin SL, et al: Effectiveness of educational interventions to improve food safety practices among older adults. *J Nutr Gerontol Geriatr* 30(4):369, 2011.

*For more information on focus groups, what they are, how they are conducted, and their usefulness to educators, consider the following source: *Conducting a focus group*, Ames, Iowa, 2009, Iowa State University Extension. Retrieved February 27, 2013. from <http://www.agmrc.org/business_development/starting_a_business/marketbusiness_assessment/articles/conducting-focus-groups>.

and growth of microorganisms. Foods dried at high temperatures, such as ready-to-eat cereals, and foods that are freeze-dried retain more flavor and color. The removal of water from a food also slows enzyme activity and destructive oxidation reactions.

- *Adding acid, sugar, salt, or chemical compounds:* Various natural and chemical additives influence the growth of bacteria and were used for centuries to protect food from spoilage before refrigeration and other modern technologies were available. Acid foods lower in pH are more resistant to the growth of bacteria, so fermentation with the production of acid was used to turn perishable milk into yogurt or cheese that could be safely stored for a longer time. Adding salt or sugar to a food controls the growth of bacteria by limiting the water available to existing microorganisms. In this way, the high sugar content of jams or jellies prevents spoilage. In earlier times, salt curing was a means of preserving meat, and pickling is still used by home and commercial food processors. Chemical compounds such as sodium benzoate or calcium propionate are added to bread and grain products to retard the growth of mold and bacteria and increase shelf life.

- *Changing the atmosphere:* A new method of food preservation involves changing the atmosphere, that is, removing the oxygen necessary for bacterial growth and enzyme activity and replacing it with carbon dioxide (CO_2) or nitrogen, which slows these activities. Modified atmosphere packaging is used for highly perishable foods such as ready-to-eat chicken pieces and salad mixes.

- *Irradiation:* Irradiation extends shelf life and increases the safety of many foods. Irradiation uses energy sources such as gamma rays, similar to microwaves, that pass through the food and safely kill harmful bacteria but have little effect on nutrients. Irradiation is used to sterilize rations for space travel and for patients who require completely germ-free food, such as those undergoing bone marrow transplants. Most spices, herbs, and seasonings are irradiated. Irradiation destroys more than 99% of any *E. coli* in ground meat and more than 99% of any *Salmonella* in fresh eggs and poultry.[66] Although this technology is safe and effective, less than one tenth of 1% of the fruits, vegetables, meat, and poultry sold in the United States is irradiated.[62] Health care facilities are the primary users of irradiated foods. The sale of irradiated food has been opposed by those who erroneously believe food becomes radioactive or expect irradiation will mask unsanitary processing or storage. Irradiation has been endorsed as safe by the Academy of Nutrition and Dietetics (formerly the American Dietetic Association), the American Medical Association, and the World Health Organization.

Chemical Additives

As consumers demand new flavors, improved textures, and increased shelf life, new additives and new uses for existing additives are being evaluated. To date, the FDA has approved about 700 additives for use in food (see discussion of the GRAS list and required review of new additives in the section

"Regulation of Food Ingredients and Food Additives"). Additives serve many functions in processed foods[67]:

- *Provide a smooth and consistent texture:* Emulsifiers in cake mixes and liquid pancake batters prevent ingredients from separating; anticaking agents prevent clumping and allow mixtures to flow freely.
- *Add nutrients to the diet:* Vitamin D is added to dried skim milk, fluid milk, and soy milk to assist in the absorption of calcium; calcium is added to juices to increase intake among those individuals who avoid milk.
- *Prevent destructive oxidation reactions:* Preservatives prevent rancidity in liquid oils and mixtures containing unsaturated fats; vitamin C or other antioxidants prevent fresh fruit such as sliced apples from turning brown.
- *Prevent microbial growth:* Calcium and sodium propionate prevent the growth of mold in bread and other baked products.
- *Add flavor or color:* Spices add to the flavor and enjoyment of food, and colors provide eye appeal; yellow coloring is added to margarine to take on the appearance of butter.

Table 9-3 lists some examples of food additives. Vitamins that act as antioxidants are sometimes added to processed foods not to increase their nutrient content but to enhance their shelf life.

The additives described previously are intentional additives that serve a specific purpose. Other substances are unintentional additives that are not added on purpose but find their way into the food by some other means, although usually in very small amounts. In Chapter 7 we noted the increasing amounts of iodine entering the food supply as a result of iodine-containing cleaning agents used in the dairy industry. The FDA is currently evaluating potential residues adsorbed from food packaging materials and containers. A case in point is bisphenol A (BPA), a chemical used in the manufacture of reusable water bottles, food containers, baby bottles, and resin-coated food cans, including those used for infant formula.[68] Trace amounts of BPA can migrate from the container into the food or water and thereby enter the body, although this transfer occurs in very small amounts. It is known that BPA is rapidly metabolized and excreted,[69] in contrast to mercury, which remains in the body for long periods. Nevertheless, manufacturers are looking for alternatives to BPA for use in infant food containers.

Nutritional Aspects of Food Processing

The effect of food processing on food nutrient content continues to concern both consumers and health advocates. In general, carbohydrates, fats, and proteins are less affected and minerals and vitamins are more affected by food processing. However, both the characteristics of the food and the processing methods used influence the stability or loss of nutrients. Effects on specific nutrients are summarized as follows:

- *Macronutrients:* The major change in carbohydrates and proteins is the Maillard or browning reaction that occurs between sugars and amino acids at high temperatures.

TABLE 9-3	EXAMPLES OF FOOD ADDITIVES AND THEIR FUNCTIONS		
TYPE	**CHEMICAL COMPOUND**	**FUNCTION**	**COMMON FOOD USES**
Anticaking agent	Calcium silicate, calcium stearate	Used to keep food dry and prevent caking if moisture is absorbed from the air; keeps item free-flowing	Table salt, powdered sugar, baking powder
Antimicrobial agent	Calcium propionate, sodium propionate	Prevent growth of mold	Bread
Antioxidants	Butylated hydroxyanisole (BHA) Butylated hydroxytoluene (BHT)	Prevents oxidation reactions and rancidity in unsaturated fatty acids	Vegetable oils, potato chips
Bleaching agent	Chlorine, benzoyl peroxide	Whiten appearance	Freshly milled wheat flour, white flour for all-purpose use or cakes
Chemical leavening systems	Sodium bicarbonate	Acts with an acid in a batter to release carbon dioxide for leavening	Double-acting baking powder for quick breads, cakes, cookies
Coloring agent	Annatto (natural) FD&C Red #3 FD&C Yellow #5 (artificial)	Make color of food items more appealing	Margarine, candy, carbonated beverages, fruit drinks
Dough conditioners	Ammonium chloride, calcium phosphate	Improves volume	Bread
Emulsifier	Lecithin, monoglycerides and diglycerides	Keeps the water-soluble and fat-soluble ingredients evenly distributed throughout a food	Margarine, cake mixes
Humectants	Propylene glycol, sorbitol	Retain moisture, prevent food from becoming hard or stiff	Soft cookies, cake frosting, marshmallow candy
Flavoring agents	Amyl acetate, methyl salicylate, essential oils, monosodium glutamate, sodium chloride (salt)	Enhance flavor or aroma of foods	Most processed foods
Preservative	Sodium nitrate (color) Sodium nitrite (food safety)	Preserves pink color in cured meats; prevents rancidity in meats and botulism	Processed meats such as frankfurters, canned foods
Sequestrant	Citric acid	Binds with metals such as iron or copper to prevent changes in flavor, color, or appearance	Wine, juice, mayonnaise
Stabilizers and thickeners	Pectin, locust bean gum, guar gum, carrageenan	Maintain appropriate food texture and mouth feel; thickener, absorb water	Jelly, ice cream, pudding, yogurt

This happens in normal baking and forms new sugar–amino acid compounds that cannot be digested or absorbed. The amino acid lysine enters into the browning reaction resulting in some loss, although in the United States, grain foods are not the major sources of lysine. Hydrogenation of liquid vegetable oils to produce solid table fats forms *trans* fatty acids that have negative effects on health. (See Chapter 4 to review fat hydrogenation.)

- *Minerals:* Major mineral losses result from the refining of cereal grains. When the germ and bran are removed from the kernel to produce a finer-textured flour or cereal, iron, along with zinc, chromium, and magnesium, is lost. Under current food enrichment standards iron is added back to refined flours and cereals, but the other minerals are not. Mineral content and bioavailability is retained with most other processing methods.

- *Vitamins:* No vitamin is completely stable to food processing, although losses vary from one to another. Vitamins are lost during the storage of fruits and vegetables through the action of enzymes and oxidation.[70] Researchers have suggested that some synthetic vitamin forms are more stable to food processing than naturally occurring forms, but in general, factors that affect vitamin losses influence all forms of a particular vitamin.[71]

- *Fat-soluble vitamins:* Vitamin A is relatively stable to heat. Fairly small amounts are lost in milk pasteurization, but holding milk at high temperatures for long periods increases losses. Vitamin E in oils is generally not affected by heat treatment or frying, but freezing rapidly destroys it. Naturally occurring vitamin D is not harmed by heat, but must be protected from light and atmospheric oxygen.[71,72]

- *Water-soluble vitamins:* Thiamin is sensitive to heat, and losses occur in baking and high-temperature processing of cereals. Thiamin is also lost in foods cooked in an alkaline medium or in large amounts of water. Light is extremely destructive to riboflavin, and riboflavin-containing foods must be stored in opaque containers to avoid loss. Riboflavin does withstand the heat treatment of pasteurization, so milk remains a good food source. Niacin and pantothenic acid are generally stable in all foods. Folate is destroyed by light, and large amounts are lost in vegetables heated to high temperatures in large amounts of water. Vitamin B_6 is sensitive to light and is lost in cooking and canning of vegetables. Long exposure to heat or hot storage causes destruction of ascorbic acid. It is best that vitamin C–containing beverages and foods be packaged with no head space, because the presence of oxygen leads to serious losses over time.[71,72]

Food processing as a concept brings forth intense emotions such that a well-known nutrition expert recently asked the question "Is 'processed' a four-letter word?"[73] Health advocates sometimes encourage avoidance of processed foods considered to be limited in nutrients, whereas food companies promote the taste, convenience, and, to the extent possible, the nutritional appropriateness of their products. Processed foods run the gamut from minimally processed, washed, and packaged fruits and salad greens, to canned or frozen fruits and vegetables, to ready-to-eat convenience foods including breakfast cereals, luncheon meats, and frozen meals.[74] Some methods of food processing remove important nutrients and fiber and reduce our intakes of important phytochemicals. Development of convenience foods sometimes involves the addition of sugar, fat, and sodium with increased kcalories and risk of chronic disease. On the other hand, processed foods with added vitamins and minerals contribute to nutritional well-being.

A USDA survey reported that added nutrients to processed food contributed 45% of the thiamin, about 25% of the riboflavin and niacin, 50% of the folate, 38% of the iron, and 59% of the vitamin D intake of all Americans ages 2 and over.[75] In fact, it is difficult to meet the recommended intake of vitamin D without fortified foods. Many minimally processed and preserved foods reduce waste and offer convenience, supporting greater use of nutrient-dense foods such as fruits and vegetables. At the same time, processed foods based on synthetic materials rather than real food offer little in the way of nutrition. A healthy diet can include both minimally processed and convenience foods if chosen carefully with an emphasis on nutrient density and variety.

TO SUM UP

Food patterns evolve from a social perspective. As our society changes, so does what we eat. Parents are working longer hours, more adults are living alone, and almost half of our food budget is spent on meals away from home. Surveys suggest the American public is becoming more conscious of nutrition and health; however, fast-food and convenience meals are the norm in many families. As more of our food comes from farmers and processors across the country and around the globe, the threat of food contamination and risk of widespread outbreaks of foodborne illness escalate. Two government agencies—the FDA and the USDA—carry responsibility for maintaining a safe and wholesome food supply. The USDA oversees meat and poultry, and the FDA regulates the processing, labeling, and formulation of all other foods, including GM foods. The nutrition label helps consumers select food to maximize their nutrient intake and avoid inappropriately high levels of kcalories, sodium, and fat. Under current laws dietary supplements are largely unregulated, putting undiscerning users at risk. The CDC monitors the incidence of foodborne illness, and several government and private agencies have joined forces to provide public and professional education promoting safe food handling. Public demand for good-tasting food, quickly and easily prepared, and with a long shelf life, has led to growing use of food additives and new processing methods. Consumers and health professionals must continue to monitor the nutrient content of processed food and implications for nutrition and health.

QUESTIONS FOR REVIEW

1. What are some social and psychological factors that influence your personal food habits? Describe some food customs or special observances in your family that involve food. Do these customs have a positive or negative influence on nutrient intake? Explain.

2. You are preparing a 15-min lesson on food safety as part of a nutrition education class for young families receiving Supplemental Nutrition Assistance Program benefits. Develop an outline for your presentation including any visuals you would use. Develop or select a brochure that would be suitable for this audience.

3. A pregnant mother who has been eating more fish to obtain a good supply of n-3 fatty acids read a newspaper article indicating that all ocean fish are contaminated with mercury. She is concerned about the safety of her baby. Review the current advisory of the FDA (www.fda.gov and Box 9-4) regarding the consumption of fish by pregnant women. How would you advise her? Develop some practical menu suggestions to help her.

4. Find a print or Internet advertisement for a new dietary supplement or health remedy and identify the population to whom it is directed. Using the criteria in Box 9-5,

evaluate this product. Does it appear to be helpful or harmful? How would you respond to a consumer seeking your advice on its use?

5. You are helping a day care provider develop a food safety program for her facility. Compile a list of 10 guidelines for the staff that will reduce the risk of foodborne illness among their children. (Visit the Fight BAC! Goes to Child Care website at http://www.fightbac.org/campaigns/fight-bac-goes-to-childcare for some ideas.)

6. Select a type of frozen entree and review the nutrition labels on three examples of that product. Make a table that lists the number of servings; kcalories per serving; grams of protein, fat, and fiber; milligrams of sodium; and %DV for calcium, iron, vitamin A, and vitamin C. Compare the relative merits and disadvantages of each. Which is the best choice based on its contribution of protein, fiber, and vitamins and minerals? Which is the poorest choice in terms of fat, kcalories, and sodium?

7. Name five methods of food preservation. Which methods destroy harmful bacteria and which merely retard their growth? What are the appropriate storage conditions for food preserved by each of these methods?

8. Visit the CDC Multistate Foodborne Outbreak Investigations website and review reported outbreaks of foodborne illness that occurred over the past year (http://www.cdc.gov/outbreaknet/outbreaks.html). What foods were involved and why/how did the outbreak occur? Which consumer groups were most affected?

REFERENCES

1. Goody CM, Drago L, editors: *Cultural food practices*, Chicago, 2010, Diabetes Care and Education Dietetic Practice Group, American Dietetic Association.
2. Kittler PG, Sucher KP, Nahikian-Nelms M: *Food and culture*, ed 6, Belmont, Calif, 2012, Wadsworth/Cengage Learning.
3. Fitzgerald A, Heary C, Kelly C, et al: Self-efficacy for healthy eating and peer support for unhealthy eating are associated with adolescents' food intake patterns. *Appetite* 63:48, 2013.
4. Bruening M, Eisenberg M, MacLehose R, et al: Relationship between adolescents' and their friends' eating behaviors: breakfast, fruit, vegetable, whole-grain and dairy intake. *J Acad Nutr Diet* 112:1608, 2012.
5. Massey A, Hill AJ: Diet and food craving: a descriptive and quasi-prospective study. *Appetite* 58(3):781, 2012.
6. Maslow AH: *Motivation and personality*, New York, 1954, Harper & Row.
7. Sloan AE: What, when and where America eats. *Food Technol* 66:21, 2012.
8. Sloan AE: The new American family. *Food Technol* 65:23, 2011.
9. Hensel K: Developing foods for an aging population. *Food Technol* 66:23, 2012.
10. International Food Information Council Foundation: *Food & Health Survey. Consumer attitudes toward food safety, nutrition, and health*, Washington, D.C., 2012, International Food Information Council Foundation. at: <www.foodinsight.org>. Retrieved on February 20, 2013.
11. Kuhn ME: Serving up convenience. *Food Tech* 64:29, 2011.
12. Sebastian RS, Enns CW, Goldman JD: *Snacking patterns of U.S. adults. What we eat in America, NHANES 2007-2008, Dietary Data Brief No 4*, Beltsville, Md., 2011, Food Surveys Research Group, U.S. Department of Agriculture. at: <http://www.ars.usda.gov/Services/docs.htm?docid=19476>. Retrieved on February 13, 2013.
13. Sebastian RS, Enns CW, Goldman JD: *My Pyramid intakes and snacking patterns of U.S. adults. What we eat in America, NHANES 2007-2008, Dietary Data Brief No 5*, Beltsville, Md., 2011, Food Surveys Research Group, U.S. Department of Agriculture. at: <http://www.ars.usda.gov/Services/docs.htm?docid=19476>. Retrieved on February 13, 2013.
14. Sebastian RS, Goldman JD, Enns CW: *Snacking patterns of U.S. adolescents. What we eat in America, NHANES 2005-2006, Dietary Data Brief No 2*, Beltsville, Md., 2010, Food Surveys Research Group, U.S. Department of Agriculture. at: <http://www.ars.usda.gov/Services/docs.htm?docid=19476>. Retrieved on February 13, 2013.
15. U.S. Department of Agriculture, Agricultural Research Service: Meals and snacks: Distribution of meal patterns and snack occasions by gender and age, in the United States, 2009-2010, Table 33, *What We Eat in America*, 2012. at: <www.ars.usda.gov/ba/bhnrc/fsrg>. NHANES 2009-2010. Retrieved on February 19, 2013.
16. Zizza CA, Tayie FA, Lino M: Benefits of snacking in older Americans. *J Am Diet Assoc* 107:800, 2007.
17. Duffey KJ, Popkin BM: Energy density, portion size, and eating occasions: contributions to increased energy intake in the United States, 1977-2006. *PLoS Med* 8(6):e1001050, 2011.
18. Neumark-Sztainer D, Wall M, Fulkerson JA, et al: Changes in the frequency of family meals from 1999 to 2010 in the homes of adolescents: trends by sociodemographic characteristics. *J Adolesc Health* 52:201, 2013.
19. Hammons AJ, Fiese BH: Is frequency of shared family meals related to the nutritional health of children and adolescents. *Pediatrics* 127(6):e1565, 2011.
20. Berge JM, MacLehose RF, Loth KA, et al: Family meals. Associations with weight and eating behaviors among mothers and fathers. *Appetite* 58:1128, 2012.
21. Merten MJ, Williams AL, Shriver LH: Breakfast consumption in adolescence and young adulthood: parental presence, community context, and obesity. *J Am Diet Assoc* 109:1384, 2009.
22. Brown D: The rise of the male cook. *J Am Diet Assoc* 107:731, 2007.
23. Hornick BA, Childs NM, Edge MS, et al: Is it time to rethink nutrition communications? A 5-year retrospective of Americans' attitudes toward food, nutrition and health. *J Acad Nutr Diet* 113(1):14, 2013.
24. Kapsak WR, Rahavi ER, Childs NM, et al: Functional foods: consumer attitudes, perceptions, and behaviors in a growing market. *J Am Diet Assoc* 111(6):804, 2011.

25. American Dietetic Association: Position of the American Dietetic Association: agriculture and food biotechnology. *J Am Diet Assoc* 106:285, 2006.

26. Massengale RD: Biotechnology: going beyond GMOs. *Food Tech* 64:30, 2011.

27. Magana-Gomez JA, de la Barca AM: Risk assessment of genetically modified crops for nutrition and health. *Nutr Rev* 67:1, 2009.

28. Davies WP: An historical perspective from the green revolution to the gene revolution. *Nutr Rev* 61(Suppl 6):S124, 2003.

29. Dubock A: Crop conundrum. *Nutr Rev* 67:17, 2009.

30. Wilkins J: Fact or fishberry? Answering consumer questions about genetically engineered foods. *ADA Times* 2(4):5, 2005.

31. U.S. Food and Drug Administration: *Report on the Food and Drug Administration's review of the safety of recombinant bovine somatotropin, CFSAN.* Updated April 23, 2009, Washington, D.C., 2009, U.S. Department of Health and Human Services. from: <www.fda.gov/AnimalVeterinary/SafetyHealth/ProductSafetyInformation/ucm130321.htm>. Retrieved February 19, 2013.

32. Vicini J, Etherton T, Kris-Etherton P, et al: Survey of retail milk composition as affected by label claims regarding farm-management practices. *J Am Diet Assoc* 108:1198, 2008.

33. U.S. Food and Drug Administration: *About FDA*, Rockville, Md., 2011, U.S. Department of Health and Human Services. from: <http://www.fda.gov/AboutFDA/default.htm>. Retrieved February 21, 2013.

34. U.S. Food and Drug Administration: *Dietary Supplement Health and Education Act of 1994*, Public Law 103-417, Rockville, Md., 2009, U.S. Department of Health and Human Services. at: <http://www.fda.gov/Regulatory Information/Legislation/FederalFoodDrugandCosmetic ActFDCAct/SignificantAmendmentstotheFDCAct/ucm148003.htm>. Retrieved on February 20, 2013.

35. U.S. Food and Drug Administration: *Dietary Supplement Safety Act: How Is FDA Doing 10 Years Later*, Rockville, Md., 2009, U.S. Department of Health and Human Services. from: <http://www.fda.gov/NewsEvents/Testimony/ucm113767.htm>. Retrieved on February 20, 2013.

36. Dimitri C, Oberholtzer L: *Marketing U.S. organic foods: recent trends from farms to consumers, EIB No 58, Economics Research Service*, Washington, D.C., 2009, U.S. Department of Agriculture. at: <http://www.ers.usda.gov/media/185272/eib58_1_.pdf>. Retrieved on February 20, 2013.

37. U.S. Department of Agriculture: *The National Organic Program, Agricultural Marketing Service*, Washington, D.C., 2013. at: <http://www.ams.usda.gov/AMSv1.0/nop>. Retrieved on February 20, 2013.

38. U.S. Food and Drug Administration: *Mercury in fish and shellfish: EPA and FDA advice for women who might become pregnant, women who are pregnant, nursing mothers, EPA-823-R-04-005*, Washington, D.C., 2004, U.S. Department of Health and Human Services and U.S. Environmental Protection Agency. at: <http://www.fda.gov/Food/FoodborneIllnessContaminants/Metals/ucm351781.htm>. Retrieved on February 20, 2013.

39. U.S. Food and Drug Administration: *Guidance for industry: a food labeling guide*, Washington, D.C., 2009, U.S. Department of Health and Human Services. at: <http://www.fda.gov/downloads/Food/GuidanceRegulation/UCM265446.pdf>. Retrieved February 20, 2013.

40. U.S. Food and Drug Administration: *Factsheet on the new proposed nutrition facts label*, Silver Spring, Md., 2014, U.S. Department of Health and Human Services. at: <http://www.fda.gov/Food/GuidanceRegulation/Guidance DocumentsRegulatoryInformation/LabelingNutrition/ucm387533.htm>. Retrieved on March 16, 2014.

41. U.S. Food and Drug Administration: *Health claims meeting significant scientific agreement (SSA)*, Washington, D.C., 2013 (last update), U.S. Department of Health and Human Services. at: <http://www.fda.gov/Food/Ingredients PackagingLabeling/LabelingNutrition/ucm2006876.htm>. Retrieved on February 20, 2013.

42. U.S. Food and Drug Administration: *Gluten-free labeling of food*, Washington, D.C., 2013, U.S. Department of Health and Human Services. at: <http://www.fda.gov/Food/GuidanceRegulation/GuidanceDocumentsRegulatory Information/Allergens/ucm362510.htm>. Retrieved August 10, 2013.

43. McLellan TM, Lieberman HR: Do energy drinks contain active components other than caffeine? *Nutr Reviews* 70(12):730, 2012.

44. Sepkowitz KA: Energy drinks and caffeine-related adverse effects. *JAMA* 309(3):243, 2013.

45. U.S. Food and Drug Administration: *Letter to manufacturers regarding botanicals and other novel ingredients in conventional foods*, Washington, D.C., 2013 (last update), U.S. Department of Health and Human Services. at: <http://www.fda.gov/Food/GuidanceRegulation/GuidanceDocumentsRegulatoryInformation/Dietary Supplements/ucm103443.htm>. Retrieved on February 20, 2013.

46. Howland J, Rohsenow DJ: Risks of energy drinks mixed with alcohol. *JAMA* 309(3):245, 2013.

47. Park S, Onufrak S, Blanck H, et al: Characteristics associated with consumption of sports and energy drinks among US adults: National Health Interview Survey, 2010. *J Acad Nutr Diet* 113(1):112, 2013.

48. Marcason W: How can I help my clients sort out the conflicting and confusing information regarding dietary supplements? *J Am Diet Assoc* 110(9):1408, 2010.

49. Centers for Disease Control and Prevention: *Estimating foodborne illness: an overview*, Atlanta, Ga, 2013, Division of Foodborne, Waterborne, and Environmental Diseases. at: <www.cdc.gov/foodborneburden/estimates-overview.html>. Retrieved on February 20, 2013.

50. American Dietetic Association: Position of the American Dietetic Association: food and water safety. *J Am Diet Assoc* 109:1449, 2009.

51. Marcason W: Is the incidence of foodborne illness in the United States changing. *J Am Diet Assoc* 111(6):966, 2011.

52. Beauchamp CS, Sofos JM: Diarrheagenic *Escherichia coli*. In Juneja VK, Fofos JN, editors: *Pathogens and toxins in foods. Challenges and interventions*, Washington, D.C., 2010, ASM Press.

53. McCabe-Sellers BJ, Beattie SE: Food safety: emerging trends in foodborne illness surveillance and prevention. *J Am Diet Assoc* 104:1708, 2004.

54. Cox NA, Richardson LJ, Musgrove MT: *Campylobacter jejuni* and other campylobacters. In Juneja VK, Sofos JN, editors: *Pathogens and toxins in foods. Challenges and interventions*, Washington, D.C., 2010, ASM Press.

55. Sneed J, Strohbehn CH: Trends impacting food safety in retail foodservice: implications for dietetics practice. *J Am Diet Assoc* 108:1170, 2008.

56. Iwamoto M, Ayers T, Mahon BE, et al: Epidemiology of seafood-associated infections in the United States. *Clin Microbiol Reviews* 23(2):399, 2010.

57. Seo KS, Bohach GA: Staphylococcal food poisoning. In Juneja VK, Sofos JN, editors: *Pathogens and toxins in foods. Challenges and interventions*, Washington, D.C., 2010, ASM Press.

58. Peck MW: *Clostridium botulinum*. In Juneja VK, Sofos JN, editors: *Pathogens and toxins in foods. Challenges and interventions*, Washington, D.C., 2010, ASM Press.

59. Centers for Disease Control and Prevention: *Norovirus*, Atlanta, Ga., 2013, National Center for Immunization and Respiratory Diseases, Division of Viral Diseases. at: <http://www.cdc.gov/norovirus/index.html>. Retrieved on February 20, 2013.

60. Painter JA, Hoekstra RM, Ayers T, et al: Attribution of foodborne illnesses, hospitalizations, and deaths to food commodities by using outbreak data, United States, 1998-2008. *Emerging Infectious Dis* 19(3):407, 2013. at: <http://wwwnc.cdc.gov/eid/article/19/3/pdfs/11-1866.pdf>. Retrieved on February 25, 2013.

61. Barak JD, Schroeder BK: Interrelationships of food safety and plant pathology: the life cycle of human pathogens on plants. *Annu Rev Phytopathol* 50:241, 2012.

62. Kuehn BM: Reports highlight new cause of pertussis, tickborne illness, and better food safety. *JAMA* 307(17):1785, 2012.

63. Partnership for Food Safety Education: Safe food handling. The Four Core Practices, Partnership for Food Safety Education, 2010. at: <http://www.fightbac.org/safe-food-handling>. Retrieved on August 10, 2013.

64. United States Department of Health and Human Services: Healthy People 2020. Topics and objectives: food safety, 2012. at: <http://www.healthypeople.gov/2020/topicsobjectives2020/overview.aspx?topicid=14>. Retrieved on February 25, 2013.

65. Parker R: *Introduction to food science*, Albany, N.Y., 2003, Delmar/Thomson Learning.

66. Parnes RB, Lichtenstein AH: Food irradiation: a safe and useful technology. *Nutr Clin Care* 7:149, 2004.

67. U.S. Department of Health and Human Services: *Food additives. Medline Plus Medical Encyclopedia, U.S. National Library of Medicine*, Rockville, Md., 2012, National Institutes of Health. at: <http://www.nlm.nih.gov/medlineplus/ency/article/002435.htm>. Retrieved on February 25, 2013.

68. U.S. Food and Drug Administration: *Update on bisphenol A (BPA) for use in food contact applications*, Silver Spring, Md., 2013 (last update), U.S. Department of Health and Human Services. at: <http://www.fda.gov/NewsEvents/PublicHealthFocus/ucm064437.htm>. Retrieved on February 25, 2013.

69. U.S. Food and Drug Administration: *FDA continues to study BPA*, Silver Spring, Md., 2013 (last update), U.S. Department of Health and Human Services. at: <http://www.fda.gov/ForConsumers/ConsumerUpdates/ucm297954.htm>. Retrieved on February 25, 2013.

70. Hotz C, Gibson RS: Traditional food-processing and preparation practices to enhance the bioavailability of micronutrients in plant-based diets. *J Nutr* 137:1097, 2007.

71. Henry CK, Chapman C, editors: *The nutrition handbook for food processors*, Boca Raton, Fla., 2002, CRC Press.

72. Finley JW, Deming DM, Smith RE: Food processing, nutrition, safety, and quality. In Shils ME, Shike M, Olson J, editors: *Modern nutrition in health and disease*, ed 10, Baltimore, Md., 2006, Lippincott Williams & Wilkins.

73. Dwyer JT, Fulgoni VL, Clemens RA, et al: Is "processed" a four-letter word? The role of processed foods in achieving dietary guidelines and nutrient recommendations. *Adv Nutr* 3(4):536, 2012.

74. Fox M: Defining processed foods for the consumer. *J Acad Nutr Diet* 112(2):214, 2012.

75. Fulgoni VL, Keast DR, Bailey RL, et al: Foods, fortificants, and supplements: where do Americans get their nutrients? *J Nutr* 141:1847, 2011.

FURTHER READINGS AND RESOURCES

Further Readings

Cappellano KL: Supporting local agriculture. Farmers markets and community-supported agriculture and gardens. *Nutr Today* 46(4):203, 2011.

[Dr. Cappellano gives us suggestions on how we can support local agriculture and increase the availability of fresh fruits and vegetables.]

Fox M: Defining processed foods for the consumer. *J Acad Nutr Diet* 112:214, 2012.

[This article helps us answer the question "What is a processed food?" and better assist consumers in making healthy choices.]

Sloan AE: What, when and where America eats. *Food Tech* 65:21, 2012.

[Dr. Sloan provides a comprehensive review of food trends among American consumers and the implications for food scientists and nutritionists.]

Websites of Interest

- U.S. Department of Health and Human Services. FoodSafety.gov is the government gateway to food safety information on appropriate food safety practices, foodborne illness, recalls of unsafe food, and concerns of vulnerable population groups: www.foodsafety.gov (materials available in English and Spanish).
- Partnership for Food Safety Education; Fight BAC! Keep Food Safe From Bacteria provides food safety materials for adults, children, and food service workers: http://www.fightbac.org/ (materials available in English and Spanish).
- International Food Information Council. This site provides consumer information on food labeling, food additives, and food ingredients: www.ific.org/.

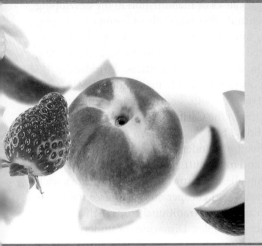

Community Nutrition: Promoting Healthy Eating

Eleanor D. Schlenker

EVOLVE WEBSITE

http://evolve.elsevier.com/Williams/essentials/

OUTLINE

Nutrition and Public Health
The Ecology of Malnutrition
Community-Based Interventions

Family Economic Needs: Food Assistance Programs
Selecting Food in the Marketplace
Health Promotion

Health and nutrition professionals have active roles in community and public health programs across the globe. Despite food shortages and famine in some regions, which result in lost years and poor quality of life, overweight and obesity and their related chronic diseases continue to rise worldwide. In this chapter we look at educational approaches and nutrition intervention programs that assist communities and individuals in adopting healthy lifestyles and food habits. Such programs include national government initiatives such as the Special Supplemental Nutrition Program for Women, Infants, and Children (WIC), which combines both food distribution and nutrition education, as well as local activities sponsored by a school or community coalition that encourage families to walk together. We look at how nutrition education and intervention programs are developed and marketed. We also consider the use of food resources to help individuals and families obtain maximum benefit from their food dollars.

NUTRITION AND PUBLIC HEALTH

Framework for Health

Our goal for nutrition is optimum health and well-being, but health can be described in various ways. Health for an individual is sometimes defined as soundness of body and mind, or freedom from disease or pain.[1] The World Health Organization (WHO) takes this a step further by including all dimensions of wellness: physical, emotional, social, environmental, and spiritual.[2] The term *public health* focuses on populations rather than individuals, although the size of the population can vary from a healthy-baby clinic to stemming the worldwide invasion of avian flu. Public health programs are directed toward preventing disease rather than curing existing disease, and emphasize positive lifestyle intervention. Public health agencies monitor the health status of the population to determine what services are needed and how they might be implemented. National and international public health agencies investigate outbreaks of disease and existing malnutrition to determine their cause and implement preventive services.

Nutrition in Public Health

Nutrition is fundamental to public health. In the 20th century, nutrient-deficiency diseases were rampant across the globe and still persist in many low-income and developing nations. In this century the quality and quantity of nutrient intake were recognized as environmental factors that contribute to the development of cardiovascular disease, diabetes, obesity, and cancer. Although these conditions are more visible as public health problems in the developed world, developing nations are coping with the "double burden" of malnutrition: nutrient-deficiency diseases and diseases of affluence such as overweight. In developing nations these patterns of disease and premature death depend largely on the prevailing social and economic conditions,[3] and what food is available. In affluent nations malnutrition is more likely the result of poor choices from the existing food supply rather than a food shortage.

Worldwide Prevalence of Malnutrition

Malnutrition as a worldwide public health problem continues to grow in scope. In developing countries about 925 million people suffer from hunger; 125 million children are underweight; and another 195 million children are stunted (low growth for their age).[4] Nearly 160 million people are living in ultra poverty, on less than 50 cents a day, and more than three fourths of them are in sub-Saharan Africa.[5] When food is available it often consists of a few staple foods. Even if adequate in energy, such a diet does not provide the variety required to supply all nutrients needed for health. Micronutrient deficiencies affect more people than do caloric deficiencies (36% vs. 12% of the estimated world population). About 25% of the world's population have low intakes of iodine, putting them at risk of goiter or cretinism, and about the same number have anemia resulting from iron or folate deficiency. One in four children in developing countries has poor vitamin A status, adding to the risk of blindness, and zinc deficiency likely contributes to poor growth status and death. Over half of child deaths occurring worldwide are associated with malnutrition.[6] Problems in food distribution, rather than a lack of available food, are often the roots of malnutrition. Close to 80% of the world's malnourished children live in countries that report food surpluses.[7] In low-income nations female-headed households are more likely to suffer severe poverty than male-headed households.[8]

Even in the midst of plenty, millions of families in the United States have insufficient supplies of food.[9] Although an estimated 85.1% of U.S. households are food secure, having access to adequate food, 14.9% experience food insecurity at least once in a year, meaning they had limited or uncertain availability of nutritionally safe and adequate food. Food-insecure households include over 50 million people; 17 million of these are children.[9] These families cope by reducing the variety of their diet or relying on a few basic foods. However, 5.7% of food-insecure households (including 5 million children) experience very low food security with reduced food intake. Household members will not eat even though they are hungry, will skip or reduce the size of a meal, and in desperate cases, will not eat for an entire day. For some families this extreme lack of food occurs in only 1 or 2 months of the year, but for one third of those with low food security, missing meals and reducing portion size is a chronic problem. Food insecurity is more likely to occur in single-parent households, households with children, those living below the poverty line, or in African-American and Hispanic households.[9] (Box 10-1 provides some screening tools to identify families who are food insecure.)

Malnutrition and Health

Food shortages affect physical and emotional health.[10] The worry of not having enough food brings depression, anxiety, and stress; malnutrition in pregnancy results in low birth weight, which puts an infant at risk. Malnutrition adds to weakness and disability among older adults, costing years of productive life.[7] At one time, energy and protein deficits were viewed as the major causes of malnutrition in the developing world; however, chronic diseases such as coronary vascular disease, diabetes, and hypertension, resulting from overweight, are expected to overtake undernutrition as the leading cause of death in low-income countries. Worldwide, 1.5 billion adults are overweight (body mass index [BMI] $\geq$ 25) with gains observed in both high-income countries and developing countries in the Caribbean, Latin America, North Africa, and the Middle East.[11]

Although difficult to understand, problems of underweight, stunting, and micronutrient deficiencies exist side by side with growing obesity. Growing focus on calorie-rich sugar crops, oil seeds, and cheaper animal-source foods has diverted attention away from traditional crops such as grains, legumes, and other vegetables. Disparities of undernutrition and obesity sometimes exist in the same family. Social norms often reflect differences in food allocation related to age or gender. High-quality foods may be given first to males responsible for the financial support of the family, or parents may indulge their children. Older adults often retain more traditional eating patterns rather than adopting new foods.[12]

Finally, undernutrition at one stage of the life cycle may hasten the development of obesity at another stage.[13] Children who experienced fetal growth retardation and underfeeding as infants are at risk of rapid and inappropriate weight gain if overfed in childhood, and rapid weight gain

---

BOX 10-1   QUESTIONS TO IDENTIFY FOOD INSECURITY

- In the past 12 months did you ever run out of food and have no money to purchase food?
- In the past 12 months did you or your children ever skip a meal because you had run out of food and had no money to purchase food?
- In the past 12 months were you or your children ever hungry but didn't eat because you didn't have enough food and had no money to purchase additional food?
- In the past 12 months did you ever cut the size of your children's meals because there wasn't enough food in the house and you had no money to purchase additional food?

Data from Hampl JS, Hall R: Dietetic approaches to U.S. hunger and food insecurity. *J Am Diet Assoc* 102:921, 2002.

KEY TERMS

hunger   A potential consequence of food insecurity resulting from prolonged, involuntary lack of food, and resulting in discomfort, illness, weakness, or pain.

food secure   An available supply of food adequate in quality and quantity to meet the nutritional needs of all family members at all times throughout the year

food insecurity   Limited or uncertain availability of food and the inability to obtain a sufficient supply of nutritionally safe, adequate, and acceptable food through socially acceptable means.

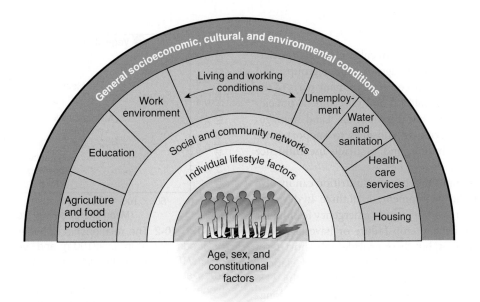

Age, sex, and
constitutional
factors

FIGURE 10-1 Relationship between the individual, the environment, malnutrition, and disease. The first layer in this figure represents personal behavior and lifestyle including dietary habits that promote or damage health; friendship patterns and community norms also influence personal behavior; the second layer indicates social and community networks that, if available, provide social support; the third layer includes structural factors such as housing, income, and access to services including health care. These three layers represent the interaction between an individual, the environment, and the development of malnutrition and disease. (Reprinted with permission from Dahlgren G, Whitehead M: *Policies and strategies to promote social equity in health*, Stockholm, 1991, Institute for Futures Studies.)

among stunted children increases their adult risk of obesity and cardiovascular risk factors. Parents in food-insecure environments in both low- and high-income countries encourage children to eat as much as possible when food is available.[13] Nutrition experts in the United States have pointed to the distribution pattern of Supplemental Nutrition Assistance Program (SNAP) benefits as a contributing factor to the current epidemic of child obesity, as it reinforces a cycle of high kcalorie consumption at the beginning of the month when benefits are received and lower consumption toward the close of the month when food provisions have been exhausted.[10] This was confirmed among families in Minnesota who spent more than 75% of their food stamp allotment within the first 2 weeks of the month.[14] Food insecurity may lead to binge eating when food is available.

THE ECOLOGY OF MALNUTRITION

From the biologic standpoint, malnutrition results from an inadequate supply of nutrients to support normal cell growth and function. However, the real ecology of malnutrition is an interconnecting set of physical, social, cultural, economic, political, and educational conditions (Figure 10-1). Each is more or less important at a given time and place for a given individual. If the adverse conditions are only temporary, then the malnutrition is short-term and quickly alleviated with no long-standing threat to life. However, chronic malnutrition

carries irreparable harm and, in severe conditions, death. For the epidemiologist, a triad of variables influences health and disease. These three variables—(1) the agent, (2) the host, and (3) the environment—also influence malnutrition.

Agent

The agent in malnutrition is a lack of food. As nutrient supplies grow short, physiologic changes begin to occur and worsen with time. Famine, poverty, war, unequal distribution of food across a region, or unwise choices from the food available all contribute to malnutrition.

Host

The host is the infant, child, or adult who is malnourished. Physical characteristics such as infectious or chronic diseases; the needs of growth, pregnancy, or lactation; or heavy physical labor increase the severity of the problem. Personal factors such as emotional problems and poverty lead to malnutrition.

KEY TERMS

ecology The relationship between an individual and his or her environment

epidemiologist A medical scientist who studies the causes, occurrence, distribution, control, and prevention of disease.

Environment

Lack of clean water, poor sanitation, cultural beliefs restricting certain foods for particular age or gender groups, and poor agricultural potential are common in many parts of the world. In all societies agricultural and government policies influence food availability and distribution. Land management and erosion, government subsidies to support price structures, water distribution, and pesticide use influence food production.

Intervention programs to relieve malnutrition can involve the host, the agent, the environment, or all three. In developing countries, programs often provide emergency feeding for those who are experiencing crop failure or have been displaced from their homes, but these provide only short-term solutions. Agencies such as the WHO, the United Nations Food and Agriculture Organization (FAO), and the U.S. Agency for International Development (AID) focus on long-term solutions to eliminate hunger, by improving agricultural practices and increasing local food production. But program success is often dependent on technological, cultural, and structural changes within the environment. Although the Green Revolution brought forth new plant species with improved nutrient content and greater yields, many staple foods of Africa's poor—cassava, sorghum, and millet—were not included. Soil conditions and lack of access to new varieties continue to discourage increased food production.[15] In many developing countries women tend small farms and gardens but are often left out of agricultural extension activities designed to increase local production. In addition, marketing influences what is grown and who eats it. Worldwide demand for sugars, oils, and animal foods has lowered production of vegetables and beans in favor of crops for export or animal feeds,[16] resulting in higher prices for traditional foods.[15]

Poverty and Food Access

In the United States, low-income families also face what seems to be the insurmountable task of obtaining enough food. They may be forced to acquire food that has been discarded by others, taking food from dumpsters despite the risk of foodborne illness.[17] They may purchase dented cans or day-old foods being sold at a reduced price. Families will fish from polluted streams despite the health risk if food is in short supply. Mothers will try to visit more than one food pantry to obtain a sufficient amount of food for their families. The question "Can low-income Americans afford a healthy diet?" remains unanswered. Although cultural and social factors as well as cost influence nutrient intake, individuals with higher incomes and more money to spend for food have higher intakes of micronutrients than those with lower incomes.[18,19]

When food budgets shrink, family purchases shift toward foods higher in kcalories and lower in cost. In many cases healthier foods are items to be dropped. While higher-income families purchase more fresh fruits and vegetables, whole grains, seafood, lean meat, and low-fat milk, lower-income

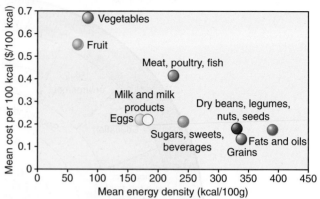

FIGURE 10-2 The relationship between the energy density of foods given in kcal/100 g and energy cost given in dollars/100 kcal for the nine major food groups. Note that fruits and vegetables have a lower energy density and a higher energy cost (more than $0.50 per 100 kcal) as compared with fats, grains, and beans that have a higher energy density and lower energy cost (about $0.20 per 100 kcal). (Reprinted with permission from Drewnowski A: The cost of US foods as related to their nutritive value. *Am J Clin Nutr* 92:1181, 2010.)

families eat more cereals, pasta, potatoes, legumes, and fatty meats. Their fruits and vegetables are often limited to iceberg lettuce, potatoes, canned corn, bananas, and frozen orange juice.[20] Figure 10-2 compares the energy density and cost of different food groups.[21] Note that grains and other starches, added sugars, and vegetable fats are the least expensive way to satisfy hunger when money is scarce. Fruits and vegetables are high in nutrients but four to five times higher in cost per 100 kcalories.[21] Vitamin C, β-carotene, potassium, and magnesium have the highest cost.[19] In general, foods associated with the greatest disease risk have the lowest cost. This may help explain why the diets of low-income families deviate from recommended guidelines and why they have the highest rates of diet-related chronic diseases.[19]

COMMUNITY-BASED INTERVENTIONS

Community Nutrition Education

Helping individuals and families make positive lifestyle changes to improve their nutrition and well-being is both an art and a science. The Dietary Reference Intakes (DRIs), the U.S. Department of Agriculture (USDA) Food Patterns, and the 2010 *Dietary Guidelines for Americans* provide the science—what nutrients and foods are needed and in what amounts—but adapting those guidelines to individuals and communities with particular food beliefs, incomes, and living situations is an art, requiring patience, sensitivity, and application of behavioral theory.

Nutrition education programs that help people understand the relationship between nutrition and health and assist them in making decisions about their food[22] can take many different forms. Community nutrition programs are sponsored by government agencies responsible for the public's health, schools, corporations, faith-based groups, health-related voluntary organizations, health care facilities, or other community groups. Target groups can include pregnant women, parents, school children, senior citizens, worksite employees, low-income families, or the general public. The SNAP and WIC programs combine food assistance with nutrition education. Other programs may offer only nutrition information, participation in health-related activities, and personal support. Such programs could include classes on healthy eating for mothers with at-risk children, community walking programs, or worksite wellness classes on weight management. The Healthy People 2020 objectives for educational and community-based programs[23] emphasize the importance of nutrition education beginning in early childhood and continuing through elementary school, high school, and college. Worksites have potential for adult health promotion programs.

Societies shape their own patterns of disease. Economic and **demographic** factors influence health among all ages.[24] Individuals new to the United States may experience difficulties in **acculturation** to a new secular and food environment.[25] As described in Figure 10-3, our task is to provide families with the information and tools for decision making that will reduce chronic disease.

Developing a Community Program

Health professionals often encounter nutrition problems in their community that trigger the need for nutrition education and intervention. Developing and implementing a program that will successfully address unmet needs requires careful and systematic planning. Program planning involves setting goals and deciding how to meet them. It speaks to the what, where, when, and how the program will be conducted. Successful program planning involves several consecutive steps, as follows[26]:

1. *Assess the needs of the target population and existing community resources.* To address individual and family needs you must know the race or ethnicity, educational level, typical household size and composition, language spoken at home, and income of the population you wish to serve. If this information is not available from your agency, it can be obtained from county or state census data. Food-related information would include the number of families receiving SNAP benefits or free or reduced-price school lunches and the availability of nearby supermarkets or grocery stores where the target group can shop. It is also important to review other local community programs or services addressing similar issues; referrals or expansion to reach the underserved might be best, rather than proposing a new program.

2. *Identify the problem.* Following your review of existing information, sort out the problem and how you might approach it. Teaching children or adults about healthy eating is of no value if your audience cannot implement what you have recommended. In a school with a large proportion of overweight children an after-school program focusing on healthy snacks and increasing physical activity might be a possible intervention. If so, you will need to cooperate with the school food service program to ensure healthy options at breakfast and lunch. If a volunteer group is providing take-home snacks for low-income children in this school, are they appropriate? If you are working with low-income mothers who receive SNAP benefits, lessons on meal planning can help ensure that food remains available for the entire month. You will need to consider whether these families have access to a supermarket that offers lower prices and a good selection or if they depend on a convenience store for their food. Is transportation a hindrance to grocery shopping?

3. *Develop realistic goals and objectives.* A goal is a general statement of what you hope will happen as a result of the program and usually does not include a specific date for completion. Objectives are specific statements describing what you plan to do; they must be measurable and include a completion date. Your action plan will be developed from these objectives. See Table 10-1 for examples of

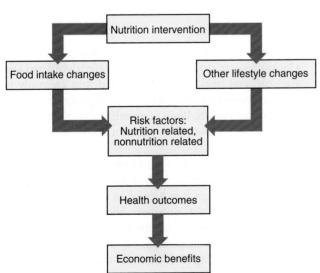

FIGURE 10-3 Model for nutrition education. The goal of community nutrition education is to bring about positive changes in food and lifestyle behaviors that lower the risk of chronic disease. (Redrawn from Olendzki MC, Tolpin HG, Buckley EL: Evaluating nutrition intervention in atherosclerosis: some theoretical and practical considerations. *J Am Diet Assoc* 79[7]:9, 1981. Reprinted with permission.)

KEY TERMS
demographics Statistical data describing a population according to age, income, gender, household composition, race, ethnic or cultural group, education, or place of residence.
acculturation The process by which newcomers to a country or region begin to adopt the practices of their neighbors; this term often refers to the adoption of new foods or food patterns by individuals moving to the United States.

TABLE 10-1	DEVELOPING SMART OBJECTIVES	
CHARACTERISTIC	**WHAT TO INCLUDE**	**EXAMPLE**
Specific (S)	What is the intended task or activity? Who is your target group?	• Increase fruit and vegetable intake of Head Start children in your community with increased servings in meals and snacks at the Head Start Center.
Measurable (M)	Are there standards available to assist in setting goals and evaluating success?	• Review current menus and snacks; calculate how many servings of fruits and vegetables are being included in meals and snacks and compare with USDA food plan recommendations for the target age group. • Review fruit and vegetable intake goals for this age group at the Healthy People 2020 website and compare with current practices.
Achievable (A)	• Is the task realistic? • Do you have sufficient resources to complete the project?	• Review food budgets within the Head Start program to determine if money is available to support purchase of more fruits and vegetables, or if funds can be reallocated among food groups to make more money available, or if it will be necessary to procure grant money to support proposed menu additions. • Identify and obtain resources needed to develop and implement in-service training for Head Start workers on greater use of fruits and vegetables in meals and snacks.
Relevant (R)	Will your target group consider this goal or activity important or worth doing?	• Develop strategies to obtain commitment of Head Start workers to the goal of increased servings of fruits and vegetables (e.g., will they support purchase of more fruit if it means fewer cookies?). • Develop a presentation describing the health status of the children served by your Head Start program (e.g., body weight, frequency of days missed because of colds or flu) and benefits of an improved diet; use with parents, Head Start workers, and potential community sponsors.
Time Frame (T)	When will project start and end?	Begin July 1 and end on June 30.

Adapted from Centers for Disease Control and Prevention, Office for State, Tribal, Local and Territorial Support, Communities of Practice Program, Resource Kit, May 2011.

Specific, Measurable, Achievable, Relevant, Time Frame (SMART) objectives.

4. *Develop an action plan.* An action plan is a blueprint for the tasks required to implement your program: who will carry out each task and the resources or assistance required. If the program will be sponsored by your agency or facility, you will need to identify other participants and gain the approval of the appropriate administrators. If you are working with another professional or community group, their responsibilities and your responsibilities must be carefully defined. If funding is required, then possible sources and procedures for obtaining resources must be noted. Procurement of teaching or handout materials or food supplies along with necessary fiscal reporting must be assigned. You and your colleagues need to consider how this program will be marketed so that announcements not only reach the target audience, but also encourage their participation. Your chosen location must be safe, comfortable, and easily accessible. Think about how you will evaluate your program and who will collect and protect the information obtained.

5. *Implement the program.* When your planning is complete, a location secured, funding in place, materials ordered and available, and responsibilities assigned, you are ready to proceed. Programs, even well-planned programs, sometimes proceed slowly. Word of mouth of a helpful program, sensitive to individual needs, can build interest and participation.

6. *Evaluate results for use in future planning.* Program evaluation can include both knowledge and behavior outcomes. Although it is helpful to know if participants have improved their nutrition knowledge, it is more important to know if they made changes in their food choices or food management. For children in the after-school class, rating the number of days they chose water or milk rather than a sugar-sweetened beverage or increased their daily steps as measured by a step counter indicates whether the program led to a potential improvement in health. For low-income mothers, the number of meals per week that included a fruit or vegetable serving or the number of days out of food before the end of the month impacts their children's well-being.

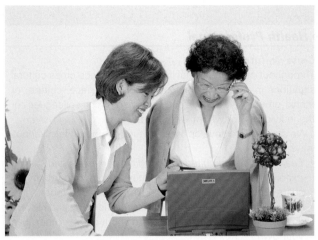

FIGURE 10-4 All ages can benefit from a community nutrition education program. Online nutrition education materials can support continued learning after the program is completed. (Copyright 2006 JupiterImages Corporation.)

Asking which lessons or activities the participants enjoyed most or found helpful is valuable for planning future programs.

Nutrition education is a process, not something that "happens to a person" and immediately changes his or her behavior. It involves small steps that over time improve nutritional status or a disease condition. Community nutrition programs demand close attention to family needs and resources, and the knowledge and practical skills required to solve food problems. As noted in Figure 10-4, persons of all ages can benefit from nutrition education.

Creating a Learning Environment

Successful community education requires attention to both the social and physical environment. It demands a relationship of trust, respect, and concern. This includes accepting people as they are and where they are in their personal development. It expects a positive environment for participation and discussion. When preparing for your teaching activity, consider the following:
- Use language appropriate to the listener.
- Present information in a way that is easily remembered.
- Provide examples that apply to the listener's personal situation.

Effective communicators develop skills in analyzing the teaching situation and responding appropriately. Careful listening and observation assist in developing a helping relationship and successful intervention. (To learn more about working with different cultures, see the Focus on Culture box, "Developing Cross-Cultural Competence: A Goal for the Health Professional.")

The physical environment is important in community education. Look for a location that is familiar to the audience, easily accessible by public transportation, and where the target group will feel comfortable. Choose a setting with adequate space, ventilation, and lighting, and free of distractions.

A community nutrition education program can consist of a few classes or involve extended individual interaction over weeks or months. For healthy individuals looking to make better food choices in the marketplace, one or two sessions may be adequate. Patients with diabetes, renal disease, or acute risk of heart disease, and those at high nutritional risk may require extended classes and follow-up to reach the program goal. (To learn more about using technology in nutrition and health education, see the Evidence-Based Practice box, "New Communication Methods: Are They Effective in Nutrition Education?")

Theories for Behavior Change

Behavioral theories provide a framework for helping us understand why people do what they do and so enable us to target our intervention strategies more effectively.[27,28] Behavior models used in nutrition education have included the health belief model, the concept of self-efficacy, and the stages of change model. We describe each of these below:
- *Health belief model:* Some individuals base their health behavior on how they perceive their vulnerability to a particular disease or condition. Such an individual would need to (1) consider himself or herself at high risk for developing a condition, (2) regard it as a serious threat to personal well-being, and (3) believe that changing his or her behavior would lessen the risk, before making a meaningful change.[29] This model also implies that any barriers to behavior change could be successfully overcome. A young woman planning a pregnancy might begin using a folate supplement to prevent a neural tube defect in her infant or an overweight older adult might begin a walking program to lower his cardiovascular risk.
- *Self-efficacy model:* This theory proposes that behavior change depends on the demands it will make on an individual and his or her perceived ability to cope with the new situation or expected behavior.[22] The greater the person's confidence in his ability to successfully perform the new task or adapt to the new situation, the more likely it is that he will implement the change. Successful interventions work by providing people with the necessary tools or resources to practice the new behavior. Helping frequent travelers develop a list of restaurant items that will fit into a lower-fat eating plan or helping mothers identify ways to add a vegetable to their evening meal increases the likelihood the goal will be achieved.
- *Stages of change:* This model was first developed to address smoking cessation[30] but has been used successfully to modify nutrition and other health behaviors.[31-33] It proposes that individuals pass through five stages of change in adopting a new behavior. How people respond to the information presented and the type of information and resources needed differ according to stage. Table 10-2 outlines the sequence and role of the health professional as applied to an individual or population.

In practice, theories of behavior change are often used together. Individuals passing through the stages of change are more likely to be successful if given tools that increase their

⊕ FOCUS ON CULTURE

Developing Cross-Cultural Competence: A Goal for the Health Professional

Consider the following situations:

- You are teaching pregnant mothers in a public health clinic and using MyPlate (choosemyplate.gov) to evaluate their food intake. A Hmong (Vietnamese) mother tells you that she never eats bread, and you are concerned about her servings from the grains group.
- You are working with an older African-American man, and he mentions that his favorite meal is his daughter's homemade Brunswick stew. What foods are included in that dish?

As a nation we are becoming increasingly diverse. To be effective educators we need to understand the food patterns of other ethnic, racial, and cultural groups, not just our own. We must acknowledge the health beliefs and values that influence individuals' food choices and nutritional status. The Hmong mother may not eat bread, but she is likely to have rice at every meal and thus more than meet her recommended servings of grains. However, she may be reluctant to take the vitamin and mineral supplements her physician recommended in the belief that they will result in a large infant and difficult delivery. The African-American man obtains important vitamins, minerals, fiber, and protein from his Brunswick stew, which is made with chicken, carrots, tomatoes, white beans, and greens.

Value Diversity

Our population includes people from different countries and cultures with different customs. At one time our society was referred to as a *melting pot,* and newcomers were expected to blend their customs and beliefs with the mainstream culture. Health care providers often imposed their beliefs and values on patients from other ethnic or cultural backgrounds. Today we strive to be a *"salad bowl,"* with each person adding a special quality to the mix.

Cross-Cultural Situations

Throughout our professional lives we experience cross-cultural situations in which we belong to a different race, culture, or ethnic group than that of our supervisors, our colleagues, or the individuals for whom we provide care.

We can begin to develop cross-cultural competence in various ways, as follows:

- *Learn about other cultures by reading, observing, and sharing experiences.* A potluck meal provides an opportunity to share foods and the cultural values surrounding food.
- *Examine your own beliefs and feelings.* Identify and resolve any stereotypes that you may hold about groups other than your own.
- *Assess how other cultures view you, and make an effort to present yourself in a positive light.* Develop verbal and nonverbal communication skills applicable to various cultural groups.
- *Consider language training as a means of preparing yourself to work with diverse populations.* Interpreters do not always understand the implications of a particular food or health custom.

Bibliography

Curry KR: Multicultural competence in dietetics and nutrition. *J Am Diet Assoc* 100:1142, 2000.

Goody CM, Drago L, editors: *Cultural food practices*, Chicago, 2010, Diabetes Care and Education Dietetic Practice Group, American Dietetic Association.

Kittler PG, Sucher KP, Nahikian-Nelms M: *Food and culture*, ed 6, Belmont, Calif., 2012, Wadsworth/Cengage Learning.

McCaffree J: Language: a crucial part of cultural competency. *J Am Diet Assoc* 108:611, 2008.

feelings of self-efficacy. As you continue to work in community education, look for clues to indicate your group's current "stage" and let this guide your intervention strategy.

Learning and Behavior

Despite our understanding of behavioral theory, the myth still prevails that an increase in knowledge will result in a change in behavior. Learning follows three basic laws:

1. Learning is *personal* and occurs in response to an individual need. People learn only what they believe will be useful to them, and they retain only what they think they will need. Children are accustomed to learning ideas or facts because they are expected to do so. Adults pay attention only to those principles for which they believe they have an immediate demand.[34] The sooner a person can put new learning to use, the more likely it will be retained. This highlights the importance of providing an opportunity to practice a behavior before the learning session is completed.

2. Learning is *developmental* and builds on prior knowledge and experience. Find out what the learner already knows and to what past experiences the new knowledge can be related.

3. Learning brings *change.* Nutrition education that focuses on learner needs and goals has the greatest chance for success. Encourage your learners to set personal goals rather than using a prescriptive approach.

The Academy of Nutrition and Dietetics recommends a total diet approach for improving nutrient intake.[35] It is the total diet, not one meal or one food, that is important. No one food is a "magic bullet" to health. The three keys are *variety, proportionality, and moderation.* Choose many different foods from each food group: Don't eat the same fruits and vegetables or the same protein foods every day. Consider proportionality: Cover half your plate with fruits and vegetables, with lesser amounts of protein and starch. Finally, encourage moderation: All foods can be included in a healthy diet if used in appropriate amounts and combined with physical activity.

EVIDENCE-BASED PRACTICE

New Communication Methods: Are They Effective in Nutrition Education?

Identify the Problem: Time commitments and transportation costs limit face-to-face nutrition education. The availability of cell phones suggests the use of telecommunication (telephone, email, or text messages) to monitor progress and offer advice when extended follow-up is needed.

Review the evidence: Two well-managed studies compared face-to-face, telephone, and email interventions for the management of weight loss in middle-aged and older men and women. Van Wier and co-workers[1] conducted a 24-month weight reduction program for nearly 1400 employees with an average BMI of 29.6. Participants received either (1) lifestyle brochures encouraging food patterns for weight reduction (the self-help group), (2) lesson modules with telephone counseling following completion of each module, or (3) web-based lesson modules with twice-weekly email messages and opportunity for counseling via email. About the same proportion of participants completed the telephone counseling and email interventions. Weight loss equaled 1.5 kg in the telephone group and 1.9 kg in the email group; the self-help group who received only one mailing lost 1.1 kg. The mean cost of the 2-year intervention was $246 per person in the email group and $279 per person in the telephone group when compared with the self-help group. Neither the telephone nor email strategy was considered to be cost-effective in terms of weight loss when compared with the self-help strategy.

Radcliff and co-workers[2] evaluated several methods of follow-up with older individuals who completed a 6-month weight control program. Here, the goal was weight maintenance rather than weight loss. Participants received either a (1) biweekly newsletter, (2) a biweekly telephone call,

or (3) were invited to a biweekly face-to-face class. The initial weight loss across the three groups was about 7% to 9% of body weight. Over the 12 months of follow-up, the newsletter group regained 3.4 kg, the telephone group, 1.3 kg, and the face-to-face class, 1.1 kg. Costs averaged $47/kg lost and not regained in the face-to-face group and $33/kg lost and not regained in the telephone and newsletter groups. Those researchers concluded that biweekly telephone calls were as effective in preventing regain as the more costly face-to-face method.

Implement the findings: Obesity management will continue to be a major focus of health care in the coming decades and cost-effective intervention methods are still to be found. One-on-one interventions, whether face to face or by telephone, are cost prohibitive if extended over long periods of time. With the growing cohort of adults for whom texting and Internet communication are a way of life, applications using these technologies need to be developed and evaluated.

References
1. van Wier MF, Dekkers JC, Bosmans JE, et al: Economic evaluation of a weight control program with e-mail and telephone counseling among overweight employees: a randomized controlled trial. *Int J Behav Nutr Phy Act* 9:112, 2012.
2. Radcliff TA, Bobroff LB, Lutes LD, et al: Comparing costs of telephone vs face-to-face extended-care programs for the management of obesity in rural settings. *J Acad Nutr Diet* 112:1363, 2012.

FAMILY ECONOMIC NEEDS: FOOD ASSISTANCE PROGRAMS

Families under economic stress often need food assistance to meet nutritional requirements. Programs funded by local communities or the federal government can supply food directly or increase food-purchasing power to provide added nutrients. Federally funded assistance programs usually target specific populations, whereas local food banks are likely to serve all age and gender groups.

U.S. Department of Agriculture Programs

The U.S. Department of Agriculture (USDA) oversees several food assistance programs that help reduce food insecurity. They are intended to increase access to food, promote a healthy diet, and implement nutrition education. It is estimated that one in four Americans participates in a food assistance program.[36] Certain programs are entitlement programs, meaning income guidelines determine eligibility and guarantee participation.

Supplemental Nutrition Assistance Program

The Supplemental Nutrition Assistance Program (SNAP), formerly known as the food stamp program, increases food-purchasing power. SNAP is an entitlement program reaching individuals and families who have incomes within 130% of the federal poverty line. In 2011, nearly 45 million people received monthly SNAP benefits at a cost of over $73 billion, making this the largest U.S. food assistance program.[36] Although SNAP makes a significant contribution to the food resources of low-income families, many recipients still run out of food before the end of the month and rely on local food pantries for help. Legislation authorizing SNAP also includes funds for nutrition education. (Lists of items that may not be purchased with SNAP benefits are found in Appendix E.)

Meal Programs

The School Nutrition Program supervised by the USDA is open to all children. Children from families who meet the federal poverty guidelines receive their lunch free or at reduced cost.[36] When it became apparent that many children were coming to school without breakfast, which seriously impeded their ability to learn, the National School Breakfast Program was put in place.[37] Children eligible for a free or reduced-cost lunch receive breakfast at the same level of payment. Local school districts, recreation departments, and nonprofit community groups that sponsor summer

TABLE 10-2   STAGES OF CHANGE MODEL FOR NUTRITION BEHAVIOR AS APPLIED TO THREE COMMUNITY SITUATIONS*

STAGE	BEHAVIORAL CHARACTERISTICS	STRATEGY	EXAMPLES
Precontemplation	Individuals have no desire or intention to change; may refuse to admit there is a problem	Focus on consciousness-raising; family support may be helpful	A. Public service announcement on need for folate prior to pregnancy B. Poster in school cafeteria about eating fruit for quick energy; add content on healthy snacks in school health class; program for parents on healthy eating for teens C. New diagnosis of elevated blood pressure by physician
Contemplation	Individuals recognize there is a problem and have given some thought to what they might do about it—at some time in the future (this category is often used for those planning to make a change in the next 6 months)	Provide information that might be helpful in addressing the problem	A. Provide printed materials describing food or supplement sources of folate in locations frequented by young women. B. Make leaflets available for pick-up in the school cafeteria suggesting a fruit snack that will fit in a backpack; hang posters advertising a website that compares the kcalories in fruit compared to other snacks C. Provide doctors' offices with printed materials on how to reduce sodium intake, recipes for herbal mixtures to replace sodium, and reputable websites for more information
Preparation	Individual is getting ready to commit to change; this stage provides the foundation for effective action	Seeks resources or tools to support change	A. Young woman checks availability of supplements when shopping; talks with pharmacist or physician about options; talks with significant other about options B. Student checks out the price of fruit and availability at the school snack shop or nearby convenience store (fruit should be available at these locations); talks with parent about putting fruit on the grocery list; looks up the kcalorie content of various fruits on the Internet C. Patient looks for low-sodium recipes on several websites; talks with physician about safety of salt substitutes; joins a class at the local hospital on healthy eating
Action	Individual has implemented at least one behavior change and is trying to practice it regularly (benchmark of 6 months or more)	Encouragement and reinforcement; progress continues despite an occasional relapse	A. Woman takes the folate supplement on most days and tries to have a good folate food source at least once a day B. Student participates in the school food service "snack special" of fresh fruit rather than chips C. Patient tries new low-sodium recipes obtained at the hospital class; adds no salt in cooking and less at the table
Maintenance	Individual has successfully implemented the behavior change for more than 6 months	Continuing encouragement and reinforcement	A. Occasional public service announcement—did you have your folate today? B. School food service continues to "spotlight" a healthy fruit to support availability C. Continued encouragement from health professional with possible improvement in medical condition; reminder poster and new recipe leaflets in doctor's office about sodium intake

- Example A—Increase folate intake among women of childbearing age to prevent neural tube defects
- Example B—Increase use of fruit as a snack among high school youth
- Example C—Reduce sodium intake to lower risk of high blood pressure among adults

education or recreation programs can apply for USDA funds to supply breakfast and lunch meals to these children. This food is especially important for those who depend on school meals for a significant portion of their nutrient intake. (Current regulations for school meals that adhere to the dietary guidelines and help to avoid inappropriate kcalorie intake can be found in Appendix E.)

WIC Program

The WIC program is administered through state health departments.[38] It provides money for food and infant formula through food vouchers or electronic credit to low-income mothers who are pregnant, postpartum, or breast-feeding, and to their infants and children up to the age of five. Both income level and nutritional risk determine eligibility. In this respect WIC differs from entitlement programs as income alone does not guarantee participation. Medical or nutritional risk must be certified by a health care professional for initial and continuing participation, and a federal budgetary ceiling caps national enrollment.

Programs for Older Americans

The Nutrition Program for the Elderly (NPE) enacted under the Older Americans Act is open to all adults age 60 and older, but services are targeted to those in greatest social and economic need. Particular attention is directed to low-income, minority, rural, and low-literacy seniors at risk for institutionalization.[39] Federal dollars are supplemented with state and local funds to meet the growing demand. Meals are served in congregate settings or home-delivered at noon on weekdays. Individuals who receive home-delivered meals must be certified as homebound by a health or social services professional or be responsible for the care of a homebound family member. Participants are encouraged to make a donation toward the cost of the meal. Home-delivered meal programs sponsored by nonprofit community groups have a set

charge but usually offer scholarships for those who cannot afford the full price.

For more information on food assistance programs and required nutrition standards, see Appendix E.

Nutrition Education Opportunities

Food assistance programs offer unique opportunities for nutrition education. Pregnant and nursing mothers participating in WIC are helped with meal planning and use of allowable WIC foods. School lunch programs present children with examples of well-balanced meals with foods from the protein, fruit, vegetable, grain, and dairy groups; breakfast always includes milk or other high-calcium food. Teachers and school health professionals can join together to provide educational experiences that connect the school meal with science and biology, social studies, and health (Table 10-3). In-school nutrition education and meals can address the growing problem of child obesity.[40] For older adults the NPE offers time before or after the meal to address nutrition topics such as limiting sodium intake, low-cost meals for one or two, or good calcium sources.

Expanded Food and Nutrition Education Program/Supplemental Nutrition Assistance Program-Nutrition Education Program

The Expanded Food and Nutrition Education Program (EFNEP)[41] and the Supplemental Nutrition Assistance Program-Nutrition Education Program (SNAP-ED)[42] funded by USDA help limited-resource families learn more about choosing a healthy diet. EFNEP is available to all families who fall below the federal poverty line, whereas SNAP-ED enrolls families receiving SNAP benefits. These programs serve youth and adults and are delivered by Cooperative Extension agents, paraprofessionals, and volunteers. Experiential lessons offer hands-on opportunities to practice skills in food preparation,

TABLE 10-3	NUTRITION EDUCATION IDEAS FOR THE SCHOOL CLASSROOM
SUBJECT	**ACTIVITIES FOR DIFFERENT GRADE LEVELS**
Language arts	Read a story about food; keep a food diary for 3 days; write an article on nutrition for the school newspaper; write a food history of your family.
Mathematics	Using food pictures count out the servings you need from each food group; calculate the kcalories, fat, protein, and carbohydrate in your lunch meal; look at the nutrition label on your favorite candy bar and using the 2000-kcalorie diet level calculate how many grams of fat you have remaining for the rest of the day.
Science	Learn about the nutrients that plants need to grow; trace the paths by which protein, carbohydrate, and fat are broken down in the digestive tract; do some simple microbiological tests before and after washing your hands.
Social studies	Research the different breads that are eaten in various countries and how they are prepared; learn which nutrients must be listed on the nutrition label and how the FDA enforces food labeling; work with the school lunch manager to have an international food day and study the culture of each country.
Art	Draw pictures of foods that we should eat every day; prepare posters advertising healthy foods offered by the school nutrition program; invent a healthy snack and prepare a package and food label.
Health	Draw a picture of a healthy meal including all of the food groups; make a plan giving you 60 min of physical activity every day; keep a food diary for one day and evaluate your intake according to the number of food servings suggested by MyPlate (choosemyplate.gov).

Ideas from Shepherd SK, Whitehead CS: *Team Nutrition's teacher handbook: tips, tools and jewels for busy educators,* Washington, D.C., 1997, U.S. Department of Agriculture.

food safety, and food budgeting. Individuals are recruited through neighborhood contacts, SNAP offices, and WIC. Group classes, media methods, one-on-one instruction, and educational mailings reach different audiences. Follow-up evaluations report that 91% of EFNEP adults increased their daily consumption of fruits and vegetables by an additional cup, and 63% of EFNEP youth began to eat a greater variety of foods.[43]

As you work in the community, it will be important to become familiar with local food assistance programs and make appropriate referrals.

Social Marketing

Social marketing principles can encourage participation in food assistance programs and adoption of appropriate nutrition behaviors. Social marketing applies commercial marketing strategies to the development of educational and public health programs.[44,45] Just as product advertising creates a need on the part of consumers for a particular food or automobile or article of clothing, so appropriate nutrition education messages influence individuals to practice healthy behaviors. Table 10-4 describes the messages prepared by a state education department to advertise their school breakfast program, targeting the needs and values of students, parents, and teachers. Social marketing sometimes addresses barriers associated with a health-related behavior. A WIC breast-feeding initiative emphasized how breast-feeding could be combined with a mother's busy lifestyle.[45] When recommending a food or lifestyle change, consider how it might better health or social well-being. (See further examples of social marketing initiatives in the Further Readings and Resources section at the close of this chapter.)

SELECTING FOOD IN THE MARKETPLACE

Helping people spend their food dollars to best advantage is integral to nutrition education. The USDA has provided various tools and meal plans to assist families with food budgeting and meal planning.

TABLE 10-4	MESSAGES FOR SOCIAL MARKETING
Marketing messages should be fitted to the target audience. The messages below were used to market a school breakfast program.	
AUDIENCE	**MESSAGE**
Students	"Breakfast at school is cool"
Parents	"Your child needs breakfast"
Teachers	"Your students will do better if they eat breakfast"

Data from Herbold N, Taylor PN: Marketing nutrition programs and services. In Edelstein S, editor: *Nutrition in public health. A handbook for developing programs and services*, Sudbury, Mass., 2006, Jones and Bartlett. Adapted from messages developed by the Massachusetts Department of Education.

Food Expenditures

The size and composition of a household influence its food budget. As household size increases, so do food costs, although age and gender make a difference. The weekly food cost of a preschooler is about half that of an adult male, and women and girls consume less food than men and boys.[46] As household income rises, the total amount of money spent for food also rises, but not proportionately. Lower-income households are forced to spend more of their income for food as compared with higher-income households (Figure 10-5).[47] Those with higher incomes may not eat greater amounts of food, but they select more expensive food, buy more prepared items, and eat in restaurants more often.

USDA Food Plans

The USDA has developed several food plans that establish the minimum amounts of money required to purchase food for a month that will meet the DRIs and *Dietary Guidelines* for each age and gender group. They are referred to as *liberal*,

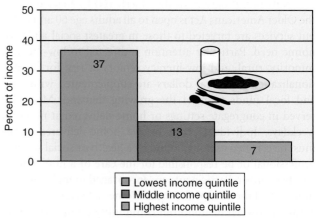

FIGURE 10-5 Proportion of income spent for food. Lower-income families must spend a greater proportion of their income on food than must higher-income families. Lower-income urban families spend 37% of their income on food compared with higher-income urban families, who spend only 7%. (Data from Blisard N, Stewart H: *Food spending in American households, 2003-04*, EIB-23, Washington, D.C., 2007, U.S. Department of Agriculture.)

KEY TERMS

poverty line The minimum amount of income required to provide food, clothing, shelter, and other basic necessities for a family of a given size and composition. This index is used to determine eligibility for government programs such as SNAP or free or reduced-cost school lunches.

paraprofessionals Individuals without a professional degree who work under the supervision of a health professional in providing nutrition education or other health or medical services; paraprofessionals are usually indigenous to the population or community they serve.

moderate, low, and thrifty, with the thrifty plan used to calculate the dollar value of SNAP benefits awarded to an individual or family.[48,49] Each food plan includes a list of grocery items expected to meet the nutritional needs of the targeted group; however, there continue to be concerns regarding the adequacy of the thrifty food plan (TFP). Food-secure households spend 121% of the TFP budget to meet their food needs, whereas food-insecure families spend about 95% of the TFP amount.[9] The USDA food plans are also criticized on the basis that they include many foods that most Americans are not accustomed to eating[20] and require prolonged preparation time that is not practical for working families.[50] To obtain the recommended daily servings of fruits and vegetables, using fresh, frozen, and canned varieties, a family would need to spend 40% of their total TFP allowance.[51] (Examples of food costs allocated by the various plans are found in Table 10-5.)

Developing a Family Food Plan

Each family has a specific amount of money they can spend for food and ideas on how to divide their food dollars. The first step is to identify food resources as well as family values and preferences related to food, because these will enter into their household food plans.

Food Resources

Food can be purchased with available dollars, produced or preserved at home, or obtained through food assistance programs. Vegetables from a home garden can be frozen or canned for later use and families in rural areas may raise animals for meat or eggs. Hunters may supplement their family's food supply with fresh meat. SNAP benefits, WIC, free or reduced-cost school meals, meal programs for older adults, or food pantries add to a family's food.

- *Access to a well-stocked grocery store* with competitive prices is essential to prudent food buying. As supermarkets move from the inner city to suburban areas that offer higher profit margins, people living in downtown urban environments who lack transportation may be forced to food shop at convenience stores with limited selection and higher prices. Older adults may have to shop at the store to which they can get a ride with a neighbor or friend. In rural areas families often drive considerable distances to find a store with a broad selection.

- *Time for food shopping and skills in food management* influence both nutrition and the food budget. Working parents and working students may not take the time to read nutrition labels. Busy adults who never learned to cook may rely on preprepared foods regardless of their nutritional value or cost. In contrast to young adults, retired persons may view store visits as a social experience, although physical limitations can make it difficult to shop and prepare meals.

- *Facilities to store and cook food* are taken for granted by individuals and families who reside in homes or apartments, but the homeless and persons who occupy single rooms lack refrigeration and cooking appliances.

Food Culture and Preferences

Food is a meaningful part of a family's relationships with one another, their neighbors, and friends. Work and school patterns influence when and where family members eat. Other characteristics, as described below, are important in developing a family food plan.

- *Family traditions:* Cultural, ethnic, and national groups have specific food patterns that they wish to continue. Sometimes it is difficult to obtain certain foods or ingredients common to their meal pattern or, if available, they are high in price.

- *Special dietary needs:* Family members observing a sodium-restricted diet or other meal plan related to a chronic condition may need special foods. Severe food-related conditions such as celiac disease require home preparation of many foods and unique ingredients.

TABLE 10-5	EXAMPLES OF USDA FOOD PLANS: AVERAGE COST OF FOOD AT HOME AT FOUR LEVELS*[†‡]			
	MONTHLY COST			
AGE-GENDER GROUPS	**THRIFTY PLAN**	**LOW-COST PLAN**	**MODERATE-COST PLAN**	**LIBERAL PLAN**
2-3–year-old child	$101.40	$128.20	$155.30	$189.00
14-18–year-old male	$169.60	$238.20	$300.00	$345.30
19-50–year-old female	$163.00	$205.60	$253.90	$323.70
Couple, 51-70 years	$360.50	$465.60	$577.00	$693.90
Couple, 19-50 years and children 6-8 and 9-11 years	$636.30	$830.30	$1036.90.	$1256.90

This file may be accessed on CNPP's home page at: <http://www.cnpp.usda.gov/USDAFoodPlansCostofFood.htm>.
*The Food Plans represent a diet at four different cost levels that meets the nutrient requirements outlined in the 1997-2005 *Dietary Reference Intakes*, 2005 *Dietary Guidelines for Americans*, and 2005 MyPyramid food intake recommendations, and assumes that all meals and snacks are prepared at home. For specific foods and quantities, see *Thrifty Food Plan, 2006* (2007) and *The Low-Cost, Moderate-Cost, and Liberal Food Plans, 2007* (2007).
[†]Costs given are for individuals in four-person families.
[‡]February 2013.

- *Amount and kind of entertaining:* Families may enjoy sharing meals or joining potluck socials with neighbors, community organizations, or religious groups.
- *Meals away from home:* Work or school schedules can require meals away from home, either a packed lunch or food purchased at that location. Families may enjoy eating out as part of their social framework.
- *Value placed on food and eating:* Food and mealtime may be an important part of a family's structure and interaction and hold high priority in allocation of resources.

Extended discussion with family members about their food resources and preferences provides a framework for developing and implementing a successful food plan.

Food Shopping
Making Choices

Food marketing is a big business, and buying family food is more complex than it may seem. Currently more than 85,000 uniquely formulated food items are available within U.S. supermarkets,[52] and a single type of food may be marketed in many different ways, each with a different price (Figure 10-6). Supermarket tours are effective strategies for developing decision-making skills and helping consumers become mindful of marketing tactics that draw attention to expensive items low in nutrients. Figure 10-7 and the Perspectives in Practice box, "Supermarket Skills," will help you hone your supermarket skills for teaching others.

Planning Ahead

To ensure a variety of foods and the number of servings recommended in the USDA Food Patterns (see Chapter 1), it is best to plan meals for the week and then develop a shopping list. This involves reviewing the food on hand and checking local newspapers or store flyers for specials on foods the family enjoys. A shopping list helps avoid impulse buying and extra trips to the store. To save time, organize grocery lists in the same order as the supermarket aisles. Individuals should

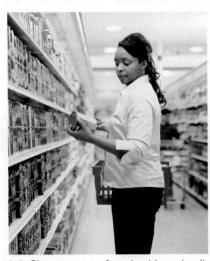

FIGURE 10-6 Shoppers are faced with a dazzling array of food choices. (From Food and Nutrition Service, U.S. Department of Agriculture and Food and Nutrition Information Center, National Agricultural Library: *Food stamp nutrition collection: photo gallery,* Beltsville, Md., 2013, U.S. Department of Agriculture. from: <grande.nal.usda.gov/viewer.php?file=fs_recipes/imgs/shopping/shopping_vertical.jpg&file_loc=shopping_vertical.jpg>. Retrieved April 3, 2013. Reprinted with permission.)

Before shopping, I:	Hardly ever	Sometimes	Most of the time
Check to see what foods I have on hand	☐	☐	☐
Plan meals to include a variety of foods from each of the major food groups	☐	☐	☐
Plan food purchases to limit amounts of fat, sugars, and sodium	☐	☐	☐
Consider how much money I have to spend on food	☐	☐	☐
Make a shopping list	☐	☐	☐
While shopping, I:			
Read ingredient labels, watching for ingredients that provide fat, sugars, and sodium	☐	☐	☐
Use nutrition labels to help select food products	☐	☐	☐
Use open dating information to ensure quality and freshness	☐	☐	☐
Use unit pricing (when available) to compare prices	☐	☐	☐
After shopping, I:			
Store foods promptly and properly to maintain their nutritive value and quality	☐	☐	☐
Place newer foods in the back of refrigerator, freezer, and cabinet shelves, so older foods will be used first	☐	☐	☐
Use perishable foods promptly to avoid food waste	☐	☐	☐

FIGURE 10-7 The Super Shopper Checklist. Most people follow a general routine when they shop for food. Have the participants in your nutrition education class check the boxes that best describe what they do before, during, and after each trip to the supermarket. If "most of the time" is their answer, they are making best use of their food dollars. (From U.S. Department of Agriculture: *Shopping for food and making meals in minutes using the dietary guidelines,* Home and Garden Bulletin No 232-10, Human Nutrition Information Center, Hyattsville, Md., U.S. Department of Agriculture.)

PERSPECTIVES IN PRACTICE

Supermarket Skills

As shoppers try to make healthy food choices, "supermarket savvy" is a pertinent topic for nutrition education. Supermarket tours help consumers not only develop more awareness of cost and nutrient quality but also recognize the marketing techniques and triggers for impulse buying.

When to shop: Advertised specials available at the beginning of the week are sometimes sold out by the end of the week. In that case ask for a "rain check" if this is an item you use. Weekdays are the best times to shop as stores are less crowded, allowing more time and space for comparison shopping. Avoid Saturdays and dinnertime through the week as stores are congested and checkout lines are long.

Wise use of coupons: Food manufacturers and grocery chains offer coupons in the newspaper, online, and in food packages. There are downsides to coupons: You may have to buy several packages or the largest size container to use your coupon or be enticed to buy something you don't need because it is "50 cents off." Also, the store brand at full price may be the equivalent or less than the national brand with a coupon. Make your shopping list first and then see if any of your coupons match; limit coupon use to those foods you use regularly.

Store layout: Displays at the ends of the aisles are set up for sale items but also are used for new or slow-moving items. Don't assume that cans or packages marked "special" are being sold at a cheaper price. Check the cost per ounce or unit to discern a true sale. National brands and more expensive items are usually placed at waist or neck level; check the prices of the items on the bottom shelf as well.

The inner aisles of a grocery store contain less expensive staples such as legumes, peanut butter, dried milk, canned tuna fish, bulk cereals, and canned vegetables and fruits. Fresh produce is usually at the front as you come in, as it

is a high-profit item and subject to impulse buying. In-store bakeries and delicatessens are also among the first counters you pass as you begin your shopping. Be alert to these incentives to buy food that you do not need or cannot afford.

Unit pricing: Unit pricing is a helpful tool for comparison shopping but be cautious when comparing a frozen with a canned product. Frozen vegetables contain little or no liquid as compared with canned vegetables that may contain as much as one-third liquid. Even if the canned item costs less per ounce, it may not be a better buy based on the actual amount of food obtained. Measure the liquid in the canned fruits and vegetables that you purchase regularly to calculate the real cost.

The USDA Cooperative Extension Service found in every state and county is a source of both print and online materials to help consumers develop food shopping skills.

Bibliography

Aase S: Supermarket trends: how increased demand for healthful products and services will affect food and nutritional professionals. *J Am Diet Assoc* 107:1286, 2007.

Kansas State Cooperative Extension Service: *We know … tips to trim food costs, MK-32,* Manhattan, Kan., 2008, Kansas State University.

United States Department of Agriculture: *Smart shopping for fruits and vegetables: 10 Tips Nutrition Education Series, DG Tip Sheet No 9,* 2011, Center for Nutrition Policy and Promotion. at: <http://www.choosemyplate.gov/foodgroups/downloads/TenTips/DGTipsheet9SmartShopping .pdf>. Accessed on March 11, 2013.

University of Kentucky Cooperative Extension Service: *Supermarket savvy, FAM-RHF 131,* Lexington, Ky., 2004, University of Kentucky College of Agriculture.

---

avoid shopping when they are hungry or rushed because then they will be more likely to buy items that they do not need or cannot afford. Limit shopping to once a week, using frozen or canned items after fresh foods have been exhausted.

Buying Wisely

Food labels contain important information about food quantity, quality, and safety, and help consumers get the best value for their food dollar. The following information on the food label and store shelf is useful when comparing prices:

- *Unit pricing:* Large packages are sometimes less expensive per unit weight than small packages, but any savings depends on how much of the product is needed and if it can be used before spoiling. If an item has an extended shelf life or is used regularly, then one large box rather than two smaller boxes is a wise choice. The unit pricing label on the store shelf indicates the true price per unit weight and can be used to compare different brands or package sizes (Box 10-2). Unit pricing tells you if the store brand costs less than the national brand for which you are also paying the cost of advertising and any special offers.

- *Open dating:* These dates indicate the freshness of an item or how soon it must be used. Box 10-3 describes the types of dating information used on food labels. Checking the "use by" date is important when considering items reduced for quick sale.

- *Package weight or volume:* Check the food label and the nutrition facts label to determine the contents of a package by weight or volume and the number of servings it contains. Deceptive packaging can suggest that the food content is greater than it actually is.

- *List of ingredients:* Ingredients are listed by weight, from the highest to the lowest, on the food label. As described in Figure 10-8, fruit drinks contain sugar, water, and flavoring but little or no juice. When purchasing bread or cereal, make certain the first ingredient is a whole grain.

- *Convenience foods:* Use comparison shopping to evaluate the relative cost and time benefit of preprepared items, as time saved may not be worth the added cost. Fresh fruits and vegetables peeled and cut into bite-sized pieces and items packaged in single servings are handy when assembling lunches or grabbing snacks, but they cut into the

BOX 10-2 UNIT PRICING

The unit price is the price per pound, ounce, quart, or serving. Unit price labels are found on the display shelves or below canned and packaged foods. Comparing unit prices can help consumers find the brand and size container that costs the least per unit.

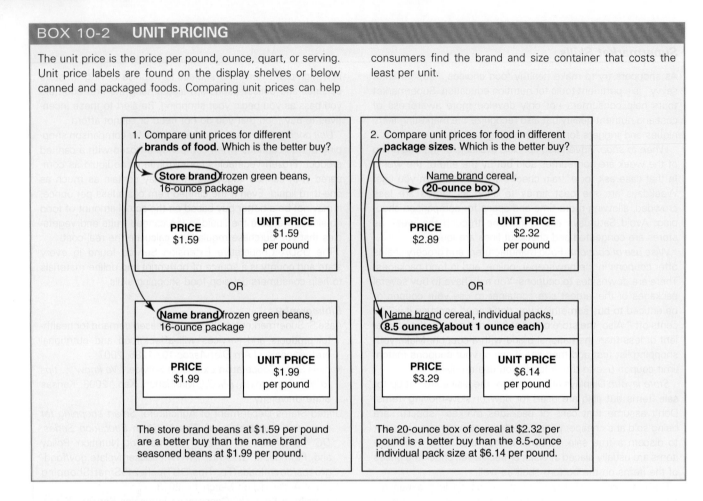

1. Compare unit prices for different **brands of food**. Which is the better buy?

Store brand frozen green beans, 16-ounce package

| PRICE $1.59 | UNIT PRICE $1.59 per pound |

OR

Name brand frozen green beans, 16-ounce package

| PRICE $1.99 | UNIT PRICE $1.99 per pound |

The store brand beans at $1.59 per pound are a better buy than the name brand seasoned beans at $1.99 per pound.

2. Compare unit prices for food in different **package sizes**. Which is the better buy?

Name brand cereal, **20-ounce box**

| PRICE $2.89 | UNIT PRICE $2.32 per pound |

OR

Name brand cereal, individual packs, **8.5 ounces** (about 1 ounce each)

| PRICE $3.29 | UNIT PRICE $6.14 per pound |

The 20-ounce box of cereal at $2.32 per pound is a better buy than the 8.5-ounce individual pack size at $6.14 per pound.

BOX 10-3 TYPES OF OPEN DATING ON FOOD LABELS

Sell by	The last date the item can be sold by the store
Best if used by	The date that indicates maximum freshness; after this date check for signs of spoilage and expect a reduced price
Expiration date or use by	The last date when active ingredients will be good (commonly used with yeast for baking); do not purchase foods after their expiration date as spoilage may have occurred even if not visible
Pack date	The date when the food was packed; this date is commonly found on canned foods; look for a recent pack date

food budget. To save money carrots could be peeled and packaged in plastic bags over the weekend for use in lunches the next week. Pancake or muffin mixes or pre-cooked meat loaves are not a prudent choice on limited food dollars. Table 10-6 provides examples of added cost to preprepared items.

Cooking Food Well

Nutrition education for meal preparers should emphasize food preparation methods that maximize food nutrient content but also promote the joy of eating. Using herbs and spices to replace salt produces good-tasting food that supports health. Broiling, grilling, or baking rather than frying reduces fat and kcalories. People eat because they are hungry and because food looks and tastes good. Recipes that are cost-effective, nutritious, and attractive help busy meal preparers, especially if they are simple and easy to remember. Many supermarket chains provide healthy recipes on their websites or in their weekly flyers that use store specials.[53] Food demonstrations or hands-on classes with tasting are effective ways to model appropriate food safety and food preparation techniques, and confirm that healthy food is good to eat. (See Box 10-4 for suggestions on planning healthy and attractive menus.)

HEALTH PROMOTION

USDA Food Pattern

The USDA Food Patterns and practical advice found on MyPlate (choosemyplate.gov) guide the development of menus that include all food groups and meet nutritional needs. Think first about fruits and vegetables and aim for a

Ingredient Listing

Ingredients are listed in order from the most to the least amount found in the product.

Grape Juice:

Grape juice, grape juice from concentrate, ascorbic acid (vitamin C). No artificial flavors or colors added

Grape Juice Drink:
(10% Grape Juice)

Water; high fructose corn syrup; sugar; grape juice concentrate; fumaric, citric, and maltic acids (provide tartness); vitamin C; natural flavor; artificial color

Powdered Grape Drink:

Sugar, citric acid (provides tartness), natural and artificial flavor, artificial color, vitamin C

This label tells you:

- Mostly grape juice and juice concentrate
- Vitamin C added

This label tells you:

- Mostly added water, syrup, and sugar
- Some grape juice
- Vitamin C added, plus other things

This label tells you:

- Mostly sugar
- No juice at all
- Vitamin C added, plus other things

FIGURE 10-8 Products with similar names can have very different ingredients and nutrient content. Read labels carefully to know what you are receiving for your money. (From U.S. Department of Agriculture: *Do you use unit prices to find the best buys? Make your food dollars count,* Program Aid No 1345, Washington, D.C., 1984, U.S. Department of Agriculture.)

TABLE 10-6   COST COMPARISONS OF HOME-PREPARED AND PREPREPARED FOODS

FOOD*	RAW INGREDIENTS	PREPREPARED	ADDITIONAL PREPARATION
Vegetables			
Carrots	Unpeeled and uncut	Small baby carrots peeled and washed	Shredded carrots
	3-oz serving (raw) at 15 cents	3-oz serving (raw) at 27 cents	3-oz serving (raw) at 60 cents
Broccoli	Frozen flowerets in family-size bag	Frozen spears in family-size bag	Frozen spears with cheese sauce
	3-oz serving at 31 cents	3-oz serving at 48 cents	3-oz serving at 90 cents
Potatoes	Fresh potatoes (from 10-lb bag; cooked and mashed with milk)	Instant mashed potatoes (milk added)	Refrigerated mashed potatoes (ready to heat)
	½ cup at 17 cents	½ cup at 24 cents	½ cup at 60 cents
Protein Foods			
Chicken	Raw chicken breasts (bone-in) at $2.79 per pound	Raw chicken breasts (boneless, skinless, and thin-sliced) at $4.99 per pound	Chicken breast cutlets (breaded and ready to heat) at $7.84 per pound
Ground beef	Ground chuck hamburger (80% lean)	Ground chuck hamburger preshaped into patties (80% lean)	Meat loaf refrigerated and ready to heat
	3-oz serving (cooked wt) at $0.87	3-oz serving (cooked wt) at $1.12	3-oz serving (heated) at $1.83
Grains			
Oatmeal	Old-fashioned oats (water added)	Quick 1-minute oats (water added)	Instant oatmeal, unflavored (water added)
	¾-cup serving at 6 cents	¾-cup serving at 6 cents	¾-cup serving (one packet) at 25 cents
Pancakes	Homemade batter	Dry pancake mix, egg and milk added	Ready to pour batter
	One 4-inch pancake at 6 cents	One 4-inch pancake at 11 cents	One 4-inch pancake at 22 cents
Sweets			
Chocolate chip cookie	Homemade cookie batter	Refrigerated cookie dough (preportioned)	Packaged cookie (in-store bakery)
	One 2 ½-inch cookie at 6 cents	One 2-inch cookie at 12 cents	One 2-inch cookie at 25 cents

*Costs based on market prices at the Kroger store in Blacksburg, Va., March 2014. Store brands used if available for all three food comparisons.

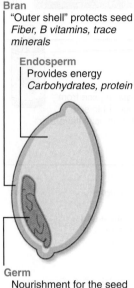

Whole grain kernel

Bran
"Outer shell" protects seed
Fiber, B vitamins, trace minerals

Endosperm
Provides energy
Carbohydrates, protein

Germ
Nourishment for the seed
Antioxidants, vitamin E, B vitamins

FIGURE 10-9 Nutrients in the bran and germ of whole grains are lost when grains are refined and the bran and germ are discarded. Current laws require that processed grains be enriched with thiamin, riboflavin, niacin, iron, and folate; however, other important nutrients such as zinc and vitamin E, also lost in processing, are not replaced. (From U.S. Department of Agriculture: *Get on the grain train: putting the guidelines into practice*, Home and Garden Bulletin No 267-2, Washington, D.C., 2002, U.S. Department of Agriculture.)

variety over the course of the week. A mix of fresh, frozen, and canned fruits and vegetables, depending on season and price, will meet financial constraints yet supply important vitamins and minerals. Home gardening or container gardening increases the availability of vegetables at reduced cost. In urban locations community gardens offer opportunities for youth and family participation.

Grain foods are well liked, relatively inexpensive, and offer many varieties for different meal plans. Whole grains are rich in fiber and especially high in trace minerals (Figure 10-9). At least three of our daily servings of grains should be whole grains.

Meat, fish, poultry, and eggs are complete proteins and supply B-complex vitamins and trace minerals. Eggs are relatively inexpensive and easy to prepare, and for most people, one egg a day is acceptable. Fish contributes omega-3 fatty acids (for a review of mercury advisories regarding fish consumption, see Chapter 9). Trimming visible fat and skin from meat and poultry reduces total fat and saturated fat. Dried beans and peas and nuts are good sources of amino acids and when combined with other plant proteins or small amounts of animal protein create a complete protein. Legumes are low in fat, high in fiber, versatile in food preparation, and easy to store. Soy protein is used to make tofu and added to chips, pasta, trail mix, and other prepared foods.

Dairy foods provide protein, calcium, and magnesium, and most milks and yogurts are fortified with vitamin D. Fat-free, low-fat, and reduced-fat milk and dairy foods are lower in kcalories and total and saturated fat. Fortified soy milk is an appropriate substitute for dairy foods.

Fats and oils supply essential fatty acids and concentrated kcalories for those with high energy needs. Polyunsaturated and monounsaturated oils are the best choices and supply vitamin E. Hydrogenated fats often include *trans* fatty acids, which are harmful to health, so consumers should check the nutrition facts label. Butter, high in saturated fat and a source of cholesterol, is best used in limited amounts. (Box 10-5 provides shopping hints for all major food groups; review Table 1-2 for detailed nutrient content of food groups.) (See the Case Study box, "Helping with Family Shopping" to apply principles of food shopping and planning.)

Food Shopping Locations
Supermarkets and Supercenters

Large grocery stores and supermarkets carry a wide variety of fresh and processed foods at reasonable prices. When several food outlets are close by, individuals can select where they want to shop or vary their location depending on the particular specials for the week. Many supercenters and convenience stores stocking groceries also sell a wide variety of nonfood merchandise.[54] Unfortunately, in many lower-income areas convenience stores make up at least two thirds of available food outlets,[55] and they often have higher prices and limited selections of healthy foods. A Florida survey reported that only 36% of convenience stores offered gallon

BOX 10-5   GETTING THE MOST FOR YOUR FOOD DOLLAR

Fruits and Vegetables

- Buy fresh fruits and vegetables in season when they cost less. Visit a farmers' market or a pick-your-own outlet to save money and enjoy a fun family activity.
- Choose produce that is firm, crisp, and free of brown or soft spots.
- Compare costs of fresh fruits and vegetables sold by weight or count. Look for the number of items in bags sold by weight.
- Check the cost of store brands versus national brands when buying canned vegetables and fruits. Avoid fancy grades that are priced higher. Grading is based on shape, size, and perfection of pieces; lower grades are equal in food value and taste.
- Compare the cost of family-size bags versus individual packages of frozen vegetables. It may be more economical to buy the family-size bag and pour out what you need. Return the unused portion to the freezer immediately to prevent thawing and loss of quality. Avoid frozen vegetables with special sauces that add to cost, fat, and sodium.
- If possible, select juice- or water-packed canned fruits rather than syrup-packed with added sugar. If using syrup-packed fruit, rinse before serving.
- If possible, select no-salt-added canned vegetables, or rinse the higher-sodium product before using.

Breads and Cereals

- Check the weight of bread loaves when comparing price, as a large loaf may not weigh more than a small loaf; higher-priced breads advertised as containing fewer kcalories may be cut into thinner slices.
- Look for whole grain breads or cereals; the word *whole* should appear first on the ingredient list. Varieties include whole wheat, whole oats, oatmeal, whole rye, or whole grain corn or corn meal. (Popped corn is an easy, whole grain snack.)
- Avoid grain products with a sugar as the first or second ingredient. It is more economical to add your own sugar to cereal and control the amount added; sugars commonly found on food labels include sucrose, fructose, molasses, honey, corn syrup, and high-fructose corn syrup (HFCS).
- Cereals providing 100% of the DRIs for many vitamins and minerals cost more; if you eat a good diet, these additional nutrients may be unnecessary. Look for those nutrients that you really need; if you eat daily multiple servings of these cereals you may be reaching the Tolerable Upper Intake Level (UL) for certain micronutrients.
- Bulgur, buckwheat, barley, and millet can be used in place of rice or potatoes; bulgur is cooked like rice and has a toast-like color and wheat flavor.

- Emphasize less-processed grains. Highly processed grains lose nutrients and fiber.

Meat, Fish, Poultry, and Eggs

- Eggs are sold according to grade and size but do not differ in nutrients. Shell color varies according to the breed of chicken but nutrients are the same.
- Check the expiration date on fresh poultry as it has a relatively short shelf life; boneless chicken is more expensive because you are paying for convenience.
- Fresh fish spoils quickly and a "fishy" odor indicates it is several days old; if fresh fish will not be used in 1 or 2 days, it is best to freeze it. Canned tuna is a good buy; water-packed tuna is lower in kcalories than oil-packed tuna.
- Lower grades of beef are less expensive and lower in fat. Beef roasts keep safely in the refrigerator for several days, but ground meat with greater exposure to the air and potential pathogens should be used in 1 to 2 days or frozen.
- Trim all visible fat from beef, pork, or ham before cooking.

Milk, Cheese, and Other Dairy Foods

- Fluid milk is sold with varying levels of fat: nonfat, 1% (low fat), 2% (reduced fat), or 3.3% (whole milk); for persons above 2 years of age, nonfat, reduced fat, or low fat is best. Canned evaporated milk with a long shelf life is available in fat and nonfat forms.
- Nonfat dried milk is low in cost and can be added to casseroles, mashed potatoes, or soups to increase their nutrient content; reconstituted nonfat dried milk mixed 1:1 with fluid milk is an economical and palatable milk for drinking.
- Families using large amounts of milk will find it economical to buy gallon jugs; be sure to check the "sell by" date when buying fluid milk (see Box 10-3).
- Natural cheeses such as cheddar or Swiss contain more calcium and vitamins and are lower in fat and sodium than processed cheeses; cheeses packaged in individual slices cost more per pound than block cheeses. Shredded cheese is higher in price than a similar weight sold in wedges or blocks.
- Cottage cheese contains less calcium than an equal measure of milk or yogurt, and is higher in sodium. Be sure to check the expiration date before purchase.

Fats and Oils

- Liquid oils are high in polyunsaturated fats and must be stored tightly closed in a cool dry place.
- Partially hydrogenated fats (soft-tub fats) are good table fats, but check the label to avoid *trans* fatty acids. Margarines with added plant sterols are higher in price.

---

sizes of low-fat milk, and the price varied from $2.22 in supermarkets to $5.09 in convenience stores. Only 7% of convenience stores carried whole wheat bread and none offered fresh vegetables.[55] When supermarkets are available in lower-income communities they are often smaller and older, have fewer checkout lines, and are open fewer hours.

Policy makers have begun to identify census tracts with high poverty rates and low food access as *food deserts*. An area in which the poverty rate reaches 20% and at least 500 people or one third of the population live at least 1 mile (if urban) or 10 miles (if rural) from the nearest supermarket or large grocery store is designated a food desert. About two

CASE STUDY

Helping with Family Shopping

Your manager at the local WIC office has asked you to assist a family with their food selection. She is concerned about the nutrient intakes of the mother and children, and their food shopping and food preparation practices. The family consists of three adults: a woman age 26, two men ages 27 and 69, and two children ages 5 and 2. Both children receive WIC food allocations. The mother goes food shopping daily, buying already prepared main dishes and any meat, dairy, and grain foods reduced for quick sale. To save money, she tries to use it all regardless of expiration or "use by" dates. She seldom buys fresh fruits and vegetables because they seem to be expensive, but fruit drinks are a family favorite.

Questions for Analysis

1. Based on the food plans developed by the USDA, what is the minimum amount of money this family must spend on food to meet their nutritional requirements?
2. Which questions would you ask this homemaker about her shopping practices?
3. What advice would you give her about food-buying practices to ensure food safety? Which family members are most vulnerable to foodborne illness? (Review Chapter 9 as needed.)
4. Which suggestions could you give her about less expensive forms of fruits and vegetables? (See Box 10-5 and Table 10-6.) Are fruit drinks a good use of her food dollars?
5. Develop a three-day menu for the family observing the USDA Food Patterns or MyPlate (choosemyplate.gov) recommendations for each food group and making use of all WIC foods available to the children. Prepare a shopping list for the purchase of needed foods. (See Appendix E for a list of WIC foods.)

thirds of food deserts are in urban locations and encompass nearly 24 million persons.[56] Individuals who lack vehicles are dependent on public transportation to food shop, and such services are scarce in rural communities. Rural residents may need to travel 20 miles or more to reach a supermarket.[57] Various city governments have begun to work with neighborhood groups to improve access to food supplies.[58] Healthy People 2020 identified the need for government incentives to encourage new food outlets in areas with low access to healthy foods.[23]

Farmers' Markets

Farmers' markets bring local produce to consumers at prices that can be lower than at supermarkets. Local fruits and vegetables are often considered to be fresher and look and taste better than similar items from a grocery store. Buying local produce also supports a local sustainable farm system.[59] WIC participants can receive vouchers to use at farmers' markets, and national initiatives are assisting older adults in accessing such outlets.

Consumer Cooperatives

Consumer cooperatives offer high-quality foods at the lowest possible price. Food cooperatives usually deal in bulk sales of whole or minimally processed foods and emphasize locally grown foods. Cooperatives usually require volunteer time from each member in addition to or in lieu of a membership fee.

Food Discount Stores

Food stores that stock fresh and processed foods, paper goods, and cleaning supplies at discount prices are growing in popularity. These stores offer few services and furnishings are sparse; however, items are usually lower in price. Processed foods sold at food discount stores may be closeouts or excess stock that is nearing its date of expiration or best use. Multiple cans or packages often make up the unit sold, so consumers must decide if the quantity being purchased can be used before spoilage occurs.

Food Banks

Food banks are warehouses that collect and store donations of food from supermarkets, food processors, food distributors, growers, and the general public. These foods are made available to soup kitchens or food pantries providing meals or groceries to those in need. Food pantries offer emergency assistance when a family is in need of food and has no resources to purchase food. Food banks across the United States distribute more than 3 billion pounds of food each year.[60] The USDA contributes over $350 million worth of commodity foods for distribution by emergency food providers.[61] (See Appendix E to learn more about commodity foods and the food items available.)

▌ TO SUM UP

Malnutrition and food shortages exist worldwide. International agencies support short-term interventions in response to famine and immediate food shortages, but also introduce agricultural interventions to increase the food supply in vulnerable locations. Such problems are complex as the increasing availability of added sugar and fats has led to growing obesity in both developed and developing nations, and some countries experience the double burden of both overweight and undernutrition. Public health interventions and community nutrition education programs help individuals and families learn to make appropriate food choices. To be successful, community education programs require careful assessment and planning. Behavioral models can help us understand how people change their behavior and assist us in developing strategies that lead to positive change. The health belief model, concept of self-efficacy, and stages of change are behavior models often used in the development of community nutrition programs. Many families under economic stress need help in obtaining the appropriate amounts and types of food. Food assistance programs add to a family's food resources and many also deliver nutrition education. Referral of clients with food needs to appropriate agencies is an important component of nutrition intervention.

QUESTIONS FOR REVIEW

1. How would you define "health"? How does it apply to nutrition education?

2. Perform a needs assessment of your county or city. Review race or ethnicity, income, age, household type, employment, language spoken at home, number of families receiving SNAP benefits, and number of children receiving school breakfast and lunch at free or reduced-cost. (a) What are food-related issues in your community? (b) What seem to be major causes of these food-related issues? (c) Which local programs exist to help meet these needs? (d) Are available programs applicable to diverse population groups? Explain. (Go to www.census.gov and select a state, then county or city to access local census statistics; state departments of education and social services post SNAP and school meal statistics according to locality; local websites are sources of available programs.)

3. Based on your needs assessment, develop a community nutrition program to address one of the issues you identified. Provide an overall goal, specific objectives, an action plan, and how you will evaluate its success. Name other health professionals or community programs or facilities that would be potential partners.

4. List the three basic principles of learning. Apply these principles to one of the following situations: (a) a low-income Hispanic mother with limited English skills whose 2-year-old son is underweight for his age or (b) a 71-year-old woman with hypertension who has been told to lower her sodium intake.

5. What is meant by food insecurity? How would you determine if a patient was food-insecure?

6. Using your local telephone directory or the Internet, compile a list of government agencies and other organizations in your community that provide food assistance. As a class project prepare a pamphlet or booklet for distribution that lists the organization, contact information, type of assistance provided, and any requirements or qualifications for receiving assistance. Distribute the booklet to local programs such as free clinics or food pantries that serve low-income families.

7. Review the various types of information provided on the food label that describe package contents, freshness, and safe handling. Develop a handout to teach these concepts to a low-literacy audience.

8. Using unit pricing, compare the cost per serving of four different ready-to-eat cereals: (a) one sugar-coated cereal, (b) one granola cereal, (c) one whole grain cereal, and (4) one cereal advertised as meeting 100% of the DRIs. Which is the most expensive per serving, and which is the least expensive per serving? Which cereal provides the best nutritional value for the money? Why?

9. Obtain a global positioning satellite (GPS) navigational device or map of your city or county. Using the telephone directory or the Internet, identify supermarkets or discount food stores and input their location. Are there neighborhoods or areas that do not have access to a large grocery store or supermarket? Visit the Food Environment Atlas maintained by the U.S. Department of Agriculture and determine if your locality has been designated a food desert (http://www.ers.usda.gov/data-products/food-environment-atlas.aspx#.UUDP1aWhCFI).

REFERENCES

1. Walker P, John M, editors: *From public health to wellbeing. The new driver for policy and action*, New York, 2012, Palgrave/Macmillan.

2. World Health Organization, Pan American Health Organization, Caribbean Private Sector Response to Chronic Diseases: *What is health and wellness? The seven dimensions of wellness*, Geneva, Switzerland, 2008, World Health Organization. at: <http://www.paho.org/english/ad/dpc/nc/7-dimensions-wellness.pdf>. Accessed on March 4, 2013.

3. Shetty PS: Food and nutrition. In Detels R, Beaglehole R, Lansang MA, et al, editors: *Oxford textbook of public health. The scope of public health*, vol 1, ed 5, New York, 2009, Oxford University Press.

4. Fanzo JC, Pronyk PM: A review of global progress toward the Millennium Development Goal 1 hunger target. *Food Nutr Bull* 32(2):144, 2011.

5. von Braun J: Food insecurity, hunger and malnutrition: necessary policy and technology changes. *New Biotech* 27(5):449, 2010.

6. Academy of Nutrition and Dietetics: Position of the Academy of Nutrition and Dietetics: nutrition security in developing nations: sustainable food, water, and health. *J Acad Nutr Diet* 113:581, 2013.

7. American Dietetic Association: Position of the American Dietetic Association: addressing world hunger, malnutrition, and food insecurity. *J Am Diet Assoc* 103:1046, 2003.

8. Tanumihardjo SA, Anderson C, Kaufer-Horwitz M, et al: Poverty, obesity, and malnutrition: an international

perspective recognizing the paradox. *J Am Diet Assoc* 107:1966, 2007.

9. Coleman-Jensen A, Nord M, Andrews M, et al: *Household food security in the United States in 2011, Economic Research Report No 141*, Washington, D.C., 2012, U.S. Department of Agriculture, Economic Research Service. Accessed at: <http://www.ers.usda.gov/publications/err-economic-research-report/err141.aspx>.

10. Dinour LM, Bergen D, Yeh M-C: The food insecurity—obesity paradox: a review of the literature and the role food stamps may play. *J Am Diet Assoc* 107:1952, 2007.

11. Finucane MM, Stevens GA, Cowan MJ, et al: National, regional, and global trends in body-mass index since 1980: systematic analysis of health examination surveys and epidemiological studies with 960 country-years and 9.1 million participants. *Lancet* 377:557, 2011.

12. Popkin BM, Adair LS, Ng SW: Global nutrition transition and the pandemic of obesity in developing countries. *Nutr Reviews* 70(1):3, 2011.

13. Kraak VI, Story M: A public health perspective on healthy lifestyles and public-private partnerships for global childhood obesity prevention. *J Am Diet Assoc* 110(2):192, 2010.

14. Bruening M, MacLehose R, Loth K, et al: Feeding a family in a recession: food insecurity among Minnesota parents. *Am J Public Health* 102(3):520, 2012.

15. Pingali PL: Green revolution: impacts, limits, and the path ahead. *Proc Natl Acad Sci U S A* 109(31):12302, 2012.

16. Popkin BM: Agricultural policies, food and public health. *EMBO Rep* 12(1):11, 2011.

17. Richards R, Smith C: The impact of homeless shelters on food access and choice among homeless families in Minnesota. *J Nutr Educ Behav* 38:96, 2006.

18. Hiza HA, Casavale KO, Guenther PM, et al: Diet quality of Americans differs by age, sex, race/ethnicity, income, and education level. *J Acad Nutr Diet* 113:297, 2013.

19. Aggarwal A, Monsivais P, Drewnoski A: Nutrient intakes linked to better health outcomes are associated with higher diet costs in the US. *PLoS ONE* 7(5):e37533, 2012.

20. Drewnowski A, Eichelsdoerfer P: Can low-income Americans afford a healthy diet? *Nutr Today* 44(6):246, 2010.

21. Drewnowski A: The cost of US foods as related to their nutritive value. *Am J Clin Nutr* 92:1181, 2010.

22. Holli BB, O'Sullivan-Maillet J, Beto JA, et al: *Communication and education skills for dietetics professionals*, ed 5, Philadelphia, Pa., 2009, Lippincott Williams & Wilkins.

23. United States Department of Health and Human Services: *Healthy People 2020: improving the health of Americans, 2020 Topics and Objectives*, Washington, D.C., 2013, U.S. Department of Health and Human Services. at: <http://www.healthypeople.gov/2020/topicsobjectives2020/default.aspx>. Accessed on August 12, 2013.

24. Centers for Disease Control and Prevention: *The burden of chronic diseases and their risk factors: national and state perspectives*, Atlanta, Ga., 2004, U.S. Department of Health and Human Services.

25. Goody CM, Drago L, editors: *Cultural food practices*, Chicago, 2010, Diabetes Care and Education Dietetic Practice Group, American Dietetic Association.

26. Moreschi JM: Planning and evaluating nutrition services for the community. In Edelstein S, editor: *Nutrition in public health. A handbook for developing programs and services*, Sudbury, Mass., 2006, Jones and Bartlett.

27. Baranowski T: Advances in basic behavioral research will make the most important contributions to effective dietary change programs at this time. *J Am Diet Assoc* 106:808, 2006.

28. Coleman MT, Pasternak RH: Effective strategies for behavior change. *Prim Care* 39(2):281, 2012.

29. Boyle MA: *Community nutrition in action: an entrepreneurial approach*, Belmont, Calif., 2003, Wadsworth/Thomson Learning.

30. Prochaska JO, Norcross JC, Diclemente CC: *Changing for good: a revolutionary six-stage program for overcoming bad habits and moving your life positively forward*, New York, 1994, Quill.

31. Hildebrand DA, Shriver LH: A quantitative and qualitative approach to understanding fruit and vegetable availability in low-income African-American families with children enrolled in an urban Head Start program. *J Am Diet Assoc* 110:710, 2010.

32. Wyker BA, Jordan P, Quigley DL: Evaluation of Supplemental Nutrition Assistance Program education: application of behavioral theory and survey validation. *J Nutr Educ Behav* 44(4):360, 2012.

33. Mays D, Gerfen E, Mosher RB, et al: Validation of a milk consumption Stage of Change algorithm among adolescent survivors of childhood cancer. *J Nutr Educ Behav* 44(5):464, 2012.

34. Kicklighter JR: Characteristics of older adult learners: a guide for dietetics practitioners. *J Am Diet Assoc* 91(11):1418, 1991.

35. Academy of Nutrition and Dietetics: Position of the Academy of Nutrition and Dietetics: total diet approach to healthy eating. *J Acad Nutr Diet* 113(2):307, 2013.

36. United States Department of Agriculture: *The food assistance landscape: FY 2011 annual report*, Washington, D.C., 2012, Economic Research Service. at: <http://www.ers.usda.gov/publications/eib-economic-information-bulletin/eib93.aspx>. Accessed on March 10, 2013.

37. Food Research and Action Center: *Federal food nutrition programs. School breakfast program*, Washington, D.C., 2012, 1875 Connecticut Ave, NW. at: <http://frac.org/federal-foodnutrition-programs/school-breakfast-program/>. Accessed on March 10, 2013.

38. U.S. Department of Agriculture: *About WIC*, Washington, D.C., 2012, Food and Nutrition Service. at: <http://www.fns.usda.gov/wic/aboutwic/>. Accessed on March 11, 2012.

39. U.S. Department of Health and Human Services: *Nutrition Services (OAA Title IIIC)*, Washington, D.C., 2012, Administration on Aging. at: <http://www.aoa.gov/AoARoot/AoA_Programs/HCLTC/Nutrition_Services/index.aspx>. Accessed on March 10, 2013.

40. Gleason PM, Dodd AH: School breakfast program but not school lunch program participation is associated with lower body mass index. *J Am Diet Assoc* 109:S118, 2009.

41. U.S. Department of Agriculture: *Expanded Food and Nutrition Education Program (EFNEP)*, Washington, D.C., 2012, National Institute of Food and Agriculture. at: <http://www.csrees.usda.gov/nea/food/efnep/efnep.html>. Accessed on March 10, 2013.

42. U.S. Department of Agriculture: *SNAP-ED*, Washington, D.C., 2009, National Institute of Food and Agriculture. at: <http://www.nifa.usda.gov/nea/food/fsne/fsne.html>. Accessed on March 10, 2013.

43. U.S. Department of Agriculture: *FY2012: NIFA—National Data*, Washington, D.C., 2013, The Expanded Food and Nutrition Education Program (EFNEP), National Institute of Food and Agriculture. at: <http://www.nifa.usda.gov/nea/food/efnep/pdf/ntl_reort_2012.pdf>. Accessed on March 10, 2013.

44. Centers for Disease Control and Prevention: *Social marketing resources*, Atlanta, Ga., 2011, Division of Nutrition, Physical Activity, and Obesity. at: <http://www.cdc.gov/nccdphp/dnpao/socialmarketing/index.html>. Accessed on March 10, 2013.

45. Herbold N, Taylor PN: Marketing nutrition programs and services. In Edelstein S, editor: *Nutrition in public health. A handbook for developing programs and services*, Sudbury, Mass., 2006, Jones and Bartlett.

46. U.S. Department of Agriculture: *Cost of food at home. U.S. average at four cost levels*, Washington, D.C., 2013, Center for Nutrition Policy and Promotion. at: <http://www.cnpp.usda.gov/usdafoodcost-home.htm>. Accessed on March 10, 2013.

47. Blisard N, Stewart H: *Food spending in American households, 2003-04, EIB-23*, Washington, D.C., 2007, Economic Research Service, U.S. Department of Agriculture.

48. U.S. Department of Agriculture, Center for Nutrition Policy and Promotion: *Thrifty food plan: 2006, CNPP-19*, Washington, D.C., 2007, U.S. Department of Agriculture. from: <www.cnpp.usda.gov/Publications/FoodPlans/MiscPubs/TFP2006Report.pdf>. Retrieved March 11, 2013.

49. U.S. Department of Agriculture, Center for Nutrition Policy and Promotion: *The low-cost, moderate-cost, and liberal food plans, CNPP-20*, Washington, D.C., 2007, U.S. Department of Agriculture. from: <www.cnpp.usda.gov/Publications/FoodPlans/MiscPubs/FoodPlans2007AdminReport.pdf>. Retrieved March 12, 2013.

50. Davis GC, Yu W: The Thrifty Food Plan is not thrifty when labor cost is considered. *J Nutr* 140:854, 2010.

51. Carlson A, Stewart H: 2011. A wide variety of fruit and vegetables are affordable for SNAP recipients, Amber Waves, December. at: <http://www.ers.usda.gov/amber-waves/2011-december/a-wide-variety-of-fruit-and-vegetables.aspx#.UT56U6WhCFI>. Accessed on March 13, 2013.

52. Wen S, Popkin BM: Monitoring foods and nutrients sold and consumed in the United States: dynamics and challenges. *J Acad Nutr Diet* 112(1):41, 2012.

53. Aase S: Supermarket trends: how increased demand for healthful products and services will affect food and nutritional professionals. *J Am Diet Assoc* 107:1286, 2007.

54. Martinez SW: *The U.S. Food marketing system: recent developments, 1997-2006, Econ Res Rep No 42*, Washington, D.C., 2007, Economic Research Service, U.S. Department of Agriculture.

55. Leone AL, Rigby S, Betterley C, et al: Store type and demographic influence on the availability and price of healthful foods, Leon County, Florida, 2008. *Prev Chron Dis* 8(6):A140, 2011. at: <http://www.cdc.gov/pcd/issues/2011/nov/10_0231.htm>. Retrieved on August 15, 2013.

56. Dutko P, Ver Ploeg M, Farrigan T: *Characteristics and influential factors of food deserts, Econ Res Rep Num 140*, Washington, D.C., 2012, Economic Research Service, U.S. Department of Agriculture.

57. Sharkey JR, Horel S: Neighborhood socioeconomic deprivation and minority composition are associated with better potential spatial access to the ground-truthed food environment in a large rural area. *J Nutr* 138:620, 2008.

58. The Food Trust: *The Food Trust*, Philadelphia, Pa, 2012, at: <www.thefoodtrust.org>. Accessed on March 12, 2012.

59. Academy of Nutrition and Dietetics: Practice paper of the Academy of Nutrition and Dietetics: promoting ecological sustainability within the food system. *J Acad Nutr Diet* 113:464, 2013.

60. Feeding America: *Network of over 200 food banks nationwide, Feeding America*, Chicago, Ill, 2012. at: <http://feedingamerica.org/>. Accessed on March 13, 2012.

61. U.S. Department of Agriculture: *The Emergency Food Assistance Program, Food and Nutrition Service Nutrition Program Fact Sheet*, 2012. at: <http://www.fns.usda.gov/fdd/programs/tefap/pfs-tefap.pdf>. Accessed on March 13, 2013.

FURTHER READINGS AND RESOURCES

Readings

Cunningham-Sabo L, Simons A: Home economics: an old-fashioned answer to a modern day dilemma? *Nutr Today* 47(3):128, 2012.

[This article points to the importance of basic cooking skills in support of a healthy diet.]

Davis JN, Ventura EE, Cook LT, et al: LA sprouts: a gardening, nutrition, and cooking intervention for Latino youth improves diet and reduces obesity. *J Am Diet Assoc* 111:1224, 2011.

Kraak VI, Story M: A public health perspective on healthy lifestyles and public-private partnerships for global childhood obesity prevention. *J Am Diet Assoc* 110(2):192, 2010.

Taft NA, Collier DN, Kolasa KM: Applying childhood obesity and cardiovascular health risk reduction guidelines: family-centered nutrition interventions. *Nutr Today* 47(5):229, 2012.

[These three articles provide examples of international, community, and family-based obesity interventions.]

Peregrin T: Picture this: visual cues enhance health education messages for people with low literacy skills. *J Am Diet Assoc* 110(Suppl 1):S28, 2010.

[This author gives suggestions for effective nutrition education with low literacy audiences.]

Websites of Interest

- Cooperative State Research, Education, and Extension Service, U.S. Department of Agriculture: *SNAP-ED Connection*. This site offers educational materials, recipes, and other resources useful when working with limited-resource audiences: http://snap.nal.usda.gov.
- Food and Nutrition Service, U.S. Department of Agriculture. This site offers links to food assistance programs, including the National School Breakfast Program, the Supplemental Nutrition Assistance Program (SNAP), and the Special

Supplemental Nutrition Program for Women, Infants, and Children (WIC): www.fns.usda.gov/fns/.
- The Food Trust. This Philadelphia-based organization brings nutrition education programs and supermarket access to inner-city neighborhoods: www.thefoodtrust.org/.

- U.S. Bureau of Census: *FedStats*. This site provides statistical data from all agencies of the federal government including population numbers and demographics, health issues, agriculture, and income parameters; data can be accessed by topic, nation, and state: www.fedstats.gov.

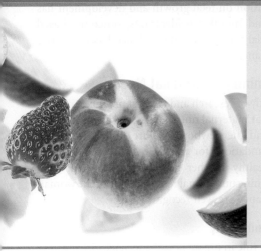

Nutrition During Pregnancy and Lactation

Sharon M. Nickols-Richardson

ⓔ EVOLVE WEBSITE

http://evolve.elsevier.com/Williams/essentials/

OUTLINE

In this chapter, we begin a three-chapter sequence on nutrition in health care throughout the life cycle. In each chapter, we will relate principles of nutrition to the remarkable process of human growth and development.

As we focus first on the beginning of new life, we examine the prenatal nutritional demands of the pregnant woman and her developing fetus, as well as maternal nutritional needs during lactation. Mother and offspring possess great adaptive abilities to meet nutritional demands during these life cycle stages.

Here, we explore the tremendous physiologic changes during pregnancy and lactation and some possible complications. You will see how vital optimal nutrition is for a successful course and outcome.

MATERNAL NUTRITION AND THE OUTCOME OF PREGNANCY

Early Medical Practice

For centuries in all cultures, a great body of folklore has surrounded pregnancy. Various traditional practices and diets have been followed, many of which have had little factual basis, and much clinical advice has been based only on supposition. For example, early obstetricians even held the notion that semistarvation of the pregnant woman was really a blessing in disguise because it produced a small baby of light weight who would be easier to deliver. To this end, they used diets restricted in kilocalories (kcalories or kcal), protein, water, and salt. Despite the lack of any scientific evidence to support such ideas, two assumptions, now known to be false, governed practice: (1) the *parasite theory* (i.e., whatever the **fetus** needs, it draws from maternal stores despite the maternal diet) and (2) the *maternal instinct theory* (i.e., whatever the fetus needs, the pregnant woman instinctively craves and consumes it).

Healthy Pregnancy

Until recently, much of the counsel given to pregnant women during the past few decades has been based more on tradition than on scientific fact. Increasing evidence indicates that positive nutritional support of pregnancy, rather than past negative restrictions born of limited knowledge and false assumptions, promotes a successful outcome with increased health and vigor of mothers and their infants. This struggle during the past few decades, particularly to define the "healthy pregnancy," has not been easy. A healthy pregnancy has often been defined by the birth weight of the newborn, because infant mortality, or death, is low for infants with birth weights of 3500 to 4500 g.[1]

The two key factors that predict infant birth weight are (1) maternal preconception weight and (2) weight gain during pregnancy.[2] Nutrition and other lifestyle factors affect maternal weight and weight gain; many of these factors, particularly nutrition, are modifiable or may be controlled by the pregnant woman. Healthy pregnancy may also be described in broader terms of *mother, infant,* and *family.* Clinicians are beginning to understand more about what this really means, especially as they observe fetal damages from malnutrition, drug abuse, and other factors. It is clear that we must assess and support more fully the quality of life of each mother and her family if we are to achieve healthy pregnancy outcomes among women.

Directions for Current Practice

Clinical observations and developing science in nutrition and medicine have provided directions for healthier pregnancies. Previous false ideas have been refuted, and a sound base for current practice has emerged. A classic report of the National Research Council (NRC) first reflected this applied scientific base and led the way. This report, *Maternal Nutrition and the Course of Human Pregnancy,* provided an undeniable, new direction for a positive approach to the management of pregnancy.[3] Indeed, continuing research has reinforced this positive direction. On the basis of the significant NRC findings, guidelines for the nutritional care of pregnant women were then issued by the American College of Obstetrics and Gynecology and the Academy of Nutrition and Dietetics (formerly known as the American Dietetic Association).[4,5] These reports continue to provide useful guidelines for physicians, nutritionists, dietitians, and nurses in their prenatal care. Nutritional guidelines for pregnancy and lactation for all nutrients are also included in the Dietary Reference Intake (DRI) recommendations published by the Food and Nutrition Board of the Institute of Medicine.[6-10] These guidelines remind us that an infant is nutritionally 9 months old at birth, even older when we consider the significance of the mother's preconception status.

The *fetal origins hypothesis* supports the notion that nutrition during gestation, or the lack thereof, sets the course for chronic disease in adulthood.[11] Development of cardiovascular disease, hypertension, obesity, type 2 diabetes, metabolic syndrome, and gestational diabetes, among other chronic diseases, has been shown in the offspring of animals for which maternal dietary intakes of macronutrients and micronutrients were manipulated, as well as in human epidemiologic studies of the relationship between infant anthropometric measurements and adult disease incidence.[12,13] In these epidemiologic studies, infant body size, shape, and weight measurements served as indicators of maternal nutrition. Changes in maternal nutrition during pregnancy require that the fetus adapt. These adaptations to nutrient supplies may lead to programming, or the mechanism (or mechanisms) through which permanent changes in organ system structures and functions occur, leading to risk of chronic disease. This hypothesis presumes that nutritional insults that occur during critical stages of embryonic and fetal development are most harmful, leading to future disease risk. The merits of the fetal origins hypothesis have been debated, and much remains to be discovered.[14] Although research regarding the influence of nutrition on fetal growth and development has unique ethical and moral considerations, outcomes-based research is essential for appropriate evidence-based practice for healthy pregnancies.

Factors Determining Nutritional Needs

An expanding body of research and the best practices of clinicians reinforce that maternal nutrition is critically important to the mother and the newborn (Figure 11-1). It lays the fundamental foundation for the successful outcome of pregnancy—a healthy mother and infant.[15] Several vital factors that determine nutritional requirements of the woman during her pregnancy are well recognized.

Age, Gravida, and Parity

Age plays a major role in pregnancy; the teenage girl adds her own growth and maturation needs to those imposed by pregnancy. In addition, the number of pregnancies (gravida) and the number of viable offspring (parity), as well as the time intervals between them, greatly influence the woman's nutrient reserves, her increased nutritional needs, and the outcome of the pregnancy.

Complex Physiologic Interactions of Gestation

Three distinct biologic entities are involved during gestation: the woman, the fetus, and the placenta, which nourishes fetal growth. Together they form a unique biologic whole. Constant metabolic interactions occur among them. Their functions, although unique, are at the same time interdependent. It is this unique biologic synergism that nourishes and sustains the pregnancy.

Basic Concepts Involved

As a result of our increased knowledge of pregnancy and nutrition, we can provide better nutritional guidance. Three basic concepts form a fundamental framework for assessing maternal nutritional needs and for planning supportive prenatal care for the woman.

KEY TERMS

fetus   The unborn offspring in the postembryonic period, after major structures have been outlined; in humans, the growing offspring from 7 to 8 weeks after fertilization until birth.

lactation   Formation and secretion of milk by mammary glands.

gestation   The period of embryonic and fetal development from fertilization to birth; pregnancy.

programming   The mechanism (or mechanisms) through which adaptations to nutrient supplies during gestation result in permanent changes in organ and body system structures and functions, potentially leading to chronic disease risk.

gravida   A pregnant woman.

parity   The condition of a woman with respect to having borne viable offspring.

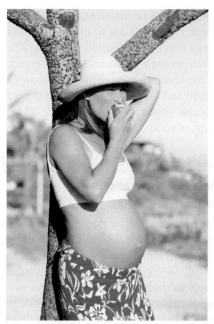

FIGURE 11-1 Adequate intake of fruits and vegetables is essential during pregnancy. (Copyright 2006 JupiterImages Corporation.)

Perinatal Concept

The prefix *peri-* comes from the Greek root meaning around, about, or surrounding. Thus the word *perinatal* refers more broadly to the scope of factors that surround a birth than merely the 9 months of the physical gestation. Certainly, as nutrition knowledge and understanding have increased, health professionals realize that a woman's life experiences surrounding her pregnancy must be considered. Her nutritional status and food patterns, which have developed during a number of years, and the degree to which she has established and maintained nutritional reserves are all important factors.

Synergism Concept

Synergism describes biologic systems in which two or more factors interact cooperatively to produce a total effect that is better and different from the original parts. Of the many biologic and physiologic examples of synergism, pregnancy is a prime case in point. Maternal organism, fetus, and placenta work synergistically to produce a system that had not existed before; this system now serves to sustain and nurture the pregnancy and its offspring. Through synergism, the physiologic systems of the mother change, and the physiologic norms of the nonpregnant woman do not apply. For example, a normal physiologic generalized edema of pregnancy is a protective response. It reflects the normal increase in total body water necessary to support the increased metabolic work of pregnancy and is associated with enhanced reproductive performance to better serve the developing offspring.

Life Continuum Concept

In a real sense, throughout her life a woman is providing for the ongoing continuum of life through the food that she eats. Each offspring obviously becomes a part of this continuing process during the pregnancy, when the mother's diet directly sustains growth and development. However, in the broader sense, the mother transfers her nutritional heritage, practices, and beliefs to her growing children, who in the next generation pass on this heritage genetically and culturally. Multigenerational factors carry forward.

HEALTH PROMOTION

Preconception Nutrition

A woman brings to each pregnancy all of her previous life experiences, including her diet and eating habits. Her general health and fitness and her state of nutrition at the time of conception are products of her lifelong dietary habits and her genetic heritage. The importance of preconception nutrition is increasingly recognized. The Maternal, Infant and Child objective included in Healthy People 2020 (see Further Readings and Resources at the end of this chapter) addresses the need for improvements in preconception nutrition and health in women in the United States.[16] Preconception counseling is an avenue to such improvements. Related to nutrition, preconception counseling may include screening for medical conditions such as iron deficiency anemia, eating disorders, drug-nutrient interactions, and genetic disorders, as well as assessment of current body weight, recent and previous weight changes, body mass index (BMI), fitness and exercise status, folate status, other nutrient intakes, eating patterns, and dietary and botanical supplement use. Evaluation of existing medical conditions such as hypertension, diabetes, thyroid disease, celiac disease, phenylketonuria (PKU), and others is important. Inquiries about the home and family environment, including income, education, safety, lead exposure, and abuse, should also be conducted during preconception counseling so that guidance, recommendations, and referrals may be thoroughly provided. Each of these nutrition and health-related factors has documented effects on pregnancy outcome, many of which are adverse. However, preconception counseling and optimal preconception nutrition may increase the odds for a healthy pregnancy and desirable infant outcome.

Infertility

Infertility is defined as the inability to conceive after 12 months of engaging in planned sexual intercourse without using methods of birth control.[17] The prevalence of infertility ranges from 6.2% to 27.5% among the population of women of reproductive ages in the United States.[18] While many factors, such as nulliparity, older age, lower educational level, and gynecologic conditions, are related to infertility, nutrition-based factors are emerging as additional contributors. For example, obesity or severe underweight in some women delays time to conception,[19,20] and dietary components, including carbohydrate, protein, and dietary fat, have been implicated in infertility.[21] An optimal diet may be necessary for fertility.

Excess Body Weight

Approximately 67% of adults in the United States are overweight, and nearly 33% are obese. Hence many women enter their pregnancies with excess body weight. This condition increases the risks of fetal mortality and malformations, excessive weight gain during pregnancy, gestational diabetes, hypertension, and preeclampsia, as well as the likelihood of preterm delivery and infant delivery by cesarean section. Pregnancy is not a time for weight loss because of the energy and nutrient requirements of the woman and fetus. Rather, a woman with excess body weight should moderately and gradually reduce her weight before pregnancy through an individualized energy-restricted diet and exercise plan. Weight gain during pregnancy should then follow recommendations based on BMI as outlined later in this chapter.

Exercise

Women who exercise before pregnancy should continue a reasonable exercise regimen during pregnancy.[22] In fact, women who engage in prenatal exercise have been shown to have health benefits compared with nonexercising women.[23] Moderate-intensity physical activity may also be beneficial to the woman and fetus, even if the woman was sedentary before conception. Each day, a pregnant woman should strive to achieve approximately 20 to 25 minutes of aerobic activity to meet a goal of approximately 150 minutes per week.[22] As the woman's body size and shape change throughout the course of pregnancy, exercise type, duration, intensity, and frequency should be adjusted to promote safety for the woman and her fetus (Figure 11-2). Physical activities that

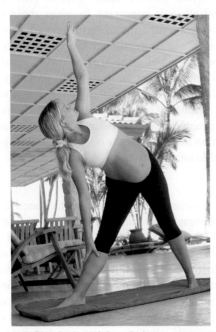

FIGURE 11-2 Physical activity during pregnancy benefits both the pregnant woman cand the fetus. (Copyright 2006 JupiterImages Corporation.)

are not recommended during pregnancy include scuba diving and those with risk of trauma to the abdominal area.[24]

The energy cost of exercise influences the kcalorie needs of the pregnant woman. Kcalories must be consumed to meet the energy cost of exercise and to promote appropriate maternal weight gain and fetal growth and development. Adequate hydration is also vital, and the woman should increase fluid intake during exercise.

NUTRITIONAL DEMANDS OF PREGNANCY

Basic Nutrient Allowances and Individual Variation

Gestation is characterized by exceedingly rapid growth and development. During this 38- to 42-week period, a single fertilized egg cell (ovum) grows into a fully developed infant weighing about 3500 g, on average. What nutrients must the woman supply to support this intense period of fetal growth and development? What must her diet provide to meet fetal nutritional demands and her own needs during this critical period?

Throughout the pregnancy an increased need exists for most of the basic nutrients, as indicated by the DRI guidelines from the Food and Nutrition Board of the Institute of Medicine (Table 11-1).[6-10] However, it is important to remember that these are guidelines; individual variances in nutrient needs must be examined for each pregnancy. Individual variations such as basal metabolic rate (BMR), BMI, physical activity, and health status must be considered. In addition, the quantitative need for nourishment of pregnant adolescents and multifetal pregnancies must be noted. Individual counseling and correct use of nutritional guidelines is imperative.[25] In considering the nutritional needs of the *healthy* pregnant woman, we will review here the macronutrients and selected micronutrients with increased needs, rationale for increased needs, and how such nutrients may be obtained from foods.

Energy Needs

The kcalories must be sufficient to perform the following two functions:

1. Supply the increased energy and nutrient demands created by the increased metabolic workload, including some maternal fat storage and fetal fat storage to ensure an optimal newborn size for survival.
2. Spare protein for tissue building.

The DRI standard recommends an additional amount of energy of approximately 340 kcal/day during the second trimester and 452 kcal/day during the third trimester of pregnancy to supply needs during this time of rapid growth.[10] Total daily kcalorie intake during middle and late pregnancy should be based on the woman's nonpregnant estimated energy requirement plus the additional energy need; it will typically increase about 15% to 20% beyond the woman's general prepregnancy need. This primary emphasis on sufficient kcalories is critical to ensure nutrient and energy needs to positively support the pregnancy. Appropriate weight gain

TABLE 11-1	DIETARY REFERENCE INTAKES PER DAY OF SELECTED NUTRIENTS FOR PREGNANCY AND LACTATION					
	NONPREGNANT GIRL		NONPREGNANT WOMAN	DURING PREGNANCY	LACTATION	
NUTRIENTS	9-13 yr 46 kg 101 lb	14-18 yr 55 kg 120 lb	19-50 yr 63 kg 138 lb	19-50 yr	(600 mL/day) first 6 mo	(750 mL/day) second 6 mo
Kilocalories	2000-2100	2300-2400	2400	No change in first trimester; +340 kcal/day for second trimester and +452 kcal/day for third trimester	+500 kcal/day (170 kcal/day from maternal stores)	+400 kcal/day
Protein (g)	34	46	46	71	71 throughout	
Calcium (mg)	1300	1300	1000	1000 throughout	1000 throughout	
Iron (mg)	8	15	18	27 throughout	9 throughout	
Vitamin A (mcg RAE)*	600	700	700	770 throughout	1300 throughout	
Thiamin (mg)	0.9	1.0	1.1	1.4 throughout	1.4 throughout	
Riboflavin (mg)	0.9	1.0	1.1	1.4 throughout	1.6 throughout	
Niacin (mg NE)†	12	14	14	18 throughout	17 throughout	
Vitamin C (mg)	45	65	75	85 throughout	120 throughout	
Vitamin D (mcg)	15	15	15	15 throughout	15 throughout	
Folic acid (mcg DFE)‡	300	400	400	600 throughout	500 throughout	

Data from Food and Nutrition Board, Institute of Medicine: *Dietary Reference Intakes for calcium, and vitamin D,* Washington, D.C., 2011, National Academies Press; Food and Nutrition Board, Institute of Medicine: *Dietary Reference Intakes for energy, carbohydrate, fiber, fat, fatty acids, cholesterol, protein, and amino acids (macronutrients),* Washington, D.C., 2005, National Academies Press; Food and Nutrition Board, Institute of Medicine: *Dietary Reference Intakes for thiamin, riboflavin, niacin, vitamin B6, folate, vitamin B12, pantothenic acid, biotin, and choline,* Washington, D.C., 1998, National Academies Press; Food and Nutrition Board, Institute of Medicine: *Dietary Reference Intakes for vitamin C, vitamin E, selenium, and carotenoids,* Washington, D.C., 2000, National Academies Press; Food and Nutrition Board, Institute of Medicine: *Dietary Reference Intakes for vitamin A, vitamin K, arsenic, boron, chromium, copper, iodine, iron, manganese, molybdenum, nickel, silicon, vanadium, and zinc,* Washington, D.C., 2000, National Academies Press.
*As retinol activity equivalents (RAEs): One RAE is equal to 1 mcg all-*trans* retinol or 12 mcg β-carotene.
†As niacin equivalents (NE), one NE is equal to 1 mg of niacin or 60 mg of tryptophan.
‡As dietary folate equivalents (DFEs), one DFE is equal to 1 mcg food folate or 0.6 mcg of folic acid from fortified food (or as a supplement consumed with food) or 0.5 mcg of a supplement taken on an empty stomach.

during pregnancy indicates whether sufficient kcalories are being provided.

Much of our knowledge regarding the importance of sufficient energy intake during pregnancy arose from records of pregnancy and infant statistics through periods of famine during World War II. Insufficient kcalorie intake during the first trimester of pregnancy was associated with infertility and increased incidence of neural tube defects and other metabolic changes, whereas inadequate kcalorie consumption in the second and third trimesters of pregnancy was associated with increased numbers of congenital abnormalities, infants of low birth weight, and infant mortality. Current famine and food insecurity in various locations around the world continue to support these earlier findings regarding the essential need for adequate kcalories during pregnancy to support an optimal infant outcome. Energy needs of pregnancy may be met through a balanced intake of macronutrients.

Protein, Fat, and Carbohydrate Needs

The total amount of protein recommended for a pregnant woman is 71 g/day, an increase of 25 g/day.[10] Protein, with its essential nitrogen, is the nutrient basic to tissue growth.

KEY TERMS
placenta Special organ developed in early pregnancy that provides nutrients to the fetus and removes metabolic waste.
synergism The joint action of separate agents in which the total effect of their combined action is greater than the sum of their separate actions.
preterm An infant that is born before the 37th week of pregnancy.
low birth weight Live-born infant weighing less than 2500 grams at birth.

Nitrogen balance studies suggest that a large amount of nitrogen is used by the woman and fetus during pregnancy and emphasize the importance of preconception maternal reserves to meet initial pregnancy needs. More protein is necessary for demands posed by the following:

- Rapid fetal growth
- Enlargement of the uterus, mammary glands, and placenta
- Increase in maternal circulating blood volume and subsequent demand for increased plasma proteins to maintain colloidal osmotic pressure and circulation of tissue fluids to nourish cells
- Formation of amniotic fluid
- Storage reserves for labor, delivery, and lactation

Milk, egg, cheese, and meat are complete protein foods of high biologic value. Protein-rich foods also contribute other nutrients, such as calcium, iron, and B vitamins. Additional protein may be obtained from legumes and whole grains, with lesser amounts in other plant sources.

An adequate supply of essential fatty acids is also vital throughout pregnancy. Tissue growth, especially the proper development of cell membranes in nerve and brain tissue, and development of organ function, notably cognition and visual acuity, require that essential fatty acids and their converted forms reach the developing fetus in sufficient amounts. Depending on individual needs, supplementation of the mother's essential fatty acid intake may be useful to maintain adequate levels.[26] However, most pregnant women may consume adequate amounts of linoleic (13 g/day) and α-linolenic (1.4 g/day) acids through consumption of canola, soybean, and walnut oils, in addition to other dietary fat sources.[10] Docosahexaenoic acid (DHA), important for visual and cognitive development, is found in salmon, mackerel, striped bass, and other fish products. Eicosapentaenoic acid (EPA), also found in fish, fish oils, flaxseed, walnuts, and canola oil, is important for blood vessel dilation, blood clotting, and reducing inflammation. Combined DHA and EPA intake of 500 mg/day is recommended.[27] Fish intake during pregnancy is encouraged, although total seafood intake should be limited to 8 to 12 oz per week, albacore tuna limited to 6 oz per week, and king mackerel, shark, swordfish, and tilefish avoided altogether to prevent methyl mercury intake during pregnancy.[28] (See Chapter 9 for more information on mercury content of fish.)

Carbohydrate intake of at least 175 g/day during pregnancy is important for an adequate supply of glucose and nonprotein energy.[10] Whole grain breads and cereals, as well as fruits and vegetables, should be consumed to meet maternal and fetal glucose needs and provide fiber for satiety and bowel regulation. Currently, popular low-carbohydrate "diets" are not recommended during pregnancy because various phases of these diets do not provide the minimum glucose load required by the maternal and fetal bodies. In general, total daily dietary kcalorie intake should comprise 15% protein, 30% fat, and 55% carbohydrate, keeping in mind the individual needs of the pregnant woman and adequate macronutrient distribution ranges.

Mineral Needs

All the major and trace minerals play roles in maternal health. Four that have special functions in relation to pregnancy deserve particular attention: (1) calcium, (2) iodine, (3) iron, and (4) zinc.

Calcium

The pregnant woman's DRI recommendation is 1000 mg of calcium per day, the same as the general recommendation for all women ages 19 to 50.[6] Calcium is the essential element for the construction and maintenance of bones and teeth. It is also an important factor in the blood-clotting mechanism and is used in normal muscle action and other essential metabolic activities. Improved absorption of calcium supplies the needs arising from the accelerated fetal mineralization of skeletal tissue during the final period of rapid growth. Dairy products are a primary source of calcium. Consumption of milk or equivalent milk foods (cheese or nonfat milk powder used in cooking) or calcium-fortified soy milk is recommended. Additional calcium is obtained in whole or fortified cereal grains and in green leafy vegetables.

Iodine

The recommendation for iodine increases by 70 mcg/day during pregnancy.[9] Iodine is vital for thyroid hormone synthesis and prevention of goiter. The need increases during gestation to support changes in maternal thyroid economy, increased maternal urinary loss, and fetal uptake of iodine. An inadequate supply of iodine to the fetus may lead to hypothyroidism in the newborn and is often associated with poor and abnormal growth, deficits in cognitive development, and poor motor function. Although infrequently encountered in the United States, infant hypothyroidism continues to be found in many developing countries. Iodine consumption is critical in the first half of pregnancy, and programs designed to provide oil- and water-based iodine supplements to women in preconception and prenatal periods in developing countries have been successful in reducing the incidence of infant hypothyroidism. Iodized salt is the primary dietary source for women in developed countries. Seafood is also a noted source of iodine.

Iron

The pregnant woman needs 27 mg of iron per day, a substantial increase beyond her general needs.[9] Some pregnant women may need supplementary iron in addition to increased dietary sources to meet the additional requirement of pregnancy. The iron cost of pregnancy is high. With increased demands for iron, often insufficient maternal stores, and inadequate provision through the usual diet, a

---

KEY TERM

amniotic fluid The watery fluid within the membrane enveloping the fetus, in which the fetus is suspended.

daily supplement of 30 to 60 mg of iron per day is generally prescribed. If a woman has iron deficiency anemia at conception, then a larger therapeutic amount of 60 to 120 mg/day of iron may be necessary to reduce the risk of a preterm delivery or low–birth-weight baby (or both).

During normal pregnancy the maternal circulating blood volume expands by 40% to 50% and may increase more with multiple fetuses. This adaptation reduces the strain on the maternal heart, minimizes hemoglobin losses at delivery, and enhances nutrient flow to the fetus. Although red blood cell mass also increases during gestation, this change does not parallel blood volume expansion, resulting in hemodilution of red blood cell mass. Thus specific guidelines are used to determine iron deficiency anemia during pregnancy (see the section on anemia later in this chapter). Maternal iron is needed to supply iron to the developing placenta and fetal liver. Adequate maternal iron stores also help protect the woman against iron losses related to blood loss at delivery.

To obtain the needed amount of iron, check the percentage of elemental iron in the iron preparation being used. For example, the commonly used compound ferrous sulfate is a hydrated salt ($FeSO_4 \cdot 7H_2O$), which contains 20% iron. It is usually dispensed in tablets containing 195, 300, or 325 mg of the ferrous sulfate compound. Each tablet, then, would contain 39, 60, or 65 mg of iron, respectively. Thus to supply a regular daily supplement of 60 mg of iron, one 300-mg tablet of ferrous sulfate is required (300 mg $FeSO_4 \cdot 7H_2O$ × 20% = 60 mg iron); for a therapeutic dose of 120 mg iron, two 300-mg tablets are required.

Problems with routine iron supplementation for pregnant women include unpleasant gastrointestinal side effects (see the Effects of Iron Supplements section later in this chapter) and less motivation to maintain a good diet. Of major concern are imbalances with other trace elements, such as zinc and copper, that compete with iron for absorption. Excess iron intake, when not needed, may actually mask inadequate pregnancy-induced hemodilution. Thus some prenatal clinics follow protocols that prescribe regular prenatal vitamins with iron at the first clinic visit, adding additional iron supplementation only if hemoglobin falls to 10.5 g/dL or less at any time during the pregnancy.

A major food source of iron is liver; however, liver intake is often avoided during pregnancy. Other food sources include meat, legumes, dried fruit, green leafy vegetables, eggs, and enriched bread and cereals (see the list of iron-containing foods in Chapter 7).

Zinc

During pregnancy the DRI recommendation for zinc increases from 8 to 11 mg/day.[9] Zinc is vital for enzymatic reactions and is essential to growth and development because of its role in deoxyribonucleic acid (DNA) and ribonucleic acid (RNA) synthesis and protein production. Inadequate zinc consumption during gestation has been associated with low birth weight and congenital malformations. Iron supplementation may inhibit zinc absorption; thus additional dietary sources of zinc are critical when maternal iron supplementation is prescribed. Seafood, eggs, and meat are primary sources of zinc.

Vitamin Needs

Increased amounts of vitamins A, B complex, and C are needed during pregnancy. If these needs are met, then sufficient amounts of vitamins E and K are also available. The recommended amount of vitamin D does not increase during pregnancy but is important to fetal skeletal development.

Vitamin A

The daily amount of vitamin A recommended for pregnancy is 770 mcg of retinol activity equivalents (RAEs), a slight increase beyond a woman's regular need.[9] For most women in the United States, no extra amount is needed. However, malnourished, underweight women and those with multiple pregnancies need more. Vitamin A is an essential factor in cell differentiation, organ formation, maintenance of strong epithelial tissue, tooth formation, and normal bone growth. Liver, egg yolk, butter and fortified margarine, dark-green and yellow vegetables, and fruits are good food sources.

Excessive consumption of retinol and retinoic acid, two forms of vitamin A, has been associated with fetal malformations such as heart, facial, and ear defects. Overconsumption is generally related to the use of supplements or medications such as Accutane. Harmful effects are most damaging during the first few months of pregnancy, again emphasizing the need for prenatal counseling and appropriate preconception nutrition.

B Vitamins

A special need exists for various B vitamins, including thiamin, riboflavin, niacin, pyridoxine, vitamin B_{12}, pantothenic acid, and folate, during pregnancy. The B vitamins are important as coenzyme factors in a number of metabolic activities related to energy production, tissue protein synthesis, and function of muscle and nerve tissue; therefore they play key roles in the increased metabolic work of pregnancy. These B vitamins are usually supplied by a well-balanced diet that is increased in quantity and quality to supply needed energy and nutrients.

A special increased metabolic need exists for the B vitamin folate during pregnancy. Folate deficiency usually occurs in conjunction with general malnutrition, making the pregnant woman in low-socioeconomic conditions especially vulnerable. A specific megaloblastic anemia caused by maternal folate deficiency sometimes occurs and warrants supplementation of the diet with folic acid. This added amount is particularly needed in situations in which such demands are increased, such as in a multiple pregnancy.

Preconception folic acid supplementation has been shown in randomized clinical trials to greatly reduce a woman's risk of bearing an infant with a neural tube defect, which is the source of the serious defects of spina bifida and anencephaly. These congenital defects in the formation of the spine develop in the first few weeks of pregnancy, when the neural tube, which forms the spinal cord, does not close completely, leaving part of one or more vertebrae of the spinal cord exposed at birth. Each year in the United States approximately 3000 infants are born with spina bifida and anencephaly, and an estimated 1500 affected fetuses are spontaneously aborted.[29] Since 1992 the U.S. Public Health Service has recommended that all women of childbearing age who are capable of becoming pregnant consume from food or supplements 400 mcg of folic acid per day to prevent such deficiencies. This recommendation continues in the latest DRI guidelines, which recommend 400 mcg/day for nonpregnant women, rising to 600 mcg/day during pregnancy and 500 mcg/day during lactation.[7] The U.S. Food and Drug Administration (FDA), acting to increase folic acid consumption nationally, mandated in 1998 that enriched cereal grain products be fortified with folic acid. These fortified foods are good sources of folic acid in addition to orange and pineapple juices, oranges, and dried beans.[30] (Review Chapter 6 for more discussion on neural tube defects and their prevention.)

Choline is emerging as a nutrient of greater importance during pregnancy.[31] Although choline malnutrition is very rare in the United States, a few epidemiologic studies have reported neural tube defects in the infants of women with subclinical choline deficiency during pregnancy.[32] The recommended intake of choline during pregnancy can be met by consuming eggs and various protein foods.

Vitamin C

Special emphasis must be given to the pregnant woman's need for ascorbic acid. Vitamin C is essential to the formation of intercellular cement material in developing connective tissues and vascular systems. It also increases the absorption of iron, which is needed for the increasing quantities of hemoglobin. The DRI standard recommends 85 mg/day for the pregnant woman, an increase of 10 mg/day beyond the regular female adult need of 75 mg/day.[8] Additional food sources such as citrus fruit and other vegetables and fruits should be included in the woman's diet.

Vitamin D

Women who have adequate exposure to sunlight probably need little additional vitamin D. During pregnancy, because of the need for calcium and phosphorus presented by the developing fetal skeletal tissue, vitamin D is needed to promote the absorption and use of these minerals. The daily recommended amount for pregnancy is 15 mcg cholecalciferol (600 IU/day), which is the same as for the nonpregnant woman.[6] Food sources include fortified milk, fortified fruit juices, egg yolk, and fortified margarine.

Dietary Patterns: General and Alternative
General Daily Food Pattern

Two useful and general principles concerning eating habits for all persons also apply during pregnancy, as follows:
1. Eat an appropriate quantity of food.
2. Eat regularly and avoid fasting or skipping meals, especially breakfast.

During pregnancy a variety of familiar foods usually supply the woman's need for added nutrients and make eating a pleasure. The increased quantities of essential nutrients needed during pregnancy may be met in many ways by planning around a daily food pattern and using key types of suggested core foods. The MyPlate resource (ChooseMyPlate.gov) offers a credible and easily accessible source for a woman to develop an eating plan appropriate for her trimester of pregnancy, age, height, prepregnancy weight, and physical activity level. Figure 11-3 displays one example of a dietary plan for a pregnant woman.

Lean meats and poultry, fish, dried beans, and nuts provide dietary protein, iron, zinc, and B vitamins for growth of muscles, bones, blood, and nerves; vegetable protein foods also contribute fiber. Fluid milk and dairy products and fortified soy milk provide dietary protein, calcium, and vitamin D to build strong bones, teeth, and healthy nerves and muscles. Grains provide carbohydrates and B vitamins for energy and healthy nerves, as well as iron for healthy blood. At least one half of these grains should be whole grain cereal and bread products to provide fiber. Vitamin C–rich fruits and vegetables assist in preventing infection and promoting healing; they also promote iron absorption and act as sources of fiber. Vitamin A–rich fruits and vegetables contribute β-carotene and vitamin A to prevent infection, promote night vision, and prevent constipation. Other fruits and vegetables contribute energy and fiber to the diet. Oils provide vitamin E and essential fatty acids.

Alternative Food Patterns

With the increasing ethnic diversity in the United States, it is especially important to use a woman's personal cultural food patterns in dietary counseling. We are ethnocentric if we rigidly adhere to a single dietary pattern for all pregnant women, because intake differs among women from various cultures, belief systems, and lifestyles. We must always remember that specific nutrients, not specific foods, are required for a successful pregnancy and that these nutrients are found in a wide variety of food choices. If we are wise, we will encourage our clients to use foods that serve their nutritional needs, whatever those foods might be (see the Case Study box, "A Baby for the Delgados"). A number of resources are available as guides for cultural, religious, and vegetarian food patterns (see Further Readings and Resources at the end of this chapter). Suggestions for improving transcultural nutrition counseling skills are also available.[33,34]

KEY TERMS

spina bifida   A congenital defect in the fetal closing of the neural tube to form a portion of the lower spine, leaving the spine unclosed and the spinal cord open in various degrees of exposure and damage.

ethnocentric   Judging the cultures of other peoples based on one's own culture.

	1st trimester	2nd trimester	3rd trimester
Grains	6 oz per day	7 oz per day	8 oz per day
Whole grains	≥ 3 oz per day	≥ 3½ oz per day	≥ 4 oz per day
Vegetables	2½ cups per day	3 cups per day	3 cups per day
Dark green	1½ cups per week	2 cups per week	2 cups per week
Red and orange	5½ cups per week	6 cups per week	6 cups per week
Beans and peas	1½ cups per week	2 cups per week	2 cups per week
Starchy	5 cups per week	6 cups per week	6 cups per week
Other	4 cups per week	5 cups per week	5 cups per week
Fruits	1½ cups per day	2 cups per day	2 cups per day
Dairy	3 cups per day	3 cups per day	3 cups per day
Protein foods	5 oz per day	6 oz per day	6½ oz per day
Seafood	8 oz per week	9 oz per week	10 oz per week
Oils	5 tsp per day	6 tsp per day	7 tsp per day
Total calories	1800 kcal per day	2200 kcal per day	2400 kcal per day
Discretionary calories	161 kcal per day	266 kcal per day	330 kcal per day

FIGURE 11-3 Food intake plan for a pregnant woman based on trimester of pregnancy, age, height, prepregnancy weight, and physical activity using the MyPlate resource (www.ChooseMyPlate.gov).

CASE STUDY

A Baby for the Delgados

Mrs. Delgado is a 19-year-old married primigravida, who tested positive for urinary human chorionic gonadotropin (hCG) 2 weeks earlier. Mrs. Delgado is 160 cm (5 feet 3 inches) tall with an average pregravid weight of 57 kg (125 lb). Her current gestational age is 6 weeks. Her history for chronic disorders and other serious health problems is negative.

During her initial nutrition interview, Mrs. Delgado indicated that the pregnancy was unplanned. She seemed especially worried about the effects of her irregular diet on the baby. As college students, she and her 21-year-old husband had erratic meals, dominated by junk food. Mrs. Delgado's 24-hour diet history revealed an inadequate intake of dark-green or red-yellow-orange vegetables and milk products, as well as meat or eggs and citrus fruits. The couple realized that these types of foods were an important part of a nutritious diet but felt inexperienced as cooks and lacked the time and money to prepare healthful meals every day.

At the end of the initial counseling session, the nutritionist told the couple about a series of prenatal group discussions conducted by members of the clinic's perinatal health team, including sessions on pregnancy, labor and delivery, and the care and feeding of the infant. These are attended primarily by a mixture of experienced parents and young, first-time parents to be and are offered as a means of introducing practical aspects of pregnancy and parenting.

The Delgados attended every prenatal group meeting and kept all consequent diet-counseling sessions. Their food choices improved in time, and Mrs. Delgado's weight gain progressed normally, to a total of 13 kg (28.5 lb) by the time of delivery. The Delgados had a healthy 4 kg (8 lb 13 oz) baby girl.

Questions for Analysis

1. What health professionals ideally should be included on the health care team caring for Mrs. Delgado? Describe the significance of each role to the outcome of her pregnancy. What are the roles of Mr. and Mrs. Delgado?
2. What nutritional deficiencies would you expect in Mrs. Delgado's diet? What practical problems would you expect her to encounter in attempting to improve her diet?
3. Write a 1-day meal plan for Mrs. Delgado, taking into account her lifestyle and schedule, as well as the amounts of nutrients considered adequate for pregnancy.
4. Write a lesson plan for a group session on nutrition during pregnancy. Include a general description, behavioral objectives, content outline, teaching methods and materials, and evaluation tool (or tools) you would use.
5. Would you encourage Mrs. Delgado to breast-feed? If so, then why? What factors would you expect might discourage her from trying? How would you discuss these factors?
6. Write a lesson plan for an infant-feeding session, addressing breast-feeding and bottle-feeding methods. Include the components listed in questions 3 and 4.

Dietary Supplements

Often, "prenatal vitamins" are prescribed for pregnant women. These supplements include a variety of vitamins and minerals and are intended to add to nutrient intake from foods rather than replace food and nutrient consumption.

Iron and folate are generally the two nutrients that require supplementation during pregnancy. Some women may need additional nutrients, however.[35] For example, pregnant women who follow vegan diets, have one or more nutritional deficiencies, smoke cigarettes, use or abuse drugs or alcohol (or both), or have multiple fetuses, need prenatal vitamin and mineral supplements that include additional nutrients.

Herbal and botanical supplement use during pregnancy is discouraged because of the potentially harmful or unknown effects on the woman and fetus. However, based on cultural and traditional medicine practices and emerging trends, pregnant women may include such products in their daily routines (see the Case Study box, "Nutrition Counseling in Pregnancy"). Several reference materials are available regarding the risks associated with use of specific herbals and botanicals during pregnancy (see Further Readings and Resources at the end of this chapter).[36,37]

WEIGHT GAIN DURING PREGNANCY

General Amount of Weight Gain

Healthy women produce healthy babies across a wide range of total weight gain. During pregnancy, therefore, the nutritional focus should always be on an individualized assessment of need and the quality of the weight gain. An average weight gain during normal pregnancy is about 11 to 16 kg (25 to 35 lb).[38] Around this average, many individual variations occur. No specific rigid norm or restriction exists to which all women should be held, regardless of individual needs; therefore such a course is obviously unwise and not evidence based. Current recommendations are therefore usually stated in terms of ranges to accommodate variances in needs. An initial base for evaluation, however, may be the average weight of the components of pregnancy as shown in Table 11-2. In addition to the components of growth and development usually attributed to a pregnancy, an important part is maternal stores. This laying down of extra adipose fat tissue is necessary for maternal energy reserves to sustain rapid fetal growth during the latter half of pregnancy, for labor and delivery, and for maintaining lactation after birth. Approximately 1.8 to 3.6 kg (4 to 8 lb) of adipose tissue is commonly deposited for these needs. The Institute of Medicine updated weight gain guidelines for pregnancy in May 2009, using the World Health Organization's (WHO)

CASE STUDY

Nutrition Counseling in Pregnancy

Ms. McLane is a 33-year-old Caucasian woman who is in her twenty-ninth week of pregnancy. This is her second pregnancy. During her first pregnancy (at age 29), she gained 24 lb during a normal pregnancy and had a delivery without complications. She is presently 165.1 cm (5 feet 5 inches) tall and weighs 81.8 kg (180 lb). Her prepregnancy weight was 72.7 kg (160 lb). Ms. McLane visited her obstetrician before her second pregnancy for prepregnancy planning. She has been consuming a healthy diet and a prenatal vitamin supplement every day. After her first visit to the obstetrician during the current pregnancy (at week 10), Ms. McLane did not return for any further appointments, because of her prior positive experience with pregnancy and belief that she "didn't need anything because the first pregnancy went so well."

Ms. McLane has a positive family history for diabetes, and her mother had gestational diabetes. Ms. McLane should have been screened for gestational diabetes between the twenty-fourth and twenty-eighth weeks of her current pregnancy; however, this was not done. She experienced frequent urination and fatigue that she reported as "different" from her first pregnancy. This prompted her to return to her obstetrician. The obstetrician completed a full examination and administered an oral glucose tolerance test. One hour after consuming a 100-g solution of glucose, Ms. McLane's blood glucose concentration was 218 mg/dL. She was scheduled for follow-up testing, and gestational diabetes was confirmed. A 2200-kcal/day diabetic diet was prescribed to allow Ms. McLane to control this condition through diet.

Ms. McLane has been referred to you for nutrition counseling. This is now the thirty-first week of her pregnancy, and she shares with you that a friend suggested that she "use some natural products to help her high blood sugar." In addition to consuming her prenatal supplement on a daily basis, she takes 500 mg of burdock root and 1 tbsp of flaxseed and drinks three cups of hot fenugreek tea per day. Her prenatal supplement contains 400 mcg of folate, 250 mg of calcium, 40 mg of iron, 100 mg of vitamin C, 5 mcg of vitamin D, 3 mg of thiamin, 3 mg of riboflavin, 4 mg of pyridoxine, 40 mcg of niacin, 10 mg of vitamin E, 5 mcg of vitamin B_{12}, 30 mg of zinc, and 10 mg of copper. Completion of a dietary intake analysis shows that Ms. McLane's kcalorie intake is 1750 per day. She reported that she has been nauseated for about 2 weeks, so she also added 300 mg of powdered ginger to each cup of the fenugreek tea. She reported some diarrhea and Braxton Hicks contractions during the last week, as well a lack of desire to be physically active.

Questions for Analysis

1. What is Ms. McLane's body mass index (BMI) based on her prepregnancy weight?
2. What is the recommended amount of weight gain for Ms. McLane based on prepregnancy weight and BMI? Has she experienced an appropriate weight gain so far?
3. Is the current level of kcalories appropriate based on her condition of gestational diabetes, BMI, and weight gain?
4. What additional information would you collect from Ms. McLane to complete a nutritional assessment?
5. How would you approach a nutritional intake plan for Ms. McLane?
6. Why would Ms. McLane's friend have recommended burdock root, flaxseed, and fenugreek? Be specific for each botanical. Are burdock root, flaxseed, fenugreek, or ginger recommended for use during pregnancy?
7. Identify at least five points that you would make during a nutrition counseling session with Ms. McLane. Discuss the priority for the first counseling session with Ms. McLane.

TABLE 11-2	APPROXIMATE WEIGHT OF COMPONENTS OF NORMAL PREGNANCY
COMPONENTS	**WEIGHT**
Fetus	3500 g (7.5 lb)
Placenta	450 g (1 lb)
Amniotic fluid	900 g (2 lb)
Uterus (weight increase)	1100 g (2.5 lb)
Breast tissue (weight increase)	1400 g (3 lb)
Blood volume (weight increase)	1800 g (4 lb) (1500 mL)
Maternal adipose tissue stores	1800-3600 g (4-8 lb)
TOTAL	10,850-12,650 g (10.9-12.7 kg; 24-28 lb)

classifications for prepregnancy BMI. The guidelines are as follows[38]:

- Normal-weight women with a BMI of 18.5 to 24.9 should gain from 11.5 to 16 kg (25 to 35 lb).
- Underweight women with a BMI of less than 18.5 should gain 12.7 to 18.1 kg (28 to 40 lb).
- Overweight women with a BMI of 25.0 to 29.9 should gain 6.8 to 11.5 kg (15 to 25 lb).
- Obese women with a BMI of 30.0 or more should gain 5.0 to 9.2 kg (11 to 20 lb).

The recommendation for adolescent girls is that they should follow the adult BMI guidelines and gain weight within the corresponding range. The recommendation for a woman carrying twins who is of normal BMI is a weight gain range of 16.8 to 24.5 kg (37 to 54 lb).[38] Overweight women carrying twins should gain 14.2 to 22.8 kg (31 to 50 lb), whereas obese women carrying twins should gain 11.5 to 19.1 kg (25 to 42 lb).[38] Compared with single-birth infants, twin-birth infants are five times more likely to be born prematurely (gestation of less than 37 weeks), nine-and-a-half times more likely to be very low birth weight (less than 1500 g), and eight-and-a-half times more likely to be low birth weight (less than 2500 g).[39]

Quality of Weight Gain

The important consideration lies in the nutritional quality of the gain. Specifically, the foods consumed should be nutrient dense, not full of empty kcalories, to meet nutrient requirements. In addition, in some cases clinicians have failed to distinguish between weight gained as a result of edema and that resulting from deposition of fat, which provides maternal stores for energy to sustain rapid fetal growth during the latter part of pregnancy and energy for lactation to follow. Analysis of the total tissue gained in an average pregnancy shows that the largest component, 62%, is water. Fat accounts for 31% and protein for 7%. Water is also the most variable component of the tissue gained, accounting for a range of 8 kg (18 lb) to as much as 11 kg (24 lb). Of the 8 kg of water usually gained, about 5.5 kg (12 lb) is associated with fetal tissue and other tissues gained in pregnancy. The remaining

2.5 kg (6 lb) accumulates in the maternal interstitial tissues.[40] Gravity causes the maternal tissue fluids to pool more in the lower extremities, leading to general swelling of the ankles, which is seen routinely in pregnant women. This fluid retention is a normal adaptive phenomenon designed to support the pregnancy and to exert a positive effect on fetal growth. Connective tissue becomes more hygroscopic as a result of the estrogen-induced changes in the ground substance and thus becomes softer and more easily distended. This facilitates delivery of the infant through the cervix and vaginal canal. In addition, the increased tissue fluid during pregnancy provides a means for handling the increased metabolic work and circulation of numerous metabolites necessary for fetal growth.

Clearly, severe kcalorie restriction is harmful to the developing fetus and the woman. It is inevitably accompanied by restriction of the vitally needed nutrients essential to the growth process. Moreover, weight reduction should never be undertaken during pregnancy. Sufficient weight gain should be encouraged with the use of a nourishing diet.

Rate of Weight Gain

On the whole, about 0.5 to 2.0 kg (1.1 to 4.4 lb) is a target for average weight gain during the first trimester for all pregnant women.[38] Thereafter, the target for average weight gain per week is 0.5 kg (1 lb) for underweight and normal-weight women, 0.3 kg (0.6 lb) for overweight women, and 0.23 kg (0.5 lb) for obese women. No scientific justification exists for routinely limiting weight gain to lesser amounts. Moreover, an individual woman who needs to gain more should not have unrealistic patterns imposed on her. It is only unusual patterns of gain, such as a sudden sharp increase in weight after the twentieth week of pregnancy that may signal abnormal water retention, which should be monitored closely, especially if it occurs in conjunction with blood pressure elevation and proteinuria. Conversely, an insufficient or low maternal weight gain during the second or third trimester increases the risk for intrauterine growth retardation.[41]

Weight Gain and Sodium Intake

A moderate amount of dietary sodium is needed for two essential reasons:

1. It is the major mineral required to control the extracellular fluid compartment.
2. This vital body water is increased during pregnancy to support its successful outcome.

Current practice usually follows a regular diet with moderate sodium intake, 1.5 to 2.3 g/day, with light use of salt to taste.[42] Limiting sodium beyond this general use is contrary to physiologic need in pregnancy and is unfounded. The NRC and professional obstetric guidelines have labeled routine salt-free diets and diuretics as potentially dangerous.[3-5] Maintaining the needed increase in circulating blood volume during pregnancy requires adequate amounts of sodium and protein, as well as adequate fluid intake to prevent dehydration and possible premature contractions.

GENERAL DIETARY PROBLEMS

Functional Gastrointestinal Problems
Nausea and Vomiting

Some general dietary problems temporarily interfere with food and nutrient intake. Most are easily resolved through dietary counseling and with medical attention and have no long-term adverse effect on the quality of maternal weight gain. Symptoms of nausea and vomiting are usually mild and short term, the so-called morning sickness of early pregnancy, because it occurs more often on arising than later in the day. At least 50% of all pregnant women, most of them in their first pregnancy, experience this condition, beginning during the fifth or sixth week of the pregnancy and usually ending about the fourteenth to sixteenth week. A number of factors may contribute to the situation. Some factors are physiologic, with causal factors based on hormonal changes that occur early in pregnancy. Another factor is low blood sugar, which can be relieved by carbohydrate foods, but will return within 2 to 3 hours after a meal. Others may be psychologic, based on situational tensions or anxieties about the pregnancy itself. Still others may be dietary problems, based on poor food habits. Simple treatment generally improves food tolerance. Frequent small low-fat meals and snacks, which are fairly dry and consist chiefly of easily digested energy-yielding foods such as carbohydrates (mainly starches), are usually more readily tolerated, such as crackers and pretzels. Some women find that fruit-flavored popsicles aid in abating nausea. In addition, it may help to avoid cooking odors as much as possible. Liquids are best taken between meals instead of with meals.

Hyperemesis

In a small number of pregnant women, about 3.5 per 1000 pregnancies, a severe form of persistent nausea and vomiting occurs that does not respond to usual treatment. This condition, *hyperemesis*, begins early in the pregnancy and may last throughout. It may develop into the more serious pernicious form of **hyperemesis gravidarum**. This persistent condition causes severe alterations in fluids and electrolytes, weight loss, and nutritional deficits, sometimes requiring hospitalization and alternative feeding by enteral or parenteral methods to sustain the pregnancy (see Chapter 19). Pyridoxine supplementation has been suggested as a preventive measure to abate nausea and vomiting, along with an increased protein and lower carbohydrate content of the diet.[43] Some prescription medications may also be useful but require physician supervision.[43] Continued personal support and reassurance are important.

Constipation

The complaint of constipation is seldom more than minor, but it contributes to discomfort and concern. Placental hormones relax the gastrointestinal muscles, and the pressure of the enlarging uterus on the lower portion of the intestine may make elimination somewhat difficult. Increased fluid intake and the use of naturally laxative foods containing dietary fiber, such as whole grains, fruits and vegetables, dried fruits (especially prunes and figs), and other fruits and juices, generally promote regularity. Laxatives should be avoided. Appropriate daily exercise is essential for overall health during pregnancy.

Hemorrhoids

A fairly common complaint during the latter part of pregnancy is that of hemorrhoids. These are enlarged veins in the anus, often protruding through the anal sphincter. This vein enlargement is usually caused by the increased weight of the fetus and its downward pressure. The hemorrhoids may cause considerable discomfort, burning, and itching. Occasionally, they may rupture and bleed under pressure of a bowel movement, causing anxiety. The problem is usually controlled by the dietary suggestions given for constipation. In addition, sufficient rest during the latter part of the day may help relieve some of the downward pressure of the uterus on the lower intestine.

Heartburn or Gastric Pressure

Pregnant women sometimes voice the related complaints of heartburn or a full feeling. These discomforts occur especially after meals and are usually caused by the pressure of the enlarging uterus crowding the stomach. Gastric reflux of some of the food mass, now a liquid chyme mixed with stomach acid, may occur in the lower esophagus, causing an irritation and a burning sensation. Obviously this common complaint has nothing to do with heart action but it receives the name because of the close proximity of the lower esophagus to the heart. The full feeling comes from general gastric pressure, lack of normal space in the area, a large meal, or gas formation. These complaints are usually remedied by dividing the day's food into a series of small meals, avoiding eating large meals at any time, and not lying down after a meal. Comfort is also improved by wearing loose-fitting clothing.

Effects of Iron Supplements

The effects of an iron supplement may include gray or black stools and sometimes nausea, constipation, or diarrhea. To help avoid food-related effects, the iron supplement should be taken 1 hour before a meal or 2 hours after it, with liquid such as water or orange juice but not with milk or tea. The absorption of iron is increased with vitamin C and decreased with milk, other dairy foods, eggs, whole grain bread and cereal, and tea. Ferrous fumarate and ferrous gluconate are alternate forms of iron supplements with good absorption properties that tend to result in less gastrointestinal distress.

KEY TERMS
hygroscopic Taking up and retaining moisture readily.
hyperemesis gravidarum Severe vomiting during pregnancy, which is potentially fatal.

HIGH-RISK PREGNANCIES

Identify Risk Factors Involved

To avoid the consequences of sustained poor nutrition during pregnancy, a first procedure is to identify women at risk. In a joint report, the American College of Obstetrics and Gynecology and the Academy of Nutrition and Dietetics issued a set of risk factors, shown in Box 11-1, that identify women with special nutritional needs during pregnancy.[5] These nutrition-related factors are based on clinical evidence of inadequate nutrition. However, rather than waiting for clinical symptoms of poor nutrition to appear, a better approach would be to identify poor food patterns that will induce nutritional problems and to prevent these problems from developing. On this basis, three types of dietary patterns predict failure to support optimal maternal and fetal nutrition: (1) insufficient food intake, (2) poor food selection, and (3) poor food distribution throughout the day. These patterns, added to the list of risk factors in Box 11-1, are much more sensitive for nutritional risk.

Plan Personal Care

Once early assessment identifies risk factors, practitioners can then give more careful attention to these women. By working closely with each woman and her personal food pattern and living situation, a food plan can be developed with her to ensure an optimal intake of energy and nutrients to support her pregnancy and its successful outcome.

Recognize Special Counseling Needs

Several special needs require sensitive counseling. These areas of need include the age and parity of the woman; any use of

BOX 11-1   NUTRITIONAL RISK FACTORS IN PREGNANCY

Risk Factors Present at the Onset of Pregnancy
- Age: <15 years old or >35 years old
- Frequent pregnancies: three or more during a 2-year period
- Poor obstetric history or poor fetal performance
- Poverty
- Bizarre or faddist food habits
- Abuse of nicotine, alcohol, or drugs
- Therapeutic diet required for a chronic disorder
- Weight: <85% or >120% of standard weight

Risk Factors Occurring During Pregnancy
- Low hemoglobin (HGB) or hematocrit (HCT): HGB <12 g/dL, HCT <35%
- Inadequate weight gain: any weight loss or weight gain of <1 kg (2 lb)/month after the first trimester
- Excessive weight gain: >1 kg (2 lb)/week after the first trimester

From American College of Obstetrics and Gynecology and American Dietetic Association Task Force on Nutrition: *Assessment of maternal nutrition*, Chicago, 1978, American College of Obstetrics and Gynecology.

harmful agents such as alcohol, cigarettes, drugs, or pica; and socioeconomic problems.

Age and Parity

Pregnancies at either age extreme of the reproductive cycle pose special problems. The Centers for Disease Control and Prevention reported that approximately 410,000 live births occurred to female teenagers during the year 2009.[44] The adolescent pregnancy carries many social and nutrition-related risks associated with increased incidence of low birth weight and perinatal mortality, among other poor outcomes. The obstetric history of a woman is expressed in terms of number and order of pregnancies, or her gravida status. A nulligravida (no prior pregnancy) who is 15 years of age or younger is especially at risk because her own growth is incomplete; therefore sufficient weight gain and the quality of her diet are particularly important.[40] Nutrients of particular concern are those for which the adolescent female requirements are greater than the adult requirements, including calcium, magnesium, phosphorus, and zinc. These nutrients are critical for growth and development of the adolescent, as well as for her fetus. Sensitive counseling provides information and emotional support; it should involve family members or other persons significant to the adolescent. On the other hand, the primigravida (an individual with her first pregnancy) who is older than 35 years of age also requires special attention. She may be more at risk for hypertension, either preexisting or pregnancy-induced, and may need more attention to the rate of weight gain and amount of sodium used, as well as any drug therapy prescribed. In addition, several pregnancies within a limited number of years leave a mother drained of nutritional resources and entering each successive pregnancy at increased risk.

Social Habits: Alcohol, Cigarettes, and Drugs

Alcohol, cigarettes, and drugs are three personal habits that may cause fetal damage and are contraindicated during pregnancy. No safe level of alcohol consumption has yet been found for pregnant women. Extensive or habitual alcohol use may lead to one of the fetal alcohol spectrum disorders known as *fetal alcohol syndrome (FAS)*, which is currently a leading cause of mental retardation.[45] FAS is characterized by growth retardation, malformed facial features, joint and limb abnormalities, cardiac defects, mental retardation, and in serious cases, death. FAS signs have been seen in tests with rats as early as the human equivalent of the third week of gestation, when most women are unaware of their pregnancies. Thus moderate-to-heavy drinking among sexually active women of childbearing age may carry potential danger. Even moderate prenatal alcohol exposure has been associated with low birth weight and has effects on a child's psychomotor and cognitive development in the absence of malformations, known as *fetal alcohol effects (FAE)*.[46]

Cigarette smoking during pregnancy is also contraindicated.[47] Harmful substances in tobacco and impaired oxygen transport cause fetal damage and special problems of placental abnormalities, leading to increased risk of spontaneous abortion (miscarriage), prematurity, low birth weight, impairment of mental and physical growth, and increased potential mortality. Counseling with women and families who smoke should stress the importance of quitting for pregnancy and beyond.

Drug use, both recreational and medicinal, also poses concerns.[48] Self-medication with over-the-counter drugs carries potential adverse effects. The use of illicit drugs is especially hazardous, exposing the developing fetus to the risks of addiction and possibly human immunodeficiency virus (HIV) from the woman's use of contaminated needles during drug injections. Dangers come not only from the drug itself or contaminated needles but also from impurities contained in illicit drugs. Evaluation of the effects of street drugs (marijuana, cocaine, heroin, methadone) on nutritional status is difficult because of multiple drug use, uncertain purity, unknown dose and timing, and inadequate nutritional status of many drug users. A high incidence of meconium staining (which could relate to fetal damage), poor prenatal weight gain, very short (less than 3 hours) or prolonged labor, operative delivery (cesarean, forceps), and other perinatal problems among marijuana users has been reported. Such outcomes indicate that it is prudent to abstain from marijuana use during pregnancy.[48,49]

Abuse from megadosing with basic nutrients such as vitamin A or use of prescription medications such as Acitretin during pregnancy may cause fetal damage as previously described (see Further Readings and Resources at the end of this chapter).[48] A number of drugs are often prescribed for female patients to treat a variety of psychologic and mental health disorders. However, if taken during pregnancy, many drugs exhibit teratogenic effects.[48] If any of these drugs are taken on a long-term basis for the treatment of serious conditions, such as clinical depression, bipolar disorder, or schizophrenia, then comprehensive medical and psychologic assessment and follow-up is needed throughout the pregnancy. Lithium has been associated with an increased risk for Ebstein's anomaly (a rare cardiovascular abnormality), goiter, and diabetes insipidus, as well as neonatal toxic disturbances such as cyanosis, hypothermia, and bradycardia. A diminished suck reflex will impede attempts to nourish the infant exposed to lithium in utero. Diazepam (Valium) is associated with an abnormal fetal heart rate. The neonate risks delivery by cesarean section, with oral-facial malformations, a depressed Apgar score, and a reluctance to feed. Rats exposed to diazepam in utero have exhibited abnormal motor skills and arousal processes. Tricyclic antidepressants (e.g., imipramine) have led to morphologic and behavioral abnormalities in rats.

Hydantoin (Dilantin, phenytoin) is used to control seizures caused by epilepsy and other conditions. Even though this drug has caused malformations in the offspring of rats, physicians are reluctant to discontinue it for their patients with epilepsy during pregnancy. This may be one case in which use of a drug prenatally is more beneficial than not using it: While up to 7% of children born to mothers using the drug develop malformations, significantly more develop malformations and developmental disabilities when the mother's epilepsy is untreated.[48] Thus with the exception of drugs used to treat individuals with seizure disorders or natural replacement therapy (e.g., insulin for persons with type 1 diabetes), drugs should be avoided at all costs during pregnancy to ensure the health of the woman and a safe and healthy outcome of the pregnancy. The nutrition counselor is well advised to keep up with the most recent findings regarding medications (prescribed, over-the-counter, and street drugs) to evaluate the nutritional status of the woman who uses them and to allow the practitioner and the woman to design a plan of action to safely eliminate the drug, preferably before conception. In addition, evaluation of herbal and botanical supplements, which are not regulated in the same manner as prescription and over-the-counter drugs, is necessary to inform the woman of potential safety issues and to counsel her appropriately.

Caffeine

Although milder in its effect (depending on the extent of use) than the agents just discussed, caffeine remains a widely used drug that can cross the placenta and enter fetal circulation. Its use at levels of 500 mg/day or greater has been associated with an increased risk of first-trimester spontaneous abortion.[50,51] Most health agencies have recommended that pregnant women limit caffeine consumption from foods, beverages (coffee, tea, cocoa, cola), and medications to less than 300 mg/day because of the many uncertainties regarding the fetal effects of maternal caffeine consumption.[52]

Pica

Pica is the craving and consumption of unusual nonfood substances such as laundry starch, clay, dirt, or ice. This practice during pregnancy is more widespread than health care workers have believed, particularly in southern regions of the United States and among specific ethnic and cultural groups. Some pica practices have been associated with iron deficiency anemia, although the direction of causality is unknown.[53,54] Where these unusual practices exist, they must be appreciated as cultural patterns that require a respectful approach and understanding by health workers who seek to negotiate appropriate behavior changes (see the Focus on Culture box, "Pica During Pregnancy: Cultural Norm of Concern").[55]

KEY TERMS

nulligravida A woman who has never been pregnant.

primigravida A woman who is pregnant for the first time.

meconium staining Resulting from fetal distress, the passing of the first stool by the fetus before birth, resulting in a green-yellow discoloration of the amniotic fluid and often the infant's skin, nailbeds, and umbilical cord at birth; harmful and potentially fatal.

teratogenic Causing malformation of an embryo, due to a teratogen (agent or substance that is teratogenic).

FOCUS ON CULTURE

Pica During Pregnancy: Cultural Norm of Concern

Pica is the ingestion of nonfood substances or food components including but not limited to clay, dirt, chalk, cornstarch, laundry starch, baking powder, baking soda, ice, and freezer frost. These substances are often craved with subsequent consumption. Approximately 20% of pregnant women engage in pica, and the prevalence of this psychobehavioral disorder is greater in rural (compared with urban) areas and in certain cultures.

Normal Cultural Behavior or Pregnancy-Induced Disorder

In a group of women from a variety of ethnic and religious backgrounds living in Kenya, more than 80% reported consumption of approximately 1 cup of soil on a daily basis. Soil intake was more common in the latter part of pregnancy. In these cultures, pica represents a cultural norm that may increase in prevalence during pregnancy.

Nearly 45% of women born and living in western Mexico engaged in pica during pregnancy, whereas only about 30% of Mexican-born women currently residing in California practiced pica during pregnancy. Although pica may be a culturally accepted norm, changes in prevalence may be induced with acculturation into a society where this behavior is less common.

Consequences of Pica and Need for Counseling

A pregnant woman who engages in pica, regardless of cultural background, should be informed about the health consequences of pica. Although it is unclear if nutrient deficiencies precipitate pica behaviors or vice versa, many pica substances are capable of binding nutrients to render them unavailable for absorption. Nutritional anemias may occur, which will have adverse effects on both mother and baby. Exposure to toxins and teratogens from nonfood substances such as battery acid or ashes is also possible. Gastrointestinal perforation, constipation, and microbial infections are additional potential outcomes of pica.

An understanding by the health care practitioner regarding factors leading to pica is vital to effecting changes in behavior. For example, the pregnant woman who believes that a nonfood substance has an essential role in the body's balance or harmony with her environment may be less willing to avoid consumption of that nonfood substance. On the other hand, a pregnant woman who consumes eggshells because of the sensory cravings associated with the texture may be amenable to substituting a crunchy food substance for this nonfood product. Inquiry regarding the history of pica in the pregnant woman is important to identify sources of pica substances and to involve other family members or cultural leaders who may support such behavior; they may need counseling to facilitate appropriate behavior changes. Such nutrition counseling must be delivered in a culturally sensitive and appropriate manner, with emphasis on the importance of behavior changes for an optimal outcome for the infant.

Bibliography

Corbett RW, Ryan C, Weinrich SP, et al: Pica in pregnancy: does it affect pregnancy outcomes? *MCN Am J Matern Child Nurs* 28(3):183, 2003.

Geissler PW, Prince RJ, Levene M, et al: Perceptions of soil-eating and anaemia among pregnant women on the Kenyan coast. *Soc Sci Med* 48(8):1069, 1999.

Mills ME: Craving more than food: the implications of pica in pregnancy. *Nurs Womens Health* 11(3):266, 2007.

Njiru H, Elchalal U, Paltiel O: Geophagy during pregnancy in Africa: a literature review. *Obstet Gynecol Surv* 66(7):452, 2011.

Rainville AJ: Pica practices of pregnant women are associated with lower maternal hemoglobin level at delivery. *J Am Diet Assoc* 98(3):293, 1998.

Simpson E, Mull JD, Longley E, et al: Pica during pregnancy in low-income women born in Mexico. *West J Med* 173(1):20, 2000.

Socioeconomic Challenges

Special counseling is required for women and young girls facing economic challenges. Numerous studies and clinical observations indicate that lack of prenatal care, often associated with racial prejudices and fears, as well as a lack of adequate financial resources, places the expectant mother in grave difficulty. Special counseling that is sensitive to personal needs is required to help plan resources for care and financial assistance. Resources include programs such as the federally funded Special Supplemental Nutrition Program for Women, Infants, and Children (WIC), described in Appendix E, as well as numerous state and local programs. An example of a community partnership program promoting prenatal care is Stork's Nest, sponsored by the March of Dimes in affiliation with a national women's organization and local community service agencies. Another successful program targeted for low-income women is BabyCare, administered by the Virginia Department of Health (see Further Readings and Resources at the end of this chapter).

COMPLICATIONS OF PREGNANCY

Anemia

Anemia is common during pregnancy. It is often associated with the normal maternal blood volume increase of 40% to 50% and a disproportionate increase in red cell mass of about 20%. Of all women in large prenatal clinics in the United States, about 10% have hemoglobin concentrations of less than 10 g/dL and a hematocrit reading less than 32%. Normal values for hemoglobin and hematocrit during pregnancy are 11.5 to 15 g/dL and 32% to 36.5%, respectively. Anemia is far more prevalent among the poor, many of whom live on diets barely adequate for subsistence. However, anemia is by no means restricted to lower economic groups.

Iron Deficiency Anemia

A deficiency of iron is by far the most common cause of anemia in pregnancy. The total iron cost of a single normal pregnancy is large—approximately 500 to 800 mg. Of this amount, the fetus uses nearly 300 mg. The remainder is used in the expanded maternal blood volume and its increased red blood cells and hemoglobin mass. This iron requirement typically exceeds the available reserves in the average woman. Thus in addition to including iron-rich foods in the diet, a daily supplement or increased therapeutic dose may be required, as previously described.

Folate Deficiency Anemia

A less common megaloblastic anemia of pregnancy results from folate deficiency. During pregnancy, the fetus is sensitive to folate inhibitors and therefore has increased metabolic requirements for folate. To prevent this anemia the DRI standard recommends 600 mcg of folate per day during pregnancy. Women with poor diets will need supplementation to reach this intake goal.

Hemorrhagic Anemia

Anemia caused by blood loss is more likely to occur during labor and delivery than during pregnancy. Blood loss may occur earlier, as a result of abortion or ruptured tubular pregnancy. Most women undergoing these physiologic problems receive blood via transfusion, and iron therapy may be indicated for adequate replacement for hemoglobin formation.

Pregnancy-Induced Hypertension
Relation to Nutrition

A number of clinicians have presented clinical and laboratory evidence that pregnancy-induced hypertension (PIH) is a disease that principally affects young women with their first pregnancy. Although the genetic and immune-related causes of PIH are becoming clearer, diet plays a role in the risk of preeclampsia. For example, diets poor in kcalories, protein, calcium, magnesium, potassium, and dietary fiber have been associated with risk of PIH.[56] Regardless of the underlying causes and multiorgan effects, nutritional support of the pregnancy is, as always, a primary concern. Certainly, as many practitioners have observed, PIH is classically associated with poverty, inadequate diet, and little or no prenatal care. Much of the PIH problem, which seems to develop early from the time of implantation of the fertilized ovum into the uterine lining, may be reduced by good prenatal care from the beginning of the pregnancy, which inherently includes attention to sound nutrition. It is this sound nutritional status, which a woman brings to her pregnancy and maintains throughout it, that provides her with optimal resources for adapting to the physiologic stress of gestation. Her fitness during pregnancy is a direct function of her past state of nutrition and her optimal nutrition throughout pregnancy.

Clinical Symptoms

PIH is defined according to its manifestations, which generally occur in the third trimester toward term. These symptoms are hypertension, abnormal and excessive edema, albuminuria, and, in severe cases, convulsions or coma, a state called eclampsia.

Treatment

Specific treatment varies according to the individual patient's symptoms and needs. Optimal nutrition is a fundamental aspect of therapy in any case. Emphasis is given to a regular diet with adequate dietary protein and calcium, as well as to a diet that is rich in fruits and vegetables, providing magnesium, potassium, and dietary fiber. Correction of plasma protein deficits stimulates the capillary fluid shift mechanism and increases circulation of tissue fluids, with subsequent correction of the hypovolemia. In addition, adequate salt and sources of vitamins and minerals are needed for correction and maintenance of metabolic balance.

Multiple Fetuses

The incidence of multifetal pregnancies has increased in recent decades and presents unique concerns. Infants born from a multifetal pregnancy are more likely to have lower-than-average birth weights and are at risk for preterm delivery.[39] Thus the nutritional needs of these women must be given special attention. Energy intake must be increased beyond the needs of a single fetus pregnancy so that the recommended weight gain for multiple fetuses is achieved. This increase in energy intake often provides for the additional nutrient demands that exist. Attention to adequate folate intake is critical to reduce risks of low birth weights and preterm delivery. Supplemental iron may be necessary to reduce the incidence of anemia, more commonly found in women with multiple fetuses. Additional calcium and vitamin D are needed with multiple fetuses to promote adequate calcium absorption for optimal bone mineralization in utero. Zinc, copper, and pyridoxine supplementation may also be required to support multifetal growth and development.

Maternal Disease Conditions

Preexisting clinical conditions in the woman further complicate pregnancy. In each case, management of these conditions is based on general principles of care related to pregnancy and to the particular disease involved. Examples of such maternal conditions are reviewed here; they are hypertension, diabetes mellitus, PKU, HIV, and eating disorders.

Hypertension

Preexisting hypertension in the pregnant woman can have considerable maternal and fetal consequences. Many of these problems can be prevented by initial screening and continued monitoring by the prenatal nurse, with referral to the clinical nutritionist for a plan of care. The hypertensive disease process begins long before signs and symptoms appear, and later symptoms are inconsistent. Risk factors for hypertension before and during pregnancy are listed in Box 11-2. Nutritional therapy centers on the following three principles:

1. Prevention of weight extremes (i.e., underweight or obesity)
2. Correction of any dietary deficiencies and maintenance of optimal nutritional status during pregnancy
3. Management of any related coexisting disease (e.g., diabetes mellitus, hyperlipidemia)

Sodium intake may be moderate but should not be unduly restricted because of its relation to fluid and electrolyte balances during pregnancy. Initial and continuing client education and a close relationship with the nurse-nutritionist care team contribute to successful management of the hypertension and prevent problems that may occur. (For a more detailed discussion of vascular disease, see Chapter 21.)

Diabetes Mellitus and Gestational Diabetes Mellitus

The management of preexisting diabetes in pregnancy presents special problems. Today, however, improved expectations for the diabetic woman's pregnancy constitute one of the success stories of modern medicine. Contributing factors to this improved outlook include advances in technology for monitoring fetal development, increased knowledge of nutrition and diabetes, and management refinements in tight blood glucose control through self-monitoring.[57,58]

During pregnancy, glycosuria is not uncommon because of the increased circulating blood volume and its load of metabolites. Routine screening protocols, typically conducted between the twenty-fourth and twenty-eighth week of gestation, are used during pregnancy to detect gestational diabetes mellitus (GDM). GDM is an intolerance of carbohydrate such that blood glucose concentration increases during pregnancy. In 95% of cases this carbohydrate or glucose intolerance resolves after delivery. Treatment during pregnancy is important because of the increased risk these women carry for fetal damage during this gestational period.[59] The most common outcome for an infant born to a mother with GDM is macrosomia, a larger than normal body size. Other infant complications include hypoglycemia, jaundice, and trauma at birth. Although GDM occurs in 2% to 13% of the pregnant population, up to 50% of women with pregnancy-induced abnormal glucose tolerance subsequently develop overt diabetes. Team management is required for adequate care of gestational and preexisting types 1 and 2 diabetes mellitus.[57,58] (See Chapter 22 for a detailed discussion of diabetes care.)

Maternal Phenylketonuria

The successful detection and management of infants with PKU through newborn screening programs in all states have ensured their normal growth and development to adulthood. PKU is a genetic metabolic disease caused by a missing enzyme for the metabolism of the essential amino acid phenylalanine. It is controlled by a special low-phenylalanine diet initiated at birth. Now a new generation of young women with PKU since birth are beginning to have children of their own. However, maternal PKU presents potential fetal hazards. Experience has shown how crucial it is for the woman to follow a strict low-phenylalanine diet before conception, to minimize risks of fetal damage in the early cell differentiation weeks of pregnancy.

Human Immunodeficiency Virus

Carefully monitored care throughout pregnancy and after birth is essential for pregnant women who are infected with HIV. Two goals are most important: (1) to reduce the rate of the disease progression in the woman through nutritional support and (2) to minimize the chance of HIV vertical transmission from mother to infant, either in the womb or after birth via breast-feeding. Poor weight gain and nutrient deficiencies during pregnancy are often found in HIV-positive patients. Although specific nutrient requirements for HIV-infected pregnant women have not been established, these patients may need up to 150% of normal pregnancy intakes of macronutrients and micronutrients. Continual individual monitoring and adjustment are essential. Infants can be infected by HIV during labor and delivery and through breast milk. Where safe alternatives to breast milk are available, such as commercial formula or banked human milk, a decision on breast-feeding depends on the HIV status of the newborn

---

BOX 11-2 RISK FACTORS FOR PREGNANCY-INDUCED HYPERTENSION

Before Pregnancy
- Nulligravida
- Diabetes
- Preexisting condition (hypertension, renal or vascular disease)
- Family history of hypertension or vascular disease
- Diagnosis of pregnancy-induced hypertension (PIH) in a previous pregnancy
- Dietary deficiencies
- Age extremes (≤ 20 years old, ≥ 35 years old)

During Pregnancy
- Primigravida
- Large fetus
- Glomerulonephritis
- Fetal hydrops
- Hydramnios
- Multiple gestation
- Hydatidiform mole

KEY TERMS
eclampsia Advanced pregnancy-induced hypertension (PIH), manifested by convulsions.
hypovolemia Abnormally decreased volume of circulating blood in the body.
preeclampsia Hypertension (blood pressure greater than 140/90 mmHg) and proteinuria (more than 300 mg protein/24-hr urine) in pregnancy; if untreated, may develop into eclampsia.

infant. In the United States the Centers for Disease Control and Prevention (CDC) and the American Academy of Pediatrics recommend HIV-positive mothers do not breast-feed when the infant is not infected.[60,61]

Eating Disorders

Eating disorders, specifically anorexia nervosa and bulimia nervosa, have been previously described (see Chapter 8). Diagnosis and treatment of these disorders in the nonpregnant state require multidisciplinary approaches, and even greater consideration with further specialized care is required for a pregnant woman with anorexia or bulimia nervosa. Anorexia nervosa is uncommon during pregnancy, because amenorrhea is a diagnostic criteria for the disorder; however, ovulation and subsequent conception has been reported.[62] Compared with anorexia nervosa, pregnancy in a woman with bulimia nervosa is more likely, because of more typical menstrual patterns, weight status, and less restrictive eating. Bulimia nervosa has been linked to spontaneous abortion, poor weight gain, low infant birth weight, premature deliveries, and congenital malformations.[63] A team approach that emphasizes nutritional needs of the growing fetus, anticipated maternal body size and shape changes, and postpartum care is critical to a successful course and outcome.[63,64]

NUTRITION DURING LACTATION

Current Breast-Feeding Trends

Data from the National Immunization Survey show that approximately 75% of mothers initiate breast-feeding.[65] Several factors contribute to this rate of breast-feeding initiation:

- More mothers are informed about the benefits of breast-feeding (Figure 11-4).[66,67]
- Practitioners recognize the ability of human milk to meet infant needs (Table 11-3) and promote immune function.[68,69]
- Maternity wards and alternative birth centers have been modified to facilitate successful lactation.

- Community support is increasingly available, even in workplaces.[70]
- Programs that promote breast-feeding are increasingly responsive to a wider range of maternal socioeconomic conditions and cultural backgrounds.[71-74]

Exclusive breast-feeding by well-nourished mothers can be adequate for periods ranging from 2 to 15 months,[75-78] although sources of iron and vitamin D are needed by the infant around 6 months of age. Exclusive breast-feeding is strongly encouraged for at least 6 months. Unfortunately, breast-feeding declines to fewer than 45% and fewer than 24% of mothers by 3 months and 6 months, respectively.[65] Solid foods are usually added to the baby's diet at about 6 months of age; the Academy of Nutrition and Dietetics' position is that breast-feeding should continue for at least the first 12 months of the infant's life.[78]

Cultural factors may influence how women in racial and ethnic groups regard breast-feeding. Hispanic and Asian

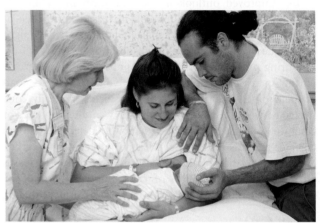

FIGURE 11-4 By teaching about the newborn and family, the nurse helps parents develop confidence in their ability to provide care for the infant. (From McKinney ES, Ashwill JW, Murray SS, et al: *Maternal-child nursing*, Philadelphia, Pa., 2000, Saunders.)

TABLE 11-3	SELECTED NUTRITIONAL COMPONENTS OF HUMAN MILK (PER 100 mL)			
MILK COMPONENT	**COLOSTRUM**	**TRANSITIONAL**	**MATURE**	**COW'S MILK**
Kilocalories	57.0	63.0	65.0	65.0
Vitamins, fat soluble				
A (mcg)	151.0	88.0	75.0	41.0
D (IU)	—	—	5.0	2.5
E (mg)	1.5	0.9	0.25	0.07
K (mcg)	—	—	1.5	6.0
Vitamins, water soluble				
Thiamin (mcg)	1.9	5.9	14.0	43.0
Riboflavin (mcg)	30.0	37.0	40.0	145.0
Niacin (mcg)	75.0	175.0	160.0	82.0
Pantothenic acid (mcg)	183.0	288.0	246.0	340.0
Biotin (mcg)	0.06	0.35	0.6	2.8
Vitamin B_{12} (mcg)	0.05	0.04	0.1	1.1
Vitamin C (mg)	5.9	7.1	5.0	1.1

mothers tend to listen to their mothers, grandmothers, and significant others more when making choices about breast-feeding, while non-Hispanic white mothers depend more on recommendations from health care providers.[79] Black women tend to have less interest in breast-feeding compared to women in other racial groups.[80] Women of all racial and ethnic groups who search for information about breast-feeding and are more highly educated are more likely to exclusively breast-feed, suggesting that socioeconomic status is correlated to infant feeding choices. Moreover, educational interventions and support systems for breast-feeding can increase the number of women intending to and who actually breast-feed.[81] Women should be educated early and continually about breast-feeding, and health care providers should seek to understand the cultural and socioeconomic influences related to breast-feeding choices among women of racial and ethnic groups.

Nutritional Needs

The physiologic needs of lactation are different from those of pregnancy, and they demand adequate nutritional support (see Table 11-1). The basic nutritional needs for lactation include the following additions to the mother's prepregnancy needs.

Energy

The recommended caloric increase is 330 kcal/day (plus 170 kcal/day from maternal stores) in the first 6 months and 400 kcal/day in the second 6 months of breast-feeding (beyond the usual adult allowance). This makes a daily total of about 2700 to 2800 kcal/day for milk production and maternal energy needs.[10] This additional energy need for the overall total lactation process is based on the following four factors:

1. *Milk content:* An average daily milk production for lactating women is 780 mL (26 oz). The energy content of human milk averages 0.67 to 0.74 kcal/g. Thus 26 oz of milk has a value of about 525 kcal.
2. *Milk production:* The metabolic work involved in producing this amount of milk is about 80% efficient and requires from 400 to 450 kcal. During pregnancy the breast is developed for this purpose, stimulated by hormones from the placenta, and forms special milk-producing cells called *lobules* (Figure 11-5). After birth the mother's production of the hormone prolactin continues this milk-production process, which the suckling infant stimulates. Thus milk production depends on the demand of the infant. The suckling infant stimulates the brain's release of the hormone oxytocin from the pituitary gland to initiate the letdown reflex for the release of the milk from storage cells to travel down to the nipple. This reflex is easily inhibited by the mother's fatigue, tension, or lack of confidence, a particular source of anxiety in the new mother. She may be reassured that a comfortable and satisfying feeding routine is usually established in 2 to 3 weeks (Figure 11-6).
3. *Maternal adipose tissue storage:* A component of the energy need for lactation (170 kcal/day in the first 6 months) is

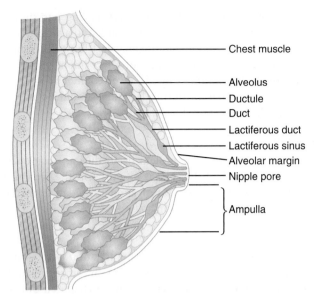

FIGURE 11-5 Structural features of the human mammary gland. (From Mahan LK, Escott-Stump S, editors: *Krause's food, nutrition, and diet therapy,* ed 11, Philadelphia, Pa., 2004, Saunders.)

Chest muscle
Alveolus
Ductule
Duct
Lactiferous duct
Lactiferous sinus
Alveolar margin
Nipple pore
Ampulla

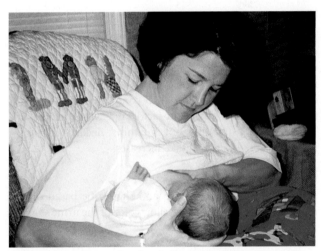

FIGURE 11-6 Breast-feeding infant and mother. (From Lowdermilk DL, Perry SE, Bobak IM: *Maternity and women's health care,* ed 7, St Louis, Mo., 2000, Mosby.)

drawn from maternal adipose tissue stores deposited during pregnancy in normal preparation for lactation to follow in the maternal cycle. Depending on the adequacy of these stores, additional energy input may be needed in the lactating woman's daily diet.

4. *Exercise:* Lactating women generally balance energy expenditure from exercise with increased energy intake and alterations in prolactin to maintain an adequate milk supply. In some women, the weight gained during pregnancy may be largely retained and contribute to obesity. Some overweight women who are breast-feeding have concerns whether a weight-loss program might endanger the growth of their infants. Research with overweight

women who were exclusively breast-feeding has shown that a diet and exercise program that led to a weight loss of around 0.5 kg/week (approximately 1 lb/week) from 4 to 14 weeks postpartum did not affect infant growth.[82] However, the mother who is involved in any specific weight-loss program during lactation should be monitored closely as should her infant.[82,83]

Protein

The recommendation for protein needs during lactation is 71 g/day during both the first 6 months and the second 6 months.[10] This is an increase of about 25 g/day from the regular needs of the adult woman.

Minerals

The DRI standard for calcium during lactation is 1000 mg/day, the same as for the nonpregnant or pregnant adult woman.[6] The amount of calcium that was required during gestation for the mineralization of the fetal skeleton is now diverted into the mother's milk production. Iron, because it is not a major mineral component of milk and because of lactational amenorrhea, need not be increased during lactation.

Vitamins

The DRI standard for vitamin C during lactation is 120 mg/day.[8] This is a considerable increase from the regular 75 mg/day for adult women. Increases beyond the mother's prenatal intake are also recommended for vitamin A because it is a constituent of milk,[9] and for the B-complex vitamins because they are involved as coenzyme factors in energy metabolism.[7] Therefore the quantities of vitamins needed invariably increase as the kcalorie intake increases.

Fluids

Ample fluid intake is needed and should be based on the mother's urine color. A pale-yellow color of the urine suggests adequate fluid intake. Beverages such as juices and milk contribute fluid and kcalories.[42]

Food Intake

Figure 11-7 displays an example of a healthy food intake pattern for a breast-feeding woman. In general, 7 to 8 oz of grains, at least one half of which are whole grains; 3 cups of vegetables; 2 cups of fruits; 3 cups of fluid milk or dairy products; 6 to 6.5 oz of lean meats, poultry, fish, dried beans, and nuts; and 6 to 7 tsp of oils per day are recommended to meet nutrient needs during lactation (www.ChooseMyPlate.gov).

Dietary Supplements

Many health practitioners recommend that women continue their prenatal nutrient supplements during lactation. Specifically, women with certain health conditions or nutrient needs may require supplements while breast-feeding.[84] For example, mothers who consume vegan diets will need vitamin-B_{12} supplements.[84,85] Individual recommendations for nutrient supplementation during lactation should be based on a full assessment of the mother's nutritional status and other environmental factors.

Women may desire to use herbal or botanical products as galactogogues (agents that stimulate breast milk production), relaxants, or analgesics. The safety for mother and infant and efficacy of such products during lactation have not been adequately evaluated in randomized, placebo-controlled trials. In general, women should not use herbals and botanicals during lactation; however, some may be appropriate for use within defined quantities.[37]

Rest and Relaxation

In addition to the increased diet, the nursing mother requires rest, moderate exercise, and relaxation. Both parents may benefit from counseling focused on reducing the stresses of their new family situation, as well as meeting their own

FIGURE 11-7 Food intake plan for a breast-feeding woman based on maternal age, height, current weight, and physical activity, infant birth date, and exclusive breast-feeding or combination feeding using the MyPlate resource (www.ChooseMyPlate.gov).

	0–6 months	7–12 months
Grains	6 oz per day	9 oz per day
Whole grains	≥ 4 oz per day	≥ 4½ oz per day
Vegetables	3 cups per day	3½ cups per day
Dark green	2 cups per week	2½ cups per week
Red and orange	6 cups per week	7 cups per week
Beans and peas	2 cups per week	2½ cups per week
Starchy	6 cups per week	7 cups per week
Other	5 cups per week	5½ cups per week
Fruits	2 cups per day	2 cups per day
Dairy	3 cups per day	3 cups per day
Protein foods	6 oz per day	6½ oz per day
Seafood	10 oz per week	10 oz per week
Oils	7 tsp per day	8 tsp per day
Total calories	2400 kcal per day	2600 kcal per day
Discretionary calories	330 kcal per day	362 kcal per day

personal needs. Postpartum depression is increasingly recognized as a specific, and sometimes very serious, condition in mothers. Ranging from "baby blues" to postpartum psychosis, the relationship of this condition with nutritional status requires further investigation.[86,87] For example, iron deficiency anemia may be a risk factor for postpartum depression (see Evidence-Based Practice box, "Iron and Postpartum Depression"). The connections among nutrient needs, postpartum depression, and breast-feeding duration will be of future interest.

Maternal Medical Conditions

Breast-feeding should be encouraged in most mothers (see the Perspectives in Practice box, "Breast-Feeding: The Dynamic Nature of Human Milk"). However, some conditions exist for which it is recommended that women in the United States not breast-feed, including HIV-positive status, active untreated tuberculosis, human T-lymphocytic virus, illicit drug use, and with specific chemotherapeutic agents. Other conditions or medications should be discussed with health practitioners.[78]

EVIDENCE-BASED PRACTICE

Iron and Postpartum Depression

Is it possible that clinical deficiencies of nutrients cause postpartum depression? Iron-deficiency anemia is common among women, particularly postpartum women because of iron losses with delivery and mobilization of iron stores to support fetal growth, development, and iron storage during the latter stages of pregnancy. An association between low hemoglobin concentration (less than 12 g/dL) and increased self-rated symptoms of depression were reported in eight postpartum women within the first month after delivery. This was significantly different from lower self-rated symptoms of depression in 29 postpartum women with hemoglobin concentration greater than 12 g/dL. In a separate study, lower plasma ferritin concentration was present in women reporting symptoms of postpartum depression. One randomized controlled trial found that self-reported depression and stress significantly decreased in 30 postpartum women with iron-deficiency anemia who were treated with 125 mg ferrous sulfate (along with folate and vitamin C), compared with 21 untreated anemic postpartum women (supplemented with only folate and vitamin C) and 30 nonanemic control women.

Questions for Analysis
1. Does this evidence suggest that postpartum women should routinely be supplemented with iron to prevent postpartum depression?
2. What additional evidence is required to establish practice guidelines regarding nutrition and prevention or treatment of postpartum depression?

Bibliography
Albacar G, Sans T, Martin-Santos R, et al: An association between plasma ferritin concentrations measured 48 h after delivery and postpartum depression. *J Affect Disord* 131(1–3):136, 2011.

Beard JL, Hendricks MK, Perez EM, et al: Maternal iron deficiency anemia affects postpartum emotions and cognition. *J Nutr* 135:267, 2005.

Corwin EJ, Murray-Kolb LE, Beard JL: Low hemoglobin level is a risk factor for postpartum depression. *J Nutr* 133:4139, 2003.

PERSPECTIVES IN PRACTICE

Breast-Feeding: The Dynamic Nature of Human Milk

Human milk is the ideal first food for human infants. Its dynamic nature changes to match growth needs. The mother's choice to breast-feed her infant depends on a number of factors, however, especially for new mothers, who often need information and counseling from early pregnancy.

Even premature infants can thrive on human milk. Mothers and physicians have sometimes been reluctant to consider breast-feeding for infants born prematurely or delivered by cesarean section, fearing that the early birth or surgical procedure may have some negative effect on the quantity or quality of human milk. This uncertainty about the nutritional quality of mother's milk has also led physicians to encourage adding formula or solid foods (or both) to the diet to make sure the infant is well fed. These practices are usually unnecessary. They often contribute to allergies, obesity, and digestive problems because of the extra stress placed on an immature gut.

Breast Milk for the Preterm Infant
The levels of nutrients in mother's milk shift according to the gestational age of the infant at birth. The preterm infant is often denied its mother's milk by some hospital workers because they think of it as mature milk having too little protein and too much lactose to meet the child's needs. An analysis of the nutritional quality of preterm milk, however, reveals energy and fat concentrations that are 20% to 30% greater, protein levels 15% to 20% greater, and lactose levels 10% lower than those found in mature milk. Premature milk can meet the preterm infant's nutritional and developmental needs, if the mother is committed to breast-feeding and/or expressing breast milk and feeding by bottle or feeding tube to her infant.

Breast Milk During Weaning
Nutrient levels continue to change with time to match changing growth patterns and developing digestive abilities. Mother's

Continued

Breast-Feeding: The Dynamic Nature of Human Milk—cont'd

milk does provide sufficient kcalories and nutrients to keep babies well fed without supplemental formula or food. Even when the infant is being weaned, the nature of human milk ensures adequate nutrients, just in case the new, solid-food diet cannot meet the child's needs. Human milk collected during gradual weaning has been found to have increased concentrations of protein, sodium, and iron. Lactose levels are lower, possibly so that increased amounts of kcalories can be supplied by fats, a more concentrated source.

Breast Milk and the Cesarean Section Infant

The quality of human milk is not influenced by the way the baby comes into the world. Many women fear that a baby born by cesarean section cannot be nursed because they think that this method of delivery delays or prevents the production of mature milk. Milk production is stimulated by the release of the placenta, which occurs whether the delivery is vaginal or not. Studies confirm that no significant difference exists in the length of time it takes for mature milk to come in after vaginal or cesarean deliveries.

Thus premature or cesarean deliveries should not discourage women from breast-feeding. Mothers should not underestimate the nutritive quality of their milk simply because it does not appear as rich and thick as cow's milk. After all, cow's milk is made for young calves, who are up and running around after birth and have a much shorter, faster growth period. For the human infant, in nutritional and immunologic terms, breast milk remains the best milk.

Mothers' Facts and Fancies About Breast-Feeding

In early counseling, mothers express a variety of concerns about breast-feeding. Following are a few such statements:

"My Breasts Aren't Big Enough"

When it comes to breast-feeding, all women are created equal. The only parts of the breast that participate in milk production are the glandular and nervous tissue and the nipple; these are basically the same in healthy women. The only difference between a size 32A and a size 42DD is the amount of fat tissue the breast contains.

"Breast-Feeding Causes Cancer"

Actually, investigators have been looking to breast-feeding as a possible means of preventing breast and ovarian cancer. Epidemiologic studies suggest a decreased risk for these cancers in women who breast-feed, but additional evidence is needed before a consensus may be reached.

"Breast-Feeding Will Ruin My Figure"

Because the caloric demand of breast-feeding exceeds that of the nonpregnant woman by about 400 to 500 kcalories, a slightly faster rate of weight loss may be expected, although hormonal adaptations may limit the extent to which weight loss is experienced during lactation. Oxytocin, the hormone manufactured to stimulate the letdown reflex, also stimulates uterine contractions, helping reduce the uterus to its prepregnancy size more rapidly.

"Breast-Feeding Is Painful"

It may be painful in the first few days or even weeks as mother and baby establish a pattern of feeding and proper latch and release techniques. Milk should not be allowed to collect in the breast to the point of engorgement, the nipples should be kept clean and dry, and a variety of feeding positions may be used while nursing to decrease the chances of having a painful experience. Mastitis is a painful infection of the breast that requires medical attention and often antibiotic treatment.

"Breast Milk Is Not Nutritious"

The thin, bluish appearance of breast milk has some women convinced that it is no more nourishing than water. Let them look at Table 11-3; they will be pleasantly surprised at how well breast milk meets the nutritional needs of the infant.

"I Will Have to Change My Diet to Breast-Feed"

Foods that were eaten during pregnancy may be consumed during lactation. Some women report that after they eat onions, cauliflower, cabbage, or other foods their infants do not like the taste of their breast milk. Other women say that eating chocolate or drinking coffee, for example, "makes their babies fussy" when breast-feeding. Scientific evidence does not discourage moderate intake of these foods or drinks. A well-balanced diet that includes a variety of colorful foods and fluids is encouraged during breast-feeding.

"I Cannot Go to Work or School if I Breast-Feed"

Breast milk can be stored for up to 5 days in the refrigerator or up to 5 months in the freezer. Many working mothers take advantage of this by expressing their milk and storing it for use by care providers. In fact, women often express milk on their breaks at school or work. (Some places of employment even have lactation rooms and provide breast pumps at the workplace.) Expressing milk not only relieves the pressure of buildup but it also allows the milk to be stored for later use at home.

Other women would like to breast-feed but are worried about special "what if" situations, such as the following:

"What if I Need a Cesarean Section?"

The method of delivery does not affect the quality or quantity of milk produced. The baby can be held in such a way (the "football hold") that he or she does not rest on the mother's abdominal stitches.

"What if the Baby Is Premature?"

Mother's milk changes to meet the infant's needs at all stages of development.

"What if the Baby Has Down Syndrome?"

Infants with Down syndrome can be nursed; however, it does require time, patience, and the use of slightly different nursing techniques. The mother should be told about the special nursing needs of infants with Down syndrome to avoid disappointment or a feeling of failure should breast-feeding become impractical for her particular living situation.

Breast-Feeding: The Dynamic Nature of Human Milk—cont'd

"What if I Have Twins?"

Believe it or not, it has been done. It takes time, patience, and good coordination to breast-feed twins, but it is possible. Triplets, however, are another matter altogether. Women have successfully nursed triplets, but often they did very little else until the babies were weaned. This mother will need emotional support, whether she attempts to nurse or, finding the amount of time and patience required overwhelming, prefers to bottle-feed.

"What if I Have Pierced Nipples or Have Had Breast Surgery?"

Nipple jewelry appears to interfere with breast-feeding; however, a mother who wishes to maintain her piercing while breast-feeding may use retainers. Women should be made aware that serious complications because of nipple piercing have been reported, requiring pharmaceutical or surgical treatments that have required up to 12 months for resolution. Very little is known about later breast-feeding successes or complications after earlier removal of a nipple piercing. Breast augmentation and reduction surgeries have shown mixed results related to successful breast-feeding; however, this issue has not been adequately investigated. One retrospective study has shown that previous breast reduction does not impair the ability to breast-feed, while a separate study found that breast-feeding success was 25% lower in women who had undergone breast augmentation. Women should be informed about the current lack of knowledge surrounding these issues but presented with guidance for decision making.

"What if I Become Pregnant?"

Some women may purposefully choose to breast-feed to avoid pregnancy, but this is not a dependable contraception method. Well-nourished women of the world tend to be more fertile and may find themselves pregnant and breast-feeding at the same time. Women who breast-feed must understand that the lack of a menstrual period during lactation (lactational amenorrhea) does not mean they cannot become pregnant. Contraceptives may be required if another pregnancy is not desired at the current time. If pregnancy occurs, then the woman should discuss appropriate infant-feeding solutions with her health care team.

Advantages and Barriers to Breast-Feeding

These factors need to be reviewed with each individual mother in her particular situation so that she can make the informed decision that is best for the infant and herself.

Many nutritional, physiologic, psychologic, and practical advantages to breast-feeding exist; six are identified as follows:

1. Human milk changes to meet changing nutrient and energy needs of the newborn and the maturing infant during the first months of life. It is always there in the correct form to meet the growing infant's needs.
2. Infants experience fewer infections because the mother transfers certain antibodies and immune properties in human

milk to her nursing infant. In addition, no exposure of the infant to infectious organisms in the environment that can contaminate preparation and equipment for bottle-feeding, especially in poorer living situations.
3. Fewer allergies and intolerances occur, especially in allergy-prone infants, because cow's milk contains a number of potentially allergy-causing proteins that human milk does not have.
4. Ease of digestion is greater with breast milk because human milk forms a softer curd in the gastrointestinal tract that is easier for the infant to digest.
5. The convenience and economy of breast milk are greater because the mother is free from the time and expense involved in buying and preparing formula, and her breast milk is always ready and sterile.
6. Breast-feeding provides psychologic bonding because the mother and infant relate to one another during feeding, regular times of rest and enjoyment, and cuddling and fulfillment.

Despite the advantages of breast-feeding, some women do have to deal with perceived barriers associated with misinformation, personal feelings of modesty, family pressures, or outside employment, among other factors. Addressing these barriers, such as the following, before delivery rather than after will increase the likelihood that the mother breast-feeds her infant:

- Misinformation, a major barrier, creates negative impressions and ideas. Women in today's world often lack positive role models in extended families or experienced friends with whom they can discuss their feelings and obtain much practical guidance. Experienced breast-feeding mothers or lactation consultants can fill this need, especially for young first-time mothers.
- Personal modesty and anxiety, or a fear of appearing immodest in breast exposure, may hinder some mothers from breast-feeding. Sensitive counseling, especially with a positive role model as described previously, can help to allay some of these personal fears. Most of women's breast-feeding is done in the privacy of the home rather than around others; therefore early support during initial experiences would be helpful.
- Family pressures, especially from the husband, not to breast-feed have strong influences on the mother, even though she may want to do so. Initial counseling and education about breast-feeding should include both parents whenever possible. Reasons for negative attitudes can be explored and misinformation clarified with sound education.
- Outside employment, with a limited maternity leave and job loss if the mother does not return to work at that time, can complicate the mother's decision, even though she may want to breast-feed her baby. However, if the mother does have the will, then it is possible to breast-feed and be employed. After breast-feeding is well established, she can regularly express milk by hand or with a breast pump into sterile disposable nursing bags to use with disposable holder, cap, and nipple ensemble. Rapid chilling and strict

Continued

PERSPECTIVES IN PRACTICE

Breast-Feeding: The Dynamic Nature of Human Milk—cont'd

sanitation are required, but it can be planned, given the commitment. Some companies provide child care facilities for their employees, recognizing that helping employees with this modern need is good business. The mother can plan occasional formula feeds to fill in with the sustained breast-feeding.

All of these approaches to breast-feeding have real rewards for the infant. In addition, they can strengthen the mother's confidence in her maternal capabilities. The importance of these intangible benefits should not be underestimated.

Bibliography

American Academy of Pediatrics Section on Breastfeeding: Breastfeeding and the use of human milk. *Pediatrics* 129(3):e827, 2012.

Chung M, Ip S, Yu W, et al: Interventions in primary care to promote breastfeeding: a systematic review. *Agency for Healthcare Research and Quality (US)* Report No.: 09-05126-EF-1, 2008.

Cruz NI, Korchin L: Breastfeeding after augmentation mammaplasty with saline implants. *Ann Plast Surg* 64(5):530, 2010.

Cruz-Korchin N, Korchin L: Breast-feeding after vertical mammaplasty with medial pedicle. *Plast Reconstr Surg* 114(4):890, 2004.

Lewis CG, Wells MK, Jennings WC: *Mycobacterium fortuitum* breast infection following nipple-piercing, mimicking carcinoma. *Breast J* 10(4):363, 2004.

Martin J: Is nipple piercing compatible with breastfeeding? *J Hum Lact* 20(3):319, 2004.

Pisacane A, Toscano E, Pirri I, et al: Down syndrome and breastfeeding. *Acta Paediatr* 92(12):1479, 2003.

Position of the American Dietetic Association: Promoting and supporting breastfeeding. *J Am Diet Assoc* 109(11):1926, 2009.

Siskind V, Green A, Bain C, et al: Breastfeeding, menopause, and epithelial ovarian cancer. *Epidemiology* 8(2):188, 1997.

Yang L, Jacobsen KH: A systematic review of the association between breastfeeding and breast cancer. *J Women Health (Larchmt)* 17(10):2008, 1635.

TO SUM UP

Pregnancy involves synergistic interactions among three distinct biologic entities: (1) the fetus, (2) the placenta, and (3) the woman. Maternal needs reflect the increasing nutritional needs of the fetus and the placenta, as well as the need to meet maternal needs and to prepare for lactation. An optimal weight gain of about 11 kg (25 lb), or more or less as needed based on prepregnancy BMI, is recommended during pregnancy to accommodate rapid growth. Even more significant than the actual weight gain is the quality of the diet.

Common problems occurring during pregnancy include nausea and vomiting, heartburn, and constipation. In most cases they are easily relieved without medication by simple, often temporary, changes in the diet. Serious problems with pregnancy may be associated with preexisting chronic maternal conditions, such as diabetes mellitus, or conditions arising as a result of the physical or metabolic demands of pregnancy, such as iron deficiency anemia and PIH. Unusual or erratic eating habits, age, parity, prepartum weight status, and low income are among the many related factors that also place the woman at risk for complications.

The Academy of Nutrition and Dietetics strongly encourages public health and clinical efforts that promote breast-feeding to optimize the indisputable nutritional, immunologic, psychologic, and economic benefits. The ultimate goal of prenatal care is a healthy infant and a mother physically capable of breast-feeding her child, should she choose to do so. Human milk provides essential nutrients in quantities required for optimal infant growth and development. It also supplies immunologic factors that offer protection against infection. Lactation requires an increase in kcalories beyond the needs of pregnancy. Adequate fluid intake is guided by the mother's natural thirst.

QUESTIONS FOR REVIEW

1. List and discuss five factors that influence the nutritional needs of the woman during pregnancy. Which factors would place a woman in a high-risk category? Why?
2. List six nutrients that are required in larger amounts during pregnancy. Describe their special role during this period. Identify four food sources of each.
3. Identify two common problems associated with pregnancy, and describe the dietary management of each.
4. List and describe the screening indicators and risk factors for hypertension and diabetes mellitus during pregnancy.
5. List and discuss five major nutritional factors of lactation.
6. Using the MyPlate resource (www.ChooseMyPlate.gov), determine a food intake plan for a 27-year-old woman who is 5 feet 5 inches tall, weighs 130 pounds, exercises for less than 30 minutes per day, and is exclusively breast-feeding her 2-month-old infant.

REFERENCES

1. Mathews TJ, MacDorman MF: Infant mortality statistics from the 2007 period: linked birth/infant death data set. *Natl Vital Stat Rep* 59(6):1, 2011.

2. Nahum GG, Stanislaw H, Huffaker BJ: Accurate prediction of term birth weight from prospectively measurable maternal characteristics. *Prim Care Update Ob Gyns* 5(4):193, 1998.

3. Food and Nutrition Board Committee on Maternal Nutrition, National Research Council National Academy of Sciences: *Maternal nutrition and the course of human pregnancy*, Washington, D.C., 1970, National Academies Press.

4. American College of Obstetricians and Gynecologists, Committee on Nutrition: *Nutrition in maternal health care*, Chicago, 1974, American College of Obstetricians and Gynecologists.

5. American College of Obstetrics and Gynecology and American Dietetic Association Task Force on Nutrition: *Assessment of maternal nutrition*, Chicago, 1978, American College of Obstetricians and Gynecologists.

6. Food and Nutrition Board, Institute of Medicine: *Dietary Reference Intakes for calcium and vitamin D*, Washington, D.C., 2011, National Academies Press.

7. Food and Nutrition Board, Institute of Medicine: *Dietary Reference Intakes for thiamin, riboflavin, niacin, vitamin B6, folate, vitamin B12, pantothenic acid, biotin, and choline*, Washington, D.C., 1998, National Academies Press.

8. Food and Nutrition Board, Institute of Medicine: *Dietary Reference Intakes for vitamin C, vitamin E, selenium, and carotenoids*, Washington, D.C., 2000, National Academies Press.

9. Food and Nutrition Board, Institute of Medicine: *Dietary Reference Intakes for vitamin A, vitamin K, arsenic, boron, chromium, copper, iodine, iron, manganese, molybdenum, nickel, silicon, vanadium, and zinc*, Washington, D.C., 2000, National Academies Press.

10. Food and Nutrition Board, Institute of Medicine: *Dietary Reference Intakes for energy, carbohydrate, fiber, fat, fatty acids, cholesterol, protein, and amino acids (macronutrients)*, Washington, D.C., 2005, National Academies Press.

11. Barker DJ: Fetal origins of coronary heart disease. *BMJ* 311(6998):171, 1995.

12. Barker DJ: The origins of the developmental origins theory. *J Intern Med* 261(5):412, 2007.

13. Skogen JC, Overland S: The fetal origins of adult disease: a narrative review of the epidemiological literature. *JRSM Short Rep* 3(8):59, 2012.

14. Rasmussen KM: The "fetal origins" hypothesis: challenges and opportunities for maternal and child nutrition. *Annu Rev Nutr* 21:73, 2001.

15. Nutrition-Cognition National Advisory Committee: *Statement on the link between nutrition and cognitive development in children*, Medford, Mass., 1998, Center on Hunger, Poverty, and Nutrition Policy, Tufts University.

16. U.S. Department of Health and Human Services: *Healthy People 2020: framework*, ed 2, Washington, D.C., 2010, U.S. Government Printing Office.

17. American College of Obstetricians and Gynecologists: Frequently asked questions, FAQ137, gynecological problems, treating infertility, August 2012. <http://www.acog.org>.

18. Thoma ME, McLain AC, Louis JF, et al: Prevalence of infertility in the United States as estimated by the current duration approach and a traditional constructed approach. *Fertil Steril* S0015-0282(12)02449:1, 2013.

19. Jungheim ES, Moley KH: Current knowledge of obesity's effects in the pre- and periconceptional periods and avenues for future research. *Am J Obstet Gynecol* 203 (6):525, 2010.

20. Rich-Edwards JM, Spiegelman D, Garland M, et al: Physical activity, body mass index, and ovulatory disorder infertility. *Epidemiol* 13(2):184, 2002.

21. Shaum KM, Polotsky AJ: Nutrition and reproduction: is there evidence to support a "Fertility Diet" to improve mitochondrial function? *Maturitas* S0378-5122(13)00020-0:1, 2013.

22. U.S. Department of Health and Human Services: *Physical activity guidelines for Americans*, ed 1, Washington, D.C., 2008, U.S. Government Printing Office.

23. De Ver Dye T, Fernandez ID, Rains A, et al: Recent studies in the epidemiologic assessment of physical activity, fetal growth, and preterm delivery: a narrative review. *Clin Obstet Gynecol* 46(2):415, 2003.

24. Committee on Obstetric Practice: ACOG committee opinion: exercise during pregnancy and the postpartum period. *Int J Gynaecol Obstet* 77(1):79, 2002.

25. Food and Nutrition Board, Institute of Medicine: *Dietary Reference Intakes: applications in dietary assessment*, Washington, D.C., 2000, National Academies Press.

26. Al MD, van Houwelingen AC, Hornstra G: Long-chain polyunsaturated fatty acids, pregnancy, and pregnancy outcome. *Am J Clin Nutr* 71(Suppl 1):285S, 2000.

27. Carlson SE: Docosahexaenoic acid supplementation in pregnancy and lactation. *Am J Clin Nutr* 89(Suppl):678S, 2009.

28. U.S. Department of Agriculture and U.S. Department of Health and Human Services: *Dietary Guidelines for Americans, 2010*, ed 7, Washington, D.C., 2010, U.S. Government Printing Office.

29. Centers for Disease Control and Prevention: Use of supplements containing folic acid among women of childbearing age: United States, 2007. *MMWR Morb Mortal Wkly Rep* 57(1):5, 2008.

30. Mosley BS, Cleves MA, Siega-Riz AM, et al: Neural tube defects and maternal folate intake among pregnancies conceived after folic acid fortification in the United States. *Am J Epidemiol* 169(1):18, 2009.

31. Corbin KD, Zeisel SH: The nutrigenetics and nutrigenomics of the dietary requirement for choline. *Prog Mol Biol Transl Sci* 108:159, 2012.

32. Sanders LM, Zeisel SH: Choline: dietary requirements and role in brain development. *Nutr Today* 42:181, 2007.

33. O'Hagan K: *Cultural competence in the caring professions*, London, 2001, Jessica Kingsley Publishers.

34. Hogan-Garcia M: *Four skills of cultural diversity competence: a process for understanding and practice*, Belmont, Calif., 1999, Brooks/Cole.

35. Allen LH: Multiple micronutrients in pregnancy and lactation: an overview. *Am J Clin Nutr* 81(Suppl 5):1206S, 2005.

36. Blumenthal M, Goldberg A, Brinckmann J: *Herbal medicine: expanded commission E monographs*, Boston, 2000, Integrative Medicine Communications.

37. *Physician's desk reference (PDR) for herbal medicine*, ed 4, Montvale, N.J., 2007, Thomson Healthcare Inc.

38. Institute of Medicine: *Weight gain during pregnancy: reexamining the guidelines*, Washington, D.C., 2009, National Academies Press.

39. Luke B, Leurgans S: Maternal weight gains in ideal twin outcomes. *J Am Diet Assoc* 96(2):178, 1996.

40. Food and Nutrition Board, Institute of Medicine: *Nutrition during pregnancy*, Washington, D.C., 1990, National Academies Press.

41. Butte NF, Hopkinson JM, Mehta N, et al: Adjustments in energy expenditure and substrate utilization during late pregnancy and lactation. *Am J Clin Nutr* 69(2):299, 1999.

42. Food and Nutrition Board, Institute of Medicine: *Dietary Reference Intakes for water, potassium, sodium, chloride, and sulfate*, Washington, D.C., 2004, National Academies Press.

43. Goodwin TM: Hyperemesis gravidarum. *Obstet Gynecol Clin North Am* 35:401, 2008.

44. Pazol K, Warner L, Gavin L, et al: Vital signs: teen pregnancy—United States, 1991-2009. *MMWR Morb Mortal Wkly Rep* 60(13):414, 2001.

45. Ikonomidou C, Bittigau P, Ishimaru MJ, et al: Ethanol-induced apoptotic neurodegeneration and fetal alcohol syndrome. *Science* 287(5455):1056, 2000.

46. Barinaga M: Neurobiology: a new clue to how alcohol damages brains. *Science* 287(5455):947, 2000.

47. Kirchengast S, Hartmann B: Nicotine consumption before and during pregnancy affects not only newborn size but also birth modus. *J Biosoc Sci* 35(2):175, 2003.

48. Briggs GG, Freeman RK, Yaffe SJ: *Drugs in pregnancy and lactation*, ed 9, Philadelphia, Pa., 2011, Lippincott Williams & Wilkins.

49. Greenland S, Richwald GA, Honda GD: The effects of marijuana use during pregnancy. II. A study in a low-risk home-delivery population. *Drug Alcohol Depend* 11(3–4):359, 1983.

50. Danish Epidemiology Science Centre at the Institute of Preventive Medicine: Does caffeine and alcohol intake before pregnancy predict the occurrence of spontaneous abortion? *Hum Reprod* 18(12):2704, 2003.

51. Signorello LB, McLaughlin JK: Maternal caffeine consumption and spontaneous abortion: a review of the epidemiologic evidence. *Epidemiology* 15(2):229, 2004.

52. Position of the American Dietetic Association: Nutrition and lifestyle for a healthy pregnancy outcome. *J Am Diet Assoc* 108(3):553, 2008.

53. Lopez LB, Ortega Soler CR, de Portela ML: Pica during pregnancy: a frequently underestimated problem. *Arch Latinoam Nutr* 54(1):17, 2004.

54. Rainville AJ: Pica practices of pregnant women are associated with lower maternal hemoglobin level at delivery. *J Am Diet Assoc* 98(3):293, 1998.

55. Boyle JS, Mackey MC: Pica: sorting it out. *J Transcult Nurs* 10(1):65, 1999.

56. Wagner LK, Leeman L, Gopman S: Preeclampsia. In Lammi-Keefe CJ, Couch S, Phillipson E, editors: *Handbook of nutrition and pregnancy*, ed 1, Totowa, N.J., 2008, Humana Press, pp 155-160.

57. Slocum J, Barcio L, Darany J, et al: Preconception to postpartum: management of pregnancy complicated by diabetes. *Diabetes Educ* 30(5):740, 2004.

58. Mensing C, Boucher J, Cypress M, et al: National standards for diabetes self-management education. *Diabetes Care* 28(Suppl 1):S72, 2005.

59. Alberico S, Strazzanti C, De Santo D, et al: Gestational diabetes: universal or selective screening? *J Matern Fetal Neonatal Med* 16(6):331, 2004.

60. Wunderlich SM: Nutritional assessment and support of HIV-positive pregnant women and their children: perspective from an industrialized country. *Nutr Today* 35(3):107, 2000.

61. Taren DL: The infant feeding and HIV transmission controversy impacts public health services. *Nutr Today* 35(3):103, 2000.

62. James D: Eating disorders, fertility, and pregnancy: relationships and complications. *J Perinatal Neonatal Nurs* 15(2):36, 2001.

63. Morrill ES, Nickols-Richardson SM: Bulimia nervosa during pregnancy: a review. *J Am Diet Assoc* 101(4):448, 2001.

64. Position of the American Dietetic Association: Nutrition intervention in the treatment of eating disorders. *J Am Diet Assoc* 111(8):1236, 2011.

65. Allen JA, Li R, Scanlon KS, et al: Progress in increasing breastfeeding and reducing racial/ethnic differences—United States, 2000-2008. *MMWR Morb Mortal Wkly Rep* 62:77, 2013.

66. Ryan AS: The resurgence of breastfeeding in the United States. *Pediatrics* 99(4):E12, 1997.

67. World Health Organization: WHO advises: ten steps to successful breast-feeding. *World Health* 2:28, 1997.

68. Schanler RJ, O'Connor KG, Lawrence RA: Pediatricians' practices and attitudes regarding breastfeeding promotion. *Pediatrics* 103(3):E35, 1999.

69. Emmett PM, Rogers IS: Properties of human milk and their relationship with maternal nutrition. *Early Hum Dev* 49(Suppl 1):S7, 1997.

70. Wright AL, Bauer M, Naylor A, et al: Increasing breast-feeding rates to reduce infant illness at the community level. *Pediatrics* 101(5):837, 1998.

71. Carmichael SL, Prince CB, Burr R, et al: Breast-feeding practices among WIC participants in Hawaii. *J Am Diet Assoc* 101(1):57, 2001.

72. Chapman DJ, Damio G, Young S, et al: Effectiveness of breastfeeding peer counseling in a low-income, predominantly Latina population: a randomized controlled trial. *Arch Pediatr Adolesc Med* 158(9):897, 2004.

73. Philipp BL, Merewood A: The baby-friendly way: the best breastfeeding start. *Pediatr Clin North Am* 51(3):761, 2004.

74. Kannan S, Carruth BR, Skinner J: Cultural influences on infant feeding beliefs of mothers. *J Am Diet Assoc* 99(1):88, 1999.

75. Kramer MS, Kakuma R: Optimal duration of exclusive breastfeeding. *Cochrane Database Syst Rev* (1):CD003517, 2002.

76. Fewtrell MS, Morgan JB, Duggan C, et al: Optimal duration of exclusive breastfeeding: what is the evidence to support current recommendations? *Am J Clin Nutr* 85(Suppl):635S, 2007.

77. American Academy of Pediatrics Section on Breastfeeding: Breastfeeding and the use of human milk. *Pediatrics* 115(2):496, 2005.

78. Position of the American Dietetic Association: Promoting and supporting breastfeeding. *J Am Diet Assoc* 109(11):1926, 2009.

79. Gibson MV, Diaz VA, Mainous AG, et al: Prevalence of breastfeeding and acculturation in Hispanics: results from NHANES 1999-2000 study. *Birth* 32(2):93, 2005.

80. Spencer BS, Grassley JS: African American women and breastfeeding: an integrative literature review. *Health Care Women Int* 34(7):607, 2013.

81. Renfrew MJ, McCormick FM, Wade A, et al: Support for healthy breastfeeding mothers with healthy term babies. *Cochrane Database Syst Rev* (5):CD001141, 2012.

82. Lovelady CA, Garner KE, Moreno KL, et al: The effect of weight loss in overweight, lactating women on the growth of their infants. *N Engl J Med* 342(7):449, 2000.

83. Butte NF: Dieting and exercise in overweight, lactating women. *N Engl J Med* 342(7):502, 2000.

84. Picciano MF: Pregnancy and lactation: physiological adjustments, nutritional requirements and the role of dietary supplements. *J Nutr* 133(Suppl 1):1997S, 2003.

85. Weiss R, Fogelman Y, Bennett M: Severe vitamin B_{12} deficiency in an infant associated with a maternal deficiency and a strict vegetarian diet. *J Pediatr Hematol Oncol* 26(4):270, 2004.

86. Brockington I: Postpartum psychiatric disorders. *Lancet* 363(9405):303, 2004.

87. Falceto OG, Giugliani ER, Fernandes CL: Influence of parental mental health on early termination of breast-feeding: a case-control study. *J Am Board Fam Pract* 17(3):173, 2004.

FURTHER READINGS AND RESOURCES

Readings

Dyer JS, Rosenfeld CR: Metabolic imprinting by prenatal, perinatal, and postnatal overnutrition: a review. *Semin Reprod Med* 29(3):266, 2011.

[Does chronic disease begin in utero? A critical evaluation of evidence to support this hypothesis is provided. Mechanisms underlying metabolic programming of disease origins during in utero development are discussed.]

Kirkwood NA: *A hospital handbook on multiculturalism and religion: practical guidelines for health care workers*, ed 2, New York, 2005, Morehouse Publishing.

Mangels R: *Everything vegan pregnancy book*, ed 1, Avon, Mass., 2011, F+W Media, Inc.

[These resources offer facts and insights about culture and religion and implications for eating during pregnancy.]

Lammi-Keefe CJ, Couch S, Phillipson E: *Handbook of nutrition and pregnancy*, ed 1, Totowa, N.J., 2008, Humana Press.

[This excellent resource provides helpful guidance for healthy pregnancies, as well as important information for identifying women at nutritional risk.]

Picciano MF, McGuire MK: Use of dietary supplements by pregnant and lactating women in North America. *Am J Clin Nutr* 89(Suppl):633S, 2009.

[Should pregnant and lactating women consume dietary supplements? This informative article reviews the current understanding of dietary supplement use in women residing in North America who are pregnant and lactating.]

Websites of Interest

- March of Dimes Birth Defects Foundation: www.marchofdimes.com.
- U.S. Department of Health and Human Services, Food and Drug Administration, Center for Food Safety and Applied Nutrition: www.cfsan.fda.gov.
- U.S. Department of Health and Human Services, Office of Disease Prevention and Health Promotion: Healthy People 2020: www.healthypeople.gov/2020/about/default.aspx.
- U.S. Department of Health and Human Services, National Institutes of Health, National Center for Complementary and Alternative Medicine: http://nccam.nih.gov.
- Virginia Department of Health, Office of Family Health Services, BabyCare: www.vahealth.org/babycare.

Nutrition for Normal Growth and Development

Sharon M. Nickols-Richardson

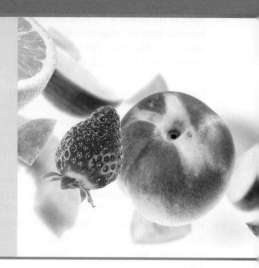

ⓔ EVOLVE WEBSITE

http://evolve.elsevier.com/Williams/essentials/

OUTLINE

Human Growth and Development
Nutritional Requirements for Growth
Stages of Growth and Development: Age-Group Needs

HEALTH PROMOTION
Children and Adolescents: Seeking Fitness

In this second chapter in our life cycle series, we look at growing infants, children, and adolescents. We consider their physical growth and their inseparable psychosocial development at each progressive stage. This unified growth and development nurture the integrated progression of the child into the adult.

Within this dual framework of physical and psychosocial development, we consider food and feeding and their vital roles in the development of the whole child. In each age-group we relate nutritional needs and the food that supplies them to the normal physical maturation and psychosocial development achieved in that stage.

HUMAN GROWTH AND DEVELOPMENT

Individual Needs of Children

Growth may be defined as an increase in body size. Biologic growth of an organism occurs through cell multiplication (hyperplasia) and cell enlargement (hypertrophy). *Development* is the associated process by which growing tissues and organs take on a more complex function. Both of these processes are part of one whole, forming a unified and inseparable sequence of growth and development. Through these changes a small, dependent newborn is transformed into a fully functioning independent adult. However, each child is a unique entity with individual needs. This is a paramount principle in working with children. Thus we must always seek to discover these individual human needs if we are to help

each child reach his or her greatest growth and development potential.[1]

Normal Life Cycle Growth Pattern

The normal human life cycle includes the following four general stages of overall growth and development: (1) infancy, (2) childhood, (3) adolescence, and (4) adulthood.

1. *Infancy:* Growth velocity is rapid during the first year of life, with the rate tapering off in the latter half of the year. At 6 months of age an infant has typically doubled its birth weight, and at 1 year he or she will likely have tripled it.

2. *Childhood:* During the latent period of childhood, after infancy and before adolescence, the growth rate slows and becomes erratic. During some periods, plateaus are reached. At other times, small spurts of growth occur. This overall growth deceleration affects appetite accordingly. At certain times, children will have little or no appetite; at other times, they will eat voraciously. Parents who know that this is a normal pattern can relax and avoid making eating a battleground with their children.

3. *Adolescence:* With the beginning of puberty, the second period of growth acceleration occurs. Because of hormonal influences, enormous physical changes take place, including growth and maturation of long bones, development of the sex characteristics, and gains in fat and muscle mass.

4. *Adulthood:* In the final stage of a normal life cycle, growth levels off on the adult plateau. Then it gradually declines during old age—the period of senescence.

Measuring Childhood Physical Growth
Growth Charts

Children grow at widely varying individual rates. In clinical practice a child's pattern of growth is compared with **percentile** growth curves derived from measurements of large numbers of children throughout the growth years. Contemporary **growth chart grids**, developed by the National Center for Health Statistics (NCHS), reflect the growth patterns of breast-fed and formula-fed infants and provide a broad baseline for evaluating growth patterns in children today.[2] These charts are based on data from nationally representative samples of children that include various racial and ethnic groups (see Further Readings and Resources at the end of this chapter). Two age intervals are presented: birth to 3 years and 2 to 20 years, with separate curves for boys and girls. A variety of grids are available to monitor growth based on weight and age, length (or stature) and age, weight-for-length (or body mass index [BMI]), and head circumference and age (see the Evolve website for *CDC Growth Charts: United States*). Head circumference is a valuable measure in infants, but it is seldom measured routinely after 3 years of age. Directions for use of these growth charts for infants and children with special growth patterns are also available.

The Centers for Disease Control and Prevention recommends that an infant's weight be measured using an infant scale (pan shaped). These may be digital or balance-beam scales. When possible, the infant should be measured in the nude. If a diaper must be worn, weight should be adjusted for the weight of this item. The infant should be gently placed lying supine in the middle of the scale. Infant weight should be recorded to the nearest 0.01 kg. If an infant has difficulty laying still, the weight of the infant may be estimated by weighing an adult holding the infant and subtracting the weight of the adult.

Stature should be measured by recumbent length. An infantometer should be used to measure the length of an infant by laying the infant supine on a horizontal backboard, with the head against the fixed head piece. Once the infant's head is gently secured at the head piece in the Frankfort horizontal plane, the infant's legs should be extended by pressing mildly on the knees. The foot piece of the infantometer should then be adjusted to rest securely at the infant's heels. Toes should be pointed upward with feet perpendicular to the foot piece, while the head, shoulders, bottom, and heels lie flat against the backboard. Length is typically measured to the nearest 0.1 cm. Two individuals are generally required to complete measures of recumbent length.

At 2 years of age and beyond, weight should be measured on a standing digital or balance-beam scale to the nearest 0.1 kg. Height should be measured by recumbent length and standing height until 4 years of age, after which standing height alone may be used for this anthropometric measurement. Standing height should be measured using a stadiometer. Feet should be flat on the floor or platform with heels together and toes adjusted outward, and body weight should be evenly distributed on both legs. Children should be facing away from the stadiometer, with the head, shoulders, bottom, and heels touching the stadiometer. The head should be aligned in the Frankfort horizontal plane. Hair should be flat. The head piece of the stadiometer should be lowered to rest firmly on the head. The child should then inhale and hold this position during the measurement. Standing height is typically measured to the nearest 0.1 cm. Repeated measurements are typically conducted and averaged at each measurement interval, with the average measurement being recorded. Infants and children should never be left alone during anthropometric measurements.

Nutrition Assessment

Practitioners use the nutrition care process to assess, evaluate, and monitor a child's growth and development, with growth charts and other clinical standards as points of reference. A number of methods and measures, including anthropometry, clinical signs, laboratory tests, and nutritional analysis, may be used as described in Chapter 16.

Motor, Mental, and Psychosocial Development
Motor Growth and Development

Gross motor skills, such as sitting, standing, walking, and running, develop within the first 18 months of life. Fine motor skills gradually develop over a longer period of time. Such control over and coordination of voluntary muscle develops in conjunction with mental, emotional, social, and cultural growth as the child interacts and reacts to sensory stimulants in the environment. Motor skills greatly influence feeding skills and energy needs of the child. For example, the pincer grasp allows toddlers to have better control when handling finger foods. Toddlers and children who are more active and spend more time walking and running generally require more energy.

Mental Growth and Development

Measures of mental growth usually involve abilities in speech and other forms of communication, as well as the ability to

---

KEY TERMS

growth velocity Rapidity of motion or movement; rate of childhood growth during normal periods of development compared with a population standard.

growth deceleration Period of decreased speed of growth at different points of childhood development.

growth acceleration Period of increased speed of growth at different points of childhood development.

percentile One of 100 equal parts of a measured series of values; rate or proportion per hundred.

growth chart grids Grids comparing stature (length), weight, and age of children by percentile; used for nutritional assessment to determine how their growth is progressing. The most commonly used grids are those of the National Center for Health Statistics (NCHS).

handle abstract and symbolic material in thinking. Young children think in very literal terms. As they develop in mental capacity, they can handle more than single ideas, and they can form constructive concepts.

Emotional Growth and Development

Emotional growth is measured in the capacity for love and affection, as well as the ability to handle frustration and anxieties. It also involves the child's ability to control aggressive impulses and to channel hostility from destructive to constructive activities.

Social and Cultural Growth and Development

The social development of a child is measured as the ability to relate to others and to participate in group living and cultural activities. These social and cultural behaviors are first learned through relationships with parents and family, and these relationships greatly influence food habits and feeding patterns. As the child's horizon broadens, relationships are developed with those outside the family, with friends, and with others in the community at school or at religious or other social gatherings. For this reason, a child's play during the early years is a highly purposeful activity.

NUTRITIONAL REQUIREMENTS FOR GROWTH

Energy Needs

During childhood, the demand for kilocalories (kcalories or kcal) is relatively great. However, much variation exists in need with age and condition. For example, the total daily energy intake of a 5-year-old child is spent in the following way:

- Approximately 50% supplies basal metabolic requirements
- Approximately 5% is used in the thermic effect of food (TEF)
- Approximately 25% goes toward daily physical activity
- Approximately 12% is needed for tissue growth
- Approximately 8% is lost in the feces

Protein Needs

Protein provides amino acids, the essential building materials for tissue growth. As a child grows, the protein requirements per unit of body weight gradually decrease. For example, during the first 6 months of life an infant requires 1.52 g of protein/kg/day.[3] This amount gradually decreases throughout childhood until adulthood, when protein needs are only about 0.8 g/kg/day.[3] Usually, the healthy, active, growing child will consume the necessary amounts of kcalories and protein if a variety of food is provided. The Acceptable Macronutrient Distribution Range (AMDR) for dietary protein for children 1 year and older is 10% to 35% of total kcalories.[3]

Essential Fatty Acid Needs

Fat kcalories are important as backup energy sources but are particularly needed to supply linoleic and α-linolenic acids, which are essential fatty acids. Linoleic acid is required for the synthesis of brain and nerve tissue and normal mental development. Infants consuming adequate amounts of breast milk or infant formula in the first 6 months of life and after complementary foods are added in the second 6 months of life are likely to meet their Adequate Intake (AI) for the essential fatty acids. Children 1 year and older may follow the AMDR of 20% to 35% of total kcalories without any adverse effect on growth and development.[3]

Carbohydrate Needs

Carbohydrates are the primary energy source and are important in sparing protein for its vital role in tissue formation. Most importantly, carbohydrates provide glucose for essential brain function.[3] The AMDR for dietary carbohydrate is 45% to 65% of total kcalories for children 1 year and older.[3]

Fiber

Many complex-carbohydrate foods also provide dietary fiber. Fiber is important to satiety and bowel regulation, and affects blood lipid and glucose concentrations, as well as the vascular system. Fiber may also provide protection against some types of cancer and overweight.[3]

Water Requirements

The infant's relative need for water is greater than that of the adult. The infant's body content of water is approximately 70% to 75% of total body weight, whereas in the adult, water contributes only 60% to 65% of total body weight. In addition, a large amount of the infant's total body water is outside of cells and more easily lost. Thus prolonged water loss because of diarrhea, as occurs among infants in developing countries given formula prepared from contaminated water, is a serious threat to life and requires immediate oral hydration therapy.[4] Rotavirus is a common cause of diarrhea in infants in many nations. Any infant who is experiencing diarrhea and fluid imbalance should be immediately examined by a health care professional. The child's water need is related to energy intake and urine concentration. Generally, an infant drinks a daily amount of water equivalent to 10% to 15% of body weight, whereas the adult's daily water intake equals 2% to 4% of body weight. A summary of approximate daily fluid needs during the growth years is provided in Table 12-1.[5] In general, infants are able to meet their water needs by consuming breast milk or infant formula. Infant formula should not be diluted with additional water as this may lead to fluid excess and electrolyte disturbances such as low serum sodium concentration, a potentially life-threatening condition.

Mineral and Vitamin Needs

Minerals and vitamins play essential roles in tissue growth and maintenance, as well as in overall energy metabolism. Positive childhood growth and development depend on an adequate amount of these essential substances. For example, rapidly growing young bones require calcium and phosphorus. A radiograph of a newborn's body would reveal a skeleton appearing as a collection of disconnected, separate bones requiring mineralization. Calcium is also needed for tooth development, muscle contraction, nerve excitation, blood coagulation, and heart muscle action. Another mineral of concern is iron, essential for hemoglobin formation and mental and psychomotor development. The healthy infant's fetal iron stores are depleted within 9 to 12 months after birth. Thus solid food additions around this time help supply needed iron. Such foods as iron-fortified cereals and meat assist in providing adequate dietary iron. The use of iron-fortified formulas and other foods by high-risk children assists in reducing the incidence of iron deficiency anemia among infants and young children.[6] In general, iron supplements are not needed during infancy.

Excess amounts of particular micronutrients are also of concern in feeding children. Excess intake is usually the result of inappropriate use of vitamin or mineral supplements and may occur because of misunderstanding, illiteracy, or carelessness. When supplements are indicated because of a specific and defined medical or nutritional condition, parents must be carefully instructed to use only the amount directed and no more. The following two nutrients pose particular hazards when consumed in excessive amounts:

1. *Vitamin A:* Symptoms of toxicity from excess vitamin A include lack of appetite, slow growth, drying and cracking of the skin, enlargement of the liver and spleen, swelling and pain in the long bones, and bone fragility.
2. *Vitamin D:* Symptoms of toxicity from excess vitamin D include nausea, diarrhea, weight loss, excess urination (especially at night), and eventual calcification of soft tissues, including the renal tubules, blood vessels, bronchi, stomach, and heart.

Summaries of the Dietary Reference Intakes (DRIs) for overall nutritional needs and growth, developed by the Food and Nutrition Board of the Institute of Medicine, are provided in Tables 12-2, 12-3, and 12-4.

STAGES OF GROWTH AND DEVELOPMENT: AGE-GROUP NEEDS

Psychosocial Development

The developmental tasks of choosing and consuming foods do not develop in a vacuum. They flow as an integral part of physical, motor, and psychosocial development. In this section we discuss food and feeding practices at each of the stages of childhood and their relationship to normal physical and psychosocial maturation. Developing neuromuscular motor skills enable the child to accomplish related physical activities involved with food. Psychosocial development influences food attitudes, behavior, patterns, and habits.

Throughout the human life cycle, food and feeding not only supply nutrients for physical and motor growth but also play a role in personal and psychosocial development. The nutritional age-group needs of children cannot be understood apart from the child's overall maturation as a unique person. A leading American psychoanalyst, Erik Erikson,[7] has contributed to our understanding of human personality and growth throughout critical periods of development. His theory of human development has come to play a significant role in our view of the human life cycle.

TABLE 12-1	APPROXIMATE DAILY FLUID NEEDS DURING GROWTH YEARS
AGE	(IN mL/KG)
0-3 mo	120
3-6 mo	117
6-12 mo	89
1-3 yr	108
4-8 yr	85
9-13 yr	67 (boys)
	57 (girls)
14-18 yr	54 (boys)
	43 (girls)

Data from Food and Nutrition Board, Institute of Medicine: *Dietary References Intakes for water, potassium, sodium, chloride, and sulfate*, Washington, D.C., 2004, National Academies Press.

TABLE 12-2	DIETARY REFERENCE INTAKES FOR ENERGY AND PROTEIN						
	AGE	WEIGHT		HEIGHT		ENERGY*	PROTEIN
Infants	0-0.5 yr	6 kg	13 lb	62 cm	24 in	438-645 kcal	9.1 g
	0.5-1 yr	9 kg	20 lb	71cm	28 in	608-844 kcal	13.5 g
Children	1-3 yr	12 kg	27 lb	86 cm	34 in	768-1683 kcal	13 g
	4-8 yr	20 kg	44 lb	115 cm	45 in	1133-2225 kcal	19 g
Male subjects	9-13 yr	36 kg	79 lb	144 cm	57 in	1530-3038 kcal	34 g
	14-18 yr	61 kg	134 lb	174 cm	68 in	2090-3804 kcal	52 g
Female subjects	9-13 yr	37 kg	81 lb	144 cm	57 in	1415-2762 kcal	34 g
	14-18 yr	54 kg	119 lb	163 cm	64 in	1718-2858 kcal	46 g

Data from Food and Nutrition Board, Institute of Medicine: *Dietary Reference Intakes for energy, carbohydrate, fiber, fat, fatty acids, cholesterol, protein, and amino acids (macronutrients)*, Washington, D.C., 2002, National Academies Press.
*Varies according to gender, body size, age, and level of physical activity.

TABLE 12-3   DIETARY REFERENCE INTAKES FOR VITAMINS

AGE	VITAMIN A (in mcg RAE)	VITAMIN D (in mcg)	VITAMIN E (in mg TE)	VITAMIN K (in mcg)	VITAMIN C (in mg)	THIAMIN (in mg)	RIBOFLAVIN (in mg)	NIACIN (in mg NE)	VITAMIN B$_6$ (in mg)	FOLATE (in mcg)	VITAMIN B$_{12}$ (in mcg)
Infants 0-0.5 yr	400	10	4	2	40	0.2	0.3	2	0.1	65	0.4
Infants 0.6-1.0 yr	500	10	5	2.5	50	0.3	0.4	4	0.3	80	0.5
Children 1-3 yr	300	15	6	30	15	0.5	0.5	6	0.5	150	0.9
Children 4-8 yr	400	15	7	55	25	0.6	0.6	8	0.6	200	1.2
Boys 9-13 yr	600	15	11	60	45	0.9	0.9	12	1	300	1.8
Boys 14-18 yr	900	15	15	75	75	1.2	1.3	16	1.3	400	2.4
Girls 9-13 yr	600	15	11	60	45	0.9	0.9	12	1	300	1.8
Girls 14-18 yr	700	15	15	75	65	1.0	1.0	14	1.2	400	2.4

From Food and Nutrition Board, Institute of Medicine: *Dietary Reference Intakes for calcium and vitamin D*, Washington, D.C., 2011, National Academies Press; Food and Nutrition Board, Institute of Medicine: *Dietary Reference Intakes for thiamin, riboflavin, niacin, vitamin B$_6$, folate, vitamin B$_{12}$, pantothenic acid, biotin, and choline*, Washington, D.C., 1998, National Academies Press; Food and Nutrition Board, Institute of Medicine: *Dietary Reference Intakes for vitamin C, vitamin E, selenium, and carotenoids*, Washington, D.C., 2000, National Academies Press; Food and Nutrition Board, Institute of Medicine: *Dietary Reference Intakes for vitamin A, vitamin K, arsenic, boron, chromium, copper, iodine, iron, manganese, molybdenum, nickel, silicon, vanadium, and zinc*, Washington, D.C., 2001, National Academies Press.
NE, niacin equivalent; *RAE*, retinal activity equivalent; *TE*, tocopherol equivalent.

TABLE 12-4   DIETARY REFERENCE INTAKES FOR MINERALS

AGE	CALCIUM (in mg)	PHOSPHORUS (in mg)	MAGNESIUM (in mg)	IRON (in mg)	ZINC (in mg)	IODINE (in mcg)	SELENIUM (in mcg)	FLUORIDE (in mg)
Infants 0-0.5 yr	200	100	30	0.27	2	110	5	0.01
Infants 0.6-1.0 yr	200	275	75	11	3	130	20	0.5
Children 1-3 yr	700	460	80	7	3	90	20	0.7
Children 4-8 yr	1000	500	130	10	5	90	30	1.0
Boys 9-13 yr	1300	1250	240	8	8	120	40	2.0
Boys 14-18 yr	1300	1250	410	11	11	150	55	3.0
Girls 9-13 yr	1300	1250	240	8	8	120	40	2.0
Girls 14-18 yr	1300	1250	360	15	9	150	55	3.0

From Food and Nutrition Board, Institute of Medicine: *Dietary Reference Intakes for calcium and vitamin D*, Washington, D.C., 2011, National Academies Press; Food and Nutrition Board, Institute of Medicine: *Dietary Reference Intakes for calcium, phosphorus, magnesium, vitamin D and fluoride*, Washington, D.C., 1997, National Academies Press. Food and Nutrition Board, Institute of Medicine: *Dietary Reference Intakes for vitamin C, vitamin E, selenium, and carotenoids*, Washington, D.C., 2000, National Academies Press; Food and Nutrition Board, Institute of Medicine: *Dietary Reference Intakes for vitamin A, vitamin K, arsenic, boron, chromium, copper, iodine, iron, manganese, molybdenum, nickel, silicon, vanadium, and zinc*, Washington, D.C., 2001, National Academies Press.

Erikson identified eight stages in human growth and a basic psychosocial developmental problem with which the individual struggles at each stage.[7] The developmental problem at each stage has a positive ego value and a conflicting negative counterpart, as follows:

1. *Infancy:* trust versus distrust
2. *Toddler:* autonomy versus shame and doubt
3. *Preschooler:* initiative versus guilt
4. *School-age child:* industry versus inferiority
5. *Adolescent:* identity versus role confusion
6. *Young adult:* intimacy versus isolation
7. *Adult:* generativity versus stagnation
8. *Older adult:* ego integrity versus despair

Given favorable circumstances, a growing child develops positive ego strength at each life stage and builds increasing inner resources and strengths to meet the next life crisis. The struggle at any age, however, is not forever won at this point. A residue of the negative remains, and in periods of stress, such as an illness, some regression is likely to occur. However, as the child gains mastery at each stage of development, assisted by significant positive and supportive relationships, integration of self-controls takes place. Changes that occur at each stage influence food intake and the interaction of the child with family members, peers, and counselors, as follows[8,9]:

- *Infant:* Infants require appropriate stimulation to thrive; they enjoy seeing different colors, engaging in verbal interactions, and being physically held. Activities such as holding objects, looking at pictures, or hearing nursery rhymes support motor and cognitive development. Their attention span is short, which can create problems at feeding time.
- *Toddler:* Toddlers grow rapidly and begin to demonstrate autonomy, with display of temper tantrums or other negative behaviors. They learn behaviors from their parents. They begin to develop language skills and can recall past experiences. Play is an important medium for self-expression and allows the child to express some control over his or her environment.
- *Preschooler:* The preschool years are a time for increasing social experiences, and children begin to interact more with other children. Preschoolers have an increased ability to express themselves and may try to exert control through demands for or refusal of certain foods.
- *School-age child:* The school-age child enters a formal learning environment, and attention span increases. At this age, children are more selective in choosing friends, and the influence of peers becomes more obvious. As the environment becomes more structured, physical activity may decline, despite the need for play and further coordination of motor skills.
- *Adolescent:* Adolescents become more autonomous in their actions and attempt to exert independence from parental control. Teens perceive themselves to be invulnerable to illness or injury, and risk-taking behaviors involving drugs or alcohol may begin. Obsession with body image may result in inappropriate nutrition practices.

Various related developmental tasks surround each of these stages. These learnings, when accomplished, contribute to successful resolution of the core problem.

Infant (Birth to 1 Year)
Physical Characteristics of a Full-Term Infant
The full-term infant is born after successful growth and development during a normal gestation period of about 40 weeks (280 days). During the first year of life the infant generally triples in weight, growing rapidly from an average birth weight of about 3.5 kg (7.5 lb) to a 1-year-old child ready to walk and weighing about 10 kg (22 lb). Thus energy requirements during this first year of tremendous growth are high.

Full-term infants have the ability to digest and absorb protein, a moderate amount of fat, and simple carbohydrates. They have some difficulty with starch because amylase, the starch-splitting enzyme, is not produced at birth. However, as starch is introduced, this enzyme begins to function. The renal system functions well in infancy, but more water relative to body size is needed than in the adult to manage the renal

solute load in urinary excretion. The first baby teeth do not erupt until about the fourth month; therefore, food must initially be liquid and later semiliquid.

Nutrition for the Full-Term Infant
The first food for infants, breast milk or infant formula, generally provides all the nutrients required by a healthy infant for the first 6 months of life. Exclusive breast-feeding can, in fact, be adequate for the first 12 months of life (with the exception of iron and vitamin D); however, most mothers choose to supplement their infants' diets with complementary foods around the sixth to seventh month.[10] Nearly all infants born in a hospital receive an injection of vitamin K shortly after birth to ensure an adequate level of this nutrient, and it is important that infants born at home also receive supplemental vitamin K. It may be necessary to provide vitamin D supplements to breast-fed infants, because breast milk may not supply adequate vitamin D to prevent deficiency and the development of rickets.[11,12] This is especially critical in the case of African-American mothers, who are less able to initiate the synthesis of vitamin D in their skin, or for mothers who wear special clothing for religious reasons that limits their skin exposure to the sun (see the Focus on Culture box, "Nutritional Rickets: Role of Culture"). It is important that breast-feeding mothers be well nourished to supply optimal levels of nutrients in their milk.[13]

Infants have limited nutritional stores from gestation, and this is especially true for iron. Around 6 or 7 months of age, semisolid foods such as iron-fortified cereals may be added to the diet to help meet increasing nutritional needs.

Psychosocial and Motor Development
The core psychosocial developmental task during infancy is the establishment of trust in others. Much of the infant's early psychosocial development is tactile in nature from touching and holding, especially with feeding. Feeding is the infant's primary means of establishing human relationships. The close mother-infant or caregiver-infant bonding in the feeding process fills the basic need to build trust. The need for sucking and the development of the oral organs—the lips and mouth—as sensory organs represent adaptations that ensure an adequate early food intake for survival. As a result, food becomes the infant's general means of exploring the environment and is one of the early means of communication. The infant has an additional "nonnutritive" sucking need that is satisfied, especially with the extra effort required

KEY TERMS
autonomy   The state of functioning independently, without extraneous influence.
renal solute load   Collective number and concentration of solute particles in a solution carried by the blood to the kidney nephrons for excretion in the urine. The particles are usually nitrogenous products from protein metabolism and the electrolyte sodium.
tactile   Pertaining to the touch.

⊕ FOCUS ON CULTURE*

Nutritional Rickets: Role of Culture

The eradication of nutritional rickets, or the vitamin D deficiency of childhood, is one of the greatest public health success stories in the United States. Fortification of cow's milk and supplementation of infant formula with vitamin D ensured the virtual disappearance of this nutritional disease by 1970. The understanding of the importance of sunlight exposure in initiating the conversion of inactive vitamin D to active vitamin D, in addition to adequate dietary intake, was monumental. Unfortunately, rickets is on the rise because of a variety of cultural and related behavioral factors.

Factors Linked to Rickets

Several studies describe causes of nutritional rickets. One study found that 46% of infants born to African-American women were vitamin D deficient at birth, whereas 10% of infants born to Caucasian women were vitamin D deficient. Vitamin D status at birth was linked to maternal vitamin D deficiency at delivery. Other common factors among such studies include exclusive and prolonged breast-feeding and inadequate sunlight exposure in infants. Although most women do not continue to breast-feed their infants beyond 6 months, certain women, primarily Caucasians of high educational and economic backgrounds, have extended periods of breast-feeding. In many cases, vitamin D supplementation is not provided to the infant; thus with an average human milk content of 68 IU/L in Caucasian women, this vitamin D source is inadequate to meet the skeletal demands for this nutrient.

Inadequate sunlight exposure of infants with darkly pigmented skin is another potential cause of rickets. For example, several case studies and larger epidemiologic investigations have shown a significant prevalence of rickets in African-American infants, even those infants residing in southern climates with an abundance of sunlight. Other reports have documented rickets in infants required to be fully covered by clothing because of religious or cultural demands.

Rickets has also been documented in infants of lactating mothers who consume vegan diets. Children who are raised on vegan diets or macrobiotic diets may also have vitamin D–deficiency disorders. Often these diets are practiced to support cultural or religious beliefs.

Prevention and Treatment of Rickets

Rickets can be easily prevented, but health care practitioners must be able to recognize the clinical signs and symptoms of rickets once developed (see Chapter 6). Dietary intake assessment is often the first indicator of underlying biochemical and clinical indicators of nutritional deficiency diseases. Screening for special diets, infant-feeding method and duration, supplementation, and behaviors related to sunlight exposure of mother and child is necessary. Vitamin D supplementation of the mother, the child, or both is typically decided on a case-by-case basis. Increased sunlight exposure is another avenue to increasing vitamin D concentration in the blood. Culturally sensitive counseling is required for prevention and treatment of nutritional rickets. Targeted public health and community interventions may also help to diminish rickets once again.

Bibliography

Bodnar LM: High prevalence of vitamin D insufficiency in black and white pregnant women residing in the northern United States and their neonates. *J Nutr* 137(2):447, 2007.

Gordon CM, Feldman HA, Sinclair L, et al: Prevalence of vitamin D deficiency among healthy infants and toddlers. *Arch Pediatr Adolesc Med* 162(6):505, 2008.

Lazol JP, Cakan N, Kamat D: 10-year case review of nutritional rickets in Children's Hospital of Michigan. *Clin Pediatr (Phila)* 47(4):379, 2008.

Lee JM, Smith JR, Philipp BL, et al: Vitamin D deficiency in a healthy group of mothers and newborn infants. *Clin Pediatr (Phila)* 46(1):42, 2007.

Wagner CL, Greer FR, American Academy of Pediatrics, Section on Breastfeeding and Committee on Nutrition: Prevention of rickets and vitamin D deficiency in infants, children, and adolescents. *Pediatrics* 122(5):1142, 2008.

*The author thanks Melissa K. Zack for her assistance in creating this box.

---

in sucking while breast-feeding. As muscular coordination involving the tongue and the swallowing reflex develops, infants gradually learn to eat a variety of semisolid foods, beginning around 6 to 7 months of age. As physical and motor maturation proceed, infants begin to show a desire for self-feeding. When these stages of development occur, the exploration of new motor skills and autonomy should be encouraged. If their needs for food and love are fulfilled in this early relationship with the mother, father, other caregivers, and family members, then trust is developed. Infants evidence this trust by an increasing capacity to wait a few minutes for feedings until they are prepared.

Breast-Feeding

The ideal food for the human infant is human milk.[10] It has specific characteristics that match the infant's nutritional requirements during the first year of life. The process of breast-feeding today, as in the past, is successfully initiated and maintained by most mothers who try. However, sometimes problems occur when getting started, as well as a high degree of variability among nursing mothers as to frequency of feedings, intake per feeding, and infant growth (see Chapter 11). Thus in providing support for mothers who want to breast-feed their babies, experienced nutritionists and nurses, many of whom are certified professional lactation consultants, advise flexibility rather than a rigid approach (see Further Readings and Resources at the end of this chapter). The World Health Organization (WHO) and the United Nations Children's Fund created the Baby Friendly Hospital Initiative (BFHI)[14,15]; this program has increased the breast-feeding initiation rate of mothers in participating hospitals.[16] Box 12-1 lists the actions that hospitals must carry out to earn

BFHI status. Many hospitals use lactation consultants to oversee compliance with the actions and to promote breast-feeding practices that are optimal, yet realistic, for mother and infant.

The mother's breasts, or mammary glands, are highly specialized secretory organs, as indicated in Chapter 11 and illustrated in Figure 11-5. They are composed of glandular tissue, fat, and connective tissue. The secreting glandular tissue has 15 to 24 lobes, each containing many smaller units called *lobules*. In the lobules, secretory cells called *alveoli* form milk from the nutrient material supplied to them via a rich capillary system. During pregnancy the breasts are prepared for lactation. The alveoli enlarge and multiply, and toward the end of the prenatal period they secrete a thin, yellowish fluid called colostrum, which contains important antibodies and proteins. Hormonal components in breast milk also enhance the maturation of the gastrointestinal tract. Typically by the end of the second week, mature milk is produced; as the infant grows, the breast milk develops, adapting in composition to meet growth needs.

Breast milk is produced under the stimulating influence of the hormone prolactin from the anterior pituitary gland. After the milk is formed in the mammary lobules by alveoli, it is carried through converging branches of the lactiferous ducts to reservoir spaces called ampullae or the lactiferous sinus located under the areola, the pigmented area of skin surrounding the nipple. Another pituitary hormone, oxytocin, stimulates the ejection of the milk from the alveoli to the ducts, releasing it to the baby. This is commonly called the *let-down reflex*. It causes a tingling sensation in the breast and begins the flow of milk. The initial sucking of the baby stimulates this reflex. The newborn rooting reflex, oral need for sucking, and basic hunger drive usually induce and maintain breast-feeding by the healthy mother.

The mother should follow the baby's lead with an on-demand schedule. The baby's continuing rhythm of need establishes feedings, usually about every 2 to 3 hours in the first few weeks after birth.[4,13] The newborn's rooting reflex and somewhat recessed lower jaw are natural adaptations for feeding at the breast. The mother can feed the baby for about 10 to 15 minutes on each breast. When the baby is satisfied, he or she can be released from the breast. The nipple should air dry to prevent irritation and soreness (see the Focus on Food Safety box, "Ensuring the Safety of Breast Milk and Infant Formula").

The mother's diet and rest are important factors in establishing lactation and breast-feeding. Figure 11-7 suggests a balanced diet to support ample milk production, including food choices from various food groups for meals and snacks (see Chapter 11). Natural thirst guides adequate fluid intake. Sufficient rest and relaxation for the mother are essential. An adequate energy intake is especially important in the early weeks to establish regular milk production. A gradual weight loss occurs as maternal fat stores are slowly depleted, but the mother should not expect a rapid return to her prepregnancy weight. Overweight mothers with a BMI between 25 and 30 kg/m^2 can lose about 1 lb/wk while successfully breast-feeding their infants by reducing energy intake by approximately 500 kcal per day and engaging in aerobic exercise on 4 days per week.[17] However, rigorous dieting should not be undertaken by breast-feeding mothers.

Breast-feeding may influence feeding behavior and taste preferences into childhood.[18] Acceptance of a wide variety of tastes and preferences for foods may occur if the infant is breast-fed. Odorous compounds, found in foods and beverages, transfer into breast milk[19]; such flavor exposure during breast-feeding often affects acceptance of same-flavored foods in childhood.[18] Studies suggest that breast-fed infants

---

BOX 12-1 PRIORITIZING BREAST-FEEDING: THE BABY FRIENDLY HOSPITAL INITIATIVE (BFHI)

Actions to Earning BFHI Status
- Write and implement a breast-feeding policy.
- Train health care personnel to support the policy.
- Tell pregnant women how to breast-feed and about its benefits.
- Assist mothers with breast-feeding their newborns in the first 30 minutes after delivery.
- Demonstrate to mothers how to breast-feed and express breast milk.
- Provide only breast milk to infants, unless contraindicated.
- Allow infant to be with mother at all times.
- Educate mothers about on-demand feeding.
- Avoid use of pacifiers or other synthetic nipples.
- Educate mothers about breast-feeding issues and finding support after leaving the hospital.

KEY TERMS

colostrum Thin yellow fluid first secreted by the mammary gland a few days before and after childbirth, preceding the mature breast milk. It contains up to 20% protein, including a large amount of lactalbumin, more minerals, and less lactose and fat than in mature milk, and immunoglobulins representing the antibodies found in maternal blood.

lactiferous ducts Branching channels in the mammary gland that carry breast milk to holding spaces near the nipple ready for the infant's feeding.

ampullae A general term for a flasklike wider portion of a tubular structure; spaces under the nipple of the breast for storing milk.

areola A defined space; a circular area of different color surrounding a central point, such as the darkened pigmented ring surrounding the nipple of the breast.

rooting reflex A reflex in a newborn in which stimulation of the side of the cheek or the upper or lower lip causes the infant to turn its mouth and face to the stimulus.

FOCUS ON FOOD SAFETY

Ensuring the Safety of Breast Milk and Infant Formula

Breast milk or formula can be a source of food-related illness in an infant if these fluids are not properly used and stored. All equipment used in the expression or pumping of breast milk, including pump components and containers, and in the preparation of formula, including scoops and containers, should be sterilized. Most equipment and bottle parts, including synthetic nipples, are dishwasher-safe and may be sterilized in this manner. Alternatively, such components may be sterilized in boiling water for 10 to 12 minutes.

Breast milk may stand at room temperature (77°F or less) for up to 6 hours. Breast milk may be stored for no more than 8 days in a 32°F to 38°F refrigerator or in a self-defrosting freezer for up to 5 months. If not used within these time frames, then breast milk should be discarded and not used to feed the infant. Some lactation consultants use the "5/5/5 rule" for breast milk handling: Use breast milk that has been at room temperature within 5 hours, store breast milk in the refrigerator for no more than 5 days, and maintain breast milk in a freezer for no more than 5 months.

Mixed or reconstituted infant formula may be stored for up to 24 hours in a 32°F to 38°F refrigerator. Formula should not be left to stand at room temperature and cannot be frozen. If mixed formula has been in the refrigerator for more than 24 hours or left at room temperature, then it should be thrown away and not used to feed the infant.

Whether a bottle contains breast milk or formula, any unused content should be discarded within 1 hour of when the infant began feeding from the bottle. Additional substances, such as (but not limited to) honey, sugar, infant cereal, soft drinks, and alcohol, should never be added to a bottle containing breast milk or infant formula.

Data from Ogundele MO: Techniques for the storage of human breast milk: implications for anti-microbial functions and safety of stored milk. *Eur J Pediatr* 159(11):793, 2000.

are less likely to become overweight as children compared with infants who are formula-fed.[20-22] Infants who develop a pattern of eating in moderation are less likely to become overweight, and breast-fed infants have more control regarding the amount of milk they consume than do formula-fed infants. Formula-fed infants may be urged to empty their bottle, even though they may turn away when they are satisfied. Force-feeding is less likely to occur in the breast-fed infant but should be avoided in all infants. Feeding should be discontinued at the first sign that the infant has had enough. Children who gain weight more rapidly during the first 4 months of life are more likely to be overweight by middle childhood.

Recent evidence suggests that breast-feeding promotes a healthy gut microbiota.[23-27] The totality of bacterial genes in the gastrointestinal tract or the gut microbiome has been suggested to play a role in short- and long-term health promotion and disease prevention. Breast-feeding appears to cultivate health-promoting gut bacteria and may serve to support the maturation of an infant's gut-associated immune system, thereby preventing diarrhea, necrotizing enterocolitis and even allergies, obesity, and diabetes.[23-27] Breast milk contains oligosaccharides, antimicrobial agents, and immunoglobulins, along with antiinflammatory factors and, of course, nutrients. Breast milk has also been shown to contain certain bacteria, which are proving to be beneficial to the gut microbiome.[23-27] When possible, infants should be breast-fed.

There are circumstances in which an infant should not receive breast milk. A growing public health issue in the United States and worldwide is the advisability of breast-feeding by mothers who are human immunodeficiency virus (HIV) positive, because breast-feeding can be a route of HIV transmission to an infant.[28] In some countries where formula is very expensive and clean water is not readily available, the risks of bottle-feeding may still outweigh the risk of HIV transmission for breast-fed infants. For the premature and low–birth-weight baby, feeding through the first year of life poses additional problems.

Bottle-Feeding

Formula feeding by bottle may be preferred by some mothers for a variety of reasons. If the mother does not choose to breast-feed or stops breast-feeding before her infant reaches the age of 1 year, then bottle-feeding of an appropriate formula is an acceptable alternative. A variety of commercial formulas that attempt to approximate the composition of human milk are available. Some of the cow's milk–based formulas are adjusted with whey protein to more nearly approximate the protein ratio in human milk.

A topic of current interest is the nutritional benefit of substantial amounts of the long-chain fatty acids arachidonic acid (ARA) and docosahexaenoic acid (DHA) provided in breast milk. These fatty acids appear to play a special role in development of the brain and tissue of the retina.[29] Based on the presence of ARA and DHA in human breast milk and the normal metabolic conversion of linoleic acid to ARA and α-linolenic acid to DHA (along with evidence linking ARA and DHA to visual acuity and cognitive development), the U.S. Food and Drug Administration (FDA) approved the addition of these long-chain polyunsaturated fatty acids to infant formula.

Special formulas have been developed for infants with allergies, lactose intolerance, diarrhea, fat malabsorption, or other problems,[30] and several types of constituent proteins and carbohydrates are used. These special formulas include cow's milk protein, soy protein, and casein hydrolysate, and elemental formulas (Table 12-5). Hypoallergenic formulas have been developed for infants who are allergic to cow's milk or commercial formulas based on cow's milk and have existing symptoms of that allergy.[30] Even partially hydrolyzed proteins can provoke an allergic response in infants with hypersensitivity to cow's milk. In the preparation of hypoallergenic formulas, all proteins are completely hydrolyzed to free amino acids. Although some infants allergic to cow's milk tolerate soy formulas, they are not hypoallergenic.

TABLE 12-5   A COMPARISON OF TYPES OF FORMULAS MANUFACTURED FOR FULL-TERM INFANTS

TYPE OF FORMULA USED		PROTEIN CONTENT	FAT CONTENT	CARBOHYDRATE CONTENT
Milk-based routine	Source:	Nonfat cow's milk	Vegetable oils	Lactose
	g/100 kcal:	2.2-2.3	5.4-5.5	10.5-10.8
	% kcalories:	9	48-50	41-43
Whey-adjusted routine	Source:	Nonfat cow's milk plus demineralized whey	Vegetable and oleo oils	Lactose
	g/100 kcal:	2.2	5.4	10.8
	% kcalories:	9	48	43
Soy isolate (cow's milk sensitivity)	Source:	Soy isolate	Vegetable oils	Corn syrup solids and/or sucrose
	g/100 kcal:	2.5	5.3-5.5	10.3-10.6
	% kcalories:	10	47-50	41-42
Casein hydrolysate (protein sensitivity, galactosemia)	Source:	Casein hydrolysate	Corn oil, other vegetable oils, and MCT	Tapioca starch and glucose, sucrose, or corn syrup solids
	g/100 kcal:	2.8	5.0-5.6	10.2-11.0
	% kcalories:	11	45-50	41-44

MCT, Medium-chain triglycerides.

In recent years the use of soy protein–based infant formulas has increased. Researchers estimate that during infancy, 36% of formula-fed infants in the United States are, at some point, given this type of formula.[31] At one time, soy protein–based formula was used primarily to feed infants who could not tolerate the protein from cow's milk or the lactose found in standard formulas. However, the use of soy protein–based formulas has been increasing among parents who wish to feed their infants vegetarian diets. In addition, soy protein–based formulas have been used in the management of babies with acute diarrhea. To ensure an appropriate complement of amino acids, soy protein–based formulas are supplemented with methionine, carnitine, and taurine. Some controversy surrounds the use of soy protein–based infant formula because of the estrogen-like effects of soy, and the American Academy of Pediatrics recommends the use of soy protein–based infant formula only for infants with galactosemia and lactase deficiency or for infants of caregivers who prefer a vegetarian eating pattern[32] (see the Evidence-Based Practice box, "Food Allergies in Children"). Soy protein–based formula is not recommended as a means of preventing food intolerances or allergies.[33]

Standards for the levels of nutrients required in infant formulas are based on requirements from the National Institute of Standards and Technology. Certified and reference levels have been established for nearly 85 nutrient-related constituents.[34]

When feeding formula, the baby should be cradled in the arm as in breast-feeding, keeping the baby's head upright as much as possible to avoid milk running into the ear canals and causing an ear infection. The close human touch and warmth are important. When the infant is obviously satisfied, extra milk should not be forced, regardless of the amount remaining in the bottle. Any remaining formula should be thrown away and not refrigerated for reuse (see the Focus on Food Safety box, "Ensuring the Safety of Breast Milk and Infant Formula"). Infants usually take the amount of formula they need. Today most infants are fed on demand versus scheduled, which works out to be about every 2 to 3 hours. Healthy infants soon establish their individual feeding patterns according to their individual growth requirements. Only infant formula and water are appropriate for bottle-feeding; other fluids such as juice, flavored drinks, and carbonated beverages should not be provided through bottles.

Breast-Feeding and Formula-Feeding Combination

Some women may desire the flexibility of both breast-feeding and formula-feeding their infants. For example, a mother working outside of the home may choose to breast-feed her infant in the morning before work and in the evening after work and use formula during the day. This combination is possible but is recommended only after an adequate supply of breast milk and infant-feeding pattern have been established. Factors to consider include infant's acceptance of a

KEY TERMS

casein hydrolysate formulas Infant formulas composed of hydrolyzed casein, a major milk protein, produced by partially breaking down the casein into smaller peptide fragments, making a product that is more easily digested.

elemental formulas Nutrition support formulas composed of single elemental nutrient components that require no further digestive breakdown and thus are readily absorbed. Infant formula produced with elemental, ready-to-be-absorbed components of free amino acids and carbohydrate as simple sugars.

synthetic nipple and formula's taste, mother's ability or need to express breast milk during the day, and growth of the infant.

Cow's Milk

Regular unmodified cow's milk is not suitable for infants for several reasons, as follows:

- It causes gastrointestinal bleeding.
- Its renal solute load is too concentrated for the infant's renal system to handle; this leaves too small a margin of safety for maintaining water balance, especially during illness, diarrhea, or hot weather.
- Early exposure to cow's milk increases the risk of developing allergies to milk proteins.
- It adversely affects nutrition status.[13] Cow's milk is low in iron, and iron status in the infant is lowered even further

by the associated gastrointestinal bleeding and blood loss caused by the cow's milk. In addition, cow's milk is a poor source of vitamins C and E and essential fatty acids. Infants have need for fat; thus they should not be fed reduced-fat milks such as nonfat or 2% fat. Low-fat or nonfat milks do not provide (1) sufficient energy to support growth requirements, which leads the infant to consume increased volumes of milk and excessive protein, and (2) sufficient linoleic acid, the essential fatty acid needed for growth and development of body tissues found in the fat portion of milk.[13] A specific form of eczema has been observed in infants deficient in linoleic acid, and a low-fat diet in infancy may impair physical and intellectual development.

To meet the special needs of infants, the American Academy of Pediatrics recommends breast milk or formula as the major food source up to 1 year of age, with a gradual addition of appropriate foods beginning at 6 to 7 months.[4] No need exists for special formulas for older infants; such formulas also present an added expense to the family.

Premature or Small-for-Gestational-Age Infants

Infants born too early or too small have many food-related difficulties to overcome and present a special challenge in feeding. A poor sucking reflex, difficulty in swallowing, small gastric capacity, reduced intestinal motility, tiring easily from eating and being handled, and increased nutrient requirements for catch-up growth all need to be considered. The health team involved in the care of premature or small-for-gestational-age infants is faced with a myriad of decisions to overcome these feeding difficulties. Whenever possible, these infants should be fed breast milk, usually fortified with additional protein, vitamins, and minerals to the levels found in special formulas developed to meet their particular needs. Delivery of breast milk or formula using tube feeding (enteral feeding) carries less risk of complications than the delivery of nutrients through the veins (parenteral feeding).

A comparison of the nutrient content of breast milk and special formulas for the premature infant is presented in Table 12-6. Formulas developed for the premature infant may have as much as 30% more protein per fluid volume than those developed for the normal infant, as well as increased amounts of calcium, zinc, and the B-complex vitamins. This enriched formula also supports catch-up growth in term infants who are small for their gestational age.[35] Nutrition support of the high-risk infant requires a team approach that includes the pediatrician, nurse, dietitian, and a lactation consultant who can assist the mother and family in developing a routine for expressing and safely storing her breast milk to feed her infant.

EVIDENCE-BASED PRACTICE

Food Allergies in Children

A food allergy is an adverse reaction to a food or food component brought on by the body's immune system. Foods that most commonly trigger an allergic and immune-based response in children include milk, eggs, wheat, soy, peanuts, and tree nuts. Other foods, such as strawberries, may result in an allergic reaction. Signs and symptoms of a food allergy include itching in the mouth, swelling in the oral cavity, tightening of the throat, difficulty breathing, abdominal pain and cramping, vomiting, diarrhea, hives, rashes, and hypotension. In extreme cases, anaphylactic shock may occur. Many children or parents of children may report food intolerances or negative reactions to foods or food components, not triggered by the body's immune system. In these cases, understanding the food-related response is important to determining the severity of the reaction, the origin of the response, and the appropriate course of treatment.

Questions for Analysis

1. What evidence is needed to distinguish a food allergy from a food intolerance?
2. What is the appropriate course of action for a child who has a suspected food allergy?

Bibliography

Gray PE, Mehr S, Katelaris CH, et al: Salicylate elimination diets in children: is food restriction supported by the evidence? *Med J Aust* 198:600, 2013.

Jackson KD, Howie LD, Akinbami LJ: Trends in allergic conditions among children: United States, 1997-2011. *NCHS Data Brief* 1, 2013.

Lau CH, Gupta RS: The pediatrician's role in the diagnosis and management of food allergy. *Pediatr Ann* 42:116, 2013.

Longo G, Berti I, Burks AW, et al: IgE-mediated food allergy in children. *Lancet* 382:1656, 2013.

Soares-Weiser K, Panesar SS, Rader T, et al: The diagnosis of food allergy: protocol for a systematic review. *Clin Transl Allergy* 3:18, 2013.

KEY TERM

small for gestational age Describes an infant with a weight below the 10th percentile for gestational age.

TABLE 12-6   NUTRITIONAL VALUE OF SELECTED SPECIAL FORMULAS AND HUMAN MILK FOR THE PRETERM INFANT

NUTRITIONAL COMPONENT	ADVISABLE INTAKE FOR BIRTH WEIGHT		HUMAN MILK CONTENT		STANDARD FORMULAS		SPECIAL PREMATURE FORMULAS	
	1.0 kg (2.2 lb)	1.5 kg (3.3 lb)	PRETERM	MATURE	ENFAMIL* SIMILAC†	ENFAMIL PREMATURE LIPIL*	SIMILAC SPECIAL CARE†	GERBER GOOD START PREMATURE‡
Kcal/dL			73.0	73.0	67.0	81.0	81.0	67.0
Protein (g/200 kcal)	3.1	2.7	2.6§	1.5	2.2	6.0	2.7	6.0
Vitamins, Fat Soluble								
D (IU/120 kcal/kg/day)	600.0	600.0	—	4.0	70.0-75.0	288.0	180.0	216.0
E (IU/120 kcal/kg/day)	30.0	30.0	—	0.3	2.0-3.0	7.6	5.0	7.2
Vitamins, Water Soluble								
Folic acid (mcg/120 kcal/kg/day)	60.0	60.0	—	8.0	9.0-19.0	48.0	45.0	54.0
C (mg/120 kcal/kg/day)	60.0	60.0	—	7.0	10.0-14.0	24.0	45.0	36.0
Minerals								
Calcium (mg/100 kcal)	160.0	140.0	40.0	43.0	63.0-78.0	197.0	180.0	164.0
Phosphorus (mg/100 kcal)	108.0	95.0	18.0	20.0	42.0-53.0	99.0	100.0	85.0
Sodium (mEq/100 kcal)	2.7	2.3	1.5‖	0.8	1.0-1.8	1.8	1.9	2.0

*Mead Johnson Nutritional Division, Evansville, Ind.
†Abbott Laboratories, Abbott Park, Ill.
‡Nestle, Vevey, Switzerland.
§Range: 1.9-2.8 g/100 kcal.
‖Range: 0.9-2.3 mEq/100 kcal.

Beikost: Solid Food Additions

Beikost feeding begins the transition from a predominantly liquid diet to a predominantly solid food diet.[36] Nutritional and medical authorities agree that for the first 6 to 7 months of life the optimal single food for the infant is human breast milk or an appropriate formula. No nutritional basis exists for introducing solid foods to an infant earlier than 6 to 7 months of age; before this age, it may contribute to overfeeding. Until then, the infant does not need any additional food and is not able to adequately handle other foods. In addition to nutritional reasons, developmental reasons exist for delaying the addition of solid foods until the age of 6 to 7 months. The following developmental tasks must have been mastered before the infant is prepared to receive solid foods:

- The infant can communicate desire and interest in food by opening his or her mouth and leaning forward or, conversely, leaning back or turning away, participating in the feeding process.
- The infant can sit up with support and has good control of the trunk and neck.
- The infant has developed the ability to move food to the back of the mouth for swallowing.

Developmental abilities to use the hands and fingers are required before self-feeding can be initiated. Self-feeding efforts begin first with a whole hand (palmar) grasp and then move to a more refined finger (pincer) grasp by the end of the first year. The first item for self-feeding may be a piece of Melba toast that can be grasped with the whole hand. As solid food is gradually added, the amount of breast milk or formula consumed is reduced accordingly. Box 12-2 lists the developmental milestones that correspond to feeding skills and practices.

Both cultural patterns and the age and educational level of the mother influence infant-feeding practices. Some of these practices, such as adding cereal to the infant's bottle to

---

KEY TERMS
palmar grasp Early grasp of the young infant, clasping an object in the palm and wrapping the whole hand around it.
pincer grasp Later digital grasp of the older infant; usually picking up smaller objects with a precise grip between thumb and forefinger.

TABLE 12-7	GUIDELINE FOR ADDING SOLID FOODS TO INFANT'S DIET DURING THE FIRST YEAR*	
WHEN TO START	**FOODS ADDED**	**FEEDING**
Months 6-9	Infant cereal	10 a.m. and 6 p.m.
	Pureed baby foods such as cooked vegetable or fruit	2 p.m.
	Zwieback or hard toast that easily dissolves	At any feeding
Months 9-10	Potato: baked or boiled and mashed or sieved	10 a.m. and 6 p.m.
	Egg yolk (at first, hard cooked and sieved or scrambled; soft boiled or poached later)	
Suggested Meal Plan for 9 Months to 1 year or Older		
7 a.m.	Milk	240 mL (8 oz)
	Infant cereal	2-3 tbsp
	Strained fruit	2-3 tbsp
	Zwieback or dry toast	
Noon	Milk	240 mL (8 oz)
	Strained vegetables	2-3 tbsp
	Chopped meat or one whole egg	
	Cooked fruit	2-3 tbsp
3 p.m.	Milk	120 mL (4 oz)
	Toast, zwieback, or crackers	
6 p.m.	Milk	240 mL (8 oz)
	Whole egg or chopped meat	
	Potato: baked or mashed	2 tbsp
	Cooked fruit	2-3 tbsp
	Zwieback or toast	

*Semisolid foods should be given immediately before milk feeding. One or 2 tsp should be given first. If food is accepted and tolerated well, then the amount should be increased to 1 to 2 tbsp per feeding. Never introduce honey or cow's milk during infancy; avoid foods and food sizes that present a choking hazard; always have adult supervision of an infant during feeding.
Note: Banana or cottage cheese may be used as substitution for any meal.

<table>
<tr><td>

BOX 12-2   DEVELOPMENTAL MILESTONES ASSOCIATED WITH FEEDING SKILLS AND PRACTICES AT APPROXIMATE AGES IN INFANCY*

- **Suckling, sucking,** swallowing—breast milk or infant formula (birth to 6 to 7 months)
- Controlled head and tongue movements, independent sitting stability, tooth eruption, controlled palmar and pincer grasps, crawling, early verbalization—breast milk or infant formula; infant cereal (iron fortified); pureed fruits, vegetables, and meats (7 to 9 months)
- Controlled chewing and grasping, additional tooth eruption, use of spoon and "sippy cup"—breast milk or infant formula; infant cereal (iron fortified); well-cooked, smooth, and softly textured vegetables; mashed or sliced fruits; infant crackers (9 to 10 months)
- Standing and sitting alone, verbalization, controlled gross motor skills, early walking—breast milk or infant formula, infant cereal (iron fortified), bite-sized foods, smooth and textured foods, some "table" foods (10 to 12 months)

*Never introduce honey or cow's milk during infancy; avoid foods and food sizes that present a choking hazard; always have adult supervision of an infant during feeding.

</td></tr>
</table>

help the baby sleep through the night, are related more to the convenience of the mother than to the benefit of the infant. It may not be in the infant's best interest to sleep through the night at a very early age or to adapt as early as possible to three meals a day. In addition, cereal displaces formula when added to the bottle. Smaller amounts of food, eaten on a more frequent basis, may contribute to the pattern of eating in moderation.

The traditional transition food is fortified infant cereal—specifically, infant rice cereal mixed with a little milk or formula—because rice cereal has the least potential for allergic reaction. Vegetables, fruits, potato, egg yolk, and finally meat can be added to the diet in a gradual sequence. No one sequence of food additions must be followed (a general guide is provided in Table 12-7). Single foods are given first, one at a time in small amounts, about 5 to 7 days apart; in this way, adverse reactions can be identified. These foods are usually offered before the milk feeding. Individual responses and

KEY TERMS
suckling Drawing milk from the breast.
sucking Drawing liquid into the mouth by suction produced from movements of the oral cavity, tongue, and lips.

needs can be a basis for choice, as food becomes a source of enjoyment and a new means of building warm family relationships. A basic goal during this time is to have the infant learn to enjoy many different foods. This is the perfect time to introduce a wide variety of foods, because infants appear to be more willing to taste new foods than are toddlers; in fact, the greater the variety of foods presented when the addition of solid food is begun, the greater the number of foods the infant will accept when they are first presented.[37] Breast-fed infants seem to be more receptive to new foods with new flavors. As stated previously, exposure to a variety of flavors in breast milk, the result of the mother's varied diet, helps prepare an infant to accept new flavors and foods.

Many commercial baby foods are prepared without the formerly used ingredients of sugar, salt, or monosodium glutamate (MSG). Some mothers prefer preparing their own baby food. This can be done by cooking and straining vegetables and fruits and forming a puree using a blender, food processor, or Foley mill. These foods can be frozen in ice cube trays or in 1-tbsp amounts on a cookie sheet. The cubes or individual portions are easily stored in plastic bags in the freezer; then a single portion can be reheated conveniently for use at a feeding. When working with mothers, it is important to stress the need for a clean environment when preparing infant foods to avoid the danger of foodborne illness.

Two foods that require special attention in infant feeding are honey and fruit juices. Honey should never be given to an infant who is younger than 1 year, because it can lead to botulism, a fatal condition in infants. Some fruit juices, including apple, pear, and prune, contain sorbitol, which can lead to diarrhea in infants and toddlers. If given, fruit juice should be limited to no more than 4 oz per day.

Summary Principles

The following two principles should guide the feeding process:
1. Nutrients are needed, not specific foods.
2. Food is a main basis of early learning.

Food not only provides physical sustenance but also fulfills other personal development and cultural needs. Good food habits are formed early in life and continue to develop as a child grows older. By the time infants are about 9 or 10 months old, they should be able to eat many family foods that are cooked, chopped, or mashed and simply seasoned, without the need for special infant foods. Throughout the first year of life, the infant's needs for physical growth and psychosocial development will be met by breast milk or formula and a variety of solid food additions, as well as a loving and trusting relationship between parents and child (Figure 12-1).

Toddler (1 to 3 Years)
Physical Characteristics and Growth

After the rapid growth of the first year, the growth rate of children slows. However, although the rate of gain is less, the pattern of growth produces significant changes in body form.

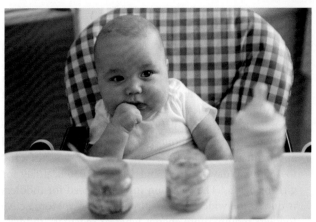

FIGURE 12-1 This child is taking a variety of solid food additions and developing wide tastes. Here, feeding serves as a source not only of physical growth but also of psychosocial development. Optimal physical development and security are evident, the result of sound nutrition and loving care. (Credit: PhotoDisc.)

The legs become longer, and the child begins losing "baby fat." Less total body water exists, and more of the remaining water is inside cells. The young child begins to look and feel less like a baby and more like a child. Energy demands are lower because of the decelerated growth rate. However, important muscle development is taking place. In fact, muscle mass development accounts for about one half of the total weight gain during this period. As the child begins to walk and stand erect, more muscle is needed to strengthen the body and support these movements. For example, a special need exists for big muscles in the back, the buttocks, and the thighs. The overall rate of skeletal growth slows, with increased deposits of mineral in existing bone rather than a lengthening of bones. The increased mineralization strengthens bones to support the increasing body weight. The child has six to eight teeth at the beginning of the toddler period. By 3 years of age, the remaining deciduous teeth have erupted.

Psychosocial and Motor Development

The psychosocial development of the toddler is pronounced. The core developmental problem they struggle with is the desire for autonomy. Each child has a profound increasing sense of self, of being a distinct and individual person apart from the parents, not just an extension of them. As physical mobility increases with increased gross and fine motor skill development, the sense of autonomy and independence grows. An expanding curiosity leads to much exploration of the environment, and increasingly the mouth is used as a means of exploring. Touch is important, providing the means of learning what objects are like. The constant use of the word "no" reflects the significant struggle between the newly emerging ego needs and the caregiver's control efforts. The child wants to do more and more, but the attention span is fairly short and interest shifts quickly from one thing to another.

Food and Feeding

Physical growth and psychosocial development during the toddler period influence nutrient needs (see Tables 12-2, 12-3, and 12-4) and food patterns (see the Perspectives in Practice box, "Feeding Toddlers and Preschoolers: Eating Is a Family Affair"), as follows:

- *Energy:* The energy requirement now increases very slowly in small spurts. At about 1 year of age, children need approximately 850 kcal/day; this rises to a range of 1160 to 1680 kcal/day for boys and 1080 to 1650 kcal/day for girls by age 3.[3] The variation in energy need for toddlers is due to the wide range of physical activity. More active toddlers require more energy, whereas sedentary toddlers do not. From ages 1 to 2, some children do not eat as much as they did in the second half of infancy. Caregivers will avoid conflict with their toddler about eating if they remember this decrease in need for kcalories is normal, resulting from a slowing in the growth rate and the child's necessary struggle for autonomy and selfhood, which often involves refusal of food. Appetite varies in the toddler; therefore food intake may be irregular, with periods of good appetite and periods of disinterest in food. Encouragement is needed from caregivers, but constant conflict with the child about eating serves no useful purpose. A small plate of snacks, including finger-food pieces of raw fruit and cheese kept in the refrigerator or a few crackers on a special colorful plate, can give the child a measure of positive control when hungry. Toddlers will eat when they are hungry. Positive early experiences help develop appropriate food acceptance patterns.[1]
- *Protein:* In relation to energy needs, protein needs are relatively increased during this stage of life. The toddler requires about 13 g of protein per day.[3] Muscle and other body tissues are growing rapidly. At least half of this protein should be of animal origin, because animal protein has high biologic value. However, toddlers who follow a balanced and well-planned ovolactovegetarian diet grow just as well and attain similar heights as their nonvegetarian counterparts.[4] Diets planned for vegan children will need to incorporate soy and legume protein and build on the complementarity of plant proteins (see Chapter 5).
- *Minerals:* Calcium and phosphorus are needed for bone mineralization. The bones are strengthening to keep pace with muscle development and increasing activity. Iron is needed to maintain adequate hemoglobin levels because the increase in body size requires an increasing blood volume. Adequate levels of zinc are necessary to support protein synthesis and cell division. The principle of increasing iron absorption from nonheme sources such as vegetables by including a small amount of heme iron from meat at the same meal (as discussed in Chapter 7) holds true for feeding the toddler.
- *Vitamins:* The fat-soluble and water-soluble vitamins are critical to macronutrient use and growth and development. A variety of food intake eaten in proportion to energy needs should provide adequate vitamins to the toddler.
- *Fiber:* Because solid foods make up a larger portion of the diet of toddlers than that of infants, constipation often becomes more prevalent. Adequate fiber of 19 g/day is recommended for children ages 1 to 3 years.[3]
- *Food choices:* About 2 to 3 cups of milk daily is sufficient for the young child's needs. Sometimes excessive milk intake, a habit carried over from infancy, excludes many solid foods from the diet. As a result, the child may lack iron and develop a so-called milk anemia. On the other hand, if a child dislikes milk as a beverage, then replacement can be made with cheese, creamed soups, puddings, or custards, or nonfat dry milk can be used in cooked cereals, mashed potatoes, meat loaf, and casseroles. Calcium-fortified foods can assist in adding calcium to the diet. Offering the child an increasing variety of foods will help to develop good food habits; food habits are learned, and little opportunity exists for learning if a child is not exposed to a wide variety of foods. Refined sweets are best avoided, reserving them for special occasions, not for habitual use or to bribe a child to eat.

Another important consideration when selecting food for the toddler is the risk of choking and death by **asphyxiation**. Foods that are round, hard, and not easily dissolved can cause choking. Such food items include hot dogs, grapes, peanut butter in globs, hard pieces of raw fruits and vegetables, hard candy, and popcorn. Risk of **aspiration** may increase with small grains, such as rice. Young children should always be supervised when eating and should eat sitting down. Running when eating can lead to choking. It is best that children not eat in a moving car unless a second adult, in addition to the driver, is available to assist if needed.

Summary Principles

The following two important principles should be emphasized when working with caregivers to guide feeding practices during this period:

1. The child needs fewer kcalories but relatively more protein and minerals for physical growth; therefore a variety of foods should be offered in appropriate portion sizes to provide key nutrients. It is important that day care providers and parents work cooperatively to support the development of good food patterns.
2. The child is struggling for selfhood as part of normal psychosocial development. This struggle is expressed in refusing food and the desire to do things for self before being fully able to do them efficiently. If caregivers are patient, offer a variety of foods in small amounts, and

---

KEY TERMS

asphyxiation   To become unconscious or dead due to an interruption in breathing caused by obstruction, such as food, noxious agent, or allergic reaction.
aspiration   Taking in of foreign matter, such as food or fluid, into the lungs.

PERSPECTIVES IN PRACTICE

Feeding Toddlers and Preschoolers: Eating Is a Family Affair

Regardless of their ages, children need the same nutrients as adults but in different amounts. The challenge for parents and caregivers is to make available appropriate and appealing foods and to set the time and place for eating. Young children must learn how to make food choices and to decide how much food they need to consume. We can help parents and caregivers develop child-feeding strategies based on the developmental needs of their young children. First, we must remind them that their children are not growing as fast as they did during the first year of life; it follows that they need less food. In addition, a child's energy needs are sporadic; therefore, periods of increased food intake will vary with periods of smaller intake. Forcing food during periods of low intake may encourage overeating or food aversion, which can lead to food intake problems later in life.

Amount of Food

Children are not ready for adult-sized portions and may be overwhelmed by large amounts of food on their plate. It is better to serve less food than children are likely to eat and have them ask for more. In planning portion sizes, a good rule of thumb is 1 tbsp of food for every year of age. When the child begins to play with the food on the plate or seems to lose interest in eating, remove the plate and provide another activity.

Feeding Frequency

Children do best with a regular feeding schedule; try to keep meals and snacks at regular times. Young children have small stomachs, and it is difficult for them to consume enough food at one meal to last them until the next meal. They may need to eat five or six times a day. Try to allow at least 1½ or 2 hours between snacks and meals. When choosing between-meal snacks, look to foods that will provide not only additional kcalories but also protein and important vitamins and minerals. Fruit, crackers, raw vegetables (as appropriate), cheese, milk, and cereal are good snacks. It is best if children are not overtired at mealtime; if possible, plan a short rest period immediately before a meal.

What Foods

Over time, it is important for the young child to learn to eat a variety of foods, although it may be necessary to offer a new food 8 to 10 times, each including at least a taste, before it will be accepted. The child should learn to eat what other family members are eating and not be provided with special foods. However, when planning meals, be sure to have one item that the child likes and will eat. In addition, children are more willing to try a new food if it is accompanied by a favorite food; try to pair such foods at the same meal. Serve dessert, if any, with the main meal rather than later; it should not assume special importance in relation to other foods. Do allow your toddler or preschooler to make some choices about foods for meals or snacks, just as older children are able to do. This develops skills in making food choices.

Avoid Forbidding Certain Foods

All foods, including sweets, can be included in a healthy diet for young children if limited in frequency and amount. It is important that children learn how to moderate their intakes of such foods. Excluding certain foods makes them more attractive and may ultimately lead to increased intake when they do become available.

Food Safety

Two major safety considerations in feeding children are avoidance of foodborne illness and the possibility of choking. Young children are very vulnerable to foodborne illness resulting from (1) foods that are not fully cooked, such as hamburger or eggs; (2) foods contaminated by contact with an unwholesome food or other source of bacteria; or (3) improperly stored food with bacterial growth. Eating such foods can lead to serious illness or even death in the young child, as occurred when preschoolers ate improperly cooked hamburger at a fast-food restaurant. Children must be taught at a young age to wash their hands thoroughly after they use the bathroom and before they touch a food. Parents should ask about food-handling and other sanitary practices when evaluating the suitability of a caregiver or a care facility.

Children younger than 4 years of age are at greatest risk for choking and death by asphyxiation. Foods most likely to cause choking are those that are round and hard and do not dissolve in saliva. Typical items that cause choking are hot dogs, grapes, peanut butter in globs, hard pieces of raw fruits and vegetables, hard candy, or popcorn. Young children should always be supervised when eating and should eat sitting down.

Social Environment at Meal Time

Try to keep mealtime as pleasant as possible. Allow enough time for the young child to eat. Having to hurry adds stress to mealtime and takes away the pleasure of eating, especially for the child who is still learning to self-feed. Be patient about spills or accidents; it takes time to develop feeding skills. Choose appropriate utensils that are unbreakable and easy for the child to grasp. Children are less likely to accept a food that was first introduced in a negative meal situation; therefore, make mealtime an enjoyable family time that reinforces positive eating behaviors. Parental modeling is an important influence in encouraging children to try new foods. Toddlers are more likely to taste a new food if they see an adult, especially a familiar adult or parent, eating it. Children model the food choices of parents and caregivers; be sure that others at the table are eating vegetables and drinking milk. Parental modeling is as important in the choice of snacks as it is at mealtime.

Bibliography

Cutler GJ, Flood A, Hannan P, et al: Multiple sociodemographic and socioenvironmental characteristics are correlated with major patterns of dietary intake in adolescents. *J Am Diet Assoc* 111(2):230, 2011.

Continued

PERSPECTIVES IN PRACTICE

Feeding Toddlers and Preschoolers: Eating Is a Family Affair—cont'd

Fisher JO, Birch LL: Restricting access to palatable foods affects children's behavioral response, food selection, and intake. *Am J Clin Nutr* 69(6):1264, 1999.

Kleinman RE, editor: *Pediatric nutrition handbook*, ed 6, Elk Grove Village, Ill., 2009, American Academy of Pediatrics.

Rodenburg G, Kremers SP, Oenema A, et al: Associations of children's appetitive traits with weight and dietary behaviours in the context of general parenting. *PLoS One* 7(12):e50642, 2012.

Scaglioni S, Arrizza C, Vecchi F, et al: Determinants of children's eating behaviors. *Am J Clin Nutr* 94(6 Suppl):2006S, 2011.

Thorpe M: Parents as role models: nutrition is a family affair. *J Am Diet Assoc* 102(1):64, 2002.

Zuercher JL, Wagstaff DA, Kranz S: Associations of food group and nutrient intake, diet quality, and meal sizes between adults and children in the same household: a cross-sectional analysis of U.S. households. *Nutr J* 10:131, 2011.

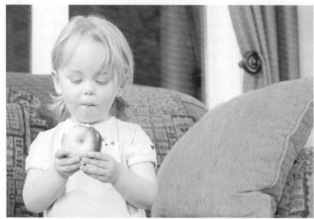

FIGURE 12-2 Fruits are an important part of the toddler's diet. (Copyright 2006 JupiterImages Corporation.)

encourage some degree of food choice and self-feeding in the child's own ceremonial manner, then eating can be a happy, positive means of development.

If we are to achieve the goal of establishing good food patterns for life, it is especially important to introduce a variety of fruits and vegetables along with grains and meats during this stage of development (Figure 12-2). A 3-year study following 72 children from the age of 2 to the age of 5 found that they ate few fruits and vegetables and that their food choices changed very little over the 3 years.[38] Only three fruits (apples, bananas, and grapes) and four vegetables (carrots, green beans, corn, and French fries) were included among lists of 19 favorite foods given by mothers and children. Macaroni and cheese, pizza, chicken, and cereal were the four top foods, and fruit drinks, carbonated beverages, milk, and apple juice were the most commonly used beverages.[39]

Preschooler (3 to 6 Years)
Physical Characteristics and Growth
As shown in normal childhood growth charts (see the Evolve website for *CDC Growth Charts: United States*), each child tends to settle into a regular genetic growth channel as physical growth continues in spurts. On occasion the child bounds with energy. Play is hard play—running, jumping,

and testing new physical resources. At other times, the child will sit for increasing periods of time engrossed in passive types of activities. Mental capacities are developing, and more thinking and exploring of the environment occurs. Energy needs and specific nutrients are shown in Tables 12-2, 12-3, and 12-4. Protein requirements continue to increase as the child grows older. Preschool children need about 13 to 19 g/day of good-quality protein,[3] as found in milk, egg, meat, cheese, legumes, and soy. They continue to need calcium and iron to support growth and to build body stores. Because vitamins A and C and folate are often lacking in the diets of preschool children, a variety of fruits and vegetables should be provided. Vitamin D, important for calcium absorption, can be obtained in fortified milk or soy products or by spending time playing outdoors in the sun.

Psychosocial and Motor Development
Each stage of development builds on the previous one. The psychosocial developmental stage for preschool children involves increased socialization and initiative. They are beginning to develop their superego—the conscience. As powers of active movement increase, they have a growing imagination and curiosity. This is a period of increasing imitation. Boys and girls may imitate adults who serve as role models. Much of this becomes evident in their play by the use of grown-up clothes and role-playing in a variety of situations. Self-feeding skills increase, and eating takes on increased social aspects. The family mealtime is an important event for socialization, because children imitate their parents and others at the table.[8] Whom a child sees as a role model may have long-term implications in respect to nutrient intake and health. For example, in nearly 200 girls of kindergarten age, the best predictor of their milk intakes was the milk intakes of their mothers. If the mother drank soft drinks rather than milk, then so did her daughter.[40]

KEY TERM

growth channel The progressive regular growth pattern of children, guided along individual genetically controlled channels, influenced by nutritional and health status.

Food and Feeding

The preschool child is beginning to form definite responses to various types of foods, as follows:

- *Vegetables and fruits:* Fruits are usually well liked. However, of all the food groups, vegetables usually are liked the least by children, yet these foods contain many vitamins and minerals needed for growth. Where space or opportunity exists, involving the young child in the planting and growing of vegetables in a small garden or in containers is an excellent way to draw the child's interest to vegetables to be tasted. Trips to the market or learning activities in the day care setting can help a child see a variety of shapes and colors in vegetables and discover new ones that can be prepared in a variety of ways. It is important to remember that children have a keen sense of taste; therefore, flavor and texture are important. Children usually dislike strong vegetables such as cabbage and onions but do like crisp raw vegetables or fruits cut in small pieces to eat as finger foods. Mixed vegetables and fruits are less tolerated than individual ones. Children also react to consistency of vegetables, disliking them when they are overcooked. Tough strings and hard pieces are difficult to chew and swallow and should be removed.

- *Milk, cheese, egg, meat, and legumes:* It is helpful if children can set their own goals of quantities of food. Portions need to be relatively small (see the Perspectives in Practice box, "Feeding Toddlers and Preschoolers: Eating Is a Family Affair"). If children can pour their own milk from a small pitcher into a small glass, then they will drink more. Smaller children like their milk served closer to room temperature, not icy cold. In addition, they prefer it in small glasses that hold about 4 to 6 oz rather than in large, adult-sized glasses. Cheese is a favorite finger food or snack; however, the major source of calcium in this age-group is milk. Egg is usually well liked if hard-cooked or scrambled. Meat should be tender and easy to cut and chew; hence, ground meat is popular. Ground meat also must be well cooked to make it safe. (To avoid the risk of foodborne illness that can be fatal in the young child, ground meat should be cooked to a temperature of 160° F, the meat should have a gray-white color, and juices should be clear.)

- *Grains:* The wide variety in which grains can be eaten adds to their appeal to children who enjoy breads, cereals, and crackers. Whole grains provide important fiber. To avoid unwanted kcalories, presweetened cereals should be used infrequently if at all.

- *Temperature:* Because children prefer their foods lukewarm and not hot, some foods may remain on their plates and become dry and gummy such that the child refuses to eat them. Thus very small portions should be served at a time.

- *Single foods:* Children usually prefer single foods to combination dishes such as casseroles or stews. Preschool is also a period of language learning. Children like to learn names of foods and to be able to recognize and name them on the basis of their shape, color, texture, and taste; these identifiable characteristics need to be retained as much as possible.

- *Finger foods:* Children like to eat food they can pick up with their fingers. Often, a variety of raw fruits and vegetables cut into finger-sized pieces and offered to children for their own selection provide a source of needed nutrition.

- *Food jags and food neophobia:* Because of developing social and emotional needs, preschool children commonly have food jags, refusing to eat all except one particular food. This may last for several days, but it is usually short lived and of no major consequence. Food neophobia, commonly referred to as picky or fussy eating, is the refusal to eat new foods. Strategies for lowering food neophobia include offering new foods with familiar foods, introducing new foods in a playful manner, and continuing to introduce new foods repeatedly.

Summary Principles

The preschool period is one of important growth for the young child. Lifetime food habits are forming. Food continues to play an important part in the developing personality, and group eating becomes significant as a means of socialization. The following two principles should be considered when interacting with preschoolers:

1. The social and emotional environment and companionship at mealtime with family, other caregivers, or other children greatly influence the young child's food intake and diet quality. The child learns food patterns at the family table and follows the examples of food eaten by parents or older siblings.[8] The child may attend a day care or preschool in which group eating occurs. Food habits of preschoolers are greatly affected by peer modeling, and food preferences develop according to what the group is eating. Children in this stage of development may begin to respond to environmental cues encouraging them to consume more food than they need. In a day care setting, it was found that 5-year-old children ate more food when presented with larger portions, whereas 3½-year-old children were not affected by portion size.[41] In light of the growing numbers of overweight children, we need to encourage parents to be alert to portion size when serving their children's food.

2. Many food preferences and tolerances are established during this period. Exposure to a wide variety of foods in appropriate portion sizes may set the stage for lifetime food habits and associated patterns of health. This stage of growth is also a time for the young child to develop appropriate physical exercise habits, and games that include activities such as skipping or jumping should be encouraged in a safe environment. Physical fitness established at an early age can lower the risk of overweight and obesity in childhood and adulthood, respectively.[42] Encouraging young children to participate in active games rather than sedentary pastimes such as watching videos or television may support appropriate food patterns as well

(see Further Readings and Resources at the end of this chapter). Even a 30-second commercial for a snack food has been shown to influence the food choices of preschool-age children.[43]

School-Age Child (6 to 12 Years)
Physical Characteristics and Growth

The school-age period preceding adolescence has been called the *latent time of growth*. During this stage, the rate of growth slows and body changes occur very gradually. However, resources are being laid down for the rapid adolescent growth that lies ahead; sometimes this has been called the *lull before the storm*. By now the body type has been established, and growth rates vary widely. Girls usually outdistance boys in the latter part of this period.

Psychosocial and Motor Development

Psychosocial development during these early school years centers on the formal learning environment and its expectations. Children have widening horizons, new school experiences, and challenging learning opportunities. They develop increased cognitive capacity and the ability to problem solve. They learn to cooperate in group activities and begin to experience a sense of adequacy and accomplishment, and sometimes the realities of competition. The child begins to move from a dependence on parental standards to those of peers (Figure 12-3). Pressures are generated for self-control of a growing body, and inappropriate concepts of body image that lead to chronic dieting or eating disorders likely take root during this period. Negative attitudes are sometimes expressed; these changes in temperament are evidence of the struggle for growing independence. It is a diffuse period of gangs, cliques, hero worship, pensive daydreaming, emotional stress, and learning to get along with other children. This is also a period during which nutrition and health concepts can be learned.

Food and Feeding

The slowed rate of growth during this period results in a gradual decline in the food requirement per unit of body

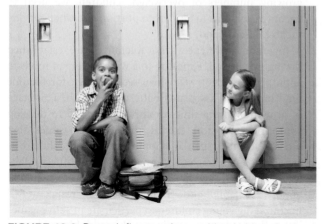

FIGURE 12-3 Peers influence the nutrition habits of school-age children. (Copyright 2006 JupiterImages Corporation.)

weight. This decline continues up to the period just before approaching adolescence. Likes and dislikes are a product of earlier years. Family food attitudes are imitated; however, increasing outside activities begin to compete with family mealtimes, and family conflicts may arise.

School and the Learning Environment

Research has established the relationship between sound nutrition and childhood learning.[42] Breakfast is particularly important for the school-age child. It *breaks the fast* of the sleep hours and prepares the child for problem solving and memory in the learning hours at school.[44] The National School Breakfast and Lunch Programs provide nourishing school meals that many children would not otherwise have (see Appendix E). Studies have documented the positive relationship between breakfast intake and school performance,[44,45] and programs to increase school breakfast participation have been implemented. School programs guided by the U.S. Department of Agriculture (USDA) help to maintain sound nutrition by implementing the 2010 *Dietary Guidelines for Americans* (see Further Readings and Resources at the end of this chapter) into child breakfast and lunch programs.[46] Schools should also take a premier role in promoting lifelong physical activity patterns in children. Health professionals must take leadership roles in their communities to ensure that school meal programs provide positive examples of nutritionally appropriate meal patterns and introduce children to new foods that they may not have tasted previously.[47,48]

The USDA released ChooseMyPlate in 2010 for food guidance in the United States. These program materials are designed to assist individuals in identifying energy needs, setting goals for food and nutrient intakes, and developing food intakes based on food groups. The My Daily Food Plan (Figure 12-4) was developed to build knowledge related to food and nutrient intake along with balance between food intake and physical activity. Classroom-based activities are available on the website of the USDA (www.teamnutrition.usda.gov/) for implementation in schools.

The school-age child has increasing exposure to positive and negative food habits. Television becomes a powerful source of food information. At the same time, positive learning opportunities can occur in the classroom when nutrition education is integrated with other activities and parents provide support and reinforcement at home. An important learning experience can be the preparation of simple meals; in an urban community, 35% of the children in third grade ate at least one meal a day that they prepared themselves or a brother or sister prepared.[49]

Although declines in physical activity no doubt have contributed to the growing number of overweight children, some researchers have also pointed to changes in eating habits. A comparison of diet surveys during the past 30 years indicated that today's children select foods that have larger portion sizes and more kcalories than foods selected by children in the past.[50] An important message to children should be to eat only when they are hungry; portion size

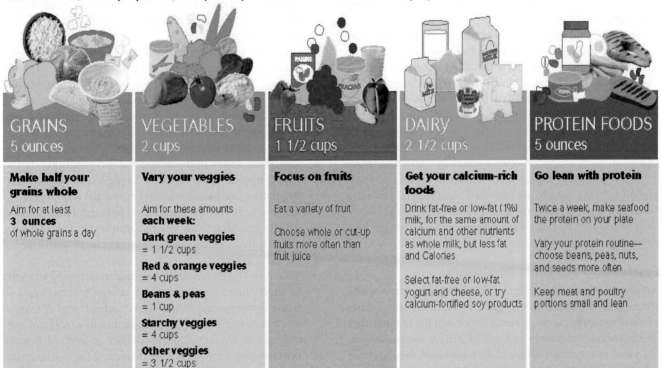

My Daily Food Plan

Based on the information you provided, this is your daily recommended amount for each food group.

GRAINS 5 ounces	VEGETABLES 2 cups	FRUITS 1 1/2 cups	DAIRY 2 1/2 cups	PROTEIN FOODS 5 ounces
Make half your grains whole Aim for at least **3 ounces** of whole grains a day	**Vary your veggies** Aim for these amounts **each week:** **Dark green veggies** = 1 1/2 cups **Red & orange veggies** = 4 cups **Beans & peas** = 1 cup **Starchy veggies** = 4 cups **Other veggies** = 3 1/2 cups	**Focus on fruits** Eat a variety of fruit Choose whole or cut-up fruits more often than fruit juice	**Get your calcium-rich foods** Drink fat-free or low-fat (1%) milk, for the same amount of calcium and other nutrients as whole milk, but less fat and Calories Select fat-free or low-fat yogurt and cheese, or try calcium-fortified soy products	**Go lean with protein** Twice a week, make seafood the protein on your plate Vary your protein routine—choose beans, peas, nuts, and seeds more often Keep meat and poultry portions small and lean

Find your balance between food and physical activity

Be physically active for at least **60 minutes** each day.

Know your limits on fats, sugars, and sodium

Your allowance for oils is **5 teaspoons** a day.
Limit Calories from solid fats and added sugars to **120 Calories** a day.
Reduce sodium intake to less than **2300 mg** a day.

Your results are based on a 1600 Calorie pattern.   Name: _____

This Calorie level is only an estimate of your needs. Monitor your body weight to see if you need to adjust your Calorie intake.

FIGURE 12-4 My Daily Food Plan. This daily food plan is intended for an 8-year-old boy of average height and weight who is physically active 30 to 60 minutes each day. (From U.S. Department of Agriculture: <http://www.choosemyplate.gov/myplate/results.html?name=undefined&age=8&gender=male&weight=56&heightfeet=4&heightinch=2&activity=low&weightN=56&heightfeetN=4&heightinchN=2&validweight=0&validheight=0&>.)

should be moderate, and the best foods are those that are relatively low in kcalories but rich in protein, vitamins, and minerals.

Sound nutrition is especially critical for the child athlete. Children ages 6 to 12 years who are engaged in athletic competition need appropriate nutritional advice from parents, coaches, and trained professionals to meet their energy, protein, and fluid needs for training and competition.[51]

Summary Principles

Growth slows during the school-age years, yet development rapidly continues. Individual- and group-learning experiences greatly influence children. The following two principles should be considered when working with school-age children:

1. Energy needs decline, but the quality of the diet is essential to provide the minerals and vitamins essential to school performance and physical demands.
2. The school and home environments must be conducive to assisting 6- to 12-year-olds with making appropriate food and activity choices. These choices should be based on sound evidence related to nutritional needs of the school-age individual.

Adolescent

Physical Characteristics and Growth

During the adolescent period, with the onset of puberty, the final growth spurt of childhood occurs. Maturation during this time varies so widely that chronologic age as a reference point for discussing growth ceases to be useful. **Physiologic**

age becomes more important in dealing with individual boys and girls. Adolescent growth accounts for wide fluctuations in physical size, metabolic rate, food needs, and even illness. These capacities can be more realistically viewed only in terms of physiologic growth, often characterized by Tanner stages of pubertal growth.[52]

The profound body changes occurring in the adolescent result from the release of estrogen and testosterone, the sex steroid hormones that regulate the development of the sex characteristics. The rate at which these body changes occur varies widely and is particularly distinct in the growth patterns that emerge between the sexes. In girls, the amount of subcutaneous fat increases, and the hip breadth widens in preparation for childbearing. This fat accumulation and change in body shape are often sources of anxiety to many figure-conscious young girls. In adolescent boys, physical growth is manifested by an increased muscle mass and long bone growth. Although the growth spurt in boys is slower than that of girls, boys soon surpass girls in weight and height.

Psychosocial and Motor Development

Adolescence is an ambivalent period marked by stresses and strains. On the one hand, teenagers look back to the securities of childhood; on the other hand, they reach for the maturity of adulthood. Emergence of a self-identity is the major psychosocial developmental task of the adolescent; the search for self, begun in early childhood, reaches its peak during these years. The profound body changes associated with sexual development and the capability of reproduction also result in changes in body image and resulting tensions in maturing girls and boys. Motor development and skilled coordination is complete.

The identity crisis of the adolescent years, largely revolving around sexual development and preparation for an adult role in a complex society, produces many psychologic, emotional, and social pressures. Although the period of most rapid physical growth is relatively short, only 2 or 3 years, the attendant psychosocial development continues during a much longer period. The pressure for peer group acceptance is strong, and fads in dress and food habits play out this theme. In addition, in a technologically developed society such as the United States, high values are placed on education and achievement. Social tensions and family conflicts are often created. These conflicts may have nutritional consequences as teenagers eat away from home more often and develop snacking patterns reflective of personal and peer group choices.

Food and Feeding

With the rapid growth of adolescence comes increased demands for energy, protein, vitamins, and minerals:

- *Energy:* Kcalorie needs increase with the metabolic demands of growth and energy expenditure. Although individual needs may vary, girls require fewer kcalories than boys, based on their smaller body size and body composition.[3] Sometimes, the large appetite, characteristic of this rapid growth period, leads adolescents to satisfy their hunger with snack foods that are high in sugar and fat and low in essential protein, vitamins, and minerals.
- *Protein:* Adolescent growth needs for protein increase to support the pubertal changes in both sexes and the developing muscle mass in boys. To sustain daily needs and to maintain nitrogen reserves, girls require 46 g/day and boys require 52 g/day.[3]
- *Minerals:* The calcium requirement for all adolescents rises to 1300 mg/day to meet the demands of bone growth. In fact, adolescence is a critical time for the development of bone mass under the influence of the increasing levels of the sex hormones, especially estrogen. Poor bone mineralization in adolescence increases vulnerability to bone fracture at later ages.[53] Menses and consequent iron losses in the adolescent girl predispose her to simple iron deficiency anemia. Young female athletes who begin training before menarche and develop secondary amenorrhea may in turn have reduced bone mineral density resulting from low estrogen levels. For all young athletes, fluid replacement in any exercise or performance period is essential.[51]
- *Vitamins:* The B vitamins are needed in increased amounts to meet the extra demands of energy metabolism and tissue development. Intakes of vitamins C and A may be low because of erratic food intake and low intake of vegetables and fruits. A high prevalence of folate deficiency exists among adolescent girls, increasing the risk of neural tube defects (NTDs) in babies born to teenage mothers (see Chapter 6 for a review of NTDs). Vitamin D deficiency is present in up to one half of all adolescents.[54] More prevalent in the winter and spring months and in African-American and Hispanic adolescent boys and girls,[55] vitamin D deficiency is associated with rickets (overt deficiency) and increased risk of developing osteoporosis, cardiovascular disease, and certain cancers later in life.[55] Use of sunscreens, purposeful avoidance of sunlight exposure, and limited intake of vitamin D–fortified milk contribute to vitamin D deficiency in adolescents. A vitamin D supplement of 10 mcg/day is recommended for adolescents who do not consume food sources of vitamin D.[56]

In the development of nutrition intervention programs for teens, it is important to consider their cultural and ethnic backgrounds, recognizing that food habits and problems may differ (see the Case Study box, "Nutrition Program for Adolescents"). We also need to consider cost when making nutritional recommendations to students or parents. Among limited-resource mothers, fruits and some vegetables were perceived as being less filling, and one mother noted it was

---

KEY TERM

physiologic age   Rate of biologic maturation in individual adolescents that varies widely and accounts more for wide and changing differences in their metabolic rates, nutritional needs, and food requirements than does chronologic age.

more important to have her son's hunger satisfied than to provide particular fruits or vegetables.[57] Nutrition counseling must be individualized, taking into consideration both cultural food preferences and other circumstances existing within the family.

Eating Habits

Physical and psychosocial pressures influence adolescent eating behavior (see the Perspectives in Practice box, "Food Habits of Adolescents: Where Do We Begin?"). By and large,

CASE STUDY

Nutrition Program for Adolescents

Amanda is a graduate student of clinical nutrition assigned to the "Save Our Senior High" project in a metropolitan community of 300,000 located in the northwestern United States. A representative of the city's educational advisory board approached her institution for assistance in developing a program that addresses three major problems faced by the majority of high school students: (1) popularity of fad diets among athletes, (2) overweight, and (3) iron deficiency anemia.

Amanda and other members of her class met with students who were learning other health professions (medicine, dentistry, nutrition, nursing, social work), as well as several student representatives from the high school, to plan the program. After they developed goals and objectives, they decided that the nutrition topics would be addressed in a series of workshops: Nutrition and Physical Fitness, Food for the Teen Years, and Snack Facts.

The program was introduced to the students through an advance bulletin distributed at the largest high school in the city, where the project was to begin. The bulletin included an article written by Amanda: "Teenage Nutrition: A Seeming Paradox." This article responded to a common concern expressed by adolescents: the apparent preoccupation of school officials with the students' food habits when they, as a group, looked and usually felt very healthy.

Amanda's article stirred a tremendous interest in the student population. Attendance at each session was high, and the discussions were lively. The evaluation results were positive. In reviewing the evaluative data and low cost of the project, the city council asked Amanda and her classmates to repeat the program at two other high schools where these problems were also prevalent. The council approached the school board about the possibility of including the project in the citywide high school curriculum for the coming year.

Questions for Analysis

1. Outline the content of Amanda's article to reflect major points that you would have included.
2. Write a class outline for each workshop, including objectives, major topics, and questions you would expect from the students. What teaching methods and materials would you expect to be most effective in each workshop?
3. What outside influences on eating habits would you expect in this student population? How effective would you expect this educational program to be in influencing a change of behavior in eating habits?
4. Aside from in-school nutrition education programs, describe possible tactics for influencing the eating habits of teenagers.

PERSPECTIVES IN PRACTICE

Food Habits of Adolescents: Where Do We Begin?

Adolescents who have entered their growth spurt seem to eat all the time. The questions for health professionals are "What are they eating?" and "How do we help them improve their choices?" Both the quantity and quality of food are important during this period of rapid growth. Lean body mass increases by about 35 kg in boys and 19 kg in girls during these years, and 45% of total bone mass is accrued. Generous supplies of iron, zinc, calcium, and essential vitamins are needed to support these changes in body size and development.

Food Intake in the Teen Years

Despite the critical nutrient needs in this life stage, national dietary surveys indicate that of all age-groups, teens have the poorest diets. Their intakes of calcium, iron, zinc, vitamin A, and folate often fall below recommended levels. Although on the average teens eat three or four servings of vegetables each day, one or two of these servings are potatoes, most likely French fries; dark-green and deep-yellow vegetables are eaten infrequently. Boys and girls between the ages of 12 and 19 years eat about one-and-a-half servings of fruit each day, and about half comes from citrus sources. From the dairy group,

boys consume only two-and-a-half servings and girls consume only one-and-a-half servings each day, which does not meet their need for calcium (1 dairy serving = 300 mg calcium). At the same time, most adolescents exceed their need for protein. Foods such as hamburgers, pizza with cheese, tacos, and milkshakes—popular among teens—are good sources of protein. Foods high in sugar such as soft drinks and candy and items high in fat, including pastries, fatty meats, and fried foods, are eaten regularly by many teens. Boys and girls obtain between 30% to 35% of their kcalories from added sugars and solid fats. Nearly one fifth of adolescents use vitamin-mineral supplements, but the supplement users have better diets and obtain increased intakes of nutrients from food. Teens also indulge in risk-taking behaviors: about one fifth smoke, one third use marijuana, and approximately one third report use of alcohol.

Lifestyle and Nutritional Behavior

Lifestyle choices in the teen years are influenced by peer pressure and teens' growing need to express their independence and make their own decisions. Teens also lead busy lives with

Continued

Food Habits of Adolescents: Where Do We Begin?—cont'd

school, sports, and jobs. Focus group interviews with teens in Minnesota indicated that (1) food taste and appeal, (2) time, and (3) convenience were the three most important factors influencing their food choices. They liked foods that looked good and chose the same foods repeatedly because they knew how they were going to taste. Foods such as pastries and other high-sugar or high-fat items were perceived as tasting better than more healthy foods such as fruits, vegetables, or dairy products. Fast-food restaurants are popular because the food is served quickly. Teens often skip breakfast. Individuals in this age-group do not want to spend time preparing food or cleaning up afterward. Food items must be easy to prepare or ready to eat, easy to eat on the go or carry in a backpack, or delivered to the house.

Unfortunately, health is often not an important personal issue at this life stage. A feeling of invulnerability and the idea that they have plenty of time in future years to worry about their health are common in teens. At the same time, body weight and appearance are major concerns for 49% of girls and 43% of boys. The need to be thin causes some adolescent girls to adopt nutritionally inadequate diets or, worse, develop anorexia or bulimia nervosa (see Chapter 8). Adolescent boys trying to increase their muscle mass or "bulk up" may resort to unproven and potentially dangerous supplements or eat high-fat foods in an effort to obtain more kcalories. When working with teens who claim to be dieting, it is necessary to talk with them individually about what kind of diet they are following. For some teens, dieting means drastically reducing their food intake or choosing foods erroneously believed to have special effects on appearance; for others, dieting refers to healthful practices like increasing their intakes of fruits and vegetables or cutting down on fats and sweets.

How Do We Help Teens Improve Their Food Choices?
Improving the food choices of this age-group will require the combined efforts of parents, health professionals, food manufacturers, restaurant personnel, and food retailers. An important message to teens is that appropriate food choices, along with regular physical activity, can help to achieve and maintain (1) a healthy weight and positive level of fitness, (2) a high energy level for school and work, and (3) an overall sense of well-being. Physical education and health teachers, nutrition educators, athletic coaches, school nurses, and parents must work together to develop programs that will reach teens at school and on the playing field.

Teens want information that they can use now, not 10 years from now. One topic of immediate use would be selecting a lower-fat or lower-kcalorie meal at a fast-food restaurant or choosing a more healthy pizza for home delivery. Snacks such as bananas, oranges, or apples; plastic containers of juice; or individual packages of ready-to-eat cereal travel well in a backpack, as do new ultrapasteurized milk drinks that do not require refrigeration. Teens should be encouraged to choose simple-to-prepare or carry-along breakfasts, such as ready-to-eat cereal or whole grain bread (or a bagel) with peanut butter. Among junior high school students, ready-to-eat cereals provided a breakfast that was lower in cost, lower in fat, and higher in

important nutrients including calcium, iron, vitamins A and D, and folate than fast-food breakfast meals, granola, or toaster pastries.

Because taste is the most important factor in food selection for teens, it is important that healthy foods taste good. School cafeteria managers need to produce good-tasting and satisfying food that is attractively served. This means that the school meal must be viewed as an extension of the school's educational mission and supported by teachers and parents. Salad bars have become popular among some teens, and salads "to go" might meet the need of taste and convenience. Recipes that are reduced in fat and sugar but pleasing in taste and texture need to be developed for quantity food programs.

Food manufacturers must be urged to improve the nutrient quality of ready-to-eat main dishes, as well as snack foods. Taste-testing parties with teens that compare lower-fat or reduced-sugar items with less-nutritious products may help to dispel the myth that healthy foods do not taste good. Many popular foods among teens, such as pizza or tacos, can be exceedingly healthy choices if attention is paid to reducing the levels of ingredients high in fat and saturated fat.

Finally, food retailers who cater to the teen audience must be urged to sell and advertise healthy foods. Some fast-food restaurants include orange juice or low-fat milk as drink options in combination meals as an alternative to soft drinks. Salads are an option at many fast-food outlets, and baked potatoes may be available as an alternative to French fries. Advertisements for soft drinks or less-healthy food items often carry the endorsements of popular sports stars. Such endorsements have been applied to foods such as milk that are important to health and well-being. Community coalitions involving health professionals, educators, and parents concerned about adolescents and their future health will be necessary to bring about needed changes.

Bibliography
Bruening M, Larson N, Story M, et al: Predictors of adolescent breakfast consumption: longitudinal findings from Project EAT. *J Nutr Educ Behav* 43(5):390, 2011.
Cutler GJ, Flood A, Hannan P, et al: Major patterns of dietary intake in adolescents and their stability over time. *J Nutr* 139(2):323, 2009.
Hur IY, Reicks M: Relationship between whole-grain intake, chronic disease risk indicators, and weight status among adolescents in the National Health and Nutrition Examination Survey, 1999-2004. *J Acad Nutr Diet* 112(1):46, 2012.
Kleinman RE, editor: *Pediatric nutrition handbook*, ed 6, Elk Grove Village, Ill., 2009, American Academy of Pediatrics.
Kuehn BM: Teen perceptions of marijuana risks shift: use of alcohol, illicit drugs, and tobacco. *JAMA* 309(5):429, 2013.
Neumark-Sztainer D, Story M, Perry C, et al: Factors influencing food choices of adolescents: findings from focus-group discussions with adolescents. *J Am Diet Assoc* 99(8):929, 1999.
Neumark-Sztainer D, Wall M, Story M, et al: Are family meal patterns associated with disordered eating behaviors among adolescents? *J Adolesc Health* 35(5):350, 2004.

boys fare better than girls. Their large appetites and the sheer volumes of food they consume usually ensure generally adequate nutrient intakes, but the adolescent girl may be less fortunate. The following two factors combine to increase concerns surrounding nutrition and food intake in adolescent girls:

1. *Physiologic sex difference:* Because sexual maturation in girls brings about increased fat deposition during the adolescent growth period and because many teenage girls are relatively inactive, it is easy for them to gain weight.
2. *Social and personal tensions:* Social pressures dictating thinness sometimes cause adolescent girls to follow unwise and self-imposed diets for weight loss. In some cases actual self-starvation regimens lead to complex and far-reaching eating disorders such as anorexia nervosa and bulimia nervosa (see Chapter 8). These problems, which can assume severe proportions, usually involve a distorted self-image and an irrational pursuit of thinness, even when actual body weight is normal or even less than age norms. In the absence of described eating disorders, constant dieting can still result in varying degrees of poor nutrition in the teenage girl at the very time in life when her body needs to be building reserves for potential reproduction. The harmful effects that bad eating habits can have on the future course of a pregnancy are clearly indicated in many studies relating preconception nutrition status to the outcome of gestation (see Chapter 11).

Summary Principles

The following two principles should be considered when intervening with food habits during adolescence:

1. Nutrient demands are high for final growth and development; therefore, the quality of the diet is vital (Figure 12-5).
2. Food choices and eating patterns may be less than optimal because of the many influential factors that affect choices during adolescence.

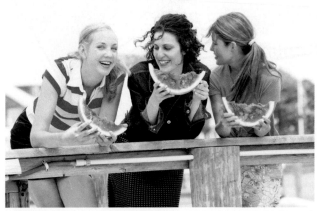

FIGURE 12-5 Fruits and vegetables help meet the high nutrient demands during adolescence. (Copyright 2006 JupiterImages Corporation.)

CHILDREN AND ADOLESCENTS: SEEKING FITNESS

The *Dietary Guidelines for Americans* 2010 provides direction for the development of a healthy diet and lifestyle for all persons age 2 and older.[58] The 2010 edition set goals not only for food patterns in all age-groups but also for appropriate physical activity. Many chronic diseases that influence well-being in later life actually begin in childhood. Thus lifestyle practices that promote healthy behaviors related to diet and physical activity must be introduced at an early age, when patterns are being developed that will continue for a lifetime.

Weight Management

Body weight and physical activity are intrinsically related. A regular pattern of exercise beginning in childhood has been shown to promote lifelong heart health and may prevent the accumulation of excess body fat. Large numbers of U.S. children are overweight.[59] Racial, ethnic, and regional differences are seen in overweight among children. Boys, African Americans, Hispanics, and those living in the Southern states are more likely to be overweight. High-energy diets, coupled with inactivity patterns leading to increased body fat, are associated with the growing incidence of type 2 diabetes in children of school age.

Body fat increases rapidly during the first year of life and then slows until about age 6, when a normal increase again occurs in the size and number of body fat cells. For some children, an inappropriate accumulation of body fat begins about this time or even earlier. Figure 12-6 displays the multifaceted nature of overweight in childhood. Attention must be given to the personal or child characteristics and risk factors, parenting skills and family dynamics, and environmental factors of the community and society that contribute to this complex problem. In general, accumulation of excess body fat can be accelerated by a high energy intake in relation to energy needs or a sedentary life pattern with low energy expenditure.[60] One approach to prevention of inappropriate accumulation of body fat in a child of any age is regular physical activity. The goal is to promote body weight gain within healthy ranges to support normal growth and development.[60] In overweight children and adolescents, the goal is to slow gains in body weight while promoting optimal growth and development.[4]

Physical Activity

Although children and adolescents are typically more active than most adults, many of them appear to be settling into a sedentary lifestyle more common among adults. We know that about one half of girls and one quarter of boys do not exercise vigorously on a regular basis.[61] Television, computer games, the Internet, and similar sedentary pastimes are

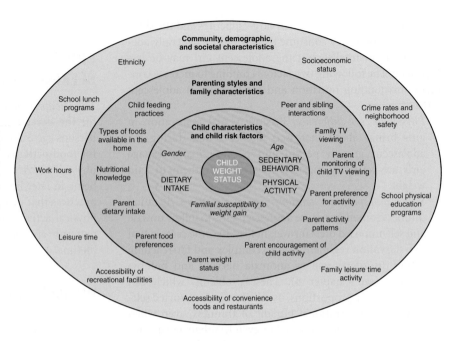

FIGURE 12-6 Ecological model of predictors of childhood overweight. (Copyright 2001 *Obesity Reviews*. From Davison KK, Birch LL: Childhood overweight: a contextual model and recommendations for future research. *Obes Rev* 2:159, 2001. Reprinted with permission.)

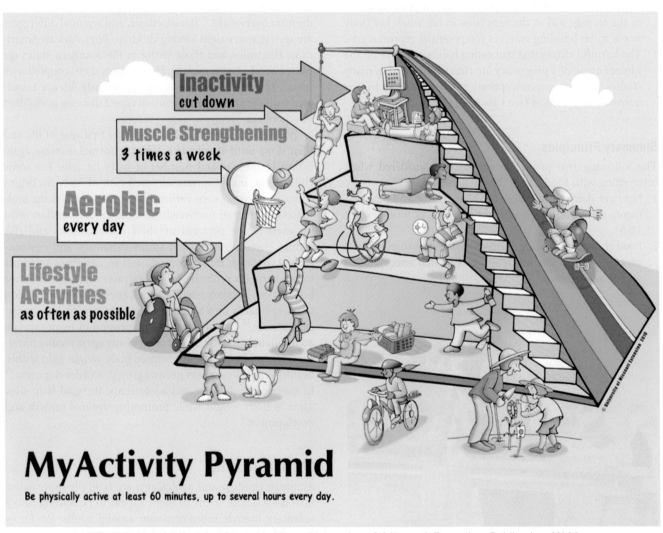

FIGURE 12-7 MyActivity Pyramid. (From University of Missouri Extension Publication N386 [Revised, September 2011]. Reprinted with permission. Available at: <www.extension.missouri .edu/publications/DisplayPub.aspx?P=n386>.)

MyActivity Pyramid

Be physically active 60 minutes, up to several hours every day.
Use these suggestions to help meet your goal:

Lifestyle Activities	Aerobic	Muscle Strengthening	Inactivity
As often as possible	**Every day**	**3 times a week**	**Cut down**

• Play outside
• Help with chores
• Take the stairs
• Pick up toys
• Walk
	• Dance
	• Skateboard
	• Tag
	• Ride your bike
	• Martial arts, like karate
	• Sports
	  ◦ Ice or field hockey
	  ◦ Basketball
	  ◦ Swimming
	  ◦ Tennis
	  ◦ Soccer
		• Tug-of-war
		• Rope climb
		• Pull-ups
		• Sit-ups
		• Push-ups
		
		Muscle-strengthening exercises help your bones get stronger so you can run and play.
			• Screen time (TV, computer, video games*)
			• Sitting longer than 60 minutes
			
			Instead of watching sports on TV, go outside and play a sport!
			
			* Video games that require physical activity may count toward your 60 minutes.

Find your balance between food and fun:
- Move more. Aim for at least 60 minutes every day.
- Walk, dance, bike, rollerblade – it all counts. How great is that!

This publication is adapted from the USDA's MyPyramid and the 2008 Physical Activity Guidelines for Americans, chapter 3. Funded in part by USDA SNAP.
Running out of money for food? Contact your local food stamp office or go online to *dss.mo.gov/fsd/fstamp*. For more information, call MU Extension's Show Me Nutrition line at 1-888-515-0016.

UNIVERSITY OF MISSOURI
Extension

■ Issued in furtherance of the Cooperative Extension Work Acts of May 8 and June 30, 1914, in cooperation with the United States Department of Agriculture. Director, Cooperative Extension, University of Missouri, Columbia, MO 65211
■ an equal opportunity/ADA institution ■ 573-882-7216 ■ extension.missouri.edu

FIGURE 12-7, cont'd

growing in popularity. Watching television for more than 2 hours per day during childhood is related to overweight and the presence of other risk factors for chronic diseases.[62] The physical activity guideline for children and adolescents is a minimum of 1 hour of aerobic, moderate- to vigorous-intensity physical activity each day.[63] Vigorous-intensity and muscle-strengthening physical activity that is weight bearing and promotes bone health should be completed at least 3 days each week.[63]

Helping Children Develop an Active Lifestyle

Parents and caregivers, schools, and communities need to work together to increase physical activity among children.[64] Children are more likely to develop an active lifestyle if parents and role models also demonstrate such behavior. Taking your teddy bear for a walk can be a meaningful activity for a preschooler who belongs to a family who walks together regularly. School games and physical education programs should focus on activities such as walking or running that allow all students to participate, rather than on games in which several students are active but the majority sit and watch. Moving away from competitive games that discourage participation by overweight or less-skilled players to such activities as kickball, dancing, or aerobics that can be done alone to music or in groups after school are worthwhile objectives for physical education. Bike riding and jumping rope are good forms of vigorous exercise. Making school facilities such as a gymnasium or walking track available to families and students after school hours might encourage an increased level of physical activity. Figure 12-7 illustrates one example of guidelines regarding activity levels for children ages 6 to 11 years.

TO SUM UP

Normal growth and development depend on nutrition to support heightened physiologic and metabolic processes. Nutrition, in turn, depends on a multitude of social, psychosocial, cultural, and environmental influences that affect individual growth potential throughout the life cycle.

Four types of growth interact during each phase of development: (1) physical, (2) mental, (3) emotional, and (4) sociocultural. Each type of growth must be evaluated when assessing the child's nutrition status and planning an effective counseling approach. Nutritional needs change with each growth period and must be individualized according to the unique growth pattern of every child.

Infants experience rapid growth. They have immature digestive systems and limited ability to absorb and excrete metabolites efficiently. Breast-feeding is preferred during the first year of life. Solid foods are not needed or adequately tolerated until an infant is 6 to 7 months old.

Toddlers (ages 1 to 3 years), preschoolers (ages 3 to 6 years), and school-age children (ages 6 to 12 years) experience the slowed and erratic latent growth of childhood. Their energy requirements per unit of body weight are not as great

as those of infants. Their nutritional needs center on protein for growth, with attendant minerals and vitamins. Social and cultural factors influence the development of food habits in these age-groups. Appropriate food behavior by parents and caregivers that can be modeled by children of these ages strongly influences the adoption of good eating habits during these periods of development.

Adolescents (ages 12 to 18 years) experience a second large growth spurt before reaching adulthood. This rapid growth involves sexual maturation and physical growth. During this period, girls increase their body proportion of fat, whereas boys increase their body proportion of muscle. Reaching peak bone mass is an important milestone for both genders during this period of development. In general, boys (who consume larger amounts of food) more easily achieve the increased kcalorie and nutrient needs of adolescence. In contrast, girls (who may feel social and peer pressure to restrict food intake to avoid weight gain) are less likely to meet their optimal nutrient requirements for growth. This pressure may also inhibit their ability to acquire the nutritional reserves necessary for later reproduction.

QUESTIONS FOR REVIEW

1. How is physical growth measured? What are the NCHS growth charts, and how are they used? What are the limitations of these charts? What are some clinical, biochemical, and dietary measures that are helpful in assessing the nutritional status of infants and children?

2. Describe the physical and psychosocial characteristics of the newborn. What are the capabilities of the newborn's digestive and renal systems, and how do they relate to infant feeding?

3. Why is breast-feeding the preferred method for feeding infants (discuss nutritional and psychosocial factors)? Describe the anatomic and hormonal components that participate in the delivery of breast milk to the nursing infant.

4. You are planning a nutrition education class to prepare pregnant mothers for breast-feeding. Outline the material that you would present, including (a) dietary needs for the new breast-feeding mother, (b) techniques for holding and feeding the baby, and (c) nipple care.

5. You are counseling a pregnant mother who has decided not to breast-feed. Describe some types of commercial formulas that would provide an appropriate alternative feeding for her infant. Describe the feeding techniques that will be important in meeting the psychosocial needs of her infant.

6. You are working with a mother whose newborn has been found to be allergic to milk proteins. What might be an appropriate food source for this infant?

7. You are working with a low-income mother who has chosen not to breast-feed. She is concerned about the

high cost of infant formula and would like to feed her infant cow's milk because it is cheaper. What would you tell her?

8. Outline a general schedule for a new mother to use as a guide for adding solid foods to her infant's diet during the first year of life; indicate both the time of addition and the items to be offered.

9. What changes in physical growth and psychosocial development influence eating habits in the (a) toddler, (b) preschool child, and (c) school-age child? How do these factors influence the nutritional needs of each age-group?

10. What factors influence the changing nutritional needs of adolescents? Who is usually at increased nutritional risk during this stage—boys or girls? Why? What nutritional deficiencies may be associated with this vulnerable age?

11. You are the director of a food service program in an elementary school and want to start a nutrition education program. You are working with a science teacher, a social studies teacher, and the school nurse to develop lessons that will connect learning in the classroom with good nutrition in the lunchroom. Visit the USDA's Food and Nutrition Information Center website for Team Nutrition (www.fns.usda.gov/tn) to find some ideas and materials that will assist you in this project. Develop a lesson plan for presentation in the science or social studies class that focuses on nutrition or food patterns, and indicate how you will connect this lesson with the lunch program.

REFERENCES

1. Chumlea WC, LaMonte M: Physical growth and maturation. In Samour PQ, King K, editors: *Handbook of pediatric nutrition*, ed 4, Sudbury, Mass., 2012, Jones & Bartlett Learning.

2. Kuczmarski RJ, Ogden CL, Grummer-Strawn LM, et al: *CDC growth charts: United States, advance data, vital and health statistics*, No. 314, Hyattsville, Md., 2000, Centers for Disease Control and Prevention.

3. Food and Nutrition Board, Institute of Medicine: *Dietary Reference Intakes for energy, carbohydrate, fiber, fat, fatty acids, cholesterol, protein, and amino acids (macronutrients)*, Washington, D.C., 2002, National Academies Press.

4. Kleinman RE, editor: *Pediatric nutrition handbook*, ed 6, Elk Grove Village, Ill., 2009, American Academy of Pediatrics.

5. Food and Nutrition Board, Institute of Medicine: *Dietary References Intakes for water, potassium, sodium, chloride, and sulfate*, Washington, D.C., 2004, National Academies Press.

6. Eden AN, Sandoval C: Iron deficiency in infants and toddlers in the United States. *Pediatr Hematol Oncol* 29(8):704, 2012.

7. Erikson E: *Childhood and society*, New York, 1963, WW Norton.

8. Savage JS, Fisher JO, Birch LL: Parental influence on eating behavior: conception to adolescence. *J Law Med Ethics* 35(1):22, 2007.

9. Salvy SJ, de la Haye K, Bowker JC, et al: Influence of peers and friends on children's and adolescents' eating and activity behaviors. *Physiol Behav* 106(3):369, 2012.

10. Position of the American Dietetic Association: Promoting and supporting breastfeeding. *J Am Diet Assoc* 109(11):1926, 2009.

11. Wagner CL, Greer FR, American Academy of Pediatrics, Section on Breastfeeding and Committee on Nutrition: Prevention of rickets and vitamin D deficiency in infants, children, and adolescents. *Pediatrics* 122(5):1142, 2008.

12. Perrine CG, Sharma AJ, Jefferds ME, et al: Adherence to vitamin D recommendations among US infants. *Pediatrics* 125(4):627, 2010.

13. Akers S, Groh-Wargo S: Normal nutrition during infancy. In Samour PQ, King K, editors: *Handbook of pediatric nutrition*, ed 4, Sudbury, Mass., 2012, Jones & Bartlett Learning.

14. Philipp BL, Merewood A: The baby-friendly way: the best breastfeeding start. *Pediatr Clin North Am* 51(3):761, 2004.

15. Chalmers B: The Baby Friendly Hospital Initiative: where next? *BJOG* 111(3):198, 2004.

16. Rosenberg KD, Stull JD, Adler MR, et al: Impact of hospital policies on breastfeeding outcomes. *Breastfeed Med* 3(2):110, 2008.

17. Lovelady C: Balancing exercise and food intake with lactation to promote post-partum weight loss. *Proc Nutr Soc* 70(2):181, 2011.

18. Beauchamp GK, Mennella JA: Early flavor learning and its impact on later feeding behavior. *J Pediatr Gastroenterol Nutr* 48(Suppl 1):S25, 2009.

19. Desage M, Schaal B, Soubeyrand J, et al: Gas chromatographic-mass spectrometric method to characterize the transfer of dietary odorous compounds into plasma and milk. *J Chromatogr B Biomed Appl* 678(2):205, 1996.

20. Philipsen NM, Philipsen NC: Childhood overweight: prevention strategies for parents. *J Perinat Educ* 17(7):44, 2008.

21. Stettler N: Nature and strength of epidemiological evidence for origins of childhood and adulthood obesity in the first year of life. *Int J Obes* 31(7):1035, 2007.

22. Hediger ML, Overpeck MD, Ruan WJ, et al: Early infant feeding and growth status of U.S.-born infants and children aged 4-71 mo: analyses from the Third National Health and Nutrition Examination Survey, 1988-1994. *Am J Clin Nutr* 72(1):159, 2000.

23. Isolauri E: Development of healthy gut microbiota early in life. *Child Health* 48(Suppl 3):1, 2012.

24. Vael C, Desager K: The importance of the development of the intestinal microbiota in infancy. *Curr Opin Pediatr* 21:794, 2009.

25. Musso G, Gambino R, Cassader M: Obesity, diabetes, and gut microbiota: the hygiene hypothesis expanded? *Diabetes Care* 33(10):2277, 2010.

26. Kalliomaki M, Collado MC, Salminen S, et al: Early differences in fecal microbiota composition in children may predict overweight. *Am J Clin Nutr* 87:534, 2008.

27. Le Huerou-Luron I, Blat S, Boudry G: Breast- v. formula-feeding: impacts on the digestive tract and immediate and long-term health effects. *Nutr Res Rev* 23:23, 2010.

28. Lawrence RM: Circumstances when breastfeeding is contraindicated. *Pediatr Clin North Am* 60(1):295, 2013.

29. Agostoni C: Role of long-chain polyunsaturated fatty acids in the first year of life. *J Pediatr Gastroenterol Nutr* 47(Suppl 2):S41, 2008.

30. American Academy of Pediatrics, Committee on Nutrition: Hypoallergenic infant formulas. *Pediatrics* 106(2 Pt 1):346, 2000.

31. Merritt RJ, Jenks BH: Safety of soy-based infant formulas containing isoflavones: the clinical evidence. *J Nutr* 134:1220S, 2004.

32. Bhatia J, Greer F: American Academy of Pediatrics Committee on Nutrition: Use of soy protein-based formulas in infant feeding. *Pediatrics* 121:1062, 2008.

33. Osborn DA, Sinn J: Soy formula for prevention of allergy and food intolerance in infants. *Cochrane Database Syst Rev* (3):CD003741, 2004.

34. Sharpless KE, Lindstrom RM, Nelson BC, et al: Preparation and characterization of standard reference material 1849 infant/adult nutritional formula. *J AOAC Int* 93(4):1262, 2010.

35. Fewtrell MS, Morley R, Abbott FA, et al: Catch-up growth in small-for-gestational-age term infants: a randomized trial. *Am J Clin Nutr* 74(4):516, 2001.

36. Fomon SJ: Infant feeding in the 20th century: formula and beikost. *J Nutr* 131(2):409S, 2001.

37. Birch LL: Development of food preferences. *Annu Rev Nutr* 19:41, 1999.

38. Skinner JD, Carruth BR, Houck KS, et al: Longitudinal study of nutrient and food intakes of white preschool children aged 24 to 60 months. *J Am Diet Assoc* 99(12):1514, 1999.

39. Nicklas TA, Baranowski T, Baranowski JC, et al: Family and child-care provider influences on preschool children's fruit, juice, and vegetable consumption. *Nutr Rev* 59(7):224, 2001.

40. Fisher J, Mitchell D, Smiciklas-Wright H, et al: Maternal milk consumption predicts the tradeoff between milk and soft drinks in young girls' diets. *J Nutr* 131(2):246, 2001.

41. Rolls BJ, Engell D, Birch LL: Serving portion size influences 5-year-old but not 3-year-old children's food intakes. *J Am Diet Assoc* 100(2):232, 2000.

42. Position of the American Dietetic Association: Nutrition guidance for healthy children ages 2 to 11 years. *J Am Diet Assoc* 108(6):1038, 2008.

43. Borzekowski DLG, Robinson TN: The 30-second effect: an experiment revealing the impact of television commercials on food preferences of preschoolers. *J Am Diet Assoc* 101(1):42, 2001.

44. Kleinman RE, Hall S, Green H, et al: Diet, breakfast, and academic performance in children. *Annu Nutr Metab* 46(Suppl 1):24, 2002.

45. Pivik RT, Tennal KB, Chapman SD, et al: Eating breakfast enhances the efficiency of neural networks engaged during mental arithmetic in school-aged children. *Physiol Behav* 106(4):548, 2012.

46. Food and Nutrition Service: Nutrition standards in the National School Lunch and School Breakfast programs. Final rule. *Fed Regist* 77(17):4088, 2012.

47. Position of the American Dietetic Association: Local support for nutrition integrity in schools. *J Am Diet Assoc* 110(8):1244, 2010.

48. Story M, Nanney MS, Schwartz MS: Schools and obesity prevention: creating school environments and policies to promote healthy eating and physical activity. *Milbank Q* 87(1):71, 2009.

49. Melnick TA, Rhoades SJ, Wales KR, et al: Food consumption patterns of elementary schoolchildren in New York City. *J Am Diet Assoc* 98(2):159, 1998.

50. Piernas C, Popkin BM: Increased portion sizes from energy-dense foods affect total energy intake at eating occasions in US children and adolescents: patterns and trends by age group and sociodemographic characteristics, 1977-2006. *Am J Clin Nutr* 94(5):1324, 2011.

51. Position of the American Dietetic Association, Dietitians of Canada, and the American College of Sports Medicine: Nutrition and athletic performance. *J Am Diet Assoc* 109(3):509, 2009.

52. Chemaitilly W, Escobar O, Witchel SF: Endocrinology. In Zitelli BJ, McIntire SC, Nowalk AJ, editors: *Atlas of pediatric physical diagnosis*, ed 6, Philadelphia, Pa., 2012, W.B. Saunders.

53. Wosje KS, Specker BL: Role of calcium in bone health during childhood. *Nutr Rev* 58(9):253, 2000.

54. Gordon CM, DePeter KC, Feldman HA, et al: Prevalence of vitamin D deficiency among healthy adolescents. *Arch Pediatr Adolesc Med* 158:531, 2004.

55. Huh SY, Gordon CM: Vitamin D deficiency in children and adolescents: epidemiology, impact and treatment. *Rev Endocr Metab Disord* 9:161, 2008.

56. Wagner CL, Greer FR: American Academy of Pediatrics Section on Breastfeeding; American Academy of Pediatrics Committee on Nutrition: Prevention of rickets and vitamin D deficiency in infants, children, and adolescents. *Pediatrics* 122:1142, 2008.

57. Hampl JS, Sass S: Focus groups indicate that vegetable and fruit consumption by food stamp-eligible Hispanics is affected by children and unfamiliarity with non-traditional foods. *J Am Diet Assoc* 101(6):685, 2001.

58. U.S. Department of Agriculture and U.S. Department of Health and Human Services. *Dietary Guidelines for Americans, 2010 (Policy Document)*, ed 7, Washington, D.C., 2010, U.S. Government Printing Office. Available at: <http://www.cnpp.usda.gov/dietaryguidelines.htm>. Retrieved July 25, 2012.

59. Ogden CL, Carroll MD, Kit BK, et al: Prevalence of obesity and trends in body mass index among US children and adolescents, 1999-2010. *JAMA* 307(5):483, 2012.

60. Thivel D, Saunders TJ, Chaput J-P: Physical activity in children and youth may have greater impact on energy intake than energy expenditure. *J Nutr Educ Behav* 45(1):e1, 2013.

61. Troiano RP, Macera CA, Ballard-Barbash R: Be physically active each day: how can we know? *J Nutr* 131(2, Suppl 1):451S, 2001.

62. Hancox RJ, Milne BJ, Poulton R: Association between child and adolescent television viewing and adult health: a longitudinal birth cohort study. *Lancet* 364(9430):257, 2004.

63. U.S. Department of Health and Human Services: *Physical activity guidelines for Americans*, ed 1, Washington, D.C., 2008, U.S. Government Printing Office.

64. Veugelers PJ, Fitzgerald AL: Effectiveness of school programs in preventing childhood obesity: a multilevel comparison. *Am J Public Health* 95(3):432, 2005.

FURTHER READINGS AND RESOURCES

Bauer KW, Larson NI, Nelson MC, et al: Socio-environmental, personal and behavioural predictors of fast-food intake among adolescents. *Public Health Nutr* 12(10):1767, 2009.

Bruening M, Eisenberg M, MacLehose R, et al: Relationship between adolescents' and their friends' eating behaviors: breakfast, fruit, vegetable, whole-grain, and dairy intake. *J Acad Nutr Diet* 112(10):1608, 2012.

Clark MA, Fox MK: Nutritional quality of the diets of US public school children and the role of the school meal programs. *J Am Diet Assoc* 109(2 Suppl):S44, 2009.

Cooke L, Fildes A: The impact of flavor exposure in utero and during milk feeding on food acceptance at weaning and beyond. *Appetite* 57(3):808, 2011.

Erinosho T, Dixon LB, Young C, et al: Nutrition practices and children's dietary intakes at 40 child-care centers in New York City. *J Am Diet Assoc* 111(9):1391, 2011.

Fitzgerald A, Heary C, Kelly C, et al: Self-efficacy for healthy eating and peer support for unhealthy eating are associated with adolescents' food intake patterns. *Appetite* 63:48, 2013.

Fletcher A, Bonell C, Sorhaindo A: You are what your friends eat: systematic review of social network analyses of young people's eating behaviours and bodyweight. *J Epidemiol Community Health* 65(6):548, 2011.

Harnack LJ, Oakes JM, French SA, et al: Results from an experimental trial at a Head Start center to evaluate two meal service approaches to increase fruit and vegetable intake of preschool aged children. *Int J Behav Nutr Phys Act* 9:51, 2012.

Howland M, Hunger JM, Mann T: Friends don't let friends eat cookies: effects of restrictive eating norms on consumption among friends. *Appetite* 59(2):505, 2012.

[Adolescents are an important target group for nutrition education. They are highly influenced by their peers and their social networks. Strategies to improve their nutrition and health behaviors may require a multidimensional approach that taps into social structures.]

Mennella JA, Trabulsi JC: Complementary foods and flavor experiences: setting the foundation. *Ann Nutr Metab* 60(Suppl 2):40, 2012.

Position of the American Dietetic Association: Local support for nutrition integrity in schools. *J Am Diet Assoc* 110(8):1244, 2010.

Position of the American Dietetic Association: Promoting and supporting breastfeeding. *J Am Diet Assoc* 109(11):1926, 2009.

Trabulsi JC, Mennella JA: Diet, sensitive periods in flavor learning, and growth. *Int Rev Psychiatry* 24(3):219, 2012.

Trout KK, Wetzel-Effinger L: Flavor learning in utero and its implications for future obesity and diabetes. *Curr Diab Rep* 12(1):60, 2012.

[These articles provide some insight into early feeding experiences and flavor preferences that may impact later food behaviors in childhood and adolescence.]

Witt KE, Dunn C: Increasing fruit and vegetable consumption among preschoolers: evaluation of color me healthy. *J Nutr Educ Behav* 44(2):107, 2012.

[Children attending day care, Head Start, or schools with a breakfast and lunch program receive a major proportion of their meals for the day at that location. This article provides some insight into the role of day care centers and schools in supporting the development of good food habits in children, as well as the role of community health professionals in supporting school food programs in the United States.]

Websites of Interest
- Centers for Disease Control and Prevention, National Center for Chronic Disease Prevention and Health Promotion, Division of Nutrition and Physical Activity: www.cdc.gov/nccdphp/dnpa.
- Centers for Disease Control and Prevention, National Center for Health Statistics: *2000 CDC Growth Charts: United States*: www.cdc.gov/growthcharts.
- U.S. Department of Agriculture, U.S. Department of Health and Human Services, *Dietary Guidelines for Americans* 2010: http://www.cnpp.usda.gov/dietaryguidelines.htm.
- International Lactation Consultant Association: www.ilca.org.
- La Leche League International: www.llli.org.
- U.S. Department of Agriculture, My Daily Food Plan: www.choosemyplate.gov/downloads/DailyFoodPlanSAMPLE.png.
- U.S. Department of Agriculture, Food and Nutrition Service, Team Nutrition: www.fns.usda.gov/tn/.
- U.S. Department of Agriculture: the MyPlate resource (www.ChooseMyPlate.gov).

CHAPTER
13

Nutrition for Adults: Early, Middle, and Later Years

Eleanor D. Schlenker

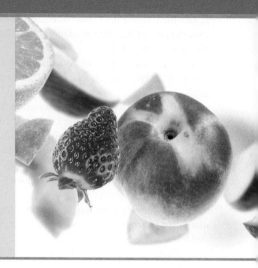

ⓔ EVOLVE WEBSITE

http://evolve.elsevier.com/Williams/essentials/

This chapter completes our three-chapter sequence on nutrition through the life cycle. After the tumultuous adolescent years come the challenges, opportunities, and concerns of adulthood and maturity.

When adolescents come of age, they have three quarters of their potential years of life still remaining. But the seeds of chronic disease that become apparent in later years are often planted before age 25, a period when risk-taking behaviors and poor attention to diet and positive health habits are commonplace. At the same time, public health interventions targeting middle-age and older adults can bring about improvements in health and life expectancy and reduce chronic disease and disability. Although life expectancy continues to rise in the United States, we still fall behind many other countries in projected years of life at both younger and older ages.[1] As we review the adult life stages—the early, middle, and later years—we will look at individual needs and the role of nutrition in promoting a favorable health advantage.

ADULTHOOD: CONTINUING GROWTH AND DEVELOPMENT

Adult Growth and Development

The adult years are distinguished by the attainment of optimal function in all body systems and achievement of reproductive capacity. Yet, adults continue to grow and develop in various ways. Upon reaching physical maturity, growth marked by increasing numbers of cells and changing body size is halted, and replication, forming new cells to replace old ones, begins. Although the general public holds that aging begins at a certain time in life, such as retirement or when a person begins to "look old," aging encompasses the whole of life as we grow and mature. Two important considerations govern the development and evolution of the physiologic, psychosocial, and nutritional components of life across adulthood:

1. *The individual:* Gradual aging occurs in all adults, but the *rate* of change is an individual characteristic.
2. *Life history:* Aging is a total life process. Experiences in one stage of life hold importance for well-being in succeeding stages.

Our genes, environment, and lifestyle influence the rate and magnitude of aging changes and progression of chronic

> **KEY TERM**
>
> **replication** To make an exact copy; to repeat, duplicate, or reproduce. In genetics, replication is the process by which double-stranded deoxyribonucleic acid (DNA) makes copies of itself with each separating strand synthesizing a complementary strand. Cell replication is the process by which living cells divide to produce exact copies of themselves.

disease as we move through the adult years. Even if family history puts us at risk, lifestyle choices and an appropriate food intake enable us to exert some control over our future health and aging. Our cultural and ethnic heritage[2] and accessibility to medical care also influence our long-term health. Each stage of adult life provides the foundation for the one that follows. Harmful health behaviors in the young adult years accelerate physiologic deterioration, while positive lifestyle patterns slow metabolic and physical changes and the progression of existing disease.

The Nature of Aging

Researchers use the term *aging* to refer to all changes that occur in an individual over time from the moment of conception until death. In the health field we usually think of aging as those changes that occur later in life and lead to increasing vulnerability, frailty, and risk of death. The term **gerontology** refers to the study of how and why aging happens and differs from the term **geriatrics**, which describes the diseases and medical conditions common to older individuals. Changes in organ systems and the functional decline that occurs with age are controlled by an individual's biologic limits to cell replication, not his age in years. In fact, **chronologic age** is the least suitable measure of human aging.

Normal Versus Successful Aging

Experts who study the aging process have defined two types of human aging: normal aging and successful aging. In normal aging, genetic and environmental influences interact to produce degenerative changes in body systems. In successful aging, regressive changes are slowed or prevented by positive lifestyle choices and health interventions. A healthy diet, regular physical activity, a positive mental outlook, appropriate health care, and avoidance of smoking are lifestyle patterns that contribute to successful aging. As we review the food intake, lifestyle patterns, and disease risk of young, middle-age, and older adults, consider areas for intervention that will promote successful aging.

ADULT STAGES: YOUNG ADULT (19 TO 40 YEARS)

Physical Characteristics and Lifestyle

After the turbulence of the adolescent years, growth levels off into adult maintenance and stability. The core psychosocial task of the young adult is building relationships outside the core family (Figure 13-1). Many young adults are continuing their education or combining classes with full-time or part-time employment. Households are established and individuals may take on the parenting role. With a changing work environment, many find it difficult to meet the expectations of education, work, and family, or effectively plan for the future. Young adults ages 18 to 44 are more likely than older adults to feel worried, nervous, or anxious,[3] and life dissatisfaction is often associated with risky health behaviors such as smoking, heavy drinking, or physical inactivity.[4]

Nutritional Needs

The growth patterns of adolescence are strengthened in the adult body. Young men have increased muscle mass and growth in the long bones, and young women develop a greater proportion of subcutaneous fat, genetically intended to support reproduction. Nutritional concerns for the young adult include energy, calcium, iron, and vitamins, as follows (Dietary Reference Intakes [DRIs] are found in Tables 13-1 to 13-3):

- *Energy:* The Recommended Dietary Allowance (RDA) for active men ages 19 to 30 is about 3000 kcal/day; for active women the RDA is about 2400 kcal/day.[5] Energy needs decrease slightly in succeeding decades. Physical activity plays an important role in maintaining energy balance (Figure 13-2).
- *Protein:* The RDA is 56 g/day for adult men and 46 g/day for adult women,[5] based on a daily need of 0.8 g/kg body weight. Young men are consuming about two times their RDA, and young women are consuming more than one and one half times their RDA.[6]
- *Minerals:* Three minerals—calcium, iron, and potassium—warrant special attention. Young adults need 1000 mg of calcium per day to ensure continued development and maintenance of peak bone mass,[7] but only 50% of men and about 25% of women in this age-group meet the goal.[8] Iron is a problem for both young men and young women, but for different reasons. Women of childbearing age must offset the iron lost through the menses, making their RDA 18 mg/day,[9] but mean intake is only about three fourths of this amount.[6] In contrast, young men have

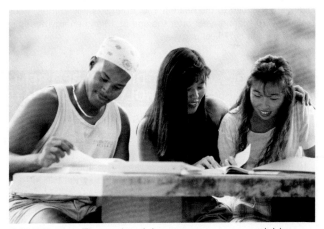

FIGURE 13-1 The early adult years center on social interaction and building networks outside of family. (Credit: PhotoDisc.)

KEY TERMS
gerontology Study of how and why aging happens.
geriatrics Describes the diseases and medical conditions common to older individuals.
chronologic age A person's age in years.

intakes more than twice their RDA of 8 mg.[6,9] Iron intake is closely related to energy intake and use of ready-to-eat cereals, bread, and beef by young men. Fruits and vegetables are major sources of potassium, and low intakes of these foods decrease the supply of this nutrient.[10]

Potassium intakes of young men and young women fall well below the DRI.[6]

- *Vitamins:* Vitamin intake is less than optimal in many young adults. Although folic acid intake from both natural and fortified sources exceeds the DRI of 400 mcg among certain young women, many do not obtain this amount.[6] Young adults who spend little time in the sun and do not use vitamin D–fortified dairy products or take supplements are low in this vitamin and less able to absorb calcium. Vitamin D status is especially critical in Hispanic and African-American populations because of increased

| TABLE 13-1 | **DIETARY REFERENCE INTAKES FOR ENERGY AND PROTEIN FOR ACTIVE ADULTS***† |

AGE (yr)	WEIGHT kg	lb	HEIGHT cm	in	ENERGY (kcal)	PROTEIN (g)
Males						
19-30	70	154	177	70	3000	56
31-50	70	154	177	70	2900	56
51-70	70	154	177	70	2700	56
≥71	70	154	177	70	2500	56
Females						
19-30	57	126	163	64	2400	46
31-50	57	126	163	64	2300	46
51-70	57	126	163	64	2100	46
≥ 71	57	126	163	64	2000	46

Data calculated from standards found in Food and Nutrition Board, Institute of Medicine: *Dietary Reference Intakes for energy, carbohydrate, fiber, fat, fatty acids, cholesterol, protein, and amino acids (macronutrients)*, Washington, D.C., 2002, National Academies Press.
*Because adults are urged to remain physically active throughout their lives, reference weights remain the same for all adult age categories.
†These energy recommendations are based on the midpoint of each age range: age 25, age 40, age 60, and age 80. Calculated values are rounded to the nearest 100. Energy needs in men decline by 10 kcal per year after the age of 19 and energy needs in women decline by 7 kcal per year.

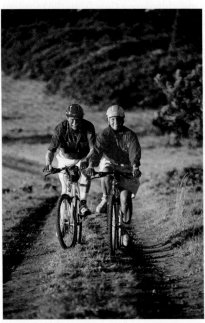

FIGURE 13-2 Energy needs vary according to level of physical activity. (Credit: PhotoDisc.)

| TABLE 13-2 | **ADULT DIETARY REFERENCE INTAKES FOR MINERALS, ELECTROLYTES, AND WATER** |

AGE (yr)	CALCIUM (mg)	PHOSPHORUS (mg)	MAGNESIUM (mg)	IRON (mg)	ZINC (mg)	IODINE (mcg)	FLUORIDE (mg)	POTASSIUM (mg)	SODIUM (mg)	WATER (L/day)
Males										
19-30	1000	700	400	8	11	150	4	4700	1500	3.7
31-50	1000	700	420	8	11	150	4	4700	1500	3.7
51-70	1000	700	420	8	11	150	4	4700	1300	3.7
≥71	1200	700	420	8	11	150	4	4700	1200	3.7
Females										
19-30	1000	700	310	18	8	150	3	4700	1500	2.7
31-50	1000	700	320	18	8	150	3	4700	1500	2.7
51-70	1200	700	320	8	8	150	3	4700	1300	2.7
≥71	1200	700	320	8	8	150	3	4700	1200	2.7

Data from Food and Nutrition Board, Institute of Medicine: *Dietary Reference Intakes for calcium, phosphorus, magnesium, vitamin D, and fluoride*, Washington, D.C., 1997, National Academies Press; Food and Nutrition Board, Institute of Medicine: *Dietary Reference Intakes for vitamin A, vitamin K, arsenic, boron, chromium, copper, iodine, iron, manganese, molybdenum, nickel, silicon, vanadium, and zinc*, Washington, D.C., 2001, National Academies Press; Food and Nutrition Board, Institute of Medicine: *Dietary Reference Intakes for water, potassium, sodium, chloride, and sulfate*, Washington, D.C., 2004, National Academies Press; *Dietary Reference Intakes for calcium and vitamin D*, Washington, D.C., 2011, National Academies Press.

TABLE 13-3 ADULT DIETARY REFERENCE INTAKES FOR VITAMINS

AGE (yr)	VITAMIN A (mcg)	VITAMIN D (mcg)	VITAMIN E (mg)	VITAMIN C (mg)	THIAMIN (mg)	RIBOFLAVIN (mg)	NIACIN (mg NE)	VITAMIN B6 (mg)	FOLATE (mcg)	VITAMIN B12 (mcg)
Males										
19-30	900	15	15	90	1.2	1.3	16	1.3	400	2.4
31-50	900	15	15	90	1.2	1.3	16	1.3	400	2.4
51-70	900	15	15	90	1.2	1.3	16	1.7	400	2.4
≥71	900	20	15	90	1.2	1.3	16	1.7	400	2.4
Females										
19-30	700	15	15	75	1.1	1.1	14	1.3	400	2.4
31-50	700	15	15	75	1.1	1.1	14	1.3	400	2.4
51-70	700	15	15	75	1.1	1.1	14	1.5	400	2.4
≥71	700	20	15	75	1.1	1.1	14	1.5	400	2.4

Data from Food and Nutrition Board, Institute of Medicine: *Dietary Reference Intakes for thiamin, riboflavin, niacin, vitamin B6, folate, vitamin B12, pantothenic acid, biotin, and choline,* Washington, D.C., 1998, National Academies Press; Food and Nutrition Board, Institute of Medicine: *Dietary Reference Intakes for vitamin C, vitamin E, selenium, and carotenoids,* Washington, D.C., 2000, National Academies Press; Food and Nutrition Board, Institute of Medicine: *Dietary Reference Intakes for vitamin A, vitamin K, arsenic, boron, chromium, copper, iodine, iron, manganese, molybdenum, nickel, silicon, vanadium, and zinc,* Washington, D.C., 2001, National Academies Press; Food and Nutrition Board, Institute of Medicine: *Dietary Reference Intakes for calcium and vitamin D,* Washington, D.C., 2011, National Academies Press.
NE, Niacin equivalent.

skin pigmentation and decreased ability to synthesize vitamin D.[7]

Food Habits

Restaurant meals are popular among busy young adults. Many eat away from home three or four times per week, and their choice of restaurant influences both food intake and body weight.[11,12] Frequent meals at fast-food restaurants that serve primarily burgers and fries were associated with a higher risk of overweight or obesity, and higher intakes of kcalories, fat, and sugar-sweetened beverages.[12] In comparison, meals at full-service restaurants were not related to body-weight status and led to increased intakes of vegetables, including dark-green and orange vegetables, whole grains, and fiber. Sharing meals with others at home increased intakes of fruits, vegetables, and milk products, and may be a way to encourage fewer fast-food meals in this age-group.[13] Adults ages 20 to 29 have the highest intakes of total sugar of any adult group,[6] likely reflecting their intakes of sweetened beverages and grains. Many young adults working 40 or more hours per week report lack of time as a barrier to healthful eating.[14]

Health and Chronic Disease

Public health leaders express concern about the worsening health profiles of young adults. Risky behaviors such as smoking, low physical activity, and alcohol abuse are not uncommon in this age group.[15] Unfortunately, the threat of chronic disease seems remote to an individual with youthful vigor. Unwanted weight gain is also associated with the young adult years. One third of adults between the ages of 20 and 39 are obese,[16] increasing their risk of diabetes, high blood pressure, and high cholesterol.[17] Changes in living arrangements and lifestyle associated with new independence make young adults vulnerable to weight gain. Body mass index

(BMI) increased by 2.5 kg/m² in men and 1.7 kg/m² in women between the ages of 18 and 25.[18] Many had established households during this 7-year interval, and living with a partner increased their likelihood of weight gain. However, attitudes and food patterns of a significant other also can have positive effects on health behavior. Young women whose significant others practiced positive behaviors were more likely to eat five or more fruits and vegetables daily and complete 3.5 hours of physical activity each week.[19]

The term *metabolic syndrome* refers to a constellation of factors including elevated BMI and waist circumference, elevated blood pressure, inappropriate blood lipid levels, and elevated blood glucose or insulin levels that contributes to chronic disease. Although we usually associate these risk factors with middle age and beyond, they are appearing in young adults with poorly chosen diets and low physical activity. Among young adults ages 19 to 38, more than 40% had at least one or two of these risk factors; more than 10% had three or more.[20] Young adults who skip breakfast are more likely to be overweight, have abdominal obesity, or elevated blood cholesterol or insulin levels than those having a ready-to-eat cereal.[21] Those eating the breakfast cereal added to their fruit, whole grain, and milk intakes.[22] Improved dietary intake along with greater physical activity could improve the risk profile associated with metabolic syndrome. (We will learn more about interventions for metabolic syndrome in Chapter 21.)

ADULT STAGES: MIDDLE ADULT (40 TO 65 YEARS)

Physical Characteristics and Lifestyle

As individuals move into their 40s, cell replication begins to slow, and men and women begin to experience age-related loss of muscle mass, a condition called *sarcopenia*.[23] Although everyone experiences some muscle loss, individuals with low physical activity lose significant amounts, whereas those practicing strength training lose lesser amounts. The resulting slow but steady decrease in basal metabolic rate (BMR) lowers energy needs, adding to the risk of overweight or obesity.[24,25] Shifts in employment can bring reductions in salary or loss of retirement benefits, wreaking havoc on personal and financial well-being, with debilitating stress. Some parents may experience the "empty nest syndrome" as their children set up their own households (Figure 13-3) and have time for their own pursuits, new hobbies, or further education. Others become caregivers to grandchildren or their aging parents who are no longer able to live independently. Economic strains are leading to more multigenerational households with parents, their adult children, and grandchildren all living under the same roof.

Nutritional Needs

Needs for particular nutrients change in the middle adult years, and intake has a critical bearing on chronic disease risk (see Tables 13-1 to 13-3).

- *Energy:* Loss of active tissue coupled with a sedentary lifestyle lowers kcalorie requirements and unless energy intake and activity level are adjusted, body fat will accrue. Healthy middle-age adults increased their waist circumference by 4 to 5 cm over 5 years.[25]
- *Minerals:* Calcium intake assumes special importance, particularly for women. Menopause and the loss of estrogen bring about a decrease in calcium absorption and an increase in bone turnover, with a net loss of bone mass and greater risk of fracture. Between ages 51 and 70 the DRI for calcium increases to 1200 mg for women but remains at 1000 mg for men.[7] Optimum intake helps preserve bone mass[26,27]; however, among women actual intakes are far less than recommended. The median intake in women is only 759 mg, although men take in

936 mg.[28] Less than 10% of women ages 51 to 70 are meeting their calcium goal. When the menses cease, iron needs in women drop from 18 to 8 mg, comparable to adult men.[9] Sodium intake declines somewhat in middle age, but women still exceed by twofold the Tolerable Upper Intake Level (UL) of 2300 mg. Men exceed the UL by almost threefold.[6]

- *Vitamins:* The RDA for vitamin D is set at 15 mcg to ensure adequate calcium absorption,[7] but vitamin D status is declining in this age-group. Lower milk consumption, increasing BMI, and more frequent use of sun protection lowers both dietary sources and skin production.[29] Vitamin E intake is below the recommended level despite the need for antioxidant protection as the aging process continues.[6] Vitamin B_6 requirements increase because aging adults use this vitamin less efficiently.[30]

Food Habits

Middle-age adults came to maturity during the early growth of the fast-food industry and more than half of middle-age adults with adolescent children report a fast-food family dinner meal at least once per week. Those with more fast-food meals had greater proportions of body fat.[31] Middle-age adults are also consumers of sugar-sweetened beverages, with men taking in on average 159 kcal and women 86 kcal per day from this source.[32] Alcohol also adds to the energy intake of both men and women. A national survey reported that on drinking days, men had 272 kcal from alcohol and women had 210 kcal; for both genders this equaled about 10% of their energy intake for the day.[33]

Intakes of protective foods are less than desirable in this age group. Less than 33% of adults ages 45 to 64 consume two or more servings of fruit each day, and less than 30% have three or more vegetables. Hispanic and African-American adults have particularly low intakes of vegetables.[34] Middle-age adults, as compared with young adults, use more dietary supplements, especially vitamins E and C, the B-complex vitamins, and calcium.[35] Supplements are important in helping many individuals meet DRI standards for vitamins C, A, D, and E.[36]

Chronic Disease Risk

The middle adult years hold the key to health in this stage of life and beyond. Those who establish positive health habits as young adults enter their middle years with a minimum of chronic disease. For those who made poor lifestyle choices, cardiovascular disease, diabetes, and cancer increase in prevalence. At least 38% of men and women in this age group have one modifiable cardiovascular risk factor and at least 22% have two or more (Box 13-1). It is estimated that 29% of U.S. adults have hypertension and 59% have a high-risk lipid profile.[37] Although the majority of those with high blood pressure are being treated with antihypertensive medication, only about half of those with high blood cholesterol are using a lipid-lowering drug.[38] The rise in body weight has helped fuel the increase in diabetes prevalence and younger age of diagnosis (46 vs. 52 years).[39]

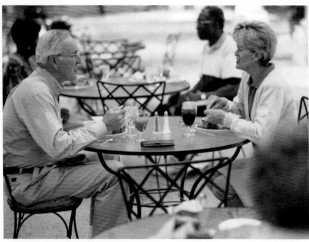
FIGURE 13-3 Middle-adult years can be a time for personal growth. (Credit: PhotoDisc.)

ADULT STAGES: OLDER ADULT (65 TO 85 YEARS)

Aging in America

The first of the baby boomer generation born between 1946 and 1964 is reaching age 65 and many are facing economic uncertainty and spiraling health care costs. As the older population grows, their personal, social, and health care needs will be felt in all our lives. The young and middle-age adults that we discussed earlier in this chapter will comprise the older population of 2050 and beyond.

Following are some personal characteristics of the older population and their potential impact on health and nutrition services:

- *Increase in life expectancy:* Life expectancy is a general measure of the overall health of a population.[40] Over the past century, life expectancy at birth rose significantly based on improved sanitation, the discovery of antibiotics, and higher standards of living (Figure 13-4). Better prevention and treatment of heart disease, cancer, and stroke, the most common causes of death in older adults, has contributed to longer life expectancies. Sixty-five-year-olds can expect to live another 19 years, and 85-year-olds another 6 to 7 years.[40] Those 85 and older are the fastest growing age cohort in the United States and will double in number over the next 25 years.
- *Ethnic and racial diversity:* Currently, 80% of the population above age 64 is Caucasian, but this will change. By 2050, 42% of the older U.S. population will be Asian, Hispanic, or African American (Figure 13-5).[40] Nutrition education programs and meal services will need to adjust to different customs, food patterns, and family roles. Growing diversity is also promoting greater interest in complementary and alternative medicine (CAM). (See the Focus on Culture box, "Cultural and Ethnic Differences in Health Practices" for related discussion.)
- *Education:* Eighty percent of older adults have completed high school, and 23% have a bachelor's degree or higher[40]; however, older racial and ethnic groups differ widely in

levels of education. Only 47% of older Hispanic adults and 65% of older African-American adults completed high school, compared with 84% of older Caucasian adults.[40] Limited ability to read or understand labels on food or medications interferes with good self-care.

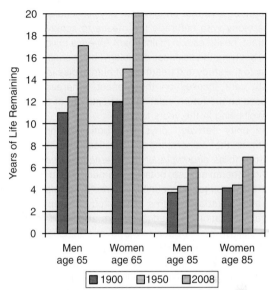

FIGURE 13-4 Life expectancy is increasing among older adults. Men age 65 can expect to live 17 more years and women age 65 can expect to live 20 more years. At age 85, older adults can expect to live another 6 to 7 years. (Data from Federal Interagency Forum on Aging-Related Statistics: *Older Americans 2012: key indicators of well-being,* Washington, D.C., 2012, U.S. Government Printing Office.)

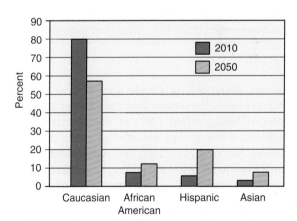

FIGURE 13-5 Percent of persons ages 65 and older according to race and ethnic group. The older population will continue to become more diverse in the coming years. (Data from Federal Interagency Forum on Aging-Related Statistics: *Older Americans 2012: key indicators of well-being,* Washington, D.C., 2012, U.S. Government Printing Office.)

BOX 13-1	**MODIFIABLE RISK FACTORS FOR HEART DISEASE AND STROKE***

High blood pressure
High total and low-density (LDL) lipoprotein cholesterol levels
Low high-density (HDL) lipoprotein cholesterol levels
Diabetes (type 2)
Tobacco use
Obesity

Data from van Eenwyk J, Bensley L, Ossiander EM, et al: Comparison of examination-based and self-reported risk factors for cardiovascular disease, Washington State, 2006-2007. *Prev Chron Dis* 9:E117, 2012.

*These risk factors can be modified through prevention, early recognition, and treatment.

KEY TERM

life expectancy The number of years a person of a given age, gender, race, or ethnic group can expect to live.

Cultural and Ethnic Differences in Health Practices

Health beliefs and practices often spring from our cultural and ethnic backgrounds. The word *health* was derived from an Anglo-Saxon word meaning *wholeness*, or the interaction of the mind and body in reaching a state of well-being.[1] Many cultures believe that bringing our physical and spiritual beings in harmony with nature is the means to achieving health. In contrast, health care in mainstream America builds on biomedicine, applying the sciences of biology, biochemistry, and physiology to the study and treatment of human diseases. Traditional health care focuses on the present, whereas biomedicine focuses on the future, relating the treatment of today to physical well-being in the years to come.[1]

The unity between physical, emotional, and psychologic health is the cornerstone of traditional health care, often referred to as *alternative* or *complementary medicine*. These healing therapies use botanical remedies and interventions such as massage or acupuncture to rectify imbalances in physical and spiritual systems. Mind-body therapies, including prayer, relaxation, or meditation, are also used to prevent or cure disease by individuals who favor traditional therapies. In a U.S. survey, nearly 4 of 10 adults reported using CAM therapy in the past 12 months.[2] Alternative treatments to improve health or relieve problem conditions are growing in favor as individuals assert more control over their own health.

East Asian traditional medicine is based on Ayurvedic medicine developed in ancient times. *Ayur* means longevity and *veda* means knowledge of; this system of medicine uses diet, herbal remedies, and meditation to realign the mind, body, and soul. Over time, Ayurvedic botanical remedies were used to treat digestive disorders, heart problems, diabetes, and urinary tract disorders, and were the foundation for many of the drugs we use today.[1]

Traditional home remedies that make use of herbs and plants have been passed down from generation to generation. Teas made from yellow root or sassafras or ginger are used to relieve stomach distress, and many families use lemon-flavored water with honey to ease the symptoms of a cold.[1] Herbal teas prepared from peppermint, chamomile, parsley, and wormwood are used to relieve diarrhea or other illnesses. Tonics made from eggnog or malt are expected to stimulate the appetite or build strength in pale children or pregnant and postpartum women. Certain alternative medicines, however, are hazardous. Preparations containing mercury or lead, brought into the United States from other countries, adversely affect fetal neurodevelopment or lead to miscarriage or premature birth if consumed during pregnancy.[3]

It is important to know not only what health strategies your patients are observing but also the source of their attitudes and beliefs. Those at greatest risk are often less likely to use biomedical preventive measures. Effective approaches must combine the strengths of biomedicine and complementary therapies.

For more information on CAM visit the website of the National Center for Alternative and Complementary Medicine: www.nccam.nih.gov/.

References
1. Kittler PG, Sucher KP, Nahikian-Nelms M: *Food and culture*, ed 6, Belmont, Calif., 2012, Wadsworth/Cengage Learning.
2. Barnes PM, Bloom B, Nahin RL: *Complementary and alternative medicine use among adults and children: United States, 2007, Natl Health Stat Report*, Hyattsville, Md., Dec 10, 2008, National Center for Health Statistics, pp 1–23.
3. Center for Disease Control and Prevention: Lead poisoning in pregnant women who used Ayurvedic medications from India–New York City, 2011-2012. *MMWR* 61(33):641, 2012.

- *Income:* About 9% of people ages 65 and older have incomes below the poverty line, and another 26% are low income, falling within 199% of the poverty threshold. However, some groups are affected more than others. African-American, Hispanic, and Asian older adults are more likely to fall below the poverty line, and older women have lower incomes than older men. Persons over age 74 are more likely to be poor.[40]
- *Living arrangements:* Because women live longer, more older women are widowed and more older men are married. Thirty-seven percent of older women live alone compared with only 19% of older men.[40] Older single Asian, Hispanic, and African-American women are more likely to live with other family members, as compared with older, single Caucasian women.[40] Only 4.1% of individuals over age 64 reside in institutional settings, although this percentage rises to 13.2% among those over age 84.[41] Older men and women who live alone often have lower incomes and less money to spend on food. They also lack help with meal preparation, and may have no support on sick days.

- *Physical disability:* As individuals age they decline in health, develop physical limitations, and require more health and community services. Chronic diseases such as heart disease, stroke, cancer, and diabetes negatively affect quality of life and contribute to decline in function and the ability to remain independent.[40] Individuals who are unable to stoop, reach over their heads, or lift 10 lb will have difficulty shopping for groceries, preparing meals, or performing housekeeping tasks (Figure 13-6).[40]

Physiologic Changes in Older Adults

The later adult years bring a gradual waning of physical vigor, work capacity, and strength. Physical changes are often minimal immediately following retirement but become more pronounced as individuals move through their 70s and 80s. Lifestyle choices, disease history, and environmental hazards coupled with each person's unique set of genes determine the rate and severity of age-related changes. As a result, older people of the same age are less alike than younger people of the same age, because each has experienced a different set of

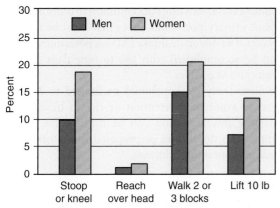

FIGURE 13-6 Percent of persons ages 65 and older who are unable to perform these tasks without help. These tasks are necessary for remaining independent. (Data from Federal Interagency Forum on Aging-Related Statistics: *Older Americans 2012: key indicators of well-being*, Washington, D.C., 2012, U.S. Government Printing Office.)

genetic and environmental influences. Some individuals are physically old at age 50, whereas others maintain an active pace into their 80s or 90s. All age-groups are susceptible to illness and disease, but in younger adults it is more likely an acute problem that runs its course in a few days or weeks. Conditions common to older adults are usually chronic and will over time impose limitations on daily activities and lifestyle.

All older adults experience ongoing changes in major organ systems. Such physiologic changes that influence nutrient utilization and nutritional status are summarized in the following sections.

Body Composition

Over time muscle loss affects functional capacity, with the potential loss of independence; reduction in bone mass adds to the risk of fracture. Even if body weight remains unchanged, the older adult has proportionately more fat.[42-44] Body fat also changes position, moving from the extremities to the trunk, especially the abdomen. This too has implications for health as abdominal fat releases excessive amounts of fatty acids, raising blood lipid and blood insulin levels.[45] Although some older adults experience weight gain, others undergo progressive weight loss, leading to frailty, disability, and diminished quality of life.[46]

Cardiovascular System

Changes in the heart and vascular system lessen their ability to deliver nutrients and oxygen to working tissues, and remove waste. The heart weakens as a pump and is less able to respond to increased demands for oxygen during strenuous physical exercise, emotional stress, or acute illness. A drop in the amount of blood pumped with each stroke reduces the blood supply to major organs such as the kidney and lungs. Major arteries including those that deliver nutrients to the heart muscle itself stiffen and narrow with atherosclerotic deposition. This stiffening limits arterial stretch when blood is delivered, and contributes to the rise in blood pressure common in older age.[47]

Renal System

Aging kidneys are less efficient and require more time to clear waste products from the blood. Urine cannot be concentrated to the same extent; thus, increased fluid is required to excrete a given amount of waste. This is why older people receiving high-protein supplements, which produce large amounts of nitrogen-containing waste, need additional fluid. Fluid balance is poorly regulated at very high or very low intakes of water and sodium.[47]

Respiratory System

The air sacs in the aging lung are less elastic, making it more difficult to move air in and out of the lungs. Other changes in the air sacs reduce the available surface area for exchange of oxygen and carbon dioxide. Widening areas of the lungs no longer participate in gas exchange, and this "dead space" is susceptible to the growth of pathogens. Smoking and air pollution contribute to loss of lung function and a reduced supply of oxygen for normal activity and periods of stress.[47]

Gastrointestinal System

Gastrointestinal changes influence secretions, muscles, and nerves involved in the digestion of food. Loss of gastric acid interferes with the absorption of vitamin B_{12} and reduces uptake of thiamin, folate, calcium, and iron.[7,9,30] Changes in nerve and muscle function contribute to constipation in frail older adults by increasing the time needed for food to pass through the lower digestive tract.

Nutritional Needs

The DRIs have two age categories for people above age 50[5]:
1. Ages 51 to 70
2. Ages 71 and older

These two categories address the physiologic changes and chronic conditions that continue to develop as aging continues. Nutrient absorption and utilization become less efficient, and this is especially apparent in times of illness or stress. Nutrient stores undergo rapid loss and are difficult to replace. At this time we know very little about the interaction between the aging process and chronic disease or how they influence nutritional needs, especially in persons age 85 and older. (The DRIs for persons above age 50 are described in Tables 13-1, 13-2, and 13-3.)

Energy and Macronutrients

- *Energy:* Energy intake continues to decline from middle to older age. The average energy intake of American women drops from 1750 kcal at ages 50 to 59 to 1525 kcal at age 70 and older. In American men kcalories decrease from about 2500 kcal to 1900 kcal in these age-groups.[6] A physically active 65-year-old man weighing 70 kg needs about

2700 kcal/day and a physically active woman of this age weighing 57 kg needs about 2100 kcal/day.[5] Beyond age 70, further declines in energy expenditure are more likely to reflect decreasing physical activity rather than further changes in lean body mass.[48]

- *Carbohydrates:* Persons of all ages should obtain 45% to 65% of their total energy from carbohydrates, with an emphasis on complex carbohydrates.[5] Diets rich in fiber reduce the need for laxatives and their potential for electrolyte disruption. Complex carbohydrates in legumes and whole grains help modulate postprandial blood glucose levels.
- *Fats:* Fat intake within the range of 20% to 35% of total kcalories[5] balances the need for essential fatty acids with the disease risk associated with high-fat diets. Obtaining more kcalories from healthy fats helps prevent weight loss in frail older adults. Fats are generally well digested and absorbed at older ages, although digestion may be slowed; dividing fat intake among all meals and snacks enhances digestion and utilization.

Protein

- *Protein:* The RDA for protein is set at 0.8 g/kg body weight for younger and older adults[5]; however, this standard remains controversial. The DRI expert committee concluded that healthy older adults use protein as efficiently as healthy younger adults and therefore have no increased need for this nutrient. However, intakes of 1.0 g/kg body weight or more are needed to support nutritional well-being and prevent age-related muscle loss, especially in frail or chronically ill elderly or when metabolic systems are less efficient[49-51]; thus clinicians recommend this higher intake for persons over age 70.[51,52] Older individuals recovering from surgery or acute illness may require as much as 1.5 g/kg for optimal recovery. For strength training, an intake of 1.2 g/kg body weight may be optimum to support muscle building.[50] Although protein intakes moderately above the RDA are believed appropriate for older adults with normal kidney function, individualized recommendations are indicated for those with kidney impairment.[49]

Minerals and Electrolytes

- *Calcium:* The calcium DRI for men above age 70 rises from 1000 to 1200 mg as a strategy to reduce bone loss and bone fracture.[7] The recommended intake for women increased from 1000 to 1200 mg at age 51 and continues at this level. Fluid milk, fortified soy milk, fortified juices, and fortified yogurt will supply vitamin D along with calcium.
- *Iron:* Following menopause, the iron requirement of women drops to 8 mg/day, and iron supplements for both genders are inappropriate unless the individual is being treated for iron deficiency anemia and supervised by a physician.[9] In older adults anemia is more likely related to vitamin B_{12} deficiency or chronic disease than to iron deficiency. (See Chapter 7 for more discussion of nutritional anemias.)

- *Potassium:* Various diuretics common to older adults bring about urinary potassium losses that must be replenished by diet. The Adequate Intake (AI) for potassium (4700 mg) can be accomplished with five to nine daily servings of fruits and vegetables.[10]
- *Sodium:* Daily intakes should be limited to 2300 mg or less[9] to avoid fluid retention or rise in blood pressure. Meeting this limitation can be difficult for frail older adults who depend on preprepared foods, often high in sodium-containing additives.

Vitamins

- *Folate:* Optimum folate helps prevent a rise in blood homocysteine levels that damage blood vessels and accelerate atherosclerosis.[30]
- *Vitamin B_6:* As an active coenzyme in protein synthesis, vitamin B_6 is important to preserve muscle mass.[30] Vitamin B_6 is stored and metabolized mainly in muscle, so the sarcopenia of aging likely changes the body's handling of this nutrient.[30]
- *Vitamin B_{12}:* Age-related decreases in gastric acid hinder the release of vitamin B_{12} from animal protein foods. Vitamin B_{12}–fortified breads and cereals or vitamin B_{12} supplements can supply the amount needed to prevent megaloblastic anemia and changes in **cognitive** function.[30]
- *Vitamin D:* To ensure adequate vitamin D levels despite reduced sun exposure and skin synthesis, the RDA increases from 15 mcg (600 IU) for those ages 51 to 70 to 20 mcg (800 IU) for persons older than age 70.[7] Older individuals who spend most of their time indoors will need vitamin D–fortified foods or supplements.[7] Older adults living in the community were obtaining about 350 IU or 40% of their DRI for vitamin D from supplements.[53]

Fluids

Dehydration is a concern for healthy and chronically ill older adults.[54,55] Physiologic changes, effects of disease, medications, and environmental circumstances predispose older people to inadequate fluid intake (Box 13-2). Changes in the hypothalamus alter the thirst mechanism such that older persons do not get thirsty and drink when or as much as they should, and aging kidneys are less able to conserve water to compensate for lower intake. Changes in total body water influence the dilution of medications. Dehydration affects alertness and cognitive function. The general recommendation of 1500 mL/day increases when outdoor or indoor temperatures rise. In patients with fever, daily fluid needs increase by 500 mL for each degree Centigrade beyond normal.[55] On the other hand, older adults are at risk of overhydration (water intoxication) when fluid intakes are inappropriately high, because excess water is less efficiently excreted.

KEY TERM

cognitive Pertaining to mental processes such as memory, judgment, and reasoning.

Older persons and their caregivers should monitor fluid intake and be alert to signs of dehydration. In long-term care facilities, responsibility for overseeing fluid intake must be assigned and those responsible must be held accountable.

BOX 13-2   RISK FACTORS FOR DEHYDRATION IN OLDER ADULTS

- Advanced age (85 years and older)
- Loss of thirst sensation
- Problems with mobility
- Confusion or cognitive changes
- Problems in swallowing
- Medications promoting fluid loss (diuretics, laxatives)
- Incontinence leading to self-imposed fluid restriction

Modified from Ferry M: Strategies for ensuring good hydration in the elderly. *Nutr Rev* 63(suppl 6):S22, 2005. Copyright 2005 International Life Sciences Institute.

Influences on Food Intake

Many physical, social, and environmental influences relating to the individual and the community converge to support the health and quality of life of older adults (Figure 13-7). Personal characteristics relating to health, relationships, and economic situation, as well as community resources such as transportation to the grocery store, safe neighborhoods for walking, or available meal programs influence nutritional and physical well-being. Various conditions and situations described below adversely affect food intake in aging adults.

- *Changes in the mouth and esophagus:* Periodontal disease, tooth loss, and poorly fitting dentures (or no dentures) make chewing and eating painful and difficult. Those with few or no teeth consume fewer portions of fruits and vegetables and have less variety in their diets.[54,56] Loss in taste, smell, or sight take away from the enjoyment of eating and influence appetite. As noted in Chapter 2, changes in salivary secretion resulting in xerostomia (dry mouth) make eating and swallowing troublesome.

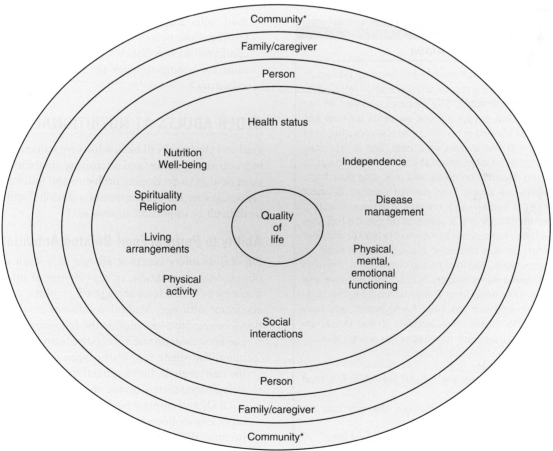

FIGURE 13-7 Personal characteristics, nearby neighbors or family caregivers, and support services available in the community help an older person remain independent. We use the term *community** to include health and supportive services at local, state, and federal levels, as well as health professionals and researchers. (American Dietetic Association: Position paper of the American Dietetic Association: nutrition across the spectrum of aging. *J Am Diet Assoc* 105:616, 2005. Reprinted with permission of the Academy of Nutrition and Dietetics, formerly the American Dietetic Association.)

Radiation treatment or stroke damaging the nerves in the head and neck, or complications of diabetes and Parkinson's disease interfere with the swallowing reflex and cause fear of choking. Aging changes in the appetite control center of the hypothalamus reduce food intake. (See the Case Study box, "An Older Woman Living Alone," to see an example of these problems.)

- *Multiple medications:* Treatment regimens involving multiple drugs (polypharmacy) often lower food intake by producing anorexia, nausea, or unpleasant tastes. Other prescription medications increase appetite, with higher food intake than is desirable. (Nutrient-medication interactions are discussed further in Chapter 18.)
- *Psychosocial distress:* Emotional loss arising from the death of a spouse, physical separation from family and friends, or fear for the future can result in depression and disinterest in food. Older African Americans who expressed a high level of dissatisfaction with their lives had poorer diets, higher in fat and lower in fruits and vegetables, although social support at mealtime appeared to overcome this disadvantage and improve overall food intake.[57] Older

CASE STUDY

An Older Woman Living Alone

Miss E is 81-years-old and lives in public housing. Her apartment kitchen has a two-unit cook top and a small refrigerator but very little storage space. She prepares and eats all her meals alone. She has always enjoyed mealtime but now has trouble with food sticking in her throat, so she cooks her food until it is very soft and seldom eats meat. She is very tired much of the time; on days when she is not well enough to fix a meal, she depends on cereal and milk. She likes fruits and vegetables but always buys canned varieties because they are easier to swallow and cost less than fresh or frozen. Miss E does her shopping at a supermarket about a half mile away. It had been her custom to walk to the market and take the bus home, but it is becoming more difficult to walk, so she rides both ways. She makes the trip twice a week so that she has fewer items to carry at one time. Because she has always liked to walk, Miss E maintained a healthy body weight, but recently she has been losing weight and now worries about her health. She wonders if she should be taking a vitamin supplement to increase her energy level.

Questions for Analysis

1. What physical changes are influencing Miss E's food intake?
2. What socioeconomic or psychologic changes may be affecting her food intake?
3. Which nutrients are likely to be low in her diet? Why?
4. What might be causing her tiredness?
5. What are your general concerns about Miss E's physical condition? What are the implications of her recent weight loss?
6. Would you recommend that Miss E begin to take a vitamin or mineral supplement? If so, then what might she take? Justify your recommendation.

patients with clinically diagnosed depression have poorer diets than those otherwise similar in age, gender, education, chronic disease, and alcohol intake.[58] Older persons living or eating alone, especially men who were unaccustomed to preparing food,[59] may not go to the trouble of planning and cooking a meal. Alcohol sometimes displaces food in the diet. Distorted body image with self-imposed food restriction (anorexia nervosa) occurs in older women and men.

- *Economic problems:* Older adults living in poverty often lack the resources to purchase the quality and quantity of food they should have. Older adults with annual incomes less than $12,000 were more likely to have diets based on fried chicken and fish, starchy vegetables, and refined grains.[60] Other low-income older adults were found to have energy intakes only 83% of that recommended.[61] Inadequate housing with nonworking appliances put older individuals at risk.
- *Chronic illness and disability:* Food shopping and meal preparation are difficult or impossible for persons who use a cane or walker, have vision loss, or no longer drive. Those who depend on others for transportation and shop irregularly are often limited in fresh fruits and vegetables and fluid milk. Inappropriately restrictive diets that forbid favorite ethnic or comfort foods lower food intake. Chronic conditions such as diabetes, with growing financial obligations for testing supplies or medications, worsen food insecurity.[62]

OLDER ADULTS AT NUTRITIONAL RISK

Frail and chronically ill older adults are vulnerable to declining nutritional status and increasing disability. Caregivers must be alert to developing problems and initiate early intervention before the progression of a downhill spiral that will be difficult or impossible to reverse.

Ability to Perform Food-Related Activities

Physical disability occurs at all ages as a result of accident, injury, disease condition, or developmental injury, but the majority of individuals are age 65 or older, and problems accelerate with age. Medical conditions resulting in functional or cognitive loss include the following:

- *Cardiovascular disease:* Congestive heart failure that results in an inadequate supply of oxygen to muscles, including the heart muscle, limits general movement and self-care.
- *Pulmonary disease:* Chronic obstructive pulmonary disease (COPD) and emphysema bring changes in the alveoli (air sacs); less air flows in and out of the lungs and breathing becomes difficult.
- *Musculoskeletal disease:* Rheumatoid arthritis is an autoimmune disorder affecting joints in the hands, arms, and feet. Such loss of movement can restrict food shopping, meal preparation, and, in severe cases, self-feeding. Osteoarthritis (degenerative joint disease) limits flexibility in hand motion and makes walking and standing difficult and painful. Osteoporosis and subsequent hip fracture

often confine the individual to a wheelchair, with loss of independence and institutionalization.

- *Neuromuscular disease:* A cerebrovascular accident (stroke) can result in irreversible paralysis and loss of movement or uncontrolled movement, presenting problems with speech, walking, self-feeding, and self-care. Individuals with cerebral palsy and spina bifida have similar problems in self-care.
- *Progressive neurologic disorders:* Individuals with advanced Parkinson's disease who have joint rigidity, body stiffness, and tremors find meal preparation and self-feeding difficult. Multiple sclerosis, myasthenia gravis, and Alzheimer's disease are other examples of neurologic disorders that affect food-related activities. (These medical conditions are discussed in greater detail in Part 3, "An Introduction to Clinical Nutrition.")

Chronic conditions with related disability often require food-related adaptations that may include assistive devices for self-feeding. The ability to self-feed has implications for physical and emotional well-being. Anger, frustration, fear, and a sense of grief can accompany the loss of this fundamental skill. When a meal is dependent on the cooperation of the feeder, it is no longer driven by the inner eating pace or rhythm of the individual being fed.[63] This lowers meal satisfaction and can influence the amount of food consumed. A variety of assistive devices can be purchased or fashioned at little or no cost to help persons with limited range of motion or poor grasp self-feed (Figure 13-8). (Activity scales used to assess an individual's ability to perform self-care and self-feeding or other tasks related to independent living and the assistance that is required, are described in the Perspectives in Practice box, "Community-Based Long-Term Care: How Do We Decide?")

Development of Overt Malnutrition

Inadequate intakes of kcalories and protein have been identified in many older adults. For reasonably healthy older adults, usual daily energy needs range from 1600 to 2200 kcal for women and 2000 to 2800 kcal for men, depending on lean body mass and level of physical activity.[5] However, many at-risk older adults take in less than these amounts, and African-American and Hispanic older adults have lower intakes than Caucasians (Table 13-4).[6,64,65] Older women in their 70s who were living independently were found to be taking in fewer than 1200 kcal per day.[60] Older adults admitted to a Veterans Affairs facility had energy intakes prior to admission as low as 62% of calculated needs.[66] Homebound older adults often have daily energy intakes below 1000 kcal.[62] Inappropriately low kcalorie intake adds to muscle weakness and frailty when dietary protein must be used for energy. Common chronic conditions such as cancer, cardiac failure, and COPD increase energy needs. Older adults are less able to regulate their energy intake to compensate for day-to-day fluctuations, so temporary reductions in food intake as a result of illness or limited food availability can become the norm, with fewer kcalories consumed and progressive weight loss.[67]

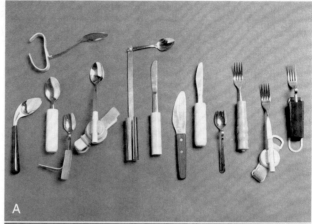

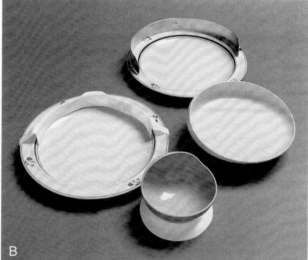

FIGURE 13-8 Various small and inexpensive aids assist individuals with disabilities in self-feeding. **A,** Utensil adaptations help with length, grasp, and range of motion. **B,** Plate guards and scoop bowls provide an edge to help place food on the utensil. (From Olson DA, DeRuyter F: *Clinician's guide to assistive technology,* St Louis, Mo., 2002, Mosby.)

Protein-energy malnutrition occurs in older adults living at home,[68] in long-term care facilities,[69,70] or in the hospital.[70] Among older patients admitted for recuperative care, only 19% were meeting their protein requirement, and 41% were taking in less than half their DRI, which contributed to their physical deterioration.[66] Although kcalorie intake was not reported in these patients it is likely that energy intake was also below optimum, resulting in the use of available protein for energy. Older adults should be encouraged to spread their protein across all meals of the day. Nutrition surveys indicate that older people consume less than 20% of their protein at breakfast, with most eaten with dinner.[71] Muscle mass is better preserved when 25 to 30 g of protein are consumed at each meal, ensuring an ongoing supply of amino acids for tissue building and maintenance. Although 10% to 35% of total kcalories is the accepted range for protein,[5] intakes at the higher end are best for older adults who consume limited kcalories.

Community-Based Long-Term Care: How Do We Decide?

At one time *long-term care* referred to medical, social, or personal services provided to individuals in skilled nursing homes or other resident facilities. Older adults who needed help with daily tasks that could not be provided by family members moved from their homes to such a facility. Today we place more emphasis on community-based long-term care, developing support services that will enable older adults to remain in their own homes or with family members. The first step is evaluating the individual's functional and cognitive capabilities that will determine a safe and appropriate level of care. Two evaluation scales used to assess an individual's ability to remain independent are the Activities of Daily Living (ADLs) and the Instrumental Activities of Daily Living (IADLs).

The following list of ADLs focus on a person's ability to manage personal care either independently, with some level of help, or not at all:

- Bathing
- Dressing
- Feeding
- Using the toilet
- Transferring between bed and chair

An older adult requiring assistance with personal care may be able to remain in the community if family, paid caregivers, or both are available on a daily basis to provide the help needed.

The following list of IADLs evaluates an individual's ability to perform housekeeping tasks and other chores required for independent living:

- Preparing meals
- Performing housecleaning chores
- Handling money and balancing a checkbook
- Shopping without help
- Using the telephone
- Leaving home without help

A person able to perform some, if not all, of these tasks may still remain independent if food-related services such as grocery shopping or home-delivered meals can be established.

Evaluations using the ADLs or IADLs are usually performed by a health professional or trained social worker. This may occur at discharge planning after a hospitalization or convalescence. They can also be requested by family members or health or social service professionals working with the older adult. Ongoing review is provided by a designated case manager who serves as the gatekeeper for professional and support services; he or she monitors any changes in physical or cognitive abilities that require an adjustment in services or level of independence that can be sustained.

TABLE 13-4	**MEAN ENERGY INTAKES OF PERSONS AGE 65 AND OLDER**	
	MEN	**WOMEN**
Caucasian	2032 kcal	1529 kcal
African American	1704 kcal	1275 kcal
Hispanic	1748 kcal	1419 kcal

Data from Bowman SA: Socioeconomic characteristics, dietary and lifestyle patterns, and health and weight status of older adults in NHANES, 1999-2002: a comparison of Caucasians and African Americans. *J Nutr Elderly* 28(1):30, 2009; and Bermudez OI, Falcon LM, Tucker KL: Intake and food sources of macronutrients among older Hispanic adults: association with ethnicity, acculturation, and length of residence in the United States. *J Am Diet Assoc* 100:665, 2000.

Underweight is a serious condition in older adults; men and women in their 60s with a BMI under 18.5 have a mortality risk more than twice that of their normal-weight counterparts.[72] Physicians recommend that older adults maintain a BMI between 22 and 27.[73,74] Problems with declining health, economic uncertainty, or social isolation can result in depression or **failure to thrive**, with low food intake, extensive loss of weight, loss of physical function, and reduced cognitive capacity.[75] The key to continued physical and mental well-being is to avoid unintentional weight loss by ensuring a sufficient intake of kcalories and protein.

Chronic Disease and Malnutrition

Medical conditions accentuate the risk of malnutrition. Immune factors called *cytokines*, released in response to chronic disease or tissue injury, not only lower food intake but also interfere with the utilization of available nutrients so that even aggressive efforts at nutrition intervention cannot always reverse continuing weight loss.[76] Congestive heart failure and cancer cause profound anorexia and wasting, referred to as *cardiac* and *cancer cachexia*. Undernutrition in the aging adult lowers immune function, slows production of red blood cells, and accelerates muscle loss.

Nutrition Screening

Nutrition screening identifies warning signs of malnutrition that initiate a downhill spiral leading to future disability and loss of independence. Nutrition screening takes place in hospitals, long-term care facilities, and the community to seek out those older adults at nutritional risk. The Self MNA (Mini Nutritional Assessment for Adults 65 Years of Age and Older) (Figure 13-9) consists of seven questions that point to

---

KEY TERM

failure to thrive   A syndrome described in older adults that is characterized by loss of body weight and deterioration in physical and cognitive function; usually caused by inadequate food intake.

BOX 13-3	NUTRITION ALERTS FOR OLDER ADULTS IN LONG-TERM CARE

- Involuntary loss of 5% of body weight in 1 month or 10% in 6 months
- Leaving 25% or more of served food uneaten over the past 7 days
- BMI ≤21

Data from Thomas DR, Ashmen W, Morley JE, et al: Nutritional management in long-term care: development of a clinical guideline. *J Gerontol A Biol Sci Med Sci* 55A(12):M725, 2000. *BMI,* Body mass index.

inadequate nutrient intake and projected weight loss.[77] It would be useful in senior centers, congregate meal sites, physicians' offices, home health programs, or home-delivered meals programs. Nutrition screening supports initiation of intervention strategies to prevent the progression to overt undernutrition. A set of warning signs for use with residents in long-term care facilities is found in Box 13-3.

Community Food Assistance Programs for Older Americans

Several tax-supported food assistance programs help older adults meet their food needs. The Supplemental Nutrition Assistance Program (SNAP) extends food-buying power, making food more accessible to adults with limited resources. However, the program that has the greatest effect on the nutritional health of older Americans is the national Elderly Nutrition Program, which provides congregate and home-delivered meals to people age 60 and older. (For more information on these programs, see Appendix E.)

Nutrient Supplementation

Healthy older adults who consume a variety of foods, including fortified foods, and meet the DRI for energy are unlikely to require nutrient supplements. However, those with low energy intakes and chronic health problems will benefit from prudent supplementation. Multiple medications, a limited variety of foods, isolation, and little social support put individuals at risk for nutrient deficiency. Nutrient supplements help replenish body stores after critical or debilitating illness.

Nutrient supplementation should be based on an individual assessment and supervised by a health care professional. Individuals who use single-nutrient supplements in addition to multivitamin-multimineral supplements are most at risk for exceeding the UL for one or more nutrients or precipitating dangerous interactions. An evaluation of dietary intake along with biochemical parameters of nutritional status should provide the basis for any supplement recommendation. Nutritional supplements should add to food, not replace it.

HEALTH PROMOTION

Healthy Food Patterns for Optimum Function

Older Americans are not only living longer but also enjoying robust and active lives. More than 75% of those ages 90 and over still live in the community, and half live alone.[78] Good nutrition and self-care can be key to slowing aging changes and chronic disease. A 16-year follow-up of more than 5000 middle-age individuals reported that those with higher scores on the Healthy Eating Index, a measure of the food servings recommended by MyPlate (ChooseMyPlate. gov), were more likely to experience *ideal aging*—free of chronic disease with high physical, mental, and cognitive function.[79] Those following a diet high in fats, sweets, refined grains, and red meat had lower odds of ideal aging, regardless of other health behaviors. Older adults are "health conscious" and more likely to make positive lifestyle and dietary changes consistent with intervention programs as compared with young and middle-age groups.[80] Older adults interviewed in a national survey were motivated to use dietary supplements with the intention of improving their bone, eye, or heart health.[81]

Although many persons ages 65 and over meet suggested servings of whole fruits, vegetables, meat, and beans,[34] they can still benefit from appropriate nutrition education. Food guides as described in Chapter 1 can be important as energy needs decline and people eat less food. Food guides promote the selection of foods from all major food groups and help ensure dietary diversity. Eating a low variety of foods, even nutrient-dense foods, results in less than the recommended intakes of kcalories and required nutrients and low body weight in older adults living independently in their communities.[82] Current public health messages that emphasize lowering fat intake, being sensitive to portion size, and selecting lower-calorie rather than higher-calorie snacks have the goal of preventing inappropriate weight gain among younger and middle-age adults. However, these messages could be having an unwanted effect on older adults, as many are consuming less food than they should.[83] Elevated blood cholesterol levels and excessive body weight become somewhat less important as risk factors for cardiovascular disease in older adults[83]; thus appropriate intakes of healthy fats or kcalories should not be compromised in an ill-advised effort to lose weight.

Physical Activity for Optimal Function

Physical activity promotes fitness and helps delay age-related changes in functional capacity. There are two types of physical activity, and each has a role in maintaining optimum health.

1. *Endurance exercise:* The rhythmic use of the large muscles in walking, running, or jogging promotes cardiovascular fitness. For many older individuals walking is a safe form of endurance exercise that supports cardiovascular health, weight management, and independent living.

Nestlé
NutritionInstitute

Self MNA®
Mini Nutritional Assessment
For Adults 65 years of Age and Older

Last name: _____   First name: _____

Date: _____   Age: _____

Complete the screen by filling in the boxes with the appropriate numbers. Total the numbers for the final screening score.

Screening

A **Has your food intake declined over the past 3 months? [ENTER ONE NUMBER]**
Please enter the most appropriate number (0, 1, or 2) in the box to the right.

0 = severe decrease in food intake
1 = moderate decrease in food intake
2 = no decrease in food intake

☐

B **How much weight have you lost in the past 3 months? [ENTER ONE NUMBER]**
Please enter the most appropriate number (0, 1, 2, or 3) in the box to the right.

0 = weight loss greater than 7 pounds
1 = do not know the amount of weight lost
2 = weight loss between 2 and 7 pounds
3 = no weight loss or weight loss less than 2 pounds

☐

C **How would you describe your current mobility? [ENTER ONE NUMBER]**
Please enter the most appropriate number (0, 1, or 2) in the box to the right.

0 = unable to get out of a bed, a chair, or a wheelchair
     without the assistance of another person
1 = able to get out of a bed or a chair, but unable to go
     out of my home
2 = able to leave my home

☐

D **Have you been stressed or severely ill in the past 3 months? [ENTER ONE NUMBER]**
Please enter the most appropriate number (0 or 2) in the box to the right.

0 = yes
2 = no

☐

E **Are you currently experiencing dementia and/or prolonged severe sadness? [ENTER ONE NUMBER]**
Please enter the most appropriate number (0, 1, or 2) in the box to the right.

0 = yes, severe dementia and/or prolonged severe sadness
1 = yes, mild dementia, but no prolonged severe sadness
2 = neither dementia nor prolonged severe sadness

☐

Please total all of the numbers you entered in the boxes for questions A-E and write that number here: ☐

FIGURE 13-9 Self MNA® Mini Nutritional Assessment *For Adults 65 years of Age and Older.* The *SELF MNA® (Mini Nutritional Assessment)* is a checklist to identify those older individuals in the community who are at nutritional risk. Forms and updates can be accessed at www.mna-elderly.com. (Reprinted with the permission of the Société des Produits Nestlé S.A., Vevey, Switzerland, Copyright 2012 Nestlé. All rights reserved.)

Now, please CHOOSE ONE of the following two questions – F1 or F2 – to answer.

Question F1

Height (feet & inches)		Body Weight (pounds)		
4'10"	Less than 91	91-99	100-109	110 or more
4'11"	Less than 94	94-103	104-113	114 or more
5'0"	Less than 97	97-106	107-117	118 or more
5'1"	Less than 100	100-110	111-121	122 or more
5'2"	Less than 104	104-114	115-125	126 or more
5'3"	Less than 107	107-117	118-129	130 or more
5'4"	Less than 110	110-121	122-133	134 or more
5'5"	Less than 114	114-125	126-137	138 or more
5'6"	Less than 118	118-129	130-141	142 or more
5'7"	Less than 121	121-133	134-145	146 or more
5'8"	Less than 125	125-137	138-150	151 or more
5'9"	Less than 128	128-141	142-154	155 or more
5'10"	Less than 132	132-145	146-159	160 or more
5'11"	Less than 136	136-149	150-164	165 or more
6'0"	Less than 140	140-153	154-168	169 or more
6'1"	Less than 144	144-158	159-173	174 or more
6'2"	Less than 148	148-162	163-178	179 or more
6'3"	Less than 152	152-167	168-183	184 or more
6'4"	Less than 156	156-171	172-188	189 or more
Group	**0**	**1**	**2**	**3**

Please refer to the chart on the left and follow these instructions:

1. Find your height on the left-hand column of the chart.

2. Go across that row and circle the range that your weight falls into.

3. Look to the bottom of the chart to find what group number (0, 1, 2, or 3) your circled weight range falls into.

Write the Group Number (0, 1, 2, or 3) here: ☐

Write sum of questions A-E (from page 1) here: ☐

Lastly, calculate the sum of these 2 numbers: ☐

Question F2   DO NOT ANSWER QUESTION F2 IF QUESTION F1 IS ALREADY COMPLETED.

Measure the circumference of your LEFT calf by following the instructions below:

Loop a tape measure all the way around your calf to measure its size.

Record the measurement in inches: _____

If Less than 12 inches, enter "0" in box to the right.

If 12 inches or Greater, enter "3" in box to the right.

© SIGVARIS   ☐

Write the sum of questions A-E (from page 1) here: ☐

Lastly, calculate the sum of these 2 numbers: ☐

Screening Score 14 points maximum

12 – 14 points:	Normal nutritional status	
8 – 11 points:	At risk of malnutrition	☐
0 – 7 points:	Malnourished	

If you score between 0 - 11, please take this form to a healthcare professional for consultation.

FIGURE 13-9, cont'd

EVIDENCE-BASED PRACTICE

Can Age-Related Loss of Muscle Mass Be Prevented?

Define the problem: Loss of muscle mass can lead to disability and loss of independence. Decreases in muscle size and strength affect the older individual's ability to walk with confidence, carry groceries, or perform household chores. Muscle fiber atrophy results from a sedentary lifestyle and is worsened by normal aging, reduced secretion of growth hormone and sex steroid hormones, and marginal protein intake. By age 70 muscle mass is half what it was at age 30, and muscle strength declines at an even faster rate. At one time it was assumed that muscle loss in older age was inevitable.

Review the evidence: Comparisons of muscle mass and muscle strength in young (age 26), middle-age (age 51), and older (age 71) men revealed that lifelong levels of strength training as well as age influence muscle gain or loss.[1] In each age-group those who participated in regular strength training had more muscle and lean body mass than those who were sedentary. In fact, older men who engaged in regular strength training had greater muscle mass and muscle strength than did untrained men who were younger. Clinicians at the Human Research Center on Aging at Tufts University developed an intervention to test if strength training could replace muscle in frail older nursing home residents age 90 or older.[2] All who completed the 8-week intervention increased their muscle mass, but more importantly, improved their ability to carry out activities of daily living (ADLs). Those who, before going through the program, needed assistance to get up from a chair or walk across the room were able to carry out those actions without help after the program. Just 9 months of strength training increased total fat-free mass in these frail older adults. However, training must continue for gains to be retained. A protein-rich meal followed by a bout of strength training increases muscle protein synthesis to the same extent in older as in younger individuals.[3]

Implement the findings: Strength training has been confirmed as a means of helping older adults retain or regain muscle strength and muscle mass; however, participants need to obtain prior approval from their health care provider, and such programs should be supervised by a trained exercise physiologist. Inactive or frail older adults must begin slowly to avoid injury. Sufficient protein is needed for muscle-building to occur, with a dietary goal of 1.0 to 1.5 g/kg body weight. A meal containing 25 to 30 g of protein after the exercise workout supports protein synthesis.[4] (A sample meal providing 25 g of protein would include one cup of reduced-fat or skim milk, a sandwich including two ounces of turkey, 2 ounces of tuna fish or two eggs, and 1 cup of baby carrots.) Community centers often offer supervised strength training programs for older adults. Guides and DVDs for beginning an exercise program are available free from the National Institute on Aging at http://go4life.nia.nih.gov/exercise-guide-video.

References

1. Sallinen J, Ojanen T, Karavirta L, et al: Muscle mass and strength, body composition and dietary intake in master strength athletes vs untrained men of different ages. *J Sports Med Phys Fitness* 48:190, 2008.
2. Fiatarone MA, Marks EC, Ryan ND, et al: High intensity strength training in nonagenarians: effects on skeletal muscle. *JAMA* 263:3029, 1990.
3. Symons TB, Sheffield-Moore M, Mamerow MM, et al: The anabolic response to resistance exercise and a protein-rich meal is not diminished by age. *J Nutr Health Aging* 15(5):376, 2011.
4. Evans WJ, Boccardi V, Paolisso G: Perspective: dietary protein needs of elderly people: protein supplementation as an effective strategy to counteract sarcopenia. *J Am Med Dir Assoc* 14(1):67, 2013.

2. *Resistance exercise:* Strength training (or *resistance training,* as it is sometimes called) is a form of exercise in which the individual pushes against or lifts a set weight. This brings about an increase in size and strength of muscle fibers, adding to the ability to perform household tasks. (The Evidence-Based Practice box, "Can Age-Related Loss of Muscle Mass Be Prevented?" examines the benefits of strength training in preventing muscle loss.) (All types of physical activity and related nutritional needs are discussed in Chapter 14.)

TO SUM UP

Nutrient needs throughout adult life respond to the ebb and flow of continuing maturation and gradual decline. In young adults nutrients support the physical body that has reached its full potential and build reserves for active living. Lifestyle patterns formed by young adults often continue throughout life, and sedentary living and unwanted weight gain are concerns. Middle age begins the period of physical decline, although changes occur slowly at the onset. Losses of muscle and bone mass influence functional capacity and threaten independent living in later years if allowed to continue unchecked. Attention to protein, calcium, and vitamin D, along with participation in endurance and resistance exercise, slows these processes. Patterns of healthy eating, regular physical activity, and avoidance of smoking or other addictive behaviors, established early in life, support successful aging and the delay of degenerative changes. Nutrient needs in advanced age are influenced by changes in body composition, organ function, and chronic disease, and often complicated by associated malnutrition and weight loss. Physical disability, poverty, chewing or swallowing problems, isolation and depression, and multiple medications lower food intake and add to nutritional risk. The Self MNA® form offers a tool to identify at-risk older adults and educate individuals and communities in preventive care.

QUESTIONS FOR REVIEW

1. Select one of the adult age-groups, and describe its physical characteristics, psychosocial development, socioeconomic status, and nutritional needs. What do you see as the most urgent topic for health promotion in this age-group? Why?

2. You are working with a 32-year-old man who lives alone. He has a demanding job with no time to exercise and eats fast-food most of the time. He has gained 15 lb over the past 2 years and is concerned about his overall health. What questions should you ask before making any diet or lifestyle recommendations? What diet and lifestyle recommendations might be compatible with his general lifestyle?

3. You are working with a middle-age adult who is overweight, sedentary, and eats mostly meat, bread, potatoes, and desserts. Does this person represent normal aging or successful aging? How would you approach this individual about his health and what suggestions would you have for improvement?

4. What is meant by the aging process? Describe how physiologic changes occurring in advanced age might influence food intake or nutritional status.

5. Discuss the economic status, ethnic and racial composition, and living arrangements of the aging population. How might these factors influence the older adult's diet or health status? What are the implications for health and support services? Describe the individual in this age-group that you would consider to be at greatest risk. Why did you choose him or her?

6. Interview a family member, neighbor, or friend who is over age 65. What are some changes in health, living arrangements, or employment/retirement that have influenced his or her lifestyle over the past 10 years? How have these changes affected his or her eating habits?

7. You are helping a 75-year-old retired couple on a limited income with their diet. Both appear to be underweight, and you suspect that their food supplies are limited. Using the USDA Food Pattern develop a 3-day menu of meals and snacks that will supply each food group in the appropriate amounts for their age, gender, and activity level. How might you increase their energy intake and still remain within the suggested ranges for the three macronutrients? (USDA Food Patterns and Calorie Recommendations can be accessed at http://www.cnpp.usda.gov/USDAFoodPatterns.htm.)

8. Distinguish between the terms *gerontology* and *geriatrics.* Go to your school library and find the *Journal of Gerontology* and the *Journal of the American Geriatrics Society.* Look for an article in each journal that discusses a nutrition problem or nutrition-related disease in older adults. Compare the articles as to the type of information presented and how they might be used.

9. Identify a food-related program for older adults in your community and interview the director to determine (a) the target audience, (b) the types and amounts of food provided, (c) any major problems associated with implementation of the program, and (d) the major successes of the program. If possible, administer the Self MNA® (Mini Nutritional Assessment) checklist to some of the participants. How would you characterize their nutritional risk?

10. Visit your local drugstore and review the liquid supplements marketed to older adults. Make a table describing four different liquid meal supplements listing (a) the cost and (b) the amounts of kcalories, protein, calcium, vitamin D, vitamin B_6, vitamin B_{12}, and folate per 1-cup serving. Using the nutrient analysis program on the Evolve website that accompanies your textbook, select a fortified cereal that would be eaten with 1 cup of milk. Compare the cost, kcalories, and designated nutrients in a 1-cup serving of the liquid supplement with the usual serving of the cereal with 1 cup of milk. Based on your findings, what would you recommend as an evening snack? Explain.

REFERENCES

1. Institute of Medicine, Woolf SH, Aron L, editors: *U.S. health in international perspective: shorter lives, poorer health,* Washington, D.C., 2013, National Academy Press.

2. Goody CM, Drago L, editors: *Cultural food practices,* Chicago, 2010, Diabetes Care and Education Dietetic Practice Group, American Dietetic Association.

3. Centers for Disease Control and Prevention: QuickStats: percentage of adults aged ≥18 years who often felt worried, nervous, or anxious, by sex and age group—National Health Interview Survey, United States, 2010-2011. *MMWR* 62(10):197, 2013.

4. Strine TW, Chapman DP, Balluz LS, et al: The associations between life satisfaction and health-related quality of life, chronic illness, and health behaviors among U.S. community-dwelling adults. *J Community Health* 33:40, 2008.

5. Food and Nutrition Board, Institute of Medicine: *Dietary Reference Intakes for energy, carbohydrate, fiber, fat, fatty acids, cholesterol, protein, and amino acids (macronutrients),* Washington, D.C., 2002, National Academies Press.

6. U.S. Department of Agriculture, Agricultural Research Service: Table 1. Nutrient Intakes from Food: Mean Amounts Consumed per Individual, by Gender and Age, in the United States, 2009-2010, What We Eat in America, NHANES 2009-2010. 2012. at: <http://www.ars.usda.gov/SP2UserFiles/Place/12355000/pdf/0910/Table_1_NIN_GEN_09.pdf>. Accessed on April 13, 2013.

7. Food and Nutrition Board, Institute of Medicine: *Dietary Reference Intakes for calcium and vitamin D,* Washington, D.C., 2011, National Academies Press.

8. U.S. Department of Health and Human Services, U.S. Department of Agriculture: *Report of the Dietary Guidelines Advisory Committee on the Dietary Guidelines for Americans*

2010, Washington, D.C., 2010, Center for Nutrition Policy and Promotion, U.S. Department of Agriculture. from: <http://www.cnpp.usda.gov/DGAs2010-DGACReport.htm>. Retrieved November 12, 2012.

9. Food and Nutrition Board, Institute of Medicine: *Dietary Reference Intakes for vitamin A, vitamin K, arsenic, boron, chromium, copper, iodine, iron, manganese, molybdenum, nickel, silicon, vanadium, and zinc*, Washington, D.C., 2001, National Academies Press.

10. Food and Nutrition Board, Institute of Medicine: *Dietary Reference Intakes for water, potassium, sodium, chloride, and sulfate*, Washington, D.C., 2004, National Academies Press.

11. Larson NI, Nelson MC, Neumark-Sztainer D, et al: Making time for meals: meal structure and associations with dietary intake in young adults. *J Am Diet Assoc* 109:72, 2009.

12. Larson N, Neumark-Sztainer D, Laska MN, et al: Young adults and eating away from home: associations with dietary intake patterns and weight status differ by choice of restaurant. *J Am Diet Assoc* 111:1696, 2011.

13. Larson N, Fulkerson J, Story M, et al: Shared meals among young adults are associated with better diet quality and predicted by family meal patterns during adolescence. *Public Health Nutr* 16(5):883, 2013.

14. Escoto KH, Laska MN, Larson N, et al: Work hours and perceived time barrier to healthful eating among young adults. *Am J Health Behav* 36(6):786, 2012.

15. National Center for Health Statistics: *Health, United States, 2008 with chartbook on the health of young adults*, DHHS Publication No 2009-1232, Hyattsville, Md., 2009, U.S. Government Printing Office.

16. Ogden CL, Carroll MD, Kit BK, et al: *Prevalence of obesity in the United States, 2009-2010, NCHS Data Brief No 82*, Atlanta, Ga., 2012, U.S. Department of Health and Human Services, Centers for Disease Control and Prevention.

17. Merten MJ: Weight status continuity and change from adolescence to young adulthood: examining disease and health risk conditions. *Obesity (Silver Spring)* 18(7):1423, 2010.

18. Burke V, Beilin LJ, Dunbar D, et al: Changes in health-related behaviours and cardiovascular risk factors in young adults: associations with living with a partner. *Prev Med* 39(4):722, 2004.

19. Berge JM, MacLehose R, Eisenberg ME, et al: How significant is the 'significant other'? Associations between significant others' health behaviors and attitudes and young adults' health outcomes. *Int J Behav Nutr Phy Act* 9:35, 2012.

20. Yoo S, Nicklas T, Baranowski T, et al: Comparison of dietary intakes associated with metabolic syndrome risk factors in young adults: the Bogalusa Heart Study. *Am J Clin Nutr* 80:841, 2004.

21. Deshmukh-Taskar P, Nicklas TA, Radcliffe JD, et al: The relationship of breakfast skipping and type of breakfast consumed with overweight/obesity, abdominal obesity, other cardiometabolic risk factors and the metabolic syndrome in young adults. The National Health and Nutrition Examination Survey (NHANES); 1999-2006. *Public Health Nutr* 3:1, 2012.

22. Deshmukh-Taskar P, Radcliffe JD, Liu Y, et al: Do breakfast skipping and breakfast type affect energy intake, nutrient intake, nutrient adequacy and diet quality in young adults? NHANES 1999-2002. *J Am Coll Nutr* 29(4):407, 2010.

23. Paddon-Jones D, Rasmussen BB: Dietary protein recommendations and the prevention of sarcopenia. *Curr Opin Clin Nutr Metab Care* 12(1):86, 2009.

24. Hall KD, Heymsfield SB, Kemnitz JW, et al: Energy balance and its components: implications for body weight regulation. *Am J Clin Nutr* 95:989, 2012.

25. Ekelund U, Brage S, Besson H, et al: Time spent being sedentary and weight gain in healthy adults: reverse or bidirectional causality. *Am J Clin Nutr* 88:612, 2008.

26. Moschonis G, Katsaroli I, Lyritis GP, et al: The effects of a 30-month dietary intervention on bone mineral density: The Postmenopausal Health Study. *Br J Nutr* 104:100, 2010.

27. Dawson-Hughes B: Commentary: a revised clinician's guide to the prevention and treatment of osteoporosis. *J Clin Endocrinol Metab* 93(7):2463, 2008.

28. Moshfegh A, Goldman J, Ahuja J, et al: *What We Eat in America, NHANES 2005-2006: Usual Nutrient Intakes from Food and Water Compared to 1997 Dietary Reference Intakes for Vitamin D, Calcium, Phosphorus, and Magnesium*, Washington, D.C., 2009, U.S. Department of Agriculture, Agricultural Research Service.

29. Looker AC, Pfeiffer CM, Lacher DA, et al: Serum 25-hydroxyvitamin D status of the U.S. population: 1988-1994 compared with 2000-2004. *Am J Clin Nutr* 88:1519, 2008.

30. Food and Nutrition Board, Institute of Medicine: *Dietary Reference Intakes for thiamin, riboflavin, niacin, vitamin B-6, folate, vitamin B-12, pantothenic acid, biotin, and choline*, Washington, D.C., 1998, National Academies Press.

31. Fulkerson JA, Farbakhsh K, Lytle L, et al: Away-from-home family dinner sources and associations with weight status, body composition, and related biomarkers of chronic disease among adolescents and their parents. *J Am Diet Assoc* 111:1892, 2011.

32. Ogden CL, Kit BK, Carroll MD, et al: *Consumption of sugar drinks in the United States, 2005-2008, NCHS Data Brief No 71*, Atlanta, Ga., 2011, U.S. Department of Health and Human Services, Centers for Disease Control and Prevention.

33. Breslow RA, Chen CM, Graubard BI, et al: Diets of drinkers on drinking and nondrinking days: NHANES 2003-2008. *Am J Clin Nutr* 97:1068, 2013.

34. Hiza HA, Casavale KO, Guenther PM, et al: Diet quality of Americans differs by age, sex, race/ethnicity, income, and education level. *J Acad Nutr Diet* 113(2):297, 2013.

35. Radimer K, Bindewald B, Hughes J, et al: Dietary supplement use by U.S. adults: data from the National Health and Nutrition Examination Survey, 1999-2000. *Am J Epidemiol* 160:339, 2004.

36. Bailey RL, Fulgoni VL, Keast DR, et al: Examination of vitamin intakes among US adults by dietary supplement use. *J Acad Nutr Diet* 112:657, 2012.

37. van Eenwyk J, Bensley L, Ossiander EM, et al: Comparison of examination-based and self-reported risk factors for cardiovascular disease, Washington State, 2006-2007. *Prev Chron Dis* 9:E117, 2012.

38. Wang H, Steffen LM, Jacobs DR, et al: Trends in cardiovascular risk factor levels in the Minnesota Heart Survey (1980-2002) as compared with the National Health and Nutrition Examination Survey (1976-2002): a partial explanation for Minnesota's low cardiovascular disease mortality. *Am J Epidemiol* 173:526, 2011.

39. Koopman RJ, Mainous AG 3rd, Diaz VA, et al: Changes in age at diagnosis of type 2 diabetes mellitus in the United States, 1988 to 2000. *Ann Fam Med* 3:60, 2005.

40. Federal Interagency Forum on Aging-Related Statistics: *Older Americans 2012: key indicators of well-being*, Washington, D.C., 2012, U.S. Government Printing Office.

41. U.S. Department of Health and Human Services: *A profile of older Americans, 2011: living arrangements*, Washington, D.C., 2012, Administration on Aging. at: <http://www.aoa.gov/AoARoot/Aging_Statistics/Profile/2011/6.aspx>. Accessed on April 12, 2013.

42. Hughes VA, Roubenoff R, Wood M, et al: Anthropometric assessment of 10-y changes in body composition in the elderly. *Am J Clin Nutr* 80:475, 2004.

43. St-Onge MP, Gallagher D: Body composition changes with aging: the cause or the result of alterations in metabolic rate and macronutrient oxidation. *Nutrition* 26(2):152, 2010.

44. Li Z, Heber D: Sarcopenic obesity in the elderly and strategies for weight management. *Nutr Reviews* 70(1):57, 2011.

45. Pi-Sunyer FX: The epidemiology of central fat distribution in relation to disease. *Nutr Rev* 62(7 Pt 2):S120, 2004.

46. American Dietetic Association: Practice paper of the American Dietetic Association: individualized nutrition approaches for older adults in health care communities. *J Am Diet Assoc* 110:1554, 2010.

47. Kane RL, Ouslander JG, Abrass IB: *Essentials of clinical geriatrics*, ed 5, New York, 2004, McGraw-Hill.

48. Blanc S, Schoeller DA, Bauer D, et al: Energy requirements in the eighth decade of life. *Am J Clin Nutr* 79:303, 2004.

49. Paddon-Jones D, Short KR, Campbell WW, et al: Role of dietary protein in the sarcopenia of aging. *Am J Clin Nutr* 87(Suppl):1562S, 2008.

50. Campbell WW, Leidy HJ: Dietary protein and resistance training effects on muscle and body composition in older persons. *J Am Coll Nutr* 26:696S, 2007.

51. Volpi E, Campbell WW, Dwyer JT, et al: Is the optimal level of protein intake for older adults greater than the recommended dietary allowance? *J Gerontol A Biol Sci Med Sci* 68(6):677, 2013.

52. Chernoff R: Protein and older adults. *J Am Coll Nutr* 23(Suppl 6):627S, 2004.

53. Murphy SP, Wilkens LR, Monroe KR, et al: Dietary supplement use within a multiethnic population as measured by a unique inventory method. *J Am Diet Assoc* 111:1065, 2011.

54. Academy of Nutrition and Dietetics: Position of the Academy of Nutrition and Dietetics: food and nutrition for older adults: promoting health and wellness. *J Acad Nutr Diet* 112:1255, 2012.

55. Ferry M: Strategies for ensuring good hydration in the elderly. *Nutr Rev* 63(6 Pt 2):S22, 2005.

56. Ervin RB: *Healthy eating index scores among adults, 60 years of age and over, by sociodemographic and health characteristics: United States, 1999-2002. Advance Data, Publication No 395*, Washington, D.C., 2008, U.S. Department of Health and Human Services.

57. Wickrama KA, Ralston PA, O'Neal CW, et al: Life dissatisfaction and eating behaviors among older African Americans: the protective role of social support. *J Nutr Health Aging* 16(9):749, 2012.

58. Payne ME, Steck SE, George RR, et al: Fruit, vegetable, and antioxidant intakes are lower in older adults with depression. *J Acad Nutr Diet* 112:2022, 2012.

59. Hughes G, Bennett KM, Hetherington MM: Old and alone: barriers to healthy eating in older men living on their own. *Appetite* 43:269, 2004.

60. Hsiao PY, Mitchell DC, Coffman DL, et al: Dietary patterns and diet quality among diverse older adults: the University of Alabama at Birmingham study of aging. *J Nutr Health Aging* 17(1):19, 2013.

61. Racine EF, Lyerly J, Troyer JL, et al: The influence of home-delivered Dietary Approaches to Stop Hypertension meals on body mass index, energy intake, and percent of energy needs consumed among older adults with hypertension and/or hyperlipidemia. *J Acad Nutr Diet* 112:1755, 2012.

62. Sharkey JP: Longitudinal examination of homebound older adults who experience heightened food insufficiency: effect of diabetes status and implications for service provision. *Gerontologist* 45:773, 2005.

63. Martinsen B, Harder I, Biering-Sorensen F: Sensitive cooperation: a basis for assisted feeding. *J Clin Nurs* 18(5):708, 2009.

64. Bowman SA: Socioeconomic characteristics, dietary and lifestyle patterns, and health and weight status of older adults in NHANES, 1999-2002: a comparison of Caucasians and African Americans. *J Nutr Elder* 28:30, 2009.

65. Bermudez OI, Falcon LM, Tucker KL: Intake and food sources of macronutrients among older Hispanic adults: association with ethnicity, acculturation, and length of residence in the United States. *J Am Diet Assoc* 100:665, 2000.

66. Dennis RA, Johnson LE, Roberson PK, et al: Changes in activities of daily living, nutrient intake, and systemic inflammation in elderly adults receiving recuperative care. *J Am Geriatr Soc* 60:2246, 2012.

67. Roberts SB, Rosenberg I: Nutrition and aging: changes in the regulation of energy metabolism with aging. *Physiol Rev* 86:651, 2006.

68. Sharkey JR: Diet and health outcomes in vulnerable populations. *Ann N Y Acad Sci* 1136:210, 2008.

69. American Dietetic Association: Position of the American Dietetic Association: individualized nutrition approaches for older adults in health care communities. *J Am Diet Assoc* 110:1549, 2010.

70. White JV, Guenter P, Jensen G, et al: Consensus statement of the Academy of Nutrition and Dietetics/American Society for Parenteral and Enteral Nutrition: characteristics recommended for the identification and documentation of adult malnutrition (undernutrition). *J Acad Nutr Diet* 112:730, 2012.

71. Berner LA, Becker G, Wise M, et al: Characterization of dietary protein among older adults in the United States: amount, animal sources, and meal patterns. *J Acad Nutr Diet* 113(6):2013.

72. Flegal KM, Graubard BI, Williamson DF, et al: Excess deaths associated with underweight, overweight, and obesity. *JAMA* 293:1861, 2005.

73. Thomas DR, Ashmen W, Morley JE, et al: Nutritional management in long-term care: development of a clinical guideline. *J Gerontol A Biol Sci Med Sci* 55A(12):M725, 2000.

74. Chau D, Cho LM, Jani P, et al: Individualizing recommendations for weight management in the elderly. *Curr Opin Clin Nutr Metab Care* 11(1):27, 2008.

75. Rocchiccioli JT, Sanford JT: Revisiting geriatric failure to thrive: a complex and compelling clinical condition. *J Gerontol Nurs* 35:18, 2009.

76. Evans WJ, Morley JE, Argiles J, et al: Cachexia: a new definition. *Clin Nutr* 27:793, 2008.

77. Huhmann MB, Perez V, Alexander DD, et al: A self-completed nutrition screening tool for community-dwelling older adults with high reliability: a comparison study. *J Nutr Health Aging* 17(4):339, 2013.

78. U.S. Bureau of Census: Census Bureau releases comprehensive analysis of fast-growing 90-and-older population, Newsroom release, November 17. 2011. at: <http://www.census.gov/newsroom/releases/pdf/cb11-194_fig2.pdf>. Accessed on April 15, 2013.

79. Akbaraly T, Sabia S, Haggar-Johnson G, et al: Does overall diet in midlife predict future aging phenotypes? A cohort study. *Am J Med* 126(5):411, 2013.

80. Winkleby MA, Cubbin C: Changing patterns in health behaviors and risk factors related to chronic diseases, 1990-2000. *Am J Health Promot* 19(1):159, 2004.

81. Bailey RL, Gahche JJ, Miller PE, et al: Why US adults use dietary supplements. *JAMA Intern Med* 173(5):355, 2013.

82. Roberts SB, Hajduk CL, Howarth NC, et al: Dietary variety predicts low body mass index and inadequate macronutrient and micronutrient intakes in community-dwelling older adults. *J Gerontol A Biol Sci Med Sci* 60A:613, 2005.

83. Diehr P, O'Meara ES, Fitzpatrick A, et al: Weight, mortality, years of healthy life, and active life expectancy in older adults. *J Am Geriatr Soc* 56:76, 2008.

FURTHER READINGS AND RESOURCES

Readings

American Dietetic Association: Food and nutrition programs for community-residing older adults: position of the American Dietetic Association, the American Society for Nutrition, and the Society for Nutrition Education. *J Am Diet Assoc* 110:463, 2010.

Anyanwu UO, Sharkey JR, Jackson RT, et al: Home food environment of older adults transitioning from hospital to home. *J Nutr Gerontol Geriatr* 30(2):105, 2011.

Bailey RL, Gahche JJ, Miller PE, et al: Why US adults use dietary supplements. *JAMA Intern Med* 173(5):355, 2013.

Rocchiccioli JT, Sanford JT: Revisiting geriatric failure to thrive: a complex and compelling clinical condition. *J Gerontol Nurs* 35:18, 2009.

[These researchers address problems of food availability and intake and potential interventions in older adults.]

Berge JM, MacLehose R, Eisenberg ME, et al: How significant is the 'significant other'? Associations between significant others' health behaviors and attitudes and young adults' health outcomes. *Int J Behav Nutr Phy Act* 9:35, 2012.

Cluskey M, Grobe D: College weight gain and behavior transitions: male and female differences. *J Am Diet Assoc* 109:325, 2009.

Escoto KH, Laska MN, Larson N, et al: Work hours and perceived time barrier to healthful eating among young adults. *Am J Health Behav* 36(6):786, 2012.

[These articles address lifestyle issues that contribute to the food patterns and long-term health of young adults.]

Breslow RA, Guenther MM, Juan W, et al: Alcoholic beverage consumption, nutrient intakes, and diet quality in the US adult population, 1999-2006. *J Am Diet Assoc* 110:551, 2010.

Li F, Harmer P, Cardinal BJ, et al: Built environment and changes in blood pressure in middle aged and older adults. *Prev Med* 48:237, 2009.

[Excessive alcohol intake and physical inactivity are lifestyle practices that influence long-term health. These articles suggest the extent of these problems and how they might be addressed.]

Hiza HA, Casavale KO, Guenther PM, et al: Diet quality of Americans differs by age, sex, race/ethnicity, income, and education level. *J Acad Nutr Diet* 113(2):297, 2013.

[These authors address various socioeconomic and demographic factors that influence food intake in adults.]

Websites of Interest

- Administration on Aging (AoA). This site describes many programs and health-related materials to assist older adults: www.aoa.gov/.
- National Institutes of Health (NIH). The NIH Health Information site contains materials on healthy lifestyles and specific diseases; individual locations focus on teens, men, and women's health: http://health.nih.gov/.
- National Institute on Aging (NIA). This site includes updates on aging research along with materials and resources available to older adults and their families: www.nia.nih.gov.
- USA.gov—Senior Citizens' Resources. This site includes many topics such as health, retirement, and grandparents raising grandchildren: www.usa.gov/Topics/Seniors.shtml.

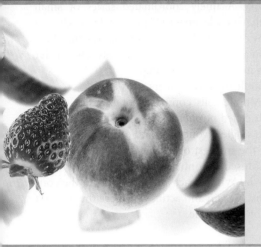

Nutrition and Physical Fitness

Staci Nix

"Good food choices will not make a mediocre athlete into a champion, but poor food choices may prevent the potential champion from realizing his/her potential."[1]

EVOLVE WEBSITE

http://evolve.elsevier.com/Williams/essentials/

Nutrition and physical fitness are integral to overall health, weight maintenance, and disease prevention. In an increasingly fast-paced and technology-dependent society, making regular physical activity part of a busy life requires commitment. Physical fitness is a vital cornerstone in the preventive approach to controlling chronic disease in modern civilization.

We examine first how nutrition provides energy for muscle action; then we apply principles to enhancing fitness and athletic performance by building a reasonable and appropriate personal exercise program for the adult.

PHYSICAL ACTIVITY, MODERN CIVILIZATION, AND CHRONIC DISEASE

Physical Fitness and Health

The Centers for Disease Control and Prevention (CDC) defines *physical activity* as any bodily movement produced by the contraction of skeletal muscles that increases energy expenditure above a basal level.[2] Examples of physical activity would be walking or riding a bike as a form of transportation, using the stairs instead of the escalator, or manual labor such as carpentry work, gardening, or farming. Physical activity differs from *exercise* based on the structure and purpose. *Exercise* is a subcategory of physical activity that is planned, structured, repetitive, and purposive in the sense that the improvement or maintenance of one or more components of physical fitness is the objective.[2] People engage in exercise for the purpose of training, competing, and keeping organs and bodily functions healthy. Examples of exercise include aerobic classes, jogging, running, swimming, cycling, weight training, tennis, and other such bouts of planned activities with the intension of improving overall physical fitness.

Physical fitness is defined by the CDC as the ability to carry out daily tasks with vigor and alertness, without undue fatigue, and with ample energy to enjoy leisure-time pursuits and respond to emergencies. Physical fitness includes a number of components consisting of cardiorespiratory endurance (aerobic power), skeletal muscle endurance, skeletal muscle strength, skeletal muscle power, flexibility, balance, speed of movement, reaction time, and body composition.[2]

Physical inactivity is a global health problem and is estimated by the World Health Organization (WHO) to contribute to 3.2 million deaths annually. There are only three risk factors for mortality with a higher prevalence worldwide: high blood pressure, tobacco use, and high blood glucose.[3]

Increased participation in regular physical activity as a part of everyday life remains a national health goal. The U.S. Department of Health and Human Services (USDHHS), in its report *Healthy People 2020* has set health-related goals for Americans in nutrition and physical fitness. The 2020 target is to reduce the percentage of adults who do not engage in any leisure-time physical activity to 32.6% or less. Current progress reports indicate that only 43.5% of adults meet the minimum recommendation of aerobic physical activity and muscle-strengthening activity on a regular basis.[4] All *Healthy People 2020* objectives are available at www.healthypeople.gov/2020/.

Health promotion, disease prevention, and disease management require attention to the related roles of nutrition and physical fitness. The U.S. Department of Agriculture (USDA) has published national dietary guidelines every 5 years since 1980. Starting with the *Dietary Guidelines for Americans 2000*,[5] a category titled "Aim for Fitness" was added. These guidelines encourage all people to practice healthy eating choices, to be physically active each day, and to aim for a healthy weight. The 2010 *Dietary Guidelines* encourage Americans to prevent and/or reduce overweight and obesity through improved eating and physical activity and to increase physical activity and reduce time spent in sedentary behaviors.[6]

Modern Developed Nations and Chronic Disease

Over time and many generations, daily life in developed nations has evolved from agriculture-based societies requiring constant physical exertion to a more sedentary standard of living. Poor nutrition and inactivity contribute to a host of illnesses, the so-called diseases of civilization, including cardiovascular disease, type 2 diabetes, metabolic syndrome, and some forms of cancer. Substantial research supports both the preventive and therapeutic roles of a healthy diet and physical activity on such chronic diseases.[7-9]

BODY IN MOTION

Nature of Energy

The term *energy* refers to the body's ability, or power, to do work. The energy required to do work takes several different forms: mechanical, chemical, electrical, radiant, and heat. Energy, like matter, can neither be created nor destroyed. It can only be changed into another form; therefore, energy is constantly cycled in the body and environment. We also speak of energy as being potential or kinetic. Potential energy is stored energy, ready to be used. Kinetic energy is active energy, being used to do work. Energy balance in physical activity requires appropriate nutrition to supply the substrate fuels, which along with oxygen and water, meet widely varying levels of energy demands for body action.

Muscle Physiology
Muscle Structure

The synchronized action of millions of specialized cells that make up our skeletal muscle mass makes possible all forms of physical activity. A finely coordinated series of small bundles within the muscle fibers (Figure 14-1) produce a smooth symphony of action through simultaneous and alternating contraction and relaxation. These successively smaller muscle structures include the following:

- *Fasciculi:* A bundle of muscle fibers.
- *Muscle fiber:* Muscle cells composed of bundles of still smaller strands called *myofibrils.*
- *Myofibril:* Each single myofibril strand of the muscle fiber is made up of the smallest of all the fiber bundles, called *myofilaments.* Muscular contraction occurs here.
- *Myosin* and *actin:* Within each myofilament are the contractile proteins, myosin and actin, which are the smallest moving parts of the muscle.

Muscle Action

Inside the muscle fiber, structures run the length of the cell that are called *myofibrils.* Myofibrils contain the contractile proteins, myosin and actin, which interact in the presence of calcium to shorten the cell (and the muscle). The muscle shortens to cause movement in different directions at the joint. When the calcium is pumped out of the surrounding fluid, the cell then relaxes to return the muscle elastically to its resting length. This alternating process of muscle contraction and relaxation can continue until muscle glycogen is depleted and muscle fatigue occurs.

Fuel Sources

Fuel sources at rest are a mix of carbohydrate and fat. During exercise, carbohydrate is the primary fuel, and with longer aerobic bouts, some fat is used. A fuel of last resort is protein, which is only used when the other fuels are exhausted. The high-energy compound driving body cells is adenosine triphosphate (ATP), the energy currency of the cell. Various forms of energy are called on for successive energy needs:

- *Immediate energy:* High-power or immediate energy demands over a short time depend on ATP being readily available within the muscle tissue. This amount is used rapidly, and a backup compound, creatine phosphate (CP), is made available. These high-energy compounds, however, will sustain exercise for only 5 to 8 seconds.
- *Short-term energy:* For anaerobic bursts like sprints and weight lifting (between 30 seconds and 2 minutes), muscle glycogen provides the only available fuel source through the lactate pathway. Although the amount of available glycogen is small, it is an important rapid source of energy for brief muscular effort.
- *Long-term energy:* Exercise continuing more than 2 minutes requires an oxygen-dependent, or aerobic, energy system. A constant supply of oxygen in the blood is necessary for continued exercise. The mitochondria, which are organelles within the cell, produce large amounts of ATP. The ATP is produced mainly from glucose and fatty acids and supplies the continued energy needs of the body (Figure 14-2).

Exercise intensity will also affect the preferred source of fuel for the active muscles. More sustained, low-intensity

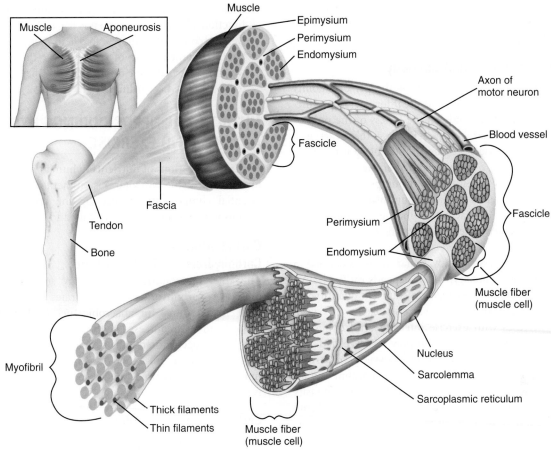

FIGURE 14-1 Skeletal muscle, showing the progressively smaller bundles within bundles. (From Thibodeau GA, Patton KT: *Anatomy & physiology,* ed 5, St Louis, Mo, 2003, Mosby.)

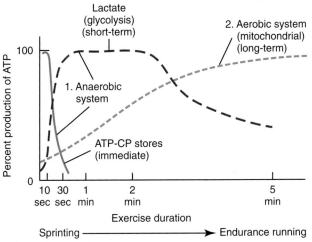

FIGURE 14-2 Contribution of the two energy systems during exercise of increasing duration. The anaerobic energy system provides adenosine triphosphate (ATP) to the working myofilaments from ATP–creatine phosphate (CP) stores and the lactate or glycolytic path. The aerobic system supplies ATP from mitochondria, which require oxygen to burn carbohydrates and fats. (Redrawn from Nieman DC: *Exercise testing and prescription,* ed 5, Boston, 2003, McGraw-Hill.)

TABLE 14-1	EFFECT OF INTENSITY ON FUEL TYPE
EXERCISE INTENSITY	**FUEL USED BY MUSCLE**
<30% VO₂max (easy walking)	Carbohydrates at first, then largely muscle fat stores with durations over 30 min
40%-60% VO₂max (jogging, brisk walking)	Fat and carbohydrate used evenly
75% VO₂max (running)	Mainly carbohydrate
≥80% VO₂max (sprinting)	Nearly 100% carbohydrate

exercises rely primarily on muscle fat stores for energy through the aerobic pathway. As intensity increases the source of energy gradually shifts to carbohydrates and makes more use of the lactate system (Table 14-1).

Nutrients become depleted during continued exercise as the body draws on its stored energy. As demands for ATP increase, the body metabolizes blood glucose and muscle glycogen to provide energy via anaerobic glycolysis. With prolonged exercise of increased intensity, however, the levels of these nutrients fall too low to sustain the body's demands. Without a resupply of nutrients, fatigue follows, and exercise cannot continue.

Oxygen Use and Physical Capacity

The most profound limit to exercise is the person's ability to deliver oxygen to the tissues and use it for energy production. This vital ability depends on the fitness of the pulmonary and cardiovascular systems. Because the heart is a muscle, aerobic exercise strengthens it, enabling it to pump more blood per beat, a capacity called *stroke volume*. The cardiac output—how much the heart pumps out in a given period of time—depends on the amount of blood per contraction and on the cardiac rate, which is the number of contractions in a given time. The following factors are influential in fitness level:

- *Cardiovascular fitness:* Cardiovascular fitness is defined in terms of aerobic capacity, which depends on the body's ability to deliver and use oxygen in sufficient quantities to meet the demands of increasing levels of exercise. Oxygen uptake increases with exercise intensity until either the demand is met or the ability to supply it is exceeded. The maximum rate the body can take in oxygen, or aerobic capacity, is called the VO_2max—the maximum uptake volume of oxygen. This capacity determines the intensity and duration of exercise that a person can perform. From the resting level, a steep rise in oxygen consumption occurs during the first 3 minutes of exercise. After approximately 6 minutes the rate levels off into a steady state, indicating equilibrium between the energy required by the exercising muscles and the aerobic energy-producing system. The aerobic capacity of an individual is measured in terms of milliliters of oxygen consumed per kilogram of body weight per minute. Thus people of differing sizes can be compared equally.
- *Genetic influence:* A person's aerobic capacity is largely determined by their genetic propensity for exercise response.[10] In other words, physiologic gains and cardiovascular adaptation from the same exercise program will vary among individuals based on their specific genetics.
- *Age:* Before puberty, lean body mass is about equal in boys and girls of comparable body size, but it increases rapidly in boys at puberty under the anabolic effect of testosterone. Maximal aerobic capacity declines gradually with age, largely as a result of age-related losses in lean body mass.
- *Body composition and gender:* Gender differences in aerobic capacity reflect differences in body composition. In general, men have a higher aerobic capacity because of their larger lean body mass, the active metabolic body tissue. These highly metabolic tissues of the body use more oxygen than other tissues such as fat. When oxygen consumption is expressed only in terms of lean body mass instead of body weight, however, men and women have a similar aerobic capacity. In general, women carry more body fat, a gender difference in body composition that serves critical biologic functions (see Chapter 8). Apart

from stored adipose tissue fuel, essential structural and functional body fat in women is 8% to 12% of their body weight (compared with 3% to 5% in men).[11] In addition, because women must, of course, carry their entire body weight as part of their total workload, their performance will be affected accordingly.

NUTRITIONAL NEEDS DURING PHYSICAL ACTIVITY AND EXERCISE

All six classifications of nutrients in human nutrition (carbohydrates, protein, fat, vitamins, minerals, and water) are essential components in meeting the body's energy and hydration needs for physical activity and exercise.

Carbohydrates
Carbohydrates as Fuel Substrate

The chief macronutrient for energy support throughout exercise is carbohydrate. Carbohydrates are the *only* available energy source for anaerobic fuel. Carbohydrate fuels come from two sources: (1) the circulating blood glucose and (2) glycogen stored in muscle and liver tissue. Liver glycogen contributes to blood glucose homeostasis, whereas muscle glycogen is used for the specific muscle in which it is stored.

Carbohydrates in the Diet

Carbohydrates are the preferred energy nutrient. Carbohydrate energy should contribute 45% to 65% of the kilocalories (kcalories or kcal) in the daily diet. Athletes competing in long endurance events should increase their energy from carbohydrates to 60% to 70% of their daily total (6 to 10 g/kg body weight).[12] Complex carbohydrates (starches) are preferable to simple carbohydrates (monosaccharides and disaccharides). Starches break down gradually and help maintain blood glucose levels more evenly (avoiding low blood glucose drops), as well as maintain glycogen storage as a constant primary fuel. Simple sugars, however, can supply important immediate energy, especially for endurance athletes requiring thousands of kcals during their events.

In prolonged bouts of intense exercise, studies have found that diets low in carbohydrate have proved to be less efficient at maintaining energy homeostasis and pace.[13,14] A low-carbohydrate diet decreases the body's capacity for work, which intensifies over time. Athletes on a low-carbohydrate diet are susceptible to fatigue, ketoacidosis, and dehydration. Conversely, a high-carbohydrate diet enhances muscle glycogen concentrations and exercise performance.[13] In addition, carbohydrate supplementation during exercise bouts improves whole-body carbohydrate oxidation and metabolic

---

KEY TERM

aerobic capacity Milliliters of oxygen consumed per kilogram of body weight per minute; influenced by body composition and fitness level.

TABLE 14-2	MODIFIED DEPLETION-TAPER PRECOMPETITION PROGRAM FOR GLYCOGEN LOADING	
DAY	**EXERCISE**	**DIET**
1	90-min period at 70%-75% VO$_2$max	Mixed diet, 50% carbohydrate (350 g)
2-3	Gradual tapering of time and intensity	Day 1 diet continued
4-5	Tapering of exercise time and intensity continues	Mixed diet, 70% carbohydrate (550 g)
6	Complete rest	Days 4 and 5 diet continued
7	Day of competition	High-carbohydrate pre-event diet

From Wright ED: Carbohydrate nutrition and exercise. *Clin Nutr* 7(1):18, 1988, with permission from Elsevier.

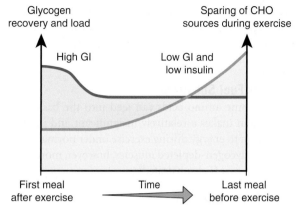

FIGURE 14-3 The relative value of high GI and low GI feedings in pursuing glycogen recovery and load or sparing of glucose sources and availability during exercise. (From Mondazzi L, Arcelli E: Glycemic index in sport nutrition. *J Am Coll Nutr* 28[Suppl]:455S–463S, 2009.)

efficiency.[15,16] Therefore athletes given carbohydrate feedings before and during exercise maintain glucose concentrations and rates of glucose oxidation necessary to exercise strenuously and delay fatigue.

Carbohydrate loading is a common practice among endurance athletes that is intended to encourage muscles to deposit maximum glycogen stores immediately before an endurance event for extra stored energy. The initial method of glycogen loading was a two-step procedure. First, athletes consumed a diet low in carbohydrates, while simultaneously exercising at high intensity; thus muscle glycogen stores were rapidly depleted. In the second step, athletes did just the opposite; they gradually decreased exercise intensity while consuming a diet high in carbohydrates (approximately 70% to 75% of total caloric intake). Table 14-2 illustrates the second phase of this procedure. Glycogen storage capacity and rates are higher after glycogen depletion; however, a substantial increase in glycogen storage will still occur without the stringent first step of this plan. The most recent paper outlining carbohydrate loading practices by Sedlock at Purdue University presents flexible strategies for the athlete to choose from to best fit their personal needs.[17] Because every gram of glycogen stored requires 2.7 mL of water, potential side effects may occur. Extra water weight in muscles may result in tight or sore muscles that could ultimately hinder performance. Athletes are encouraged to experiment with carbohydrate loading before their competitive events to ensure comfort and personal benefits.

The benefits of using the glycemic index (GI) (see Chapter 3) as a guide for choosing what types of carbohydrate foods to consume before, during, and after exercise is inconclusive. However, some researchers believe that there may be an advantage in choosing high-GI foods while muscle glycogen stores are recovering and then gradually moving to a diet of low-GI foods to spare glucose during long endurance events (Figure 14-3).[18]

Fat
Fat as Fuel Substrate
Fatty acids serve as a fuel source from dietary intake and adipose tissue. In the presence of oxygen, fatty acids are oxidized to provide energy. The rate at which this can occur is determined in part by the rate of mobilization of fatty acids from storage, but not all stored fat is alike. The body stores fat in two ways: (1) depot fat in adipose tissue, which is destined for transport back and forth to other tissues as needed for energy, and (2) essential fat in metabolically active tissue, such as bone marrow, heart, lungs, liver, spleen, kidneys, intestines, muscles, and nervous system, which is reserved in these places for necessary structural and functional use only. Although storage depot fat in men and women is roughly comparable, essential fat reserves are significantly different; they are about three times greater in women.

Fat in the Diet
Fat, as a fuel substrate, is drawn from the body's adipose tissue in response to increasing activity of the enzyme hormone-sensitive lipase (HSL). HSL activity rises as blood insulin levels decrease, allowing for the mobilization of fatty acids throughout the body. It is not necessary to specifically consume extra fat to maintain the body's adipose tissue, because excess kcalories from all macronutrients will be converted to fat and stored. On the other hand, a moderate level of fat is necessary in the diet for the absorption of fat-soluble vitamins and to ensure adequate intake of the essential fatty acids (linoleic and α-linolenic acids). An extremely low fat intake can be medically dangerous by creating a deficiency of the essential fatty acids. The standard recommendation that 20% to 35% of kcalories come from fat, per the Acceptable Macronutrient Distribution Range (AMDR), is ample for most healthy individuals. Athletes requiring a larger percent of kcalories from carbohydrates and protein will subsequently consume a lower percentage of kcalories from fat. However,

because the total number of kcalories consumed is more than the average person, the absolute amount of fat consumed is still adequate at 15% to 25% of total kcalories.[12]

Protein

Protein as Fuel Substrate

Although some amino acids can feed into the basic energy cycle, protein makes a relatively insignificant and inefficient contribution to energy during exercise under normal circumstances. In glycogen-depleted muscles, however, more protein will be used as a fuel substrate.[19]

Protein in the Diet

A daily intake of 0.8 to 1 g of protein/kg of body weight is sufficient to meet the general needs of the physically active person. This amounts to the recommended daily dietary intake for adults, with 10% to 35% of the kcalories in the diet coming from protein. It is accepted that the optimal dietary protein intake for athletes is more than the generally active person (in the range of 1 to 2 g/kg); however, the exact amount is unclear.[20,21] As athletes increase their total kcalorie intake to meet elevated energy needs, a balanced varied diet will provide proportionally more protein and may be adequate to cover the additional needs.[1]

There is no indication that protein or amino acids from dietary supplements are necessary to meet needs or are superior to whole food forms of protein. A well-balanced diet can easily meet dietary protein needs for the active person and the athlete (see Chapter 5). Excess protein in the diet cannot be stored in the body as amino acids; thus protein is converted to fat, and the amine portion (nitrogen) must be excreted.

Micronutrients

Vitamins and Minerals as Catalytic Cofactors

Vitamins and minerals cannot be used as fuel substrates. They are not oxidized or expended in the process of energy production. Vitamins and minerals are, however, essential as catalytic cofactors in enzyme reactions.

Vitamins and Minerals in the Diet

Increased physical exertion during exercise or athletic training does not require a greater intake of vitamins and minerals beyond current recommendations. A well-balanced diet will supply adequate amounts of vitamins and minerals, and exercise may improve the body's efficient use of them. Because athletes, for example, have an increased dietary need for energy, their larger kcalorie intake from high-quality food sources will boost their general intake of vitamins and minerals. If, however, an athlete is restricting calories, vitamin and mineral deficiencies are a possibility. Energy-restricting behaviors often result in avoidance of animal products such as meat and dairy, which are particularly rich sources of calcium, iron, and zinc.

On the opposite end of the spectrum, multivitamin and mineral supplementation does not improve physical performance in healthy athletes who eat a well-balanced diet.

Furthermore, the potential side effects of toxicity are well known (see Chapters 6 and 7).

Hydration: Water and Electrolytes

Water and Dehydration

Controlled studies in experimental settings have shown that dehydration limits exercise capacity in endurance- and resistance-training activities. However, the real-world application and interpretations from these studies are limited.[22,23] The effects of dehydration depend on many factors, such as testing environment, psychologic stressors, intensity and duration of exercise, body temperature, level of fitness, and preexercise state of hydration (see the Case Study box, "Fluid and Energy Needs for Endurance Athletes"). In cases of severe dehydration, athletes may experience problems such as cramps, delirium, vomiting, hypothermia, and hyperthermia. By establishing euhydration before athletic events, and consuming fluid replacement beverages during events as thirst indicates, these problems can be prevented. Adequate fluid intake and access to rehydration fluids should be planned for all types of athletes, not just individuals who participate in endurance events. Some strategies to increase fluid intake by athletes are provided in Box 14-1.

Cause of Dehydration. ATP production results in significant heat release within the working muscle. During moderate-intensity physical activity, most individuals maintain a body temperature within a desirable range. However, during intense exercise, or exercise in hot environments, heat production may exceed the body's acceptable temperature

CASE STUDY

Fluid and Energy Needs for Endurance Athletes

Jamie is a 25-year-old man training for an ultramarathon race of 50 miles. He is 5 feet 10 inches tall and currently weighs 170 lb. On his long runs of more than 3 hours, he has been drinking water, approximately 30 oz, and consuming one GU (an energy supplement containing 100 kcal from simple sugar) at the 2-hour mark. Jamie is coming to you for advice because he is becoming increasingly weak and nauseous toward the end of his runs. He reports feeling light-headed and irritable on his long training days. Jamie states that he is eating an egg salad sandwich with two hard-boiled eggs mixed with 3 tbsp of mayonnaise on whole wheat bread about 20 minutes before his run.

Questions for Analysis

1. What sources of fuel is Jamie predominately using in this type of exercise?
2. How much fluid should he be consuming during a 3-hour run?
3. Based on his weight, how many calories and grams of carbohydrate should Jamie consume during his run?
4. On what time schedule would you recommend that he consume his fluid and carbohydrate?
5. What would you recommend regarding Jamie's preexercise meal?

range for performance and the body's heat tolerance capacity.[24] Sweating is our primary mechanism for dissipating body heat. The major source of fluid loss in sweat is plasma fluid. High-intensity or long-endurance events (especially in hot climates) can cause the loss of several liters of water as sweat to regulate body temperature. Unless this fluid is replaced, consequences from dehydration and heat illness may result.

Prevention of Dehydration. To prevent dehydration, athletes are advised to (1) establish euhydration at least several hours before activity; (2) drink during exercise to avoid excessive water loss, defined as 2% to 3% body weight loss from water; and (3) replace fluid loss after completion of exercise.[23,25] The American College of Sports Medicine recommends that athletes develop a customized fluid replacement program catering to their needs and preferences (e.g., fluid temperature, taste preferences).[25] Measuring weight before and after activity is an easy and appropriate method to estimate fluid loss in sweat. Water volume and weight are equivalent (i.e., 16 oz of water = 1 lb of weight); thus one can assume that weight lost during activity is equivalent to the volume of water lost. Hydration with fluids containing glucose and sodium reduces urinary fluid loss. Therefore, during longer events (particularly those lasting more than 2 hours), fluids with mild solutions of sodium are recommended to help reduce fluid loss and prevent dehydration.[26]

Sodium

In the 1960s researchers believed that sodium losses exceeded water loss during vigorous activity with substantial sweat production. However, sweat is more dilute than internal fluids, and thus we lose proportionately more water than sodium. In most instances, sodium losses are replaced with the athlete's next meal. However, for ultraendurance events lasting more than 3 hours, fluid replacements including sodium are fundamental in preventing sodium losses and reducing the risk of **hyponatremia**.[27] Therefore, the current recommendations state that during longer and more demanding endurance events, especially in warm or humid

environments, a mild sodium and glucose (20 to 50 mmol/L sodium and 4% to 8% glucose solution) sports drink that has rapid gastric emptying and intestinal absorption times may be beneficial.[25] A number of specialty sports drinks are now available with replacement electrolytes (see the Evidence-Based Practice box, "Sorting Out the Sports Drinks Saga").

NUTRITION AND ATHLETIC PERFORMANCE

Exercise and Energy

Exercise raises the body's kcalorie expenditure and has the additional benefit of helping to regulate appetite to meet these needs. Table 14-3 gives some examples of the amount of kcalories spent in various activities. The building of glycogen reserves is important for athletes such as long-distance runners who compete in endurance events and need a steady supply of energy within the muscle. When exercise levels rise from mild or moderate amounts up to strenuous levels, kcaloric needs also rise to supply needed fuel.

Active people, even athletes, require no more dietary fat than their inactive counterparts. Carbohydrate is the preferred fuel and is the critical food for the active person—not only before an exercise period but also during the recovery phase. The complex carbohydrate forms (i.e., starches) sustain energy needs and supply added fiber, vitamins, and minerals. Thus the recommended composition of energy nutrients

TABLE 14-3	APPROXIMATE ENERGY EXPENDITURE PER HOUR DURING VARIOUS ACTIVITIES	
---	---	
ACTIVITY	**KCALORIES PER HOUR***
Sleeping	63
Lying/sitting, awake	70
Standing, relaxed	84
Rapid typing, sitting	105
Dressing and undressing	140
Walking slowly (24 min/mile)	210
Water aerobics	280
High-impact aerobics	490
Football, flag/touch	560
Walking very fast (12 min/mile)	560
Stair, treadmill	630
Swimming, vigorous effort	700
Running (8 min/mile)	875

From Nix S: *Williams' basic nutrition & diet therapy,* ed 14, St Louis, Mo., 2013, Elsevier.
*For an adult weighing 70 kg (154 lb).

BOX 14-1	STRATEGIES FOR SPORTS TEAM MEMBERS TO INCREASE FLUID INTAKE

- Establish a regular schedule; drink during warm-up exercises and between periods of play.
- Give each player a sports squeeze bottle.
- Supply players with a sports drink that tastes good during exercise.
- Make available a choice of fluids to drink.
- Offer cool fluids.
- Avoid carbonated beverages because athletes tend to drink less when the beverage is carbonated.

From Palumbo CM: Nutrition concerns related to the performance of a baseball team. *J Am Diet Assoc* 100(6):704, 2000. Copyright with permission from the American Dietetic Association.

KEY TERM

hyponatremia Serum sodium less than 135 mEq/L; a relative excess of body water compared with sodium.

EVIDENCE-BASED PRACTICE

Sorting Out the Sports Drinks Saga

Problem: Sorting through the many available sports drinks and the plethora of claims that accompany each one is no easy task. Ultimately we need to answer these questions: How much and what kind of a sports drink is needed during physical activity and exercise?

The first well-known commercially available sports drink was a solution called *Gatorade,* a beverage its developers named for their university's football team. They reasoned that if they analyzed the sweat of their players, they could then replace the lost minerals and water in a drink containing some flavoring, coloring, and sugars to make it acceptable, and it would taste better and have more benefits than plain water. Although Gatorade is beneficial for some athletes, most do not need it during general exercise.

However, what endurance athletes do need, especially in hot weather, is water and fuel in the form of carbohydrates. For athletes losing substantial amounts of water and sodium through sweat, electrolyte replacement is also an important consideration. Hyponatremia, although rare, can be fatal. The most common cause of hyponatremia in endurance athletes results from excess sodium loss through sweat combined with fluid replacement of plain water. Water dilutes the plasma sodium even more, exacerbating the condition. Thus sports drinks with simple carbohydrates and electrolytes are beneficial for endurance athletes.

Simply adding sugar to water holds it in the stomach longer, where it is not available for immediate cellular needs. To meet the body's requirements during long events, a second category

of sports drinks is available, containing glucose polymers instead of sugar, as well as less sodium. These short chains of about five glucose molecules—maltodextrins—are produced in the breakdown of starch. These drinks are less concentrated and are only slightly sweetened and flavored. In addition, they leave the stomach rapidly, thus making them ideal as a continuing fuel source for the endurance athlete.

Another category of sports drinks on the market adds large amounts of vitamins and minerals to their solutions. All of these extra vitamins do not help an athlete's performance, and on a hot day a perspiring athlete could easily consume a megadose in four or five bottles. Athletes who eat well-balanced diets with enough kcalories to maintain energy balance do not need additional vitamin or mineral supplementation.

As a general guide, it is worth the time to sort out the costs and claims made by sports drink manufacturers. These products are not for everyone. Although special sports drinks may meet the needs of athletes competing in physically demanding endurance events, they are not required by those participating in less demanding sports activities. Water is the best solution for regular needs, and it costs far less.

Bibliography

American College of Sports Medicine, American Dietetic Association, Dietitians of Canada: Joint position statement: nutrition and athletic performance. *Med Sci Sports Exerc* 41(3):709, 2009.

to support physical activity in highly active people is as follows[12]:

- *Carbohydrate:* 6 to 10 g/kg body weight per day
- *Protein:* 1.2 to 1.4 g/kg of body weight per day for endurance athletes and 1.2 to 1.7 g/kg body weight per day for resistance- and strength-training athletes
- *Fat:* 20% to 35% of total kcalories

Pregame and Training Meals

Protein and fat delay the emptying of the stomach, and neither contributes to the glycogen stores needed during exercise. Therefore the ideal pregame meal is approximately 200 to 300 g of carbohydrate that is eaten about 3 to 4 hours before the event, allowing adequate time for digestion and absorption.[12] A sample meal is illustrated in Box 14-2. This meal should be high in complex carbohydrates, moderate in protein, and with little fat or fiber. Good food choices include pasta, bread, bagels, muffins, and cereal with nonfat milk or milk substitute. Throughout the period of vigorous training, a high-carbohydrate diet with 500 to 600 g/day is recommended, such as that illustrated in Table 14-4. Small amounts of foods or drinks that contain carbohydrates may be consumed briefly before the event without affecting performance for most athletes. All athletes should experiment with their own level of tolerance during training sessions.

BOX 14-2   SAMPLE PREGAME MEAL

This sample pregame meal includes approximately 234 g of carbohydrates, is high in complex carbohydrates, and is low in protein, fat, and fiber:

- 1½ cups cooked spaghetti (332 kcal, 65 g carbohydrate)
- ¾ cup tomato sauce (135 kcal, 20 g carbohydrate)
- 1 slice French bread, large (281 kcal, 55 g carbohydrate)
- 1 baked potato, large (278 kcal, 63 g carbohydrate)
- 1 cup apple juice (125 kcal, 31 g carbohydrate)

Energy During Exercise

For activities lasting less than 1 hour, most athletes do not need exogenous sources of energy during the exercise period. However, performance is enhanced during longer endurance events with the interval consumption of carbohydrates. The American College of Sports Medicine, the Academy of Nutrition and Dietetics (formerly American Dietetic Association), and the Dietitians of Canada recommend eating or drinking 0.7 g of carbohydrate per kilogram of body weight per hour (approximately 30 to 60 g/hour) during long events.[12] It is most effective to consume equal amounts of the preferred food every 15 to 20 minutes throughout the event rather than consuming the entire 30 to 60 g at once. Athletes should

TABLE 14-4 HIGH CARBOHYDRATE DIET

MENU	CARBOHYDRATE
Breakfast	
1 orange, 2⅝-in diameter	16 g
1 cups plain oatmeal, cooked, regular and quick	55 g
1 cup skim milk	12 g
1 oat bran muffin, medium	55 g
1 tbsp jam	14 g
Snack	
½ cup seedless raisins	57 g
Lunch	
Lettuce salad	
1 cup romaine lettuce	2 g
½ cup garbanzo beans	23 g
½ cup tomatoes, chopped	4 g
2 tbsp French dressing	5 g
2 cups macaroni and cheese	87 g
1½ cups apple juice	42 g
Snack	
2 slices whole wheat bread	23 g
2 tbsp peanut butter	6 g
1 tbsp honey	17 g
Dinner	
½ turkey breast, no skin	0 g
1¾ cups mashed potatoes, with whole milk	65 g
1 cup peas and onions	16 g
¾ cup fruit salad (banana, pineapple, papaya, guava)	43 g
1 cup skim milk	12 g
Snack	
1 cup cranberry juice, unsweetened	31 g
1 banana, small	23 g
TOTAL	**608 g**

Data from U.S. Department of Agriculture, Agricultural Research Service: *National nutrient database for standard reference,* Release 25, Washington, D.C., 2013, U.S. Government Printing Office. Available at: <www.nal.usda.gov/fnic/foodcomp/search/index.html>. March 29, 2013.

experiment with various forms of glucose before competition to determine what is best tolerated. A large variety of sports drinks, gels, and other forms of carbohydrates are available from which the athlete may choose. The food of choice should provide carbohydrates primarily from glucose, with little or no fat, protein, or fiber.

Energy After Exercise: Recovery

Proper nutrition is not only important to the athlete before and during exercise, but it also plays a major role in recovery after the event. It is well accepted that fluid and carbohydrates consumed within 30 minutes after a glycogen-depleting endurance event will result in better glycogen synthesis and muscle recovery than if those same replacement nutrients were consumed 2 hours or more after the event.[12] Beverages of 6% glucose concentration are adequate during this period, but higher concentrations may be consumed, depending on the tolerance of the athlete. For athletes taking only a short break between events (e.g., triathletes), foods and beverages ingested should be limited to primarily carbohydrate-containing substances. For athletes recovering for longer periods of time, a replacement meal or beverage containing 1.2 g of carbohydrate per kilogram of body weight (over several hours) results in an increased rate of muscle glycogen recovery.[28]

Myths and Misinformation

Athletes and their coaches are particularly susceptible to myths and claims about foods and dietary supplements, relentlessly searching for the competitive edge (see the Focus on Culture box, "The Winning Edge—or Over the Edge?"). Knowing this, marketers unremittingly exploit this hunt. Manufacturers sometimes make distorted and false claims about products. For example, pangamic acid was marketed as "vitamin B$_{15}$," although it is not a vitamin at all and carried claims about its ability to enhance oxygen transport during exercise, to lessen muscle fatigue, and to increase endurance. Naturally, if such a compound existed, then it would be of interest to athletes and their trainers. However, scientific research has exposed these claims as unfounded.[29,30] Nevertheless, products and advertisements still appear for "vitamin B$_{15}$," although it is currently illegal to distribute pangamic acid in the United States.

Training and Precompetition Abuses Among Athletes
Weight-Control Measures

The sport of wrestling has a long history of widely fluctuating weight patterns among its athletes. Wrestlers often restrict food and fluid intake to qualify for a weight classification that is less than their off-season weight, seeking to gain advantages in strength, speed, and leverage over a smaller opponent. This practice of "making weight" still seems to be an ingrained tradition that produces large, frequent, and rapid weight-loss and regain cycles, with methods such as dehydration, food restriction, and loss of food and fluid through induced vomiting and use of laxatives and diuretics. Such disordered eating affects normal growth, and progressive dehydration impairs regulation of body temperature and cardiovascular function. Other sports such as bodybuilding and gymnastics often follow similar routines, especially before competition. In sports that favor lean bodies, it is not uncommon for young preadolescent girls, who wish to maintain a small body size in the face of advancing age, to reduce food intake and body fat and sometimes develop eating disorders.[31] As a result, a cascade of events may follow: impaired growth, delayed puberty, induced amenorrhea from low estrogen levels, disruption or delay in bone density

FOCUS ON CULTURE

The Winning Edge—or Over the Edge?

Athletes, their coaches, and our entire culture have become increasingly aware that the percentage of body fat versus the percentage of lean body mass is an influential factor on athletic performance. Each extra pound of body fat an athlete carries into competition is nonproductive weight. It is the muscles, the lean body mass, that provide the strength, agility, and endurance required to win.

Because of this, athletes strive to achieve as low a percentage of body fat as possible while still maintaining good health. In reaching for such a goal, however, many young athletes develop an abhorrence of body fat, resulting in food aversion and the undertaking of excessive weight-loss regimens. These self-generated excesses are commonly reinforced by those surrounding the young athletes: coaches, teammates, and parents. Such an all-consuming focus may result in compulsive behaviors, driving the athlete to set unrealistic goals, and leading to abusive weight loss.

Such excessive voluntary weight losses in young athletes are not usually the result of chronic emotional problems, as with other psychologic eating disorders. The reasons typically are more superficial, resulting from an accumulation of immediate and short-term goals and concerns. These athletes usually respond well to counseling and can reverse the excessive behavior with the support of concerned friends and teammates.

Yet for a few individuals, compulsive fixation on lean body mass and the loss of body fat becomes obsessive and enduring. Unfortunately our mass media culture reinforces the view that the most desirable attributes of beauty are slimness in women and physical prowess in men. When a susceptible individual enters a time of stress in search of a firm identity, he or she may turn toward cultural and media stereotypes to provide a positive self-concept. For women this stress is usually encountered during adolescence, when some young women think being physically attractive is the key to social acceptance. For men the sense of self is more closely tied to their vocational and sexual effectiveness, both of which some men relate to their physical abilities. Thus the test of a man's abilities tends to occur more often in adulthood, which may result in his preoccupation with physical fitness as a way to deny any decline in strength or ability. Such long-term compulsive fixation on body image in susceptible individuals may result in disordered eating that requires extensive counseling.

Compulsive dieting, as in anorexia nervosa, is a serious psychologic disorder; compulsive training, on the other hand, is seen by society as a positive personality trait showing dedication. In reality, both may be symptomatic of unstable self-concepts and attempts to establish a firm sense of identity. They are perceptual disorders: anorexia nervosa victims always see themselves as overweight; compulsive exercisers always see themselves as out of shape. For these individuals, no goal, once attained, is sufficiently satisfying. Such striving, often despite physical indications against it, has resulted in permanent disabilities and even death.

The danger of athletic pressure leading to eating disorders was highlighted by the 1994 death from anorexia nervosa of 22-year-old Christy Henrich, a world-class American gymnast. At 4 feet 10 inches (147 cm) and 95 lb (43 kg), Christy won a silver medal at the 1989 U.S. National Championships. She was known as a perfectionist who pushed herself hard, a characteristic that, when extreme, is often associated with eating disorders in athletes. She felt compelled to lose more weight and at times limited herself to only an apple a day even while continuing to train. Because of her eating disorder, she eventually lost the strength to perform and was forced to retire from competition. She weighed only 60 lb (27 kg) when she died. Although her death marked the first time an American gymnast had died from an eating disorder, such problems are widely known in competitive women's gymnastics, especially at the national and international levels.

It should be noted that such risk factors are not true for all competitive athletes, nor are such risk factors confined to competitive athletes. Caucasian female athletes reported the highest prevalence of disordered eating and the lowest level of self-esteem in a 2004 study examining the cultural and ethnic differences in collegiate athletes. However, a 2012 study found that athletes were no more likely to suffer from disordered eating, body dissatisfaction, or self-esteem issues than the sedentary female college student. The researchers reported that body shame was a consistent predictor of disordered eating in all college females, regardless of athletic standing.

Bibliography

Jankauskiene R, Pajaujiene S: Disordered eating attitudes and body shame among athletes, exercisers and sedentary female college students. *J Sports Med Phys Fitness* 52(1):92–101, 2012.

Johnson C, Crosby R, Engel S, et al: Gender, ethnicity, self-esteem and disordered eating among college athletes. *Eat Behav* 5(2):147–156, 2004.

Obituary: Christy Henrich 1972-1994, Int Gymnast. *Int Gymnast* 36(10):1994.

development, and even osteoporosis.[32] A similar pattern has been observed among young long-distance runners, cheerleaders, and dancers.[33]

Drug Abuse

From ancient Greek runners and discus throwers in the first Olympian contests to top competitors from around the world in current Olympic events, athletes have experimented with

KEY TERMS
amenorrhea The absence of menses (menstrual cycle) entirely or no more than three periods in a year; associated with lower-than-normal estrogen levels in women.
osteoporosis Abnormal thinning of bone, producing a porous, fragile, latticelike bone tissue of enlarged spaces that is prone to fracture or deformity.

various ergogenic aids in their eternal search for the competitive edge or the perfect body. Modern athletes—from professional football players to their aspiring high school counterparts—are doing the same thing, trying to find the magic potion in everything from bee pollen and seaweed to freeze-dried liver flakes, gelatin, amino acid supplements, and ginseng. Such efforts have been worthless in most cases but fortunately not particularly harmful. However, in the case of anabolic-androgenic steroids, human growth hormone, and insulin-like growth factor, which are now epidemic in the sporting world, great danger and even death may lie ahead for the user.[34] These dangers include cardiovascular health risk, impaired liver function, disturbances in normal steroid production, increased aggression and hostility, mood disturbances, and additional disturbances in psychologic and dermatologic conditions.[35]

The use of legal pharmacologic agents in an illegal manner has created a black market network, which adds criminal jeopardy and street preparation impurities to the drug's inherent dangers. Abuse of anabolic steroids in the United States has moved from its early use among bodybuilders and invaded almost all areas of athletics, beginning as early as adolescence.[36] In addition, other abuses amplify the dangers of steroids. For example, diuretics are often abused by athletes to rapidly lose water weight and to dilute the urine in attempt to mask the use of other banned substances during drug screenings.[37]

Risks for Female Athletes

Some female athletes who enter highly competitive and demanding sports face health risks related to anemia and low bone mineral density (BMD) if their diets do not adequately meet their nutrient needs. These risks are especially prevalent for women athletes in sports with intensive training and endurance events, such as gymnastics and running. Highly skilled dancers in the performing arts world often face similar risks.

Sports Anemia and Iron Deficiency Anemia

Normal hemoglobin (Hb) values are approximately 12 to 15.5 g/dL for women and 13.5 to 17.5 g/dL for men. Iron deficiency anemia is defined as hemoglobin levels less than these ranges. As baseline plasma volume increases with aerobic training, the concentration of hemoglobin (found within red blood cells) is reduced as a percentage of total blood. Such a situation is more appropriately referred to as *sports anemia* rather than iron deficiency anemia, because the total volume of red blood cells is normal. Additional iron intake, whether through food or supplementation, is not needed in sports anemia. However, care must be taken to appropriately distinguish sports anemia from other forms of true anemias.

True iron deficiency anemia is typically a result of inadequate iron in the diet, decreased iron absorption, or increased iron losses. Absolute and functional levels of iron deficiency are particularly of concern for elite athletes.[38]

Reduced hemoglobin in an athlete's blood means reduced oxygen-carrying capacity with negative implications for aerobic capacity and the ability to sustain an exercise workload.[39] Accordingly, one of the first implications for iron deficiency anemia is exertional fatigue. Unless a woman is experiencing amenorrhea, she will have cyclic menstrual loss of iron. Some iron is lost in profuse sweating and occasionally because of intravascular hemolysis, which is the rupture of red blood cells caused by the stresses of heavy exercise. Neither sweat nor intravascular hemolysis is believed to be a major contributor to iron loss. Regular evaluation of dietary iron intake and iron status among athletes is warranted.

Low Bone Mineral Density

An inadequate diet, intentionally or not, combined with an interrupted menstrual cycle can lead to low BMD (osteopenia). In some cases the bone loss may progress to a state of osteoporosis at an abnormally young age. It has been called the *female athlete triad* (Figure 14-4) because of the three contributing factors: (1) inadequate energy availability, (2) menstrual dysfunction, and (3) bone loss. While this disorder is notable in female athletes, it is also found in the general population at a high rate as well.[40] The Perspectives in Practice box, "The Female Athlete Triad: How Performance and Social Pressure Can Lead to Low Bone Mass," illustrates the contributing factors that ultimately lead to injury.

An estimated 40% to 60% of a woman's normal BMD for her lifetime is created during adolescence, when her sex hormone estrogen becomes active. Diet and hormones must work together. An adequate amount of calcium must exist in the diet, as well as normal functioning of the female estrogen cycle that stimulates osteoblastic activity (bone growth). Unfortunately, many young females restrict their diets in an effort to control their weight, growth, and body fat, with resulting inadequate dietary energy and calcium. Some may have more profound eating disorders, such as anorexia nervosa. At the same time, intense athletic training in women can lead to primary or secondary amenorrhea. Amenorrhea is more common in athletes than in nonathletes; it is especially prevalent among aesthetic, endurance, and weight-class sports.[33] When athletic training begins before normal menarche, the onset of puberty and its associated growth and

---

KEY TERMS

ergogenic Tendency to increase work output; various substances that increase work or exercise capacity and output.

osteopenia Below-normal level of bone mineral density, which increases the risk of stress fractures; the bone thinning is not as severe as that found in osteoporosis.

primary amenorrhea Amenorrhea delay of menarche past the age of 16.

secondary amenorrhea Cessation of the normal menstrual cycle after menarche.

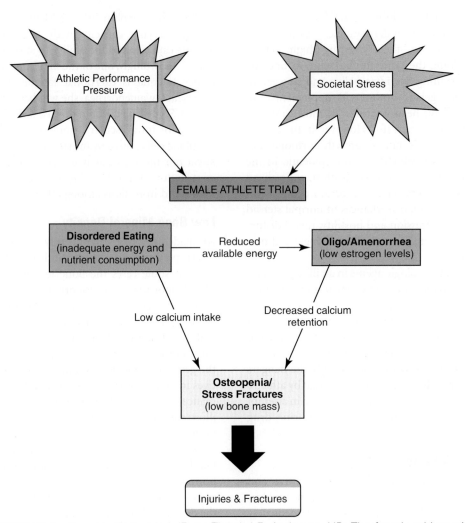

FIGURE 14-4   Female athlete triad. (From Thrash LE, Anderson JJB: The female athlete triad: nutrition, menstrual disturbances, and low bone mass. *Nutr Today* 35[5]:168, 2000, with permission from Lippincott Williams & Wilkins.)

developmental patterns may be delayed. Such delays include the secondary sex characteristics shaping the female figure. When the menstrual cycle is delayed or interrupted, normal estrogen levels are depressed. As a result, these young women athletes are at a high risk for low BMD and stress fractures.[41] Injuries and fractures can interrupt or permanently end an athletic career, and bone mineral loss may be irreversible and become a lifelong risk.

HEALTH PROMOTION
BUILDING A PERSONAL EXERCISE PROGRAM

Exercise is a critical component in health promotion and disease prevention. The current *Physical Activity Guidelines for Americans* state the following[42]:

Children and Adolescents: Participate in 60 minutes (1 hour) or more of physical activity daily.

- Most of the 60 or more minutes a day should be either moderate- or vigorous-intensity aerobic physical activity, and should include vigorous-intensity physical activity at least 3 days a week. Table 14-5 describes the classifications of exercise intensity.
- As part of their 60 or more minutes of daily physical activity, children and adolescents should include muscle-strengthening physical activity on at least 3 days of the week.
- As part of their 60 or more minutes of daily physical activity, children and adolescents should include bone-strengthening physical activity on at least 3 days of the week. (See Chapter 12 for more information about children and physical activity.)

Adults: Avoid inactivity. Some physical activity is better than none, and adults who participate in any amount of physical activity gain some health benefits.

- For substantial health benefits, adults should do at least 150 minutes (2 hours and 30 minutes) a week of

The Female Athlete Triad: How Performance and Social Pressure Can Lead to Low Bone Mass*

The female athlete triad consists of three health afflictions: (1) disordered eating with energy restriction, (2) menstrual disturbances, and (3) osteopenia (low bone mass) or even osteoporosis. Low bone mineral density (BMD) is the leading cause of stress fractures and injuries throughout the body, some of which may be irreversible. In addition, recent research indicates the triad is associated with compromised endothelial function indicating an increased risk for cardiovascular disease. Women in top physical form may be more susceptible to social and performance pressure leading to disordered eating habits and exercise regimens. The dilemma facing women athletes today is how to maintain optimal physical performance while not provoking health risks.

Women who participate in competitive endurance sports, such as rowing or long-distance running, or who are judged partially on physical appearance, such as in ice skating, diving, gymnastics, or dancing, are more likely to be preoccupied with their weight and to have self-image issues. Social and competitive pressure for a woman to be thin can contribute to her sense of imperfection (for both athletes and nonathletic females). These demands and pressures can lead to disordered eating patterns, which in combination with strenuous exercise may result in low energy availability. This drop in energy will be followed by a drop in performance as the athlete loses focus and concentration and is fatigued. Some women develop psychologic eating disorders, such as bulimia nervosa, characterized by binge eating followed by compensatory mechanisms; or anorexia nervosa, characterized by the refusal or inability to consume sufficient calories for daily requirements. These disorders may, in turn, progress to additional health problems including depression, seizures, cardiac arrhythmia, myocardial infarction, or other health complications. The seriousness of the eating disorder is linked to the amount of stress and concern the woman feels over her body image, combined with the amount of emphasis placed on weight by the woman, her trainers, and her coaches. Athletes often equate leanness with performance, and some are willing to go to great lengths to satisfy perfectionist needs.

Poor caloric intake and disordered eating may lead to menstrual irregularity. Amenorrhea is the suppression of menstrual cycles to a level of zero to three menses a year, and primary amenorrhea is the repression of all menstrual cycles until after age 16. In some highly competitive sports, adolescent females may actually strive to delay the onset of puberty to maintain small, childlike physiques. Some women experience oligomenorrhea, which are sporadic cycles that occur three to nine times a year. The levels of estrogen and progesterone that regulate menses can be affected by metabolism, intensive exercise, dieting, or stress.

Menstrual irregularities are related to low bone density. Before the age of 30, bone density reaches its peak, and it is vital for young women to strive for dense bones in early adulthood to maintain healthy bone density later in life. If the density of bones is compromised, then osteopenia occurs; if severe enough, it can be a signal of future osteoporosis. Porous bones increase the likelihood of stress fractures and injuries, and women are more likely to incur such injuries than men.

Some studies, however, indicate that weight-bearing activities, such as gymnastics, seem to actually improve bone density, even perhaps in vertebrae, and they may help prevent density decreases later in life. Nonetheless, the problem facing women athletes who are eating improperly is that the decline in BMD is amplified as menstrual cycles continue to be erratic. Weight-bearing sports will not overcome the tendency for participants to have low BMD if diet and exercise levels are not balanced.

The primary goal of treatment is to reestablish energy balance by increasing caloric intake, decreasing exercise, and/or weight gain as needed. Nutrient supplementation may be indicated to maximize bone growth and avert endothelial dysfunction involving calcium, vitamin D, vitamin K, and folic acid. Hormone replacement therapy and oral contraceptive pills have been used as a treatment modality in the past. However, when used alone, neither will improve BMD nor address the underlying metabolic problems. Education and further research are needed to find the optimal course.

The best course of action is to have women athletes monitor their diets to ensure adequate caloric intake and sufficient micronutrient consumption. The prevention of osteoporosis later in life depends on habits of the individual and the modification of factors that can lead to the triad of eating disturbances, menstrual irregularity, and low bone density. Body weight is individual, depending on height and skeletal structure, and one specific weight goal should not exist for all female athletes.

The societal and competitive pressures that cause the initial step in this three-step process must be addressed. Asking female athletes to sacrifice their health for an unrealistic body image projected on them by others (as well as their coaches' and trainers' desire for vicarious victory) must not alter what constitutes acceptable eating habits. In today's weight-conscious society, the emphasis must not be on a perfect image, size, or body but rather on the perfect balance of health and training. The female athlete's skeletal integrity, and potentially her cardiovascular function, suffers as she resorts to drastic measures in her aspiration for an overly lean physical image.

The need to educate trainers, athletes, and health professionals about the consequences of neglected nutrition is imperative. Young female athletes must understand that deprivation of life's essential nutrients does significant bodily harm.

Bibliography

Duckham RL, Peirce N, Meyer C, et al: Risk factors for stress fracture in female endurance athletes: a cross-sectional study. *BMJ Open* 2(6):2012.

Hoch AZ, Papanek P, Szabo A, et al: Association between the female athlete triad and endothelial dysfunction in dancers. *Clin J Sport Med* 21(2):119–125, 2011.

Nattiv A, Loucks AB, Manore MM, et al: American College of Sports Medicine position stand. The female athlete triad. *Med Sci Sports Exerc* 39(10):1867–1882, 2007.

Zach KN, Smith Machin AL, Hoch AZ: Advances in management of the female athlete triad and eating disorders. *Clin Sports Med* 30(3):551–573, 2011.

*With contribution from Meredith Catherine Williams.

TABLE 14-5	CLASSIFICATION OF EXERCISE INTENSITY		
INTENSITY	% MAXIMUM HEART RATE	%VO₂MAX	PERCEIVED EXERTION
Light	57-63	37-45	Very light to fairly light
Moderate	64-76	46-63	Fairly light to somewhat hard
Vigorous	77-95	64-90	Somewhat hard to very hard

Adapted from Garber CE, Blissman B, Deschenes MR: American College of Sports Medicine position stand. Quantity and quality of exercise for developing and maintaining cardiorespiratory, musculoskeletal, and neuromotor fitness in apparently healthy adults: guidance for prescribing exercise. *Med Sci Sports Exerc* 43(7):1334–1359, 2011.

moderate-intensity, or 75 minutes (1 hour and 15 minutes) a week of vigorous-intensity aerobic physical activity, or an equivalent combination of moderate- and vigorous intensity aerobic activity. Aerobic activity should be performed in episodes of at least 10 minutes, and preferably, it should be spread throughout the week.

- For additional and more extensive health benefits, adults should increase their aerobic physical activity to 300 minutes (5 hours) a week of moderate intensity, or 150 minutes a week of vigorous intensity aerobic physical activity, or an equivalent combination of moderate- and vigorous-intensity activity. Additional health benefits are gained by engaging in physical activity beyond this amount.
- Adults should also do muscle-strengthening activities that are moderate or high intensity and involve all major muscle groups on 2 or more days a week, as these activities provide additional health benefits.

Older Adults: The guidelines for adults also apply to older adults. In addition, the following guidelines are just for older adults:

- When older adults cannot do 150 minutes of moderate-intensity aerobic activity a week because of chronic conditions, they should be as physically active as their abilities and conditions allow.
- Older adults should do exercises that maintain or improve balance if they are at risk of falling.
- Older adults should determine their level of effort for physical activity relative to their level of fitness.
- Older adults with chronic conditions should understand whether and how their conditions affect their ability to do regular physical activity safely.

Exercise and Disease Prevention
Coronary Heart Disease

Exercise reduces risks for heart disease in several ways related to heart function, blood cholesterol levels, and oxygen transport:

- *Heart muscle function:* Exercise, especially aerobic conditioning, strengthens the heart, thereby enabling the heart to pump more blood per beat (stroke volume). A heart strengthened by exercise has an increased aerobic capacity; that is, the heart can pump more blood per minute without an undue increase in the heart rate. Therefore exercises that rely primarily on the aerobic oxygen system for energy

such as walking, jogging, and workouts on light cardiopulmonary exercise machines improve heart function.
- *Blood lipid levels:* Aerobic exercise programs improve blood lipid profiles by lowering total cholesterol (TC), low-density lipoproteins (LDL), the TC/high-density lipoprotein (HDL) ratio, and triglycerides. When aerobic training is combined with a prudent diet, the improvements in lipid profile are even more significant.[43]
- *Oxygen-carrying capacity:* Exercise also enhances the circulatory system by increasing the oxygen-carrying capacity of the blood. As training continues, a person's VO₂max will improve, thus increasing the efficiency of oxygen use and uptake.

Hypertension

The risk for cardiovascular complications increases continuously with increasing levels of blood pressure. Hypertension is indicated when the systolic blood pressure is greater than 140 mm Hg, the diastolic blood pressure is greater than 90 mm Hg, or both. Exercise is one of the most effective nondrug treatments for treating and reducing the risk of hypertension.[44,45] Even for persons with moderate to severe hypertension, exercise has proven to be an important adjunct to drug therapy, offsetting adverse drug effects and lowering medication requirements. Normal rises in blood pressure occur during dynamic (e.g., walking, cycling) and resistance (i.e., strength training) exercise. Both forms of exercise are beneficial for individuals with hypertension. However, exercisers should avoid holding their breath during the exertion phase of heavy weight lifting to prevent severe stress on the cardiovascular system, especially those with diagnosed hypertension.

Diabetes

Resistance and endurance-type exercise programs help maintain glucose homeostasis in patients with impaired glucose tolerance and type 2 diabetes.[46] Physically active lifestyles are especially beneficial for individuals with type 2 diabetes to reduce the risk of chronic complications associated with the disease.[47] Exercise improves the action of a person's naturally produced insulin by increasing the sensitivity of insulin receptor sites on cells. In managing type 1 diabetes mellitus, the type of exercise and when it is done must be balanced with food and insulin to prevent reactions caused by drops in blood glucose. (See Chapter 22 for a more detailed discussion of diabetes.)

Weight Management

While exercise alone is not generally sufficient to obtain or maintain weight loss, it is an important aspect of a healthy lifestyle that, when implemented together, does favor fitness and a healthy weight. Together with a well-planned diet, physical activity, planned exercise, or both help with energy balance and increased energy output (see Chapter 8).[48] Fat is used efficiently as the fuel source for muscles during lower-intensity (30% to 60% VO_2max) aerobic exercise such as walking, jogging, swimming, and light cycling.

Stress Management

Exercise helps reduce stress-related eating. It also provides a physical outlet for working off the hormonal physiologic effects of catecholamines and corticoid hormones produced in the body by stress, thus helping to reduce a major risk factor in the development of chronic disease.[49]

Bone Disease

Weight-bearing exercises improve bone mineralization, thus reducing the risk of bone weakness and of potential osteoporosis.

Mental Health

Extended aerobic exercise stimulates the production of brain opiates, which are substances called *endorphins*. These natural substances decrease pain (this is how aspirin works, by stimulating production of endorphins) and improve the mood, including an exhilarating kind of "high."

Assessment of Personal Health and Exercise Needs

Many kinds of exercise exist. Choosing the best form depends on individual health, personal needs, the aerobic benefits involved, and personal enjoyment.

Assessing Health and Personal Needs

In planning an exercise program, it is important to assess individual health status, personal needs, present level of fitness, and resources available. Discussing an exercise program with a medical practitioner is always recommended, and getting a medical clearance before beginning an exercise program is especially important for older individuals and those with chronic disease. It is wise to start slowly and build gradually rather than risk injury and discouragement. Moderation and consistency are key.

Beginning a Program

Many options exist regarding where, what, when, and how one exercises. It is important to evaluate these options before committing to any one routine. A golden rule for success is that if a person enjoys the activity they are doing, then they are much more likely to make it part of their everyday schedule. Some individuals benefit from joining a fitness facility where they feel encouraged by others. Others, however, may shy away from fitness facilities for fear of discomfort. Keeping the following questions in mind while designing an exercise program can be helpful:

1. Which is better, a fitness facility or a home program?
   - Is external encouragement helpful in maintaining a regular exercise schedule? Is company and interaction with others desirable during exercise, or is exercising alone preferable?
   - Is sticking to a schedule ideal and easy, or is it more realistic to work around other obligations and exercise when and where possible?
   - Is a fitness facility located near home or work? Is it affordable?
   - Is the office or home in an area that can provide uninterrupted bouts of exercise?
2. What type of exercise best fits the needs of you or your client?
   - It is important for everyone to determine independently what he or she *likes* to do. If the exercise chosen is not fun, then the patient or client will soon stop doing it, making it of no benefit. Encourage someone who has little exposure to various forms of physical activity to experiment with a variety of activities before committing to one.
   - While exercising at a fitness facility, would your client or patient enjoy aerobic workouts on a bike, on a treadmill, or in a group class?
   - If your client or patient is considering exercising at home, you can ask other questions: Do you live in an area where you can run, walk, or bike? If not, then do you have access to a stationary bike, treadmill, or other aerobic machine? Try to choose an activity that he or she can stick with throughout the year, or choose a variety of activities that can be alternated during various seasons. For instance, perhaps swimming or biking in the summer, whereas running or participating in aerobic classes would work in the winter.
   - For strength training, fitness facilities usually provide an assortment of free weights and resistance machines. Always encourage your client or patient to ask for help if he or she is not sure how to correctly perform any exercise. Resistance training can be done effectively at home as well, with a combination of resistance bands, small hand weights, or even cans of beans!

Frequency, Intensity, and Duration

To achieve aerobic benefits from exercise, it is recommended that individualized exercise prescriptions meet the following levels of intensity and duration[50]:

- *Frequency:* 5 or more days per week of moderate exercise, or 3 or more days per week of vigorous exercise, or a combination of moderate and vigorous exercise on 3 to 5 days per week.
- *Intensity:* Moderate and/or vigorous intensity is recommended for most adults (see Table 14-5).
- *Duration:* 30 to 60 minutes per day (150 minutes per week) of purposeful moderate exercise, or 20 to 60 minutes per day (75 minutes per week) of vigorous exercise, or a

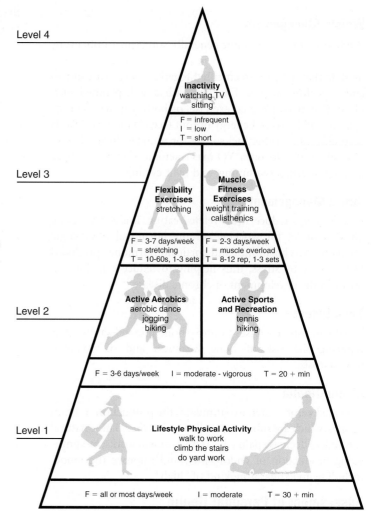

FIGURE 14-5 Physical Activity Pyramid. (Adapted with permission from Corbin CB, Lindsey R: *Fitness for life*, ed 5, Champaign, Ill., 2005, Human Kinetics, pp 64.)

combination of moderate and vigorous exercise per day is recommended for most adults. Less than 20 minutes per day of exercise can be beneficial, especially in previously sedentary persons. If exercise is broken into short periods, the accumulated duration should be 30 minutes or more daily in bouts of 10 minutes or more each period.

Types of Exercise

Many types of exercise exist from which a participant may choose. Many of them are enjoyable and healthful but do not reach aerobic levels. For example, golf is a passion for many and gets them outdoors, but it is far too slow and sporadic to be aerobic. It is best to have a variety of exercises in any exercise plan (Figure 14-5). Even though many sports do not reach aerobic levels, if they are enjoyable they should be included.

Aerobic Exercise

Forms of exercise that can be sustained at a necessary level of intensity to provide aerobic benefits include such activities as swimming, running, jogging, bicycling, and aerobic dancing routines and workouts (Table 14-6). The exercise performed should be regular, purposeful, continuous and rhythmic in

TABLE 14-6	EXAMPLES OF AEROBIC EXERCISES FOR PHYSICAL FITNESS*
TYPE OF EXERCISE	**AEROBIC FORMS**
Ball playing	Handball
	Racquetball
	Squash
Bicycling	Stationary
	Touring
Dancing	Aerobic routines
	Ballet
	Disco
Jumping rope	Brisk pace
Running or jogging	Brisk pace
Skating	Ice-skating
	Roller-skating
Skiing	Cross-country
Swimming	Steady pace
Walking	Brisk pace

*Maintained at aerobic level for at least 30 minutes total.

nature, and involve the major muscle groups.[50] Perhaps the simplest and most popular form of stimulating exercise is walking. If the pace is fast enough to elevate the pulse and maintain it, then walking can be an excellent form of aerobic exercise. Walking is convenient, available, and appropriate for most people; in addition, it requires no equipment other than good walking shoes.

Resistance Exercise

Resistance types of exercises are designed to increase muscle strength and endurance. An ideal program would consist of several exercises with 8 to 12 repetitions of each, focusing on the major muscles of the body, performed 2 to 3 days per week. For an individual whose primary goal is to gain strength and power, the repetitions should be of high intensity (60% to 80% of 1 rep max). For improved endurance, a lower weight should be used that will allow at least 15 to 20 repetitions before muscle fatigue.[50]

Weight-bearing exercises, such as walking, jogging, aerobic dancing, or jumping rope, are important for bone structure and strength. In each of these exercises, muscles are working against gravity. Bones will adapt to the environment and load put on them during weight-bearing exercises to build more bone cells and increase bone density.

Flexibility Exercises and Stretching

Flexibility exercises and stretching are recommended for all age groups. Selecting a variety of stretches that target each of the major muscle-tendon units is ideal to help maintain joint mobility, stability, and balance. Stretching and holding the stretch for 10 to 60 seconds at a point of tightness is recommended at least 2 to 3 days a week.[50]

TO SUM UP

The energy molecule of the body is ATP, and the powerhouse of the cell is the mitochondrion. The cell's depot of energy is creatine phosphate. These two high-energy phosphate compounds are in limited supply. They can produce energy for a brief initial period only and need to be replenished for exercise to continue. This added supply is produced by anaerobic glycolysis, with energy made available for continued exercise by the body's aerobic system. The process of glycolysis metabolizes only carbohydrate substrate, furnished by either blood glucose or stored glycogen. Dietary carbohydrate is necessary to replenish these fuel sources. Protein contributes little to energy for exercise, whereas the body's ability to burn fat as fuel depends on the level of fitness and intensity of exercise. The higher the body's efficiency in using oxygen, the more fatty acids will contribute to the energy supply. Even in the best-trained athletes, fatty acid oxidation must be accompanied by glucose metabolism.

Contrary to popular belief, exercise does not require an increased intake of vitamins or minerals. The body's increased needs are well supplied by a normal healthy diet. Exercise increases the body's need for kcalories and water. Cold water taken in small, frequent amounts is the best way to prevent dehydration in most athletic events and exercise. In most cases, electrolytes lost in sweat are replaced by a diet of adequate quality and quantity. A mild saline and glucose solution (4% to 8%) may supply fluid and fuel to sustain energy during longer endurance events. Some athletes use harmful practices such as food and fluid deprivation for controlling weight, as well as such ergogenic aids as illegal steroid drugs for bulking muscles.

The optimal diet for the athlete is moderate in protein and fat, with 6 to 10 g/kg of body weight per day coming from carbohydrates. The pregame meal should be small, having little or no protein or fat and relying mainly on complex carbohydrates.

The health benefits of general and aerobic exercise are numerous. Excellent aerobic exercises include sustained fast walking, swimming, jogging, running, and aerobic dancing or workouts. Approach any exercise sensibly, and choose those activities that are enjoyable.

QUESTIONS FOR REVIEW

1. What are the component muscle structures, and how do they produce muscular action?
2. What type of substrate fuel does the body use for immediate energy needs? For short-term needs? For long-term needs?
3. How does oxygen relate to physical activity capacity and aerobic effect?
4. Outline the nutrition and physical fitness principles to discuss with an athlete. Plan a diet for this client that would meet nutrient and energy needs.
5. Why is fluid balance vital during exercise periods? How is water and electrolyte balance achieved?
6. Describe the short-term and long-term consequences of female athlete triad.

REFERENCES

1. Maughan RJ, Shirreffs SM: Nutrition for sports performance: issues and opportunities. *Proc Nutr Soc* 71(1):112–119, 2012.
2. Centers for Disease Control and Prevention: Physical activity, glossary of terms, 2011. Available from: <www.cdc.gov/physicalactivity/everyone/glossary/>.
3. World Health Organization: *Global health risks: mortality and burden of disease attributable to selected major risks*, Geneva, 2009, World Health Organization.
4. U.S. Department of Health and Human Services: *Healthy people 2020*, Washington, D.C., 2010, U.S. Government Printing Office.

5. U.S. Department of Agriculture: *Dietary Guidelines for Americans 2000*, ed 5, Washington, D.C., 2000, U.S. Government Printing Office.

6. U.S. Department of Agriculture: *Dietary Guidelines for Americans 2010*, Washington, D.C., 2010, U.S. Government Printing Office.

7. Roberts CK, Barnard RJ: Effects of exercise and diet on chronic disease. *J Appl Physiol* 98(1):3–30, 2005.

8. Leung FP, Yung LM, Laher I, et al: Exercise, vascular wall and cardiovascular diseases: an update (Part 1). *Sports medicine* 38(12):1009–1024, 2008.

9. Yung LM, Laher I, Yao X, et al: Exercise, vascular wall and cardiovascular diseases: an update (part 2). *Sports Medicine* 39(1):45–63, 2009.

10. Timmons JA: Variability in training-induced skeletal muscle adaptation. *J Appl Physiol* 110(3):846–853, 2011.

11. American College of Sports Medicine: *ACSM's resource manual for guidelines for exercise testing and prescription*, ed 5, Baltimore, Md., 2006, Lippincott Williams & Wilkins.

12. Rodriguez NR, DiMarco NM, Langley S: Position of the American Dietetic Association, Dietitians of Canada, and the American College of Sports Medicine: Nutrition and athletic performance. *J Am Diet Assoc* 109(3):509–527, 2009.

13. Green HJ, Ball-Burnett M, Jones S, et al: Mechanical and metabolic responses with exercise and dietary carbohydrate manipulation. *Med Sci Sports Exerc* 39(1):139–148, 2007.

14. Rauch HG, St Clair Gibson A, Lambert EV, et al: A signalling role for muscle glycogen in the regulation of pace during prolonged exercise. *Br J Sports Med* 39(1):34–38, 2005.

15. Harger-Domitrovich SG, McClaughry AE, Gaskill SE, et al: Exogenous carbohydrate spares muscle glycogen in men and women during 10 h of exercise. *Med Sci Sports Exerc* 39(12):2171–2179, 2007.

16. Dumke CL, McBride JM, Nieman DC, et al: Effect of duration and exogenous carbohydrate on gross efficiency during cycling. *J Strength Cond Res* 21(4):1214–1219, 2007.

17. Sedlock DA: The latest on carbohydrate loading: a practical approach. *Curr Sports Med Rep* 7(4):209–213, 2008.

18. Mondazzi L, Arcelli E: Glycemic index in sport nutrition. *J Am Coll Nutr* 28(Suppl):455S–463S, 2009.

19. Gibala MJ, Peirce N, Constantin-Teodosiu D, et al: Exercise with low muscle glycogen augments TCA cycle anaplerosis but impairs oxidative energy provision in humans. *J Physiol* 540(Pt 3):1079–1086, 2002.

20. Phillips SM: Dietary protein requirements and adaptive advantages in athletes. *Br J Nutr* 108(Suppl 2):S158–S167, 2012.

21. Phillips SM, Van Loon LJ: Dietary protein for athletes: from requirements to optimum adaptation. *J Sports Sci* 29(Suppl 1):S29–S38, 2011.

22. Maughan RJ: Investigating the associations between hydration and exercise performance: methodology and limitations. *Nutr Rev* 70(Suppl 2):S128–S131, 2012.

23. Goulet ED: Dehydration and endurance performance in competitive athletes. *Nutr Rev* 70(Suppl 2):S132–S136, 2012.

24. Hillman AR, Vince RV, Taylor L, et al: Exercise-induced dehydration with and without environmental heat stress results in increased oxidative stress. *Appl Physiol Nutr Metab* 36(5):698–706, 2011.

25. Sawka MN, Burke LM, Eichner ER, et al: American College of Sports Medicine position stand. Exercise and fluid replacement. *Med Sci Sports Exerc* 39(2):377–390, 2007.

26. Shirreffs SM, Sawka MN: Fluid and electrolyte needs for training, competition, and recovery. *J Sports Sci* 29(Suppl 1):S39–S46, 2011.

27. Anastasiou CA, Kavouras SA, Arnaoutis G, et al: Sodium replacement and plasma sodium drop during exercise in the heat when fluid intake matches fluid loss. *J Athl Train* 44(2):117–123, 2009.

28. Howarth KR, Moreau NA, Phillips SM, et al: Coingestion of protein with carbohydrate during recovery from endurance exercise stimulates skeletal muscle protein synthesis in humans. *J Appl Physiol* 106(4):1394–1402, 2009.

29. Herbert V: Pangamic acid ("vitamin B_{15}"). *Am J Clin Nutr* 32(7):1534–1540, 1979.

30. Currell K, Moore DR, Peeling P, et al: A-Z of nutritional supplements: dietary supplements, sports nutrition foods and ergogenic aids for health and performance—part 28. *Br J Sports Med* 46(1):75–76, 2012.

31. Rosen DS: Identification and management of eating disorders in children and adolescents. *Pediatrics* 126(6):1240–1253, 2010.

32. Ozier AD, Henry BW: Position of the American Dietetic Association: nutrition intervention in the treatment of eating disorders. *J Am Diet Assoc* 111(8):1236–1241, 2011.

33. Nattiv A, Loucks AB, Manore MM, et al: American College of Sports Medicine position stand. The female athlete triad. *Med Sci Sports Exerc* 39(10):1867–1882, 2007.

34. Rogol AD: Drugs of abuse and the adolescent athlete. *Ital J Pediatr* 36:19, 2010.

35. Hartgens F, Kuipers H: Effects of androgenic-anabolic steroids in athletes. *Sports Med* 34(8):513–554, 2004.

36. Mulcahey MK, Schiller JR, Hulstyn MJ: Anabolic steroid use in adolescents: identification of those at risk and strategies for prevention. *Phys Sportsmed* 38(3):105–113, 2010.

37. Cadwallader AB, de la Torre X, Tieri A, et al: The abuse of diuretics as performance-enhancing drugs and masking agents in sport doping: pharmacology, toxicology and analysis. *Br J Pharmacol* 161(1):1–16, 2010.

38. Reinke S, Taylor WR, Duda GN, et al: Absolute and functional iron deficiency in professional athletes during training and recovery. *Int J Cardiol* 156(2):186–191, 2012.

39. Dellavalle DM, Haas JD: Iron status is associated with endurance performance and training in female rowers. *Med Sci Sports Exerc* 44(8):1552–1559, 2012.

40. Coelho GM, Soares Ede A, Ribeiro BG: Are female athletes at increased risk for disordered eating and its complications? *Appetite* 55(3):379–387, 2010.

41. Duckham RL, Peirce N, Meyer C, et al: Risk factors for stress fracture in female endurance athletes: a cross-sectional study. *BMJ Open* 2(6):2012.

42. Centers for Disease Control and Prevention: *Physical activity guidelines for Americans*, Washington, D.C., 2008, U.S. Department of Health and Human Services.

43. Kelley GA, Kelley KS, Roberts S, et al: Efficacy of aerobic exercise and a prudent diet for improving selected lipids and lipoproteins in adults: a meta-analysis of randomized controlled trials. *BMC Med* 9:74, 2011.

44. Ranković G, Djindjić N, Ranković-Nedin G, et al: The effects of physical training on cardiovascular parameters, lipid disorders and endothelial function. *Vojnosanit Pregl* 69(11):956–960, 2012.

45. National Institutes of Health; National Heart, Lung, and Blood Institute; National High Blood Pressure Education Program: *The Seventh Report of the Joint National Committee on Prevention, Detection, Evaluation, and Treatment of High Blood Pressure*, Bethesda, Md., 2004, National Institutes of Health.

46. van Dijk JW, Manders RJ, Tummers K, et al: Both resistance- and endurance-type exercise reduce the prevalence of hyperglycaemia in individuals with impaired glucose tolerance and in insulin-treated and non-insulin-treated type 2 diabetic patients. *Diabetologia* 55(5):1273–1282, 2012.

47. Colberg SR, Sigal RJ, Fernhall B, et al: Exercise and type 2 diabetes: American College of Sports Medicine and the American Diabetes Association: joint position statement. Exercise and type 2 diabetes. *Med Sci Sports Exerc* 42(12):2282–2303, 2010.

48. Donnelly JE, Blair SN, Jakicic JM, et al: American College of Sports Medicine position stand. Appropriate physical activity intervention strategies for weight loss and prevention of weight regain for adults. *Med Sci Sports Exerc* 41(2):459–471, 2009.

49. Tsatsoulis A, Fountoulakis S: The protective role of exercise on stress system dysregulation and comorbidities. *Ann N Y Acad Sci* 1083:196–213, 2006.

50. Garber CE, Blissmer B, Deschenes MR, et al: American College of Sports Medicine position stand. Quantity and quality of exercise for developing and maintaining cardiorespiratory, musculoskeletal, and neuromotor fitness in apparently healthy adults: guidance for prescribing exercise. *Med Sci Sports Exerc* 43(7):1334–1359, 2011.

FURTHER READINGS AND RESOURCES

Readings

Garber CE, Blissmer B, Deschenes MR, et al: American College of Sports Medicine position stand. Quantity and quality of exercise for developing and maintaining cardiorespiratory, musculoskeletal, and neuromotor fitness in apparently healthy adults: guidance for prescribing exercise. *Med Sci Sports Exerc* 43(7):1334–1359, 2011.

[This position stand paper provides guidelines for individualized exercise prescription for healthy adults.]

Rodriguez NR, DiMarco NM, Langley S: Position of the American Dietetic Association, Dietitians of Canada, and the American College of Sports Medicine: Nutrition and athletic performance. *J Am Diet Assoc* 109(3):509–527, 2009.

[This joint position statement emphasizes the importance of nutrition in physical activity, athletic performance, and recovery from exercise. The experts specifically address nutrient and fluid needs, body composition, supplements and ergogenic aids, and the roles and responsibilities of health care professionals.]

Websites of Interest

- American College of Sports Medicine: www.acsm.org.
- National Coalition for Promoting Physical Activity: www.ncppa.org.
- U.S. Department of Health and Human Services, *Physical Activity and Health: A Report of the Surgeon General*: www.cdc.gov/nccdphp/sgr/sgr.htm.

The Complexity of Obesity: Beyond Energy Balance

Allan Higginbotham

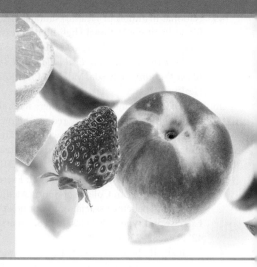

ⓔ EVOLVE WEBSITE

http://evolve.elsevier.com/Williams/essentials/

OUTLINE

Realities of Obesity
Energy Intake, Energy Expenditure, and Development
  of Obesity
Obesity as a Disease

Beyond Energy Balance
Epidemiologic Model
Overview of Treating the Disease of Obesity
Health Promotion

In this chapter, we look at the complex issue of obesity. In recent years the prevalence of obesity has grown to epidemic proportions. Linked as a risk factor for many chronic disorders in the United States, the magnitude of this health care problem and its effect on the health care system is immense.

We are living in a time when the number of overweight individuals is increasing more rapidly than ever before. This chapter is intended to help you understand this problem. Using an epidemiologic model of the interactions between environmental agents and the human host to explain obesity, we explore food, medications, physical inactivity, toxins, and viruses as environmental agents that act on the genetically programmed host to disturb energy balance and cause obesity. Large portion size, high fat intake, sugar-sweetened beverages, and labor savings innovations all play a role in the toxic environment that leads to obesity. The genetic, physiologic, and psychologic responses of the host determine whether or not this "toxic environment" will produce obesity. Reversing the current trends of obesity requires a new look at the limits of the energy balance concept and a better understanding of how environmental factors acutely and chronically change responses of the susceptible host so that obesity is manifested.

REALITIES OF OBESITY

During the early part of the twentieth century, the prevalence of obesity increased slowly; however, around 1980 it began to increase more rapidly.[1-4] As illustrated in Figure 15-1, the rise in the rate of obesity has continued to the present time. In the period between 2009 and 2010, the prevalence of obesity was 35.7%.[1]

Although historically a greater percentage of women have been obese, the latest data indicate no significant difference in prevalence between men and women at any age. Overall, adults aged 60 and over are more likely to be obese than younger adults. Among men there was no significant difference in obesity prevalence by age. Among women, however, 42.3% of those ages 60 and over are obese compared with 31.9% of women ages 20 to 39.[1] Moreover, African-American (59%) and Hispanic women (41%) have a higher prevalence of obesity than Caucasian women (33%). This racial disparity is larger in women than in men.[2] Overweight is also higher among people who make less money and have less education than it is among those who have a higher education and income.[3] Children are also affected by obesity. The prevalence was about 5% in 1960 but has increased to 17% in 2010.[1,5]

Obesity increases the risk of developing many chronic diseases including type 2 diabetes mellitus, coronary heart disease, hypertension, gallbladder disease, certain forms of cancer, and sleep-breathing disorders.[4] Prominent among these is type 2 diabetes mellitus. This disease most often occurs in overweight or obese adolescents and adults and presages a bleak future, particularly for children as the complications of blindness, heart disease, renal failure, and amputation disable them in the next 20 or so years. Through the development of chronic diseases, being overweight reduces life expectancy and shortens life span by 3 to 7 years for a 40-year-old individual with a body mass index (BMI) of 30 or more.

Obesity increases the cost of health care, which has now been estimated to be as high as $147 billion per year. Moreover, in the United States roughly one half of the costs are paid by Medicare and Medicaid, suggesting that taxpayers foot the bill for much of the costs of obesity.[5,6] The frequency of hospital and medical office visits increases with increasing body weight. The use of drugs and surgery to treat the complications associated with obesity also increases.

Fortunately, risks associated with obesity are generally ameliorated by modest weight loss. A weight loss of 5% to 10% of initial body weight is sufficient to reduce the development of diabetes in people with prediabetes by up to 58%.[7] Weight loss that is maintained is an effective treatment for hypertension. Risks from abnormal blood lipids (dyslipidemia) are also reduced with weight loss.[8]

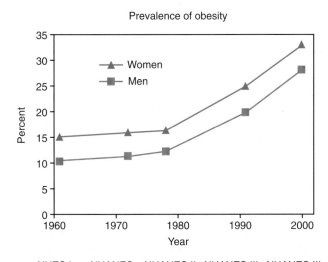

FIGURE 15-1 Graph illustrating the prevalence of obesity. The upper line shows the prevalence of obesity for women and the lower line for men, using data from several surveys of obesity done by the U.S. government beginning in the years 1960 to 1962. Obesity rose slowly from 1960 until approximately 1980, when the rate for men and women began to increase. (Data from National Center for Health Statistics: *National Health and Nutrition Examination Survey I, 1960-1962* and *National Health and Nutrition Examination Surveys 1970-1974, 1976-1980, 1988-1994, and 1999-2000,* Hyattsville, Md., 1960–2000, Centers for Disease Control and Prevention.)

For children and adults, a social stigma is associated with a weight problem.[9] Overweight children are less liked as playmates and tend to view themselves less favorably than normal-weight children. Children are often teased at school by being labeled "fatty" and other derogatory terms. Such disparaging remarks often jeopardize feelings of self-confidence. Many overweight children and adults are traumatized by the stigma of obesity. Adults experience prejudice in social and economic situations. Measures of quality of life show that the obese score lower on many scales and that weight loss improves their quality of life (see the Focus on Culture box, "Antifat Bias: The Last Acceptable Form of Cultural Discrimination").

To tackle the hazards of obesity for children, adolescents, and adults, we need to adopt effective strategies for prevention and, where prevention fails, for treatment of obesity.

ENERGY INTAKE, ENERGY EXPENDITURE, AND DEVELOPMENT OF OBESITY

One easy way to view the problem of obesity is with the aid of a teeter-totter, a childhood toy. On one side is the amount of food we eat expressed in calories (joules). On the other side is the energy we expend during the day for our various activities, which includes the energy needed to heat our bodies and keep them at 37°C (98.6°F), the energy needed to keep our hearts beating, our brains working, our kidneys filtering blood, our intestines digesting food, and all other essential body processes whether we are awake or not. Energy is also used for physical activity when we sit, stand, walk, run, or do other activities. When the two sides of the teeter-totter are in balance, that is, when the energy on one side is equal to the energy on the other side, we are in "energy balance." As long as we are in energy balance, we will not gain or lose weight. Overweight develops when the energy on the intake side is more than on the expenditure side, which can occur because energy intake rises, because energy expenditure falls, or both. The conservation of energy implied by the energy balance equation is often referred to as the *First Law of Thermodynamics* applied to human energy consumption and expenditure. This law was first demonstrated for human beings more than 100 years ago, and no reason exists to doubt that it provides the overall framework for understanding the way in which obesity develops. However, as we will show, the problem of obesity lies in the details of the relation of energy intake and energy expenditure.

OBESITY AS A DISEASE

Obesity is a disease. What do we mean by this? A disease has several components. First, it has a cause. As noted previously, this is the result of an imbalance between energy intake and energy expenditure. It has clinical signs and symptoms such as increased amount of fatness that is usually visible to the eye. No one would have difficulty distinguishing between an overweight and normal-weight

⊕ FOCUS ON CULTURE

Antifat Bias: The Last Acceptable Form of Cultural Discrimination

Our culture idealizes slimness and denigrates obesity. Discrimination based on weight bias has been recognized in many different areas of our society, including representation of obese persons in our culture. Common stereotypes of obese persons include the following:

- Warm
- Dependable
- Gluttonous
- Lazy
- Stupid
- Worthless

Popular messages in the media promote fat jokes and idealization of thin women and muscular men. Unfortunately, it appears that it is socially acceptable in the United States to assume that obese people are fully responsible for their condition. Do health care professionals, however, who are trained to understand that obesity is caused by hereditary and environmental factors and is not merely a function of personal behavior (e.g., overeating, lack of exercise), express this same bias? Regrettably, research shows that health professionals are not immune to overt or inherent antifat bias. The very people who are responsible for caring for individuals who are obese demonstrated the following attitudes toward obese patients[1-8]:

- Family practice physicians described obese patients with negative terms such as *lacking self-control.*
- Physicians reported that they would feel more negatively toward overweight patients and spend less time with them but would order more tests.
- Nurses reported the following:
  - Feeling uncomfortable caring for obese patients
  - Being "repulsed" by obese persons
  - Having a preference not to care for obese patients
- Medical students described obese patients as follows:
  - Less attractive
  - More depressed
  - Less compliant

- Registered dietitians and dietetic students reported negative attitudes toward obese individuals.
- Overweight and obese women are less likely to be screened for cervical and breast cancer.

Thus it appears the physical and psychologic consequences of obesity may stem from not only Western culture's weight-related bias and stigma but also from the biases of health professionals. Obviously, Schwartz and colleagues[6] were right when they said, "Much more work is needed to understand and ameliorate this bias."

How about you? Are you part of the solution or part of the problem?

References

1. Bagley CR, Conklin DN, Isherwood RT, et al: Attitudes of nurses toward obesity and obese patients. *Percept Mot Skills* 68:954, 1989.
2. Hebl MR, Xu J: Weighing the care: physicians' reaction to the size of a patient. *Int J Obes Relat Metab Disord* 25:1246, 2001.
3. Loomis GA: Attitudes and practices of military family physicians regarding obesity. *Mil Med* 166:121, 2001.
4. Maroney D, Golub S: Nurses' attitudes toward obese persons and certain ethnic groups. *Percept Mot Skills* 75:387, 1992.
5. Oberrieder H, Walker R, Monroe D, et al: Attitude of dietetics students and registered dietitians toward obesity. *J Am Diet Assoc* 95:914, 1995.
6. Schwartz M, Chambliss HO, Brownell KD, et al: Weight bias among health professionals specializing in obesity. *Obes Res* 11:1033, 2003.
7. Teachman BA, Gapinski KD, Brownell KD, et al: Demonstrations of implicit anti-fat bias: the impact of providing causal information and evoking empathy. *Health Psychol* 22:68, 2003.
8. Wigton RS, McGaghie WC: The effects of obesity on medical students' approach to patients with abdominal pain. *J Gen Intern Med* 16:262, 2001.

---

individual walking down the street. Obesity also has a "**pathology**," by which we mean the presence of some unique features that allow one to diagnose it under a microscope, at an autopsy examination, or by defined blood tests. For obesity this is the enlarged fat cell.

All forms of obesity have as one characteristic an enlargement of the individual fat cells all over the body. The adult human has close to 60 billion fat cells. As people gain weight, the first change in these cells is to enlarge to accommodate the extra fat. As the cells reach their maximal size, additional cells may be recruited to store the extra fat. Fat cells are very remarkable. They not only store vast amounts of energy for later use, but they are also part of the larger endocrine cellular system that secretes products into the bloodstream that have effects elsewhere. In the case of fat cells, many secreted products can affect blood clotting

(plasminogen activator inhibitor-1 [PAI-1]), the removal of fats from the blood (lipoprotein lipase), inflammation (interleukin-1 [IL-1], interleukin-6 [IL-6], tumor necrosis factor-α [TNF-α]), blood pressure (angiotensinogen), and energy balance (**leptin**). The release of this latter hormone—leptin—is an important signal from the fat cells to the brain about the amount of body fat. Circulating levels of leptin are directly related to amount of body fat. Until the amount of body fat reaches a "critical" level in women, menstruation does not occur. In many women who are ballet dancers or gymnasts, with small amounts of body fat, menstrual periods cease because leptin levels are too low. The many hormones produced and secreted from the fat cells in the body produce the **pathophysiologic** responses that lead to the associated diseases we described previously. Thus obesity can be described as an endocrine disease.

BEYOND ENERGY BALANCE

There is no doubt that obesity results from energy imbalance and that we can predict the magnitude of the weight change over time if we know the net energy balance. However, it is what the energy balance concept does not tell us that is most important in dealing with obesity. The first law of thermodynamics does not tell us anything about the regulation of food intake or the way in which genes are involved in this process. It does not help us to understand why men and women distribute fat in different places on their bodies or to understand how fat distribution changes with age. The first law of thermodynamics also does not help us to understand why some drugs produce weight gain, whereas others produce weight loss, or why weight loss stops after a period of treatment with diet or medication. Understanding these mechanisms will allow us to tackle the epidemic of obesity.

One problem with the concept of energy balance is that we are never in complete energy balance for any length of time. To study energy balance, healthy men were housed in small, sealed rooms so that their respiratory gasses could be measured to determine energy expenditure (respiration calorimetry). Food intake and exercise were manipulated to get as close as possible to zero energy balance—that is, when energy intake equals energy expenditure.[10,11] In fact, the difference was rarely closer than 50 kcal/day, or about 2.5% out of an intake of 2000 kcal/day. The values of energy imbalance for these healthy men ranged from 50 to 150 kcal/day. Had these differences been maintained for 1 year, these men would be expected to gain about 2.5 kg (5.5 lb) at the smaller error and 7.5 kg (16.5 lb) at the larger error.

To keep from gaining weight, we must make "corrective" responses in energy intake or energy expenditure to counterbalance the error that occurred on previous days. These corrective responses around a weight of relative stability make it look as though "weight regulation" exists. For some people the oscillations around this balance point can keep weight stable for many years. For others a slow upward drift occurs in this regulatory point, and weight is gradually gained. If you are fortunate enough to have robust corrective responses, then you can maintain a stable weight over many years. If it is not stable, then the following two strategies are available:

1. *Conscious control:* This method is exhibited in some people who have a pattern of eating called *restrained eating.*
2. *Regular weighing:* This second and perhaps best way to maintain weight over a long period is to weigh oneself regularly at the same time of day on an accurate scale and address weight increases in a timely fashion by adjusting energy intake.

Because we are never in energy balance, we need to view energy balance as an ideal, not a realistic goal to be obtained by counting calories.

From the perspective of energy balance, the solution to obesity should be simple: eat less and exercise more. The truth of this advice was shown by Kinsell and colleagues[12] for overweight individuals housed in a metabolic ward and provided with all their food. During the course of several months,

---

KEY TERMS

overweight A body mass index (BMI) of 25 or greater (weight [kg]/height^2 [m^2])

obesity An excess amount of body fat. A body mass index (BMI) of 30 or greater (weight [kg]/height^2 [m^2]). Three subclasses of obesity are defined as follows:

- Class 1 = BMI 30-34.9 kg/m^2
- Class 2 = BMI 35-39.9 kg/m^2
- Class 3 = BMI >40 kg/m^2

prevalence This term relates the number of individuals with a particular condition at a particular time to the total number of people. If 10 people were overweight in a population of 1000, then this would indicate a prevalence of 1%.

diabetes mellitus A disease defined by a high level of glucose in the blood, which often appears in the urine if it is high enough. Two general types of diabetes mellitus exist: type 1, which refers to the disease normally diagnosed in younger individuals (younger than 30 years of age) in which the pancreas cannot produce enough insulin and thus not enough circulating insulin exists, and type 2, which refers to the disease normally diagnosed in older individuals who are often overweight or obese and in which more than enough circulating insulin exists but relatively poor response to this insulin occurs.

body mass index (BMI) Body weight in kilograms divided by the height in square meters (kg/m^2). It can be calculated from pounds and inches as 703 × body weight in pounds ÷ by the height in inches squared. This measurement is the common method used to define overweight and obesity.

prediabetes A condition also known as *impaired glucose tolerance* and defined as a fasting glucose between 100 and 126 mg/dL and a blood glucose between 140 and 199 mg/dL 2 hours after ingestion of 75 g of glucose.

stigma A mark or identification marking. In this context it is an increased body fat that is obvious to the viewer and that elicits emotional feelings, which are usually negative.

calories The amount of heat energy needed to raise the temperature of water from 14°C to 15°C. Because this is a small unit, we usually use *kilocalories*, which are 1000 of these small calories (see also *joule*).

joules Units of energy. The International System of Units uses joules in place of calories to refer to food energy, and most nutrition journals require its use instead of calories (1 kcal = 4.184 kilojoules [kJ], often rounded to 4.2 kJ for ease in calculation). A 1000-kcal diet would be equivalent to a 4200-kJ or 4.2-MJ (megajoule) diet.

KEY TERMS

pathology The science of disease. Changes that reflect disease can be in organs (e.g., liver disease), tissues (e.g., skin disease), cells, or parts of cells.

leptin A peptide of 167 amino acids that is produced primarily in fat cells and released into the blood to circulate as a hormone to the brain to tell the body about long-term regulation of body fat.

pathophysiologic Term referring to the processes by which the disease develops.

these patients ate diets with 1200 kcal/day. After the initial rapid weight loss because of rebalancing body fluids, subsequent weight loss was linear and was not affected by wide variations in fat, carbohydrate, and protein content of the diet. More recent studies using foods tagged with a nonradioactive isotopic carbon-13 showed that weight loss increased in relation to how well subjects adhered to a diet.[13] Thus it is adherence to diets, not diets themselves, which make the difference.

Another limitation to the concept of energy balance as the cause of obesity is the implication that if you are getting fatter, then it is your fault. You need only to control your calorie intake (food) and calorie expenditure to control the problem, which implies that we should blame our children for their obesity. This notion seems grossly inappropriate. If obesity were easily controlled by moderating calorie intake, then the U.S. military would not discharge up to 5000 men and women yearly for failing to meet its weight standards. If loss of livelihood is not sufficient motivation to lose weight, then the problem must be more complex.

In the very rare instance of leptin deficiency in humans, the cure of obesity involves treatment with leptin. This concept demonstrates a genetic basis for some obesity, more than simply lack of willpower.[14] Although simple in theory, applying the ideas of energy balance and calorie counting to body weight control has proven unsuccessful. More than 95% of people using dietary, behavior, and lifestyle approaches to lose weight regained it within less than 5 years.[15]

EPIDEMIOLOGIC MODEL

The current epidemic can be viewed from the perspective of an epidemiologic model shown in Figure 15-2. Food, low physical activity, drugs, viruses, and toxins are the environmental agents that facilitate the development of obesity. One or more of these factors acting on a susceptible host can produce obesity. Using this model, we can approach

the problem by manipulating either the environment or the host.

Environmental Agents
Food and Its Costs as a Major Environmental Agent
Several components of our food supply may be important in determining whether or not obesity develops. The first of these is the size of food packages and restaurant portions. Convincing evidence indicates that when larger portion sizes are provided, more food is eaten. Portion sizes have dramatically increased in the past 40 years[16] and now need reduction. Sugar-sweetened beverages that contain 10% high fructose corn syrup (HFCS) are available in 12-, 20-, 32-, and 44-oz containers and provide 150, 250, 400, or 550 kcal if the entire drink is consumed. Prepackaged foods list the calories per serving, but the package often contains more than one serving, encouraging consumption of more than the recommended serving size.

Patterns of food consumption have changed during the past 30 years. The most striking change from 1970 to 2010 has been the rising consumption of HFCS.[17] HFCS is now used as the caloric sweetener in almost all soft drinks, as well as in reconstituted juice drinks and many solid foods. The rise in HFCS consumption occurred over the same time interval as the rapid rise in the prevalence of obesity.[18] On the one hand, this relationship may be strictly coincidental. However, on the other hand, it may not be (Figure 15-3). Fructose is sweeter than either glucose or sucrose, a molecule that is a combination of fructose and glucose. In addition, HFCS is a solution of fructose and glucose as separate molecules, and thus it differs in osmotic properties from a solution with the same concentration of sucrose.[19]

The intake of sugar-sweetened beverages has been related to the epidemic of obesity.[17-19] Ludwig, Peterson, and Gortmaker[20] reported that the intake of soft drinks was a predictor of initial BMI in children in the Planet Health Study. They also showed that higher soft drink consumption predicted an

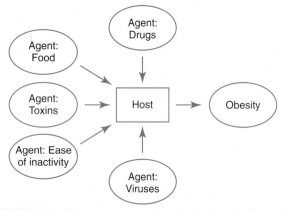

FIGURE 15-2 Epidemiologic model of obesity. In this model the agent that produces obesity is "food" or food-related products. If food is in limited supply, then obesity does not develop. The food that is ingested interacts with the host. In a susceptible host the toxic effects of food produce obesity, the disease.

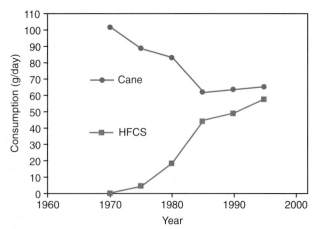

FIGURE 15-3 The consumption of high-fructose corn syrup (HFCS) and sugar (sucrose) over the years when the obesity epidemic developed. (Copyright 2005, George A. Bray, Baton Rouge, La.)

increase in BMI; during nearly 2 years of follow-up, those with the highest soft drink consumption at baseline had the highest increase in BMI. A Danish study[21] showed that individuals who consumed calorically sweetened beverages during 10 weeks gained weight, whereas subjects drinking the same amount of artificially sweetened beverages lost weight. In one study, children who were focusing on reducing intake of "fizzy" drinks and replacing them with water showed slower weight gain than those not advised to reduce the intake of fizzy drinks.[22] These studies strongly suggest that calorie-containing soft drinks could play a role in the epidemic of obesity. If so, then their consumption should be curtailed, particularly for very young children, and for schoolchildren, for whom beverages are a ready source of energy with few other nutrients.

Dietary fat is another component that may be related to the epidemic of obesity.[23,24] Fats contain more than twice the energy of carbohydrates (9 kcal/g). Foods combining fat and sugar may be a particular problem because they are often very palatable and usually inexpensive.[25] The Leeds Fat Study shows that people who were high-fat consumers have an increased incidence of obesity.[26] Providing palatable low-fat foods is important.

Several studies now show that when infants were given breast milk as the sole source of nutrition for more than 3 months, their risk of obesity was significantly reduced at the time of entry into school and in adolescence compared with infants who were not breast-fed or who were breast-fed for less than 3 months.[27,28] The composition of the breast milk may be important. Over the past 50 years the proportion of n-6 fatty acids in human milk has increased, reflecting changes in dietary fat composition. The amount of n-3 fatty acids in breast milk has remained constant. A higher amount of n-6 fatty acids provides prostaglandin derivatives that stimulate fat cell proliferation in infants.[27,29,30] This is a concept that needs further evaluation. The rate of weight gain between ages of 2 and 12 years also predicts future obesity; those children who gain the most weight have the highest risk of becoming obese. Monitoring weight change early can be predictive of future obesity.

Calcium intake is another dietary factor that may be related to the development of obesity in children and adults. The level of calcium intake in population studies is inversely correlated with the risk of being overweight. In other epidemiologic studies and in feeding trials, higher dietary calcium is associated with reduced BMI or reduced incidence of insulin resistance.[31,32] Calcium supplementation does not appear to be as effective as calcium from dairy products and other foods.

The cost of food is another factor in the cause of obesity. The price of items we buy influences our choices and the amount we buy. During the period from 1960 to 1980 the price of food rose more slowly than the other components in the consumer price index. Real wages also rose, providing additional money for consumption, some of which could buy a wider variety of healthy foods such as fresh fruits and vegetables, fish, and dairy products. This period was a time when

the rise in the prevalence of obesity was slow. However, between 1983 and 2009 the relative cost increase in these food items was much faster than the foods with higher energy density, which contain more fat and sugar. In this period the price of fresh fruits and vegetables rose 190%, fish by 100%, and dairy products by 82%. Contrast this with sugar and sweets, which increased 66%; fats and oils, 70%; and carbonated beverages, 32%.[5] This means that your food dollar will buy relatively more food energy if the foods contain more sugar and fat or are carbonated beverages.

Low Levels of Physical Activity

Epidemiologic data show that low levels of physical activity and watching more television predict higher body weight.[33] Recent studies suggest that individuals in American cities where they had to walk more tended to weigh less than those living in other cities. Low levels of physical activity also increase the risk of early mortality. The Aerobic Center Longitudinal Study was carried out with more than 80,000 individuals over a period of 35 years. Several studies based on this cohort addressed both the independent and combined effects of adiposity and fitness on death rate. These studies demonstrated that low fitness resulted in a greater risk of mortality than fatness, whereas fitness diminished the impact of fatness on mortality.[34] It is thus better to be thin than fat and to be physically active rather than inactive.

Drugs and Chemicals That Produce Weight Gain

Several drugs can cause weight gain, including a variety of hormones and psychoactive agents.[35] The degree of weight gain is generally not sufficient to cause substantial obesity, except occasionally in patients treated with high-dose corticosteroids, as well as some psychoactive drugs such as valproate. These drugs can also cause insulin resistance and increase the risk of developing type 2 diabetes mellitus.

Cessation of smoking is another environmental agent that will affect body fat stores. Partially mediated by nicotine withdrawal, a weight gain of 1 to 2 kg (2.2 to 4.4 lb) is seen in the first few weeks and is often followed by an additional 2- to 3-kg weight gain over the next 4 to 6 months, resulting in an average weight gain of 4 to 5 kg or more.[36]

Viruses as Environmental Causes of Obesity

The injection of several viruses into the central nervous system (CNS) produces obesity in mice. Recent findings of antibodies to one of the adenoviruses (Ad-36) in larger amounts in obese humans raises the possibility that viruses

---

KEY TERMS

incidence The number of new cases of a particular condition that develop over time. If among 1000 people, 10 people who were not overweight initially become overweight in 1 year, then the incidence rate would be 10 cases per 1000 person-years.

energy density The amount of energy or calories in a food compared with the weight of the food.

are involved in some cases.[37] The adenoviral syndrome can be replicated in nonhuman primates and is characterized by modest obesity and a low circulating cholesterol concentration. Further studies are needed to establish that a syndrome of obesity associated with low concentrations of cholesterol clearly exists in human beings. If so, then this would enhance the value of the epidemiologic model.

Toxins

In experimental animals, exposure in the neonatal period to monosodium glutamate (MSG), a common flavoring ingredient in food, produces obesity. A similar effect of reduction in glucose can also produce obesity, suggesting that the brain of the growing animal, and possibly that of human beings, may respond with damage to the "metabolic sensors" that regulate food needs. In human beings, we know that body fat stores many "toxic" chemicals that are mobilized with weight loss. The metabolic rate can be reduced by organochlorine molecules[38] and conceivably prolonged exposure to many chlorinated chemicals in our environment has affected metabolic pathways and energy metabolism.

Host
Genetic Factors

Several kinds of research indicate that genetic factors are important in regulating body weight and in whether we develop obesity. The first is family studies. For more than 75 years we have known that individuals from families with overweight parents are likely to be overweight. In contrast, individuals from families in which the parents are lean are likely to be lean. Adoption studies in which children are traced to their birth families show that the children are more like their biologic parents than like the parents who adopted them. Finally, studies in identical and nonidentical twins provide the icing on the cake, so to speak. When identical twins that have been reared in separate families from birth are identified, they are found to be more like each other than are nonidentical twins similarly reared apart. From these data we can place the role of genetic factors between 35% and 70% of the inheritance of obesity, meaning that if one individual in a given environment becomes overweight, it is highly likely that his or her identical twin would also become overweight. If one twin resists obesity, then the other identical twin would be very likely to resist obesity as well.

Further insight into the genetic causes of obesity has come from the cloning of several genes that produce obesity in human beings. Leptin, identified in 1994, was the first of these important gene products to be identified. As noted previously, it is produced in adipose tissue and secreted into the blood in relation to the amount of body fat.[39] Leptin-deficient individuals are massively obese from childhood. When they are treated with leptin, food intake falls and body fat is mobilized until body weight is nearly normalized, indicating that this is an important metabolic pathway for which the gene has been identified. This genetic defect is extremely rare, and most obese people have an appropriate level of circulating leptin for their size, indicating that there is an error in leptin

signaling either with the leptin receptor or a downstream pathway.

The most common single gene defect in obese children and adults is in the melanocortin-4 receptor, a key regulator of food intake.[39,40] When this receptor is inactive, food intake is nearly as high as when leptin is deficient. When this receptor is only partially inactivated, the food intake is only modestly beyond control levels.

Several other rare genetic defects have been identified in the regulatory process for controlling food intake that, when abnormal, lead to obesity. These basic biologic insights tell us that body fat has important regulation that is largely, if not completely, independent of willpower.

Intrauterine Imprinting

Several intrauterine events may lead to obesity later in life, probably because of fetal imprinting as a result of early exposure that affects brain plasticity. The Dutch winter famine of 1945 showed that starvation of infants *in utero* could affect long-term postnatal weight status. Another example is the infants of mothers who smoked during pregnancy; these infants have an increased risk of becoming overweight during their first three decades of life when compared with infants of mothers who did not smoke during pregnancy.[41] Similarly, infants of mothers who have diabetes are at higher risk of developing obesity than infants born to mothers who did not have diabetes during pregnancy.[42] Infants who are small for their birth date are at higher risk of developing central adiposity and diabetes than normal-weight infants. Finally, experimental studies teach us that exposure to high levels of insulin during the period of brain plasticity can lead to obesity later in life.

Physiologic Control

To maintain a stable body weight over time, the body must correct daily errors in energy balance. A number of physiologic factors are known to disturb this correction. Overall, low metabolic rate may also predict future weight gain,[43] but conversely, a high rate of carbohydrate oxidation, as measured by a high respiratory quotient (RQ) predicts future weight gain.[44] One explanation is that when carbohydrate oxidation is higher than carbohydrate intake, carbohydrate stores are depleted, and we must eat to replace them. Obese individuals who have lost weight are less effective in increasing fat oxidation in the presence of a high-fat meal than normal-weight individuals, and this may be one reason why they are so susceptible to weight regain.

Fat cells in our body serve two major functions: (1) They store and release fatty acids ingested from food or from liver or fat cells, and (2) they secrete many important hormones and chemicals. The discovery of leptin catapulted the

---

KEY TERM
insulin Hormone produced by the pancreas that lowers blood glucose by enhancing its entry into cells.

fat cell into the arena of endocrine cells.[45] In addition to leptin, the fat cell secretes a variety of other peptides (lipoprotein lipase, adipsin [complement D], complement C, adiponectin, TNF-α, IL-6, PAI-1, angiotensinogen, bradykinin, and resistin). The fat cell also releases other metabolites such as lactate, fatty acids, glycerol, and prostacyclin. Our understanding of fat cells as important endocrine cells continues to expand.

Production of cortisol from inactive cortisone in fat cells by the enzyme 11β-hydroxysteroid dehydrogenase type 1 may be important in determining the quantity of visceral adipose tissue.[46] Changes in this enzyme may contribute to the risk menopausal women face in developing more visceral fat. High levels of this enzyme keep the quantity of cortisol in visceral fat high, providing a fertile environment for the development of new fat cells.

Increased visceral fat seems to result in a high level of proinflammatory cytokines. The ratio of visceral fat is proportional to the risk for development of metabolic and cardiovascular problems associated with obesity. Interestingly, if a substantial amount of visceral fat is surgically removed, then insulin resistance is immediately improved.[47]

Information about hunger and satiety comes from the gastrointestinal (GI) tract, where several peptides signal the body to stop or start eating. Ghrelin has received recent attention because, in contrast to other GI hormones, it stimulates food intake.[48] Levels of ghrelin are low in obesity, except for Prader-Willi syndrome, suggesting that it may play a role.

The brain is a receiver, transducer, and transmitter of information about hunger and satiety. Several neurotransmitter systems are involved in regulation of food intake.[49] Serotonin receptors modulate the quantity of food eaten and macronutrient selection, and their loss through genetic targeting produces obesity. Peptide neurotransmitters also play a very important role in the regulation of feeding. Sleep deprivation is one way to enhance the release of peptides that produce hunger.[50,51] In young men allowed to sleep only 4 hours per night for 2 days, leptin decreased and ghrelin increased relative to the pattern seen with 10 hours of sleep on each of 2 nights.

OVERVIEW OF TREATING THE DISEASE OF OBESITY

Prevention of the Current Epidemic

The epidemic of obesity occurs on a genetic background that has not changed significantly in the past 100 years and certainly not since the epidemic began 30 years ago. Nonetheless, it is clear that genetic factors play a critical role in the susceptibility of becoming obese in a "toxic environment."[52] One analogy is that "genes load the gun and a permissive or toxic environment pulls the trigger." Modification of environmental factors that act on our ancient genes must be the strategy to prevent the disease. The belief that this can be done by the individual alone is to miss the argument of how environmental factors have acted on these genes to produce the current

epidemic, with major emphasis on the imprinting of the plastic brain of the growing child and adolescent.

We argue that the first law of thermodynamics has lulled us into the uncomfortable position of believing that individuals, through willpower, increased food choices, or more places to exercise can overcome the current epidemic of obesity. Cognitive approaches relying on individual commitment and resolve have been unsuccessful in stemming the epidemic, and nothing suggests that they will be more successful in the future.

We also argue that it is what the first law of thermodynamics does not tell us that is important. In this context it is the unconscious host systems on which environmental factors operate that produces the disease. If the vending machines now in schools contained beverages with no added sugar or HFCS, then available calories would be reduced. We have argued that the exposure of young children to HFCS may produce detrimental imprinting of the brain, making obesity more likely and more difficult to control.

At least three preventive strategies are available to deal with the epidemic: (1) education, (2) regulation, and (3) modification of the food supply. Education in the school curriculum about good nutrition and healthy weight would be beneficial in helping all children learn how to select appropriate foods. School breakfast and lunch programs should match the educational messages.

It is unwise to rely on educational strategies alone, because they have not prevented the obesity epidemic. Regulation is a second strategy. Regulating an improved food label would be one good idea. Regulations on appropriate serving sizes in packages and nutrition information provided by restaurants might be part of the solution. Headway is being made in these areas due to public pressure.

Modification in some components of the food system is a third and most important strategy. Because the energy we eat comes from food, we need to modify this system to provide less energy density if we are to succeed in combating the epidemic of obesity.

Treatment of Overweight People When Prevention Fails

A detailed discussion of treatment for obesity is beyond the scope of this chapter, but a few general comments about the major approaches are essential because they involve food intake and exercise. Although prevention is unlikely to be successful by relying solely on individual initiative, treatment requires individual initiative. For any change to occur, the individual must be ready for change. This idea of "stages of change" is a key component of any individual approach. The overweight person must be aware that he or she has a problem and must have moved beyond the stage of precontemplation (i.e., the stage of denial before a person is willing to do something about a problem) and into a stage of contemplation and then to action. When overweight individuals are in this state, they are ready to move forward. Their options are diet, exercise, behavioral therapy, medication, and surgery. These are the principal approaches available to those who have a weight problem that they want to address. The use of diet, exercise, and behavioral therapy are appropriate for all levels of overweight.

Dietetic professionals can play an important role in all of these approaches. First, the educated dietetic professional needs to be keenly aware of the complexity of the obesity problem. The dietitian obviously cannot alter the genetic makeup of an individual but is able to address the environmental aspects that serve to exacerbate the situation. Simply handing out diet sheets will not work. Helping obese patients requires attention to their overall diet history, current eating and activity patterns, and behavioral obstacles that either cause problems or prevent change. Although quick weight loss may be a patient's immediate desire, permanent lifestyle changes should be the primary objective. Tips for addressing this have been outlined by Bray and Champagne (Box 15-1).[53] Finally, the dietitian can be an instrument of change by appealing to policymakers to modify environmental conditions such as the school vending machine situation cited previously.

Diet

Popular diets have been published for more than 150 years; obviously, if any diet were significantly better than the others, it would have "won the battle" and the others would have disappeared. Popular diets can be grouped into several categories: low-energy (calorie) diets, low-fat diets, low-carbohydrate diets, and high-protein diets. A summary of data abstracted by the U.S. Department of Agriculture (USDA) is shown in Table 15-1.

Several popular diets, including the Atkins Diet (low carbohydrate), the Ornish (low fat), Weight Watchers, and the Zone diet (high protein), were recently compared and found to produce comparable weight loss, suggesting that none of these diets is better than the other.[54] A randomized clinical trial that compared reduced-calorie diets with different macronutrient targets (low or high fat, average or high protein, low or high carbohydrate) determined that any type of reduced-calorie diet can be effective in achieving weight loss.[55]

Exercise

Increased movement, both modest and vigorous, is a way to increase energy expenditure that will burn fat deposits. Human beings expend approximately two thirds of their energy with basal activities, including maintaining body temperature, and only approximately one third in various activities. Thus to expend a significant number of calories through exercise takes time. As a rule of thumb, approximately 100 kcal are expended for each mile walked. If it takes 15 minutes to walk a mile, then you could expend up to

---

BOX 15-1 PRACTICE POINTS FOR THE CLINICAL DIETITIAN

- *Focus on personal history:* More than ever, the personal history of the patient is a critical focus area for the dietitian in clinical practice who deals with patients diagnosed with the metabolic syndrome. In particular, assessment of past dietary habits using a valid food frequency questionnaire is warranted. The current dietary practices of the patient can help to highlight target areas; collecting a food record for as many days as the patient is willing to keep it will be instrumental in future counseling efforts.

- *Obtain thorough information:* Encouraging the patient to provide as much dietary information as possible will make a measurable difference in the accuracy of the dietary data for evaluation purposes. Remember to focus on the fact that no judgments will be formed; you are simply identifying areas of diet for which you will be targeting change.

- *Assess exercise habits:* Physical activity patterns are useful for designing the total lifestyle program. The dietitian may choose to collect a physical activity questionnaire from the patient and, in addition, provide the patient with an activity monitor to assess actual physical activity steps for a more accurate appraisal of daily activity levels.

- *Customize:* For increased success, dietary treatment needs to be highly individualized. It may be helpful to include a variety of weight-loss strategies, such as meal replacements (for quicker initial weight loss), slightly higher protein diets, low-fat diets, and perhaps even a Mediterranean diet approach. An important point to remember: What works for one patient may not necessarily be ideal for another.

- *Consult the physician:* Working with the patient's physician to provide the ideal combination of diet, physical activity suggestions, behavior changes, and medication (if prescribed by the physician) is key to the patient's success.

- *Follow-up:* Regular evaluations to monitor patient progress are key to weight management by the physician and the dietitian in clinical practice.

Data from Bray GA, Champagne CM: Obesity and the metabolic syndrome: implications for dietetics practitioners. *J Am Diet Assoc* 104:86, 2004.

TABLE 15-1 FEATURES OF THE MAJOR DIETS USED BY AMERICANS

TYPE OF DIET	CALORIES	FAT, g (%)	CARBOHYDRATE, g (%)	PROTEIN, g (%)
Typical American diet	2200	85 (35)	274 (50)	82 (15)
High-fat, low-carbohydrate diet	1400	94 (60)	35 (10)	105 (30)
Moderate-fat diet	1450	40 (25)	218 (60)	54 (15)
Low-fat and very-low-fat diet	1450	16-24 (10-15)	235-271 (65-75)	54-72 (15-20)

Modified from Freedman MR, King J, Kennedy E: Popular diets: a scientific review. *Obes Res* 9(Suppl):1S, 2001, with permission from NAASO, The Obesity Society.

400 kcal in an hour of brisk walking. From a practical point of view it is often easier to eat 400 kcal less than to exercise for the extra 400 kcal. Despite the relatively large effort to burn a considerable amount of energy with physical activity, people who exercise more have been shown to have greater weight-loss maintenance than did those who exercised less.[56] This observation may be due to an increase in lean mass with the physically active, which would increase basal energy expenditure.

Behavioral Therapy

Since their introduction in 1967, behavioral approaches to helping overweight individuals focus on the issues that revolve around eating have been a cornerstone in the treatment of obesity. These techniques are adapted from psychologic learning theory, in which rewarding appropriate behavior tends to reinforce that behavior. The process involves familiarity with the activities associated with learning and providing consequences of eating, as well as rewards that reinforce appropriate behaviors. Among the successful techniques in this area are self-monitoring, increased physical activity, and eating a lower-fat diet. People who are successful at maintaining a lowered body weight over time use these and other techniques.

Medication

Currently only six medications are approved by the U.S. Food and Drug Administration (FDA) for the treatment of obesity. These include five drugs that have only been approved for short-term use (**benzphetamine** [Didrex], **diethylpropion** [Tenuate], **phendimetrazine** [Adipost, Anorex-SR, Appecon, Bontril PDM, Bontril Slow Release, Melfiat, Obezine, Phendiet, Plegine, Prelu-2, Statobex], **phentermine** [Adipex-P, Fastin, Ionamin, Obenix, Obephen, Oby-Cap, Oby-Trim, Panshape M, Phentercot, Phentride, Pro-Fast HS, Pro-Fast SA, Pro-Fast SR, Teramine, Zantryl], and a combination of phentermine and **topiramate** [Qsymia]) and two drugs that have been approved for longer-term use—**orlistat** (Alli, Xenical) and **lorcaserin** (Belviq).

Researchers believe that all of the drugs except for orlistat work by modifying the neurotransmitters in the CNS. Some of these drugs work in part by binding to molecules on the surface of brain cells (neurons) that transport neurotransmitters back into these neurons after they have been secreted. Because the short-term drugs are related to the addictive drug amphetamine, albeit quite indirectly, the U.S. government regulates their use through the Drug Enforcement Administration (DEA). Topiramate was originally sold as an anticonvulsant medication that was found to have the side effect of weight loss by increasing feelings of fullness, making foods taste less appealing, and increasing energy expenditure. In clinical studies with these drugs, the weight loss is approximately 4 to 5 kg (8.8 to 11 lb) more than with placebo controls after 6 to 12 months of treatment. To be eligible for use of medications, an individual needs to have a BMI greater than 30 kg/m², unless associated problems exist, such as diabetes, heart disease, high blood pressure, or other

problems that would benefit from weight loss. In that case, the lower limit for use of medications may be 27 kg/m² (see the Diet-Medications Interactions table, "Drugs Used to Treat Obesity").

Orlistat contrasts with these centrally acting drugs. It works in the intestine to block an enzyme called *lipase*, which is produced and secreted from the **pancreas**. At clinically used doses, it blocks digestion of approximately one third of the dietary fat. This dietary fat then passes through the intestinal tract and exits the body in the feces. When used improperly, this drug can produce significant GI tract symptoms. In clinical studies this drug produces 2 to 4 kg (4.4 to 8.8 lb) more weight loss than placebo-treated groups and appears to be slightly less effective than the other types of drugs.[57]

Surgery

Use of bariatric surgery for treatment of obesity has expanded greatly with the rising obesity rate.[58] Several different types of operations are currently in use for treatment of

---

KEY TERMS

benzphetamine One of the appetite-suppressant drugs that has been approved for more than 30 years for short-term use but that is regulated by the U.S. Drug Enforcement Agency (DEA) because of potential for addictive abuse (trade name, Didrex).

diethylpropion One of the appetite-suppressant drugs that has been approved for more than 30 years for short-term use but that is regulated by the DEA because of potential for addictive abuse (trade name, Tenuate).

phendimetrazine One of the appetite-suppressant drugs that has been approved for more than 30 years for short-term use but that is regulated by the DEA because of potential for addictive abuse; trade names, Adipost, Anorex-SR, Appecon, Bontril PDM, Bontril Slow Release, Melfiat, Obezine, Phendiet, Plegine, Prelu-2, and Statobex.

phentermine One of the appetite-suppressant drugs that has been approved for more than 30 years for short-term use but that is regulated by the DEA because of potential for addictive abuse; trade names, Adipex-P, Fastin, Ionamin, Obenix, Obephen, Oby-Cap, Oby-Trim, Panshape M, Phentercot, Phentride, Pro-Fast HS, Pro-Fast SA, Pro-Fast SR, Teramine, and Zantryl.

orlistat Drug (trade name, Xenical) that partially blocks pancreatic lipase, thus decreasing digestion of dietary fat. It is available by prescription and over the counter; trade names, Alli and Zenical.

lorcaserin Drug (trade name, Belviq) approved as an appetite suppressant in 2012 that works through a serotonergic pathway.

pancreas Gland located near the duodenum and small intestine that has two sets of cells: (1) acinar cells, which secrete digestive enzymes into the intestine, and (2) beta cells, which produce and secrete insulin into the blood.

topiramate Originally used as an anticonvulsant, drug was approved in 2012 to be used in combination with phentermine for weight loss under the trade name Qsymia.

DIET-MEDICATIONS INTERACTIONS

Drugs Used to Treat Obesity

Generic Name	Trade Name	Mechanism of Action	Food-Drug Interactions
Benzphetamine	Didrex	Appetite suppressant, stimulates CNS and decreases appetite (similar to amphetamine); short-term use only	Alcohol may increase the dizziness effects of this medicine.
Diethylpropion	Tenuate, Tenuate Dospan		
Phendimetrazine	Adipost, Anorex-SR, Appecon, Bontril PDM, Bontril Slow-Release, Melfiat, Obezine, Phendiet, Plegine, Prelu-2, Statobex		A reduced-calorie diet must be followed while using an appetite suppressant to lose weight. In addition, to keep the lost weight from returning, changes in diet and exercise must be continued after the weight has been lost.
Phentermine	Adipex-P, Fastin, Ionamin, Obenix, Obephen, Oby-Cap, Oby-Trim, Panshape M, Phentercot, Phentride, Pro-Fast HS, Pro-Fast SA, Pro-Fast SR, Teramine, Zantryl		
Phentermine/ Topiramate	Qsymia	Appetite suppressant, makes foods taste less appealing, and increases energy expenditure	Alcohol produces several interactions with this medication.
Orlistat	Alli, Xenical	Blocks fat from being absorbed in intestine	This drug prevents the absorption of some dietary fat. It should be taken during the meal or within 1 hour of eating and may decrease absorption of fat-soluble vitamins from food. A multivitamin supplement should be taken once a day at least 2 hours before or after taking orlistat.
			The diet should contain no more than 30% of calories as fat; more fat in the diet will increase side effects.
			Patients who have diabetes mellitus may need to have their insulin or oral hypoglycemic agents adjusted.
			Patients may experience gas with leaky bowel movements, inability to hold bowel movements, increased bowel movements, oily bowel movements, and oily spotting of underclothes.
Lorcaserin	Belviq	Works on serotonergic system	A reduced-calorie diet must be observed in conjunction with the medication to lose weight and keep it off.
			Extreme caution is warranted with other serotonergic drugs such as antidepressants or antipsychotics.

obesity. Usually the stomach is restricted, part of the small intestine is bypassed, or both. To be eligible for surgical intervention, an overweight individual needs to have a BMI greater than 40 kg/m², unless the person has associated diseases such as diabetes, heart disease, sleep apnea, or osteoarthritis, in which case the BMI for considering therapy can be lowered to 35 kg/m². Gastric bypass is associated with the near-elimination of type 2 diabetes and improvements in cardiovascular risk factors, sleep apnea, and quality of life. Side effects include dumping syndrome, which produces nausea, flushing, bloating, and extreme diarrhea. Weight loss after surgery is greatest over the first 12 months and continues until about 18 months. Patients lose an average of 60% of excess weight after gastric bypass and 40% after gastric restriction. At 2 years after surgery, 30% of patients have regained some weight.[59] Weight regain is associated with reduced remission of type 2 diabetes. Bariatric surgery patients should participate in nutrition education and support group programs to ameliorate weight regain. More data are needed on the long-term effects of bariatric surgery.

HEALTH PROMOTION

Our lives are constrained by the laws of nature—gravity, momentum, and thermodynamics—with which we have been dealing in this chapter. The strategies we take to deal with the influence of these laws on our lives include education, regulation, and product design. Deaths from the effects of the laws of momentum produced by automobile accidents provide a glimpse into the strategies we could use to minimize this effect. They also provide insights into the strategies that may be needed to deal with the epidemic of obesity. Although the laws of momentum or the laws of thermodynamics cannot be changed, their effect on producing automobile accidents and obesity can be mitigated. This goal can be achieved through better education about driving and about nutritional needs to prevent obesity. Just as educating drivers about the dangers of speeding and not wearing seatbelts may not always cause a change in behavior, educating people about the dangers of being overweight and energy balance may not affect the diet of many people. Education can be complemented in the case of cars by regulations that require seat belts, air bags, and other safety devices. In the case of obesity it can be complemented by limiting access to large portion sizes and to high-energy–density foods, as well as creating an environment in which physical activity is more prevalent. Finally, product design to make cars safer partly addresses the driving problem, just as modifying the types of foods that are available and food prices may help to combat the obesity epidemic by redesigning the food environment.

TO SUM UP

Obesity is a chronic, relapsing disease characterized by an accumulation of excess body fat caused by habitual consumption of more energy than is used. Normally, physiologic systems hold the body in energy balance, but environmental factors such as food, medications, physical inactivity, toxins, and viruses can interact with the host's genetic predisposition to gain weight. Obesity is a major health issue because it increases the risk for many other chronic diseases (especially type 2 diabetes), raises health care costs, and may produce psychologic stress. The increased prevalence of obesity in the past few decades has been attributed to a "toxic environment" of abundant high-energy foods with little need for physical activity. Reversing this trend requires a better understanding of how environmental factors affect the development of obesity and a redesigning of these factors.

QUESTIONS FOR REVIEW

1. Why is obesity considered to be a disease?
2. What are the psychologic, pathologic, and financial effects of obesity?
3. Why are adipose cells considered to be endocrine cells?
4. Explain how portion sizes may contribute to obesity.
5. How does high fructose corn syrup contribute to obesity?
6. What is the function of leptin?
7. What have twin studies shown about obesity?
8. What are three prevention strategies for dealing with the obesity epidemic?
9. What is the most effective popular diet?
10. What criteria must a person meet to qualify for weight loss surgery?

Acknowledgments

The author wishes to thank George A. Bray and Catherine M. Champagne for their contributions to this chapter in the previous edition.

REFERENCES

1. Ogden CL, Carroll MD, Kit BK, et al: Prevalence of obesity in the United States, 2009-2010. *NCHS Data Brief* 1, 2012.
2. Flegal KM, Carroll MD, Kit BK, et al: Prevalence of obesity and trends in the distribution of body mass index among US adults, 1999-2010. *JAMA* 307:491, 2012.
3. Wang Y, Beydoun MA: The obesity epidemic in the United States–gender, age, socioeconomic, racial/ethnic, and geographic characteristics: a systematic review and meta-regression analysis. *Epidemiol Rev* 29:6, 2007.
4. Kopelman PG: Obesity as a medical problem. *Nature* 404:635, 2000.
5. Finkelstein EA, Strombotne KL: The economics of obesity. *Am J Clin Nutr* 91:1520S, 2010.
6. Trogdon JG, Finkelstein EA, Hylands T, et al: Indirect costs of obesity: a review of the current literature. *Obes Rev* 9:489, 2008.
7. Knowler WC, Barrett-Connor E, Fowler SE, et al: Reduction in the incidence of type 2 diabetes with lifestyle intervention or metformin. *N Engl J Med* 346:393, 2002.

8. Unick JL, Beavers D, Bond DS, et al: The long-term effectiveness of a lifestyle intervention in severely obese individuals. *Am J Med* 126(236):242, 2013.

9. Puhl RM, King KM: Weight discrimination and bullying. *Best Pract Res Clin Endocrinol Metab* 27:117, 2013.

10. de Jonge L, Nguyen T, Smith SR, et al: Prediction of energy expenditure in a whole body indirect calorimeter at both low and high levels of physical activity. *Int J Obes Relat Metab Disord* 25:929, 2001.

11. Smith SR, de Jonge L, Zachwieja JJ, et al: Concurrent physical activity increases fat oxidation during the shift to a high-fat diet. *Am J Clin Nutr* 72:131, 2000.

12. Kinsell LW, Gunning B, Michaels GD, et al: Calories do count. *Metabolism* 13:195, 1964.

13. Lyon XH, Di VV, Milon H, et al: Compliance to dietary advice directed towards increasing the carbohydrate to fat ratio of the everyday diet. *Int J Obes Relat Metab Disord* 19:260, 1995.

14. Licinio J, Caglayan S, Ozata M, et al: Phenotypic effects of leptin replacement on morbid obesity, diabetes mellitus, hypogonadism, and behavior in leptin-deficient adults. *Proc Natl Acad Sci U S A* 101:4531, 2004.

15. Stern JS, Hirsch J, Blair SN, et al: Weighing the options: criteria for evaluating weight-management programs. The Committee to Develop Criteria for Evaluating the Outcomes of Approaches to Prevent and Treat Obesity. *Obes Res* 3:591, 1995.

16. Young LR, Nestle M: Reducing portion sizes to prevent obesity: a call to action. *Am J Prev Med* 43:565, 2012.

17. Bray GA, Popkin BM: Calorie-sweetened beverages and fructose: what have we learned 10 years later. *Pediatr Obes* 8:242, 2013.

18. Morgan RE: Does consumption of high-fructose corn syrup beverages cause obesity in children? *Pediatr Obes* 8:249, 2013.

19. Stanhope KL, Schwarz JM, Havel PJ: Adverse metabolic effects of dietary fructose: results from the recent epidemiological, clinical, and mechanistic studies. *Curr Opin Lipidol* 24:198, 2013.

20. Ludwig DS, Peterson KE, Gortmaker SL: Relation between consumption of sugar-sweetened drinks and childhood obesity: a prospective, observational analysis. *Lancet* 357:505, 2001.

21. Raben A, Agerholm-Larsen L, Flint A, et al: Meals with similar energy densities but rich in protein, fat, carbohydrate, or alcohol have different effects on energy expenditure and substrate metabolism but not on appetite and energy intake. *Am J Clin Nutr* 77:91, 2003.

22. James J, Thomas P, Cavan D, et al: Preventing childhood obesity by reducing consumption of carbonated drinks: cluster randomised controlled trial. *BMJ* 328:1237, 2004.

23. Astrup A, Ryan L, Grunwald GK, et al: The role of dietary fat in body fatness: evidence from a preliminary meta-analysis of ad libitum low-fat dietary intervention studies. *Br J Nutr* 83(Suppl 1):S25–S32, 2000.

24. Bray GA, Popkin BM: Dietary fat intake does affect obesity! *Am J Clin Nutr* 68:1157, 1998.

25. Drewnowski A, Rehm CD: Energy intakes of US children and adults by food purchase location and by specific food source. *Nutr J* 12:59, 2013.

26. Blundell JE, Macdiarmid JI: Fat as a risk factor for overconsumption: satiation, satiety, and patterns of eating. *J Am Diet Assoc* 97:S63–S69, 1997.

27. Beyerlein A, Toschke AM, von Kries R: Breastfeeding and childhood obesity: shift of the entire BMI distribution or only the upper parts? *Obesity* 16:2730, 2008.

28. von Kries R, Koletzko B, Sauerwald T, et al: Breast feeding and obesity: cross sectional study. *BMJ* 319:147, 1999.

29. Young BE, Johnson SL, Krebs NF: Biological determinants linking infant weight gain and child obesity: current knowledge and future directions. *Adv Nutr* 3:675, 2012.

30. Muhlhausler BS, Ailhaud GP: Omega-6 polyunsaturated fatty acids and the early origins of obesity. *Curr Opin Endocrinol Diabetes Obes* 20:56, 2013.

31. de Oliveira Freitas DM, Stampini Duarte Martino H, Machado Rocha Ribeiro S, et al: Calcium ingestion and obesity control. *Nutr Hosp* 27:1758, 2012.

32. Huang L, Xue J, He Y, et al: Dietary calcium but not elemental calcium from supplements is associated with body composition and obesity in Chinese women. *PLoS One* 6:e27703, 2011.

33. Erik LC, Poulton R, Welch D, et al: Programming obesity and poor fitness: the long-term impact of childhood television. *Obesity (Silver Spring)* 16:1457, 2008.

34. Hainer V, Toplak H, Stich V: Fat or fit: what is more important? *Diabetes Care* 32(Suppl 2):S392–S397, 2009.

35. Heal DJ, Gosden J, Jackson HC, et al: Metabolic consequences of antipsychotic therapy: preclinical and clinical perspectives on diabetes, diabetic ketoacidosis, and obesity. *Handb Exp Pharmacol* (212):135, 2012.

36. O'Hara P, Connett JE, Lee WW, et al: Early and late weight gain following smoking cessation in the Lung Health Study. *Am J Epidemiol* 148:821, 1998.

37. Esposito S, Preti V, Consolo S, et al: Adenovirus 36 infection and obesity. *J Clin Virol* 55:95, 2012.

38. Tremblay A, Chaput JP: About unsuspected potential determinants of obesity. *Appl Physiol Nutr Metab* 33:791, 2008.

39. Zhang Y, Scarpace PJ: The role of leptin in leptin resistance and obesity. *Physiol Behav* 88:249, 2006.

40. O'Rahilly S, Farooqi IS, Yeo GS, et al: Minireview: human obesity–lessons from monogenic disorders. *Endocrinology* 144:3757, 2003.

41. Toschke AM, Ehlin AG, von Kries R, et al: Maternal smoking during pregnancy and appetite control in offspring. *J Perinat Med* 31:251, 2003.

42. Dabelea D, Pettitt DJ, Hanson RL, et al: Birth weight, type 2 diabetes, and insulin resistance in Pima Indian children and young adults. *Diabetes Care* 22:944, 1999.

43. Astrup A, Gotzsche PC, van de Werken K, et al: Meta-analysis of resting metabolic rate in formerly obese subjects. *Am J Clin Nutr* 69:1117, 1999.

44. Zurlo F, Lillioja S, Esposito-Del Puente A, et al: Low ratio of fat to carbohydrate oxidation as predictor of weight gain: study of 24-h RQ. *Am J Physiol* 259:E650–E657, 1990.

45. Spiegelman BM, Flier JS: Obesity and the regulation of energy balance. *Cell* 104:531, 2001.

46. Hochberg Z, Friedberg M, Yaniv L, et al: Hypothalamic regulation of adiposity: the role of 11beta-hydroxysteroid dehydrogenase type 1. *Horm Metab Res* 36:365, 2004.

47. Esposito K, Giugliano G, Scuderi N, et al: Role of adipokines in the obesity-inflammation relationship: the effect of fat removal. *Plast Reconstr Surg* 118:1048, 2006.

48. Altman J: Weight in the balance. *Neuroendocrinology* 76:131, 2002.

49. Blundell JE, Goodson S, Halford JC: Regulation of appetite: role of leptin in signalling systems for drive and satiety. *Int J Obes Relat Metab Disord* 25(Suppl 1):S29–S34, 2001.

50. Van Cauter E, Holmback U, Knutson K, et al: Impact of sleep and sleep loss on neuroendocrine and metabolic function. *Horm Res* 67(Suppl 1):2, 2007.

51. Spiegel K, Tasali E, Penev P, et al: Brief communication: sleep curtailment in healthy young men is associated with decreased leptin levels, elevated ghrelin levels, and increased hunger and appetite. *Ann Intern Med* 141:846, 2004.

52. Rankinen T, Zuberi A, Chagnon YC, et al: The human obesity gene map: the 2005 update. *Obesity (Silver Spring)* 14:529, 2006.

53. Bray GA, Champagne CM: Obesity and the metabolic syndrome: implications for dietetics practitioners. *J Am Diet Assoc* 104:86, 2004.

54. Dansinger ML, Gleason JA, Griffith JL, et al: Comparison of the Atkins, Ornish, Weight Watchers, and Zone diets for weight loss and heart disease risk reduction: a randomized trial. *JAMA* 293:43, 2005.

55. Sacks FM, Bray GA, Carey VJ, et al: Comparison of weight-loss diets with different compositions of fat, protein, and carbohydrates. *N Engl J Med* 360:859, 2009.

56. Anderson JW, Konz EC, Frederich RC, et al: Long-term weight-loss maintenance: a meta-analysis of US studies. *Am J Clin Nutr* 74:579, 2001.

57. Rodgers RJ, Tschop MH, Wilding JP: Anti-obesity drugs: past, present and future. *Dis Model Mech* 5:621, 2012.

58. Noria SF, Grantcharov T: Biological effects of bariatric surgery on obesity-related comorbidities. *Can J Surg* 56:47, 2013.

59. Hsu LK, Benotti PN, Dwyer J, et al: Nonsurgical factors that influence the outcome of bariatric surgery: a review. *Psychosom Med* 60:338, 1998.

Introduction to Clinical Nutrition

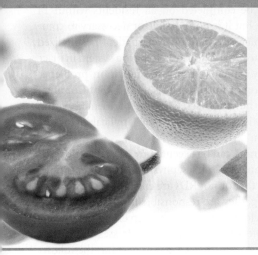

Nutrition Assessment and Nutrition Therapy in Patient Care

Ritamarie Little

OUTLINE

Role of Nutrition in Clinical Care

Nutrition Screening and Assessment

Nutrition Diagnosis

Nutrition Intervention: Food Plan and Management

Evaluation: Quality Patient Care

In this chapter, we focus on the Nutrition Care Process (NCP), which is the foundation of nutrition therapy. Information gathered during nutrition assessment is used to establish goals for nutrition intervention. Once interventions are initiated, monitoring and evaluation function as the point of reference from which to determine efficacy of treatment.

Nutrition assessment is defined as a "process used to evaluate nutritional status, identify disorders of nutrition, and determine which individuals need nutrition instruction and/or nutrition support."[1] Because no single test measures nutritional status, nutrition assessment draws from numerous indexes to provide a complete picture of nutritional health.[2]

ROLE OF NUTRITION IN CLINICAL CARE

Nutrition therapy plays an essential role in disease management, health care, and preventive health care and should be provided by a qualified nutrition professional.[2,3] Comprehensive nutrition assessment provides the necessary foundation for appropriate nutrition therapy based on identified needs. Nutrition assessment and nutrition therapy promote multiple goals: assisting patients in recovery from illness or injury, helping persons maintain follow-up care to promote health, and helping to control health care costs.[4] Registered dietitians (RDs) use their expertise and skills to make sound clinical judgments and to work effectively with the clinical care team. These professionals provide an essential component for successful management of the patient's plan of care.

Nutritional Status

Nutritional status can be established by measuring indicators of nutrient stores. Variations of nutrient stores result in changes in nutritional status when nutrient needs and nutrient use are increased or alterations in nutrient intake occur. Inadequacy or excess of a particular nutrient produces physiologic alteration in the body.[2]

Malnutrition

Many patients are malnourished when admitted to the hospital, whereas others may develop malnutrition during their hospital stay.[5] Hospitalized patients with hypermetabolic and physiologic stress of illness or injury can be at risk for malnutrition from increased nutritional needs. Hospital operating guidelines that provide for nutrition screening on admission, combined with follow-up monitoring, will identify patients at malnutrition risk and provide essential medical nutrition therapy.[2] However, potential problems arising from hospital routines may contribute to a lack of adequate nourishment in some cases, including the following:

- Highly restricted diets remaining on order and unsupplemented too long
- Unserved meals because of interference of medical procedures and clinical tests
- Unmonitored patient appetite

Each injured or ill patient is a unique person and requires special treatment and care. A formidable array of staff persons

BOX 16-1 BODY MASS INDEX

Calculating BMI

$$BMI = \frac{Weight\ (kg)}{Height^2\ (m)}\ or\ BMI = \frac{Weight\ (lb)}{Height^2\ (in)} \times 704.5$$

Example: An individual weighs 65 kg (143 lb) and is 1.7 m (5 feet 7 inches) tall. BMI = $65/(1.7)^2$ = 22.5 kg/m^2

Classification of BMI
Underweight: <18.5
Normal: 18.5-24.9
Overweight: 25.0-29.9
Obese: ≥30.0
Extreme obesity: ≥40.0

From Moore MC: *Pocket guide to nutrition assessment and care,* ed 6, St Louis, Mo., 2009, Mosby.

seek to determine needs and implement what each patient requires as appropriate care. When individual human needs are met with personal care, within the context of carefully developed care protocols, patients will not feel intimidated and powerless.

Undernutrition: Undernutrition subsequent to insufficient intake; altered digestion; or absorption of protein, energy, or both (calories); is called *protein-energy malnutrition (PEM)* or *protein-calorie malnutrition (PCM).* Characteristics include weight loss, fat loss, muscle wasting and weakness, impaired immune function, poor wound healing, and reduction of protein synthesis.[1]

Overnutrition: More than two thirds of American adults are overweight or obese,[6] making these conditions the two most common forms of overnutrition.[1] Overweight is defined as body mass index (BMI) greater than 25 and obesity as BMI greater than 30 (Box 16-1). Both are associated with a number of health risks including coronary heart disease, type 2 diabetes mellitus, certain cancers (breast, endometrial, colon), hypertension, dyslipidemia, stroke, gallbladder disease, liver disease, sleep apnea, osteoarthritis, and infertility.[7]

NUTRITION SCREENING AND ASSESSMENT

Patients at nutritional risk need to be identified to allow provision of high-quality nutrition care.[8] Poor nutritional status may create complications that may lead to increased morbidity and mortality, length of stay, and cost of care.[9] Identification of nutrition risk is accomplished through the process of nutritional assessment. However, before patients can be assessed, they must first be identified. Identification takes place through the process of nutrition screening, the entry into the NCP (Box 16-2).[10,11]

Nutrition Screening

Nutrition screening is defined as "the process of identifying characteristics known to be associated with nutrition problems with the purpose of identifying individuals who are malnourished or at nutritional risk."[8,11] In long-term care,

assessments must be completed on all residents within 14 days of admission, but it is not possible or necessary to complete a full nutrition assessment on every patient hospitalized in acute care. It is necessary, however, to have a system in place to quickly identify patients at risk for nutrition problems, such as malnutrition or nutritional risk.[2] The Joint Commission requires that nutrition screening be performed within 24 hours of inpatient admission when applicable for the patient's condition.[12]

Nutrition screening can be executed by RDs, dietetic technicians, dietary managers, nurses, physicians, or other trained personnel.[2,8,9] Whether or not RDs are engaged in performing nutrition screening, they are responsible for providing input regarding the development of suitable screening parameters to make certain the screening process addresses the correct parameters.[8] The nutrition screening process has the following characteristics[13]:

- May be completed in any setting
- Facilitates completion of early intervention goals
- Includes collection of relevant data on risk factors and interpretation of data for intervention and treatment
- Determines need for a nutrition assessment
- Is cost-effective

Each facility or setting is responsible for determining the most appropriate mechanism for screening patients. It is important to identify patients at nutritional risk.[14] Once individuals are identified, a nutrition assessment can be performed, and personalized intervention can then be planned and implemented.[1] Certain criteria are used for nutrition screening[1,14]:

- Weight (i.e., BMI greater than 25 or less than 18.5)
- Unintentional weight loss of 10% or more of usual body weight within 6 months or less than 5% of usual body weight in 1 month
- Nausea and vomiting
- Chewing and swallowing ability
- Diagnosis or presence of chronic disease
- Increased metabolic requirements (e.g., trauma, burns, systemic infection)
- Food allergies
- Diet
  - Altered intake (e.g., recent surgery, serious illness, parenteral or enteral nutrition)
  - Inadequate intake expected to continue 7 days or longer
- Laboratory data (i.e., albumin, hematocrit)

If patients have been hospitalized for an extended length of time, they should be rescreened.[14] It is vital that a patient at nutritional risk is referred to an RD who will conduct the nutrition assessment, make nutrition diagnoses, and provide nutrition care.

Nutrition Assessment

Nutrition assessment is "a systematic approach to collect, record, and interpret relevant data from patients, clients, family members, caregivers and other individuals and groups. [It] is an ongoing, dynamic process that involves initial data

BOX 16-2   THE ACADEMY OF NUTRITION AND DIETETICS' NUTRITION CARE PROCESS

Definition of the Nutrition Care Process

Providing nutrition care using the Nutrition Care Process (NCP) from the Academy of Nutrition and Dietetics (AND) (formerly the American Dietetic Association [ADA]) begins when a patient is recognized as being at nutritional risk and requires additional support to attain or maintain positive nutritional status. The NCP is defined as "a systematic problem-solving method that dietetics professionals use to critically think and make decisions to address nutrition-related problems and provide safe and effective quality nutrition care." It is composed of the following four separate but interrelated and associated steps:

1. Nutrition assessment
2. Nutrition diagnosis
3. Nutrition intervention
4. Nutrition monitoring and evaluation

Each step builds on the preceding one, but the process is not necessarily linear. The International Dietetics and Nutrition Terminology is a standardized language used to describe the results of each step of the model. Standardized language allows for appropriate, accurate, ongoing, relevant, and timely documentation of nutrition care. Figure 16-1 provides a visual illustration of the NCP model.

Step 1: Nutrition Assessment

Techniques such as those outlined in the chapter are used to systematically obtain information necessary to determine or reassess whether or not a nutrition problem (or diagnosis) exists. If so, then the problem is diagnosed using a PES (problem, etiology, signs and symptoms) statement in step 2 of the NCP (see Figure 16-1).

Step 2: Nutrition Diagnosis

Before nutrition intervention can take place, the nutrition problem (or problems) must be identified. This is accomplished with the nutrition diagnosis. Standardized language is used to make the nutrition diagnosis clear to other nutrition and health care professionals. When the nutrition problem has been identified, it is labeled with a specific, standardized diagnostic term. The nutrition diagnosis statement or PES statement is organized in three distinct parts: (1) the problem (P); (2) the etiology, or cause, of the problem (E); and (3) the signs and symptoms associated with the problem (S). Typically, nutrition diagnoses fall into three categories or domains:

1. Intake
2. Clinical
3. Behavioral-environmental

The following is an example of how a nutrition diagnosis is written:

A disordered eating pattern is *related to* harmful beliefs about food and nutrition *as evidenced by* the reported use of laxatives after meals and statements that calories are not absorbed when laxatives are used.

Step 3: Nutrition Intervention

Intervention begins once the nutritional diagnosis is identified. It is generally aimed at the etiology (E) of the nutrition diagnosis

and is directed at reducing or eradicating effects of the signs and symptoms (S). Nutrition interventions are intended to modify a nutrition-related problem and comprise two interconnected components: (1) planning and (2) implementation. Nutrition diagnoses are prioritized in the planning component, whereby implementation is the "action phase." The plan is communicated and carried out, data continue to be collected, and nutrition interventions are revised as necessary. Four categories or domains of nutrition intervention have been identified:

1. Food and/or nutrient delivery
2. Nutrition education
3. Nutrition counseling
4. Coordination of care

Step 4: Nutrition Monitoring and Evaluation

The point of this step in the NCP is to measure improvement made by the patient in meeting nutrition care goals. Patients' progress is examined by determining if the nutrition intervention is being executed and by providing evidence that the intervention *is* or *is not* altering the patients' nutritional status. Nutrition monitoring and evaluation terms are organized into four categories or domains:

1. Food- and nutrition-related history
2. Biochemical data, medical tests, and procedures
3. Anthropometric measurements
4. Nutrition-focused physical findings

In summary, the NCP allows for continuous treatment alteration. As patients' conditions change, so do diagnoses, plans, and interventions. If patients do not respond to interventions, then new interventions can be developed for them. However, it is important to remember that any and all nutrition interventions should be planned in consultation with patients, as well as with their caregivers or significant others. For more detailed information regarding the NCP, please refer to the Bibliography below.

BIBLIOGRAPHY

American Dietetic Association: *International Dietetics and Nutrition Terminology (IDNT) Reference Manual. Standardized language for the nutrition care process,* ed 4, Chicago, 2013, American Dietetic Association.

American Dietetic Association: Nutrition Care Process and Model Part 1: The 2008 Update. *J Am Diet Assoc* 108:1113, 2008.

American Dietetic Association: Nutrition Care Process Part II: Using the International Dietetics and Nutrition Terminology to document the Nutrition Care Process. *J Am Diet Assoc* 108:1287, 2008.

Lacey K, Pritchitt E: Nutrition Care Process and model: ADA adopts road map to quality care and outcomes management. *J Am Diet Assoc* 103(8):1061, 2003.

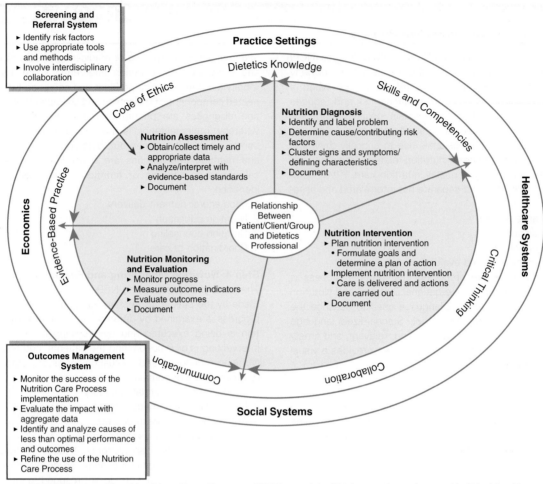

FIGURE 16-1 The Nutrition Care Process (NCP) model. (Redrawn from Lacey K, Pritchitt E: Nutrition Care Process and model: ADA adopts road map to quality care and outcomes management. *J Am Diet Assoc* 103[8]:1061, 2003, with permission from the American Dietetic Association [ADA].)

collection as well as continual reassessment and analysis of the patient's/client's status compared to specified criteria."[10] The fundamental purpose of nutrition assessment in general clinical practice is to determine the following three factors:

1. Overall nutritional status of the patient
2. Current health care needs—physical, psychosocial, and personal (see Diet-Medications Interactions box, "Assess Your Knowledge of Food-Drug Interactions")
3. Related factors influencing these needs in the person's current life situation

The first step in nutrition assessment, as with assessing any situation to determine needs and actions, is to collect pertinent information, which will act as a database, for use in identifying needs. The clinical dietitian, assisted by other health care team members as needed, uses several basic types of activities for nutrition assessment of patients' needs, as follows:

• Anthropometric data
• Biochemical tests
• Clinical observations

• Diet evaluation and personal histories (i.e., medical, social, medications) (See the Focus on Culture box, "Cultural Stereotyping: Melting Pot or Salad Bowl?")

Each part of this approach is important because no single parameter directly measures individual nutritional status or determines problems or needs. Further, the overall resulting impression must be interpreted within the context of the patient's own social and health factors, because these factors have the potential to alter his or her nutritional requirements. The procedures outlined here provide a good base in general practice.

Anthropometric Measurements

Anthropometric measurements are measurements of body size, weight, and proportions. These measurements can be used to assess nutritional status, as well as growth and development of infants and children; they are useful tools for monitoring the effects of nutritional intervention.[9]

Weight. One of the most important measurements in nutritional assessment is body weight. It is used to predict

DIET-MEDICATIONS INTERACTIONS

Assess Your Knowledge of Food-Drug Interactions

Medications can treat and cure many health problems, but they must be taken properly to be effective. Many medications interact with foods, beverages, alcohol, and caffeine to make them less effective or cause dangerous side effects. Assess your knowledge of food-drug interactions by answering the following questions:

1. No risk of food-drug interactions exist when taking over-the-counter medications.
   a. True.
   b. False.

2. Your neighbor, Greta, has serious allergies. Her physician prescribed an antihistamine to control her symptoms. Which of the following labels might appear on her prescription bottle?
   a. Take on an empty stomach.
   b. Take with food.
   c. Take only at bedtime.
   d. Take with coffee.

3. The previously mentioned label is on Greta's prescription antihistamine because:
   a. Effectiveness is increased when taken on an empty stomach.
   b. Effectiveness is increased when taken with food.
   c. The drug is metabolized more efficiently when taken at bedtime.
   d. Caffeine enhances absorption of the medication.

4. Your other neighbor, Abdul, has a horrible headache from studying too hard last night. He asks you if he should take his over-the-counter nonsteroidal antiinflammatory drug (NSAID) on an empty stomach or with a meal. He should take the NSAID with food because:
   a. These medications can irritate the stomach.
   b. Food will increase effectiveness.
   c. It is easier to remember to take them with a meal.

5. Combining NSAIDs or acetaminophen with alcohol will:
   a. Decrease stomach irritation.
   b. Increase risk of liver damage.
   c. Protect the liver from the effects of alcohol.
   d. Have no effect whatsoever.

6. Your cousin Vinny is dining on a super-sized meal at the local fast-food restaurant. Which of the following prescription medications should he avoid taking with the meal because high-fat meals may increase levels in the body?
   a. Hydrochlorothiazide (diuretic)
   b. Tetracyclines (antibiotic)
   c. NSAIDs
   d. Some forms of theophylline (bronchodilator)

7. Grandma Minnie takes a diuretic to control hypertension. Her physician told her this drug could cause hypokalemia. Which of the following foods should she eat on a regular basis to avoid hypokalemia?
   a. Hamburgers and hot dogs
   b. Twinkies and Ding Dongs
   c. Low-fat dairy products
   d. Bananas, oranges, and potatoes

8. Uncle Joe is taking captopril (an angiotensin-converting enzyme [ACE] inhibitor) for his high blood pressure. He cannot remember if his physician told him to take the captopril with a meal or on an empty stomach. What can you tell him?
   a. Take it with meals to increase absorption.
   b. Take it 1 hour before or 2 hours after meals so as to not affect absorption.
   c. Take it with breakfast but not with dinner.

9. Your roommate's cousin's uncle is taking a "statin" medication to lower serum cholesterol. Which of the following statements is true about statin medications?
   a. Avoid drinking large amounts of alcohol because it may increase risk of liver damage.
   b. Take with breakfast to enhance absorption.
   c. Take with the evening meal to decrease absorption.

10. High doses of vitamin E may prolong clotting time and increase risk of bleeding. Large doses of vitamin E should be avoided when taking which of the following drugs?
    a. Warfarin (anticoagulant)
    b. Lovastatin (3-hydroxy-3-methylglutaryl coenzyme A [HMG-CoA] reductase inhibitor)
    c. Furosemide (diuretic)
    d. NSAIDs

11. Your cousin Bunny is taking oral contraceptives. Which of the following drugs may decrease effectiveness of "the pill," thereby increasing her chance of pregnancy?
    a. Anticoagulants
    b. NSAIDs
    c. Antibiotics
    d. Antidepressants

12. Bunny's pet turtle, Speedy, died. She wants to take St. John's wort because her roommate told her it would help with her depression. Are there any problems with her taking St. John's wort while she is taking oral contraceptives?
    a. No. St. John's wort is an herb and sold at the Universal Nutrition Center at the mall. Herbal and dietary supplements cannot be sold if they are not safe.
    b. Yes. St. John's wort will decrease effectiveness of the oral contraceptives.

13. Mr. Wilson is very excitable and nervous. Which of the following might be an explanation for this?
    a. He took Cipro (quinolone) with his morning coffee.
    b. He took penicillin at breakfast, which included yogurt.
    c. He took aspirin on an empty stomach.
    d. He just received a call from the Internal Revenue Service (IRS) to schedule an audit of last year's tax return.

14. Curt is taking tetracycline to control acne. Which of the following should he avoid?
    a. Dairy products
    b. Antacids
    c. Vitamins containing iron
    d. All of the above

Continued

⬥ DIET-MEDICATIONS INTERACTIONS

Assess Your Knowledge of Food-Drug Interactions—cont'd

15. Your favorite aunt, Constance, takes a monoamine oxidase inhibitor (MAOI). Her pharmacist cautioned her about eating foods high in tyramine (an amino acid). Why?
    a. MAOIs combined with tyramine cause hiccups.
    b. A rapid, potentially fatal decrease in blood pressure can occur.
    c. A rapid, potentially fatal increase in blood pressure can occur.
    d. None of the above will happen. Her pharmacist is mistaken.

16. Your nervous neighbor, Biff, takes alprazolam (Xanax), an antianxiety drug. He was told he should not take the Xanax with Mountain Dew. Why?
    a. Carbonation in the soft drink will enhance effects of the Xanax.
    b. Carbonation in the soft drink will decrease effects of the Xanax.
    c. Caffeine in Mountain Dew may lessen the antianxiety effect of Xanax.
    d. Caffeine in the Mountain Dew may enhance the antianxiety effect of Xanax.

17. Kevin just found out his stomach pain is being caused by excess acid production that caused an ulcer. His physician prescribed a histamine blocker and told him to avoid alcohol. Why?
    a. Alcohol is a gastric irritant, which will make it more difficult for the stomach to heal.
    b. Alcohol decreases the effectiveness of the histamine blocker.
    c. Alcohol increases the effectiveness of the histamine blocker.

d. Kevin's physician does not want any of her patients to drink alcohol.

18. Grandpa Moe takes digoxin for his heart condition. Your cousin Sunshine brought him ginseng on her last visit. Should he take ginseng with the digoxin?
    a. Yes. Herbal products are natural and safe.
    b. No. Ginseng falsely elevates plasma digoxin levels.
    c. It does not matter.

19. Trixie has a bad case of poison ivy. The physician gave her a prescription for Medrol, a corticosteroid to stop the itching. She cannot remember if the physician told her to take the Medrol on an empty stomach or with food. Can you help her?
    a. It does not matter if Trixie takes it on an empty stomach or not.
    b. Trixie should take the medicine on an empty stomach to decrease stomach irritation.
    c. Trixie should take the Medrol with food or milk to decrease stomach upset.

20. Great Uncle John takes nitroglycerin (nitrate) for chest pain. Which of the following can add to the blood vessel–relaxing effect of nitrates and cause dangerously low blood pressure?
    a. Milk and dairy products
    b. Fruits and vegetables
    c. Alcohol
    d. Meats and cheeses

Answers: 1. b; 2. a; 3. a; 4. a; 5. b; 6. d; 7. d; 8. b; 9. a; 10. a; 11. c; 12. b; 13. a; 14. d; 15. c; 16. c; 17. a; 18. b; 19. c; 20. c.

🌐 FOCUS ON CULTURE

Cultural Stereotyping: Melting Pot or Salad Bowl?

Do all Southerners eat grits? Do all those who practice the Jewish religion follow orthodox food laws? Do all people of Hispanic origin eat tortillas and beans? Should you address your patient informally (by his or her first name) or more formally (e.g., Mrs. Garcia or Mr. Sato)? If your patient does not look you in the eye while talking, is he or she being deceitful or showing respect? Why do you need to know the answer to these questions and others?

The population of the United States is growing increasingly culturally diverse. Between 2000 and 2010, the Hispanic population grew by 43% and the Asian population grew by 45.6%. Almost 25% of the total population is non-Anglo American. By 2043, while non-Hispanic Caucasians will be the largest single ethnic group, no group will make up a majority of the population. By 2060, minority groups, which now make up 37% of the total population, will grow to 57% of the total U.S. population. So what does this mean to you?

In terms of nutrition assessment and nutrition counseling, cultural diversity is a fact. Cultural competency is a necessity. Cultural competency is more than recognizing and accepting cultural diversity. It is a skill critical to all dietitians and health care professionals. What good does it do to conduct a nutrition assessment or provide nutrition education if the patient's cultural background is not considered? Culture includes language, lifestyle, values, beliefs, and attitudes. These and other elements of culture influence how patients might experience illness, how they might access health care, and how they get well.

To deliver culturally competent care, dietitians and health care providers must understand beliefs, values, traditions, and cultural practices. Consider the following differences in the dominant American cultural **paradigm**, the Anglo-American culture, and more traditional cultural populations:

Cultural Stereotyping: Melting Pot or Salad Bowl?—cont'd

Anglo American	More Traditional Cultures	What This May Mean to You
Personal control of environment	Fate	Many traditional cultures believe fate, God, or other supernatural factors determine a person's destiny and directly influence health. The way they eat and exercise cannot have any influence on whether or not they develop complications of diabetes, for example.
Change	Tradition	Tradition and continuity are valued more than change. A reverence for the past takes precedence over efficiency of striving.
Time dominates	Human interaction dominates	Personal relationships determine self-worth and take priority over time schedules—promptness is not always a priority.
Human equality	Hierarchy, rank, status	In some cultures, health care professionals are more highly respected than other professionals. This may result in patients being less forthcoming if they disagree with a health care professional.
Individualism, privacy	Group or family welfare	Decision making about health issues may be a family affair.
Self-help	Birthright inheritance	Individuals may not believe they can help themselves in terms of their health.
Competition	Cooperation	Cooperation is preferred to competition.
Future orientation	Past orientation	Preventive care may not be a priority.
Action taking, goal setting, work oriented, informal approach preferred	"Being" orientation	Informality (e.g., calling people by their first names) is associated with rudeness in many traditional cultures. Clarify the patient's preference early.
Directness, openness, honesty	Formality	Individuals may not "volunteer" information.
Practicality, efficiency	Idealism, spiritualism	Idealism is stressed over practicality or expedience.

There was a time when minorities in the United States tended to imitate the dominant middle-class culture, but this is no longer the case. Individual and cultural expression are becoming desirable. It is an expression of respect to learn about different cultures, to develop flexibility in how to approach clients and patients, and to develop cultural competency.

How Culturally Competent Are You?*

1. When the patient and dietitian come from different cultural backgrounds, the nutrition history obtained may not be accurate.
   a. True.
   b. False.
2. Which of the following are the correct ways to communicate with a patient through an interpreter?
   a. Making eye contact with the interpreter when you are speaking, then looking at the patient while the interpreter is telling the patient what you said.
   b. Speaking slowly, pausing between words.
   c. Asking the interpreter to further explain the patient's statement to get a more complete picture of the patient's condition.
   d. None of the above.
3. Which of the following statements is *not* true?
   a. Friendly (nonsexual) physical contact is an important part of communication for many Latin-American people.
   b. Many Asian people think it is disrespectful to ask questions of a health care professional.

c. Most people of African heritage are either Christian or follow a traditional religion.
d. Eastern Europeans are highly diverse in terms of customs, language, and religion.
4. Which of the following is good advice for a health care professional attempting to use and interpret nonverbal communication?
   a. The provider should recognize that a smile may express unhappiness or dissatisfaction in some cultures.
   b. To express sympathy, a health care professional can lightly touch a patient's arm or pat the patient on the back.
   c. If a patient will not make eye contact with a health care professional, then it is likely the patient is hiding the truth.
   d. When a language barrier exists, the provider can use hand gestures to bridge the gap.
5. Some symbols—a positive nod of the head, a pointing finger, a "thumbs-up" sign—are universal and can help bridge the language gap.
   a. True.
   b. False.
6. A female Muslim patient may avoid eye contact, physical contact, or both because:
   a. She does not want to spread germs.
   b. Muslim women are taught to be submissive.
   c. Modesty is very important in Islamic tradition.
   d. She does not like the health care professional.

Continued

FOCUS ON CULTURE

Cultural Stereotyping: Melting Pot or Salad Bowl?—cont'd

7. When a patient is not compliant with prescribed nutrition therapy after several visits, which of the following approaches is *not* likely to lead to compliance?
   a. Involving family members.
   b. Repeating the instructions very loudly and several times to emphasize the importance of the nutrition therapy.
   c. Agreeing to a compromise in the recommended nutrition therapy.
   d. Spending time listening to discussions of folk and alternative remedies.

8. If a family member speaks English and the patient's native language and is willing to act as interpreter, then this is the best possible solution to the problem of interpreting.
   a. True.
   b. False.

9. Which of the following is *true?*
   a. People who speak the same language have the same culture.
   b. The people living in the African continent share the main features of African culture.
   c. Cultural background, diet, religious, and health practices, as well as language, can differ widely within a given country or part of the country.
   d. An alert health care professional can usually predict a patient's health behaviors by knowing what country he or she comes from.

10. Out of respect for a patient's privacy, the health care professional should always begin a relationship by seeing an adult patient alone and drawing the family in as needed.
    a. True
    b. False

Answers: 1. a; 2. d; 3. c; 4. a; 5. b; 6. c; 7. b; 8. b; 9. c; 10. b.

Bibliography

Betterley C: *Increasing cultural competency of nutrition educators through travel study programs* Unpublished paper, 2001.

Brannon C: Cultural competency—values, traditions, and effective practice. *Today's Dietitian* 6(11):14, 2004. from: <www.todaysdietitian.com/newarchives/td_1104p14.shtml>. Retrieved March 13, 2009.

Curry KR: Multicultural competence in dietetics and nutrition. *J Am Diet Assoc* 100:1142, 2000.

Stein K: Moving cultural competency from abstract to act. *J Am Diet Assoc* 110:S21, 2010.

U.S. Census Bureau: *Census 2010 data for the United States*, Washington, D.C., 2010, U.S. Government Printing Office. from: <www.census.gov>. Retrieved March 11, 2013.

*Quiz modified from Management Sciences for Health and the U.S. Department of Health and Human Services, Health Resources and Administration, Bureau of Primary Healthcare: *The provider's guide to quality & culture*, Boston, 2008, Management Sciences for Health. Retrieved March 11, 2013. from: www.erc.msh.org/mainpage.cfm?file=1.0.htm&module=provider&language=English.

energy expenditure in prediction equations (see the Evidence-Based Practice box, "What is the Best Prediction Equation to Determine Energy Needs?").[9] Hospitalized patients should be weighed at consistent times—for example, before breakfast after the bladder has been emptied. Clinic patients should be weighed without shoes in light, indoor clothing or an examining gown. For accuracy, use regular clinic beam scales with nondetachable weights (Figure 16-2). Additional weight attachment is available for use with very obese persons. Metric scales with readings to the nearest 20 g provide specific data; however, the standard clinic scale is satisfactory. Scales should be checked frequently and calibrated every 3 or 4 months for continued accuracy. The weight of nonambulatory (unable to stand or walk) individuals can be measured using a bed or chair scale (Figure 16-3).

After careful reading and recording of the patient's weight, ask about usual body weight. Interpret the patient's present weight in terms of the percentage of usual body weight. Check for any recent weight loss: 1% to 2% in the past week, 5% during the past month, 7.5% during the previous 3 months, or 10% in the past 6 months are significant. Unintentional weight loss greater than these rates can be severe. Unexplained weight loss is a problem with persons of any age. It is particularly important in older adults, because it may be a clue to depression or a wasting disease such as cancer and

needs to be on record and followed up. Values charted in the patient's record should indicate the percentage of weight change.

Length and Stature. Measurements of length and stature (height) are easily obtained anthropometric measures. They are the most sensitive indicators of growth and development in infants and children.[9]

If possible, use a fixed measuring stick or tape on a true vertical flat surface. Have the patient stand as straight as possible, without shoes or hat, heels together, and looking straight ahead. Heels, buttocks, shoulders, and head should be touching the wall or vertical surface of the measuring rod. Read the measure carefully, and compare it with previous recordings. Children younger than 2 years should be measured using a stationary headboard and movable footboard (Figure 16-4). Note growth of children or the diminishing height of adults. Metric measures of height in centimeters provide a smaller unit of measure than inches.

> **KEY TERM**
>
> **paradigm** A pattern or model serving as an example; a standard or ideal for practice or behavior based on a fundamental value or theme.

EVIDENCE-BASED PRACTICE

What is the Best Prediction Equation to Determine Energy Needs?

Assessment of energy needs is a necessary component in the Nutrition Care Process (NCP). Indirect calorimetry is the "gold standard" for determining resting metabolic rate (RMR) and is accurate within 5% in most cases. However, because indirect calorimetry is not always available, prediction equations are commonly used to determine RMR.

The four prediction equations most commonly used in clinical practice are as follows:

Mifflin-St. Jeor

Men $\quad$ RMR = (9.99 × wt in kg) + (6.25 × ht in cm) − (4.92 × age in yr) + 5

Women $\quad$ RMR = (9.99 × wt in kg) + (6.25 × ht in cm) − (4.92 × age in yr) − 161

Harris-Benedict

Men $\quad$ RMR = 66.47 + (13.75 × wt in kg) + (5.0 × ht in cm) − (6.75 × age in yr)

Women $\quad$ RMR = 665.09 + (9.56 × wt in kg) + (1.84 × ht in cm) − (4.67 × age in yr)

Owen

Men $\quad$ RMR = 879 + (10.2 × wt in kg)

Women $\quad$ RMR = 795 + (7.18 × wt in kg)

World Health Organization/Food & Agriculture Organization/United Nations University (WHO/FAO/UNU)

Weight Only (Age [yr])

Men

18-30	15.3 × wt in kg + 679
31-60	11.6 × wt in kg + 879
>60	13.5 × wt in kg + 487

Women

18-30	14.7 × wt in kg + 496
31-60	8.7 × wt in kg + 829
>60	10.5 × wt in kg + 596

Weight & Height (m) (Age [yr])

Men

18-30	(15.4 × wt in kg) − (27 × ht in m) + 717
31-60	(11.3 × wt in kg) + (16 × ht in m) + 901
>60	(8.8 × wt in kg) + (1128 × ht in m) − 1071

Women

18-30	(13.3 × wt in kg) + (34 × ht in m) + 35
31-60	(8.7 × wt in kg) − (25 × ht in m) + 865
>60	(9.2 × wt in kg) + (637 × ht in m) − 302

Of the four equations listed previously, the Mifflin-St. Jeor equation was found to be the most accurate in estimating basal metabolic rate (BMR). The oldest prediction equation in clinical use, Harris-Benedict, was found to systematically overestimate basal energy expenditure (BEE) by at least 5%. The Owen equation underestimates RMR about 21% of the time and overestimates RMR 6% of the time. Accuracy of the WHO/FAO/UNU equations could not be evaluated because of how the equations have been validated. For more details about the research of these prediction equations, please refer to the Frankenfield manuscripts cited in the bibliography.

Bibliography

Food and Agricultural Organization/World Health Organization/United Nations University: *Energy and protein requirements. Report of a Joint FAO/WHO/UNU expert consultation*, World Health Organization Technical Report Series 724, Geneva, Switzerland, 1985, WHO.

Frankenfield DC, Muth ER, Rowe WA: The Harris-Benedict studies of human basal metabolism: history and limitations. *J Am Diet Assoc* 98(4):439, 1998.

Frankenfield D, Roth-Yousey L, Compher C: Comparison of predictive equations for resting metabolic rate in healthy nonobese and obese adults: a systematic review. *J Am Diet Assoc* 105(5):775, 2005.

Harris JA, Benedict FG: *A biometric study of basal metabolism in man*, Washington, D.C., 1919, Carnegie Institute of Washington. Pub No 279.

Mifflin MD, St Jeor ST, Hill LA, et al: A new predictive equation for resting energy expenditure in healthy individuals. *Am J Clin Nutr* 51:241, 1990.

Owen OE, Holup JL, Dalessio DA, et al: A reappraisal of the caloric requirements of men. *Am J Clin Nutr* 46:875, 1987.

Owen OE, Kavle E, Owen RS, et al: A reappraisal of caloric requirements in healthy women. *Am J Clin Nutr* 44:1, 1986.

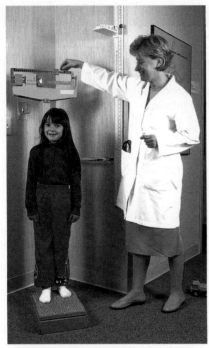

FIGURE 16-2 Balance beam scale. (From Jarvis C: *Physical examination and health assessment,* ed 6, St. Louis, Mo., 2012, Elsevier Saunders.)

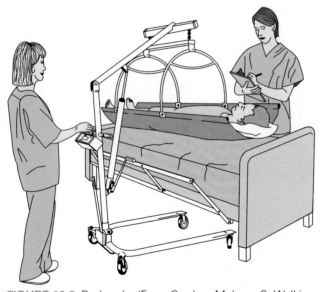

FIGURE 16-3 Bed scale. (From Grodner M, Long S, Walkingshaw BC: *Foundations and clinical applications of nutrition: a nursing approach,* ed 5, St Louis, Mo. 2012, Elsevier.)

Although it is always preferable to obtain standing measurements,[9] this is not always possible. Several alternative measures can provide values for estimating height and weight of persons confined to bed:

- *Knee height* (Figure 16-5) has been shown to correlate well with stature.[17-19] Measurement is taken with the person lying in the supine position. The left leg is measured with knee and ankle at a 90-degree angle using a specialized

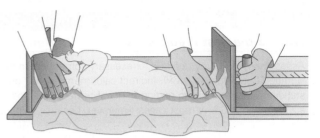

FIGURE 16-4 Measuring a baby's stature. (From Mahan LK, Escott-Stump S: *Krause's food, and the nutrition care process,* ed 13, Philadelphia, Pa., 2012, Elsevier Saunders.)

sliding caliper. Measurements are then entered into one of the following validated equations[15,17]

Men:

$$\text{Stature (cm)} = [2.02 \times \text{knee height (cm)}]$$
$$- (0.04 \times \text{age}) + 64.19$$

Women:

$$\text{Stature (cm)} = [1.83 \times \text{knee height (cm)}]$$
$$- (0.24 \times \text{age}) + 84.88$$

- To estimate height of a nonambulatory person who has no skeletal abnormalities or contractures, *recumbent bed measurement* can be taken by marking the base of the heels and top of the crown on the bed sheet (Figure 16-6) on which the patient is resting in a straight line. The distance between these two lines can be measured with a tape measure.
- *Arm span* measurement taken from sternal notch to the longest finger on the dominant hand is reliable in individuals with no contractures, spinal deformities, and who can fully extend their arms. To estimate stature, multiply the number obtained by 2.[15,20]

Body Mass Index. BMI is a ratio of weight to height and has been correlated with overall mortality and nutritional risk.[2,15] It does not estimate body composition (lean body mass or adiposity); however, it is a reliable indicator of total body fat (see Box 16-1), which is related to the risk of disease.[16] Although BMI measurements are valid for men and women, they do have some limits[15,16]:

- BMI has not been validated in acutely ill patients.
- BMI may overestimate body fat in individuals who have a muscular build.
- BMI may underestimate body fat in older adults and others who have lost muscle mass.

Standardized growth charts for children can be found on the Centers for Disease Control and Prevention (CDC) website (www.cdc.gov/nchs/about/major/nhanes/growthcharts/clinical_charts.htm). These growth charts show percentile rankings of height and weight for age and weight for height, as well as BMI for age.[1]

Waist Circumference. Waist circumference is inexpensive, easy to perform, and assesses abdominal fat content.

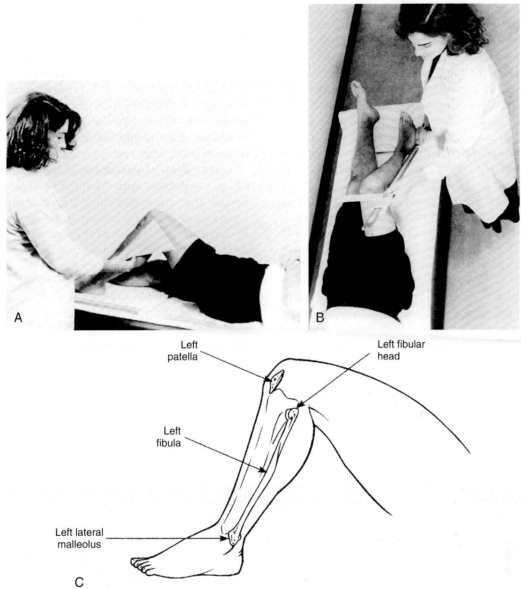

FIGURE 16-5 Knee height measurement. (From Lee RD, Nieman DC: *Nutritional assessment,* ed 4, Boston, 2007, McGraw-Hill.)

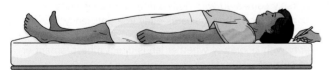

FIGURE 16-6 Recumbent bed length. (From Lee RD, Nieman DC: *Nutritional assessment,* ed 4, Boston, 2007, McGraw-Hill.)

BMI and waist circumference highly correlate with obesity and risk for disease, and both should be used to classify overweight and obesity, as well as to estimate disease risk.[1,15,21] Circumference greater than 40 inches in men and greater than 35 inches in women indicates risk for disease. It should be noted that visceral adiposity may vary among racial and ethnic groups.[1]

Biochemical (Laboratory) Measurements

Biochemical (or laboratory) tests are a useful adjunct in measuring and managing nutritional status, but their use can be problematic.[9] Precise interpretation necessitates awareness of the appropriate test, as well as nutritional and nonnutritional factors that have the potential to alter blood chemistries. Significant nonnutritional factors to be considered include disease processes, treatments, procedures, medications, and hydration status.[22] The most commonly used methods for assessing and monitoring nutritional status and planning nutrition care in clinical practice are listed here. General ranges for normal values are given in standard texts.

Protein Assessment. Usually, biochemical assessment of protein status has been undertaken from the standpoint of two protein compartments: (1) somatic and (2) visceral proteins.[9] Somatic protein is found within skeletal muscle, and visceral proteins are found in body organs, red blood cells, white blood cells, and serum proteins. Both protein pools are metabolically active, meaning the body can tap into these stores if necessary.[9] Obviously use of any proteins stored in the body means the protein is no longer available for bodily functions like synthesis of antibodies, hormones, and other vital components. Additionally, no single laboratory test or group of tests is sensitive, specific, or both for protein malnutrition. Evaluation of serum proteins necessitates simultaneous assessment of nutrient intake, physical findings, and clinical condition.[22]

Serum Proteins. Serum protein concentrations can be helpful in determining protein status, risk of medical complications, and response to nutritional intervention with limitations.[9,22] A number of factors other than inadequate protein intake affect serum protein concentrations (Table 16-1).

Somatic Proteins. Somatic proteins can be measured using anthropometric measures such as midarm muscle area, midarm circumference, and overall body weight.[2] A laboratory test that can be used for estimating body muscle mass is 24-hour urinary creatinine excretion.[10]

When assessing biochemical measurements, it is important to consider that a review of serial laboratory data is recommended. Direction and speed of change are more important than static value. Improvement in nutrition parameters does not always confer clinical benefit. Treat the person, not the laboratory value.[22]

Clinical Observations and Nutrition Physical Assessment

Certain information used to assess nutritional status is taken from physical examinations performed by physicians and nurses. Furthermore, RDs perform nutritional physical examinations to assess patients for signs and symptoms consistent with malnutrition or specific nutrient deficiency.[2] Techniques used in nutritional physical examinations are summarized in Table 16-2.

Clinical Signs of Malnutrition. Careful attention to physical signs of possible malnutrition provides an added dimension to the overall assessment of general nutritional status. A guide for a general examination of such signs is given in Table 16-3. A careful description of any such observations is documented in the patient's medical record.

Dietary Assessment

Collecting Information. A careful nutrition history, including nutrition information related to living situation and other personal, psychosocial, and economic problems, is a fundamental part of nutrition assessment. Obtaining accurate information about basic food patterns and actual dietary intake is not simple because some individuals misreport or underreport what they eat. Each method of diet evaluation has particular strengths and limitations.[9] However, a sensitive practitioner may obtain useful information by using one or more of the basic tools described in Table 16-4.

TABLE 16-1	**LABORATORY MEASURES OF SERUM PROTEINS**	
SERUM PROTEIN	**FUNCTION**	**COMMENTS**
Albumin *Normal:* 3.5-5.0 g/dL *Depletion:* Mild: 3.0-3.4 g/dL Moderate: 2.4-2.9 g/dL Severe: <2.4 g/dL Half-life ~ 14-20 days	Maintains plasma oncotic pressure, carrier for small molecules	Not sensitive or specific for acute protein malnutrition or response to nutrition therapy; affected by hydration status, disease state, clinical condition Can be used as prognostic indicator of morbidity, mortality, and severity of illness
Transferrin *Normal:* 200-400 g/dL *Depletion:* Mild: 150-200 mg/dL Moderate: 100-149 mg/dL Severe: <100 mg/dL Half-life ~ 8-10 days	Binds iron in plasma and transports to bone marrow	Inversely correlated with body's iron stores; elevated concentration often indicates early iron deficiency Will decrease during acute illness Verify with laboratory whether lab is direct measurement or calculated
Prealbumin (transthyretin, thyroxin-binding prealbumin) *Normal:* 16-40 mg/dL *Depletion:* Mild: 10-15 mg/dL Moderate: 5-9 mg/dL Severe: <5 mg/dL Half-life ~ 2-3 days	Carrier protein for thyroxin Combined with retinol-binding protein, transports vitamin A	Influenced less by intravascular fluid volume Not affected as early or as significantly with liver disease (compared with albumin) More likely to be reflection of recent dietary intake than accurate indicator of nutritional status

Adapted from (compiled from components in tables and text) Moore MC: *Pocket guide to nutrition assessment and care,* ed 6, St Louis, Mo., 2009, Mosby; Lee RD, Nieman DC: *Nutritional assessment,* ed 4, Boston, 2007, McGraw-Hill; Thompson CW: Laboratory assessment. In Charney P, Malone AM, editors: *ADA pocket guide to nutrition assessment,* ed 2, Chicago, 2009, American Dietetic Association.

TABLE 16-2 NUTRITIONAL PHYSICAL EXAMINATION

TECHNIQUE	SKILL	PURPOSE
Inspection	Systematic visual inspection	Monitor changes to normal features
Auscultation	Using a stethoscope and naked ear to identify deviations from standard sounds	Evaluate sounds produced by heart, lungs, and gastrointestinal (GI) tract such as bowel sounds
Palpation	Examination of the body using touch	Reveal conditions that have nutritional implications such as abdominal tenderness, ascites, distention, peripheral edema, nail integrity, and skin turgor
Percussion	Use of sound to distinguish deviations from standard sounds created by presence of body organs and cavities	Identify gastric air bubble, intestinal air, or fluid present in lungs

Data from Nelms MN, Sucher K, Long S: *Understanding nutrition therapy and pathophysiology,* Belmont, Calif., 2007, Wadsworth.

TABLE 16-3 CLINICAL SIGNS OF NUTRITIONAL STATUS

AREA OF CONCERN	POSSIBLE DEFICIENCY	POSSIBLE EXCESS
Hair		
Dull, dry, brittle	Pro	
Easily plucked (with no pain)	Pro	
Hair loss	Pro, Zn, biotin	Vit A
Flag sign (loss of hair pigment in strips around head)	Pro, Cu	
Head and Neck		
Bulging fontanel (infants)		Vit A
Headache		Vit A, D
Epistaxis (nosebleed)	Vit K	
Thyroid enlargement	Iodine	
Eyes		
Conjunctival and corneal xerosis (dryness)	Vit A	
Pale conjunctiva	Fe	
Blue sclerae	Fe	
Corneal vascularization	Vit B_2	
Mouth		
Cheilosis or angular stomatitis (lesions at corners of mouth, Figure 16-7, A)	Vit B_2	
Glossitis (red, sore tongue)	Niacin, folate, vit B_{12}, and other B vit	
Gingivitis (inflamed gums)	Vit C	
Hypogeusia, dysgeusia (poor sense of taste, distorted taste)	Zn	
Dental caries	Fluoride	
Mottling of teeth		Fluoride
Atrophy of papillae on tongue	Fe, B vit	
Skin		
Dry, scaly	Vit A, Zn, EFAs	Vit A
Follicular hyperkeratosis (resembles gooseflesh)	Vit A, EFAs, B vit	
Eczematous lesions	Zn	
Petechiae, ecchymoses	Vit C, K	
Nasolabial seborrhea (greasy, scaly areas between nose and lip)	Niacin, vit B_{12}, B_6	
Darkening and peeling of skin in areas exposed to sun	Niacin	
Poor wound healing	Pro, Zn, vit C	
Nails		
Spoon-shaped nails (see Figure 16-7, B)	Fe	
Brittle, fragile	Pro	

Continued

TABLE 16-3   CLINICAL SIGNS OF NUTRITIONAL STATUS—cont'd

AREA OF CONCERN	POSSIBLE DEFICIENCY	POSSIBLE EXCESS
Heart		
Enlargement, tachycardia, failure	Vit B$_1$	
Small heart	Energy	
Sudden failure, death	Se	
Arrhythmia	Mg, K, Se	
Hypertension	Ca, K	
Abdomen		
Hepatomegaly	Pro	Vit A
Ascites	Pro	
Musculoskeletal Extremities		
Muscle wasting (especially temporal area)	Energy	
Edema	Pro, vit B$_1$	
Calf tenderness	Vit B$_1$ or C, biotoin, Se	
Beading of ribs, or "rachitic rosary" (child)	Vit C, D	
Bone and joint tenderness	Vit C, D, Ca, P	
Knock-knee, bowed legs, fragile bones	Vit D, Ca, P, Cu	
Neurologic		
Paresthesias (pain and tingling or altered sensation in the extremities)	Vit B$_1$, B$_6$, B$_{12}$, biotin	
Weakness	Vit C, B$_1$, B$_6$, B$_{12}$, energy	
Ataxia, decreased position and vibratory senses	Vit B$_1$, B$_{12}$	
Tremor	Mg	
Decreased tendon reflexes	Vit B$_1$	
Confabulation, disorientation	Vit B$_1$, B$_{12}$	
Drowsiness, lethargy	Vit B$_1$	Vit A, D
Depression	Vit B$_1$, biotin, B$_{12}$	

Data from Moore MC: *Pocket guide to nutrition assessment and care,* ed 6, St Louis, Mo., 2009, Mosby, pp 60–63.
Ca, Calcium; *Cu,* copper; *EFAs,* essential fatty acids; *Fe,* iron; *K,* potassium, *Mg,* magnesium; *Na,* sodium; *P,* phosphorus; *Pro,* protein; *Se,* selenium; *Vit,* vitamin(s); *Zn,* zinc.

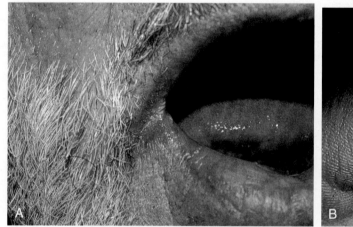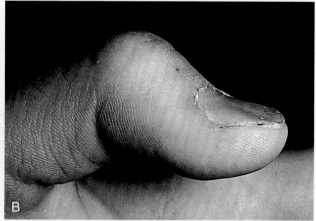

FIGURE 16-7 Examples of findings in malnourished states: **A,** Cheilosis or angular stomatitis; **B,** spoon-shaped nails. (From Moore MC: *Pocket guide to nutrition assessment and care,* ed 6, St Louis Mo., 2009, Mosby.)

Evaluation of Dietary Intake. Valid patient care planning requires analysis of all nutrition data collected. On this basis, problems requiring solutions can be identified. A detailed analysis of all available nutrition information helps determine nutrition diagnosis, any primary or secondary nutritional disease, and any underlying nutrition-related conditions.

Medical tests used for nutrition assessment are generally reliable in persons of any age, but conditions in older adult patients may interfere and need to be considered in evaluating test results. For example, laboratory values are affected by hydration status, presence of chronic diseases, changes in organ function, and drugs. Nutrition assessment is an

TABLE 16-4	STRENGTHS AND LIMITATIONS OF TECHNIQUES USED TO MEASURE DIETARY INTAKE		
TECHNIQUE	**BRIEF DESCRIPTION**	**STRENGTHS**	**LIMITATIONS**
24-hour food record	Trained interviewer asks respondent to recall, in detail, all food and drink consumed during a period of time in the recent past.	Requires <20 min to administer Inexpensive Easy to administer Can provide detailed information on types of foods consumed Low respondent burden More objective than dietary history Does not alter usual diet Useful in clinical settings	One recall rarely illustrative of typical intake Underreporting and overreporting problems Dependent on memory Omissions of sauces, dressings, and beverages can lead to low estimates of energy intake Data entry sometimes labor intensive
Food record or diary	Respondents record, at the time of consumption, the identity and amounts of all foods and beverages consumed for a period of time, usually ranging from 1 to 7 days.	Does not rely on memory Can provide detailed intake data Can provide information about eating habits Multiple-day data more representative of usual intake Reasonably valid up to 5 days	Requires high degree of cooperation Subject must be literate Takes more time to obtain data Act of recording may alter usual intake
Food frequency questionnaires	Respondents indicate how many times a day, week, month, or year they usually consume foods using a questionnaire consisting of a list of approximately >150 foods or food groups that are important contributors to the population's intake of energy and nutrients.	Can be self-administered Machine readable Modest demand on respondents Relatively inexpensive May be more representative of usual intake than a few days of diet records	May not represent usual food or portion sizes chosen by respondent Intake data can be compromised when multiple foods are grouped within single listings Depends on ability of respondent to describe diet
Diet history	Respondents are interviewed by a trained interviewer about number of meals eaten per day, their appetites, their food dislikes, the presence or absence of nausea and/or vomiting, the use of nutritional supplements and/or herbal products, cigarette smoking, as well as habits related to sleep, rest, work, and exercise.	Assesses usual nutrient intake Can detect seasonal changes Data on all nutrients can be obtained Can correlate well with biochemical measures	Lengthy interview process Requires highly trained interviewers May overestimate nutrient intake Requires cooperation of respondent with ability to recall usual diet

Modified from Lee RD, Neiman DC: *Nutrition assessment,* ed 4, Boston, 2007, McGraw-Hill.

important part of the general health care of everyone, especially older adults. Health outreach programs for older persons, such as those in rural areas, can use brief, easily administered tools for screening and assessing nutritional status and risk of malnutrition as part of geriatric care.

NUTRITION DIAGNOSIS

Nutrition diagnosis is not to be confused with medical diagnosis. Medical diagnosis is a disease or pathologic condition that can be treated or prevented, and the diagnosis does not change as long as the condition exists.[8] Nutrition diagnosis is "a food and nutrition professional's identification and labeling of an existing nutrition problem that the food and

nutrition professional is responsible for treating independently."[10] Nutrition diagnoses provide a mechanism for dietetics practitioners to document the link between nutrition assessment and nutrition intervention and to set realistic and measurable expected outcomes for patients. Identifying diagnoses also assists dietetics practitioners in establishing priorities when planning nutrition care.[23] More than one nutrition diagnosis is possible, and nutrition diagnoses change as patients' nutritional needs change.[8,10] Each nutrition diagnosis should be accompanied by an intervention and monitoring strategy.[10] Nutrition diagnoses are dependent on evidence-based practice and standardized language.[2,8] More information on evidence-based practice is available for Academy of Nutrition and Dietetics (AND) members (formerly the American Dietetic Association [ADA] at www .adaevidencelibrary.com/default.cfm.

More than 60 nutrition diagnoses have been developed through use of standardized language and are grouped into three categories: (1) intake, (2) clinical, and (3) behavioral-environmental. Standardized language provides a means for dietetics professionals to communicate with each other, as well as with other health care professionals. It is a fundamental part of the Nutrition Care Process (NCP) and assists dietetics professionals in better documenting nutrition care.[23] See Box 16-2 for more in-depth information and to determine how a nutrition diagnosis is written.

NUTRITION INTERVENTION: FOOD PLAN AND MANAGEMENT

Basic Concepts of Nutrition Therapy

Nutrition therapy is always based on normal nutritional requirements and personal needs for each particular patient. It is modified only as the specific disease in the specific individual necessitates. When planning and counseling for nutrition care, this is an important initial fact to grasp and impart to patients and clients. For example, it is a great source of encouragement to the parents of a child newly diagnosed with diabetes to know the food plan will be based on individual growth and development needs and will make use of regular foods.

Disease Application

Principles of a nutrition therapy will be based on modifications of nutritional components of the normal diet as a particular disease condition may require. These changes may include the following types of modifications:

- *Nutrients:* modification of one or more of the basic nutrients—protein, carbohydrate, fat, minerals, and vitamins
- *Energy:* modification in energy value as expressed in kilocalories (kcalories or kcal)
- *Texture:* modification in texture or seasoning, such as liquid or low residue

Individual Adaptation

Nutrition therapy may be theoretically correct and have well-balanced food plans, but if these plans are unacceptable to the patient, they will not be followed. A workable plan for a specific person must be based on individual food habits within the specific personal life situation. This can be achieved only through careful planning with the patient, or with the parents of a child who requires a special diet, based on an initial interview to obtain a diet history, knowledge of personal food habits, living conditions, and food security. In this way, diet principles can be understood and motivation secured. Regardless of the problems, nutrition therapy is valid only to the extent that it involves this kind of knowledge, as well as these particular skills and insights. Individual adaptations of the diet to meet individual needs are imperative for successful therapy.

Routine House Diets

A schedule of routine "house" diets, based on some type of cycle menu plan, is usually used in hospitals for patients who do not require a special diet modification. According to general patient need and tolerance, the diet order may be liquid (clear liquid), soft (in texture), and regular (a full, normal-for-age diet) (Table 16-5).

Managing the Mode of Feeding

Depending on the patient's condition, the clinical dietitian may manage nutrition therapy by using any one of the following four feeding modes.

1. *Oral diet.* As long as possible, of course, regular oral feeding is preferred. Supplements are added if needed. According to the patient's condition, he or she may need assistance in eating.
2. *Enteral nutrition and tube feeding.* If a patient is unable to eat but the gastrointestinal (GI) tract can be used, enteral delivery, or tube feeding, may provide needed nutrition support. A number of commercial formulas are available.
3. *Peripheral nutrition.* If the patient cannot take in food or formula via the GI tract, intravenous feeding is used. Solutions of dextrose, amino acids, vitamins, and minerals, with lipids as appropriate, can be fed through peripheral veins when the need is not extensive or long term.
4. *Total parenteral nutrition.* If the patient's nutritional need is great and support therapy may be required for a longer time, parenteral feeding through a large central vein is needed. Placement of this catheter is a special procedure. More concentrated special solutions can be used and monitored by a nutrition support team. Formulas are determined by the dietitian and physician, and they are prepared by trained pharmacists. This specialized nutrition support method was originally used only in hospitals, but advances in total parenteral nutrition (TPN) administration now allow its use in many health care settings and even at home with some patients.

EVALUATION: QUALITY PATIENT CARE

General Considerations

When the NCP is carried out, patient care activities need to be considered in terms of nutrition diagnosis and treatment objectives, as well as the extent to which each of the care activities helps to meet the particular goals of the patient and family. This evaluation is continuous and thorough, and it requires careful, objective documentation (see the Case Study box, "Nutrition Assessment and Therapy for

---

KEY TERMS

enteral A mode of feeding that uses the gastrointestinal (GI) tract; oral or tube feeding.

parenteral A mode of feeding that does not use the GI tract; instead it provides nutrition by intravenous delivery of nutrient solutions.

TABLE 16-5   ROUTINE HOSPITAL DIETS

FOOD	CLEAR LIQUID	SOFT	REGULAR
Soup	Clear fat-free broth, bouillon	Same, plus all cream soups	All
Cereal		Cooked cereal, cornflakes, rice, noodles, macaroni, spaghetti	All
Bread		White bread, crackers, melba toast, zwieback	All
Protein foods		Eggs (not fried), mild cheese, cottage and cream cheese, fowl, fish, sweetbreads, tender beef, veal, lamb, liver, bacon, gravy	All
Vegetables		Potatoes (baked, mashed, creamed, steamed, scalloped), tender cooked whole bland vegetables, fresh lettuce, tomatoes	All
Fruit and fruit juices	Fruit juices (as tolerated), flavored fruit drinks	Same, plus cooked fruit (peaches, pears, applesauce, peeled apricots, white cherries), ripe peaches, pears, bananas, orange and grapefruit sections without membrane	All
Desserts and gelatin	Fruit-flavored gelatin, fruit ices, and Popsicles	Same, plus plain sponge cakes, plain cookies, plain cake, puddings, pie made with allowed foods	All
Miscellaneous	Soft drinks (as tolerated), coffee and tea, decaffeinated coffee and tea, cereal beverages (e.g., Postum), sugar, honey, salt, hard candy, Polycose (Ross Laboratories), residue-free supplements	Same, plus mild salad dressings	All

CASE STUDY

Nutrition Assessment and Therapy for a Patient with Cancer

Esther is a 160-cm (5 feet 4 inches) tall, medium-frame, 43-year-old patient recovering from a gastrectomy performed 8 days ago to treat gastric cancer. Her weight has dropped gradually for the past 4 months, from an average of 59 kg (130 lb) before her illness began. She continues to observe a full-liquid diet, consuming 60 to 120 mL (2 to 4 oz) of milk every few hours, plus one or two soft-boiled eggs each day. Today Esther informed the nutritionist that she consumed a total of 721 mL (24 oz) of milk and two eggs.

In reviewing Esther's records, the clinical dietitian found the following nutrition assessment data: weight, 46.8 kg (103 lb); triceps skinfold, 10 mm; and midarm circumference, 17 cm. Laboratory values include serum albumin, 3 g/dL; total iron-binding capacity (TIBC), 230 mcg/dL; lymphocytes, 1200 cells/mm^3 (23%); hematocrit, 35%; and hemoglobin, 10.5 g/dL. Urinalysis (24 hours) included blood urea nitrogen, 16 g; and creatinine, 1.75 g.

After reviewing the data, the clinical dietitian calculated nitrogen balance, transferrin, and creatinine-height index, which were recorded on the patient chart. Basal energy expenditure (BEE) needs, as well as the kcalories and protein needed to overcome catabolism, were also calculated, along with estimates for additional vitamin and mineral requirements.

The clinical dietitian noted the physician had ordered chemotherapy for the patient, continuing after discharge, and recommended use of total parenteral nutrition (TPN), also to be continued after discharge, as a means of meeting Esther's nutritional needs. In addition, the clinical dietitian planned ways

of meeting any feeding problems that often accompany chemotherapy, such as sore mouth, nausea, and food intolerances. Observing a carefully prepared protocol developed by the hospital nutrition support team, Esther and her husband were instructed in procuring and using the home TPN treatment. The clinical dietitian also provided follow-up counseling for Esther and her husband at the office and in the group sessions for cancer patients and their families.

Questions for Analysis

1. Use a nutrition assessment data summary sheet from your hospital (or design your own) to record pertinent data given in this case study. What additional data would you collect? How would it be obtained?
2. For each test listed on your data sheet, explain what it measures and how that information contributes to an understanding of Esther's status.
3. What specific nutritional needs (nutrition diagnoses) can you identify in this case? List them in order of priority.
4. Calculate Esther's nitrogen balance and transferrin for day 8. Why are these indexes important to assessing her nutritional status?
5. What is Esther's creatinine-height index? How does it reflect her nutritional status?
6. What nutrition problems do you expect Esther to experience after discharge? How could they be resolved? What community agencies might contribute to her sense of well-being after discharge?

a Patient with Cancer"). It seeks to validate care while it is being given, as well as determine the effectiveness of a particular course of care. Various areas need to be investigated, as follows:

- *Estimate the achievement of nutrition therapy goals:* What is the effect of diet or mode of feeding on the illness or patient's situation? Does a need exist for any change in nutrient ratios of diet or formula as originally calculated, in meal distribution pattern, or in feeding mode?
- *Judge the accuracy of intervention actions:* Does a need exist to change any of the NCP components? For example, is it necessary to change the type of food or feeding equipment, environment for meals, procedures for counseling,

or types of learning activities for nutrition education and self-care procedures?
- *Determine the patient's ability to follow the prescribed nutrition therapy:* Do any hindrances or disabilities exist that prevent the patient from observing the treatment plan? What is the effect of nutrition therapy on the patient, family, or staff? Were the necessary nutrition assessment procedures for collecting nutrition data carried out correctly? Do patient and family understand the information given for self-care? Have community resources required by the patient and family been available and convenient for use? Has any needed food assistance program been sufficient to meet needs for the patient's ongoing care?

TO SUM UP

The basis for an accurate assessment of the patient's nutritional needs begins with the individual patient and family. Physical, psychologic, social, economic, and cultural factors in and out of the clinical setting all play a role in evaluating the patient's health status and any possible problems with the nutrition care plan.

Nutrition assessment is based on a broad foundation of pertinent data, including food and drug uses and values. Effectiveness of an assessment based on analysis of these data depends on effective communication with the patient, family members, and significant others in the development of an appropriate care plan, as well as with other members

of the health care team. The patient's medical record is a basic means of communication among health care team members.

Nutrition therapy, based on a combination of personal and physiologic needs of the patient, requires a close working relationship among nutrition, medical, and nursing staff in the health care facility. The nurse's schedule offers many opportunities to reinforce nutrition principles of the diet. Nutrition therapy does not end with the patient's discharge. Outpatient nutrition services, appropriate social services, and food resources in the community help meet the continuing needs of patients and their families.

QUESTIONS FOR REVIEW

1. Identify and discuss possible effects of various psychologic factors on the outcome of nutrition therapy.
2. Outline a general procedure for assessing the nutritional needs of a 65-year-old widower hospitalized with coronary heart disease. Include the appropriate community agencies that you would refer the patient to for follow-up care, services, and information.
3. Describe commonly used anthropometric procedures, as well as laboratory and urine tests for nutritional status

information, in terms of the significance of the measure or test (i.e., what is being measured, what the results tell you).
4. Select several clinical signs used to assess nutritional status, and describe what each sign shows in a malnourished person and why.
5. Describe the nature and purpose of quality assurance plans for standards of nutrition care.

REFERENCES

1. Moore MC: *Pocket guide to nutrition assessment and care*, ed 6, St Louis, Mo., 2009, Mosby.
2. Nelms M: Assessment of nutrition status and risk. In Nelms MN, Sucher K, Long S, editors: *Understanding nutrition therapy and pathophysiology*, Belmont, Calif., 2007, Wadsworth.
3. American Dietetic Association: Position of the American Dietetic Association: integration of medical nutrition therapy and pharmacotherapy. *J Am Diet Assoc* 110:950, 2010.
4. Wolf AM, Siadaty M, Yaeger B, et al: Effects of lifestyle intervention on health care costs: Improving Control with

Activity and Nutrition (ICAN). *J Am Diet Assoc* 107:1365, 2007.
5. Fessler TA: Malnutrition: a serious concern for hospitalized patients. *Today's Dietitian* 10(7):44, 2008.
6. Weight-Control Information Network: *Overweight and obesity statistics*, Bethesda, Md., 2012, National Institute of Diabetes and Digestive and Kidney Diseases. from: <www.win.niddk.nih.gov/statistics/index.htm>. Retrieved March 20, 2013.
7. Centers for Disease Control and Prevention: *Overweight and obesity: causes and consequences*, Atlanta, Ga., 2012, Centers for Disease Control and Prevention. from: <www.cdc.gov/obesity/adult/causes/index.html>. Retrieved March 20, 2013.

8. Lacey K, Pritchitt E: Nutrition Care Process and model: ADA adopts road map to quality care and outcomes management. *J Am Diet Assoc* 103(8):1061, 2003.

9. Lee RD, Nieman DC: *Nutritional assessment*, ed 6, Boston, 2012, McGraw-Hill.

10. American Dietetic Association: Nutrition Care Process and Model Part 1: The 2008 Update. *J Am Diet Assoc* 108:1113, 2008.

11. American Dietetic Association: ADA's definitions for nutrition screening and nutrition assessment. *J Am Diet Assoc* 94:838, 1994.

12. The Joint Commission: *Standards FAQ Details: Nutritional, Functional and Pain Assessments and Screens*, Oakbrook Terrace, Ill., 2008, The Joint Commission. from: <http://www.jointcommission.org/standards_information/jcfaq.aspx?ProgramId=39>. Retrieved March 20, 2013.

13. Identifying patients at risk: ADA's definitions for nutrition screening and nutrition assessment. *J Am Diet Assoc* 94(8):838, 1994.

14. Charney P, Marian M: Nutrition screening and nutrition assessment. In Charney P, Malone AM, editors: *ADA pocket guide to nutrition assessment*, ed 2, Chicago, 2009, American Dietetic Association.

15. Lefton J, Malone AM: Anthropometric assessment. In Charney P, Malone AM, editors: *ADA pocket guide to nutrition assessment*, ed 2, Chicago, 2009, American Dietetic Association.

16. National Heart, Lung, and Blood Institute: *Obesity education initiative*, Bethesda, Md., 2012, National Heart, Lung, and Blood Institute, National Institutes of Health. from: <www.nhlbi.nih.gov/health/public/heart/obesity/lose_wt/risk.htm>. Retrieved May 19, 2014.

17. Chumlea WC, Guo SS, Steinbaugh ML: Prediction of stature from knee height for black and white adults and children with application to mobility-impaired or handicapped persons. *J Am Diet Assoc* 94:1385, 1994.

18. Cockram DB, Baumgartner RN: Evaluation of accuracy and reliability of calipers for measuring recumbent knee height in elderly people. *Am J Clin Nutr* 52:397, 1990.

19. Muncie HI, Sobal J, Hoopes JM, et al: A practical method of estimating stature of bedridden female nursing home patients. *J Am Geriatr Soc* 35:285, 1987.

20. Mitchell CO, Lipschitz DA: Arm length measurement as an alternative to height in the nutrition assessment of the elderly. *JPEN J Parenter Enteral Nutr* 6:226, 1982.

21. American Dietetic Association Evidence Analysis Library: *Adult weight management guidelines*, Chicago, 2014, American Dietetic Association. from: <www.adaevidencelibrary.com>. Retrieved May 19, 2014.

22. Thompson CW: Laboratory assessment. In Charney P, Malone AM, editors: *ADA pocket guide to nutrition assessment*, ed 2, Chicago, 2009, American Dietetic Association.

23. American Dietetic Association: *International Dietetics and Nutrition Terminology (IDNT) reference manual. Standardized language for the nutrition care process*, ed 4, Chicago, 2013, American Dietetic Association.

FURTHER READINGS AND RESOURCES

Readings

American Dietetic Association: Position of the American Dietetic Association: integration of medical nutrition therapy and pharmacology. *J Am Diet Assoc* 103(10):1363, 2003.

American Dietetic Association: Position of the American Dietetic Association: ethical and legal issues in nutrition, hydration, and feeding. *J Am Diet Assoc* 108(5):873, 2008.

Websites of Interest

- Nestle Nutrition, Clinical Resources and Tools. This site provides tools and resources to help identify, assess, and select appropriate products to address the nutrition challenges of patients: www.nestle-nutrition.com/Clinical_Resources/Default.aspx.

- U.S. Department of Agriculture, Food and Nutrition Information Center, Dietary Analysis and Intake Calculators. This site, hosted by the Food and Nutrition Information Center (FNIC) at the National Agricultural Library (NAL), provides links to numerous diet-analysis tools: http://fnic.nal.usda.gov/dietary-guidance/interactive-tools

Metabolic Stress

Joyce Gilbert

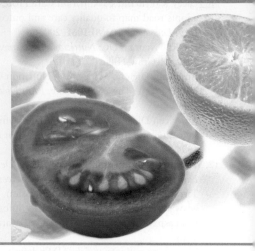

ⓔ EVOLVE WEBSITE

http://evolve.elsevier.com/Williams/essentials/

OUTLINE

Nutritional Needs of General Surgery Patients
Nutritional Concerns for Patients Undergoing Alimentary Canal Surgery

Nutritional Needs in Thermal Injuries
HEALTH PROMOTION
Immunonutrition

In this chapter, various surgical procedures are discussed, with a focus on surgical procedures and situations that could have a large nutritional consequence, particularly thermal injuries (or burns). An understanding of the surgical procedure performed, with knowledge of nutritional and absorptive function and capacity of the alimentary tract, is imperative to providing optimal nutrition care of surgery patients (see the Focus on Culture box, "Physiologic Changes Related to the Aging Process That Can Affect Surgery"). An understanding of the body's response to metabolic stress is also important when determining optimal timing and type of nutrition intervention for the patient.

NUTRITIONAL NEEDS OF GENERAL SURGERY PATIENTS

Preoperative Nutrition

The nutritional needs of surgery patients vary based on several factors, including the patient's disease process, other comorbidities, and baseline nutritional status. Many general surgery patients are adequately nourished preoperatively and therefore do not have any special nutrient requirements (see the Perspectives in Practice box, "Energy and Protein Requirements in General Surgery Patients"). The disease itself often lends to poor nutrient intake and a hypermetabolic state that places the patient at nutritional risk. Malnutrition is associated with altered immune function, poor wound healing, and

increased morbidity and mortality rates.[1] Researchers estimate that more than 50% of hospitalized patients are malnourished on hospital admission and hospital discharge.[2-5] For optimal outcome a malnourished patient should be nutritionally repleted for 7 to 10 days before surgery, if time permits.[6] Unless the gastrointestinal (GI) tract is nonfunctional, nutrient provision should be provided enterally rather than parenterally.[7] Following are some guidelines:

- *Energy:* Adequate calories should be consumed to prevent loss of endogenous stores of carbohydrate, fat, and protein. Carbohydrates should constitute the majority of calories (50% to 60%). A minimum of approximately 150 g of carbohydrates per day is needed for central nervous system (CNS) function.
- *Protein:* Most patients do not have excessive preoperative protein requirements, but body stores should be assessed. Adequate protein status is imperative to facilitate optimal wound healing.
- *Vitamins and minerals:* Any deficiency state such as anemia should be corrected. Electrolytes and fluids should be normalized and in balance with correction of dehydration, acidosis, or alkalosis.

One often-overlooked factor is the use of medicinal herbs. Many patients do not think to disclose the ingestion of herbal supplements when they are asked about medications during the preoperative interview, but some of these substances can complicate surgery. (Some common herbal supplements that can cause complications during surgery are

FOCUS ON CULTURE

Physiologic Changes Related to the Aging Process That Can Affect Surgery

Physiologic Change	Effects	Potential Postoperative Complications
Cardiovascular		
↓ Elasticity of blood vessels	↓ Circulation to vital organs	Shock (hypotension), thrombosis with pulmonary emboli, delayed wound healing, postoperative confusion, hypervolemia, decreased response to stress
↓ Cardiac output	Slower blood flow	
↓ Peripheral circulation		
Respiratory		
↓ Elasticity of lungs and chest wall	↓ Vital capacity	Atelectasis, pneumonia, postoperative confusion
↓ Residual lung volume	↓ Alveolar volume	
↓ Forced expiratory volume	↓ Gas exchange	
↓ Ciliary action	↓ Cough reflex	
Fewer alveolar capillaries		
Urinary		
↓ Glomerular filtration rate	↓ Kidney function	Prolonged response to anesthesia and drugs, overhydration with intravenous fluids, hyperkalemia, urinary tract infection, urinary retention
↓ Bladder muscle tone	Stasis of urine in bladder	
Weakened perineal muscles	Loss of urinary control	
Musculoskeletal		
↓ Muscle strength	↓ Activity	Atelectasis, pneumonia, thrombophlebitis, constipation or fecal impaction
Limitation of motion		
Gastrointestinal		
↓ Intestinal motility	Retention of feces	Constipation or fecal impaction
Metabolic		
↓ γ-Globulin level	↓ Inflammatory response	Delayed wound healing, wound dehiscence or evisceration
↓ Plasma proteins		
Immune System		
Fewer killer T cells	↓ Ability to protect against invasion by pathogenic microorganisms	Wound infection, wound dehiscence, pneumonia, urinary tract infection
↓ Response to foreign antigens		

From Keeling AW, Muro A, Long BC: Preoperative nursing. In Phipps WJ, Cassmever VL, Sands JK, editors: *Medical-surgical nursing: concepts and clinical practice,* ed 5, St Louis, Mo., 1995, Mosby.

listed in the Diet-Medications Interactions box, "Medicine or Poison?")

Immediate Preoperative Period

Typical dietary preparation for surgery involves giving nothing by mouth 8 to 12 hours before surgery. The rationale is to ensure the stomach is empty of food and liquids to prevent vomiting or aspiration during surgery or anesthesia recovery. In an emergency situation, gastric suction is used to remove stomach contents. With surgery involving the GI tract, food and fecal matter may interfere with the procedure itself and cause contamination. Therefore, before lower GI surgery, a low-residue diet may be prescribed to reduce fecal residue. Although restricting dietary intake may decrease the risks associated with anesthesia, it can also impair the patient's ability to respond to the metabolic stress of surgery. To reduce surgical stress and postoperative complications the use of an enhanced recovery after surgery (ERAS) protocol is important.[8] An ERAS protocol attenuates the surgical stress response and accelerates postoperative recovery.[9]

Postoperative Nutrition

Nutrient provision in the postoperative period depends on several factors, including the surgical procedure performed

and anticipated time to resumption of oral intake, complications of surgery and postoperative clinical status, and preoperative nutritional status. The well-nourished patient undergoing elective surgery will typically resume oral feeding by postoperative day 3 to 7, depending on return of bowel function. In this situation, supplemental nutrition in the form of enteral and parenteral nutrition is not indicated. The malnourished patient who is undergoing elective or emergency surgery and not anticipated to be able to meet his or her nutritional needs orally for a period of 7 to 10 days should receive specialized nutrition support.[6] This nutrition support should be provided enterally rather than parenterally to minimize incidence of complications.[6] Duration of this therapy will then depend on the patient's clinical status and transition to an adequate oral dietary consumption.

Energy Requirements

In the immediate postoperative period, especially in the critically ill, the goal of nutrition support is maintenance of current lean body mass, not repletion, and should serve as an adjunct to other critical therapies. Numerous factors are present that limit the effectiveness of exogenously administered nutritional substrates in preventing catabolism regardless of the level of support. It should not be expected to

PERSPECTIVES IN PRACTICE

Energy and Protein Requirements in General Surgery Patients

The nutritional needs of general surgery patients vary based on several factors, including the patient's disease process, other comorbidities, surgery to be performed, and baseline nutritional status. For example, compare the following patient situations.

Adequately Nourished Preoperative Patient

For the patient with normal energy and nitrogen balance, approximately 25 kcal/kg/day and 0.8 to 1.0 g/kg/day of protein should maintain these balances.

Adequately Nourished Postoperative Patient

If no complications have occurred after surgery, then energy requirements remain about the same—25 kcal/kg/day. Protein requirements increase slightly because of increased metabolism and need for wound healing in the postoperative period to 1.0 to 1.1 g/kg/day.

Adequately Nourished Stressed Patient

This patient is assumed to have adequate nutrient stores; therefore replenishment is not the goal. Metabolic stress increases metabolic and catabolic rates, making energy and protein needs elevated. Energy needs are estimated at 25 to 30 kcal/kg/day; protein needs, 1.2 to 1.5 g/kg/day. Postoperatively the patient should be reassessed, and protein needs may increase up to 2 g/kg/day.

Nutritionally Depleted Nonstressed Patient
Upcoming Surgery: Gastrointestinal Tract Resection Resulting from Obstruction

Because of reduced dietary intake, this patient's nutrient stores (mostly glycogen and fat) may be depleted. In the nonstressed state, protein stores are spared for the most part. Energy needs are similar to those of the nourished preoperative patient at 25 kcal/kg/day. However, protein needs are slightly elevated to 1.0 to 1.2 g/kg/day. Postoperatively this patient's energy needs will remain near the same at 25 kcal/kg/day, but protein needs are increased to 1.2 to 1.5 g/kg/day.

Nutritionally Depleted Stressed Patient

This patient has elevated requirements for energy and protein because of cytokine and hormonal shifts causing a hypermetabolic and hypercatabolic state. Energy needs are 25 to 30 kcal/kg/day, with caution to avoid overfeeding. Overfeeding in a hypermetabolic state can result in hyperglycemia, hypercarbia, hepatic steatosis, and overall immune suppression. Protein needs are elevated to 1.5 to 2.0 g/kg/day. Postoperatively the nutrient needs remain about the same. At this point the goal is to minimize loss of lean body mass, not to replenish it. Once the patient is stable and anabolic, calories can be increased to 35 kcal/kg/day as needed for rehabilitation.

Bibliography

ASPEN Board of Directors and the Clinical Guidelines Task Force: Guidelines for the use of parenteral and enteral nutrition in adult and pediatric patients. *J Parent Enteral Nutr* 26:1SA, 2002.

Frankenfield D: Energy and macrosubstrate requirements. *American Society for Enteral and Parenteral Nutrition: The science and practice of nutrition support: a case-based core,* ed 3, Dubuque, Iowa, 2001, Kendall/Hunt.

---

convert a catabolic, septic patient into an anabolic state at this time. Many undesirable metabolic complications can occur in attempting to do so, such as hypercapnia, hyperglycemia, hypertriglyceridemia, hepatic steatosis, and azotemia.[7,10-13] Once the hypermetabolic process is corrected, anabolism is favored and repletion can occur.

Multiple methods are available for determining energy requirements. Indirect calorimetry involves actual measurement of energy expenditure and remains the "gold standard."[14] However, many disadvantages to this method exist, including increased cost, the potential for improperly trained personnel, inaccurate readings in patients with an FiO_2 (fraction of inspired oxygen) of 50% or more, the possibility of malfunctioning chest tubes and endotracheal tubes, and the occurrence of bronchopleural fistulas. Because of these flaws, many institutions do not have the technology available and rely on predictive equations. Predicting energy needs can be difficult because of uncertainties regarding multiple factors of energy expenditure (Table 17-1).[15] Predictive equations (Box 17-1) may overestimate energy needs for those mechanically ventilated and sedated, and neuromuscular paralysis

EXTENT OF BODY RESERVES OF NUTRIENTS

NUTRIENT	TIME REQUIRED TO DEPLETE RESERVES IN WELL-NOURISHED INDIVIDUALS
Amino acids	Several hours
Carbohydrate	13 hours
Sodium	2-3 days
Water	4 days
Zinc	5 days
Fat	20-40 days
Thiamin	30-60 days
Vitamin C	60-120 days
Niacin	60-180 days
Riboflavin	60-180 days
Vitamin A	90-365 days
Iron	125 days (women), 750 days (men)
Iodine	1000 days
Calcium	2500 days

From Guthrie HA: *Introductory nutrition,* ed 7, St Louis, Mo., 1989, Mosby.

DIET-MEDICATIONS INTERACTIONS

Medicine or Poison?

"Poisons and medicines are oftentimes the same substances given with different intents."

Peter Mere Latham (1789-1875)

Medicinal herbs and pharmaceutical drugs: Both can be therapeutic at one dose and toxic at another. Patients may not think to include herbal supplements when reporting medications used during the preoperative interview. Possible surgical complications vary depending on the herbal supplement used. Following are some common herbal supplements that may cause surgical complications.

Herb	Common Uses	Possible Surgical Complication
Danshen (*Salvia miltiorrhiza*)	Antibacterial, antihepatotoxin, mild sedative, antiinflammatory	May cause bleeding
Dong quai (*Angelica sinensis*)	Menstrual disorders, menopause	May cause bleeding (interferes with warfarin)
Echinacea (*Echinacea purpurea*)	Prevent and treat common cold, treat infections, enhance wound healing	May interfere with effectiveness of immunosuppressant drugs given to prevent transplant rejection; may interfere with body's immune functioning after surgery; could impair wound healing
Ephedra* (Ma huang, herbal ecstasy, Chinese ephedra)	Sinus congestion, weight loss (ephedrine/caffeine)	May cause cardiovascular problems (increased heart rate, arrhythmias, heart attack or stroke); interaction with anesthesia can lead to abnormal heartbeat. For patients taking maintenance doses of monoamine oxidase inhibitors (MAOIs), interaction with anesthesia and MAOIs may result in life-threatening hypertension and coma
Feverfew (*Tanacetum parthenium*)	Migraine headaches (prophylaxis), rheumatoid arthritis (RA)	May cause bleeding
Garlic (*Allium* spp.)	Atherosclerosis, hyperlipidemia, hypertension, antithrombotic effects, chemoprevention, insect repellant, antimicrobial	May cause bleeding or interfere with normal clotting
Ginkgo (*Ginkgo biloba*)	Alzheimer's disease and non-Alzheimer's dementia, ordinary age-related memory loss, improving memory and mental function in the young, intermittent claudication, premenstrual syndrome, altitude sickness, tinnitus	May cause bleeding
Ginseng (*Panax ginseng*)	Enhancing immunity, improving mental activity, diabetes, athletic performance	May cause bleeding (interferes with warfarin)
Goldenseal (*Hydrastis canadensis*)	Antimicrobial, expectorant	May cause or worsen hypertension
Kava (*Piper methysticum*)	Anxiety	May enhance sedative effects of anesthesia
Licorice† (*Glycyrrhiza glabra*)	Peptic ulcer disease, expectorant/antitussive	May increase blood pressure
St. John's wort (*Hypericum perforatum*)	Major depression of mild to moderate severity, polyneuropathy	Can increase or decrease effect of some drugs used during and after surgery
Valerian (*Valeriana officinalis*)	Insomnia, anxiety	May interfere with effects of anesthesia

NOTE: Different herbs stay in the body for different lengths of time. An individual taking herbs may need to stop taking them 1 or 2 weeks before surgery.

Bibliography

Bratman S, Girman AM: *Mosby's handbook of herbs and supplements and their therapeutic uses*, St Louis, Mo., 2003, Mosby.

Escott-Stump S: *Nutrition and diagnosis-related care*, ed 6, Philadelphia, Pa., 2007, Lippincott Williams & Wilkins.

Fugh-Berman A: Herb-drug interactions. *Lancet* 355:134, 2000.

Kuhn MA, Winston D: *Winston and Kuhn's: Herbal therapy and supplements: a scientific and traditional approach*, ed 2, Philadelphia, Pa., 2007, Lippincott Williams & Wilkins.

Mayo Clinic Staff: *Herbal supplements and surgery: what you need to know*, Rochester, Minn., 2003, Mayo Foundation for Medical Education and Research. from: <www.mayoclinic.com>. Retrieved August 14, 2005.

*Ephedra was banned by the U.S. Food and Drug Administration (FDA) in December 2003.
†Most licorice candy contains little or no herbal licorice. Consumers should consult the product ingredients. "Licorice flavoring" is safer than "licorice extract" or "natural licorice" for these purposes.

can decrease energy requirements by as much as 30%.[16-18] Calculated results are only as accurate as the variables used in the equation. Obesity and resuscitative water weight complicate use of these equations and lead to a tendency for overfeeding.[19] It is unclear as to whether ideal body weight (IBW) or actual body weight should be used in predictive energy equations. It has been reported that obese patients should receive 20 to 30 kilocalories (kcalories or kcal)/kg IBW per day,[20] as well as use of adjusted body weight, particularly in those weighing more than 130% IBW.[21] Predictive equations have been developed to account for obesity, using actual body weight, as well as trauma, burns, and ventilatory status.[21] Patino and colleagues[22] reported a hypocaloric-hyperproteinic nutrition regimen provided during the first days of the flow phase of the adaptive response to injury, sepsis, and critical illness. The regimen consists of a daily supply of 100 to 200 g of glucose and 1.5 to 2.0 g of protein per kilogram IBW. Overall, energy requirements for surgery patients range from 20 to 35 kcal/kg usual body weight per day.[23]

Protein Requirements

Dietary protein is required to build new and maintain existing body tissue and has many functions in the body. Protein can also be oxidized directly for adenosine triphosphate (ATP) and is critical to the body's ability to perform gluco-

neogenesis. Therefore protein is an important energy substrate in addition to its role in tissue building and repair.

Protein requirements in the surgical patient are typically elevated, particularly in the critically ill. Increased requirements are the result of the need for tissue synthesis and wound healing, maintenance of oncotic pressure, adequate blood volume, maintenance of immune function, and energy substrate. Stressed critically ill patients require protein in the range of 1.5 to 2.0 g/kg/day.[22] Achieving positive nitrogen balance is nearly impossible immediately after metabolic insult, but after the primary insult is controlled or resolved, positive nitrogen balance is feasible. Protein requirements do not decrease with increasing age. Short-term inadequate protein intake in older adults has been shown to change skeletal muscle transcript levels that may lead to muscle wasting.[24] Reduction in lean body mass and obligatory loss of protein during physiologic stress increase protein requirements for critically ill older patients to requirements similar to those for younger patients.[25,26] Protein tolerance,

TABLE 17-1	INFLUENCES ON RESTING ENERGY EXPENDITURE
CLINICAL CONDITION	**REE (%)***
Elective uncomplicated surgery	Normal
Major Abdominal, Thoracic, and Vascular Surgery	
ICU + mechanical ventilation	105-109 ± 20-28
Cardiac Surgery	
ICU + mechanical ventilation	119 ± 21
Multiple Injury	
ICU + mechanical ventilation	138 ± 23
Spontaneous ventilation	119 ± 7
Head and Multiple Injury	
ICU + mechanical ventilation	150 ± 23
Head Injury	
ICU + spontaneous ventilation	126 ± 14
ICU + mechanical ventilation	104 ± 5
Infection	
Sepsis + spontaneous ventilation	121 ± 27
ICU + septic shock + mechanical ventilation	135 ± 28
Sepsis + mechanical ventilation	155 ± 14
Septic shock + mechanical ventilation	102 ± 14
Multiple injury + sepsis + mechanical ventilation + TPN	191 ± 38

Modified from Chiolero R, Revelly JP, Tappy L: Energy metabolism in sepsis and injury. *Nutrition* 13(suppl):45S, 1997, with permission from Elsevier.
ICU, Intensive care unit; *REE,* resting energy expenditure; *TPN,* total parenteral nutrition.
*Values are percentage of reference value (±SD).

BOX 17-1	SELECTED METHODS FOR ESTIMATING ENERGY REQUIREMENTS

Harris-Benedict Basal Energy Expenditure (BEE) Equation

$$\text{Male: } 66.5 + 13.8(W) + 5.0(H) - 6.8(A)$$

$$\text{Female: } 655.1 + 9.6(W) + 1.9(H) - 4.7(A),$$

where W is weight (in kilograms); H, height (in centimeters); and A, age (in years).

NOTE: To predict total energy expenditure (TEE), add an injury/activity factor of 1.2 to 1.8 depending on the severity and nature of illness.

Ireton-Jones Energy Expenditure Equations (EEEs)
Spontaneously Breathing Patients

$$EEE(s) = 629 - 11(A) + 25(W) - 609(O)$$

Ventilator-Dependent Patients

$$EEE(v) = 1784 - 11(A) + 5(W) + 244(G) + 239(T) + 804(B),$$

where EEE is given in kcal/day; v, ventilator dependent; s, spontaneously breathing; A, age (in years); W, body weight (in kilograms); G, gender (female = 0, male = 1); V, ventilator support (present = 1, absent = 0), T, diagnosis of trauma (present = 1, absent = 0); B, diagnosis of burn (present = 1, absent = 0); and O, obesity >30% more than ideal body weight (IBW) (from 1959 Metropolitan Life Insurance tables; present = 1, absent = 0).

KEY TERM

sepsis Presence in the blood or other tissues of pathogenic microorganisms or their toxins; conditions associated with such pathogens

as opposed to protein requirement, often determines amount of protein delivered. Onset of azotemia (i.e., impaired renal or hepatic function) signals the need to reduce protein delivery. Most studies that examined graded protein intakes in septic, injured, or burned patients have found no protein-sparing benefit to giving protein in excess of the previous recommendations.[27]

Fluid Requirements

Water is the medium within which all systems and subsystems function. It is necessary in digestion, absorption, transport, and use of nutrients, as well as in elimination of toxins and waste products. Total body fluid can be compartmentalized into two reservoirs: intracellular and extracellular. The intracellular compartment includes all water within the cell membrane and provides the environment for the metabolic reactions that take place in cells. The extracellular compartmental water includes all water external to cell membranes and allows nutrients to flow into cells and cellular waste products to return to the bloodstream. Water also provides structure to cells and is a vital component of thermoregulation. Water is the most abundant substance in the human body, accounting for approximately 60% of body weight of men and 50% of body weight of women. The majority of water intake comes from ingested fluid and food; a small amount is produced as a by-product of metabolic processes, primarily carbohydrate metabolism. The main source of water loss is in the form of urine. However, sizable amounts are also lost insensibly through skin and respiratory tract. Smaller amounts of water are lost in sweat and feces (Table 17-2).

Normal body water requirements can be estimated using a variety of methods. The National Research Council (NRC) recommends 1 mL/kcal energy expenditure for adults with average energy expenditure living under average environmental conditions. Fluid requirements increase with several conditions, including fever, high altitude, low humidity, profuse sweating, watery diarrhea, vomiting, hemorrhage, diuresis, surgical drains, and loss of skin integrity (e.g., burns, open wounds).

Therefore fluid balance is of vital concern after surgery. Patients often receive large volumes of fluid intraoperatively. These volumes are normally eliminated postoperatively, but occasionally the patient may require diuretics to facilitate this. Typically, surgical patients are provided with intravenous fluids until oral intake is resumed and tolerated to maintain fluid balance. Daily weight measurement of the patient provides a guideline for fluid balance.

Vitamin and Mineral Requirements

Adequate levels of vitamins and minerals are very important for optimal postoperative recovery. Vitamin C serves many functions in the body. In addition to being an antioxidant, it is required for synthesis of collagen (the structural protein found in skin, bone, tendon, and cartilage), carnitine, and neurotransmitters, as well as for immune-mediated and antibacterial functions of white blood cells. Vitamin C is also required for the scar tissue, which aids in wound healing. Iron is an essential component of the following: (1) hemoglobin, which is necessary for oxygen transport; (2) myoglobin, which is necessary for muscle iron storage; (3) and in cytochromes, which transport electrons through the respiratory chain resulting in the oxidative production of cellular energy. Vitamin K is essential in the blood-clotting cascade by activating inactive clotting factors resulting in the formation of fibrin. Surgical patients with elevated enteric losses (e.g., ostomy, stool, fistula) are at risk for several trace element deficiencies (e.g., zinc, copper). If losses exceed 800 mL/day, then extra supplementation of micronutrients should be considered. Various GI operations may also place a surgical patient at risk for several micronutrient deficiencies, depending on the amount of remaining small intestine, the location of bowel resection, and the functional status of remaining GI tract.[1]

Diets
Oral Diet

The preferred route of nutrient delivery is for the patient to be able to consume adequate nutrients through an oral diet. Fortunately the majority of surgical patients can accomplish this by postoperative day 7 at the latest. Routine intravenous fluids are intended to provide hydration and electrolytes, not energy and protein requirements. For example, 1 L of routine intravenous fluids of a 5% dextrose solution provides 50 g of dextrose, with an energy value of only 170 kcal; no protein is provided. If adequate calories and protein are not consumed, then the patient's diet may be supplemented. Often the addition of between-meal feedings that consist of soft, high-protein foods is adequate. However, sometimes commercially available oral supplements may be provided because they are a concentrated source of energy, protein, and vitamins and minerals.[28] Not all patients tolerate these supplements, because they tend to be very sweet and patients develop taste

TABLE 17-2	NORMAL DAILY FLUID GAINS AND LOSSES IN ADULTS		
FLUID GAINS		**FLUID LOSSES**	
Sensible		*Sensible*	
Food	1000 mL	Urine	1500 mL
Fluid	1200 mL	Feces	100 mL
		Sweat	50 mL
Insensible		*Insensible*	
Oxidative metabolism	350 mL	Skin	500 mL
		Lungs	400 mL
Total	2550 mL	Total	2550 mL

Reprinted from Gottschlich MM, Fuhrman M, Hammond K, Holcombe B, Seidner D. *The science and practice of nutrition support: A case-based core curriculum.* Dubuque, Iowa, 2001, Kendall/Hunt, p. 55.

fatigue. Every effort should be made to maximize the patient's diet for his or her diet preferences to improve inadequate dietary consumption.

Routine Postoperative Diets

A diet order is typically prescribed postoperatively once the patient exhibits adequate bowel function (e.g., flatus, bowel sounds present). Historically the first diet order is a clear liquid diet (Box 17-2). This diet contains hyperosmolar fluids, calories from primarily simple sugars, very little protein, and a fair amount of sodium and chloride. Because this diet is incomplete and very unpalatable, patients should be advanced to either a full liquid or soft/regular diet as soon as the clear liquid diet is tolerated. These diets are complete diets in that calorie, protein, and vitamin and mineral requirements can be met if adequate amounts are consumed. Recently this historical diet progression after GI surgery was challenged.[29] Patients randomized to a regular diet as their first postoperative diet after abdominal surgery had equal tolerance and improved nutrient intake compared with those receiving a clear liquid diet.

Specialized Nutrition Support

If an oral diet is not tolerated or feasible, then enteral or parenteral nutrition may be provided. Enteral nutrition is indicated for patients with an adequately functional GI tract and oral nutrient intake that is insufficient to meet estimated needs.[6] Enteral nutrition maintains nutritional, metabolic, immunologic, and barrier functions of the intestines; it is less expensive and safer than parenteral nutrition.[30] A series of studies of patients with GI cancer suggests parenteral nutrition increased the overall risk of postoperative complications by 10%. However, parenteral nutrition administered 7 to 10 days before surgery decreases postoperative complications by approximately 10%. Wound healing and surgical recovery may be impaired if parenteral nutrition is not begun within 5 to 10 days after surgery in patients unable to eat or tolerate enteral feeding. Although enteral nutrition is the preferred route of nutrient delivery, it is not innocuous. Some situations exist in which enteral feeding is not feasible (Box 17-3), and therefore parenteral nutrition should be used. Expected length of therapy, clinical condition, risk of aspiration, and medical expertise usually determine route of administration and type of access for tube feedings. Multiple methods for obtaining enteral access exist (Box 17-4), all of which carry various levels of required expertise, risk, and expense. Nasoenteric or oroenteric tubes are generally used when therapy is anticipated to be of short duration (e.g., less than 4 weeks) or for interim access before placement of a long-term device. Long-term access requires a percutaneous or surgically placed feeding tube. It is not always clear when enteral nutrition will be tolerated. If the needs of the individual are not met enterally, then parenteral nutrition may be implemented for either full nutrient provision or concurrently with enteral delivery to provide the balance of nutrients not tolerated.

The majority of postoperative surgical patients can tolerate a standard enteral formulation that provides their energy and protein requirements. Recent research studies have evaluated use of "immune-enhancing" enteral formulas in postoperative GI cancer patients, trauma patients, and patients with critical illness. These formulas are supplemented with various

---

BOX 17-2	TYPICAL FOODS IN POSTOPERATIVE DIETS

Clear Liquid
- Broth
- Clear juice (apple, grape, cranberry)
- Gelatin
- Sodas (Sprite, ginger ale)
- Tea
- Coffee

Full Liquid
- Juice (any)
- Milk
- Milkshakes
- Ice cream
- Cream soups
- Thinned oatmeal, corn grits
- Scrambled eggs (in some institutions)
- Oral liquid nutritional supplements (e.g., Ensure, Boost)

Soft/Regular
- Juice
- Canned fruits
- Cooked vegetables
- Soft meats (baked chicken, stews, roasts)
- Scrambled eggs
- Pancakes, biscuits, muffins
- Soups
- Soft sandwiches (egg, tuna, chicken salad, turkey, ham and cheese)
- Soft starches (mashed potatoes, pasta, rice)
- Milk, tea, coffee
- Ice cream
- Puddings, yogurt
- Soft desserts (cake, pies, soft cookies)

BOX 17-3	INDICATIONS FOR PARENTERAL NUTRITION

Indications
- Bowel obstruction
- Persistent intolerance of enteral feeding (e.g., emesis, diarrhea)
- Hemodynamic instability
- Major upper gastrointestinal (GI) bleed
- Ileus
- Unable to safely access intestinal tract

Relative Indications
- Significant bowel wall edema
- Nutrient infusion proximal to recent GI anastomosis
- High-output fistula (>800 mL/day)

BOX 17-4 METHODS OF ENTERAL ACCESS

Short Term (<4 weeks)
Nasoenteric Feeding Tube
- Spontaneous passage
- Bedside prokinetic agent

Active Passage
- Bedside assisted
- Endoscopic
- Fluoroscopic
- Operative

Long Term (>4 weeks)
Percutaneous Feeding Tube
- Percutaneous endoscopic (percutaneous endoscopic gastrostomy [PEG])
- Gastric (PEG)
- Gastric/jejunal (PEG/jejunostomy)
- Direct jejunal (direct percutaneous endoscopic jejunostomy [DPEJ])

Laparoscopic
- Gastrostomy
- Jejunostomy

Surgical
- Gastrostomy
- Jejunostomy

immune-enhancing nutrients, including L-arginine, L-glutamine, omega-3 fatty acids, nucleic acids, and various vitamins and minerals. When these diets were used in these surgical populations, decreases in infectious complications and hospital length of stay were noted.[6,31]

NUTRITIONAL CONCERNS FOR PATIENTS UNDERGOING ALIMENTARY CANAL SURGERY

The digestive tract is a metabolically active organ involved in digestion, absorption, and metabolism of many nutrients; therefore various surgical interventions involving the GI tract can result in **malabsorption** and **maldigestion** and nutritional deficiencies (Table 17-3).

Head and Neck Surgery

These patients often present for surgery malnourished because of their disease state. Many times surgical intervention is required because of a tumor that may be inhibiting the patient's ability to chew and swallow normally. Typically, loss of this ability is what makes the patient seek medical attention. Patients with head and neck cancer usually have a long history of alcohol and tobacco use, which may also affect optimal nutritional status.

TABLE 17-3 COMMON GASTROINTESTINAL OPERATIONS AND NUTRITIONAL CONSEQUENCES

LOCATION	POTENTIAL CONSEQUENCES
Esophagus	
Resection/replacement	Weight loss because of inadequate intake
Gastric pull-up	↑ Protein loss because of catabolism
Colonic interposition	May require enteral/parenteral nutrition until oral intake appropriate
	Antidumping diet; may malabsorb fat/fat-soluble vitamins, simple sugars, and various vitamins/minerals
	Early satiety because of reduced storage capacity (gastric pull-up)
Stomach	
Partial gastrectomy/vagotomy	Early satiety because of reduced storage capacity
	Delayed gastric emptying of solids because of stasis
	Rapid emptying of hypertonic fluids
Total gastrectomy	Weight loss because of dumping/malabsorption, early satiety, anorexia, inadequate intake, unavailability of bile acids and pancreatic enzymes because of anastomotic changes
	Malabsorption may lead to anemia, metabolic bone disease, protein-calorie malnutrition
	Bezoar formation
	Vitamin B_{12} deficiency because of lack of intrinsic factor
Intestine*	
Proximal	Malabsorption of vitamins/minerals (Ca^{2+}, Mg^{2+}, iron, vitamins A and D)
Gastric bypass	Protein-calorie malnutrition from malabsorption because of dumping, unavailability of bile acids and pancreatic enzymes because of anastomotic changes
	Bezoar formation
Distal	Malabsorption of vitamins or minerals (water soluble—folate, vitamins B_{12}, C, B_1, B_2, pyridoxine)
	Protein-calorie malnutrition because of dumping
	Fat malabsorption
	Bacterial overgrowth if ileocecal valve resected
Colon	Fluid and electrolyte (K^+, Na^+, Cl^-) malabsorption

*Note that consequences may occur only with extensive disease process and resection.

Depending on the patient's treatment, optimization of nutrition preoperatively is ideal. This also depends on the individual's disease progression and ability to swallow. Many times preoperative treatment involves radiation, chemotherapy, or both to reduce the tumor size. In these situations, the ability to swallow may worsen because of negative side effects of these therapies. Ideally, placement of a percutaneous endoscopic gastrostomy (PEG) feeding tube can be performed to allow for nutrition, hydration, and medication administration to maintain or improve (or both) nutritional status preoperatively. The patient may also still be able to swallow soft foods or liquids, which should be maximized for caloric and protein density. If a PEG tube is not placed preoperatively, then it can be placed intraoperatively or a nasoenteric tube may be placed. These feeding tubes are then used postoperatively until the patient is able to resume an oral diet.

Esophageal Surgery

Several medical conditions affecting the esophagus can prevent swallowing and thus nutrient intake. Common conditions include corrosive injuries and perforation, achalasia, gastroesophageal reflux disease (GERD), and partial or full obstruction caused by cancer, congenital abnormalities, or strictures. These conditions usually require surgical intervention involving removal of a segment or the entire esophagus (see the Case Study box, "The Patient with Esophageal Cancer"). The esophageal tract is then replaced with either the stomach (gastric pull-up) or the intestine (colonic and jejunal interposition). A gastric pull-up procedure involves drawing the stomach up to the esophageal stump, causing displacement of the stomach into the thoracic cavity. This procedure results in a reduction of stomach volume capacity, with potential delayed gastric emptying and dumping syndrome (Figure 17-1). The colonic and jejunal interposition procedure involves forming a new conduit by anastomosing the selected portion of bowel between the esophagus and stomach. Complications after this procedure include swallowing difficulties, strictures, and leakage at the anastomotic site.

Preoperative nutrition for these patients may be a tolerated oral diet (often liquids because of dysphasia and obstruction). If a patient is unable to consume his or her full nutrient needs orally, then a feeding tube may be placed if the esophagus is not obstructed. A PEG tube is not indicated if a gastric pull-up procedure is to be performed, because the stomach is used to make the esophageal conduit and a hole resulting from a gastrostomy tube would be contraindicated. These patients may require preoperative parenteral nutrition if the esophagus is obstructed. Intraoperatively, a jejunal feeding tube may be placed to allow for postoperative enteral nutrition until the anastomosis heals and oral intake is resumed. If enteral access is not obtained intraoperatively, then parenteral nutrition is indicated because these patients may not resume oral intake for 7 to 10 days.

For patients with chronic GERD, a Nissen fundoplication procedure may be performed. This is the most commonly performed antireflux procedure operation for patients with

gastroesophageal reflux refractory to medical management. This procedure involves wrapping the stomach around the base of the esophagus, near the lower esophageal sphincter; this places pressure and narrows the lower esophageal opening to prevent reflux (Figure 17-2). Patients are typically placed on a pureed diet for 2 weeks after this procedure, with small frequent meals, no gulping of liquids, and crushed or liquid medications. After this time solid foods are gradually added to the diet with future avoidance of bread products, nuts, and seeds, because these can become lodged in the lower esophagus and cause an obstruction.

Gastric Surgery

A number of nutrition problems may develop after gastric surgery, depending on the type of surgical procedure and the patient's response. Several indications exist for gastric surgery, including tumor removal, ulcer disease, perforation, hemorrhage, Zollinger-Ellison syndrome, gastric polyposis, and Ménétrier's disease (giant hypertrophic gastritis). A vagotomy is often performed to eliminate gastric acid secretion. Vagotomy at certain levels can alter the normal physiologic function of the stomach, small intestine, pancreas, and biliary system. Total gastric and truncal vagotomy procedures impair proximal and distal motor function of the stomach. Digestion and emptying of solids are retarded, whereas emptying of liquids is accelerated.[32] These vagotomy procedures are commonly accompanied by a drainage procedure (antrectomy or pyloroplasty) that helps the stomach to empty. Nutrition complications associated with vagotomy and pyloroplasty

---

KEY TERMS
malabsorption Malabsorption is a syndrome in which normal products of digestion do not traverse the intestinal mucosa and enter the lymphatic or portal venous branches.
maldigestion Maldigestion, which may be clinically similar to malabsorption, describes defects in the intraluminal phase of the digestive process caused by inadequate exposure of chyme to bile salts and pancreatic enzymes. Clinical symptoms of malabsorption include diarrhea, steatorrhea, and weight loss. Laboratory signs include depressed serum fat-soluble vitamin levels, accelerated prothrombin time, hypomagnesemia, and hypocholesterolemia. Patients with symptoms of malabsorption should have a laboratory workup to determine the presence and level of nutrient loss.
gastroesophageal reflux disease (GERD) Describes symptoms that result from reflux of gastric juices, and sometimes duodenal juices, into the esophagus. Symptoms include substernal burning (heartburn), epigastric pressure sensation, and severe epigastric pain. Prolonged and severe GERD can lead to esophageal bleeding, perforation, strictures, Barrett's epithelium, adenocarcinoma, and pulmonary fibrosis (from aspiration). Conservative dietary therapy involves weight reduction; restriction of carbonated beverages, caffeine, fatty foods, peppermint, chocolate, and ethanol; small frequent meals; and wearing of loose clothing to promote symptomatic relief.

CASE STUDY

The Patient with Esophageal Cancer

Kevin is a 54-year-old accountant seen by his family physician for pain with swallowing and difficulty swallowing solid foods for the past 6 weeks. This has resulted in continued weight loss and fatigue. Kevin was referred to the gastrointestinal (GI) medicine service for further evaluation. After a series of tests that included endoscopy and biopsy, Kevin was found to have esophageal cancer with the tumor lying in the midesophagus. He was then referred to the GI surgery service for surgical evaluation.

A medical history revealed that Kevin smoked two packs of cigarettes per day, drank three martinis per day, and was cachectic. A referral was sent to the dietitian for nutritional evaluation and recommendations for optimizing his nutritional status for surgery. A nutrition history revealed that during the past 6 weeks, Kevin's diet had progressively decreased in consistency to the point where he could tolerate only liquids and some soft solid foods such as mashed potatoes, oatmeal, and applesauce. At a height of 178 cm (5 feet 10 inches), Kevin's weight had dropped from 80 kg (176 lb) to 63 kg (139 lb), leaving him at 79% of his usual body weight. His blood work revealed a serum albumin level of 3.0 g/dL and prealbumin of 13.2 mg/dL. He no longer could stand long enough to make himself a meal and had to take a bath rather than shower because he became too tired. Kevin was not currently taking any medications because he could not swallow them. His current diet order was a full liquid diet.

Assessment of calorie and protein requirements estimated that Kevin required approximately 1800 kcal (basal energy expenditure + 25%) and 75 to 95 g of protein (1.2 to 1.5 g/kg) daily. Because he could eat some solid foods, the dietitian

changed him to a soft diet. The dietitian modified Kevin's diet so that it contained soft, high protein–containing solids and liquids that Kevin stated he could eat and ordered a 48-hour calorie count. A liquid multivitamin was also provided. Kevin was now able to eat enough calories and protein for 14 days preoperatively that he gained 3 kg (7 lb); his albumin increased to 3.1 g/dL, and prealbumin increased to 17 mg/dL.

Kevin underwent an esophagectomy with a gastric pull-up. A feeding jejunostomy tube was placed intraoperatively. Kevin was started on low-rate enteral feedings on postoperative day 2, which were gradually advanced to his goal requirements during the next 2 days. He was not allowed to eat until postoperative day 7 after a swallowing study for anastomotic evaluation. Once Kevin's diet was initiated and tolerated, his tube feedings were provided nocturnally because he was not able to consume 100% of his nutritional needs orally. He was discharged home with an oral postgastrectomy diet and nocturnal tube feedings to provide about 50% of his nutritional needs for 10 days, at which time his nutrition would be reevaluated.

Questions for Analysis

1. Evaluate the preoperative nutrition assessment data. Why were the particular energy and protein assessment factors chosen?
2. What dietary modifications accompany a postgastrectomy diet?
3. Why was Kevin placed on a postgastrectomy diet when his stomach was not resected?
4. At what point should his enteral tube feedings be discontinued?

KEY TERMS

dumping syndrome   Constellation of postprandial symptoms that result from rapid emptying of hyperosmolar gastric contents into the duodenum. The hypertonic load in the small intestine promotes reflux of vascular fluid into the bowel lumen, causing a rapid decrease in the circulating blood volume. Rapid symptoms of abdominal cramping, nausea, vomiting, palpitations, sweating, weakness, reduced blood pressure, tremors, and osmotic diarrhea occur. Symptoms of early dumping begin 10 to 30 minutes after eating; late dumping syndrome occurs 1 to 4 hours after a meal. Late dumping is a result of insulin hypersecretion in response to the carbohydrate load dumped into the small intestine. Once the carbohydrate is absorbed, the hyperinsulinemia causes hypoglycemia, which results in vasomotor symptoms such as diaphoresis, weakness, flushing, and palpitations. Individuals who have undergone gastrointestinal (GI) surgery resulting in a reduced or absent gastric pouch are more prone to dumping syndrome.

anastomosis   A surgical joining of two ducts to allow flow from one to the other.

sphincter   A circular band of muscle fibers that constricts a passage or closes a natural opening in the body (e.g., lower esophageal sphincter, pyloric sphincter).

Zollinger-Ellison syndrome   A condition characterized by severe peptic ulceration, gastric hypersecretion, elevated serum gastrin, and gastrinoma of the pancreas or the duodenum. Total gastrectomy may be necessary.

gastric polyposis   An abnormal condition characterized by the presence of numerous polyps in the stomach.

Ménétrier's disease (giant hypertrophic gastritis)   Rare disease characterized by large folds of nodular gastric rugae that may cover the wall of the stomach, causing anorexia, nausea, vomiting, and abdominal distress.

vagotomy   Cutting of certain branches of the vagus nerve, performed with gastric surgery, to reduce the amount of gastric acid secreted and lessen the chance of recurrence of a gastric ulcer.

---

include dumping syndrome, steatorrhea, and bacterial overgrowth.

A total gastrectomy involves removal of the entire stomach. A storage reservoir may be created using a section of jejunum. A subtotal or partial gastrectomy involves removal of a

portion of the stomach accompanied by a reconstructive procedure. A Billroth I (gastroduodenostomy) involves an anastomosis of the proximal end of the intestine (duodenum) to the distal end of the stomach (Figure 17-3). A Billroth II (gastrojejunostomy) involves an anastomosis of the stomach

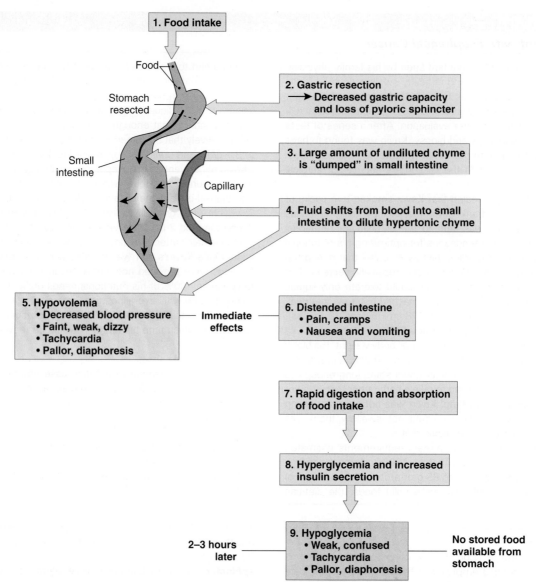

FIGURE 17-1 Dumping syndrome (postgastrectomy). (From Gould BE: *Pathophysiology for health professions*, ed 2, Philadelphia, Pa., 2002, Saunders.)

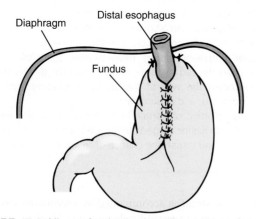

FIGURE 17-2 Nissen fundoplication. (From Lewis SM, Heitkemper MM, Dirksen SR: *Medical-surgical nursing: assessment and management of clinical problems*, ed 5, St Louis, Mo., 2000, Mosby.)

to the side of the jejunum, which creates a blind loop (Figure 17-4). Any gastric surgery carries some potential for development of malnutrition. Common consequences include weight loss, dumping syndrome, malabsorption, anemia, and metabolic bone disease. Dumping syndrome, epigastric fullness, nausea, and vomiting often occur in the early postoperative period. These symptoms are managed with dietary modifications and antiemetic medications.[32]

Generally after gastric surgery, small, frequent oral feedings are resumed according to the patient's tolerance (Box 17-5). For the first 2 weeks after surgery, soft, bland foods with a low fiber content should be consumed in small portions. Simple sugars, lactose, and fried foods should be avoided; beverages should be consumed at least 30 minutes before and after meals; and foods high in complex carbohydrates and protein should be emphasized. Generally these diet modifications are necessary only for the short term

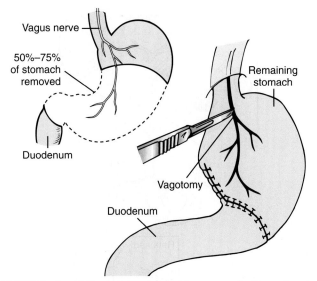

FIGURE 17-3 Billroth I (gastroduodenostomy). (From Lewis SM, Heitkemper MM, Dirksen SR: *Medical-surgical nursing: assessment and management of clinical problems*, ed 5, St Louis, Mo., 2000, Mosby.)

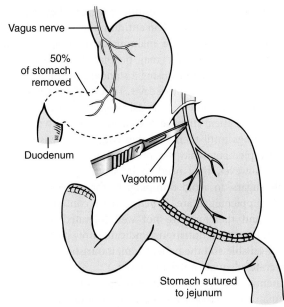

FIGURE 17-4 Billroth II (gastrojejunostomy). (From Lewis SM, Heitkemper MM, Dirksen SR: *Medical-surgical nursing: assessment and management of clinical problems*, ed 5, St Louis, Mo., 2000, Mosby.)

BOX 17-5   POSTGASTRECTOMY ANTIDUMPING DIET

Principles of the Diet

After surgery some discomfort or diarrhea may occur. Therefore to reduce the likelihood of those symptoms, a healthy, nutritionally complete diet should be observed. Each person may react to food differently. Foods should be reintroduced into the diet slowly.

Steps of the Diet

1. Intake of complex carbohydrates is unlimited (e.g., bread, vegetables, rice, potatoes).
2. Intake of simple sugars (e.g., sugar, candy, cake, pies, jelly, honey) should be kept to a minimum. Artificial sweeteners may be used.
3. Fat intake should be moderate (30% of total calories).
4. Protein (e.g., meats, legumes) consumption should be unlimited because it helps with wound healing.
5. Milk contains lactose, which may be hard to digest. Introduce milk and milk products slowly several weeks after surgery.
6. Eat small, frequent meals, approximately six meals per day, to avoid loading the stomach.
7. Limit fluids to 4 oz (½ cup) during mealtimes. This prevents the rapid movement of food through the upper gastrointestinal (GI) tract.
8. Drink fluids 30 to 45 minutes before and after eating to prevent diarrhea.
9. Relatively low-roughage foods and raw foods are allowed as tolerated after postoperative day 14.
10. Eat and chew slowly.
11. Avoid extreme temperatures of foods.

Sample Menu
Breakfast
Scrambled egg, 1
Toast, 1 slice

Margarine, 1 tsp
Low-sugar jelly, 1 tsp
Banana, 1 small

Midmorning Snack
Canned fruit, water packed, ½ cup
Graham crackers, 2 squares

Lunch
Bread, 2 slices
Ham, 2 oz
Cheese, 1 oz
Mustard, 2 tsp
Canned fruit, water packed, ½ cup
Yogurt, sugar free, 4 oz

Midafternoon Snack
Saltine crackers, 3 squares
Peanut butter, 1 tbsp

Dinner
Chicken breast, 3 oz
Mashed potatoes, ½ cup
Green beans, ½ cup
Margarine, 2 tsp
Yogurt, sugar free, 4 oz

Evening Snack
Pudding, sugar free, ½ cup
Vanilla wafers, 3 pieces

because most patients can resume a regular diet. However, some individuals may need an antidumping diet indefinitely. For individuals who were malnourished preoperatively, a small bowel feeding tube may be placed intraoperatively. Low-rate enteral feedings using a standard formulation may be initiated on postoperative day 1. Tube feedings are adjusted according to the patient's clinical progress and tolerance of an oral diet. Patients may be discharged home with nocturnal tube feedings until their oral diet consumption is optimal. Oral supplements may be provided to increase nutrient intake; however, they need to be isotonic, containing no simple sugars, to avoid dumping. Unfortunately, most oral liquid supplements are hyperosmolar, containing simple sugars, and therefore are not well tolerated after gastric surgery. Parenteral nutrition is indicated only if enteral access is not available and the patient is malnourished and not able to tolerate adequate nutrients orally.

Anemia is a common consequence of gastric surgery. Anemia can be attributed to a deficiency or malabsorption of one or more nutrients, including iron, vitamin B_{12}, and folate. Assimilation of vitamin B_{12} requires liberation of the vitamin from protein and binding of the vitamin to intrinsic factor, both of which occur in the stomach. Failure of either of these reactions to occur results in vitamin B_{12} malabsorption, which, with time, produces anemia.[32] Total gastrectomy patients require periodic intramuscular vitamin B_{12} injections. Metabolic bone disease can be a late complication of gastric surgery. The cause of metabolic bone disease varies with the surgical procedure. The Billroth II procedure is associated with more complications than the Billroth I, because it bypasses the duodenum and upper jejunum (the site of calcium absorption). Procedures that destroy the pylorus can result in rapid gastric emptying, which may contribute to development of metabolic bone disease. Rapid gastric emptying not only reduces absorption time but also, when fats are malabsorbed, can lead to formation of insoluble calcium soaps.[32] Fat malabsorption can also lead to vitamin D malabsorption, which leads to impaired metabolism of calcium and phosphorus.

Intestinal Surgery

Surgical resections of the small and large intestine are usually well tolerated. If excessive amounts of bowel are removed, then nutritional consequences can arise, depending on the location resected. If more than 50% of the small intestine is removed, then short-bowel syndrome may occur. This syndrome is characterized by severe diarrhea or steatorrhea, malabsorption, and malnutrition, depending on the amount of remaining small intestine, the site of the resection, and the functional status of the remaining GI tract. Often the patient may require long-term parenteral nutrition to maintain his or her nutritional status and fluid and electrolyte balance (see Chapter 19).

Pancreaticoduodenectomy (Whipple Procedure)

In cases of ampullary, duodenal, and pancreatic malignancies, a pancreaticoduodenectomy may be performed. This

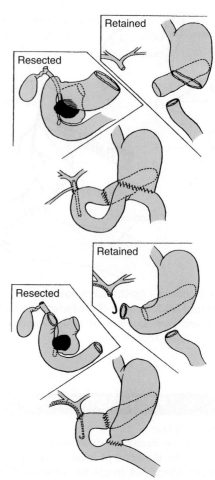

FIGURE 17-5 Whipple procedure. (From Hardy JD, editor: *Hardy's textbook of surgery,* ed 2, Philadelphia, Pa., 1988, Lippincott Williams & Wilkins.)

procedure, one of the most difficult and technically demanding in GI surgery, involves resecting the distal stomach, distal common duct, pancreatic head, and duodenum. Three anastomoses must be performed: (1) pancreaticojejunostomy, (2) choledochojejunostomy, and (3) gastrojejunostomy (Billroth II). In the past few years a pyloric-sparing Whipple procedure has become more prominent, resulting in a Billroth I anastomosis. This procedure carries fewer postoperative nutritional concerns than the other, which results in a Billroth II anastomosis (Figure 17-5).

Ileostomy and Colostomy

In cases of intestinal lesions, obstruction, or inflammatory bowel disease of the entire colon or when diversion of fecal matter is required, an ileostomy or a colostomy may be the treatment of choice. These procedures involve creation of an artificial anus on the abdominal wall by incision into the colon or ileum and bringing it out to the surface, forming a stoma (Figure 17-6). A pouch is placed externally over the stoma to collect fecal matter. In general, patients with ostomies should eat regular diets. Foods that are gas forming or difficult to digest may be avoided to reduce undesired side effects. In the case of high-output ostomies (more than 800 mL/day), patients may need to avoid hypertonic, simple sugar–containing liquids and foods; fatty foods; and foods with a high amount of insoluble fiber to reduce outputs.

Bariatric Surgery

In the past several years, surgery for treatment of obesity has become more prevalent. Probably the most common procedure for weight loss in the world is the vertical banded gastroplasty (VBG), or gastric stapling (Figure 17-7, *A*). This technique is performed under general anesthesia and requires about 4 to 5 days in the hospital postoperatively. The VBG procedure limits food intake by creating a small pouch (½ oz) in the upper stomach, with a narrow outlet (½ inch) reinforced by a mesh band to prevent stretching. The pouch fills quickly and empties slowly with solid food, producing a feeling of fullness. Overeating results in pain or vomiting, thus restricting food intake. This procedure is preferred for those people who engage in "bulk" or "binge" eating. The disadvantage of this procedure is that weight loss is not as great as that with other procedures. It does not restrict the intake of high-caloric liquids, and the pouch can stretch with overeating. As a result, 20% of people do not lose weight, and

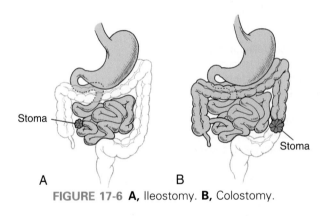

Stoma

A   B

FIGURE 17-6 A, Ileostomy. **B,** Colostomy.

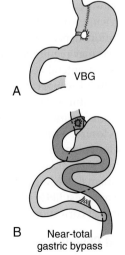

VBG

A

B   Near-total
       gastric bypass

FIGURE 17-7 A, Vertical banded gastroplasty (VBG). **B,** Roux-en-Y gastric bypass.

only half of people lose at least 50% of their excess weight with a VBG.

The Roux-en-Y gastric bypass (see Figure 17-7, *B*) is a combination of gastric stapling and intestinal bypass. It promotes weight loss by (1) restricting the amount of food a person can ingest by reducing the holding capacity of the stomach and (2) interfering with complete absorption of nutrients by shortening the length of small intestine through which the food travels. Unlike the VBG, this procedure discourages intake of high-calorie sweets by producing nausea, diarrhea, and other unpleasant symptoms. With this procedure a small gastric pouch (15 mL) is made near where stomach and esophagus meet. The small pouch and remainder of the stomach are divided from each other with staples. An opening is made in the pouch where a portion of the small intestine is connected. This new connection between the pouch and the small intestine is called a *Roux-en-Y limb*. Food then travels down the esophagus and bypasses nearly all of the stomach and first 2 feet of small intestine. Complications related to gallstones, which tend to form during rapid weight loss, can be prevented by removal of the gallbladder. This procedure is intended for people who "graze" during the day on high-calorie and sugar-containing foods, and eat large amounts. Box 17-6 lists a sample meal plan after gastric bypass surgery.

Like any major abdominal operation, these **bariatric** surgical procedures carry risks such as bleeding, infection, bowel blockage because of scar tissue formation, hernia through the incision, and anesthesia risks. The most serious risk is leakage of fluid from the stomach or intestines, which can result in abdominal infection and reoperation. Additional risks are directly related to being obese; these include blood clots in legs or lungs, pneumonia, and cardiac complications. Less immediate risks are ulcers in the stomach or intestine, dumping syndrome, **bezoar** formation, obstruction of stoma, and malnutrition from too-rapid weight loss and loss of vitamins and minerals. Some people (10% to 15%) experience some complications from the gastric bypass; death may occur from complications in 1% to 2% of patients. Because this procedure is not risk free, strict criteria for eligibility should be made. Generally, candidates are those who have at least 100-lb excess body weight (or a body mass index [BMI] of 40 kg/m^2 or greater) and have significant obesity-related medical problems and for whom all other serious attempts at weight reduction have failed. A thorough medical and

---

KEY TERMS

bariatric   A term used to describe the field of medicine that focuses on the treatment and control of obesity and diseases associated with obesity.

bezoar   A hard ball of hair or vegetable fiber that may develop within the stomach and intestines; can cause an obstruction, requiring removal. Formed because of reduced gastric motility, decreased gastric mixing and churning, and reduced gastric secretions.

BOX 17-6   POSTOPERATIVE DIET FOR GASTRIC BYPASS PROCEDURE FOR MORBID OBESITY

Stage I: clear liquids—Begin once liquids allowed; continue for two to three meals

Stage II: gastric bypass—Begin after clear liquids tolerated; liquids continue for 3 to 4 weeks

Stage III: pureed—Begin after postoperative week 4; continue for 1 to 2 weeks

Stage IV: soft, solids—Begin after postoperative week 6; continue indefinitely

Gastric Bypass Liquids
- Nonfat milk
- Blenderized soups
- 100% fruit juice (diluted ½ water and ½ juice)
- Vegetable juice (e.g., V8, tomato)
- Sugar-Free Carnation Instant Breakfast powder mixed with nonfat milk
- Grits, oatmeal, cream of wheat, mashed potatoes (thinned down enough that it could go through a straw)
- Nonfat, sugar-free milkshakes
- Thinned baby food
- Sugar-free drinks (e.g., sodas, tea)

Eating Guidelines
- Small meals: each feeding should be 4 oz total (½ cup)
- Six to eight feedings per day to consume adequate nutrients
- An hour between meals and drinking fluids
- Eat slowly/chew food well; each feeding should last at least 30 minutes
- Avoid sugars (i.e., sucrose, honey, corn syrup, fructose) and sugar-containing beverages, foods, and candy
- Low-fat foods only (avoid fried foods, gravies, excessive margarine, butter, high-fat meats, and breads)
- Eat high-protein foods (e.g., milk, yogurt, soft meats, eggs)
- Avoid soft, calorie-dense foods (e.g., ice cream, chocolate, cheese, cookies)

- Avoid obstructive foods (e.g., tough, fibrous red meat; bread made from refined flour; celery; popcorn; nuts; seeds; membranes of citrus fruits)
- Take daily complete multivitamin (liquid or chewable)
- Calcium supplements (1500 mg/day)

Sample Menu (After 8 Weeks)
Breakfast
Banana, ¼ medium
Scrambled egg, 1 egg
Toast, white, ½ slice
Margarine, ½ tsp

Morning Snack
Graham crackers, 2
Pudding, sugar free made with nonfat milk, ½ cup

Lunch
Broiled chicken breast, 2 oz
Carrots, boiled, ¼ cup
Margarine, 1 tsp
Pasta salad, ¼ cup

Afternoon Snack
Canned fruit, water packed, ½ cup

Dinner
Baked or broiled fish, 2 oz
Green beans, ¼ cup
Potato, baked, ½ small
Margarine, ½ tsp

Evening Snack
Cheese, American, 1 oz
Saltine crackers, 2 squares

NOTE: Consume nonfat milk or yogurt between meals, throughout the day. Eat and drink no more than 2 to 3 oz at a time for a daily total of 2 cups.

---

nutritional-behavioral evaluation is necessary to determine eligibility.

Other Related Problems
Enteric Fistulas

Enteric fistulas are abnormal communications between a portion of the intestinal tract and another organ (internal) or between the intestinal tract and the surface of the body (external or enterocutaneous).[32] The most common sites of origin are the pancreas and the large and small intestines. The majority of enteric fistulas result from surgical wound dehiscence or necrosis from bowel ischemia. Inflammatory bowel disease, cancer, trauma, and radiation to the abdomen can also lead to fistula development.

Several metabolic complications can arise as a result of an enteric fistula, including fluid and electrolyte losses, malnutrition, and sepsis. A retrospective analysis of patients with small bowel fistulas found a lower mortality rate, increased

spontaneous fistula closures, and increased rate of surgical closures in those receiving parenteral nutrition.[33] The route of nutrition intervention depends on the location of the fistula. Proximal fistulas may require that a patient be placed on parenteral nutrition if enteral access distal to the fistula cannot be achieved. This is because eating, and thus nutrients in the proximal bowel, stimulates GI secretions, thereby complicating fistula management and the likelihood of spontaneous fistula closure. Fistulas located in the distal bowel, particularly the colon, may have low output (less than 500 mL/day) and thus allow for oral intake of low-residue or even elemental feedings. High-output fistulas (more than 500 mL/day) most likely will not close spontaneously and require surgical correction.

Chylous Ascites and Chylothorax

Chylous leaks into the peritoneal and thoracic cavities can follow surgical injury or trauma to the lymphatic ducts and

TABLE 17-4   EBB AND FLOW PHASES

	EBB PHASE	FLOW PHASE
Hormonal and nonhormonal	↑ Glucagon ↑ Adrenocorticotropic hormone (ACTH)	↑ Counterregulatory hormones (epinephrine, norepinephrine, glucagon, cortisol) ↑ Insulin ↑ Catecholamines ↑ Cytokines (tumor necrosis factor-α [TNF-α], interleukin [IL]-1, -2, and -6)
Metabolic	Circulatory insufficiency, ↑ heart rate (vascular constriction) ↓ Digestive enzyme production ↓ Urine production	Hyperglycemia ↓ Protein synthesis/amino acid efflux ↑ Gluconeogenesis ↑ Glycogenolysis ↑↑ Urea nitrogen excretion/net (−) nitrogen balance
Clinical outcomes	Hemodynamic instability	Fluid and electrolyte imbalances Mild metabolic acidosis ↑ Resting energy expenditure (REE)

Data from Cresci G, Martindale R: Nutrition in critical illness. In Berdanier C, editor: *Handbook of nutrition and food*, Boca Raton, Fla., 2002, CRC Press; Cresci G: Metabolic stress. In Matarese L, Gottschlich M, editors: *Contemporary nutrition support practice*, ed 2, Philadelphia, Pa., 2003, Saunders.

obstruction because of cancer or congenital anomalies. Leakage of chyle into the abdominal or thoracic cavity can cause ascites, pleural effusions, abdominal pain, anorexia, hypoalbuminemia, hyponatremia, hypocalcemia, hypocholesterolemia, and elevated alkaline phosphatase.[32] Chylous leaks may resolve with conservative management, although surgical repair can be required to ligate the duct. Conservative management involves reducing the chyle flow, which is normally 1500 to 5500 mL/day. Dietary intake (fat and fluid), blood pressure, and portal blood flow contribute to the production of chyle. Dietary manipulation is the main means of reducing chyle flow. Because dietary long-chain triglycerides (LCTs) are incorporated into chylomicrons, restriction of these fats in the diet is imperative. Depending on severity of the chyle leak and patient's response, the patient may be allowed oral dietary intake with no LCTs, enteral feeding with no LCTs, or parenteral nutrition. Medium-chain triglycerides (MCTs) are allowed enterally because these are absorbed directly via the portal vein, not the lymphatic system. A diet without or limited to less than 4% of calories as LCTs is not advised for more than 10 to 14 days because it lacks essential fatty acids (linoleic and linolenic acid), causing the patient to develop a deficiency. Resolution of lymphatic leaks conservatively can take up to 6 weeks; therefore adequate nutrition during this period is important to maintain nutritional status.

NUTRITIONAL NEEDS IN THERMAL INJURIES

Patients with trauma and burns exhibit similar metabolic alterations as previously described, but metabolic alterations often occur to a much greater extent. Few traumatic injuries result in a hypermetabolic state comparable to that of a major burn. An understanding of the cause of metabolic response and implications for nutritional requirements is necessary with traumatic and burn injuries for a nutrition care plan to

be designed to minimize the effects of hypermetabolism and hypercatabolism, as well as for support immunocompetence to be developed.

Metabolic Response to Injury

Stressed patients undergo several metabolic phases as a series of ebb and flow states reflecting a patient's response to the severity of the stress. The initial ebb phase occurs immediately after injury and is associated with shock. If the injured patient survives, then the ebb phase evolves into the flow phase. Table 17-4 lists hormonal, metabolic, and clinical outcome comparisons between the two phases.

Clinical efforts in the ebb phase are focused on maintaining heart action and blood circulation. The flow state is a hyperdynamic phase in which substrates are mobilized for energy production while increased cellular activity and hormonal stimulation are noted. An energy expenditure distinction exists for each phase, making the goals of nutrition therapy variable depending on the stage in question. During the ebb phase a decrease in metabolic needs occurs. Typically, because of hemodynamic instability and need for resuscitation, nutrition intervention is not pursued during this phase. The flow phase brings hypermetabolism, yielding increased proteolysis and nitrogen loss, accelerated gluconeogenesis, hyperglycemia and increased glucose use, and retention of salt and water. Mobilization of protein, fat, and glycogen is believed to be mediated through release of cytokines such as tumor necrosis factor-α (TNF-α); interleukin (IL)-1, -2, and -6; and counterregulatory hormones such as epinephrine,

> **KEY TERM**
> chyle   The fat-containing, creamy white fluid that is formed in the lacteals of the intestine during digestion; it is transported through the lymphatics and enters the venous circulation via the thoracic duct.

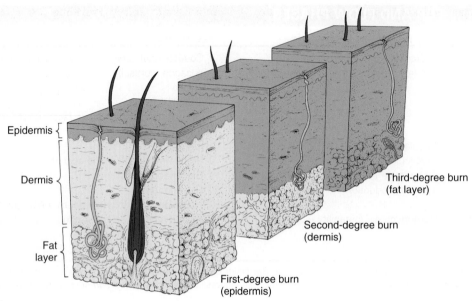

Epidermis

Dermis

Fat layer

First-degree burn (epidermis)

Second-degree burn (dermis)

Third-degree burn (fat layer)

FIGURE 17-8 Depth of skin area involved in burns.

norepinephrine, glucagon, and cortisol. Circulating levels of insulin are also elevated in most metabolically stressed patients, but responsiveness of tissues to insulin, especially skeletal muscle, is severely blunted. Researchers believe this relative insulin resistance to be caused by the effects of the counterregulatory hormones. The hormonal milieu normalizes only after the injury or metabolic stress has resolved. As long as the patient is in a hyperdynamic catabolic state, optimal nutrition support is needed but can only at best approach zero nitrogen balance in attempts to minimize further protein wasting.

Burn Wounds

Size and depth of the burn wound affect its healing process and overall prognosis (Figure 17-8). Burns are usually classified by degree using the **rule of nines**, as follows:

1. *First-degree burns:* **erythema** involving cell necrosis above the basal layer of the epidermis
2. *Second-degree burns:* erythema and blistering, and necrosis within the dermis
3. *Third-degree burns:* full-thickness skin loss, including fat layer
4. *Fourth-degree burns:* exposed bone and tendon

Burns of first- and second-degree depths generally reepithelialize without surgical intervention. Third-degree burns will not heal independent of excision and grafting. Fourth-degree burns typically involve the use of muscle flaps because skin grafting onto bone is not a viable therapy option.

Extent of the burn directly affects fluid resuscitation, surgical needs, immunocompetence, metabolic sequelae, and nutrition intervention. Second- and third-degree burns covering 15% to 20% or more of the total body surface area (TBSA), or 10% in children and older adults, usually cause extensive fluid loss and require intravenous fluid and electrolyte replacement therapy. Burns of severe depth covering more than 50% of the TBSA are often fatal, especially in infants and older adults. Thermal injury permits the loss of heat, water, nitrogen, whole proteins, and micronutrients through the open wound. Loss of the protective skin barrier allows microorganisms to access subcutaneous tissue and potentiates systemic infectious processes, contributing to the postburn hypermetabolic state. Loss of plasma volume and electrolytes through the open wound predispose the burned patient to acid-base imbalance and cardiovascular, pulmonary, and renal instability. Adequate fluid and electrolyte resuscitation during the first 24 to 48 hours of postburn hypovolemia is essential for hemodynamic stability. Extensive fluid shifts, unique to burn injury, drive the characteristic edema process of resuscitation by increasing intracellular and interstitial fluid volumes. Fluids given during the resuscitative period should be titrated in accordance with urine output to prevent overresuscitation and underresuscitation. The replacement of extracellular sodium chloride, most commonly in the form of **lactated Ringer's solution**, is obligatory for successful resuscitation.[34]

> **KEY TERMS**
> **rule of nines**   Describes the percentage of the body surface represented by various anatomic areas. For example, each upper limb, 9%; each lower limb, 18%; anterior and posterior trunk, each 18%; head and neck, 9%; and perineum and genitalia, 1%.
> **erythema**   Redness of the skin produced by coagulation of the capillaries.
> **lactated Ringer's solution**   Sterile solution of calcium chloride, potassium chloride, sodium chloride, and sodium lactate in water administered to replenish fluid and electrolytes.

In addition, certain herbs and botanicals have been suggested for use in patients with thermal injuries. (For an outline of these herbs and additional information on their efficacy, safety, and possible interaction with other drugs, see the Complementary and Alternative Medicine [CAM] box, "Feel the Burn?")

Nutrition Therapy After Burn Injury

Thermal injury induces hypermetabolism of varying intensity and duration depending on extent and depth of the body surface affected, presence of infection, and efficacy of early treatment. Energy requirements peak at approximately postburn day 12 and typically slowly normalize as the percentage of open wound decreases with reepithelialization or skin grafting.

Energy

Burn patients require individualized nutrition plans to provide optimal energy and protein to accelerate muscle and protein synthesis and minimize proteolysis. Numerous predictive equations are used to estimate energy needs. Several studies have reviewed the accuracy of predictive equations in determining energy requirements in burn patients. Consensus indicates that predictive equations tend to overestimate energy expenditure; therefore the preferred method of determining energy requirements is by using indirect calorimetry. If indirect calorimetry is not available in the clinical situation, then resting energy expenditure (REE) can be estimated at 50% to 60% more than the Harris-Benedict equation for burns of more than 20% of TBSA.[32]

Carbohydrate

During the flow phase of metabolic stress, hyperglycemia is present because of the increased glucagon-to-insulin ratio that activates gluconeogenesis. Tissue insulin resistance further exacerbates glucose intolerance. Despite these metabolic aberrations, carbohydrate should be the primary energy source provided for the burned patient. For burns exceeding 25% TBSA, carbohydrate should comprise 60% to 65% of the calories.[34] Patients should be monitored closely for hyperglycemia and glucosuria with exogenous insulin provided to maintain blood glucose levels at less than 180 mg/dL.[6] Complications of hyperglycemia include osmotic diuresis with resulting dehydration and hypovolemia, lipogenesis, fatty liver, and carbon dioxide (CO_2) retention inhibiting ventilatory weaning.

Protein

Trauma, burns, and sepsis initiate a cascade of events that leads to accelerated protein degradation, decreased rates of synthesis of selected proteins, and increased amino acid catabolism and nitrogen loss. Clinical consequences of these metabolic alterations can increase morbidity and mortality rates of patients, causing serious organ dysfunction and impaired host defenses. Therefore trauma and burn patients require increased amounts of protein in attempts to minimize endogenous proteolysis, as well as to support the large losses from wound exudate. Providing 20% to 25% of calories as protein to those with burns of greater than 25% TBSA promotes improved nutrition laboratory values, immunity, nitrogen balance, and survival.[35] Overall recommendations are to provide protein in the amount of 1.5 to 2.0 g/kg body weight, but rarely up to 3.0 g/kg body weight per day in an attempt to minimize protein losses. Providing these increased levels of protein requires continuous monitoring of fluid status, blood urea nitrogen, and serum creatinine because of high renal solute load. In addition to the quantity of protein provided, protein quality is also significant. The use of protein of high biologic value is preferred for burn patients. Consumption of whey protein has been recommended more than the use of casein because of whey's its beneficial effects on burned children, improvement in tube-feeding tolerance, enhanced solubility at low gastric pH, increased digestibility, and improved nitrogen retention. Pharmacologic doses of the single amino acids arginine and glutamine have also been explored regarding their benefit in critical illness and burns.

Fat

Lipid is an important component of a trauma or burn patient's diet for many reasons; at 9 kcal/g it is an isosmotic concentrated energy source for these patients. Dietary lipid is also a carrier for fat-soluble vitamins, as well as a provider of the essential fatty acids linoleic and linolenic acid. Even though lipids are required in critical illness, excess lipid can be detrimental. Excessive lipid administration has been associated with hyperlipidemia, fatty liver immunosuppression, and impaired clotting ability. For burn and multiple trauma patients, the recommended amount of total fat delivery is 12% to 15% of total calories. A minimum of 4% of calories in the diet should consist of essential fatty acids to prevent deficiencies, which often equates to about 10% of total calories as fat because most sources do not solely contain essential fatty acid. Formulations supplemented with fish oil, a rich source of omega-3 fatty acids (eicosapentaenoic acid [EPA] and docosahexaenoic acid [DHA]) and canola oil (α-linolenic acid) are of particular interest for their potential antiinflammatory and immune-enhancing benefits.[36]

Vitamins and Minerals

Micronutrients function as coenzymes and cofactors in metabolic pathways at the cellular level. With increased energy and protein demands associated with traumatic and burn injury, one would also expect an increased need for vitamins and minerals. In addition, increased nutrient losses from open wounds and altered metabolism, absorption, and excretion would also be suspect for requirements beyond that of the Recommended Dietary Allowance (RDA). Various vitamins and minerals have also been found to aid with wound healing, immune function, and other biologic functions. Unfortunately, little concrete data are available to support exact requirements during these hypermetabolic states. However, in addition to a daily multivitamin, burn patients may benefit from additional vitamin A (5000 IU/1000 kcal of enteral

COMPLEMENTARY AND ALTERNATIVE MEDICINE (CAM)

Feel the Burn?

The following herbs and botanical supplements have been suggested for use with thermal injury.

Herb/Botanical and Use in Burns	Efficacy	Safety Issues	Drug Interactions
Aloe (*Aloe vera*) Aloe is a topical gel used to heal burns and reduce burn pain.	It may help heal abrasions and burns; research indicates aloe significantly delays healing of deep surgical wounds.	It produces an occasional allergic reaction and may lower blood glucose levels. Aloe is considered safe, but comprehensive safety studies are lacking.	None are known. Aloe gel may be a useful adjuvant therapy when combined with hydrocortisone acetate cream. If gel is taken internally, then it can reduce absorption of many medications.
Echinacea (*E. purpurea, E. pallida, E. angustifolia*) Echinacea is used topically to enhance wound healing.	Several research studies have provided evidence that various *Echinacea* species can significantly reduce the duration and severity of illness, but little demonstration of efficacy in wound healing is reported.	Oral Echinacea causes few side effects; most common reports include bad taste and minor GI symptoms.	*E. angustifolia* (the most popular species in North America) root might inhibit cytochrome P_{450} 3A4 (CYP3A4).
Garlic (*Allium* spp.) Garlic is used orally and topically to fight infections.	Little research, if any, is available to substantiate this claim.	Garlic is on the FDA's GRAS list. Raw garlic taken in excessive doses can cause numerous symptoms such as stomach upset, heartburn, nausea, vomiting, diarrhea, flatulence, facial flushing, rapid pulse, and insomnia. Topical garlic can cause skin irritation, blistering, even third-degree burns.	When taken with anticoagulants, NSAIDs, antiplatelet agents, or other herbs that exert anticoagulation effects (feverfew, ginkgo), garlic may increase bleeding time. Blood glucose level may be decreased with hypoglycemic agents.
Gotu kola (*Centella asiatica*) Gotu kola is used in Europe as treatment for scarring.	No substantial evidence exists to support this claim.	Rare allergic reactions occur to topical gotu kola.	None are known.
Plantain (*Plantago ovata, P. psyllium, P. lanceolata, P. major*) Plantain is used topically for skin inflammation.	Efficacy has not been validated scientifically.	Plantain is safe; long-term use shows no toxicity.	None are known.
St. John's wort (*Hypericum perforatum*) Hypericum tincture or oil is used topically for inflammation and burns.	It speeds healing of burns.	Noted side effects are related to ingestion of the herb.	Interactions are related to ingestion of the herb.

Bibliography

Bascom A, Breiner MA, Brigs M, et al: *Professional guide to complementary and alternative therapies*, Springhouse, Pa., 2001, Springhouse.

Bratman S, Girman AM: *Mosby's handbook of herbs and supplements and their therapeutic uses*, St Louis, Mo., 2003, Mosby.

Escott-Stump S: *Nutrition and diagnosis-related care*, ed 6, Philadelphia, Pa., 2007, Lippincott Williams & Wilkins.

Kuhn MA, Winston D: *Winston and Kuhn's: Herbal therapy and supplements: a scientific and traditional approach*, ed 2, Philadelphia, Pa., 2007, Lippincott Williams & Wilkins.

FDA, Food and Drug Administration; *GI,* gastrointestinal; *GRAS,* generally recognized as safe; *NSAIDs,* nonsteroidal antiinflammatory drugs.

nutrition), vitamin C (500 mg twice daily), and zinc (45 mg elemental zinc per day).

Nutrient Delivery

Oral intake is generally adequate in children and adults with burns of less than 25% TBSA and in young children and infants with less than 15% TBSA. Adequate oral intake can be achieved by providing patient food preferences; high-calorie, high-protein supplements; and modular calorie and protein enhancement of foods.[34] However, patients with burns of greater than 25% TBSA often require enteral tube feeding. Gastric feedings are frequently interrupted in burn patients for multiple reasons such as the presence of gastric ileus, dressing changes, physical therapy, prone positioning, respiratory treatments, and surgery. Enteral feeding is well tolerated in burn patients when delivered in the small intestine because the small bowel maintains its absorptive capacity. Therefore a nasoenteric feeding tube is preferred. Small bowel feeding may also reduce incidence of aspiration. Enteral nutrient delivery should be initiated as soon as possible after injury (during the resuscitative period). Early enteral feedings, within the first 6 hours after the burn, have been shown to decrease the level of catabolic hormones, improve nitrogen balance, maintain gut mucosal integrity, lower the incidence of diarrhea, and decrease hospital stay.[37] A full-strength, intact protein formula at low rate (20 to 30 mL/h) advanced by 5 to 20 mL/h to the desired volume is typically tolerated.[34] Parenteral nutrition is indicated only if enteral nutrition is not tolerated or grossly inadequate, because it has been associated with metabolic and immunologic complications.[37] Whenever possible, low-rate enteral feedings should accompany parenteral nutrition to prevent villous atrophy.

HEALTH PROMOTION
IMMUNONUTRITION

It is known that malnutrition leads to suppressed immune responses. Providing nutrition support using standard enteral formulations has shown improvements in various clinical indexes of nutritional status when adequate calories and protein are given; however, a lack of demonstrated effect is seen on morbidity and mortality. During the past 20 years the field of immunology has exploded and expanded into nearly every area of medicine, including nutrition. Certain dietary components have been classified as *immune-enhancing nutrients*. Compared with standard nutrients, an immune-enhancing nutrient is a substance that provides positive effects on the immune system when provided in certain quantities. A distinct attribute of immune-enhancing agents is a modulation of the humoral and cellular immune function resulting in a reduction of systemic inflammatory response syndrome (SIRS) and postoperative infection rates.[38] Of the many immune-enhancing nutrients identified in human clinical trials, the ones that appear to be most beneficial are L-arginine, L-glutamine, nucleotides, omega-3 fatty acids (EPA and DHA), and various vitamins and minerals (zinc and vitamins A, E, and C). Several special enteral nutrient formulations have been categorized as immune-enhancing formulations (IEFs). Each of these formulas contains various combinations or levels (or both) of these immune-enhancing nutrients.[39]

Immune-Enhancing Formulations

Glutamine is known to be a major fuel source for rapidly dividing cells such as enterocytes, reticulocytes, and lymphocytes. In normal metabolic states, glutamine is a nonessential amino acid. However, during times of metabolic stress, glutamine is implicated as being conditionally essential because it is needed for the maintenance of gut metabolism, structure, and function. Despite the accelerated skeletal muscle release of amino acids, blood glutamine levels are not increased after burns. In fact, decreased plasma glutamine levels have been reported after severe burn, multiple trauma, or multiple organ failure.[40]

A number of studies have shown beneficial effects with supplemental glutamine, its precursors (ornithine α-ketoglutarate, α-ketoglutarate), or glutamine dipeptides (alanine-glutamine, glycine-glutamine). These studies deliver glutamine in pharmacologic doses of 25% to 35% of the dietary protein. Supplemental glutamine has been shown to have multiple benefits that include increased nitrogen retention and muscle mass, maintenance of the GI mucosa and its permeability, preserved immune function and reduced infections, and preserved organ glutathione levels. These protective effects of glutamine supplementation could have significant effects on morbidity and mortality rates in trauma and burn patients. Research continues on the safety and cost-effectiveness of glutamine supplementation in trauma and burns.

Arginine, like glutamine, is considered a conditionally essential amino acid. Arginine is the specific precursor for nitric oxide production, as well as a potent secretagogue for anabolic hormones such as insulin, prolactin, and growth hormone. Under normal circumstances, arginine is considered a nonessential amino acid because it is adequately synthesized endogenously via the urea cycle. However, research suggests that during times of metabolic stress, optimal amounts of arginine are not synthesized to promote tissue regeneration or positive nitrogen balance.

Studies in animals and humans have investigated the effects of supplemental arginine in various injury models. Positive outcomes from supplementation include improved nitrogen balance, wound healing, and immune function, as well as increased anabolic hormones (insulin and growth hormone). The outcomes are of special interest in the post-trauma and postburn patient during the flow phase, when enhancement of these processes would yield the greatest advantage. However, despite these positive effects, caution with excessive arginine supplementation is warranted in burn patients because of its potential adverse effects on nitric oxide production.

Even though lipids are required, excess lipid can be detrimental. Excessive lipid administration has been associated with hyperlipidemia, fatty liver immunosuppression, and impaired clotting ability. All long-chain fatty acids share the same enzyme systems because they are elongated and desaturated with each pathway competitive in nature based on substrate availability. Dietary fatty acids modulate the phospholipid cell membrane composition and the type and quantities of eicosanoids produced. Prostaglandins of the 3 series (PGE_3) and series 5 leukotrienes have proved to be antiinflammatory and immune-enhancing agents. In addition, PGE_3 is a potent vasodilator. These concepts have received considerable attention for the potential of n-3 fatty acids to enhance immune function and reduce acute and chronic inflammation.

In most standard enteral formulations, the fat source is predominantly n-6 fatty acids, with a portion coming from MCTs. Formulations supplemented with fish oil, a rich source of n-3 fatty acids (EPA and DHA) and canola oil (α-linolenic acid), are available. Clinical trials using these formulations have shown positive benefits in patients with psoriasis, rheumatoid arthritis (RA), burns, sepsis, and trauma. Researchers believe these results are caused by alterations in eicosanoid and leukotriene production, with decreased arachidonic acid metabolites (e.g., PGE_2), as well as increased production of the less biologically active trienoic prostaglandins and pentaenoic leukotrienes.

Clinical Outcomes with Immune-Enhancing Formulas
Trauma Outcomes

IEFs have been used in trauma patients and are associated with decreased incidence of intraabdominal abscess, multiple organ failure, infections, and SIRS, as well as decreased hospital length of stay and days of therapeutic antibiotic use.

Intensive Care Unit and Sepsis Outcomes

The intensive care unit population involves a very heterogeneous group, making data interpretation difficult. This population involves differing severity and pathologic processes of various disease states. Studies conducted with this population contain differences in study design and methods of reporting data, adding to the complexity of comparing results between investigations. A few studies have been conducted with various diagnoses, such as cardiac failure, pulmonary failure, transplantation, trauma, and GI surgery. Positive outcomes in the form of decreased incidence of infections, requirement for mechanical ventilation, incidence of bacteremia, and length of stay were reported when using IEFs.

Surgery Outcomes

Research in surgical populations using IEFs has been performed with preoperative, postoperative, or combined nutrition therapies. The majority of procedures performed in these studies involved upper GI cancer or head and neck cancer surgery. Significantly improved outcomes in the IEF groups include fewer infections and wound complications, decreased severity of complications, and shorter postoperative and hospital length of stay.[41]

Other Populations (Burns, Head Injury, Human Immunodeficiency Virus and Acquired Immunodeficiency Syndrome)

In patient populations comprising those with burns, head injury, or human immunodeficiency virus and acquired immunodeficiency syndrome, the study of the use of IEFs is limited. Currently only two studies investigating the effect of IEFs on immune function and nutritional status of patients with acquired immunodeficiency syndrome (AIDS) have been published. Improved weight gain was found in one of the studies when IEF was provided (but not in the other study).[42] Burn patients appear to benefit when provided with IEFs, exhibiting decreased infections and length of hospital stay. Head injury patients theoretically should benefit from IEFs because of severe hypermetabolism and the likelihood of infectious complications. However, no clinical data are available to support this theory. More research using IEFs in these populations is needed.

TO SUM UP

The nutritional status of the patient should be addressed before the patient is even considered for surgery. If the patient has any nutrient deficiencies, these should be corrected before surgery if time allows. Postoperatively the patient should be provided with nutrition as soon as feasible to improve surgical outcomes.

Postoperative nutrition may be supplied in a number of ways. The oral route is preferred; however, often it is not feasible or adequate to support metabolic needs. Enteral or parenteral nutrition may be provided for those unable to achieve adequate nutrient intake and absorption orally. Enteral feeding is preferred to parenteral feeding. Because alimentary tract surgery often alters the flow of nutrients, resulting in several potential metabolic and nutrition complications, postoperative diets are described to help minimize these effects.

QUESTIONS FOR REVIEW

1. Discuss the requirements for energy, protein, vitamins and minerals, and the means of providing them during the various stages of surgery (preoperative, immediately preoperative, postoperative).

2. Describe potential nutritional consequences that may result after surgery of the head and neck, esophagus, stomach, and intestine.

3. Develop a menu plan for a patient undergoing gastric bypass surgery for morbid obesity; include all phases of the diet progression.

4. Describe metabolic alterations that occur during metabolic stress.

5. Develop a nutrition care plan for a patient who has sustained third-degree burns covering 40% TBSA.

REFERENCES

1. Klein S, Kinney J, Jeejeebhoy K, et al: Nutrition support in clinical practice: review of published data and recommendations for future research directions. *JPEN J Parenter Enteral Nutr* 21:133, 1997.

2. Vitello J: Prevalence of malnutrition in hospitalized patients remains high. *J Am Coll Nutr* 12:589, 1993.

3. Naber T, Schermer T, De Bree A: Prevalence of malnutrition in nonsurgical hospitalized patients and its association with disease complication. *Am J Clin Nutr* 66:1232, 1997.

4. Coats K, Morgan SL, Bartolucci AA, et al: Hospital-associated malnutrition: a reevaluation 12 years later. *J Am Diet Assoc* 93:27, 1993.

5. Kelly I, Tessier S, Cahill A, et al: Still hungry in hospital: identifying malnutrition in acute hospital admissions. *Q J Med* 93:93, 2000.

6. A.S.P.E.N. Board of Directors: Guidelines for the use of parenteral and enteral nutrition in adult and pediatric patients. *JPEN J Parenter Enteral Nutr* 26:1SA, 2002.

7. VA TPN Cooperative Study: Perioperative total parenteral nutrition in surgical patients. *N Engl J Med* 325:525, 1991.

8. Gustafsson O, Ljungqvist O: Perioperative nutritional management in digestive tract surgery. In Toulson M, Correia D, Gassull M, editors: *Nutrition and the gastrointestinal tract*, ed 5, Baltimore, 2011, Lippincott Williams & Wilkins.

9. Ren L, Zhu D, Wei Y, et al: Enhanced recovery after surgery (ERAS) program attenuates stress and accelerates recovery in patients after radical resection for colorectal cancer: a prospective randomized controlled trail. *World J Surg* 36(2):407–414, 2012.

10. Cerra B, Benitez MR, Blackburn GL, et al: Applied nutrition in ICU patients: a consensus statement of the American College of Chest Physicians. *Chest* 111:769, 1997.

11. Klein C, Stanek G, Willes C: Overfeeding macronutrients to critically ill adults: metabolic complications. *J Am Diet Assoc* 98:795, 1998.

12. Pomposelli JJ, Baxter JK, Babineau TJ, et al: Early postoperative glucose control predicts nosocomial infection rate in diabetic patients. *JPEN J Parenter Enteral Nutr* 22:77, 1998.

13. Pomposelli JJ, Bistrian BR: Is total parenteral nutrition immunosuppressive? *New Horiz* 2:224, 1994.

14. Flancbaum L, Choban PS, Sambucco S, et al: Comparison of indirect calorimetry, the Fick method, and prediction equations in estimating the energy requirements of critically ill patients. *Am J Clin Nutr* 69:461, 1999.

15. Chiolero R, Revelly JP, Tappy L: Energy metabolism in sepsis and injury. *Nutrition* 13(Suppl):45S, 1997.

16. Frankenfield DC, Rowe WA, Smith JS, et al: Validation of several established equations for resting metabolic rate in obese and nonobese people. *J Am Diet Assoc* 103:1152, 2003.

17. Frankenfield DC, Roth-Yousey L, Compher C: Comparison of predictive equations for resting metabolic rate in healthy nonobese and obese adults: a systematic review. *J Am Diet Assoc* 105:775, 2005.

18. Barton RG: Nutrition support in critical illness. *Nutr Clin Pract* 10:129, 1994.

19. Cutts M, Dowdy RP, Ellersieck MR, et al: Predicting energy needs in ventilator-dependent critically ill patients: effect of adjusting weight for edema or adiposity. *Am J Clin Nutr* 66:1250, 1997.

20. Marik P, Varon J: The obese patient in the ICU. *Chest* 113:492, 1998.

21. Ireton-Jones CS, Turner WW Jr, Liepa GU, et al: Equations for estimation of energy expenditures in patients with burns with special reference to ventilatory status. *J Burn Care Rehabil* 13:330, 1992.

22. Patino J, de Pimiento SE, Vergara A, et al: Hypocaloric support in the critically ill. *World J Surg* 23:553, 1999.

23. Cresci GA, Martindale RG: Nutrition support in trauma. In *American Society for Enteral and Parenteral Nutrition: The science and practice of nutrition support: a case-based core*, ed 3, Dubuque, Iowa, 2001, Kendall/Hunt.

24. Thalacker-Mercer A, Fleet JC, Craig BA, et al: Inadequate protein intake affects skeletal muscle transcript profiles in older humans. *Am J Clin Nutr* 85:1344, 2007.

25. Campbell WW, Crim MC, Dallal GE, et al: Increased protein requirements in elderly people: new data and retrospective reassessments. *Am J Clin Nutr* 60:501, 1994.

26. Campbell WW, Johnson CA, McCabe GP, et al: Dietary protein requirements of younger and older adults. *Am J Clin Nutr* 88:1322, 2008.

27. Dabrowski G, Rombeau J: Practical nutritional management in the trauma intensive care unit. *Surg Clin North Am* 80:92, 2000.

28. Keele AM, Bray MJ, Emery PW, et al: Two-phase randomized controlled clinical trial of prospective oral dietary supplements in surgical patients. *Gut* 40:343, 1997.

29. Jeffery KM, Harkins JB, Cresci GA, et al: The clear liquid diet is no longer a necessity in the routine postoperative management of surgical patients. *Am Surg* 62:167, 1996.

30. Lipman T: Grains or veins: is enteral nutrition really better than parenteral nutrition? A look at the evidence. *JPEN J Parenter Enteral Nutr* 22:167, 1998.

31. Heyland DK, Novak F, Drover JW, et al: Should immunonutrition become routine in critically ill patients? A systematic review of the evidence. *JAMA* 286:944, 2001.

32. Sullivan M, Alonso E: Gastrointestinal and pancreatic disease. In Matarese L, Gottschlich M, editors: *Contemporary nutrition support practice*. Philadelphia, Pa., 1998, Saunders.

33. Himal HS, Allard JR, Nadeau JE, et al: The importance of adequate nutrition in closure of small intestinal fistulas. *Br J Surg* 61:724, 1974.

34. Mayes T, Gottschlich M: Burns and wound healing. In *American Society for Enteral and Parenteral Nutrition: The science and practice of nutrition support: a case-based core*, ed 3, Dubuque, Iowa, 2001, Kendall/Hunt.

35. Alexander JW, MacMillan BG, Stinnett JD, et al: Beneficial effects of aggressive protein feeding in severely burned children. *Ann Surg* 192:505, 1980.

36. Khorram-Sefat R, Behrendt W, Heiden A, et al: Long-term measurements of energy expenditure in severe burn injury. *West J Med Surg* 23:115, 1999.

37. Rose J, Shires T, Langer B, et al: Advances in burn care. In Cameron J, editor: *Advances in surgery*, vol 30, Chicago, 1996, Mosby-Year Book.

38. Cerantola Y, Hubner M, Grass F, et al: Immunonutrition in gastrointestinal surgery. *Br J Surg* 98:37, 2010.

39. Hillhouse J: Immune-enhancing enteral formulas: effect on patient outcome. *Support Line* 23:16, 2001.

40. Martindale R, Cresci G: The use of immune enhancing diets in burns. *JPEN J Parenter Enteral Nutr* 25(Suppl):S24, 2001.

41. Sax H: Effect of immune enhancing formulas in general surgery patients. *JPEN J Parenter Enteral Nutr* 25(Suppl):S19, 2001.

42. Schloerb P: Immune-enhancing diets: products, components, and their rationales. *JPEN J Parenter Enteral Nutr* 25(Suppl):S3, 2001.

FURTHER READINGS AND RESOURCES

Readings

Cerra FB: How nutrition intervention changes what getting sick means. *JPEN J Parenter Enteral Nutr* 14(Suppl 5):164, 1990.
[*This article provides a good review of three basic factors that influence what is observed at an ill patient's bedside when considering the effects of nutrition intervention: (1) the disease process inherent in the metabolic response to injury, (2) the presence of starvation, and (3) the presence of the nutrition intervention.*]

Hustler DA: Nutritional monitoring of a pediatric burn patient. *Nutr Clin Pract* 6:11, 1991.
[*This experienced dietitian-specialist on a burn center team provides a case report of a young boy who sustained mostly full-thickness burns on 56% of his total body surface area (TBSA). She describes in detail the challenge of initial evaluation and therapy, constant close monitoring, and appropriate responses to changing needs.*]

Tynes JJ, Austhof SI, Chima CS, et al: Diet tolerance and stool frequency in patients with ileoanal reservoirs. *J Am Diet Assoc* 92(7):861, 1992.
[*This brief report of a survey of patients with ileoanal reservoirs provides helpful background information about this recently developed alternative surgical procedure to the ileostomy, with practical guidance for nutritional management and patient counseling.*]

Websites of Interest

• American Academy of Physical Medicine and Rehabilitation. This is the website of the only organization exclusively serving physicians who specialize in physical medicine and rehabilitation: www.aapmr.org.

• American Botanical Council. The American Botanical Council is an independent, not-for-profit research and education organization dedicated to providing accurate and reliable information for consumers, healthcare practitioners, researchers, educators, industry, and the media: www.herbalgram.org.

• National Center for Complementary and Alternative Medicine. Lead agency of the U.S. government for scientific research on diverse medical and health care systems, practices, and products not generally considered part of conventional medicine: www.nccam.nih.gov/.

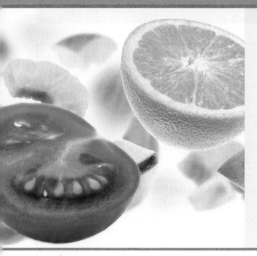

Drug-Nutrient Interactions

Joyce Gilbert

@ EVOLVE WEBSITE

http://evolve.elsevier.com/Williams/essentials/

OUTLINE

Drug-Nutrient Problems in Modern Medicine	Nutrition-Pharmacy Team
Drug Effects on Food and Nutrients	*HEALTH PROMOTION*
Food and Nutrient Effects on Drugs	"The Pain Reliever Doctors Recommend Most"

In this chapter, which continues our clinical nutrition sequence, we look briefly at some main effects of combining food and nutrients with drugs. We will see how these interactions affect nutrition therapy.

Today consumers are generally better informed about drug misuse. However, many are dangerously uninformed or misinformed about the specific drugs they may be taking, especially in relation to the food they eat.

All members of the health care team must have knowledge of drug actions and nutrition to make the wisest and most effective use of drugs and nutrition therapy. Here we examine some of these drug-nutrient effects and how these interactions affect nutrition therapy and education.

DRUG-NUTRIENT PROBLEMS IN MODERN MEDICINE

Problem Significance: Causes, Extent, and Effects

Medications and food interact in various ways. Various nutrients interfere with the medication's absorption and efficacy. In addition, medications can disturb ingestion, digestion, and absorption of nutrients. During this century, unprecedented medical progress has resulted in decreased childhood mortality rates and increased life expectancy. As we live longer, the incidence of chronic diseases such as cardiovascular disease,

type 2 diabetes mellitus, hypertension, and arthritis will continue to increase, often in a comorbid manner. Furthermore, treatment of these and other chronic diseases often involves long-term use of medications, often resulting in polypharmacy, in addition to alternative and herbal therapies (see the Focus on Culture box, "Are We Speaking the Same Language?").[1] To this we can then add the large volume of nonprescription drugs that Americans purchase without a physician's guidance (Figure 18-1).

Drug Use and Nutritional Status
Drug Administration

Drugs are administered several different ways. The administration route depends on the chemical properties of the drug, desired effect, and patient characteristics that affect administration of the drug. Drug administration routes are described in Table 18-1.

Older Adults at Risk

All of us, at any age, risk harmful drug-drug or drug-nutrient interactions. However, older adults are particularly vulnerable, and this will only become more prevalent. Today, adults older than age 65 represent approximately 14% of the U.S. population. It is projected this number will increase to 20% to 22% by 2050.[2] Older adults take a much larger percentage of prescription and nonprescription medications than their younger counterparts (Figure 18-2). Several factors

⊕ FOCUS ON CULTURE

Are We Speaking the Same Language?

Consider the following prescription label directions written half in English and half in Spanish:

Aplicarse once cada dia til rash is clear.

What does it mean to you? If you do not read Spanish, then it probably does not mean much (although you can pick out the words *once* and *til rash is clear*). In addition, if you study this phrase hard enough, then you might figure out it says something about using the medication once a day until the rash is gone.

If you read Spanish, then the meaning may be entirely different. *Once* means eleven in Spanish. If this is a mild topical medication, then perhaps no permanent harm would result if you used it 11 times a day. However, if this is an oral medication, then the results could be fatal.

Many people using prescription or over-the-counter (OTC) medications, herbal products, or vitamin and mineral supplements use a language other than English as their primary language. Foreign-born individuals make up 11% of the U.S. population. The majority of immigrants are of Hispanic origin. Although many members of these groups have good reading and writing skills in their native languages, they do not possess the same skills in English. How then are they supposed to read and understand directions regarding how to take medications or supplements? How can they adhere to a prescribed medical regimen if they are unable to read the label? This language barrier may make the individuals more susceptible to food-drug interactions.

Another barrier to health is literacy. More than 40% of patients with chronic illnesses are functionally illiterate. Almost 25% of all adult Americans read at or below a fifth-grade level, whereas medical information is typically written at a tenth-grade level or greater. The National Adult Literacy Survey (NALS) found almost 25% of patients with inadequate functional health literacy did not know how to take medications.

Limited health literacy and language barriers have many consequences. Patients who do not understand prescription directions and instructions for preventive care and self-care may make the following mistakes:

- Incorrect doses (e.g., improper infant formula preparation and feeding)
- Incorrect schedules of administration (e.g., four times a day versus four pills at one time)
- Incorrect routes of administration (e.g., teens who have misunderstood directions for contraceptive jelly and have eaten it on toast every morning to prevent pregnancy)

Low health literacy risk groups include pediatric patients, older adult patients, and patients with language barriers. Pediatric patients are at increased risk of incorrect doses. Older adult patients take multiple medications, which increases risk for errors. In addition, patients older than age 60 may have hearing loss, memory loss, short attention span, and low energy levels, thus exacerbating the problems. Patients who speak English as their second language are vulnerable to misinterpretation of information.

Following are some solutions to this problem:

- Provide written materials in several languages and at a fifth-grade reading level or lower.
- Offer small amounts of information at a time.
- Avoid using "medical speak" (medical terms that are used every day in the clinical setting but are unfamiliar to patients).
- Employ a multilingual staff.
- Have patients repeat instruction to ensure the message was received and understood.
- Use identifiers such as time-of-day references (e.g., "Take one tablet in the morning when you wake up and the second tablet at bedtime.").
- Use visual images when possible.

Bibliography

Hardin LR: Frontline pharmacist: counseling patients with low health literacy. *Am J Health Syst Pharm* 62:364, 2005.

Institute for Safe Medication Practices: Hospitals need to take action now to reduce threat of medication errors with magnesium sulfate, *ISMP Medication Safety Alert!*, March 12, 1997. from: <www.ismp.org/MSAarticles/calendar/Mar97.html>. Retrieved April 11, 2009.

Institute for Safe Medication Practices: To promote understanding, assume every patient has a health literacy problem, *ISMP Medication Safety Alert!*, October 31, 2001. from: <www.ismp.org/MSAarticles/calendar/Oct01.html#Oct31, 2001>. Retrieved April 11, 2009.

Literacy Partners of Manitoba: *Literacy and health resources*, Manitoba, Canada, 2005, Literacy Partners of Manitoba. from: <www.health.mb.literacy.ca/health.htm>. Retrieved April 11, 2009.

National Institute for Literacy: *Literacy fact sheets: scope of the literacy need*, Washington, D.C., 2001, National Institute for Literacy. from: <http://factfinder.census.gov/servlet/DatasetMainPageServlet?_program=ACS&_submenuid=&_lang=en&_ts=%29>. Available at: <www.nifl.gov>. Retrieved July 1, 2010.

U.S. Census Bureau: *Profile of selected social characteristics: 2000, Census 2000 supplementary survey summary tables*, Washington, D.C., 2001, U.S. Government Printing Office.

Wallendorf M: Literally literacy. *J Consum Res* 27:505, 2001.

contribute to an increased risk among older adults, including the following[3]:

- They are likely to be taking more drugs for longer periods to control chronic diseases.
- Their drugs are likely to be more toxic.
- They respond to drugs with increased variability.
- They have less capability of handling drugs efficiently.

- Their nutritional status is more likely to be deficient.
- They are more likely to make increased errors in self-care because of illness, mental confusion, or lack of drug information.

As a result of these problems, concerned physicians, nutritionists, pharmacists, and nurses are increasingly working together as a team to provide drug and nutrition education

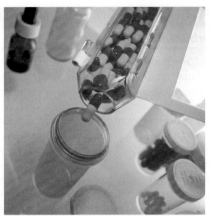

FIGURE 18-1 Prescription and nonprescription drugs have become part of American life. (Copyright 2006 JupiterImages Corporation.)

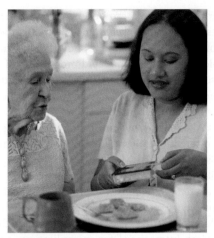

FIGURE 18-2 Older adults make up a large percentage of those taking prescription and nonprescription medications in the United States.

TABLE 18-1	DRUG ADMINISTRATION ROUTES
ADMINISTRATION ROUTE	**CHARACTERISTICS**
Oral	Requires ability to swallow and absorb the medication
Sublingual	Medication placed under tongue to dissolve; absorbed quickly across mucous membrane
Buccal	Medication placed in cheek to dissolve; absorbed quickly across mucous membrane
Parenteral	Injection in circulatory system
Subcutaneous (SC)	Injection under the skin
Intradermal (ID)	Injection under outermost layer of skin
Intramuscular (IM)	Injection into muscle
Intraperitoneal (IP)	Injection into peritoneal cavity
Intravenous (IV)	Injection into a vein
Topical	Applied to skin
Inhalation	Medication breathed into respiratory system
Ophthalmic	Placement of medication into eye
Otic	Placement of medication into ear
Epidural	Placement of medication into spinal fluid
Intrathecal	Placement of medication into membrane surrounding central nervous system (CNS)

Data from Nelms M: Pharmacology. In Nelms MN, Sucher K, Long S, editors: *Understanding nutrition therapy and pathophysiology*, Belmont, Calif., 2007, Wadsworth.

and therapy on a more sound basis. A number of drug-nutrient interactions demand this type of teamwork in patient care.[1]

Nutritional Status

Poor nutritional status can have a major effect on risk for complications of drug-nutrient reactions. Nutrient-drug mechanisms that influence nutritional status include those affecting the following:

- Stimulated or suppressed appetite
- Decreased intestinal absorption
- Increased renal excretion
- Competition or displacement of nutrients for carrier protein sites
- Interference with synthesis of a necessary enzyme, coenzyme, or carrier
- Hormonal effects on genetic systems
- Drug delivery system
- Components in drug formulation

In general, drugs are grouped according to primary action. In the following sections, we review the various effects of drugs on food and nutrients and the effects of food and nutrients on drugs. In each case we give some examples for your reference in patient care.

DRUG EFFECTS ON FOOD AND NUTRIENTS

Drug Effects on Food Intake

Appetite Changes

The following drugs may stimulate appetite, weight gain, or both[4]:

- *Antihistamines:* These drugs can lead to marked increase in appetite and subsequent weight gain. Cyproheptadine hydrochloride (Periactin) is an antihistamine also used as an appetite stimulant.
- *Antianxiety drugs:* Some drugs in this classification may lead to hyperphagia, or excessive eating. Some of these drugs include chlordiazepoxide hydrochloride (Librium), diazepam (Valium), and alprazolam (Xanax).
- *Tricyclic antidepressants:* Tricyclic antidepressants and most antipsychotic drugs such as amitriptyline hydrochloride (Elavil), olanzapine (Zyprexa), chlorpromazine hydrochloride (Thorazine), and clozapine (Clozaril) may promote appetite and lead to significant weight gain.

- *Insulin:* Hypoglycemia can occur in persons with type 1 diabetes if food is not taken immediately after their insulin injection (see Chapter 22). If some food is not readily available to counteract the rapid progression of the unrelieved severe hypoglycemia, then coma and death occur. If excess food is consumed to avoid or treat hypoglycemia, then weight gain may occur.

- *Steroids:* Anabolic steroids, including testosterone, promote nitrogen retention, increased lean body mass, and subsequent weight gain.

The following drugs may depress appetite[4]:

- *Selective serotonin reuptake inhibitors (SSRIs):* This class of antidepressants may cause anorexia and weight loss; an example is fluoxetine (Prozac). (See the Case Study box, "Drug-Herb Interaction," for an application of the use of SSRIs.)

- *Amphetamines:* These drugs act as stimulants to the central nervous system (CNS) and have the effect of depressing the desire for food, thus leading to marked loss of weight. For this reason, they have been used in the past as appetite-depressant drugs in the treatment of obesity. However, long-term use of these drugs for such treatment has caused problems, such as addiction. For this reason, amphetamines are rarely used now for this purpose. Children taking amphetamines show dose-dependent growth retardation.

- *Alcohol:* Abuse of alcohol can lead to loss of appetite, reduced food intake, and malnutrition. The anorexia, or loss of appetite, can stem from various effects of alcoholism such as gastritis, hepatitis, cirrhosis, ketosis, pancreatitis, alcoholic brain syndrome, drunkenness, and withdrawal symptoms. The resulting reduced food intake can then lead to malnutrition, which further complicates the anorexia.

Taste and Smell Changes

Drugs such as the tricyclic antidepressant amitriptyline (Elavil) may impair salivary flow, causing dry mouth along with a sour or metallic taste.[4] The antibiotic clarithromycin (Biaxin) is secreted into saliva, causing a bitter taste.[4] Antibiotics such as tetracycline may suppress natural oral bacteria, resulting in oral yeast overgrowth or candidiasis. Metronidazole (Flagyl), an antibiotic, may cause dysgeusia (abnormal or impaired sense of taste) by causing a metallic taste in the mouth.[4] Antineoplastic medications (cisplatin or methotrexate) may damage rapidly growing cells, causing stomatitis, glossitis, or esophagitis (or a combination of these problems)[4] (see the Perspectives in Practice box, "Counseling Patients About Potential Food-Medication Interactions").

Gastrointestinal Effects

Many drugs can affect the stomach and cause nausea, vomiting, bleeding, or ulceration; intestinal peristalsis; or changes in intestinal flora. Nonsteroidal antiinflammatory drugs (NSAIDs) such as aspirin (acetylsalicylic acid [ASA]), ibuprofen (Advil, Motrin), and naproxen (Aleve, Anaprox) cause stomach irritation.[4] Sometimes the irritation is so

CASE STUDY

Drug-Herb Interaction

Ivanna is a 20-year-old exchange student from Germany. She lives with three roommates and is in her junior year at the local university. Ivanna is seeking medical attention at the urging of her roommates, who report her mood has become increasingly depressed during the past two semesters. She has become withdrawn and moody but is otherwise a healthy young woman. She is 5 feet 11 inches tall and weighs 160 lb on admission.

Ivanna reports a 5-lb weight loss in the past 3 months. She takes oral contraceptives, smokes ½ pack of cigarettes per day, and drinks four to five beers on the weekends. Her mother has been treated for depression with St. John's wort by the family physician in Germany for the past 10 years. Her admitting diagnosis is depression. Physician's orders are as follows: Zoloft, 50 mg every day, referral to house psychologist for counseling, and nutrition consult for her poor eating habits.

Questions for Analysis

1. Ivanna's physician ordered Zoloft to treat her depression. Zoloft is a selective serotonin reuptake inhibitor (SSRI). Are there any pertinent nutritional considerations when using this medicine?
2. How do SSRIs work?
3. During the diet history, you ask Ivanna if she uses any over-the-counter (OTC) vitamins, minerals, or herbal supplements. She tells you her mother suggested she try *Hypericum perforatum* (St. John's wort) because in Germany it is prescribed to treat depression. Ivanna did as her mother suggested, because it is available without prescription in the United States. What is St. John's wort?
4. How is St. John's wort used in the United States?
5. How does St. John's wort work as an antidepressant?
6. Does St. John's wort have any side effects?
7. How is St. John's wort regulated in the United States? How is it used in Europe?
8. What is your immediate concern regarding Ivanna's use of St. John's wort?

Data from Nelms MN, Long S, Lacey K: *Medical nutrition therapy: a case study approach*, ed 3, Belmont, Calif., 2008, Wadsworth.

severe as to cause sudden and serious gastric bleeding.[4] Anticholinergic medications (antipsychotics, antidepressants, antihistamines) slow peristalsis, resulting in constipation. Ciprofloxacin (Cipro) is an antibiotic that can allow for the overgrowth of *Clostridium difficile*, resulting in pseudomembranous colitis.[4]

Drug Effects on Nutrient Absorption and Metabolism
Nutrient Absorption

A number of drugs can increase nutrient absorption and thus benefit nutritional status. For example, cimetidine (Tagamet), a gastric antisecretory agent, helps patients with bowel

Counseling Patients About Potential Food-Medication Interactions

- Provision of relevant medication information: drug name, drug indications, duration of therapy
- Information detailing how to take the medication
- Probable side effects and dietary suggestions to lessen symptoms
- Nutritional difficulties that may develop, particularly if dietary intake is poor
- Dietary alteration that may change drug action
- Food and beverages to avoid or consume in moderation while taking the medication
- Implications of alcohol ingestion
- Potential for interactions involving medications and vitamin and mineral supplements (or other food supplements)
- Significance of staying on a special diet prescription for treatment of medical condition
- Individualization of dietary prescription to that person only
- Consultation with prescribing physician before modifying drug or diet prescription
- Consultation with a registered dietitian (RD) for in-depth nutrition information
- Consultation with a registered pharmacist (RPh) for questions regarding drug action or possible side effects

Data from Pronsky ZM: *Food medication interactions,* ed 15, Birchrunville, Pa., 2008, Food-Medication Interactions.

resection in several ways.[4] The drug reduces gastric acid and volume output; it also lowers duodenal acid load and volume and reduces jejunal flow.[4] It maintains the pH of secretions and decreases fecal fat, nitrogen, and volume, thus improving absorption of macronutrients.[4] This drug is therefore helpful in the treatment of various gastrointestinal (GI) disorders, including peptic ulcer disease (see Chapter 20).[4] On the other hand, prolonged use of cimetidine may cause decreased absorption of vitamin B_{12}, thiamin, and iron.[4]

A number of drugs can contribute to primary malabsorption. Questran (antihyperlipidemic, bile acid sequestrant [cholestyramine]) binds vitamins A, D, E, and K in the GI tract, preventing absorption of these nutrients.[4] Colchicine, a drug used in the treatment of gout, leads to vitamin B_{12} deficiency, causing megaloblastic anemia.[4] Alcohol abuse can provoke malabsorption of thiamin and folic acid, causing peripheral neuritis and anemia.[4] Laxatives can produce severe malabsorption, leading to conditions such as osteomalacia.[4]

Secondary malabsorption may also be drug induced. For example, the antibiotic neomycin causes tissue changes in the intestinal villi, precipitates bile salts, prevents fat breakdown by inhibiting pancreatic lipase, and decreases bile acid absorption.[4] These effects can lead to steatorrhea and failure to absorb the fat-soluble vitamins A, D, E, and K.[4] Malabsorption of vitamin D in turn leads to a calcium deficiency. Other drugs cause malabsorption of folic acid or impair its use. Methotrexate, for example, used in cancer chemotherapy, is a folic acid antagonist that impairs the intestinal absorption

of calcium.[4] Summaries of medications that affect food and nutrients can be found in Table 18-2.

Mineral Depletion

Certain drugs can lead to mineral depletion through induced GI losses or renal excretion[5]:

- *Diuretics:* Diuretic drugs are intentionally used to reduce levels of excess tissue water and sodium, but they may also result in loss of other minerals, such as potassium, magnesium, and zinc. Potassium deficiency brings weakness, anorexia, nausea, vomiting, listlessness, apprehension, and sometimes diffuse pain, drowsiness, stupor, and irrational behavior. However, potassium-retaining diuretics such as spironolactone, as well as overuse of potassium supplementation, may cause the opposite effect of hyperkalemia.
- *Chelating agents:* Penicillamine attaches to metals and can lead to the deficiency of such key trace elements as zinc and copper.
- *Alcohol:* Abuse of alcohol can lead to diminished levels of potassium, magnesium, and zinc.
- *Antacids:* These commonly used OTC medications are of concern because they can produce phosphate deficiency, with symptoms of anorexia, malaise, **paresthesia**, profound muscle weakness, and convulsions, as well as calcification of soft tissues from the prolonged hypercalcemia.
- *Aspirin:* Salicylates such as ASA (aspirin) can induce iron deficiency by causing low-level blood loss from erosions in the stomach or intestinal tissue when taken incorrectly (see the Health Promotion section for discussion).

Vitamin Depletion

Certain drugs act as metabolic antagonists and can cause deficiencies of the vitamins involved.

- *Vitamin antagonists:* Various drugs have been used successfully to treat disease because they are antagonists of certain vitamins and thus can control key metabolic reactions in which that vitamin is involved. For example, warfarin (Coumadin) anticoagulants inhibit regeneration of vitamin K, which is necessary for blood clotting. In addition, some cancer chemotherapy drugs such as methotrexate have multiple antagonist effects on folate metabolism, thus inhibiting the synthesis of cell reproduction substances—deoxyribonucleic acid (DNA) and ribonucleic acid (RNA)—and protein. In a similar manner, the antimalaria drug pyrimethamine inhibits the action of folate in protein synthesis.

Special Adverse Reactions

Several reactions are related to specific drug interactions with particular nutrients, as follows:

- *Monoamine oxidase inhibitors (MAOIs):* These antidepressant drugs can increase the vascular effect of simple **vasoactive** amines, such as tyramine and dopamine, from food.[5] The resulting tyramine syndrome is marked by headache, pallor, nausea, and restlessness. With increased

TABLE 18-2   MEDICATIONS AFFECTING FOOD AND NUTRIENTS

DRUG CLASS	EXAMPLES	ACTION	NUTRIENTS AFFECTED	HOW TO AVOID
Alcohol, particularly excessive use	Beer, wine, spirits	Increases turnover of some vitamins; substitution of alcohol for food	Vitamin B_{12}, folate, and magnesium	Limit alcohol consumption to <2 drinks per day for men, <1 drink per day for women
Analgesic, NSAID, and antiinflammatory agents	Salicylates (aspirin), ibuprofen (Motrin, Advil), naproxen (Anaprox, Aleve, Naprosyn), acetaminophen (Tylenol)	Increases loss of vitamin C and competes with folate and vitamin K	Vitamin C, folate, vitamin K	Increase intake of foods high in vitamin C, folate, and vitamin K; take with 8 oz water
Antacid agents	Aluminum antacids, H_2 blockers	Inactivates thiamin; decreases absorption of some nutrients	Thiamin (B_1)	Foods containing thiamin (B_1) should be consumed at a different time; depends on antacid; possibly magnesium, phosphorus, iron, vitamin A, and folate Take antacid after meals; take iron, magnesium, or folate supplements separately by 2 hours; take separately from citrus fruit or juices or calcium citrate by 3 hours
Antiulcer agents (histamine blockers)	Ranitidine (Zantac), cimetidine (Tagamet), famotidine (Pepcid)	Decreases vitamin absorption	Vitamin B_{12}	Consult physician or RD regarding vitamin B_{12} supplementation
Antibiotic agents	Tetracycline, ciprofloxacin (Cipro)	Chelation of minerals; ingestion with caffeine may increase excitability and nervousness	Calcium, magnesium, iron, and zinc; caffeine	Take tetracycline at least 1 h before or 2 h after a meal; do not take with caffeine-containing products
Antineoplastic agents	Methotrexate	Causes mucosal damage, which may cause decreased nutrient absorption	Folate and vitamin B_{12}, (also see Antibiotic Agents)	Consult physician or RD regarding supplementation
Anticholinergic agents	Amitriptyline (Elavil), chlorpromazine (Thorazine)	Saliva thickens and loses ability to prevent tooth decay	Fluids	Increase intake of fluids
Anticonvulsant agents	Phenobarbital, phenytoin (Dilantin)	Increases metabolism of folate (possibly leading to megaloblastic anemia), vitamin D (especially in children), and vitamin K	Folate, vitamin D, and vitamin K	Increase folate, vitamins D and K intake
Antidepressant agents	Lithium carbonate, Lithane, Lithobid, Lithonate, Lithotabs, Eskalith	May cause metallic taste, nausea, vomiting, dry mouth, anorexia, weight gain, and increased thirst	Fluids	Drink 2-3 L of water per day and take with food, consistent sodium intake
Antihyperlipidemic agents	Cholestyramine (Questran), colestipol (Colestid)	Binds bile salts and nutrients	Fat-soluble vitamins (A, D, E, K), folate, vitamin B_{12}, and iron	Include rich sources of these vitamins and minerals in diet

TABLE 18-2	MEDICATIONS AFFECTING FOOD AND NUTRIENTS—cont'd			
DRUG CLASS	EXAMPLES	ACTION	NUTRIENTS AFFECTED	HOW TO AVOID
Antituberculosis agents	Isoniazid (INH)	Inhibits conversion of vitamin B$_6$ to active form	Vitamin B$_6$	Vitamin B$_6$ supplementation is necessary to prevent deficiency and peripheral neuropathy
Corticosteroid agents	Prednisone, Solu-Medrol, hydrocortisone	Increases excretion	Protein, potassium, calcium, magnesium, zinc, vitamin C, and vitamin B$_6$	Increase intake of foods high in protein, potassium, calcium, magnesium, zinc, vitamin C, and vitamin B$_6$
Loop diuretic agents	Furosemide (Lasix)	Increases mineral excretion in urine	Potassium, calcium, magnesium, zinc, sodium, and chloride	Include fresh fruits and vegetables in diet
Thiazide diuretic agents	Hydrochlorothiazide (HCTZ)	Increases excretion of most electrolytes, but enhances reabsorption of calcium	Potassium, calcium, magnesium, zinc, sodium, chloride, and calcium	Increase intake of foods high in potassium, calcium, magnesium, zinc, sodium, and chloride
Potassium-sparing diuretic agents	Triamterene (Dyrenium)	Hyperkalemia	Potassium	Avoid potassium-based salt substitutes
Laxative agents	Fibercon, Mitrolan	Decreases nutrient absorption	Vitamins and minerals	Consult physician or RD regarding supplementation
Sedative agents	Barbiturates	Increases metabolism of vitamins	Folate, vitamin D, vitamin B$_{12}$, thiamin, and vitamin C	Increase intake of foods high in folate, vitamin D, vitamin B$_{12}$, thiamin, and vitamin C
Mineral oil	Agoral Plain	Decreases absorption	Fat-soluble vitamins (A, D, E, K), β-carotene, calcium, phosphorus, and potassium	Take 2 h apart from food and fat-soluble vitamins
Oral contraceptive agents	Estrogen/progestin	May cause selective malabsorption or increased metabolism and turnover	Vitamin B$_6$ and folate	Increase foods high in B$_6$ and folate

Data from Anderson J, Bland SE: Drug-food interactions. *J Pharm Soc Wisc* 28, Nov/Dec 1998; Bobroff LB, Lentz A, Turner RE: *Food/drug and drug/nutrient interactions: what you should know about your medications,* Gainesville, 1994, University of Florida Cooperative Extension Service, Institute of Food and Agricultural Science. Available at: <www.edis.ifas.ufl.edu>; Food and Drug Administration/National Consumers League: *Food & drug interactions,* Washington, D.C., U.S. Government Printing Office. from: <www.nclnet.org/Food%20&%20Drug.pdf>. Retrieved April 11, 2009.
NSAID, Nonsteroidal antiinflammatory drug; *RD,* registered dietitian.

absorption, symptoms may escalate to apprehension, sweating, palpitations, chest pain, fever, and increased blood pressure, at times, although rarely, to the extent of hypertensive crisis and stroke.

- *Flushing reaction:* A number of drugs react with alcohol to produce a **flushing reaction** along with **dyspnea** and headache. CNS depressants, including hypnotic sedatives, antihistamines, phenothiazines, and narcotic analgesics, may cause a loss of consciousness if taken in combination with alcohol. Extreme caution must be exercised with these medications, and patients should be alerted to the dangers of mixing them with alcohol.

- *Hypoglycemia:* Drugs such as chlorpropamide (Diabinese) and similar oral medications used to control type 2 diabetes mellitus are hypoglycemic agents. They precipitate a rapid release of insulin, which may provoke a hypoglycemic reaction. This response of a rapidly reduced blood

KEY TERMS

paresthesia Abnormal sensations such as prickling, burning, and crawling of skin.
vasoactive Having an effect on the diameter of blood vessels.

glucose level is especially strong when the drugs are used with alcohol. Symptoms of hypoglycemia include weakness, mental confusion, and irrational behavior. If not treated, then loss of consciousness can follow.

- *Disulfiram reaction:* The drug disulfiram, commonly called Antabuse, is used in the treatment of alcoholism. It combats alcohol consumption by producing extremely unpleasant side effects when taken with alcohol. Within 15 minutes, flushing ensues, followed by headache, nausea, vomiting, and chest or abdominal pain. Other drugs, including aldehyde dehydrogenase inhibitors, may have a similar effect.

FOOD AND NUTRIENT EFFECTS ON DRUGS

Physiologic Factors in Drug Absorption

Absorption of drugs is a complex matter. Physiologic events are important in a number of ways.

Solution

Before an orally administered tablet or capsule can dissolve, it must first disintegrate. The absorption of the drug, either from solution in acid gastric secretions or in the more alkaline medium of the intestine, may be more or less complete, depending on its degree of solubility (see the Evidence-Based Practice box, "Grapefruit 'Juices' Certain Medications"). Food may affect eventual drug absorption at any of these points. Table 18-3 provides some examples of drugs that are better used when taken without food and those that should be taken with food. The drug then passes through the intestinal mucosa and liver circulation before entering systemic circulation. In the systemic blood circulation system, it may be subject to metabolism, deactivation, and elimination through the so-called first-pass mechanism.

Stomach-Emptying Rate

Composition of the diet affects the rate at which food enters the small intestine from the stomach. Slow emptying of food from the stomach has the effect of doling out small portions of a drug, creating more optimal saturation rates on the absorptive sites in the small intestine. Fats, high temperatures, and solid meals prolong the time the food stays in the stomach. Food usually increases secretion of bile, acid, and gut enzymes. It also enhances intestinal motility and splanchnic blood flow. Certain food particles may adsorb drugs.

Clinical Significance

Whether these physiologic events have clinical significance depends on the extent of the effect and nature of the drug. A small change in absorption is critical for a drug with a steep dose response curve but perhaps unnoticeable for a drug with a wide range of effective concentrations. In general, the amount of absorption is clinically more important than the rate of absorption, because it has increased effect on the steady-state plasma concentration of the drug after multiple doses.

KEY TERMS
flushing reaction   Short-term reaction resulting in redness of neck and face.
dyspnea   Labored, difficult breathing.
disulfiram   White to off-white crystalline antioxidant; inhibits oxidation of the acetaldehyde metabolized from alcohol. It is used in the treatment of alcoholism, producing extremely uncomfortable symptoms when alcohol is ingested after oral administration of the drug.

EVIDENCE-BASED PRACTICE

Grapefruit "Juices" Certain Medications

Almost all oral drugs are subject to first-pass metabolism. That is, any substance the body views as a toxin (e.g., drugs, alcohol) goes through the liver via hepatic portal circulation, thus removing some of the active substance from blood before it enters general circulation. This means a fraction of the original dose of the drug will not be "available" to systemic circulation because it has undergone biotransformation. In other words, the bioavailability of the drug has been altered, or lowered. One mechanism responsible for this is an enzyme system found in the intestinal wall and liver. The cytochrome P_{450} 3A4 (CYP3A4) system, specifically CYP3A4-mediated drug metabolism, is responsible for first-pass metabolism of many medications. Most medications are lipid soluble and readily absorbed. To eliminate toxins (i.e., drugs) from the body, however, the CYP3A4 system either breaks them down in the gut or changes the drug into a more water-soluble version in the liver, allowing it to be eliminated via urine.

Where does grapefruit juice come into play? Grapefruit juice blocks the CYP3A4 enzyme in the wall of the small intestine, thus increasing the bioavailability of the drug. This means an increased serum drug level, which may cause unpleasant consequences, including side effects, toxicity, or both.

What is it in grapefruit juice that does this? The precise chemical nature of the substance responsible for inhibiting the gut wall CYP3A4 enzyme is unknown, but it is believed that more than one component present in grapefruit juice may contribute to the inhibitory effect on CYP3A4.

A single glass (8 oz) of grapefruit juice has the potential to increase bioavailability and enhance beneficial or adverse effects of a broad range of medications. These effects can persist up to 72 hours after grapefruit consumption, until more CYP3A4 has been metabolized. Interactions have been found between grapefruit juice and drugs, as outlined in the following table.

Grapefruit "Juices" Certain Medications—cont'd

Interactions Between Grapefruit Juice and Medications

Category	Generic Name	Brand Name	Effect
Antihypertensive (calcium channel blockers) agents	Felodipine	Plendil	Flushing, headache, tachycardia, decreased blood pressure
	Nifedipine	Procardia, Adalat	
	Nimodipine	Nimotop	
	Nisoldipine	Sular	
	Nicardipine	Cardene	
	Isradipine	Dyna Circ	
	Verapamil	Calan, Isoptin	Same as previously stated plus bradycardia and AV block
Nonsedating antihistamine agents	Astemizole	Hismanal	No studies available; recommendation is to avoid taking grapefruit juice with astemizole
Immunosuppressant agents	Cyclosporine	Neoral, Sandimmune, SangCya	Kidney toxicity, increased susceptibility to infections
	Tacrolimus	Prograf	
Statin (HMG-CoA reductase inhibitors) agents	Atorvastatin	Lipitor	Headache, GI complaints, muscle pain, increased risk of myopathy
	Lovastatin	Mevacor	
Caffeine	Simvastatin	Zocor	Nervousness, overstimulation
Antianxiety, insomnia, or antidepressant agents	Buspirone	BuSpar	Increased sedation
	Diazepam	Valium	
	Alprazolam	Xanax	
	Midazolam	Versed	
	Triazolam	Halcion	
	Zaleplon	Sonata	
	Carbamazepine	Tegretol	
	Clomipramine	Anafranil	
	Trazodone	Desyrel	
Protease inhibitor agents	Saquinavir	Fortovase, Invirase	Doubles bioavailability, resulting in increased efficacy or toxicity depending on dose and patient variability
Sexual dysfunction agents	Sildenafil	Viagra	Delayed absorption (takes longer to become effective)

Medications Considered Safe for Use with Grapefruit

	Cetirizine	Zyrtec, Reactine	
	Fexofenadine	Allegra	
	Fluvastatin	Lescol	
	Loratadine	Claritin	
	Pravastatin	Pravachol	

Bibliography

Bailey DG, Malcolm J, Arnold O, et al: Grapefruit juice-drug interactions. *Br J Clin Pharmacol* 46(2):101, 1998.

Guo L, Fukuda K, Ohta T, et al: Role of furanocoumarin derivatives on grapefruit juice–mediated inhibition of human CYP3A activity. *Drug Metab Dispos* 28:766, 2000.

Ho PC, Saville DJ: Inhibition of human CYP3A4 activity by grapefruit flavonoids, furanocoumarins and related compounds. *J Pharm Pharm Sci* 4(3):217, 2001.

Hyland R, Roe EGH, Jones BC, et al: Identification of the cytochrome P450 enzymes involved in the N-demethylation of sildenafil. *Clin Pharmacol* 51:239, 2000.

Jetter A, Kinzig-Schippers M, Walchner-Bonjean M: Effects of grapefruit juice on the pharmacokinetics of sildenafil. *Clin Pharmacol Ther* 71(1):21, 2002.

Kane GC, Lipsky JJ: Drug-grapefruit juice interactions. *Mayo Clin Proc* 75:933, 2000.

Pronsky ZM: *Food medication interactions*, ed 15, Birchrunville, Pa., 2008, Food-Medication Interactions.

Schmiedlin-Ren P, Edwards DJ, Fitzsimmons ME, et al: Mechanisms of enhanced oral availability of CYP3A4 substrates by grapefruit constituents. *Drug Metab Dispos* 25(1):1228, 1997.

University of Illinois Chicago College of Pharmacy Drug Information Center: *Grapefruit juice interactions*, Chicago, 2005, University of Illinois. from: <https://www.uic.edu/pharmacy/services/di/grapefru.htmwww.uic.edu/pharmacy/services/di/grapefru.htm>. Retrieved July 1, 2010.

AV, Atrioventricular; *GI,* gastrointestinal; *HMG-CoA,* 3-hydroxy-3-methylglutaryl coenzyme A.

TABLE 18-3   FOODS AND NUTRIENTS AFFECTING MEDICATIONS

DRUG CLASS	EXAMPLES	USE	ACTION	FOOD/NUTRIENTS	HOW TO AVOID
Alcohol, particularly excessive use	Beer, wine, spirits	Lower inhibitions, CNS depressant	Slows absorption	Food	Consume alcohol with food or meals
Analgesic and NSAID agents	Salicylates (aspirin), ibuprofen (Motrin, Advil), naproxen (Anaprox, Aleve, Naprosyn), acetaminophen (Tylenol)	Pain and fever	Alcohol ingestion increases hepatotoxicity, liver damage, or stomach bleeding	Alcohol	Limit alcohol intake to <2 drinks per day for men, <1 drink per day for women
Antiulcer agents (histamine blockers)	Cimetidine (Tagamet)	Ulcers	Increased blood alcohol levels, reduced caffeine clearance	Alcohol, caffeine-containing foods and beverages	Limit caffeine intake; limit alcohol intake to <2 drinks per day for men, <1 drink per day for women
Antibiotic agents	Ciprofloxacin (Cipro)	Infection	Decreases absorption	Dairy products	Avoid dairy products
Anticoagulant agents	Warfarin (Coumadin)	Blood clots	Reduced efficacy, increased anticoagulation	Vitamins K and E (supplements) may reduce efficacy, alcohol and garlic may increase anticoagulation	Consistent intake of foods high in vitamin K: broccoli, spinach, kale, turnip greens, cauliflower, Brussels sprouts; avoid high dose of vitamin E (400 IU or more)
Antineoplastic agents	Methotrexate	Cancer	Increased hepatotoxicity with chronic alcohol use	Alcohol	Avoid alcohol
Antiemetic agents	Amitriptyline HCl (Elavil), chlorpromazine HCl (Thorazine)	Antidepressant; antipsychotic/antiemetic	Increased sedation	Alcohol	Avoid alcohol
Anticonvulsant agents	Phenobarbital	Seizures, epilepsy	Increased sedation	Alcohol	Avoid alcohol
Antidepressant agents: MAOIs	Phenelzine (Nardil), tranylcypromine (Parnate)	Depression, anxiety	Rapid, potentially fatal increase in blood pressure	Foods or alcoholic beverages containing tyramine	Avoid beer; red wine; American processed, cheddar, bleu, Brie, mozzarella, and Parmesan cheeses; yogurt; sour cream; beef or chicken liver; cured meats such as sausage and salami; game meats; caviar; dried fish; avocados; bananas; yeast extracts; raisins; sauerkraut; soy sauce; miso soup; broad (fava) beans; ginseng; caffeine-containing products (colas, chocolate, coffee, tea)

Drug category	Drug examples	Condition	Effect	Food	Recommendation
Antihistamine agents	Fexofenadine (Allegra), loratadine (Claritin), cetirizine (Zyrtec), astemizole (Hismanal)	Allergies	Increases drowsiness and slows mental and motor performance	Alcohol	Use caution when operating machinery/driving
Antihypertensive agents	ACE-inhibitors, angiotensin II receptor antagonists, β-blockers, verapamil HCl	Hypertension	Reduced effectiveness	Natural licorice (Glycyrrhiza glabra) and tyramine-rich foods	Avoid these foods
Antihyperlipidemic agents (HMG-CoA reductase inhibitors) or statin agents	Atorvastatin (Lipitor), lovastatin (Mevacor), pravastatin (Pravachol), sinvastatin (Zocor)	High serum LDL cholesterol	Enhances absorption, increases risk of liver damage	Food/meals, alcohol	Lovastatin should be taken with evening meal to enhance absorption; avoid large amounts of alcohol
Antiparkinsonian agents	Levodopa (Dopar, Larodopa)	Parkinson's disease	Decreased absorption	High-protein foods (eggs, meat, protein supplements), vitamin B_6	Spread protein intake equally in 3-6 meals per day to minimize reaction; avoid vitamin B_6 supplements or multivitamin supplement in doses <10 mg
Antituberculosis agents	Isoniazid (INH)	Tuberculosis	Reduced absorption with foods, increased hepatotoxicity and reduced INH levels with alcohol	Alcohol	Take on empty stomach, avoid alcohol
Bronchodilator agents	Theophylline (Slo-Bid, Theo-Dur)	Asthma, chronic bronchitis, emphysema	Increased stimulation of CNS; alcohol can increase nausea, vomiting, headache, and irritability	Caffeine, alcohol	Avoid caffeine-containing foods/beverages (chocolate, colas, teas, coffee); avoid alcohol if taking theophylline medications
Corticosteroid agents	Prednisolone (Pediapred, Prelone), methylprednisolone (Solu-Medrol), hydrocortisone	Inflammation/itching	Stomach irritation	Food	Take with food or milk to decrease stomach upset
Hypoglycemic agents	Chlorpropamide (Diabinese), metformin (Glucophage)	Diabetes	Severe nausea and vomiting	Alcohol	Avoid alcohol

Data from Bland SE: Drug-food interactions. *J Pharm Soc Wisc* 28, Nov/Dec 1998; Bobroff LB, Lentz A, Turner RE: *Food/drug and drug/nutrient interactions: what you should know about your medications*, Gainesville, 1994, University of Florida Cooperative Extension Service, Institute of Food and Agricultural Science. Available at: <www.edis.ifas.ufl.edu>; Brown CH: Overview of drug interactions. *US Pharm* 25(5), 2000. from: <www.uspharmacist.com>. Retrieved April 11, 2009; Food and Drug Administration/National Consumers League: *Food & drug interactions*, Washington, D.C. U.S. Government Printing Office. from: <www.nclnet.org/Food%20&%20Drug.pdf>. Retrieved April 11, 2009.
ACE, Angiotensin-converting enzyme; *CNS,* central nervous system; *HMG-CoA,* 3-hydroxy-3- methylglutaryl coenzyme A; *LDL,* low-density lipoprotein; *MAOIs,* monoamine oxidase inhibitors; *NSAID,* nonsteroidal antiinflammatory drug.

Effects of Food on Drug Absorption
Increased Drug Absorption
In summary, the following five basic circumstances contribute to increased absorption of a drug:

1. *Dissolving characteristics:* When a drug does not dissolve rapidly after it has been taken, the time it remains in the stomach with food is prolonged. This increased time in the stomach may increase its effective dissolution and consequent absorption. In some instances, the drug may not dissolve properly because of either the drug or gastric pH, and it is excreted, thus decreasing absorption of the drug.
2. *Gastric-emptying time:* Delayed emptying of food from the stomach can have the effect of doling out small portions of a drug, creating more optimal saturation rates on the absorption sites in the small intestine.
3. *Nutrients:* Some nutrients can promote absorption of certain drugs. For example, high-fat diets increase absorption of the antifungal drug griseofulvin. This drug is fat soluble, and high-fat diets stimulate the secretion of bile acids, which aid in absorption of the drug. Vitamin C, as well as gastric acid, enhances iron absorption. Recent studies indicate that citrus fruit reduced lipoprotein oxidation in persons who consumed a high-saturated fat diet.[6] Anticoagulant drugs interact with dietary factors, and a consistent dietary intake of vitamin K is important.[7,8] Folic acid supplementation is needed when phenytoin is used for seizure control in patients with epilepsy.[9]
4. *Blood flow:* Food intake increases splanchnic blood flow carrying any ingested drugs. This direct circulation to abdominal visceral organs stimulates absorption and results in an increased availability of the accompanying drugs.
5. *Nutritional status:* In addition to the presence of specific nutrients, nutritional status may also affect the bioavailability of certain drugs in different ways. For example, the antibiotic chloramphenicol is absorbed more slowly in children with protein-energy malnutrition, but elimination of the drug is slower in well-nourished children. In both cases the effect is a net increased bioavailability of the drug.

Decreased Drug Absorption
Absorption of some drugs is delayed or reduced by the presence of food:

- *Aspirin:* Absorption of aspirin is reduced or delayed by food. It should be taken on an empty stomach with ample water, preferably cold (see the Health Promotion section for discussion).
- *Tetracycline:* Nutritional status may also have an effect on drug absorption. For example, tetracycline absorption is impaired in malnourished individuals. Absorption of this commonly used antibiotic is also hindered when it is taken with milk, as well as with antacids or iron supplements. The drug combines with these materials to form new insoluble compounds that the body cannot absorb, causing loss of the minerals involved, that is, calcium or iron.[6]

- *Phenytoin:* The presence of protein inhibits absorption of phenytoin. Carbohydrate increases its absorption, but fat has no effect.

Effects of Food on Drug Distribution and Metabolism
Carbohydrates and Fat
Dietary carbohydrates and fat, especially their relative quantities, influence liver enzymes that metabolize drugs. For example, the presence of fat increases the activity of diazepam (Valium). Fat increases the concentration of the unbound active drug by displacing it from binding sites in plasma and tissue protein.

Licorice
Licorice, a sweet-tasting plant extract used in making chewing tobacco, candy, and certain drugs, causes sodium retention and increased hypertension.[10] A person being treated for hypertension needs to avoid any natural licorice-containing product. The active ingredient in licorice is glycyrrhizic acid, which is named for its natural plant source, *Glycyrrhiza glabra*, meaning sweet root, a member of the legume family. An analog of this active part of licorice is marketed under the trade names Biogastrone and Duogastrone, which are widely used, especially in Europe, for healing gastric ulcers, but hypertension is a side effect.

Indoles
Indoles in cruciferous vegetables (e.g., cabbage, Brussels sprouts, broccoli, cauliflower) (Figure 18-3) can speed up the rate of drug metabolism. They apparently induce mixed-function oxidase enzyme systems in the liver.

Cooking Methods
The method of cooking foods may alter rate of drug metabolism. Charcoal broiling, for example, increases hepatic drug metabolism through enzyme induction.

Vitamin Effects on Drug Action
Vitamin Effects on Drug Effectiveness
Pharmacologic doses or large megadoses beyond nutritional need of vitamins decrease blood levels of drugs when vitamins interact with the drugs. For example, large doses of folate or pyridoxine can reduce the blood level and

> **KEY TERMS**
> **indoles** Compounds produced in the intestines by the decomposition of tryptophan; also found in the oil of jasmine and clove.
> **cruciferous** Bearing a cross; botanical term for plants belonging to the botanical family Cruciferae or Brassicaceae, the mustard family, so-called because of crosslike four-petaled flowers; name given to certain vegetables of this family, such as broccoli, cabbage, Brussels sprouts, and cauliflower.

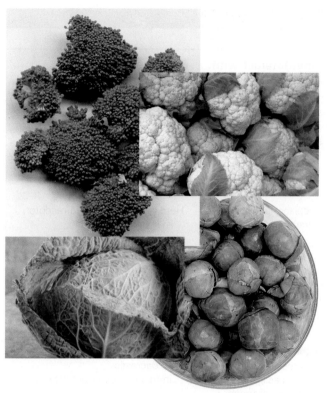

FIGURE 18-3 Examples of cruciferous vegetables. (Copyright 2006 JupiterImages Corporation.)

effectiveness of anticonvulsive drugs such as phenytoin (Dilantin) or phenobarbital that are used for seizure control. Unwise self-medication with large drug-level doses of vitamins can cause severe toxic complications (see the Complementary and Alternative Medicine [CAM] box, "At Least It's Natural!"). On the other hand, vitamins themselves may become important medications when used as part of the medical treatment for a secondary deficiency induced by a childhood genetic or metabolic disease. Such is the case with biotin in treating certain organic acidemias or with riboflavin in treating certain defects in fatty acid metabolism.

Control of Drug Intoxication

Riboflavin is useful in treating boric acid poisoning. Boric acid combines with the ribitol side chain of riboflavin and is excreted in the urine. In addition, vitamin E combats pulmonary oxygen toxicity. Premature human infants at risk for development of bronchopulmonary dysplasia by oxygen treatment have been protected by vitamin E administration during the acute phase of respiratory distress requiring oxygen treatment.

NUTRITION-PHARMACY TEAM

A decade or so ago, hospitalized patients as a whole were less severely ill than they are today. Now, however, as a reflection

COMPLEMENTARY AND ALTERNATIVE MEDICINE (CAM)

At Least It's Natural!

The U.S. Food and Drug Administration (FDA) does not regulate herbal remedies and dietary supplements, so the purity, potency, and safety of these products can and do vary. Manufacturers' claims of efficacy and safety are not subject to the same rigorous testing mandatory for medications. It is likely for herbs and dietary supplements to be contaminated with other herbs, pesticides, herbicides, and other products during growth, harvesting, preparation, and storage. Moreover, active chemical components in the herb may not be standardized. This leads to dissimilar potencies from lot to lot or even from capsule to capsule within the same lot. Safety, toxicity, and the likelihood of adverse interactions with other medications or treatments frequently have not been tested, particularly in children. Patients who are contemplating use of herbs and dietary supplements should proceed with caution and seek out products only from reliable manufacturers.

The reason many people give for using herbal remedies and food supplements is based in tradition (e.g., the Chinese have been using it for thousands of years!), as well as in their belief in the extensive and aggressive marketing claims that tout certain herbal remedies as "miracle cures," regardless of the lack of scientific data available to support such statements. Many turn to herbal remedies because they are considered natural and therefore seen as harmless. However, it is important to remember that hemlock, nightshade, mistletoe berries, belladonna, and poison ivy are all "natural" plants. What many do not realize is that the term *natural* is not synonymous with *safe*—especially when they combine herbs with medications.

Herb	Traditional Use*	Drug(s) that Interact with the Herb	Adverse Effects/Drug Interactions
Chamomile (English) (*Chamaemelum nobile, Matricaria recutita*)	Indigestion, reduce tension, and induce sleep; eczema, irritation of mucous membranes after chemotherapy or radiation (for cancer)	Anticoagulants: heparin, warfarin (Coumadin) Benzodiazepines: alprazolam (Xanax), chlordiazepoxide (Librium), diazepam (Valium), flurazepam (Dalmane), lorazepam (Ativan), temazepam (Restoril), triazolam (Halcion)	May increase bleeding time Binds to benzodiazepine receptors, which may alter effect of drug

Continued

🌼 COMPLEMENTARY AND ALTERNATIVE MEDICINE (CAM)

At Least It's Natural!—cont'd

Herb	Traditional Use*	Drug(s) that Interact with the Herb	Adverse Effects/Drug Interactions
		Central nervous system (CNS) depressants: alcohol, anticonvulsants, antiemetics, antihistamines, antipsychotics, antivertigo drugs, barbiturates, hypnotics, opioids, tricyclic antidepressants, paraldehyde (Paral)	May add to sedative effect
Chasteberry (*Vitex agnus-castus*)	Premenstrual syndrome (PMS), menopausal symptoms, amenorrhea, and other menstrual irregularities; fibrocystic breasts	Hormone replacement therapy, oral contraceptives	Herb binds to estrogen receptor, may counteract oral contraceptives
Dong quai (*Angelica sinensis*)	Menstrual irregularities, menopausal complaints	Anticoagulants	May increase bleeding time; if using concurrently, then obtain prothrombin time and International Normalized Ratio (INR) to rule out interactions
Echinacea (*Echinacea angustifolia, E. pallida, E. purpurea*)	Decrease duration of colds	Immunosuppressants: azathioprine, basiliximab, cyclosporine, daclizumab, interferon, muromonab CD3, mycophenolate, sirolimus, tacrolimus, corticosteroids	May decrease immunosuppressant effect
Ma huang, ephedra (*Ephedra sinica, E. equisetina, E. intermedia*)	Bronchodilator, decongestant, CNS stimulant, diuretic	Amitriptyline (Elavil) Anticonvulsants General anesthetics Caffeine and other xanthine alkaloids Monoamine oxidase inhibitors (MAOIs) Antihypertensives: angiotensin-converting enzyme (ACE) inhibitors, α-blockers, angiotensin II receptor blockers, β-blockers, calcium channel blockers, diuretics Insulin/oral hypoglycemic agents Methylphenidate (Ritalin) Morphine Oxytocin (Pitocin)	Drug may decrease hypertensive effect of ephedrine Sympathomimetic effects, which may interfere with drug Concurrent use may result in arrhythmias Increased effects and potential toxicity Increased sympathomimetic effects May decrease effectiveness of drug caused by stimulant effect Possible hyperglycemia with concurrent use May displace drug from adrenergic neurons, which may decrease effectiveness of drug Increases analgesic effect Possible hypertension
Evening primrose oil (*Oenothera biennis L*)	PMS, eczema, diabetic neuropathy, fibrocystic breasts, rheumatoid arthritis (RA)	Phenothiazines: chlorpromazine (Thorazine), fluphenazine (Prolixin), prochlorperazine (Compazine), promethazine hydrochloride (Phenergan) Anticoagulants	May increase risk of seizures May increase risk of bleeding
Ginkgo (*Ginkgo biloba*)	Improved blood flow, protection against free-radical damage, attention-deficit hyperactivity disorder (ADHD), dementia, macular degeneration, mental performance	Aspirin or Coumadin	May increase risk of bleeding

COMPLEMENTARY AND ALTERNATIVE MEDICINE (CAM)

At Least It's Natural!—cont'd

Herb	Traditional Use*	Drug(s) that Interact with the Herb	Adverse Effects/Drug Interactions
Ginseng American (*Panax quinquefolius*) Panax or Asian (*Panax ginseng*)	ADHD, stress reduction, chronic fatigue syndrome, fibromyalgia, age-related memory loss, menopausal cloudy thinking	Insulin/oral hypoglycemic agents Oral contraceptives/hormone replacement therapy General anesthetics Caffeine and other stimulants Immunosuppressants MAOIs	May enhance hypoglycemic effect May alter effectiveness of exogenous hormones Should be discontinued 7 days before surgery; herb increases risk of hypoglycemia and bleeding Red ginseng (steamed) may be additive to stimulant effect Ginseng has immunostimulant activity and should not be used concurrently Potentiates phenelzine, causing manic symptoms
Kava (or kava-kava) (*Piper methysticum*)	Sleep disorders, antianxiety, tension headaches, menopausal anxiety, fibromyalgia	Alprazolam (Xanax) Alcohol, tranquilizers (barbiturates), and antidepressants Antiparkinsonian drugs	Synergistic CNS activity of alprazolam May potentiate action May increase tremors and make medications less effective May reduce intestinal absorption
Senna (*Cassia senna*)	Laxative, weight loss	Any drug Antiarrhythmics Corticosteroids Digoxin/cardiac glycosides Diuretics	May reduce intestinal absorption May potentiate drug May cause hypokalemia May increase effects May interfere with potassium-sparing effect
St. John's wort	Depression, seasonal affective disorder	Theophylline and β$_2$-agonists Selective serotonin reuptake inhibitors (SSRIs)	Possibility of increased anxiety Serotonin syndrome (sweating, agitation, tremor)
Valerian (*Valeriana officinalis*)	Sleep disorders, ADHD, menstrual cramps	Sedatives, barbiturates, CNS depressants, general anesthetics, thiopental	May intensify effects

Data from Kemper K, Gardiner P, Chan E: "At least it's natural." Herbs and dietary supplements in ADHD. *Contemp Pediatr* 9:116, 2000. from <www.contemporarypediatrics.com>. Retrieved April 11, 2009; Kemper K, Gardiner P, Conboy LA: Herbs and adolescent girls: avoiding the hazards of self-treatment. *Contemp Pediatr* 3:133, 2000. from <www.contemporarypediatrics.com>. Retrieved April 11, 2009; Kuhn MA, Winston D: *Herbal therapy and supplements. A scientific and traditional approach*, ed 2, Philadelphia, Pa., 2007, Lippincott Williams & Wilkins. *Not an exhaustive listing.

of our more complex medical system and economic reform efforts, patients who are hospitalized are more acutely ill. They are more at risk for nutritional deficits and more likely to develop malnutrition, which leads to increased lengths of stay and increased costs. The task of monitoring food and drug interactions is complex and requires team responsibilities. Coordinating the pharmacy, food service, and clinical nutrition minimizes adverse drug-nutrient interactions (Table 18-4).

Hospitals and other health care facilities concentrate on key processes and functions, such as drug-nutrient interactions in this case, rather than traditional strictly compartmentalized tasks of departments. Current standards continue to focus on departmental or service roles, but this is changing because of economic necessity, as well as philosophy of care. This changing focus is being shaped, for example, in the work of The Joint Commission.[11]

The Joint Commission's accreditation manual reflects the philosophy that key functions often involve different disciplines coming together as partners with clearly defined responsibilities. The team of clinical dietitians and clinical pharmacologist is clearly one of these partnerships. Current guidelines mandate monitoring of drug therapy and counseling with patients about adverse drug-nutrient interactions.[11]

HEALTH PROMOTION

"THE PAIN RELIEVER DOCTORS RECOMMEND MOST"

Aspirin (Figure 18-4) has a venerable history. Being a buffered form of salicylic acid, it is a modified version of an ancient folk remedy of willow bark that had been used for many hundreds of years for fever, aches, and pain. However,

TABLE 18-4   ADVERSE DRUG REACTIONS CAUSED BY ALCOHOL AND SPECIFIC FOODS

TYPE OF REACTION	DRUGS	ALCOHOL/FOODS	EFFECTS
Flushing	Chlorpropamide (diabetes), griseofulvin, tetrachloroethylene	Alcohol	Dyspnea, headache, flushing
Disulfiram reaction	Aldehyde dehydrogenase inhibitors: disulfiram (Antabuse), calcium carbamide, metronidazole, nitrofurantoin, sulfonylureas	Alcohol, foods containing alcohol	Abdominal and chest pain, flushing, headache, nausea and vomiting
Hypoglycemia	Insulin-releasing agents: oral hypoglycemic drugs	Alcohol, sugar, sweets	Mental confusion, weakness, irrational behavior, unconsciousness
Tyramine reaction	Monoamine oxidase inhibitors (MAOIs): antidepressants such as phenelzine, procarbazine, isoniazid (isonicotinic acid hydrazide)	Foods containing large amounts of tyramine: cheese, red wines, chicken liver, broad beans, yeast	Cerebrovascular accident, flushing, hypertension

Modified from Roe DA: Interactions between drugs and nutrients. *Med Clin North Am* 63:985, 1979; Roe DA: *Diet and drug interactions,* ed 2, New York, 1979, AVI Books.

TABLE 18-5   IS THERE A DIFFERENCE IN PAIN RELIEVERS?

ANALGESIC	EFFECTS PAIN RELIEF	FEVER REDUCTION	OTHER EFFECTS	TRADE NAMES
Aspirin (acetylsalicylic acid [ASA])	✓	✓	Antiinflammatory Reduces blood clotting Gastric irritation May cause Reye's syndrome in children with viral infection Allergic reaction	Ascriptin, Bayer, Bufferin, Ecotrin
Acetaminophen	✓	✓	Large doses can injure the liver or kidneys Use by persons who have three or more alcoholic drinks per day may cause liver damage	Tylenol
Ibuprofen	✓	✓	Antiinflammatory Gastric irritation Reduces blood clotting Worsens existing kidney problems	Advil, Motrin IB
Naproxen sodium	✓	✓	Antiinflammatory Reduces blood clotting Worsens existing kidney problems	Aleve
Ketoprofen	✓	✓	Antiinflammatory Gastric irritation Use by persons who have three or more alcoholic drinks per day may cause gastric bleeding	Orudis, Orudis KT

Data from Mayo Clinic Staff: *Over-the-counter pain reliever guide: compare before choosing,* Rochester, Minn., 2005, Mayo Foundation for Medical Education and Research. MayoClinic.com (www.mayoclinic.com).

the acetyl group in ASA makes aspirin easier on the stomach than willow bark.

Aspirin is an analgesic agent, an effect enhanced in combination with caffeine[12] that is used for the relief of minor aches and pains. Its mechanism of action is through inhibition of certain prostaglandins (see Chapter 4). The prostaglandins have a profound influence on a spectrum of physiologic functions, including blood clotting, blood pressure, inflammatory process, contraction of voluntary muscles, and transmission of nerve impulses (Table 18-5).

Studies implicate aspirin in alleviating many disorders, dangers, and discomforts, including the following:

- Risk of repeated transient ischemic attacks (TIAs), or little strokes, is reduced by 50% in men (but not in women) who have already had one.
- Many studies indicate aspirin is effective in reducing risk for myocardial infarction.
- Aspirin is one of the most effective antiinflammatory drugs and is effective in long-term treatment of arthritis.

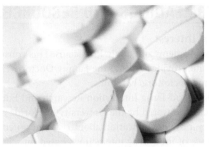

FIGURE 18-4 Aspirin remains one of the most popular pain relievers in the United States. (Copyright 2006 JupiterImages Corporation.)

- Aspirin may play a role in inhibiting spread of some cancers through its action of inhibiting production of prostaglandin E_2.
- Aspirin's effect as an anticoagulant is important in treatment of phlebitis and other clot-related disorders.
- Aspirin may be effective in promoting sleep. Many scientists now believe aspirin is as effective as most prescription sedatives, and it has far fewer and less serious side effects.

It is important to remember aspirin is a drug. Many of the benefits of aspirin stem from its systemic, wide-reaching effects on metabolism, which may have unforeseen, short- and long-term detrimental results. We do know that aspirin is to be strictly avoided by persons with hemophilia. In addition, allergic reactions to aspirin can be severe. Aspirin seems to be implicated in asthma. Children are especially vulnerable to side effects and should not be given aspirin without a physician's instructions.

Aspirin is an irritant to the stomach and intestine. Its continuous use is associated with low-level chronic loss of iron caused by mucosal erosion. This can lead to iron deficiency anemia. Aspirin has been linked to birth defects, especially when it is taken later in the course of pregnancy. It increases risk of infant and neonatal mortality, low birth weight, and intracranial hemorrhage.

The best way to take aspirin is on an empty stomach with a full glass of water. This is important: absorption of aspirin is facilitated by a large volume of liquid and inhibited by the presence of food. In addition, taking aspirin—especially on an empty stomach—without a large fluid intake invites erosion of the stomach lining.[13] However, aspirin should never be taken when using alcohol because it increases the bioavailability of alcohol, raising the blood concentration and thus the effect of alcohol on brain centers.[14]

TO SUM UP

Drugs can have multiple effects on the body's absorption, metabolism, retention, and nutrient status. They can provoke adverse reactions in combination with certain foods and can influence appetite, either repressing it or artificially stimulating it. Drugs can either increase an individual's absorption of nutrients or, more commonly, decrease absorption, sometimes leading to clinical deficiencies. Drugs can also induce mineral and vitamin deficiencies by their mode of action.

Just as drugs affect our use of food, food affects our use of drugs. Food can affect the absorption of drugs in a variety of ways. Foods also have an effect on subsequent distribution and metabolism of drugs. Vitamins may interfere with drug effectiveness, especially if they are taken in large doses. On the other hand, large doses of specific vitamins can be effective in countering certain toxicity conditions or a specific secondary deficiency induced by a genetic disease.

QUESTIONS FOR REVIEW

1. Name four ways food may affect drug use, and give examples of each.
2. If your patient were using a prescribed MAOI such as tranylcypromine sulfate (Parnate), what foods would you instruct the patient to avoid?
3. What is the most effective way to take aspirin? With what type of liquid should it be taken? Should it be taken with or without food? Why?
4. What foods would you suggest to a hypertensive patient on the diuretic drug hydrochlorothiazide (HCTZ) as good sources of potassium replacement?
5. Outline suggestions you would discuss with a patient experiencing a drug-induced taste loss. How would you explain the cause of the taste loss?

REFERENCES

1. Cresci G: Patient history. In Charney P, Malone AM, editors: *ADA pocket guide to nutrition assessment*, ed 2, Chicago, 2009, American Dietetic Association.
2. U.S. Census Bureau: *Profiles of general demographic characteristics*, Washington, D.C., 2006, U.S. Government Printing Office. from: <www.census.gov/>. Retrieved April 11, 2009.
3. Nelms M: Pharmacology. In Nelms MN, Sucher K, Long S, editors: *Understanding nutrition therapy and pathophysiology*, Belmont, Calif., 2007, Wadsworth.
4. Pronsky ZM: *Food medication interactions*, ed 15, Birchrunville, Pa., 2008, Food-Medication Interactions.

5. Merriman SH: Monoamine oxidase drugs and diet. *J Hum Nutr Diet* 12:21, 1999.

6. Harats D, Chevion S, Nahir M, et al: Citrus fruit supplementation reduces lipoprotein oxidation in young men ingesting a diet high in saturated fat: vitamin E presumptive evidence for an interaction between vitamins C and E in vivo. *Am J Clin Nutr* 67(2):240, 1998.

7. Harris JE: Interaction of dietary factors with oral anticoagulants: review and applications. *J Am Diet Assoc* 95(5):580, 1995.

8. Booth SL, Charnley JM, Sadowski JA, et al: Dietary vitamin K and stability of oral anticoagulation: proposal of a diet with constant vitamin K content. *Thromb Haemost* 77(3):408, 1997.

9. Lewis DP, Van Dyke DC, Willhite LA, et al: Phenytoin-folic acid interaction. *Ann Pharmacother* 29(7/8):726, 1995.

10. Morris DJ, Davis E, Latif SA, et al: Licorice, chewing tobacco, and hypertension. *N Engl J Med* 322:849, 1990.

11. The Joint Commission: *2012 Comprehensive accreditation manual for hospitals: the official handbook (CAMH)*, Oakbrook Terrace, Ill., 2012, The Joint Commission.

12. Schachtel BP, Fillingim MD, Lane AC, et al: Caffeine as an analgesic adjuvant. *Arch Intern Med* 151:733, 1991.

13. Koch PA, Schultz CA, Wills RJ, et al: Influence of food and fluid ingestion on aspirin bioavailability. *J Pharm Sci* 67(11):1533, 1978.

14. Roine R, Genry RT, Munõz RH, et al: Aspirin increases blood alcohol concentration in humans after ingestion of ethanol. *JAMA* 264(18):2406, 1990.

FURTHER READINGS AND RESOURCES

Websites of Interest

- American Academy of Family Physicians. This consumer-focused site provides links to the Family Doctor website: www.familydoctor.org/121.xml.
- Center for Food-Drug Interaction Research and Education. This site, cosponsored by the University of Florida and Tufts University, provides education about risk and potential significance of food-drug interactions based on scientifically founded evidence: http://www.druginteractioncenter.org/.
- Grapefruit-Drug Interactions. Created for pharmacists and other allied health professionals, this page is designed to provide up-to-date information in the large body of research on grapefruit-drug interactions: www.powernetdesign.com/grapefruit/.
- Medline Plus. This site has gathered facts from the National Library of Medicine, National Institutes of Health, and other government agencies and health-related organizations to provide information on thousands of prescription and over-the-counter medicines: www.nlm.nih.gov/medlineplus/druginformation.html.
- Rx List: The Internet Drug List, sponsored by WebMD. This site provides food-drug interaction information for consumers and health professionals: www.rxlist.com/.
- U.S. Pharmacist. *U.S. Pharmacist* is a monthly journal dedicated to providing up-to-date, authoritative, peer-reviewed clinical articles relevant to contemporary pharmacy practice in a variety of settings: www.uspharmacist.com/.

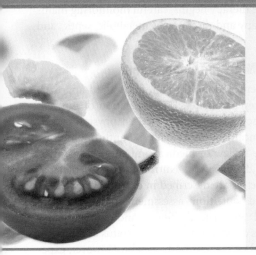

CHAPTER

19

Nutrition Support: Enteral and Parenteral Nutrition

Pamela Charney

ⓔ EVOLVE WEBSITE

http://evolve.elsevier.com/Williams/essentials/

OUTLINE

Nutrition Assessment
Enteral Nutrition Versus Parenteral Nutrition
Enteral Tube Feeding in Clinical Nutrition
Enteral Tube Feeding Formulas
Enteral Tube Feeding Delivery Systems
Monitoring the Tube-Fed Patient

Parenteral Feeding in Clinical Nutrition
Parenteral Solutions
Parenteral Nutrition Delivery System
Home Nutrition Support
HEALTH PROMOTION
Troubleshooting Diarrhea in Tube-Fed Patients

In this chapter, we look at alternate modes of feeding to provide nutrition support for patients with special needs. We examine ways of feeding when the gastrointestinal (GI) tract can be used—enteral nutrition (EN) given orally or through a feeding tube. Then we review nutrient feeding directly into a vein when the GI tract cannot be used—parenteral nutrition (PN).

Malnutrition, preexisting and hospital-induced, is a serious concern in hospitalized patients, especially those with critical illness or injury. Nutrition care provided by a skilled nutrition support team or clinician can have a positive effect on patient survival and recovery. This chapter will examine EN and PN support formulas, solutions, and delivery systems for use in hospital and home.

NUTRITION ASSESSMENT

Nutrition Support and Degree of Malnutrition

It is an easier task to maintain nutrition than to replenish body stores from malnutrition. The effect of starvation on the body, even during relatively brief periods, is well documented.[1] The small amount of glycogen stored in the liver is a crucial immediate energy source. Glycogen breakdown for fuel begins 2 to 3 hours after a meal, and glycogen stores are depleted after 30 hours of fasting in the absence of metabolic

stress. Release of amino acids from body tissue proteins begins after 4 to 6 hours of fasting to provide a source of blood glucose. In addition, fatty acids are mobilized from the body's adipose tissues to provide keto acids as a principal fuel for heart, brain, and other vital organs. As adaptation to starvation occurs, the body relies less on amino acids from protein for fuel and uses more ketones from fat to meet metabolic needs. This reduces nitrogen losses and preserves lean body mass. During critical illness this adaptation to insufficient energy to meet needs does not occur. Severely ill patients rely heavily on large amounts of glucose and protein for fuel. They often have elevated insulin levels, which inhibit the mobilization of fat for energy production, and thus increase reliance on amino acids from protein with a urinary nitrogen loss of 10 to 15 g/day or more that continues unchecked. Critical illness can lead to severe depletion of lean body mass. Nutrition provided during critical illness reduces but does not reverse the process.

For example, two healthy people are hiking in the mountains and get lost. They have a limited supply of food but adequate water available from mountain streams. Hiker #1 is severely injured in a fall while the two are searching for the way back to civilization. Both have an inadequate food supply to meet their energy needs. Hiker #2 will initially use glycogen

419

stores followed by breakdown of lean body mass and fat for energy needs. However, after several days the body will decrease its use of protein for energy and start relying on fat so that lean body mass is preserved as long as possible. This is the adaptation to starvation. Hiker #1 will not adapt to starvation. He will continue to use protein for energy and rely much less on fat for fuel and thus will lose more lean body mass during the period of inadequate energy supply than Hiker #2.

Any medical treatment has less chance of success if the patient is malnourished. The patient who becomes malnourished during hospitalization (iatrogenic malnutrition) has been referred to as *the skeleton in the hospital closet,* with several reports of general malnutrition among hospitalized patients.[2-6] Lack of adequate nutrition to meet metabolic demands is increasingly recognized as a serious concern in medical and surgical patients. Malnutrition is the end result when nutrient intake does not meet nutrient needs over some period of time. Braunschweig and colleagues[6] reported that as many as 54% of patients admitted to the hospital were malnourished, and 31% of these patients declined nutritionally during hospitalization.

In addition, many medical and surgical diagnoses are associated with nutritional risk through impact on nutrient requirements, ability to consume nutrients, or by changing nutrient metabolism. Deterioration of a patient's nutritional status during hospitalization may contribute to increased length of hospital stay, development of comorbidities, and increased cost.[6] Persons with underlying chronic disease or traumatic injury, and older adults are particularly at risk. Thus assessment, monitoring, and reassessment of nutritional status become important parts of overall care, especially for hospitalized patients (see Chapter 16). For the severely malnourished patient, especially those facing problems such as organ failure or extensive surgery, adequate and consistent provision of nutrition support is indicated. The guiding principle for provision of nutrition support is "if the gut works, then use it." Studies have shown when patients are fed appropriately enterally rather than parenterally, they experience fewer infectious complications and shorter lengths of stay, and recover more rapidly.[7-9]

Regulatory agencies such as The Joint Commission require that nutrition screening be completed within 24 hours of hospital admission. The purpose of the initial nutrition screen should be to identify potential nutrition diagnoses, including malnutrition. When risk for nutrition problems is identified through the admission nutrition screen, the registered dietitian (RD) should be consulted.

The RD conducts the initial nutrition assessment and performs ongoing monitoring of nutritional status. Initial assessment data supply the necessary basis for (1) identifying patients who require nutrition intervention, (2) determining an appropriate nutrition support route (i.e., **enteral** or **parenteral**), (3) calculating the patient's nutrient requirements, (4) determining specific formulations to meet those requirements, and (5) identifying measurable nutrition-related outcomes for determining if the nutrition care plan is appropriate

and effective. Once therapy begins, careful monitoring maintains optimal therapy and discourages metabolic, septic, and GI complications.

Guidelines for Nutrition Assessment

Nutrition assessment is done through a standard approach and includes six key parameters: (1) evaluation of nutrient intake and adequacy, (2) nutrition-focused physical assessment, (3) biochemical laboratory data, (4) anthropometrics, (5) comprehensive review of medical and surgical histories, and (6) nutrition diagnosis.[10,11] Nutrition assessment techniques and parameters are described in detail in Chapter 16. However, standard nutrition assessment parameters are adversely affected by critical illness and inflammatory response. Weight is often affected by fluid status and may no longer reflect usual or current body weight. However, experienced nutrition support RDs are able to evaluate the patient's "dry weight" by an accounting of the fluid volume infused (1 L of water weighs 1 kg). There are no laboratory values that accurately reflect nutrition status. Clinicians must rely primarily on subjective global assessment (Box 19-1) and astute clinical judgment to perform and interpret assessment of nutritional status.[5,12] Subjective global assessment focuses on history and physical examination.[5] This technique eliminates the ambiguity and nonspecific, nonsensitive nature of laboratory values during critical illness and inflammation.

BOX 19-1 SUBJECTIVE GLOBAL ASSESSMENT COMPONENTS

History
- Change in weight
- Change in dietary intake
- Gastrointestinal (GI) symptoms
- Functional capacity
- Nutritional requirements of disease

Physical Assessment
- Loss of subcutaneous fat
- Muscle loss
- Fluid retention
- Ankle and sacral edema
- Ascites

Data from Detsky AS, McLaughlin JR, Baker JP, et al: What is subjective global assessment of nutritional status? *JPEN J Parenter Enteral Nutr* 11(1):8, 1987. Reprinted with permission of SAGE Publications.

KEY TERMS

enteral A feeding modality that provides nutrients, either orally or by tube feeding through the gastrointestinal (GI) tract.

parenteral A feeding modality that provides nutrient solutions intravenously rather than through the gastrointestinal (GI) tract.

History

History includes all aspects of the patient's health: weight change, nutrient intake, GI function and symptoms, functional capacity, and diagnosis and its nutritional effect. The clinician should identify whether the patient has experienced an intentional or nonintentional weight change from normal or usual weight and the time frame during which the weight change occurred. Quantifying weight loss is not always easy, particularly if the patient has lost lean body mass but weight is unchanged because the patient is retaining fluid as occurs with end-stage liver, heart, and kidney diseases. Current or actual body weight (ABW) and height are interpreted according to changes from usual body weight (UBW) and the percent of recent weight change:

$$\text{Percent UBW} = \text{ABW} \div \text{UBW} \times 100$$
$$\text{Percent weight change} = [(\text{UBW} - \text{ABW}) \div \text{UBW}] \times 100$$

The amount of recent weight change is compared with values associated with malnutrition (Table 19-1).

Changes in appetite and dietary intake must be assessed to identify overall nutrient adequacy of the diet and potential contributing factors for reported weight loss. It is important to identify diet modifications observed and nutritional supplements consumed by the patient. The clinician must verify whether nutritional supplements are being taken in addition to meals or used as a meal replacement. It should be remembered that it is not enough to simply order these supplements: They must be consumed, and when consumed they must not take the place of food. GI function determines the ability to assimilate nutrients. The presence of nausea, vomiting, diarrhea, and anorexia inhibits nutrient intake and availability. Assessment of functional capacity of the patient determines whether the patient can perform activities of daily living (ADLs), completely or in part, or if the patient is bedridden and totally dependent on others for care. Medical and surgical history entails examination of the past and current medical problems and enables the clinician to identify potential risks for nutrient inadequacies, deficiencies, excesses, and toxicities.

TABLE 19-1	CATEGORIZATION OF SEVERITY OF WEIGHT LOSS BY PERCENTAGE OF WEIGHT LOST OVER TIME	
TIME PERIOD	**SIGNIFICANT WEIGHT LOSS (%)**	**SEVERE WEIGHT LOSS (%)**
1 week	1-2	>2
1 month	5	>5
3 months	7.5	>7.5
6 months	10	>10

Modified from the American Society for Parenteral and Enteral Nutrition (A.S.P.E.N.): Nutritional and metabolic assessment of the hospitalized patient. *JPEN J Parenter Enteral Nutr* 1(1):11, 1977. Reprinted with permission of SAGE Publications.

Physical Examination

During the physical assessment the clinician looks for signs of muscle and fat wasting. Inspection of the upper body can identify temporal, clavicular, and torso wasting of skeletal muscle mass and subcutaneous fat. Signs of edema and ascites indicate inability to keep fluid in the vascular space with subsequent interstitial fluid accumulation. Physical signs and symptoms are then correlated to the patient's disease process and current medical condition.

Basal Energy Expenditure

Over 200 different formulas have been proposed for use in estimating energy requirements. At this time, if indirect calorimetry is not available the Mifflin-St. Jeor regression equation is recommended for use in most care settings. Daily energy requirements are estimated by combining basal energy expenditures (BEEs), disease and injury energy needs, and physical activity (see Chapter 8).

The Mifflin-St. Jeor equation uses measures of weight in kilograms, height in centimeters, and age in years to calculate resting energy expenditure (REE):

$$\text{Women: REE} = (10 \times \text{wt}) + (6.25 \times \text{ht}) - (5 \times \text{age}) - 161$$
$$\text{Men: REE} = (10 \times \text{wt}) + (6.25 \times \text{ht}) - (5 \times \text{age}) + 5^{14}$$

For example, the REE for a 35-year-old woman, weighing 60 kg (132 lb), standing 165 cm (5 feet 5 inches) is calculated as follows:

$$(10 \times 60) + (6.25 \times 165) - (5 \times 35) - 161$$
$$= 600 + 1031 - 175 - 161 = 1295 \text{ kcal/day}$$

The term *REE* is often used interchangeably with BEE in discussing basal energy needs. In general, energy provision to critically ill patients should not exceed 20% beyond the BEE/REE. However, metabolic conditions such as severe burns or head injury create energy needs up to 50% to 100% beyond BEE.

Energy requirements for hospitalized patients on nutrition support vary with amount of metabolic stress but generally range from 20 to 35 kcal/kg.[15] Regardless of the calculation used to estimate energy expenditure, it is important to monitor the effect of nutrients provided to determine changes needed to maintain or replete the patient. Energy and nutrients are adjusted based on patient tolerance and desire versus actual response to nutrient provision. Remember that estimations of energy requirements are simply that—an estimation. Frequent follow-up and feeding adjustments ensure that desired therapeutic goals are met more so than which formula is utilized to estimate requirements.

The more malnourished a patient is, the more carefully resumption of nutrition should be done. Refeeding syndrome is a life-threatening response to overaggressive provision of energy to a patient who has been chronically starved. Hallmark symptoms of refeeding are a shift of electrolytes from blood into the cell, resulting in decreased blood levels of potassium, phosphorus, and magnesium, along with increased blood glucose levels and fluid retention.[16] The end result can be cardiac collapse and death. Refeeding syndrome is entirely preventable through early identification of risk combined with appropriate monitoring of serum electrolyte levels with replacement as needed.

Critically ill patients with major trauma, sepsis, and inflammation demonstrate catabolism (i.e., breakdown of body tissue) resulting in a net loss of body mass. When protein is broken down, the nitrogen component of amino acids is released and excreted in urine. Nitrogen lost in urine can be as high as 15 to 30 g over 24 hours. This can result in a negative nitrogen balance if the patient is losing more nitrogen in urine than is provided from protein in the diet. Catabolic periods with losses of lean body mass are inevitable after trauma and extensive surgery. The catabolic process increases nutrient demand and requirements. Initiating nutrition support in these patients reduces, but does not eliminate, negative nitrogen balance that occurs after traumatic injury or critical illness.

Nitrogen Balance

Nitrogen balance studies are calculations that estimate the amount of catabolism. The patient's intake of protein (nitrogen) is subtracted from nitrogen output through urinary and insensible losses:

$$Nitrogen\ balance = Nitrogen\ intake - Nitrogen\ loss$$

$$Nitrogen\ intake = Protein\ intake \div 6.25*$$

$$Nitrogen\ loss = Urinary\ urea\ nitrogen + 4^\dagger$$

For example, a patient receiving 50 g of protein per day in an enteral tube feeding is getting 8 g of nitrogen per day (50 g ÷ 6.25 = 8 g). If that individual's nitrogen losses are 10 g per 24 hours (6 g in urine per nitrogen balance study + 4 g of insensible losses), then the patient's nitrogen balance is −2 g/24 hours. Increasing protein in the enteral tube feeding to more than 62.5 g protein per day will result in a positive nitrogen balance.

However, nitrogen balance calculation is not accurate with renal failure or retained nitrogen such as elevated blood urea nitrogen (BUN). Other sources of nitrogen such as blood products, as well as the loss of nitrogen from wounds, stool, nasogastric suction, and bleeding, must also be taken into account when calculating nitrogen balance. The 4 g of insensible nitrogen loss may not be an accurate estimate and could affect the accuracy of the results. Measurement of urinary urea nitrogen requires an accurate 24-hour urine collection. Accurate 24-hour urine collections are very difficult to obtain in clinical settings, even in patients who have urinary catheters in place. Because of this and the expense associated with measurement of urinary urea nitrogen (UUN), routine use of nitrogen balance cannot be recommended in clinical practice.

---

*6.25 g of protein yields 1 g nitrogen.
†Estimated insensible losses of nitrogen.

Hepatic Proteins as Nutrition Indicators

In the past, serum levels of the hepatic transport proteins, albumin, transferrin, and prealbumin, were used to determine the patient's nutritional status. During critical illness, hepatic production of albumin, transferrin, and prealbumin is decreased in favor of increased production of acute phase reactants required for survival.[12,17] A decreased serum value of albumin, prealbumin, or transferrin therefore signifies an inflammatory process (or how sick the patient is) and does not provide information about the patient's nutritional status or response to nutrition therapy. These proteins are better used as prognostic indicators of the patient's risk of complications (morbidity) and death (mortality). It is no longer recommended that serum hepatic transport protein levels be used to assess nutritional status or to monitor response to nutrition support.

Management of Nutrition Support Patients

Management of nutrition support is ideally performed by an official interdisciplinary nutrition support committee or team composed of designated members from the departments of medicine, surgery, nutrition, nursing, and pharmacy.[18] Each team member should be certified in nutrition support by an accrediting body such as the National Board of Nutrition Support Certification and the Board of Pharmaceutical Specialties. The American Society for Parenteral and Enteral Nutrition (A.S.P.E.N.) has developed standards of practice for nutrition support professionals and interdisciplinary nutrition support competencies.[19-23] However, in many facilities, nutrition support management is overseen by an informal collection of interested clinicians, a sole nutrition support practitioner, or no one person in particular. Standards of The Joint Commission and the Accreditation Manual for Hospitals (AMH) have focused on key multidisciplinary processes that ensure performance of nutrition screening and assessment to promote quality patient outcomes.[24] (For additional considerations surrounding nutrition support, see the Focus on Culture box, "What's Religion Got to Do with It?")

Baseline nutrition data obtained before starting nutrition support provide a means of measuring effectiveness of treatment. At designated periods during therapy, certain tests are repeated to monitor the patient's course and reduce metabolic complications. Specific protocols vary in different medical centers. However, a general guide for standard monitoring data is summarized in Box 19-2.[25]

Generally, clinicians give primary importance to the following three major monitoring parameters: (1) serial weights to determine the adequacy of total energy provision and to monitor fluid status, (2) physical examination for micronutrient adequacy and changes in body fat and muscle mass, and ultimately (3) improvement in functional status.

All baseline and monitoring data are recorded in the patient's chart, along with all enteral and parenteral solution orders.

No evidence-based "rules" exist for the time to start nutrition support with either EN or PN. Determination of when

What's Religion Got To Do with It?

"That was not a natural death. It was an imposed death," said Cardinal Renato Martino, a top Vatican official. "When you deprive somebody of food and water, what else is it? Nothing else but murder." In this impassioned statement, the cardinal was referring to the landmark battle over the life of Terri Schiavo after her death after nearly 2 weeks without any nutrition support. Over 15 years had passed since Terri Schiavo had suffered severe brain damage stemming from heart failure and had relied on EN for survival ever since. The legal decision to stop her tube feeding created a national uproar and sparked many debates over end-of-life issues, including nutrition support. The Catholic Church fervently opposed the legal action taken and was especially vocal in the events surrounding Terri Schiavo's death because she was Catholic.

What role does religion have in issues such as nutrition support? In this section we will encapsulate beliefs of three religions, focusing on end-of-life issues, particularly nutrition support.

Catholicism

Because Catholics believe they are stewards of their bodies and life is to be respected, the act of withholding nutrition support is not something to be taken lightly. However, bodily life is not to be maintained at all costs. The late Pope John Paul II wrote: "Certainly there is a moral obligation to care for oneself and allow oneself to be cared for, but this duty must take account for concrete circumstances. It needs to be determined whether the means of treatment available are objectively proportionate to the prospects for improvement."

In short, withdrawal of nutrition support is not condemned, but rather only recommended when quality of life is so low nutrition is of absolutely no benefit. Although it is hard to know where the point of "no benefit" is, it is the duty of a Catholic to promote a social order in which a certain level of responsibility exists for those who are marginalized or in a vegetative state. Each case merits special consideration, and in most cases nutrition is considered a basic form of care likened to warmth and cleanliness.

Judaism

According to Judaism, life possesses an intrinsic value as a divine gift of creation. As in Catholicism, humans are thought to be only a temporary steward of the body and therefore must treat the body with utmost respect and sensitivity. Jewish law mandates humans must do everything in their power to heal themselves when ill and must also strive to save the lives of others. This obligation, however, applies only to those therapies that have a reasonable chance of success, and although some believe tube feeding is equivalent to medical treatments, Jewish tradition disagrees with this opinion. According to Jewish authorities, nutrition in any form is a basic human need and should be provided to all patients unless feeding itself causes suffering. Consequently, Jewish law further accentuates feeding must be done in a kind and compassionate manner, emphasizing the importance this religion places on nourishment.

Islam

Not unlike the other religions mentioned in this section, in Islam humans are thought of as stewards of their bodies, which are viewed as a gift from God. Sanctity of life is a monumental principle, and every moment of life is deemed precious and must be preserved. Even so, death is believed to be a natural part of life, and treatment does not have to be provided if it merely prolongs the final stages of a terminal illness. Nutrition support—especially EN—is considered part of basic care rather than a treatment; therefore it is a religious obligation to provide nourishment unless such an act shortens life.

Religion and end-of-life issues like nutrition support are complicated and sensitive matters that must be approached with understanding and tolerance. People from different religious backgrounds can have varying views on this subject that can drastically affect the choice of care provided. The Terri Schiavo case brought to life a plethora of issues that will not likely be resolved any time soon; however, when dealing with nutrition support cases, it is important to consider the implications that the patient's religion can have for your decisions and actions.

Bibliography

Associated Press: Vatican: Schiavo's death "cruel." *Fox News* March 31, 2005. (News broadcast.)

Clarfield AM, Gordon M, Markwell H, et al: Ethical issues in end-of- life geriatric care: the approach of three monotheistic religions—Judaism, Catholicism, and Islam. *J Am Geriatr Soc* 51:1149, 2003.

Cooley M: Faith, ethics help many in agonizing dilemma. *The Spokesman-Review* A1, 2005.

Huggins C: *Survey finds physicians willing to allow patients' religion to trump medical advice*, New York, August 9, 2005, Reuters Health. (News release.)

Jotkowitz A, Clarfield A, Slick S: The care of patients with dementia: a modern Jewish ethical perspective. *J Am Geriatr Soc* 53:881, 2005.

Sunshine E: Sunshine, Truncating Catholic tradition: Florida bishops avoid full consideration of ethical issues in Schiavo case. *Natl Cathol Report* 41:23, 2005. from: <http://www.natcath.com/NCR_Online/archives2/2005b/040805/040805k.php>. Retrieved December 22, 2005.

to initiate nutrition support depends on the patient's nutritional status and the anticipated time period before oral diet can be resumed and tolerated. The A.S.P.E.N. guidelines[7] recommend that nutrition support should be considered when the patient has had an inadequate oral intake for 7 to 14 days or the patient's oral intake is anticipated to remain inadequate for 7 to 14 days. A 5- to 10-day timeline is recommended for critically ill patients. Other guidelines available to identify when to feed are the "rule of five" and amount of weight loss. The rule of five states that if a patient has had no food for 5 days and is unable to tolerate an oral diet for an additional 5 days, nutrition support should be considered to reduce the risk of developing malnutrition. The weight-loss rule stratifies patients according to the percentage of weight loss of their usual total body weight over a designated period (see Table 19-1). Patients who have undergone severe weight loss and are unable to tolerate oral nutrition for 5 to 7 days or longer are candidates for nutrition support.

ENTERAL NUTRITION VERSUS PARENTERAL NUTRITION

Debate continues concerning evidence-based effectiveness of PN and EN support. Questions focus on what constitutes early EN, how to select the most appropriate enteral tube feeding formula according to each patient's specific disease state, what is the preferred method of formula delivery, and which factors contribute to enteral tube feeding–related complications, such as diarrhea or respiratory problems.[26,27] In all cases when the GI tract is functioning, EN support should be used to restore or maintain an optimal state of nutrition. PN should be reserved for patients with a nonfunctional GI tract or an inadequately functional GI tract that prevents the patient from meeting nutrient needs enterally. In some cases the patient can take some enteral feeding, but impairment in either digestive or absorptive capacity requires supplementation with parenteral therapy. The Veterans Affairs Cooperative Study showed perioperative nutrition support was beneficial for severely malnourished patients but contributed to increased complications in mild to moderately malnourished patients.[28] The GI tract should always be the first choice

for nutrition support. Figure 19-1 provides an algorithm for determining the route of nutrition support.[7]

PN is associated with serious complications, as shown in Box 19-3. Reliance on PN when the GI tract is functional can contribute to disuse of the GI tract with subsequent bacterial overgrowth, hepatic abnormalities, deterioration of GI integrity with subsequent migration of intestinal bacteria into the systemic circulation, and sepsis. Patients reliant solely on PN are at risk for septic and hepatic complications that can

BOX 19-3 COMPLICATIONS ASSOCIATED WITH PARENTERAL NUTRITION

Catheter-Related Complications
- Air embolism
- Catheter embolization
- Catheter occlusion
- Improper tip location
- Phlebitis
- Pneumothorax
- Sepsis
- Venous thrombosis

Gastrointestinal (GI) Complications
- Fatty liver
- Gastric hyperacidity
- GI atrophy
- Hepatic cholestasis

Metabolic Complications
- Acid-base imbalance
- Electrolyte abnormalities
- Essential fatty acid deficiency
- Fluid imbalance
- Glucose intolerance
- Metabolic bone disease
- Mineral abnormalities
- Overfeeding
- Refeeding syndrome
- Triglyceride elevation

BOX 19-2 CLINICAL PARAMETERS TO MONITOR DURING NUTRITION SUPPORT

Daily intake and output (I/O)
Daily weights
Physical examination
Temperature, pulse, respirations
Laboratory parameters:
- Acid-base status
- Blood urea nitrogen (BUN)
- Complete blood cell count (CBC)
- Creatinine
- Electrolytes
- Glucose
- International Normalized Ratio (INR)
- Liver function tests
- **Osmolarity**, serum and urine
- Platelet count
- Prothrombin time (PT)
- Triglyceride level
- Urinary urea nitrogen
- Urine specific gravity
- Vitamins and minerals

KEY TERM

constitutive proteins Albumin, prealbumin, transferrin. Plasma proteins often used to assess the response to nutrition support. Serum levels are nonspecific and nonsensitive to nutritional status or requirements.

KEY TERM

osmolarity The number of millimoles of liquid or solid in a liter of solution; parenteral nutrition (PN) solutions given by central vein have an osmolarity around 1800 mOsm/L; peripheral parenteral solutions are limited to 600 to 900 mOsm/L (dextrose and amino acids have the greatest effect on a solution's osmolarity).

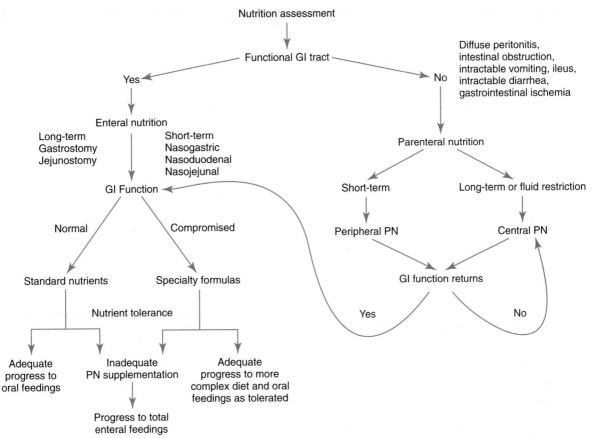

FIGURE 19-1 Route of administration of specialized nutrition support. (Reprinted from A.S.P.E.N. Board of Directors: *Clinical pathways and algorithms for delivery of parenteral and enteral nutrition support in adults,* Silver Spring, Md., A.S.P.E.N, 1998, p. 5.)

contribute to morbidity and mortality. The GI tract is the body's largest immune organ. (To learn more about probiotics and how they contribute to EN and PN, see the Evidence-Based Practice box, "Probiotics.") GI disease that prevents or reduces use of the GI tract may itself contribute to adverse effects often associated with PN. Therefore it may not be the route of feeding, but rather the inability to use the gut that increases infectious and metabolic complications.[29] Some adverse effects of PN may be related to inability to provide all necessary nutrients parenterally. Parenteral solutions are not as "complete" (i.e., they do not contain the wide variety of nutrients) as enteral formulas or an oral diet because of the complexity of adding all the nutrients found in nature to an intravenous solution.

ENTERAL TUBE FEEDING IN CLINICAL NUTRITION

Modes of Enteral Nutrition Support

Many patients with a functioning GI tract do not or cannot eat a sufficient amount of nutrients by mouth to restore, repair, or maintain physiologic systems or body tissues. The first option for providing adequate nutrition should be to deliver nutrients orally. The patient can be given small, frequent, nutrient-dense meals with an oral liquid nutritional supplement. If oral intake remains suboptimal despite attempts to increase nutrient intake with nutritional supplements and diet changes, then enteral tube feeding can be initiated to meet nutrient and energy requirements. If it is not feasible to use the GI tract for feeding or if the GI tract cannot effectively provide consistent and adequate nutrition, then PN may be an appropriate feeding modality. Therefore the following questions must be answered:

- Does the patient require nutrition support?
- What is the optimal route of feeding: oral, tube feeding, or parenteral?
- Will the enteral route alone be sufficient to meet nutrient and energy requirements?
- What type of formula is needed, and how should it be provided?
- Does the patient require long-term nutrition support?

Oral Diet

When a patient does not consume a nutritionally complete diet, the energy value of foods in the oral diet can be increased according to patient tolerance and preference with added sauces, seasonings, and dressings. Frequent, less bulky,

EVIDENCE-BASED PRACTICE

Probiotics

The popularity of probiotics has increased greatly in recent years, but the truth is that probiotics have been the subject of research for some time now. In fact, probiotics have been researched so often that a joint effort by the Food and Agriculture Organization of the United Nations (FAO) and World Health Organization (WHO) established guidelines for the evaluation of probiotics in food in October 2001.[1]

Probiotics have been defined as "live microorganisms that, when administered in adequate amounts, confer a health benefit on the host."[1] Some of the confirmed positive consequences of ingested probiotics include enhanced lactose digestion for individuals with lactose intolerance, reduced incidence of sepsis, and enhanced hepatic function for patients with alcohol-related or hepatitis C–related cirrhosis to name just a few.[1,3] The negative side effects of probiotic ingestion are, at best, rare and limited to individuals with underlying medical conditions.[1]

Intestinal microflora survive by consuming very small amounts of indigestible food that people eat. The waste products of the microflora can be beneficial, including the production of vitamin K and medium-chain fatty acids, which the host can use.[4] During periods of fasting, or when the diet does not supply sufficient nutrition for the microflora, they decrease in number.

Periods of fasting and decreased gastric motility are often found hand in hand with patients on PN or EN. Decreased gastric motility is a common and serious problem in critically ill patients as well. The decreased motility can affect EN efforts, resulting in atrophy of intestinal mucosa, sepsis, and multiple organ failure. Although probiotics have not been found to effectively reverse the effects of inhibited gastric motility, they have been proven effective in managing all forms of diarrhea. To understand the importance of effectively managing diarrhea, see the *Case Study* box at the end of this chapter.

Because of the nature of numerous procedures performed in hospitals, many patients are, at least in the short term, left in a fasting state for the purpose of surgical preparation, as well as for other reasons. Probiotics have been shown to have beneficial effects on patients during fasting periods, and

administration of probiotics can help maintain nutritional status, including enhanced recovery from malnutrition and reduced mucosal atrophy, at least in animal models.[2]

However, probiotics may have little clinical significance in critically ill patients. In one study the probiotic *Lactobacillus plantarum* 299v was enterally fed to critically ill patients.[4] A significantly delayed attenuation of systemic inflammatory response (SIRS) was found in the treatment group versus the probiotic group, although the design of the study could not confirm this delayed attenuation was caused by the probiotics.

The end result of the study concluded that probiotics may play a hand in delaying SIRS but could not reduce morbidity or mortality in critically ill patients.

In the end, consumer acceptance and researcher curiosity is spurring the demand for more research into the beneficial effects of probiotics. Probiotics are being studied at an increasing rate, and research is showing promising results; however, not enough consistent information is available to make a professional recommendation to use probiotics in the treatment of patients on EN or PN. Perhaps with more time, probiotics may find a place in assisting those on EN or PN, but for now, we will simply have to accept that probiotics only have a place in the intestines of the healthy.

References

1. *FAO/WHO guidelines for the evaluation of probiotics in food. Joint FAO/WHO Working Group report on drafting guidelines for the evaluation of probiotics in food*, London, Ontario, 2002, pp 1–11.
2. Dock DB, Latorraca MQ, Aguilar-Nacimento JE, et al: Probiotics enhance recovery from malnutrition and lessen colonic mucosal atrophy after short-term fasting in rats. *Nutrition* 20:473, 2004.
3. O'Brien A, Williams R: Nutrition in end-stage liver disease: principles and practice. *Gastroenterology* 134:1729, 2008.
4. McNaught CE, Woodcock NP, Anderson AD, et al: A prospective randomized trial of probiotics in critically ill patients. *Am J Clin Nutr* 24:211, 2005.

concentrated small meals may be helpful so that the patient is not overwhelmed or discouraged by a tray full of food. If a patient is on a modified diet (e.g., a low-fat, low-sodium, or diabetic diet), then liberalization of the diet as much as is medically feasible can help improve oral intake. For example, changing from a regimented 1800-kcal diabetic diet to a carbohydrate-counting diet allows the patient more flexibility in food selection. In some cases it may be necessary to liberalize to an unrestricted or regular diet to increase oral intake. Depending on the patient's condition and food preferences, an oral liquid nutritional supplement, commercially available or made in-house, can be provided with or between meals. However, taste fatigue can happen fairly rapidly when patients are receiving two to six cans of an

oral nutritional supplement per day. Patients may use their nutritional supplements as meal replacements, therefore not increasing overall energy and nutrient intake. It is important to offer nutritional supplements in a variety of flavors and textures to maintain adequate consumption. Some facilities, particularly those specializing in long-term care, have found that dispensing oral nutritional supplements in small amounts of 30 to 60 mL during times when medications are administered improved oral nutritional supplement intake and nutrient delivery.[30,31]

Enteral Tube Feeding

If a sufficient oral intake of nutrients and energy is not possible, then the next option is EN by tube feeding, either as a supplement to oral dietary intake or as the sole source of nutrition.

Indications for Enteral Tube Feeding

A.S.P.E.N. has published guidelines for indications for nutrition support.[7] Enteral tube feeding is indicated for patients who are (or who are likely to become) malnourished and unable or unwilling to consume adequate nutrition by mouth. Factors that affect the decision to provide enteral tube feeding include the patient's preadmission nutritional status, risk for malnutrition based on current disease or condition, ability to consume a nutritionally complete oral diet, and functional status of the GI tract. Research found no benefit to aggressive early enteral tube feeding for patients who were not malnourished versus those who waited 6 days to begin an oral diet.[32]

ENTERAL TUBE FEEDING FORMULAS

Complete Enteral Tube Feeding Formulas
Blenderized Formulas

Prior to the availability of commercial enteral formulas, the first enteral formulas were created by blenderizing regular diets and using broth or gravy to thin the mixture enough to flow through feeding tubes. Today the majority of enteral tube feedings in health care facilities are given with a defined, commercially prepared enteral tube feeding formula. However, financial or personal reasons may motivate a patient or family to use blenderized formulas for home enteral tube feeding. Although emotional comfort may be achieved by using home-prepared food, its use does create problems (see the Complementary and Alternative Medicine [CAM] box, "Homemade Enteral Formulas: A Recipe for Trouble?").

COMPLEMENTARY AND ALTERNATIVE MEDICINE (CAM)
Homemade Enteral Formulas: A Recipe for Trouble?

Home-based enteral nutrition (EN) support is a common and safe practice that has been in existence for decades. Many people have benefited from the freedom and medical support it provides, and they can maintain a healthy nutritional status in spite of the fact they cannot consume an oral diet. Advancements in pumps, tubes, and placement of tubes are all contributing factors to the success rate of home tube feeding, but another major improvement of note is the development of enteral feeding solutions. Over the years, commercial enteral feeding solutions have grown to encompass many brands and formulas specialized for nutrient needs or even a particular disease state. Most formulas can supply total nutrition to the recipient of EN support and cause few side effects if administered and calculated correctly. Therefore with all of the options commercially available, why would someone want to make "homemade" enteral solutions? More importantly, is it safe to do so?

In the past, homemade enteral solutions were a widely used and accepted entity for EN support at home and even in hospitals. Many individuals considered homemade solutions a more economical and personally fulfilling feeding method. Home caretakers such as mothers, fathers, or spouses believed making the solutions was a more affectionate and devoted method as opposed to simply opening a can. Even so, current consensus directs the consumer away from these homemade solutions, not only because of the advancements in commercial formulas but also because of potential problems with homemade solutions.

As mentioned previously, commercial formulas are nutritionally complete and specialized for a wide array of nutritional and disease states. These commercial feedings are also consistent in their formulation and, as such, are easily quantifiable to readily meet the recipient's needs. Conversely, homemade solutions of varying composition have no exact method of quantification or verification of their nutritional content. Furthermore, these solutions are not tested for digestive and absorptive properties as commercial solutions are, which can lead to a host of problems such as dehydration, constipation, vitamin deficiency, and even severe malnourishment.

Sanitation is a critical variable to consider when dealing with nutrition support and choosing an enteral feeding solution. Its importance cannot be overstated. Although no way exists to totally avoid contamination of enteral feeding, the use of commercially prepared solutions can considerably limit the chance of a health risk. Points of potential contamination such as preparation, cooking, and blenderizing are all omitted, leaving the caretaker with less of a chance of exposing the recipient to a potentially serious bacterial or viral infection; this can be especially important for those who have an altered immune system. In addition, commercially available formulas lessen the workload of the administer and guard the recipient from clogs associated with underblenderized feedings.

For the vast majority of those receiving EN support, commercially available enteral tube feeding solutions are the appropriate choice. Recently there has been a resurgence of use of home blenderized enteral formulas. Caregivers who are using home blenderized enteral formulas should be educated regarding safe practices.

Bibliography

Duperret E, Trautlein J: *Homemade tube feeding formula ... two dietitians' perspective*, Tucson, Ariz., November 20, 2003, Mealtime Notions, LLC. from: <http://www.mealtimenotions.com/GuestOpinions/GuestOpinion1HomemadeTubeFeedingFormula.htm>. Retrieved December 22, 2005.

Malone A: Enteral formula selection: a review of selected categories. *Pract Gastroenterol* 29(6):44, 2005.

Mokhalalati JK, Druyan ME, Shott SB, et al: Microbial, nutritional and physical quality of commercial and hospital prepared tube feedings in Saudi Arabia. *Saudi Med J* 25(3):331, 2004.

Stanley D: Forward. *JPEN J Parenter Enter Nutr* 25(Suppl 5):S2, 2002.

Sullivan MM, Sorreda-Esguerra P, Platon MB, et al: Nutritional analysis of blenderized enteral diets in the Philippines. *Asia Pac J Clin Nutr* 13(4):385, 2004.

These problems involve its physical form, which could cause tube clogging, an increased risk of bacterial contamination, and inconsistent nutrient adequacy based on the foods chosen and preparation techniques used. The blenderized formula must be given into the stomach and requires a normal GI tract to digest and absorb the nutrients contained in the formula. Use of blenderized formulas has decreased over the past 20 years with the proliferation of commercially available enteral tube feeding formulas.

Commercial Enteral Tube Feeding Formulas

In contrast to homemade enteral formulas, commercial enteral tube feeding formulas provide sterile, nutritionally complete, homogenized solutions suitable for small-bore enteral feeding tubes. Enteral tube feeding formulas are available as polymeric, semielemental or oligomeric, and elemental or monomeric formulas (Table 19-2).[33] It is important to keep abreast of products currently available because new formulations and enteral tube feeding products are constantly being developed. Polymeric enteral tube feeding formulas require digestion and are available with and without fiber. Macronutrients and micronutrients of a polymeric tube feeding formula can be modified for specific needs of patients with various disease states. Semielemental or oligomeric tube feeding formulas are partially digested or hydrolyzed. Smaller molecules increase the **osmolality** of the formula. Elemental or monomeric tube feeding formulas are completely predigested and require only absorption for assimilation into the body. These formulas have the highest osmolality, lowest viscosity, and worst taste of all enteral tube feeding formulas. Enteral tube feeding formulas will also vary according to nutrient density from 1 to 2 kcal/mL. More concentrated formulas are designed for patients with fluid intolerance, such as those with renal, hepatic, or cardiac failure, as well as for patients who desire less volume or fewer feedings per day. However, if patients who receive a concentrated enteral tube feeding formula do not have fluid restrictions, it is imperative to provide adequate water so that they do not become dehydrated.

Nutrient Components
Carbohydrates

Approximately 50% to 60% of the energy in the American diet comes from carbohydrates, starches, and sugars. Carbohydrates are the body's primary energy source (see Chapter 3). Although large starch molecules are well tolerated and easily digested by most patients, their relative insolubility creates problems in enteral tube feeding formulas. Thus smaller sugars formed by partial or complete breakdown of cornstarch and other glucose polymers are common tube feeding formula components (see Table 19-2).[33] Very few enteral tube feeding formulas contain lactose, because lactose intolerance is common among hospitalized patients. Tube feeding formulas can also contain soluble and insoluble fiber. Considerable controversy exists as to the benefit of providing fiber in enteral tube feeding formulations.[26,33] Insoluble fiber increases stool volume and thus is used to treat problems with gastric motility such as constipation or diarrhea. Soluble fiber has been promoted to improve blood sugar control, reduce serum cholesterol levels, and maintain colon health. The focus on maintaining normal intestinal bacteria has resulted in increased research and availability of prebiotics and probiotics given with or in enteral tube feeding formulas. Prebiotics, nondigestible food components, provide fuel to enhance repletion of normal bacteria found in the GI tract, whereas probiotics, live nonpathogenic microbes, are designed to repopulate by providing "good" bacteria directly to the GI tract.[34] The strain of probiotic and combination of strains most effective depends on the therapeutic intent (see Evidence-Based Practice box, "Probiotics" for more information).

Protein

Protein content of standard enteral tube feeding formulas is designed to maintain body cell mass and promote tissue synthesis and repair (see Chapter 5). Biologic quality of dietary protein depends on its amino acid profile, especially its relative proportions of essential amino acids. To supply these needs, the following three major forms of protein are used in nutrition support enteral tube feeding formulas: (1) intact proteins, (2) hydrolyzed proteins, and (3) crystalline amino acids (see Table 19-2).[33]

1. *Intact proteins:* Intact proteins are the complete and original forms as found in foods, although protein isolates such as lactalbumin and casein from milk are intact proteins that have been separated from their original food source. These larger polypeptides and proteins must be broken down further (digested) before they can be absorbed.

2. *Hydrolyzed proteins:* Hydrolyzed proteins are protein sources that have been broken down by enzymes into smaller protein fragments and amino acids. These smaller products—tripeptides, dipeptides, and free amino acids—are absorbed more readily into the blood circulation.

3. *Crystalline amino acids:* Pure crystalline amino acids are readily absorbed, particularly when combined in a mix of dipeptides and tripeptides. The small size of the amino acid results in an increase in osmolality of the formula. Amino acids result in a bitter-tasting formula. If an elemental tube feeding formula is used as an oral supplement, then it requires flavoring aids or special preparation methods to improve taste (e.g., pudding, frozen slush, Popsicle). However, despite flavorings, the taste can still be unacceptable to a sick patient or can quickly lead to taste fatigue and refusal by the patient.

KEY TERM

osmolality   The ability of a solution to create osmotic pressure and determine the movement of water between fluid compartments; determined by the number of osmotically active particles per kilogram of solvent; serum osmolality is 280 to 300 mOsm/kg.

TABLE 19-2 CATEGORIES AND MACRONUTRIENT SOURCES FOR VARIOUS TYPES OF ENTERNAL FORMULAS

TYPE OF FORMULA	PROTEIN SOURCES	CARBOHYDRATE SOURCES	FAT SOURCES	kcal/mL	PROTEIN CONTENT	NONPROTEIN CALORIE-TO-NITROGEN RATIO	EXAMPLES
Intact (Polymeric)	Calcium and magnesium caseinates Sodium and calcium caseinates Soy protein isolate Calcium potassium caseinate Delactosed lactalbumin Egg white solids Beef Nonfat milk	Maltodextrin Corn syrup solids Sucrose Cornstarch Glucose polymers Sugar Vegetables Fruits Nonfat milk	Medium-chain triglycerides Canola oil Corn oil Lecithin Soybean oil Partially hydrogenated soybean oil High-oleic safflower oil Beef fat	1-2	30-84 g/L	75-177 : 1	Boost (No) Compleat (No) Fibersource (No) Isocal (No) Isosource (No) Jevity (R) Nutren (Ne) Osmolite (R) Resource (No) TwoCal HN (R) Ultracal (No)
Hydrolyzed (Oligomeric or Monomeric)	Enzymatically hydrolyzed whey or casein Soybean or lactalbumin hydrolysate Whey protein Soy protein hydrolysate	Hydrolyzed cornstarch Sucrose Fructose Maltodextrin Tapioca starch Glucose oligosaccharides	Medium-chain triglycerides Sunflower oil Lecithin Soybean oil Safflower oil Corn oil Coconut oil Canola oil Sardine oil	1-1.33	21-52.5 g/L	67-282 : 1	Advera (R) AlitraQ (R) Criticare HN (No) Crucial (Ne) Peptamen (Ne) Perative (R) Tolerex (No) Vital HN (R) Vivonex Plus (No)
Modular Protein	Low-lactose whey and casein Calcium caseinate Free amino acids	—	—	**Per 100 g** 370-424	**Per 100 g** 75-88.5	—	Casec (No) ProMod (R) Resource Protein Powder (No)
Carbohydrate	—	Maltodextrin Hydrolyzed cornstarch	—	Per 100 g 380-386			Moducal (No)
Fat	—	—	Safflower oil Polyglycerol esters of fatty acids Soybean oil Lecithin Medium-chain triglycerides Fish oil	Per 1 tbsp 67.5-115			MCT Oil (No) Microlipid (No)

Modified from Gottschlich MM, Shronts EP, Hutchins AM: Defined formula diets. In Rombeau JL, Rolandelli RH, editors: *Clinical nutrition: enteral and tube feeding,* ed 3, Philadelphia, Pa., 1997, Saunders.
Ne, Nestle; *No,* Novartis; *R,* Ross.

Fat

The major roles of fat in an enteral tube feeding formula are to supply a concentrated energy source, essential fatty acids, and a transport mechanism for fat-soluble vitamins. Major forms of fat used in standard formulas are butterfat in milk-based mixtures; vegetable oils from corn, soy, safflowers, or sunflowers; medium-chain triglycerides (MCTs); and lecithin (see Table 19-2).[33] Vegetable oils supply a rich source of the essential fatty acids—linoleic and linolenic acids. Researchers continue to examine outcomes related to enteral tube feeding formulas containing various combinations of short-chain fatty acids, medium-chain fatty acids, and omega-3 fatty acids (see Chapter 4).[35,36]

Vitamins and Minerals

Standard whole-diet commercial tube feeding formulas provide 100% of the Recommended Dietary Allowance (RDA) and Dietary Reference Intake (DRI) for vitamins and minerals when the formula is provided at a specific volume per day. The volume required to provide the RDA-DRI varies with each tube feeding formula and the nutrient requirements of the patient. Delivery of a reduced volume and use of diluted formulas may require supplementation with vitamin and mineral preparations. Patients with nutrient deficiencies may require supplementation of specific vitamins and minerals in addition to the standard vitamin and mineral composition of the enteral tube feeding formula. Several enteral tube feeding formulas are designed for specific patient populations and contain micronutrients designed to meet the requirements of the particular disease state or condition.

Physical Properties

After selecting a tube feeding formula according to the patient's nutritional requirements and GI function, the clinician must consider physical properties of the formula that can affect tolerance. Individual intolerance is reflected in delayed gastric emptying, abdominal distention, cramping and pain, diarrhea, or constipation. A factor often evaluated when a patient demonstrates intolerance is osmolality of the enteral tube feeding formula. Osmolality is based on concentration of the formula and defined as number of osmotic particles per kilogram of solvent (water), energy-nutrient density, and residue content. However, no evidence indicates that enteral tube feeding formula osmolality is the primary contributor to formula intolerance. Enteral tube feeding formulas can approximate 700 mOsm, whereas some medications are 4000 mOsm or more. Signs and symptoms of enteral tube feeding intolerance, of which diarrhea is the most common, are more often related to inappropriate tube feeding techniques or drug interactions.

Medical Foods for Special Needs

Certain tube feeding formulas designed for special nutrition therapy are called **medical foods**. The U.S. Food and Drug Administration (FDA) first recognized the concept of medical

foods as distinct from drugs in 1972, when the first special formula was developed for treatment of the genetic disease phenylketonuria (PKU) in newborns (see Chapter 12). The definition of medical foods remained rather murky as medical research developed an increasing number of special formulas. The Orphan Drug Act has defined *medical food* as a food that is formulated to be consumed or administered enterally under the supervision of a physician and that is intended for the specific dietary management of a disease or condition for which distinctive nutritional requirements, based on recognized scientific principles, are established by medical evaluation. The Orphan Drug Act was subsequently incorporated into the reformed Nutrition Labeling and Education Act of 1990.

An explosion of specialty enteral tube feeding formulas has occurred over the past 10 years. Several products are available in each category of disease- or condition-specific formulation: (1) end-stage renal disease, (2) hepatic disease, (3) pulmonary disease, (4) diabetes mellitus, (5) malabsorption syndromes, (6) immunoincompetence, (7) oncology, and (8) metabolic stress. Every patient with one of the previous diagnoses does not need a specialty tube feeding formula. Indications for specialty tube feeding formulas are limited to a small subset of patients within each disease state classification for which a specialty formula is designed. Considerable debate exists regarding the treatment value and cost-effectiveness of specialty tube feeding formulas; therefore scientific evidence to support their use is needed before use can be recommended.[26]

Modular Enteral Tube Feeding Formulas

Commercially available, nutritionally complete enteral formula products for tube feeding are designed with a fixed ratio of nutrients to meet general standards for nutritional needs. However, some patients' particular needs are not met by these standard fixed-ratio tube feeding formulas, and they require an individualized modular formula. An individual formula, composed completely of modular components, is planned, calculated, prepared, and administered with the expertise of the RD. Modular enteral components are listed in Table 19-2. However, the more common use of modular components is the addition of carbohydrate, fat, or protein to a commercial formula to individualize the calorie and protein content of the formula for the patient. For example, additional protein powder can be added to increase the amount of protein per liter, or more carbohydrate or fat can be added to increase energy concentration. Other modular nutrients such as fiber and probiotics or prebiotics can also be added to the feeding regimen but should be given separately through the feeding tube and not added directly to the

---

KEY TERM

medical foods Specially formulated nutrient mixtures for use under medical supervision to treat various metabolic diseases.

commercial tube feeding formulation. Every component added to an enteral tube feeding formula can increase the osmolality and viscosity of the formula and contribute to feeding intolerance, bacterial contamination, or clogging of the feeding tube.

Blue food dye is often added to tube feeding formulas to detect aspiration of formula into the trachea and lungs. Concern exists as to safety, specificity, and sensitivity of blue dye in identifying aspiration in tube-fed patients.[38-40] The addition of blue food dye increases risk of bacterial contamination, false-positive occult stool test, discoloration of the skin and body fluids, and death. In addition, no standardization exists for how much food dye to add per liter of tube feeding formula, with formula hues ranging from pale to cobalt blue. Methylene blue should not be added to tube feeding formulas because it can adversely affect cellular function.[41] Colored dyes are not diagnostic for aspiration, are potentially harmful, and should not be added to tube feedings.[40] Nonrecumbent positioning (elevating the head of the bed 30 to 40 degrees) is an evidence-based method for aspiration prevention and should be emphasized in all tube-fed patients.[40]

ENTERAL TUBE FEEDING DELIVERY SYSTEMS

Tube Feeding Equipment

Nasoenteric Feeding Tubes

Small-bore nasoenteric feeding tubes, generally from 8 to 12 French, made of softer, more flexible polyurethane and silicone materials have replaced former large-bore stiff tubing. Small-bore feeding tubes are more comfortable for patients and permit the infusion of commercially available enteral tube feeding formulas. Nasoenteric tubes can be inserted into either the stomach or beyond the pyloric valve into the small intestine. (Figure 19-2).[42] Distal placement of a feeding tube beyond the ligament of Treitz into the jejunum is often preferred for patients with a history or risk of aspiration, impaired gastric emptying, depressed gag reflex, neurologic impairment, and critical illness.[27] Feeding tube insertion can be done blindly at the bedside or using radiographic visualization. Placement of a feeding tube should be performed by experienced, trained personnel. Feeding tube placement is an invasive procedure and carries the risk of misplacement into the lungs or brain, as well as perforation of the GI tract. During placement, aspirates of GI contents can be checked for pH and enzyme concentration, as well as visually inspected to reduce the number of radiographs required to determine when the desired location has been reached.[43] However, no tube feeding should be infused until feeding tube placement is confirmed by radiography.

Tube Feeding Enterostomies

Nasoenteric tube placement is usually indicated for short-term therapy. However, for enteral feeding anticipated to last more than 3 to 4 weeks, surgically or endoscopically placed enterostomies are preferred[42] (see Figure 19-2), as follows:

- *Esophagostomy:* A cervical esophagostomy can be placed at the level of the cervical spine to the side of the neck after head and neck surgeries for cancer or traumatic injury. This removes the discomfort of a nasoenteric tube, and the entry point can be concealed under clothing.
- *Gastrostomy:* A gastrostomy tube is surgically or endoscopically placed in the stomach if the patient is not at risk for aspiration and has normal gastric motility.
- *Jejunostomy:* A jejunostomy tube is surgically or endoscopically placed past the ligament of Treitz in the jejunum, the middle section of the small intestine. This procedure is indicated for patients with neurologic impairment, a risk or history of aspiration, an incompetent gag reflex, or gastric dysfunction. Gastric dysfunction can be related to gastric atony, gastroparesis, gastric cancer, gastric outlet obstruction, or gastric ulcerative disease.

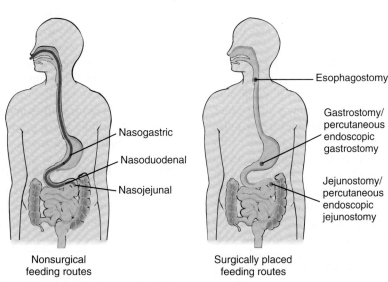

FIGURE 19-2 Types of enteral feeding routes. (From Rolin Graphics in Grodner M, Anderson SL, DeYoung S: *Foundations and clinical applications of nutrition: a nursing approach,* ed 2, St Louis, Mo., 2000, Mosby.)

Care and Maintenance of Enteral Feeding Tubes

Enteral feeding tubes should be flushed routinely with water to maintain patency and prevent clogging. Tap water is generally sufficient. If concern exists regarding safety of the water source or if the patient is immunosuppressed, then sterile water may be used to flush the feeding tube. Standard flushing volumes are 30 mL of water every 4 hours during continuous feedings. Water flushes for intermittent and bolus enteral feedings are a minimum of 30 mL immediately after each feeding. The amount of water flushed through the tube is adjusted according to the patient's fluid requirements and tolerance. Larger fluid volumes will be needed for patients who cannot drink water for hydration; smaller fluid volumes are needed for patients on fluid restrictions.

General Comfort Tips for Patients with Nasoenteric Tube Feedings

- *Thirst, oral dryness:* Lubricate lips, chew sugarless gum, brush teeth, rinse mouth frequently with water, and suck lemon drops occasionally. If a small amount of water by mouth is permitted, then let ice cubes melt in the mouth to soothe mouth and esophagus.
- *Tube discomfort:* Gargle with a mixture of warm water and mouthwash, gently blow the nose, and clean the tube regularly with water-soluble lubricant. If discomfort persists, then pull the tube out gently, clean it, and reinsert a new tube. (Many long-term users of tube feeding have learned to pass their own nasogastric tubes.)
- *Tension, fullness:* Relax and breathe deeply after each tube feeding infusion.
- *Loud stomach noises:* Take feedings in private.
- *Limited mobility:* Change positions in bed or chair, and walk around the house or hospital corridor. Perform range-of-motion exercises while confined to bed.
- *General gustatory distress with feeding:* Warm or chill the tube feeding formula, but avoid making the formula too cold because that increases risk of diarrhea.
- *Persistent hunger:* Chew a favorite food, then spit it out; chew gum; or suck lemon drops.
- *Inability to drink:* Rinse the mouth frequently with water or other liquids.

Ideally no medications should be put down small-bore feeding tubes because medications are a primary contributor to feeding tube clogs. However, the reality of life often requires administration of medications via feeding tubes. Flush with 30 mL of water before and after medication administration. Each medication should be administered separately with 5 mL of water flushed through the tube between each medication. Check with a pharmacist when determining which medications are compatible with administration through a feeding tube (see the Diet-Medications Interactions box, "Drug-Nutrient Interactions"). Medications should never be added directly to the tube feeding formula because of the risk of drug-nutrient interactions. Warm water, a 30- to 60-mL syringe, and a pumping action can be used to dislodge a clog within the feeding tube. No evidence supports the use of other liquids such as soft drinks or juices to declog feeding tubes.[44] A pancreatic enzyme and bicarbonate mixture may be effective against formula clogs but will not dissolve medication clogs.[45]

Tube Feeding Containers and Pumps

The enteric tube feeding system includes the formula container, connection tubing, and often an infusion pump. A variety of tube feeding containers and feeding sets is available. Tube feeding formulas can be administered by syringe, gravity drip, or a volumetric pump. A pump may be needed for more accurate control, which is essential for tube feedings given directly into the small intestine, tube feedings infused at slow rates, and tube feedings using more **viscous** formulas. Critically ill patients should also be tube fed by volumetric pump to increase tolerance to EN support.

Tube feeding delivery systems are categorized as either *open* or *closed*. An open delivery system involves pouring a volume of formula from a can or mixing bowl (or container) into an empty tube feeding bag, syringe, or infusion container. The infusion bag or container is reopened and refilled periodically with more formula. Clean technique is required when decanting the tube feeding formula into the bag and when handling the tubing connections. Formula hang time is limited to 8 hours or less.[24,46] Hang time is further reduced if additives such as protein powder are placed into the formula. The tube feeding infusion bag should be rinsed with sterile water before initial filling and subsequent refilling with formula.[24] The tube feeding administration set, tubing and infusion bag, should be changed every 24 hours. The primary benefit of the open system is the ability to modulate the tube feeding formula.

The closed system is composed of a sterile vessel that is purchased prefilled with tube feeding formula. The container is spiked and connected to an infusion pump. Hang time is expanded to 24 to 48 hours (refer to manufacturer's guidelines for hang time of product being used). Benefits of the closed system are a reduction of time, labor, and contamination risk.[47,48] Caveats of the closed system are its increased cost and the inability to modulate the formula. Regardless of the system used, good hand washing is essential to reduce bacterial contamination. Clinicians working with patients on tube feedings need to be familiar with different delivery systems, types of enteral feeding tubes, and features of enteral feeding pumps to determine which products are preferable for their facility and patient population.

Infusion of Enteral Tube Feeding

Tube feedings can be provided via bolus, intermittent, or continuous infusion through a feeding tube. Patients can progress from one infusion modality to another as their

---

KEY TERM

viscous Physical property of a substance dependent on the friction of its component molecules as they slide by one another; viscosity.

DIET-MEDICATIONS INTERACTIONS

Drug-Nutrient Interactions

Even though enteral nutrition (EN) support is becoming rather ordinary, relatively few clinical studies are available that document drug-nutrient interactions associated with enteral feeding solutions. This relates to the fact that administration of drugs through a feeding tube should be considered a last resort, but it can also be linked to the theory that interactions are so common and varied they are simply not reported. However, potential consequences of interactions should not be taken lightly. Use of EN support poses many pharmaceutic and dietary complications that can physically interfere with administration of nutrition, alter the bioavailability of a given drug, or cause long-term vitamin and mineral deficiencies.

Physical interferences with nutrition support are problems related to manipulation of the delivery system of nutrition support or the drug before it enters the body. Physical interferences are the most commonly reported problems and include but are not limited to occlusion of the feeding tube related to medication administration, manipulation of solid-dose forms of drugs, and exposure of photosensitive drugs to light for extended periods of time. No medication is formulated to be administered in combination with EN support; therefore the composition can sometimes alter viscosity of enteral feeding solutions and cause occlusion of the feeding tube. Furthermore, when crushing a solid-dose pill for administration through a feeding tube, there is a risk of occlusion, and the bioavailability of the medication and its time release properties will be altered considerably. Any type of drug added to a feeding solution will have longer exposure to ultraviolet light than if taken orally, which in some cases can compromise therapeutic effects.

The recipient of EN support is able to obtain total nutrition from his or her enteral feeding solutions; however, composition of these enteral feeds differ considerably from orally fed diets. Enteral feeds contain increased concentrations of proteins, vitamins, and minerals, which can bind drugs or alter the mechanism by which they are metabolized. Closely related, but resulting in a more long-term effect, are vitamin and mineral binding. Chronic problems such as osteoporosis can develop over time as a result of an interaction that goes unnoticed. The following is a brief list of some classically noted drug-nutrient interactions related to EN support.

Drug	Interaction	Possible Remedy
Phenytoin	Probable cause of interaction is the binding of phenytoin to caseinate proteins found in enteral feeds, preventing its absorption from the gastrointestinal (GI) tract.	Withhold feedings for 2 hours after administration of phenytoin. Increased dose might be in order.
Quinolones	Concurrent administration of a quinolone and enteral feed could compromise antimicrobial efficiency. This is related to the divalent cations found in enteral nutrition (EN) formulas.	Withhold feedings 1 hour before and 1 hour after administration of quinolones. Increase dose when converting from intravenous to oral form.
Warfarin	Decreased bioavailability of this drug results from high binding of warfarin to proteins found in EN. In addition, vitamin K was formerly found to reverse anticoagulant effects of warfarin, but most current enteral feeds contain little or no vitamin K.	Avoid concurrent administration of warfarin and EN solutions. Choose EN supplements that contain limited vitamin K content.

Working as a team with physicians, nurses, speech pathologists, and pharmacists can substantially reduce interactions stemming from EN support. By educating those who administer and prescribe medications, risks involved can be controlled and monitored correctly.

Bibliography

A.S.P.E.N. Board of Directors: Section IX: drug nutrient interactions. *JPEN J Parenter Enter Nutr* 26:1, 2002.

British Association for Parenteral and Enteral Nutrition, The British Pharmaceutical Nutrition Group: *Drug administration via enteral feeding tubes: a guide for general practitioners and community pharmacists*, Redditch, UK, 2001, BAPEN.

Finch C, Self T: Medication and enteral tube feedings: clinically significant interactions. *J Crit Illn* 16:20–21, 2001.

Fitzgerald M: What do I need to know about drug interactions with enteral feeding? *Medscape Nurses* 7:1, 2005. from: <http://www.medscape.com/viewarticle/498270>. Retrieved July 1, 2010.

medical condition changes. All enteral tube feedings should be initiated at full strength. Tolerance to tube feeding has not been shown to be improved with dilution of the formula.[49] Enteral tube feedings should be introduced gradually and progressed per patient tolerance. Gastric tube feedings can be given as bolus, intermittent, or continuous feedings. Small bowel tube feedings are given as continuous feedings.

Bolus tube feeding is generally initiated with 120 to 240 mL of formula every 3 to 4 hours and increased by 60 to 240 mL every 8 to 12 hours, depending on the level of illness and tolerance. The infusion period is relatively short, 10 to 20 minutes, and is infused through a syringe or from a bag by the flow of gravity.[50] The infusion should not exceed 40 to 60 mL/min. Gravity infusion is controlled by a roller clamp, raising or lowering the formula container, or advancing the plunger into the syringe.

Intermittent tube feedings are similar to bolus feedings but are given over a longer time period of 30 to 60 minutes every 3 to 6 hours. The enteral tube feeding formula is placed in a bag with rate controlled by a roller clamp. This method is used to provide periodic gastric feedings to patients who do not tolerate the more rapid infusion of a bolus feeding. The maximum amount of formula given by bolus or intermittent feedings varies from 240 to 500 mL per feeding and is based on patient tolerance and requirements.

Continuous tube feedings are provided over a defined period, with the formula infused by gravity or pump. Continuous feedings can be given over 24 hours or cycled over a shorter period, such as 8 to 20 hours per day. Enteral tube feeding tolerance is generally better in critically ill patients who are fed continuously regardless of whether fed into the stomach or small bowel.

All patients fed through a feeding tube should have the head of the bed elevated 30 to 45 degrees to reduce the risk of aspiration.[51] Patients fed with a tube into the small bowel can still aspirate gastric contents and may require concomitant gastric decompression during small bowel feeding.[52] Patients who must lie flat or in Trendelenburg's position should have enteral feedings stopped.

MONITORING THE TUBE-FED PATIENT

Monitoring of the tube-fed patient should focus on transitioning to an oral diet and reducing or eliminating dependency on tube feeding. All patients being nourished by tube feeding should be carefully monitored for signs and symptoms of enteral tube feeding intolerance. Tolerance to enteral tube feeding is determined by GI signs of vomiting, abdominal distention or bloating, and frequency and consistency of bowel movements. If problems occur, then the tube feeding formula may need to be replaced, the infusion rate adjusted, or the method of administration changed until tolerance improves and symptoms subside. In most instances the tube feeding formula itself is not the causative agent for the intolerance. Residual volume and diarrhea are two parameters that are often used to determine tolerance to tube feeding. Both are terms that have no standardized definition within each institution, much less nationwide standard definitions.

Diarrhea is generally defined by the person cleaning it up and can be based on volume, frequency, or consistency of the stools (or a combination of these factors). Fourteen definitions of diarrhea are found in the literature.[53] Commonly used definitions are more than three stools per day or more than 500 mL of stool per day for 2 consecutive days.[54] Each health care facility should define diarrhea and then create an algorithm or protocol for treatment to reduce unnecessary interruptions of enteral feeding.[54] The most common cause of diarrhea in the tube-fed patient is medications, primarily antibiotics and medications containing sorbitol (see the Health Promotion section later in this chapter for a discussion).

The interpretation of *residual volume* is also often determined by caregiver experience and not evidence-based guidelines. Enteral feeds are interrupted for gastric residual volumes ranging from 50 to 200 mL.[55] A research study defined acceptable residual volume as less than 200 mL with a nasogastric tube and less than 100 mL with a gastrostomy tube.[56] The authors suggested high residual volumes be correlated with the presence of physical signs of intolerance before stopping enteral feeding. Another study found that if patients were given a prophylactic prokinetic agent, then a residual volume of 250 mL was tolerated.[57] The A.S.P.E.N. Guidelines[7] and the Canadian Clinical Practice Guidelines[58] state a high residual volume is more than 200 mL for two consecutive checks and more than 250 mL, respectively. In contrast, according to a survey of intensive care unit (ICU) nurses, the nurses believed a residual volume greater than 100 mL was excessive.[59] A patient with a history of aspiration or reflux is at risk of aspiration even with low gastric residuals; therefore residual volumes do not always correlate with risk of aspiration.

GI aspirates that contain gastric enzymes and hydrochloric acid (HCl) required for digestion, electrolytes, enteral formula, and fluid should be returned to the patient after determining the volume. However, if doing so would make the patient uncomfortable or if the volume removed exceeds 300 mL, then the residuals should be discarded and rechecked in 1 to 2 hours. The feeding tube should be flushed with 30 mL water after checking and returning residuals to be sure gastric contents with digestive enzymes are no longer within the lumen of the feeding tube. Patient tolerance of tube feeding formula, state of hydration, and nutritional response to tube feeding should be monitored using data collected from a variety of sources, including laboratory, anthropometric, physical and clinical assessment, and nursing records. Protocols for enteral tube feeding can provide guidelines for troubleshooting problems and improve nutrient delivery.[60,61]

Clinical and Laboratory Parameters to Monitor

Blood glucose levels should be monitored daily or more frequently in patients who have diabetes or are at risk for diabetes. It is important not to overfeed patients on nutrition support. Historically insulin has been provided as needed to maintain serum glucose level at less than 200 mg/dL. However, a growing body of evidence indicates that glycemic control between 110 mg/dL[62] and 140 mg/dL[63] can significantly reduce mortality and morbidity in ICU patients.

Daily weights, compared with a baseline weight before start of the tube feeding, along with daily input and output measures, are essential for an accurate assessment of patient tolerance and nutrient adequacy. Routine monitoring also includes serum tests for potassium, sodium, chloride, carbon dioxide (CO_2), creatinine, as well as BUN and complete blood count (CBC), along with periodic tests for urine specific gravity. Sudden weight changes can indicate fluid imbalance and need to be investigated. (See Box 19-2 for a list of nutrition support monitoring parameters.)

Hydration Status

Signs of volume deficit or dehydration include weight loss, poor skin turgor, dry mucous membranes, and low blood pressure from decreased blood volume. Patients also demonstrate increased serum levels of sodium, albumin, hematocrit, and BUN, as well as elevated urine specific gravity levels. Severe dehydration is critical and life threatening. Fluid requirements can be estimated by several available formulas, such as 1 mL of water per kcalorie or 30 to 35 mL/kg. Water content of the enteral tube feeding formula and the amount of water given with medications and routine flushing of the feeding tube, as well as the patient's medical condition, are taken into consideration when determining the patient's fluid requirements. Fluids must be monitored for adequacy and adjusted as necessary to attain and maintain adequate hydration. Patients with large fluid losses from fistulas, ostomies, and drains may require intravenous hydration in conjunction with enteral tube feeding nutrition.

Signs of volume excess or overhydration include weight gain, edema, jugular vein distention, elevated blood pressure, and decreased serum levels of sodium, albumin, BUN, and hematocrit. Patients with renal, cardiac, and hepatic impairment may require less fluid than other patients.

Documentation of the Enteral Nutrition Tube Feeding

The patient's medical record is an essential means of communication among members of the health care team. The health care team is involved in actions and documentation related to (1) all ongoing nutritional analyses of actual tube feeding formula intake; (2) tolerance of the formula and any complications; (3) desired versus actual outcomes; (4) recommendations for adjustments in tube feeding formula, routine tube flushing, and method and rate of delivery; and (5) education of patient and family.

PARENTERAL FEEDING IN CLINICAL NUTRITION

PN should be reserved for patients who are unable to receive adequate nutrition via the enteral route. A.S.P.E.N. has published general guidelines to determine when PN support is appropriate.[7] Indications and contraindications for PN are listed in Box 19-4.

Basic Technique

Guidelines for ordering PN are given in Box 19-5, and an example of a basic PN solution is given in Box 19-6. PN refers to any intravenous feeding method. Nutrients are infused directly into the blood when the GI tract cannot or should not be used. The following two parenteral routes are available (Figure 19-3)[64]:

1. *Central parenteral nutrition (CPN):* A large central vein is used to deliver concentrated solutions for nutrition support. Osmolarity of central vein parenteral formulas can be as high as 1700 to 1900 mOsm/L. High formula

---

BOX 19-4   INDICATIONS AND CONTRAINDICATIONS FOR PARENTERAL NUTRITION

Indications
1. Nonfunctional gastrointestinal (GI) tract
   a. Obstruction
   b. Intractable vomiting or diarrhea
   c. Short-bowel syndrome
   d. Paralytic ileus
2. Inability to adequately use GI tract
   a. Slow progression of enteral nutrition (EN)
   b. Limited tolerance of EN
3. Perioperative condition
   a. Severely malnourished
   b. Nothing by mouth (NPO) for at least 1 week before surgery

Contraindications
1. No central venous access
2. Grim prognosis when parenteral nutrition (PN) will be of no benefit
3. EN is an alternative means of support

Conditions Previously Treated with PN that Benefit from Enteral Feeding
1. Inflammatory bowel disease
2. Pancreatitis

Modified from Fuhrman MP: Parenteral nutrition. *Dietitian's Edge* 2(1):53, 2001.

BOX 19-5   GUIDELINES FOR ORDERING PARENTERAL NUTRITION

1. Determine that the patient has central intravenous access.
2. Identify amount of energy, protein, and fluid desired.
3. Determine desired distribution of dextrose and lipids.
4. Indicate additives desired.
   a. Vitamins
   b. Minerals
   c. Electrolytes
   d. Medications
   e. Sterile water
5. Determine infusion rate based on compounded volume and time of infusion.

---

osmolarity requires infusion of the formula into a large vessel with rapid blood flow. A central line generally originates from the subclavian, internal jugular, or femoral vein, with the tip in the superior vena cava, right atrium of the heart, or inferior vena cava. Central line access can also be achieved with a peripherally inserted central catheter (PICC) that is inserted in the basilic vein, with the tip in the superior vena cava or right atrium.

2. *Peripheral parenteral nutrition (PPN):* A smaller peripheral vein, usually in the distal arm or hand, is used to deliver

less-concentrated solutions for periods less than 14 days. Osmolarity of PPN is limited to 900 mOsm/L or less to reduce risk of thrombophlebitis in smaller vessels of the upper distal extremities.[65]

Parenteral Nutrition Development

The pioneering work of American surgeons such as Jonathan Rhodes and Stanley Dudrick in the late 1960s propelled PN from theory into reality.[66] In the proceeding years, development of the surgical technique, equipment, and solutions to meet nutritional requirements of catabolic illness and injury, as well as development of certain antibiotics and diuretics, led to its widespread use and continuing development.[26,67] PN was preferentially used to treat critically ill patients until a resurgence in EN in the 1990s, when more was learned about the importance of maintaining GI integrity. PN is associated with potentially serious mechanical, metabolic, and GI complications (see Box 19-3). PN should be used judiciously to minimize the risks involved. PPN can be used in many cases as a viable alternative for brief periods for patients without central vein access.[68]

Basic factors govern decisions about use of PN: availability and functional capacity of the GI tract, prognosis, and availability of central intravenous access.[7] The cost of PN is generally more than that of enteral feeding, and institutions has demonstrated cost savings when inappropriate use of PN have been decreased.[69,70] Patients must have central intravenous access to receive PN, with one port designated exclusively for PN. Thus careful assessment of each situation should weigh benefits and burdens of providing PN for nutrition support.

Indications for PN include inability to access or the malfunction of the GI tract. Patients may have inadequate absorption of nutrients in the GI tract because of reduced bowel length or inflammation. Examples of indications for PN are obstruction, fistula, severe inflammation, intractable vomiting or diarrhea, or GI bleeding (see Box 19-4). If the GI tract is functional but the patient cannot or will not consume sufficient nutrients orally, then enteral tube feeding should be considered. Many conditions that had been previously thought to be an indication for PN are treated with enteral tube feeding, such as pancreatitis, severe malnutrition, ileus, and coma.

BOX 19-6	EXAMPLE OF A BASIC PARENTERAL NUTRITION FORMULA FOR A 65-kg PATIENT PROVIDING APPROXIMATELY 25 kcal/kg AND 1.2 g PROTEIN PER KILOGRAM

Base Solution

70% Dextrose	350 mL	245 g	833 kcal
10% Amino acids	800 mL	80 g	320 kcal
20% Lipid	250 mL	50 g	500 kcal
TOTAL	**1400 mL**		**1653 kcal**

Additives

Standard Electrolytes	Amount per day
Sodium chloride	20 mEq
Sodium acetate	50 mEq
Potassium chloride	30 mEq
Potassium phosphate	30 mEq (20 mmol phosphorus)
Calcium gluconate	10 mEq
Magnesium sulfate	10 mEq
Multivitamin preparation	10 mL
Trace element preparation	1 mL

Medications

Regular insulin	Only with hyperglycemia
H₂-antagonists	Dose depends on H₂-antagonist and renal functions
Famotidine 40 mg	

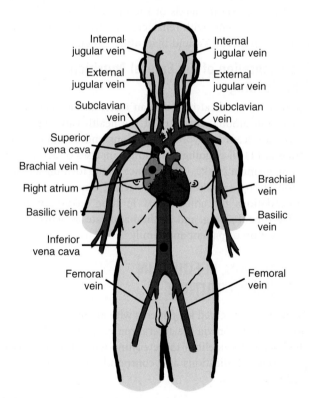

FIGURE 19-3 Sites of central venous access for parenteral nutrition (PN). (From Fuhrman MP: Management of complications of parenteral nutrition. In Matarese LE, Gottschlich MM, editors: *Contemporary nutrition support practice: a clinical guide,* Philadelphia, Pa., 1998, Saunders.)

KEY TERM

fistula Abnormal connection between two internal organs, an internal organ and the skin, or an internal organ and a body cavity.

Candidates for Parenteral Nutrition

PN should be reserved for patients unable to receive or tolerate adequate nutrients via the enteral route. On the basis of these general considerations, a number of clinical situations suggest a need for aggressive PN support:

- *Preoperative nutrition intervention:* This measure may benefit moderately to severely malnourished patients who can receive nutrition support for a minimum of 7 to 14 days preoperatively.[7] PN should be given only if EN support is not feasible or tolerated. The Veterans Affairs Cooperative Study[28] demonstrated the greatest benefit of perioperative PN was experienced by severely malnourished patients. Third-party payers do not routinely pay for preoperative nutrition support.
- *Postoperative surgical complications:* Complications that often result in initiation of PN are prolonged paralytic ileus and obstruction; stomal dysfunction; short-bowel syndrome; enterocutaneous, biliary, or pancreatic fistula; chylothorax; chylous ascites; and peritonitis. However, reports exist of successful enteral feeding with short-bowel syndrome, fistula, and chylous leaks when patients are given an elemental or semielemental, low-fat enteral formula.[71-73] PN is not indicated in patients who can resume EN within 7 to 10 days postoperatively.[7]
- *Bowel inflammation:* Intractable gastroenteritis, regional enteritis, ulcerative colitis, extensive diverticulitis, and radiation enteritis may require PN if the GI inflammation is severe and prolonged.[7] Studies have shown that in some cases enteral feeding can be feasible and beneficial in diseases with bowel inflammation.[74]
- *Malabsorption:* Nutrient losses and interference with nutrient absorption occur with chemotherapy and radiation therapy. The malabsorption that is associated with severe GI inflammation, acute severe pancreatitis, and massive burns can exceed the ability to meet nutrient requirements enterally.

Peripheral Parenteral Nutrition

Generally, decisions to use PPN instead of CPN are based on energy demands, anticipated time of use, and availability of intravenous access. Characteristics of PPN include caloric value generally less than 2000 kcal/day, of which 50% to 60% is provided by lipids; infusion volume of 2 to 3 L (dilution of the formula is required for peripheral vein tolerance); and use of infusion for less than 14 days.[68] PPN cannot be used when the patient has problems with fluid retention or hyperlipidemia.

PARENTERAL SOLUTIONS

Parenteral Nutrition Prescription

The PN prescription and plan of care are based on the calculation of basic nutritional requirements plus additional needs resulting from the patient's level of illness or injury, malnutrition, and physical activity. An example of a basic PN formula is shown in Box 19-6. The same principles of nutrition therapy are applied whether the patient is fed enterally or parenterally. Nutritional needs are fundamental—energy, protein, electrolytes, minerals, and vitamins. Guidelines are available that address PN labeling, compounding, formulations, stability, and filtering.[75] The guidelines are designed to reduce errors and complications in prescribing, preparing, labeling, and infusing parenteral solutions.

Preparation of the Parenteral Nutrition Solution

A variety of PN component solutions exist, with varying concentrations and nutrient compositions. Standard components of PN can include dextrose, lipids, amino acids, electrolytes, vitamins, minerals, and medications. Although PN is compounded with modular components and hence there is an ability to adjust dextrose, lipid, and protein independent of each other, the energy provided to meet estimated or measured energy needs should include total energy (kcalories) from carbohydrate, fat, and protein (Table 19-3). Estimated and measured energy equations are based on total energy (kcalories) requirements.

Protein-Nitrogen Source

Nitrogen is supplied by essential and nonessential crystalline amino acids in the PN solution. Standard commercial amino acid solutions range in concentration from 3% to 20%. Standard amino acid solutions are appropriate for almost all adult patients receiving PN. Protein has an energy value of 4 kcal/g (see Table 19-3) and usually provides 10% to 20% of the total energy provided in PN.

In addition to standard amino acid solutions, three types of specialized amino acid solutions have been formulated for specific disease states. The two disease-specific formulas are more expensive than standard solutions, and their effectiveness has not been demonstrated. One type is enriched with the branched-chain amino acids (BCAAs) isoleucine, leucine, and valine, and is designed for patients with liver failure. A renal failure formula contains only essential amino acids to prevent the development of hyperuremia. Neither disease-specific formula has been found to improve outcomes in these patient populations.[7] Infusion of BCAA may be beneficial in a very small population of patients with

TABLE 19-3	CALORIC VALUE PER MILLILITER OF PARENTERAL COMPONENTS	
NUTRIENT	**CONCENTRATION (%)**	**kcal/mL**
Dextrose	70.0	2.38
	50.0	1.85
Lipids	30.0	3.0
	20.0	2.0
	10.0	1.1
Amino acids	15.0	0.6
	10.0	0.4
	8.5	0.34

chronic hepatic encephalopathy that is unresponsive to drug therapy.[7] The third type of specialized amino acid formula is designed specifically for the needs of pediatric patients and is selected based on the age and nutrient requirements of the child.

Carbohydrate-Dextrose

Dextrose is the most common and least expensive source of energy used for PN support. Dextrose is available in concentrations ranging from 2.5% to 70%. Hypertonic solutions of 50% to 70% dextrose are often used in PN formulations and provide 50 or 70 g of dextrose per 100 mL, respectively. Glucose used in PN support is commercially available as dextrose monohydrate ($C_6H_{12}O_6H_2O$), which has an energy value of 3.4 kcal/g versus the energy value of 4 kcal/g of dietary glucose ($C_6H_{12}O_6$). The caloric values of dextrose solutions are given in Table 19-3. The initial dextrose content of PN should not exceed 200 g. Gradual introduction of dextrose enables the clinician to evaluate blood sugar response and, if necessary, institute insulin therapy. The amount of dextrose provided is increased to goal according to patient tolerance and should not exceed 5 mg/kg/min.

Glycerol is another form of carbohydrate used in parenteral solutions. It provides 4.3 kcal/g and is available as a component along with amino acids in a commercially available PPN solution.

Fat-Lipids

Lipid emulsions provide a concentrated energy source, 9 kcal/g, as well as the essential fatty acids linoleic and linolenic acid. A minimum of 4% to 10% of the daily energy intake should consist of fat to prevent essential fatty acid deficiency. Lipids are available in 10% (1.1 kcal/mL), 20% (2 kcal/mL), and 30% (3 kcal/mL) products (see Table 19-3). A 500-mL bottle of 10%, 20%, or 30% fat emulsion provides 550, 1000, and 1500 kcal, respectively. Commercial lipid emulsion products consist of soybean and safflower oils combined or soybean oil alone. The content of lipid in a parenteral solution is usually limited to 20% to 30% of total energy because lipids have been reported to adversely affect the immune system.[76] However, infusion of lipids over 24 hours may limit this adverse effect. Research on alternative lipid sources includes forms such as short-chain fatty acids, medium-chain fatty acids, omega-3 fatty acids, and blended or structured lipids. However, these alternatives are not available for commercial use in the United States. Lipid emulsions can be infused separately through the Y-port of the intravenous catheter (piggybacked) or combined with the dextrose and amino acid base in what is called a *total nutrient admixture* (TNA) or *3-in-1*.[75]

Electrolytes

The body maintains a balance of fluid and electrolytes in intracellular and extracellular spaces of all tissues to maintain homeostasis (see Chapter 7). Electrolyte status is affected by disease state and metabolic condition of the patient. Electrolytes in PN formulas are based on normal electrolyte balance with adjustments according to individual patient requirements. Electrolytes should be routinely monitored to determine electrolyte requirements in PN.

In general, basic electrolyte recommendations are shown in Table 19-4, with chloride and acetate balanced among the salts. Commercial amino acid formulations are available with or without added electrolytes. Amounts of electrolytes present in the amino acid solution must be taken into account when calculating additions of electrolytes for a specific patient. Guidelines for electrolyte management include the following:

1. Identify and correct any preexisting deficits before initiating PN.
2. Determine the cause of electrolyte abnormalities.
3. Replace excessive fluid and electrolyte losses.
4. Monitor and assess electrolyte status daily.

Depending on requirements for electrolyte replacement, it may be necessary to give additional electrolytes outside the PN, because limitations exist regarding what can be added to a parenteral solution based on solution stability and compatibility.[72] Selected electrolytes can be omitted from the parenteral solution when serum levels exceed normal values, such as potassium and phosphorus with renal failure. Electrolyte levels should be checked in all patients before starting PN and routinely throughout PN therapy.

Vitamins

Vitamin requirements are based on normal standards (see Chapter 6), with adjustments made according to metabolic states that require either more or less of a specific vitamin. All patients on PN should receive vitamins daily. Serum levels of vitamins should be monitored in patients requiring long-term PN or when deficiencies or excesses are suspected.

The Nutrition Advisory Group of the American Medical Association has established guidelines for parenteral administration of 12 vitamins: A, D, E, thiamin, riboflavin, niacin, pantothenic acid, pyridoxine, folic acid, biotin, cyanocobalamin, and ascorbic acid (see Table 19-4).[77] Multivitamin infusion preparations based on these guidelines are commercially available. Vitamin K has not historically been a component of any injectable vitamin formulation for adults. The FDA mandated changes in parenteral vitamin formulations that included addition of 150 mcg of vitamin K to injectable multivitamin preparations.[78] It will be important to monitor International Normalized Ratio (INR) levels, particularly for patients on anticoagulation therapy started or stopped on PN containing vitamin K. An injectable multivitamin preparation without vitamin K is also available.

KEY TERM

admixture   A mixture of ingredients that each retain their own physical properties; a combination of two or more substances that are not chemically united or that exist in no fixed proportion to each other.

TABLE 19-4	MICRONUTRIENTS AND PARENTERAL NUTRITION FOR ADULTS
MICRONUTRIENTS	**STANDARD DAILY AMOUNTS**
Electrolytes	
Potassium (K)	1-2 mEq/kg
Sodium (Na)	1-2 mEq/kg
Phosphate (HPO$_4$)	20-40 mmol
Magnesium (Mg)	8-20 mEq
Calcium (Ca)	10-15 mEq
Acetate	Balance with chloride to maintain acid-base balance
Chloride	Balance with acetate to maintain acid-base balance
Vitamins	
Vitamin A	3300 IU
Vitamin D	200 IU
Vitamin E	10 IU
Vitamin K	150 mcg
Thiamin (B$_1$)	6 mg
Riboflavin (B$_2$)	3.6 mg
Niacin (B$_3$)	40 mg
Folic acid	600 mcg
Pantothenic acid	15 mg
Pyridoxine (B$_6$)	6 mg
Cyanocobalamin (B$_{12}$)	5 mcg
Biotin	60 mcg
Ascorbic acid (vitamin C)	200 mcg
Trace Elements	
Chromium	10-15 mcg
Copper	0.3-0.5 mcg
Iodine	Not routinely provided 50 mcg for pregnant women
Iron	Not routinely provided 25-50 mg per month without blood loss
Manganese	60-100 mcg
Selenium	20-60 mcg
Zinc	2.5-5.0 mg
Molybdenum	Not routinely provided

Data from Fuhrman MP: Complication management in parenteral nutrition. In Matarese LE, Gottschlich MM, editors: *Contemporary nutrition support practice: a clinical guide,* ed 2, Philadelphia, Pa., 2003, Saunders; Task force for the revision of safe practices for parenteral nutrition: Safe practices for parenteral nutrition. *JPEN J Parenter Enteral Nutr* 28(suppl):S39, 2004; American Medical Association, AMA Department of Foods and Nutrition: Multivitamin preparations for parenteral use: a statement by the Nutrition Advisory Group. *JPEN J Parenter Enteral Nutr* 3:258, 1979; Parenteral multivitamin products; drugs for human use; drug efficacy study implementation; amendment (21 CFR 5.70). *Fed Register* 65:21200, 2000; Expert Panel for Nutrition Advisory Group, AMA Department of Foods and Nutrition: Guidelines for essential trace element preparations for parenteral use. *JAMA* 241:2051, 1979.

Trace Elements

The American Medical Association has set guidelines for the addition of four trace elements in PN solutions: zinc, copper, manganese, and chromium (see Table 19-4).[79] Trace element preparations are available with combinations of the afore-mentioned four trace elements only, the standard four plus selenium, or the standard four plus selenium, molybdenum, and iodine. Each trace element is also available as a single injectable mineral product. A growing amount of literature demonstrates the importance of providing selenium to PN patients who are critically ill[80,81] and those who require long-term PN.[82] Iron is not routinely added to PN because of incompatibility with intravenous lipids, as well as the potential adverse effects of iron dextran. Other forms of intravenous iron have less adverse effects but are not approved for addition to the PN solution. Intravenous iron should only be given to patients with iron deficiency anemia and administered apart from the PN admixture or added to a 2-in-1 PN solution.[75] A dose of 25 to 50 mg of iron dextran once a month should be sufficient to meet iron needs in a patient without blood loss.[75]

Patients on long-term PN without trace element supplementation are at risk for micronutrient deficiencies.[82,83] In addition, reports exist of excess trace element levels with infusion of standard trace element preparations.[84] Patients who require long-term PN should be routinely monitored for potential trace element deficiencies and toxicities.

Medications

Medications often added to PN include insulin, H$_2$-antagonists, heparin, metoclopramide, and octreotide. Inclusion of these medications and others will depend on each institution's guidelines and protocols for addition of medications to PN solutions. Many issues exist concerning compatibility, bioavailability, efficacy, interactions, and safety when including medications in PN solutions. Consult a pharmacist whenever considering the addition of a medication to PN solutions.

PARENTERAL NUTRITION DELIVERY SYSTEM

Equipment

Strict aseptic technique throughout PN administration by all health care personnel is absolutely essential. This includes (1) solution preparation by the pharmacist, (2) surgical placement of the venous catheter by the physician, (3) care of the catheter site and all external equipment, and (4) administration of the solution by the nurse. At every step of the PN process, strict infection control is a primary responsibility of all health care professionals.

Venous Access

Surgical placement of the venous catheter is done by the physician at the bedside or in a surgical suite, using local or general anesthesia. Intravenous catheters are available with single, double, triple, or quadruple lumens. Inconsistent data exist as to whether the number of lumens contributes to the risk of catheter-related infection.[85-87] Catheters are also categorized as either *temporary* or *permanent*. Temporary catheters involve a direct percutaneous puncture into a major vessel and are used short-term during hospitalization. Permanent catheters are designed for long-term use and are available as implanted ports, tunneled catheters, and PICCs. The tip of a central venous catheter is located in the inferior or superior vena cava, which leads directly into the heart (see Figure 19-3).[64] Placement of the catheter tip in the vena cava allows infusion of concentrated solutions, five times the concentration of blood plasma, to be infused at a rate of 2 to 3 mL/min. Hypertonic solutions are immediately diluted by the large blood flow of 2 to 5 L/min in the vena cava.

Catheter-related sepsis is a serious complication, particularly with the increase in colonization of resistant strains of microorganisms that limit available treatment options. Antibiotic-impregnated catheters and dressings are available and are associated with reduced catheter-related septic complications.[88-90] Filters (0.22 μm) on intravenous catheter tubing prevent infusion of not only particulate matter but also certain microorganisms.[75] However, a larger filter (2.1 μm) that is less effective against microorganisms must be used with PN containing lipids. Clinicians must use aseptic technique when inserting and caring for intravenous catheters.

Solution Infusion and Administration

Volumetric infusion pumps should be used to deliver the parenteral solution at a constant rate to prevent metabolic complications. Protocols for external delivery system tubing changes are provided by infection control guidelines. Routine flushing of intravenous catheters is recommended to maintain catheter patency. Needleless intravenous access devices reduce risk of needlestick injuries but can increase risk of catheter-related infections. According to the Intravenous Nurses Society standards of practice, needleless devices should be changed every 24 hours, the injection port should be disinfected with alcohol before accessing, and all junctions should be secured with Luer-Lok, clasps, or threaded devices.[91]

Infusion of PN is generally over 24 hours, particularly in the critically ill. PN is usually cycled for patients at home or who need "time off" during hospitalization for physical therapy or other routine activities. PN can be cycled over 10 to 12 hours if desired and if the patient can tolerate the larger volume over a shorter period. The rate of infusion is based on the final compounded volume and length of time the infusion is to be given. Administration of PN should be adjusted based on the patient's response and tolerance to the regimen (see the Perspectives in Practice box, "Parenteral Nutrition Administration"). When PN is being discontinued, the infusion rate should be cut by one half for 1 hour and then stopped. Abrupt interruption of PN infusion may require hanging 10% dextrose to prevent possible rebound hypoglycemia.[75]

PERSPECTIVES IN PRACTICE

Parenteral Nutrition Administration

Of all the various ways of nourishing the human body—normal eating, liquid diets, enteral nutrition (EN), and parenteral nutrition (PN)—PN requires the highest level of skilled and precise administration. A risk of potentially life-threatening complication and infection exists. Trained nutrition support clinicians are central to the success of PN. The nutrition support nurse administers the PN solution according to the nutrition support team protocol, monitoring the entire PN system frequently to see that it is operating accurately.

Specific clinical protocols will vary somewhat, but they usually include the following points:

- *Schedule carefully:* PN volume can vary from 1 to 3 L and should be infused with an infusion pump. The infusion rate is based on the total volume of the compounded solution.
- *Monitor closely:* Note metabolic effects of glucose and electrolytes. Blood glucose levels should not exceed 200 mg/dL during initiation of PN and should not exceed 110 to 150 mg/dL when the patient is stable on the formula. First-day formulas generally contain no more than 200 g dextrose. Monitor glycemic tolerance closely, particularly the first couple of days, as the feeding is advanced. Electrolyte status and glucose levels should be determined before and throughout PN administration. Increase energy provision only as patient tolerates macronutrient content.
- *Make changes cautiously:* Monitor and report the effect of all changes, and proceed slowly.
- *Maintain a constant rate:* Keep to the correct hourly infusion rate, with no "catch-up" or "slow-down" effort to meet the original volume order.
- *Discontinue PN:* Reduce the rate by one half for 1 hour before discontinuing. If patient has had insulin added to PN and is not receiving enteral tube feeding, then monitor for rebound hypoglycemia (check serum glucose 2 hours after stopping PN infusion).

Monitoring

Complications of PN include catheter, GI, and metabolic problems (see Box 19-3). In the hands of well-trained PN clinicians, risks can be minimized and complications controlled.[92] Specific evidence-based protocols, updated periodically, guide continuing assessment and monitoring.[93] Every patient on PN should undergo a routine nutrition reassessment with adjustments made in the feeding regimen according to the patient's metabolic and nutritional needs. Every effort should be made to transition the patient from PN to enteral tube feeding or oral diet whenever feasible or appropriate. Providing at least a portion of energy via the GI tract may help reduce the adverse effects associated with PN.[64]

HOME NUTRITION SUPPORT

Patients who are discharged with home nutrition support and those who started on nutrition support while in the home require special consideration. Several factors must be evaluated to ensure that the home environment is safe and the patient and family are able and willing to accept the responsibility of home infusion therapy. The home should have refrigeration, running water, electricity, and adequate storage for supplies. The patient and family must be capable of and willing to learn techniques required to administer and manage the feeding access. It is also important that the patient and family accept responsibility to comply with the infusion regimen so that the patient receives nutrients as prescribed. Ongoing communication occurs among the patient, physician, and home infusion provider, but ultimately the patient must self-manage the therapy and work closely with the home nutrition support team. The Oley Foundation (www.oley.org) provides a network of support for patients on chronic, long-term home enteral and parenteral therapies. Reimbursement for services must be confirmed before sending a patient home on nutrition support. The process can require additional diagnostic testing and documentation in order for the patient to qualify, particularly when Medicare is the source of reimbursement.

Home Enteral Tube Feeding
Patient Selection
Developments in enteral tube feeding formulas and portable, lightweight infusion equipment have simplified home tube feeding and made it easier to manage. As a result, the number of patients who receive home tube feeding continues to grow as a means of cutting hospital costs and allowing earlier family support at home. The success of home infusion of enteral tube feeding relies on the education and training of patient and family.[94]

Teaching Plan
Educating the patient and family for home infusion of enteral tube feeding is a team responsibility. This team may be hospital based or affiliated with the home infusion company that will manage the patient's care after discharge. The RD, nurse, and pharmacist develop and carry out a teaching plan, which includes topics and related tasks in preparing patients and families for discharge on home enteral feeding (Box 19-7).[89] The goal is to promote self-care and monitoring.

The hospital or home infusion company should provide a teaching manual with illustrations to guide the teaching-learning process and that can be used as a reference at home. The teaching plan should start as soon as the decision for home tube feeding is made. A social worker identifies and, if possible, resolves any personal, psychosocial, safety, or economic issues with home infusion.

Finally, the teaching plan should allow sufficient time before discharge for the patient and family to demonstrate competency in administering the tube feeding formula and recording all necessary information about formula and fluid intake, formula tolerance, and complications. Directions for recording information are included in the home infusion manual. Records are reviewed regularly by the home nutrition support team and the patient's physician.

BOX 19-7 HOME ENTERAL TUBE FEEDING EDUCATION TOPICS AND TASKS

- Which enteral formulation is used and why
- How to prepare the tube feeding formula for infusion
- How to infuse the formula through the feeding tube
- How to correctly use and troubleshoot problems with the equipment
- How much water and how often to flush the feeding tube
- How to care for the tube site
- How to recognize tube feeding formula intolerance
- How to avoid and treat complications
- How to give medications and other separate nutrients through the feeding tube
- When to call the physician or home infusion provider

Follow-up Monitoring
The plan for follow-up monitoring should be guided by specific protocols developed by the home infusion provider for laboratory, clinical, and home nutrition assessments. The home nutrition support team checks the patient's progress and works with the patient and family to troubleshoot any problems that arise and make required adjustments in the formula or tube feeding plan. Whenever feasible and appropriate, the RD works closely with the patient and family to transition from tube feeding to oral intake. A study by Silver and colleagues[95] reported older adults who received home enteral tube feeding with no consistent clinical follow-up experienced complications associated with unscheduled health care visits and readmissions to the hospital. This study demonstrated the potential for improving outcomes with more frequent monitoring, reassessment, and intervention by a home nutrition support team that includes an RD.

Home Parenteral Nutrition
The patient sent home with PN requires education and training on the provision of PN in the outpatient setting. In the hands of knowledgeable and capable patients and their families, home PN allows mobility and independence. Equipment used in the home is small and portable, fitting in a backpack and allowing patients to resume normal activities. The patient and family must be trained to use aseptic technique for adding micronutrients and medications to the solution and for accessing the intravenous catheter or port. Special equipment, solutions, and guidelines for training and supervising patients and families have been developed and are successfully used by hundreds of patients. Ongoing assessment of GI function must be performed to determine if the patient is ready to transition to enteral feedings (either oral or via feeding tube). Patients are also monitored closely for the development of complications associated with long-term PN infusion.

A study in complex inflammatory bowel disease patients demonstrated home PN could be successfully used to delay or avoid surgery.[96] The study also found anxiety about managing PN at home decreased for most of the patients after 1 week at home.

HEALTH PROMOTION
TROUBLESHOOTING DIARRHEA IN TUBE-FED PATIENTS

Diarrhea is one of the most common complications associated with tube feeding, yet the reported incidence ranges widely, from as little as 2% to as much as 70% in general patient populations to as high as 80% in ICU patients. Questions that relate to this wide variance and that plague investigators apparently center on definition and cause. However, the ultimate bottom line for patients, their families, and health insurers is the cost of the clinical search for the cause of diarrhea in these patients and the appropriate method of treatment. Although clinicians search for an effective treatment, diarrhea results in reduced energy intake, dehydration, electrolyte abnormalities, and skin breakdown. Diarrhea also causes the patient discomfort, embarrassment, and frustration.

Problem of Definition

Several definitions of enteral feeding–related diarrhea have been used in the literature. However, little agreement exists concerning which definition most accurately reflects diarrhea that requires intervention. Common definitions include output of more than 500 mL on 2 consecutive days or more than three stools per day. From a nursing standpoint, collection and measurement of stool outputs are much less desirable than tracking the number of occurrences. However, the true definition of diarrhea may need to reflect consistency and volume and not just the number of stools per 24 hours. Most institutions do not have a standard definition for diarrhea; therefore in most cases, diarrhea is defined by the person cleaning it up. Diagnosis of the cause of diarrhea and subsequent treatment consume time and health care resources. Meanwhile the patient is losing fluid, electrolytes, and nutrients through uncontrolled stool output. This can further exacerbate impaired nutritional status. Diarrhea not only takes a physical and nutritional toll on the patient but also has a psychologic effect of embarrassment and humiliation from an inability to control bodily functions and the loss of privacy.

A recently reported case of unexplained diarrhea in a tube-fed patient illustrates the difficult—and often expensive—search for the cause (see the Case Study box, "Case of the Costly Chase").

Factors Contributing to Diarrhea

Reported causes of diarrhea in tube-fed patients also vary. The finger of blame for diarrhea usually is aimed at the tube feeding formula. This results in manipulation of the formula—selection and concentration and infusion methods—usually to no avail because feeding intolerance is generally a manifestation, not the cause, of diarrhea. A variety of causes for diarrhea have been reported. The most common contributors to diarrhea in tube-fed patients are medications or some aspect of the patient's condition. However, many times a combination of events or therapies (not a single contributor) results in diarrhea.[53,54,87-100]

Formula

Tube feeding formula osmolality or concentration and rate of delivery are often blamed for instigating diarrhea. However, reports have shown no increase in the incidence of diarrhea when the formula concentration varied widely from 145 to 430 mOsm/L, and no significant association has been made between malabsorption and formula osmolality or rate of delivery. Formulas that provide more than 30% of total kcalories as fat have been associated with an increased incidence of diarrhea, whereas those providing 20% fat rarely were involved. Further study of fat composition is needed, specifically comparing medium-chain triglycerides (MCTs) versus long-chain triglycerides (LCTs) and omega-3 versus omega-6 fatty acids. Studies of the role of fiber in tube feedings have had conflicting results. No consistency is seen in the types and amount of fiber in enteral tube feeding formulas. Soluble fiber can increase colonic absorption of water. However, when the fiber given to a patient is increased rapidly, the patient will experience flatulence, abdominal distention, and constipation. Reviewers have found that studies thus far have been few, the models used have been variable, limitations were substantial, and the conclusions of investigators were mixed. In general, the amount and type of fiber in enteral formulas are not significant enough to prevent or contribute to diarrhea.[53,54,97-100]

Bacterial Contamination

Studies have shown the more manipulation and additives, such as modular components, that are added to an enteral formula, the more likely the formula will become contaminated. Tube feeding formula hang time, open versus closed delivery systems, and preparation technique can affect the risk of bacterial contamination of the enteral tube feeding formula. Formula added to open delivery systems should hang no longer than 8 hours (and for even shorter periods of time if additives are combined with the formula). Closed systems that use containers prefilled with formula can hang 24 to 48 hours. The fewer times any system is handled and opened, the less chance exists for contamination. Commercial formula manufacturers are making formulas now that contain microbial inhibitors to reduce the risk of bacterial contamination of the enteral formula itself.[53,54,97-100]

Infusion Method

Intragastric feedings are associated with an increased incidence of diarrhea. Infusion of a large amount of energy into the stomach stimulates the colon to secrete water, sodium,

Case of the Costly Chase

A reported case of unexplained diarrhea in a tube-fed patient illustrates the difficult, and often costly, search for the cause. Max was a 55-year-old man who had had an aortic aneurysm and undergone emergency surgery to repair it. In the intensive care unit (ICU), the postoperative course was complicated by respiratory problems requiring ventilator assistance. He was administered a bronchodilator drug, theophylline, in tablet form, crushed and administered by nasogastric tube with water. When Max was started on an enteral tube feeding with an isotonic formula, crushed theophylline tablets were changed to a sugar-free theophylline solution. Within a day Max began to have progressive abdominal distention and continuous liquid diarrhea. To rule out an abdominal catastrophe related to the aneurysm or surgery, a computed abdominal tomography scan, an aortogram, and colonoscopy were performed, but all of these studies produced normal results.

Despite stopping the enteral tube feeding, the distention and diarrhea continued. Stool specimens were tested for fecal leukocytes, parasites, and *Clostridium difficile* toxin, and an enteric pathogen culture was prepared. All were nondiagnostic. Extensive additional serum and urine tests, as well as a sigmoidoscopy with rectal biopsy, gave no clue. Then stool electrolytes and osmolality measures suggested an osmotic diarrhea. Because Max was not receiving enteral tube feedings, his physicians thought a secretory bacterial toxin was probably causing continuing diarrhea, so the previous studies were repeated to confirm the osmotic nature of the diarrhea. In addition, all medications were reviewed, but none appeared to be the cause.

Because the continued diarrhea prohibited enteral tube feeding and Max needed to be fed, parenteral nutrition (PN) was ordered. This move immediately brought an automatic nutrition support service consultation, which included assessment of medications. This evaluation revealed that the sugar-free theophylline solution was 65% sorbitol.

Sorbitol is a polyhydric alcohol used as a sweetener in many sugar-free products such as dietetic foods and chewing gum. Because sorbitol is considered an "inactive" ingredient, the package label and insert contained no information about it. Sorbitol content was obtained by contacting the manufacturer.

Fortunately for Max, however, the nutrition support team did know the components of the medication and found the hidden culprit. The registered dietitian (RD) knew sorbitol in larger doses acted as a laxative. Calculations of the regular daily amount of theophylline Max was taking showed he was receiving nearly 300 g of sorbitol daily when the usual laxative dose was only 20 to 50 g. The nutrition support team immediately recommended that this sorbitol-sweetened solution of theophylline be discontinued and a sorbitol-free form of the medication be used instead. Almost immediately the diarrhea began to decrease, and in 3 days it was gone.

The extent of this costly chase was revealed in Max's hospital bill. He had continued to receive the faulty drug for almost half of his 3-month hospital stay, during which time the diarrhea prevented enteral tube feeding and he had to have the more expensive PN. The PN cost $5000 more than enteral feedings would have cost for the same period. In addition, all the extensive investigations to find the cause of the diarrhea cost $5300, which together with the indirect costs for extra days of care and supplies made a total hospital bill of about $200,000.

Causes of diarrhea in tube-fed patients are many, but in the hands of a skilled nutrition support team, the formula is seldom one of them. It is often found in the medications. Just remember what this medication's hidden ingredient—sorbitol—cost Max.

Data from Wong K: The role of fiber in diarrhea management. *Support Line* 20:16, 1998.

and chloride with resulting inability of the colon to absorb nutrients.[53,54,97-100]

Patient's Condition

Malnourished or critically ill patients are more susceptible to mucosal tissue breakdown and malabsorption leading to diarrhea. Hypoalbuminemia has also been reported to be a potential cause of diarrhea because of its effect on reducing colloidal osmotic pressure within blood vessels, which could lead to edema of the intestinal mucosa, malabsorption, and diarrhea. However, no correlation has been found between patients with hypoalbuminemia and incidence of diarrhea. Patients with pancreatic insufficiency, celiac disease, short-bowel syndrome, fecal impaction, diabetes mellitus, or GI inflammation are at increased risk for diarrhea.[53,54,97-100]

Medications

Multiple medications routinely given to hospitalized patients have been related to diarrhea. Antibiotics are most often associated with GI side effects. However, patients more susceptible to developing diarrhea are those who are critically ill and on multiple medications. Extensive treatment with antibiotics and disuse of the GI tract contribute to a change in the bacterial milieu of the intestine, with proliferation of the enteric pathogen *Clostridium difficile*. Other medications associated with development of diarrhea are H_2-blockers, lactulose or laxatives, magnesium-containing antacids, potassium and phosphorus supplements, antineoplastic agents, and quinidine. Medications are often hyperosmolar and require dilution before infusion through a feeding tube. In general, drug reactions may relate to the metabolically active agent or to another ingredient added for its physical properties in the form of the drug, such as tablet or liquid (as the case in the *Case Study* box illustrates). Probiotics, nonpathogenic lactic acid bacteria, are receiving more attention as a potential treatment of diarrhea and as a means of preventing bacterial overgrowth and *C. difficile* infections.[53,54,97-100]

TO SUM UP

For patients with functioning GI tracts, EN support has proved to be a potent tool against present or potential malnutrition. EN support is achieved by an oral diet with nutrient-dense supplementation or alternately by tube feeding when the patient cannot, will not, or should not eat. Commercial tube feeding formulas with or without modular enhancement provide complete nutrition when provided in adequate amounts. Enteral tube feeding can be provided through nasoenteric or enterostomy feeding tubes with an open or closed delivery system. Tubing and container adaptations and development of small, mobile infusion pumps, together with a comprehensive teaching plan for patient and family and follow-up monitoring by a clinical team, allow many patients the option of home tube feeding.

For patients with a dysfunctional GI tract, PN is a life-sustaining therapy. This feeding method depends heavily on biomedical technology for the development of tubes, bags, pumps, and other equipment for feeding nutrients directly into the vein. The route of entry may be a large central vein for intravenous feeding over a long period or a smaller peripheral vein for feeding less-concentrated solutions for a shorter period. Home PN is successfully used by many patients with the support of family, friends, and a home nutrition support team.

QUESTIONS FOR REVIEW

1. Describe several types of patient situations in which enteral tube feeding may be indicated. What nutrition assessment procedures may help to identify these individuals?
2. Describe nutrient components of a typical complete polymeric enteral formula. How does it differ from a modular formula? How does it differ from a semielemental and an elemental formula?
3. Define PN, and identify examples of conditions in which it would be used.

The following questions apply to the case of a man referred to nutrition support services. Imagine you are caring for this patient.

While on a long transport haul as a truck driver, a previously healthy 45-year-old man was in an accident in which he sustained a severe abdominal injury that required extensive surgical repair and left the GI tract unavailable for use for an undetermined period. He is referred to the nutrition support team for PN. Early in this care he asks you how this feeding works.

4. How would you describe and explain the PN feeding process?
5. What nutrition assessment parameters would be beneficial in identifying his risk of developing malnutrition and his tolerance of parenteral therapy?
6. List typical components of a basic PN formula he may require, and describe the purpose of each to help reassure him of its adequacy and importance.
7. Sufficient energy (kcalorie) intake is essential to immediately meet his metabolic needs after surgery. Assume a normal preinjury weight (175 lb) and height (70 inches) and an added stress factor of 1.2 times his BEE. Calculate his total energy requirement, using the Harris-Benedict equation and the Mifflin-St. Jeor equation. Compare the results.
8. Define hepatic proteins, and describe why they are not appropriate indicators of nutritional status. How can you monitor the effectiveness of the PN formula in meeting his nutrition support needs for recovery?

REFERENCES

1. Borum PR: Nutrient metabolism. In Gottschlich MM, Fuhrman T, Hammond K, editors: *The science and practice of nutrition support: a case-based core curriculum*, Dubuque, Iowa, 2001, Kendall/Hunt Publishing.
2. Butterworth CE: The skeleton in the hospital closet. *Nutr Today* 9:4, 1974.
3. Bistrian BR, Blackburn GL, Hallowell E, et al: Protein status of general surgical patients. *JAMA* 230:858, 1974.
4. Naber T, Schermer T, de Bree A, et al: Prevalence of malnutrition in nonsurgical hospitalized patients and its association with disease complications. *Am J Clin Nutr* 66:1232, 1997.
5. Detsky AS, McLaughlin JR, Baker JP, et al: What is subjective global assessment of nutritional status? *JPEN J Parenter Enteral Nutr* 11(1):8, 1987.
6. Braunschweig C, Gomez S, Sheean PM, et al: Impact of declines in nutritional status on outcomes in adult patients hospitalized for more than seven days. *J Am Diet Assoc* 100:1316, 2000.
7. A.S.P.E.N. Board of Directors and the Clinical Guidelines Task Force: Guidelines for the use of parenteral and enteral nutrition in adult and pediatric patients. *JPEN J Parenter Enteral Nutr* 26:1SA, 2002.
8. Moore FA, Feliciano DV, Andrassy RJ, et al: Early enteral feeding, compared with parenteral, reduces postoperative septic complications: the results of a meta-analysis. *Ann Surg* 216:172, 1992.
9. Lipman TO: Grains or veins: is enteral nutrition really better than parenteral nutrition? A look at the evidence. *JPEN J Parenter Enteral Nutr* 22:167, 1998.
10. Shopbell JM, Hopkins JB, Shronts EP, et al: Nutrition screening and assessment. In Gottschlich MM, Fuhrman T,

Hammond K, editors: *The science and practice of nutrition support: a case-based core curriculum*, Dubuque, Iowa, 2001, Kendall/Hunt Publishing.

11. Lacey K, Pritchett E: Nutrition care process and model: ADA adopts road map to quality care and outcomes management. *J Am Diet Assoc* 103:1061, 2003.

12. Fuhrman MP, Charney P, Mueller CM, et al: Hepatic proteins and nutrition assessment. *J Am Diet Assoc* 104:1258, 2004.

13. Reference deleted in proofs.

14. Mifflin MD, St. Jeor ST, Hill LA, et al: A new predictive equation for resting energy expenditure in healthy individuals. *Am J Clin Nutr* 51(2):241, 1990.

15. Frankenfield DC, Rowe WA, Smith JS, et al: Validation of several established equations for resting metabolic rate in obese and nonobese people. *J Am Diet Assoc* 103:1152, 2003.

16. Crook MA, Hally V, Panteli JV, et al: The importance of the refeeding syndrome. *Nutrition* 17:632, 2001.

17. Vanek VW: The use of serum albumin as a prognostic or nutritional marker and the pros and cons of IV albumin therapy. *Nutr Clin Pract* 13:110, 1998.

18. Meyer J, Lund D, Smith J, et al: Benefits of a nutrition support service in an HMO setting. *Nutr Clin Pract* 16:25, 2001.

19. American Society for Parenteral and Enteral Nutrition Board of Directors: Standards of practice for nutrition support nurses. *Nutr Clin Pract* 16:56, 2001.

20. American Society for Parenteral and Enteral Nutrition Board of Directors: Standards of practice for nutrition support pharmacists. *Nutr Clin Pract* 14:275, 1999.

21. American Society for Parenteral and Enteral Nutrition Board of Directors: Standards of practice for nutrition support physicians. *Nutr Clin Pract* 18:270, 2003.

22. American Society for Parenteral and Enteral Nutrition Board of Directors: Standards of practice for nutrition support dietitians. *Nutr Clin Pract* 15:53, 2000.

23. Board of Directors, American Society for Parenteral and Enteral Nutrition: Interdisciplinary nutrition support core competencies. *Nutr Clin Pract* 14:331, 1999.

24. The Joint Commission Board of Directors: *Comprehensive accreditation manual for hospitals*, Oakbrook Terrace, Ill., 2014, The Joint Commision.

25. Fuhrman MP: Parenteral nutrition: a clinician's perspective. *Diet Edge* 2(1):53, 2001.

26. Charney P: Enteral nutrition: indications, options and formulations. In Gottschlich MM, Fuhrman T, Hammond K, editors: *The science and practice of nutrition support: a case-based core curriculum*, Dubuque, Iowa, 2001, Kendall/Hunt Publishing.

27. Roth JL, Clohessy S: Administration of enteral nutrition: initiation, progression, and transition. In Rolandelli RH, editor: *Clinical nutrition: enteral and tube feeding*, ed 4, Philadelphia, Pa., 2005, Saunders.

28. Veterans Affairs Total Parenteral Nutrition Cooperative Study Group: Perioperative total parenteral nutrition in surgical patients. *N Engl J Med* 325:525, 1992.

29. Jeejeebhoy KN: Total parenteral nutrition: potion or poison? *Am J Clin Nutr* 74:160, 2001.

30. Lewis DA, Boyle K: Nutritional supplement use during medication administration: selected case studies. *J Nutr Elder* 17(4):53, 1998.

31. Turic A, Gordon KL, Craig LD, et al: Nutrition supplementation enables elderly residents in long-term care facilities to meet or exceed RDAs without displacing energy or nutrient intakes from meals. *J Am Diet Assoc* 98:1457, 1998.

32. Watters JM, Kirkpatrick SM, Norris SB, et al: Immediate postoperative enteral feeding results in impaired respiratory mechanics and decreased mobility. *Ann Surg* 266:369, 1997.

33. Charney P, Russell M: Enteral formulations: standard. In Rolandelli RH, editor: *Clinical nutrition: enteral and tube feeding*, ed 4, Philadelphia, Pa., 2005, Saunders.

34. Matarese LE, Seidner DL, Steiger E, et al: The role of probiotics in gastrointestinal disease. *Nutr Clin Pract* 18:507, 2003.

35. Gadek JE, DeMichele SJ, Karlstad MD, et al: Effect of enteral feeding with eicosapentaenoic acid, α-linolenic acid, and antioxidants in patients with acute respiratory distress syndrome. *Crit Care Med* 27:1409, 1999.

36. Consensus recommendations from the U.S.: Summit on Immune-Enhancing Enteral Therapy. *JPEN J Parenter Enteral Nutr* 25:S61, 2001.

37. Reference deleted in proofs.

38. Metheny NA, Clouse RE: Bedside methods for detecting aspiration in tube-fed patients. *Chest* 111:724, 1997.

39. Maloney JP, Halbower AC, Fouty BF, et al: Systemic absorption of food dye in patients with sepsis. *N Engl J Med* 343:1047, 2000.

40. Maloney JP, Ryan TA: Detection of aspiration in enterally fed patients: a requiem for bedside monitors of aspiration. *JPEN J Parenter Enteral Nutr* 26:S34, 2002.

41. Maloney J, Metheny N: Controversy in using blue dye in enteral tube feeding as a method of detecting pulmonary aspiration. *Crit Care Nurse* 22:84, 2002.

42. Moore MC, editor: *Enteral nutrition. Mosby's pocket guide series: nutritional care*, ed 4, St Louis, Mo., 2001, Mosby.

43. Metheny NA, Stewart BJ, Smith L, et al: pH and concentration of bilirubin in feeding tube aspirates as predictors of tube placement. *Nurs Res* 48(4):189, 1999.

44. Metheny N, Eisenberg P, McSweeney M, et al: Effect of feeding tube properties and three irrigants on clogging rates. *Nurs Res* 37:165, 1988.

45. Sriram K, Jayanthi V, Lakshmi RG, et al: Prophylactic locking of enteral feeding tubes with pancreatic enzymes. *JPEN J Parenter Enteral Nutr* 21(6):353, 1997.

46. Marian M, Carlson SJ: Enteral formulations. In Merritt R, DeLegge MH, Holcombe B, editors: *A.S.P.E.N. nutrition support practice manual*, Silver Spring, Md., 2005, American Society for Parenteral and Enteral Nutrition.

47. Vanek VW: Closed versus open enteral delivery systems: a quality improvement study. *Nutr Clin Pract* 15:234, 2000.

48. Herlick SJ, Vogt C, Pangman V, et al: Comparison of open versus closed systems of intermittent enteral feeding in two long-term care facilities. *Nutr Clin Pract* 15:287, 2000.

49. Keohane PP, Attrill H, Love M, et al: Relation between osmolarity of the diet and gastrointestinal side effects in enteral nutrition. *BJM* 288:678, 1984.

50. Lysen LK: Enteral equipment. In Matarese LE, Gottschlich MM, editors: *Contemporary nutrition support practice: a clinical guide*, ed 2, Philadelphia, Pa., 2003, Saunders.

51. Ibáñaez J, Peñafiel A, Raurich JM, et al: Gastroesophageal reflux in intubated patients receiving enteral nutrition: effect of supine and semirecumbent positions. *JPEN J Parenter Enteral Nutr* 16:419, 1992.

52. Cogen R, Weinryb J, Pomerantz C, et al: Complications of jejunostomy tube feeding in nursing facility patients. *Am J Gastroenterol* 86:1610, 1991.

53. Mobarhan S, Demeo M: Diarrhea induced by enteral feeding. *Nutr Rev* 53:67, 1995.

54. Fuhrman MP: Diarrhea and tube feeding. *Nutr Clin Pract* 14:83, 1999.

55. Kirby DF, Delegge MH, Fleming CR, et al: American Gastroenterological Association technical review on tube feeding for enteral nutrition. *Gastroenterology* 108:1282, 1995.

56. McClave SA, Snider HL, Lowen CC, et al: Use of residual volume as a marker for enteral feeding tolerance: prospective, blinded comparison with physical examination and radiographic findings. *JPEN J Parenter Enteral Nutr* 16(2):99, 1992.

57. Pinilla JC, Samphire J, Arnold C, et al: Comparison of gastrointestinal tolerance to two enteral feeding protocols in critically ill patients: a prospective, randomized trial. *JPEN J Parenter Enteral Nutr* 25:81, 2001.

58. Heyland DK, Dhaliwal R, Drover JW, et al: Canadian clinical practice guidelines for nutrition support in mechanically ventilated, critically ill adult patients. *JPEN J Parenter Enteral Nutr* 27:355, 2003.

59. Mateo MA: Nursing management of enteral tube feeding. *Heart Lung* 25:318, 1996.

60. Spain DA, McClave SA, Sexton LK, et al: Infusion protocol improves delivery of enteral tube feeding in the critical care unit. *JPEN J Parenter Enteral Nutr* 23:288, 1999.

61. Heyland DK, Dhaliwal R, Day A, et al: Validation of the Canadian clinical practice guidelines for nutrition support in mechanically ventilated, critically ill adult patients: results of a prospective observational study. *Crit Care Med* 32:2260, 2004.

62. van den Berghe G, Wouters P, Weekers F, et al: Intensive insulin therapy in critically ill patients. *N Engl J Med* 345:1359, 2001.

63. Krinsley JS: Effect of an intensive glucose management protocol on the mortality of critically ill adult patients. *Mayo Clin Proc* 79:992, 2004.

64. Fuhrman MP: Complication management in parenteral nutrition. In Matarese LE, Gottschlich MM, editors: *Contemporary nutrition support practice: a clinical guide*, ed 2, Philadelphia, Pa., 2003, Saunders.

65. Mirtallo JM: Introduction to parenteral nutrition. In Gottschlich MM, Fuhrman T, Hammond K, editors: *The science and practice of nutrition support: a case-based core curriculum*, Dubuque, Iowa, 2001, Kendall/Hunt Publishing.

66. Dudrick SJ, Wilmore DW, Vars HM, et al: Can intravenous feeding as the sole means of nutrition support growth in the child and restore weight loss in an adult? *Ann Surg* 169:974, 1969.

67. Klein S, Kinney J, Jeejeebhoy K, et al: Nutrition support in clinical practice: review of published data on recommendations for future directions. *JPEN J Parenter Enter Nutr* 21(3):133, 1997.

68. Stokes MA, Hill GL: Peripheral parenteral nutrition: a preliminary report on its efficacy and safety. *JPEN J Parenter Enteral Nutr* 17(2):145, 1993.

69. Trujillo ED, Young LS, Chertow GM, et al: Metabolic and monetary costs of avoidable parenteral nutrition use. *JPEN J Parenter Enteral Nutr* 23:109, 1999.

70. Speerhas RA: Five year follow-up of a program to minimize inappropriate use of parenteral nutrition. *JPEN J Parenter Enteral Nutr* 25:S4, 2001.

71. Tulsyan N, Abkin AD, Storch KJ, et al: Enterocutaneous fistulas. *Nutr Clin Pract* 16:74, 2001.

72. Byrne TA, Veglia L, Celio M, et al: Beyond the prescription: optimizing the diet of patients with short bowel syndrome. *Nutr Clin Pract* 15:306, 2000.

73. Spain DA, McClave SA: Chylothorax and chylous ascites. In Gottschlich MM, Fuhrman T, Hammond K, editors: *The science and practice of nutrition support: a case-based core curriculum*, Dubuque, Iowa, 2001, Kendall/Hunt Publishing.

74. Kelly DG, Nehra V: Gastrointestinal disease. In Gottschlich MM, Fuhrman T, Hammond K, editors: *The science and practice of nutrition support: a case-based core curriculum*, Dubuque, Iowa, 2001, Kendall/ Hunt Publishing.

75. Task force for the revision of safe practices for parenteral nutrition, et al: Safe practices for parenteral nutrition. *JPEN J Parenter Enteral Nutr* 28(Suppl):S39, 2004.

76. Seidner DL, Mascioli EA, Istfan NW, et al: Effect of long-chain triglyceride emulsions on reticuloendothelial system function in humans. *JPEN J Parenter Enteral Nutr* 13:614, 1989.

77. American Medical Association, AMA Department of Foods and Nutrition: Multivitamin preparations for parenteral use: a statement by the Nutrition Advisory Group. *JPEN J Parenter Enteral Nutr* 3:258, 1979.

78. Parenteral multivitamin products; drugs for human use; drug efficacy study implementation; amendment (21 CFR 5.70). *Fed Regist* 65:21200, 2000.

79. Expert Panel for Nutrition Advisory Group, AMA Department of Foods and Nutrition: Guidelines for essential trace element preparations for parenteral use. *JAMA* 241:2051, 1979.

80. Forceville X, Vitoux D, Gauzit R, et al: Selenium, systemic immune response syndrome, sepsis, and outcome in critically ill patients. *Crit Care Med* 26:1536, 1998.

81. Angstwurm MAW, Schottdorf J, Schopohl J, et al: Selenium replacement in patients with severe systemic inflammatory response syndrome improves clinical outcome. *Crit Care Med* 27:1807, 1999.

82. Cohen HJ, Brown MR, Hamilton D, et al: Glutathione peroxidase and selenium deficiency in patients receiving home parenteral nutrition: time course for development of deficiency and repletion of the enzyme activity in plasma and blood cells. *Am J Clin Nutr* 49:132, 1989.

83. Fuhrman MP, Herrmann V, Masidonski P, et al: Pancytopenia following removal of copper from TPN. *JPEN J Parenter Enteral Nutr* 24:361, 2000.

84. Masumoto K, Suita S, Taguchi T, et al: Manganese intoxication during intermittent parenteral nutrition: report of two cases. *JPEN J Parenter Enteral Nutr* 25:95, 2001.

85. Pemberton L, Lyman B, Lander V, et al: Sepsis from triple- vs single-lumen catheters during total parenteral nutrition in surgical or critically ill patients. *Arch Surg* 121:591, 1986.

86. Farkas J, Liu N, Bier P, et al: Single- versus triple-lumen central–catheter-related sepsis: a prospective randomized study in a critically ill population. *Am J Med* 93:277, 1992.

87. Savage AP, Picard M, Hopkins CC, et al: Complications and survival of multilumen central venous catheters used for total parenteral nutrition. *Br J Surg* 80:1287, 1993.

88. Maki DG, Stolz SM, Wheler S, et al: Prevention of central venous catheter-related bloodstream infection by use of an antiseptic-impregnated catheter: a randomized, controlled trial. *Ann Intern Med* 127:257, 1997.

89. Veenstra DL, Saint S, Sullivan SD, et al: Cost-effectiveness of antiseptic-impregnated central venous catheters for the prevention of catheter-related bloodstream infection. *J Am Med Assoc* 282:554, 1999.

90. Centers for Disease Control and Prevention: Guidelines for the prevention of intravascular catheter-related infections. *MMWR Morb Mortal Wkly Rep* 51(RR–10):1, 2002.

91. Intravenous Nurses Society: Infusion nursing standards of practice. *J Intraven Nurs* 23(Suppl 6):S1, 2000.

92. Dodds ES, Murray JD, Texler KM, et al: Metabolic occurrences in total parenteral nutrition patients managed by a nutrition support team. *Nutr Clin Pract* 16:78, 2001.

93. Klein CJ, Stanek GS, Wiles CE, et al: Nutrition support care map targets monitoring and reassessment to improve outcomes in trauma patients. *Nutr Clin Pract* 16:85, 2001.

94. American Society for Parenteral and Enteral Nutrition Board of Directors: Standards for home nutrition support. *Nutr Clin Pract* 14:151, 1998.

95. Silver HJ, Wellman NS, Arnold DJ, et al: Older adults receiving home enteral nutrition: enteral regimen, provider involvement, and health care outcomes. *JPEN J Parenter Enteral Nutr* 28:92, 2004.

96. Evans JP, Steinhart AH, Cohen Z, et al: Home total parenteral nutrition: an alternative to early surgery for complicated inflammatory bowel disease. *J Gastrointest Surg* 7:562, 2003.

97. Bowling TE: Enteral-feeding-related diarrhea: proposed causes and possible solutions. *Proc Nutr Soc* 54:579, 1995.

98. Ringel AF, Jameson GL, Foster ES: Diarrhea in the intensive care patient. *Crit Care Clin North Am* 11:465, 1995.

99. Wong K: The role of fiber in diarrhea management. *Support Line* 20:16, 1998.

100. Williams MS, Harpter R, Magnuson B, et al: Diarrhea management in enterally fed patient. *Nutr Clin Pract* 13:225, 1998.

FURTHER READINGS AND RESOURCES

American Society for Parenteral and Enteral Nutrition Board of Directors and Task Force on Standards for Specialized Nutrition Support of Hospitalized Adult Patients, Standards for Specialized Nutrition Support: Adult hospitalized patients. *Nutr Clin Pract* 17:384, 2002.

A.S.P.E.N. Board of Directors and the Clinical Guidelines Task Force: Guidelines for the use of parenteral and enteral nutrition in adult and pediatric patients. *JPEN J Parenter Enteral Nutr* 26(Suppl):1SA, 2002.

Heyland DK, Dhaliwal R, Drover JW, et al: Canadian clinical practice guidelines for nutrition support in mechanically ventilated, critically ill adult patients. *JPEN J Parenter Enteral Nutr* 27:355, 2003.

Task Force for the Revision of Safe Practices for Parenteral Nutrition and the A.S.P.E.N. Board of Directors: Safe practices for parenteral nutrition. *JPEN J Parenter Enteral Nutr* 28(Suppl):S30, 2004.

Websites of Interest

- The American Society for Parenteral and Enteral Nutrition (A.S.P.E.N.). An interdisciplinary organization involved in provision of clinical nutrition therapies including parenteral and enteral nutrition: www.nutritioncare.org.
- Academy of Nutrition and Dietetics. The world's largest organization of food and nutrition professionals committed to improving the nation's health and advancing the profession of dietetics through research, education, and advocacy: www.eatright.org.
- CIGNA Medicare. This site offers free Medicare training for clinicians regarding Medicare qualifications for home enteral and parenteral nutrition: www.cignamedicare.com/webtraining.
- Dietitians in Nutrition Support. Dietetic practitioners integrating the science of enteral and parenteral nutrition to provide appropriate nutrition support to individuals in inpatient and outpatient settings: www.dnsdpg.org.
- The Oley Foundation. This nonprofit organization provides information and psychosocial support of consumers of home parenteral and enteral nutrition: www.oley.org.

Gastrointestinal Diseases

Dorothy Chen-Maynard

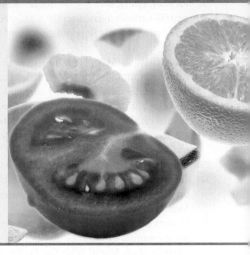

ⓔ EVOLVE WEBSITE

http://evolve.elsevier.com/Williams/essentials/

In this chapter, we consider diseases of the gastrointestinal (GI) tract and surrounding accessory organs—the liver, gallbladder, and pancreas. In health, digestion and absorption of food are accomplished through a series of intimately interrelated actions among and within these organ systems. To the extent disease or malfunction at any point interferes with this finely interwoven process, adequate nutrition is provided either through quantitative or qualitative modifications to food.

The GI tract is a sensitive mirror of the individual human condition. Its physiologic function often reflects physical and psychologic conditions. In this chapter, these basic functions, healing process, nutrition therapy indicated, and individuals' personal needs will be discussed. The Complementary and Alternative Medicine box, "Alternative Treatments for Diseases of the Gastrointestinal Tract," outlines the effectiveness of alternative treatments for diseases of the GI tract.

DIGESTIVE PROCESS

When food is taken into the mouth, the act of eating stimulates the GI tract into accelerated action. Throughout the digestive process, highly coordinated systems and interactive functions respond (Figure 20-1). Secretory functions provide the necessary environment and agents for chemical digestion. Peristalsis and gravity move the food mass along. Nutrients are absorbed into circulation and carried to cells that take up what is needed to nourish the body. Emotional factors influence overall individual response pattern. This highly individual and interrelated functional network forms the basis for nutrition therapy in disease.

After food is taken into the mouth and masticated (forming a bolus), swallowing occurs, allowing the bolus to pass from the laryngopharynx into the esophagus entrance at the upper esophageal sphincter (UES) (Figure 20-2). Food is pushed through the esophagus by gravity and involuntary muscular movements, called *peristalsis,* controlled by the medulla oblongata. Circular muscle fibers contract, constricting the esophageal wall, thereby squeezing the bolus toward the stomach. The lower esophageal sphincter (LES) muscle at the entry to the stomach forms a controlling valve, relaxing to receive the bolus and then closing to hold each bolus for some initial digestive action of enzymes. Stomach cells produce enzymes to partially break down food particles and other secretions to protect themselves from being broken down. Passage of food from mouth to stomach takes about 4 to 8 seconds.

Chyme (semiliquid mass) is released by the stomach through the pyloric sphincter into the duodenum, the first section of the small intestine, where most digestion occurs. A number of small intestine and accessory organ conditions may interfere with normal food passage and digestive

COMPLEMENTARY AND ALTERNATIVE MEDICINE (CAM)

Alternative Treatments for Diseases of the Gastrointestinal Tract

What Is Known from the Scientific Evidence About CAM Modalities for Gastrointestinal Disorders?

No well-documented herbal treatments exist for gastrointestinal (GI) disorders, although use of probiotics to treat Crohn's disease shows some promise.

What CAM Therapies Might Be Used to Treat Gastrointestinal Disorders?

Gastrointestinal Disorder	Herb	Scientific Name	Active Ingredient	Efficacy	Side Effects and/or Risks
Cirrhosis	Milk thistle (plant)	*Silybum marianum*	Silymarin (found in the fruit)	Results are inconsistent.	It is generally well tolerated but can cause laxative effects and allergic reactions in people allergic to ragweed, chrysanthemum, marigold, and daisy.
Crohn's disease	Fish oil	Docosahexaenoic acid (DHA), eicosapentaenoic acid (EPA), omega-3 fatty acids, omega-3 oils		Results are mixed as to whether or not fish oil helped keep the disease controlled in patients who were in remission.	Possible risk of bleeding complications.
Dyspepsia	Curcumin	*Curcuma longa*	Polyphenol	It stimulates contraction of the gallbladder; it provides full or partial relief of symptoms.	It could present risks in individuals with gallbladder disease. Maximum safe doses in individuals with severe hepatic or renal disease are not known.
Hepatitis C virus (HCV)	Milk thistle (plant)	*Silybum marianum*	Silymarin (found in the fruit)	Although some benefits might be seen, none are definitively beneficial in treating HCV.	See above.
	Licorice root (plant)	*Glycyrrhiza glabra*	Glycyrrhizin	Injectable form might have antiviral properties in vitro and has the potential for reducing some of short-term effects, such as fatigue and GI functions, and long-term complications of chronic HCV in patients who do not respond to interferon. It does not reduce the amount of HCV in patients' blood. (http://nccam.nih.gov/health/licoriceroot)	Licorice intake over a long period of time can lead to hypertension, salt and water retention, swelling, depletion of potassium, headache, and/or sluggishness. In addition, it can worsen ascites and can interact with certain drugs (diuretics, digitalis, antiarrhythmic agents, and corticosteroids) (see Chapter 18).
	Thymus extract (gland)	(Should not be confused with the prescription drug thymosin α₁)	Peptides from thymus glands of cows or calves sold as dietary supplements	Very little research exists, but no studies found the product beneficial for patients with HCV.	Thrombocytopenia (a drop in number of platelet cells in blood) is possible. Concern exists regarding possible contamination from diseased animal parts (people on immunosuppressive drugs should use caution).

Continued

COMPLEMENTARY AND ALTERNATIVE MEDICINE (CAM)

Alternative Treatments for Diseases of the Gastrointestinal Tract—cont'd

Gastrointestinal Disorder	Herb	Scientific Name	Active Ingredient	Efficacy	Side Effects and/or Risks
	Schisandra (plant)	*Schisandra chinensis, S. sphenanthera*	Extracts from its fruits	Some antioxidant effects are possible. No reports exist regarding the safety and effectiveness of using schisandra alone to treat HCV in humans.	It is found as an ingredient in herbal formulas and considered generally safe. In some patients it may cause heartburn, acid indigestion, decreased appetite, stomach pain, or allergic skin rashes.
	Colloidal silver	Silver	Metallic element	Silver has no known function in the human body and is not an essential mineral supplement. Claims of silver "deficiency" in the body are unfounded.	Silver builds up in body tissues: argyria—a bluish gray discoloration of the body, especially skin, other organs, deep tissues, nails, and gums. Argyria is not treatable or reversible. Other possible complications include neurologic problems (e.g., seizures), kidney damage, stomach distress, headaches, fatigue, and skin irritation. It might interfere with absorption of the following drugs: penicillamine, quinolones, tetracyclines, and thyroxine. Not safe to use.
Irritable bowel syndrome (IBS)	Peppermint oil	*Mentha piperita*	Menthol	It provides antispasmodic properties and might provide some relief from crampy abdominal pain.	Enteric-coated peppermint is believed to be reasonably safe in healthy adults; nonenteric-coated peppermint oil can cause heartburn. Maximum doses in individuals with severe hepatic or renal disease are not known.
	Probiotics	*Lactobacillus plantarum*	Acidophilus	Evidence of efficacy is mixed; it might reduce intestinal gas and pain.	No known safety issues exist.
	Flaxseed	*Linum usitatissimum*	Lignans, α-linolenic acid	It helps relieve constipation, abdominal pain, and bloating.	It is not associated with any significant adverse effects.
Nausea	Ginger	*Zingiber officinale*		It is as effective for motion sickness as standard pharmaceutical agents. In addition, it is effective in reducing nausea in pregnancy.	No drug interactions are known. Ginger should be used with care in patients using anticoagulant or antiplatelet agents.

COMPLEMENTARY AND ALTERNATIVE MEDICINE (CAM)

Alternative Treatments for Diseases of the Gastrointestinal Tract—cont'd

Gastrointestinal Disorder	Herb	Scientific Name	Active Ingredient	Efficacy	Side Effects and/or Risks
Peptic ulcer disease (PUD)	Licorice, deglycyr-rhizinated (DGL)	*Glycyrrhiza glabra*	DGL is a specially processed form of licorice that does not produce pseudohyper-aldosteronemia.	No evidence indicates that DGL eradicates *Helicobacter pylori*; it may protect gastric lining from NSAID-induced gastritis. It is no more effective than antacids in providing relief.	It may reduce testosterone levels in men. The maximum safe doses in those with severe hepatic or renal disease are not known. Licorice appears to potentiate topical and oral corticosteroids. It should be used with caution in patients taking thiazide or loop diuretics and/or digitalis.
	Probiotics	*Lactobacillus plantarum*	Acidophilus	It exerts inhibitory action on *H. pylori* but not enough to eradicate the bacterium. It may be a useful adjunct to standard antibiotic therapy.	See above.
Ulcerative colitis (UC)	Probiotics	*Escherichia coli* spp.	Nonpathogenic strain of *E. coli*	It can prevent acute attacks of UC as effectively as mesalazine.	See above.
	Essential fatty acids	DHA, EPA, omega-3 fatty acids, omega-3 oils	Fish oils	It might be helpful for reducing symptoms of UC; regular use does not appear to help prevent disease flare-ups.	See above.
	Essential fatty acids	Omega-6 fatty acid GLA	Evening primrose oil	Somewhat beneficial in preventing flare-ups.	See above.

Data from National Center for Complementary and Alternative Medicine: *CAM and hepatitis C: a focus on herbal supplements*, NCCAM Pub No D422, Bethesda, Md., 2008, NCCAM. from: <http://nccam.nih.gov/health/hepatitisc/hepatitiscfacts.htm>. Retrieved May 15, 2014; Bratman S, Girman AM: *Mosby's handbook of herbs and supplements and their therapeutic use*, St Louis, Mo., 2003, Mosby. *GLA,*γ-linolenic acid; *NSAID,* nonsteroidal antiinflammatory drug.

processes and create malabsorption problems. These overall conditions vary widely from brief periods of functional discomfort to serious disease and complete obstruction. In making nutrition therapy recommendations for food choices and feeding mode, the dietetics practitioner will take into account the degree of dysfunction.

PROBLEMS OF THE MOUTH AND ESOPHAGUS

Mouth Problems

Teeth and jaw muscles in the mouth work together to break down food into a form that can be easily swallowed.

Conditions that interfere with this process interfere with nutritional intake.

Tissue Inflammation

Tissues of the mouth often reflect a person's basic nutritional status. In malnutrition, tissues of the mouth deteriorate and become inflamed and are more vulnerable to local infection or injury, causing pain and difficulty with eating. These conditions (Figure 20-3) in the oral cavity include (1) gingivitis, inflammation of the gums, involving the mucous membrane with its supporting fibrous tissue circling the base of the teeth (see Figure 20-3, *A*); (2) stomatitis, inflammation of the oral mucosa lining the mouth (see Figure 20-3, *B*);

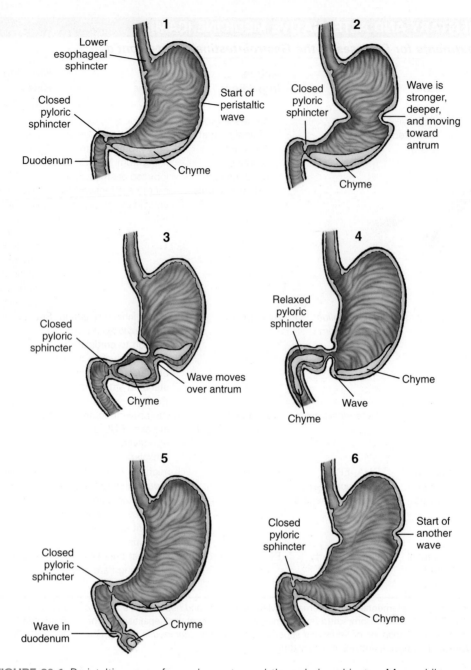

FIGURE 20-1 Peristaltic waves force chyme toward the pyloric sphincter. Meanwhile, a small amount of chyme is squirted into the duodenum, and the remainder is forced back into the stomach, where further mixing occurs. (From Monahan FD, Neighbors M: *Medical-surgical nursing: foundations for clinical practice*, ed 2, Philadelphia, Pa., 1998, Saunders.)

FIGURE 20-2 Parts of the mouth, pharynx, and esophagus involved in the swallowing process. (From Wardlaw GM, Insel PM: *Perspectives in nutrition*, ed 2, New York, 1993, McGraw-Hill.)

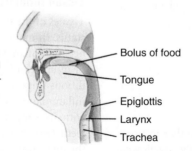
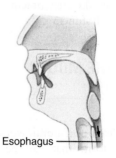
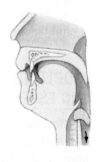

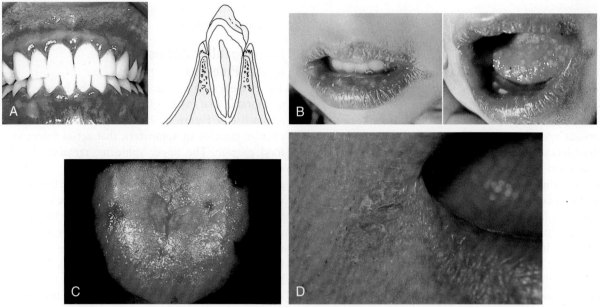

FIGURE 20-3 Tissue inflammation of the mouth. **A,** Gingivitis. **B,** Stomatitis. **C,** Glossitis. **D,** Cheilosis. (**A** from Murray PR, Rosenthal KS, Pfaller MD: *Medical microbiology,* ed 2, St Louis, Mo., 1994, Mosby; **B** from Doughty DB, Broadwell-Jackson D: *Gastrointestinal disorders,* St Louis, Mo., 1993, Mosby; **C** courtesy Hoffbrand AV, Pettit JE, Vyas P: *Color atlas of clinical hematology,* ed 4, Philadelphia, Pa., 2010, Saunders; **D** from Lemmi FO, Lemmi CAE: *Physical assessment findings,* Philadelphia, Pa., 2000, Saunders.)

(3) glossitis, inflammation of the tongue (see Figure 20-3, *C*); and (4) cheilosis, a cracking and dry scaling process at the corners of the mouth affecting the lips and corner angles, making opening the mouth to receive food difficult (see Figure 20-3, *D*).

These oral tissue problems may also be nonspecific and unrelated to nutritional factors. In some cases, gingivitis and stomatitis occur in mild form in relation to another disease or stress. Occasionally a severe form of acute necrotizing ulcerative gingivitis occurs. It is caused by a specific infectious bacterium, *Fusobacterium nucleatum,* often in conjunction with the spirochete *Treponema vincentii*; it is also known as *Vincent's disease,* from the Paris physician Henri Vincent (1862-1950), who first identified the disease process. Gums around the bases of teeth become puffy, shiny, and tender, overlapping the teeth margins. Affected gums often bleed, especially during tooth brushing. This serious condition destroys gum tissue and supporting tissues of the teeth and requires a course of antibiotic treatment.

Mouth pain in these conditions often causes decreased food intake. Maintaining adequate nutritional intake then becomes a major problem. Generally patients are given high-protein, high-energy (Calorie or kcal) liquids and then soft foods, usually nonacidic and without strong spices so as to avoid irritation. Temperature extremes may also be avoided if they cause pain. Gradually foods are increased according to toleration, and foods are often supplemented with vitamins and minerals. In severe disease, use of a mouthwash containing a mild topical local anesthetic before meals helps relieve the pain of eating.

Dental Problems

The incidence of dental caries has recently been reduced in children and young adults. However, it is still present in many children and older adults, especially those unable to afford regular dental care, and causes tooth loss and chewing problems. In older adults, periodontal disease is a major cause of tooth loss. If dental caries is untreated or if dental hygiene is poor, then gum tissue at the base of the teeth becomes damaged and pockets form between the gums and the teeth. Dental plaque forms from a sticky deposit of mucus, food particles, and bacteria. Plaque hardens into calculus, a mineralized coating developed from plaque and saliva. These hardened particles then collect in pocket openings at the base of the teeth where bacteria attack periodontal tissue. The result is bacterial erosion of bone tissue surrounding affected teeth and subsequent tooth loss. Preventive care through daily dental care with fluoridated toothpaste, careful flossing, and periodic plaque removal by a dental professional forms the best approach. Extensive tooth loss leads to the need for tooth replacement with dentures. In many older adults these dentures become ill fitting, especially when weight loss occurs, and hinder adequate chewing. All of these dental problems need to be reviewed as part of the physical assessment in any patient's nutrition history so that food textures and forms can be adjusted to individual needs.

Salivary Glands and Salivation

Disorders of the salivary glands affect eating because saliva carries an amylase that begins starch breakdown and is vital in moistening food to facilitate chewing. Problems may arise from infection, such as infection with the mumps virus that attacks the parotid gland. Other problems come from excessive salivation, which occurs in numerous disorders affecting the nervous system, such as Parkinson's disease, and from local disorders such as mouth infections or injury. Problems may arise from any disease or drug that causes overactivity of the parasympathetic division of the autonomic nervous system, which controls the salivary glands.

Conversely, lack of salivation, which causes xerostomia (dry mouth), may be a temporary condition caused by fear, salivary gland infection, or action of anticholinergic drugs that hinder the normal action of neurotransmitters. Clients with dry mouth best tolerate moist, soft foods with added gravies and sauces. Permanent xerostomia is rare but does occur in Sjögren's syndrome, a symptom complex of unknown cause thought to be an abnormal immune response. It occurs in middle-aged or older women and is marked by dry mouth and enlargement of the parotid glands; it is often associated with rheumatoid arthritis (RA) or radiation therapy. Difficulty occurs in swallowing and speaking; problems also include tooth decay and interference with taste. Salty foods dry the mouth and should be avoided. Chewing gum or sucking on sugarless candy can increase salivary secretions. Extreme mouth dryness may be partially relieved by spraying the inside of the mouth with an artificial saliva solution.

Swallowing Disorders

Most people take swallowing for granted. Each day we eat, chew, and swallow without giving it a second thought. However, the process of swallowing involves highly integrated actions of mouth, pharynx, and esophagus (see Figure 20-2). Swallowing difficulty, known medically as *dysphagia*, is a fairly common problem arising from many causes, including stroke, aging, developmental disabilities, and nervous system diseases. It may be only temporary, such as a piece of food lodged in the back of the throat, for which the abdominal thrust is appropriate first aid, or it may be involved with insufficient production of saliva and xerostomia. Such dysfunctional swallowing often causes individuals to aspirate food particles, in turn causing coughing and choking episodes. Dysphagia is of concern for many reasons. Foods may enter the trachea and aspirate into the lungs, allowing bacteria to multiply, leading to pneumonia. Clients with dysphagia are usually referred to a special interdisciplinary team that includes a physician, speech pathologist, nurse, clinical dietitian, physical therapist, and an occupational therapist, with special training in swallowing problems. Thin liquids are the most difficult food form to swallow. Depending on the level of dysphagia, liquids may need to be thickened. Thickening agents include baby rice, commercially prepared thickeners, potato flakes, or mashed potatoes. Levels of thickness include

thick (yogurt or pudding consistency) and medium thick (nectar consistency).

Esophageal Problems
Central Problems

The esophagus is a long, muscular tube lined with mucous membranes that extends from the pharynx, or throat, to the stomach (see Figure 20-2). It is bounded on both ends by circular muscles, or sphincters, that act as valves to control food passage. The upper sphincter remains closed except during swallowing, thus preventing airflow into the esophagus and stomach. Disorders along the tube that may disrupt normal swallowing and food passage include esophageal spasm (uncoordinated contractions of the esophagus), esophageal stricture (a narrowing caused by a scar from previous inflammation, ingestion of caustic chemicals, or a tumor), and esophagitis (an inflammation). These problems hinder eating and require medical attention through dilation, stretching procedures, or surgery to widen the tube, or drug therapy.

Lower Esophageal Sphincter Problems

Defects in the operation of the LES muscles may come from changes in smooth muscle itself or from nerve-muscle hormonal control. In general, these LES problems arise from spasm, stricture, or incompetence.

Achalasia

If the LES does not relax normally when presented with food during swallowing, the uncommon condition of achalasia (*a* meaning without and *chalasia* meaning relaxation) occurs. A primary esophageal motility ailment, achalasia is characterized by absence of esophageal peristalsis and failure of the LES to relax on swallowing. These aberrations bring about a functional obstruction at the gastroesophageal junction. Signs and symptoms characterizing achalasia are dysphagia (most common), regurgitation, chest pain, heartburn, and weight loss.[1]

The exact cause of achalasia is unknown, but it is thought to be an autoimmune disorder, infectious agent, or both.[1] Medical intervention and treatments are outlined in Table 20-1. Nutritional requirements of patients with achalasia vary with severity of the disease and approach to treatment. Generally, nutrient-dense liquids and semisolid foods, taken at moderate temperatures, in small quantities, and at frequent intervals are usually tolerated by patients with achalasia.[2]

Gastroesophageal Reflux Disease

Gastroesophageal reflux disease (GERD), backflow or regurgitation of gastric contents from the stomach into the esophagus, is a very common disease. Regurgitation of acid gastric contents into the lower part of the esophagus creates constant tissue irritation because the wall of the esophagus is not protected from the acid of the stomach. During reflux, many patients feel a burning sensation behind the sternum that radiates toward the mouth, producing the most common symptom of GERD: heartburn (pyrosis), which is unrelated

TABLE 20-1	MEDICAL INTERVENTIONS AND TREATMENT OF ACHALASIA
TYPE	**DESCRIPTION AND EFFICACY**
Pharmacologic: calcium channel blockers, nitrates, phosphodiesterase inhibitors	This intervention is used to reduce LES pressure and is of limited value.
Mechanical: dilation by pneumatic balloons	This intervention involves esophageal dilation to decrease LES pressure. It is successful in decreasing LES pressure in 42% to 85% of patients.
Botulism toxin: Botox	This intervention decreases LES pressure by blocking the release of neurotransmitters at presynaptic cholinergic nerve endings. The best results have been seen in patients with vigorous achalasia. Effective duration of treatment varies but takes 6 to 12 months in most patients.
Surgical: esophageal myotomy	This intervention—surgery—is considered to be the primary treatment. The procedure involves controlled division of muscle fibers of the lower esophagus and proximal stomach, followed by a partial fundoplication to prevent reflux. It relieves symptoms in 80% to 100% of patients.

Data from Pohl D, Tutuian R: Achalasia: an overview of diagnosis and treatment. *J Gastrointest Liver Dis* 16(3):297, 2007.
LES, Lower esophageal sphincter.

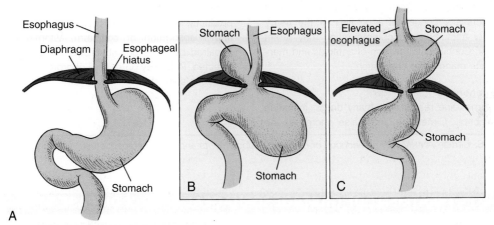

FIGURE 20-4 Hiatal hernia compared with normal stomach placement. **A,** Normal stomach. **B,** Paraesophageal hernia (esophagus in normal position). **C,** Esophageal hiatal hernia (elevated esophagus).

to disease of the heart (see the Diet-Medications Interactions box, "Potential Food Interactions with Drugs Used to Treat Heartburn"). Additional symptoms of GERD include acid indigestion and regurgitation, which often have a negative effect on quality of life.[2]

Other less common symptoms include iron deficiency anemia with chronic bleeding and aspiration, which may cause cough, dyspnea, or pneumonitis. Sometimes substernal pain radiates into the neck and jaw or down the arms. Acid reflux may be worsened by a hiatal hernia, pregnancy (estrogen and progesterone have been shown to reduce LES pressure), obesity, pernicious vomiting, or nasogastric tubes. A number of drugs also lower LES pressure, causing GERD and heartburn to be a side effect of drugs used in the treatment of other conditions.

Acid and pepsin cause tissue erosion with symptoms of substernal burning, cramping, pressure sensation, or severe pain.[2] Symptoms are aggravated by lying down or any increase of abdominal pressure, such as that caused by tight clothing. The condition is related to (1) a nonfunctioning gastroesophageal sphincter, (2) frequency and duration of the acid reflux,

KEY TERMS
abdominal thrust   A first-aid maneuver to relieve a person who is choking from blockage of the breathing passageway by a swallowed foreign object or food particle. Standing behind the person, clasp the victim around the waist, placing one fist under the sternum (breastbone) and grasping the fist with the other hand. Then make a quick, hard, thrusting movement inward and upward.
achalasia   Failure to relax the smooth muscle fibers of the gastrointestinal (GI) tract at any point of juncture of its parts; especially the failure of the esophagogastric sphincter to relax when swallowing, as a result of degeneration of ganglion cells in the wall of the organ. The lower esophagus also loses its normal peristaltic activity. Also called *cardiospasm.*
pyrosis   Heartburn.

and (3) inability of the esophagus to produce normal secondary peristaltic waves to prevent prolonged contact of the mucosa with the acid pepsin. A hiatal hernia (Figure 20-4) may or may not be present. The most common complications of GERD are stenosis and esophageal ulcer.

Data from Bratman S, Girman AM: *Mosby's handbook of herbs and supplements and their therapeutic use*, St Louis, Mo., 2003, Mosby.

💊 DIET-MEDICATIONS INTERACTIONS

Potential Food Interactions with Drugs Used to Treat Heartburn

Drugs and nutrients share related characteristics in the body. They are most often absorbed from the same sites in the intestine. Both can alter physiologic processes, and both can be toxic in high doses. Drugs used to treat heartburn, gastroesophageal reflux disease (GERD), and peptic ulcer disease (PUD) are commonly used. Many are available without prescription. Following is a discussion of common drug-nutrient and herb-drug interactions.

Antacids and Alginates

Antacids may have an effect on absorption of vitamins and iron. Antacids should be taken at least 2 hours before or after iron preparations. The effect of aluminum-containing antacids may be decreased by high-protein meals. Prolonged antacid use, along with excessive consumption of calcium, may cause high calcium levels and result in serious metabolic disease. Antacids may impair folate absorption, which may increase the risk of neural tube defects and congenital anomalies of the heart, palate, and urinary tract. Folate supplementation may offset this increased risk. Concurrent ingestion of antacids and manganese may reduce manganese absorption.

H₂-Receptor Antagonists

The H₂-blocker cimetidine reacts with many drugs, including caffeine and alcohol. Cimetidine may also increase the likelihood of alcohol intoxication. H₂-blockers decrease the body's ability to excrete caffeine; consequently, large quantities of caffeine may cause tremors, insomnia, or heart palpitations. Folate absorption or use may be impaired by H₂-blockers, which may increase risk of neural tube defects and congenital anomalies of heart, palate, and urinary tract. Folate supplementation may offset this increased risk.

H₂-blockers may impair iron absorption through effects on the pH of the digestive tract. H₂-blockers may also impair absorption of selenium. Vitamin B_{12} from food is impaired by H₂-blockers, but absorption of B_{12} supplements is not affected. Magnesium supplements can interfere with absorption of H₂-blockers. Magnesium supplements should be taken at least 2 hours before or after this medication.

Proton Pump Inhibitors

Proton pump inhibitors (PPIs) may hinder absorption of iron products, thus lessening their effectiveness. PPIs may also impair absorption of selenium. Vitamin B_{12} from food is impaired by PPIs, but absorption of B_{12} supplements is not affected. PPIs may potentiate phototoxic effects of *Hypericum* (St. John's wort).

TABLE 20-2 TREATMENT OF GASTROESOPHAGEAL REFLUX DISEASE STAGES

CATEGORY	RECOMMENDED TREATMENTS
Mild heartburn only (occasional bouts for >1 week)	Early low-fat dinners Elevation of head of bed H₂-antagonist >6 weeks and alkali antacids prn PPIs single dose >6 weeks
Moderately severe heartburn (months of daily symptoms of heartburn/chest pressure) or poor response to H₂-receptor antagonist	
Recurrence and persistence of moderately severe GERD symptoms (rapid recurrence of symptoms after course of PPI therapy; occasional odynophagia/dysphagia)	Gastroenterology consultation; endoscopy and biopsy of esophageal-gastric junction for Barrett's metaplasia Recurrent courses of PPI therapy
Severe, persistent GERD symptoms (daily symptoms, often with odynophagia; dysphagia)	Continuous PPI therapy (often two capsules per day) Add cisapride Consider referral for laparoscopic fundoplication
Recalcitrant GERD symptoms (persistent daily/nightly symptoms with regurgitation; odynophagia, dysphagia, poor response to full drug therapy)	Maximal PPI therapy and cisapride Laparoscopic fundoplication

Data from Gray GM: *Gastro-esophageal reflux disease (GERD): the spectrum of esophagitis, Barrett's, dysphagia, and cancer*, New York, 1996-2010, interMDnet Corporation. from: <http://www.cyberounds.com/cmecontent/art104.html?pf=yes>. Retrieved May 14, 2014.
GERD, Gastroesophageal reflux disease; *PPIs*, proton pump inhibitors; *prn*, as needed.

Treatment of GERD is aimed at one or more aspects that cause or continue symptoms (Table 20-2). Nutrition therapy plays only a minor role in the management (Box 20-1) of GERD, and none of the dietary measures can be classified as *evidence-based treatment*.

Hiatal Hernia

The esophagus normally enters the chest cavity at the hiatus, an opening in the diaphragm membrane, and immediately joins the upper portion of the stomach. A hiatal hernia occurs when a portion of the upper part of the stomach at this entry point of the esophagus protrudes through the hiatus alongside the lower portion of the esophagus (see Figure 20-4). Food is easily held in this herniated area of the stomach and mixed with acid and pepsin; then it is regurgitated back up into the lower part of the esophagus. Gastritis can occur in this herniated portion of the stomach and cause bleeding and anemia. Reflux of gastric acid contents causes symptoms similar to those described earlier.

A regular diet of choice using frequent small feedings for comfort is usually tolerated. In addition, because obesity is often associated with hiatal hernia, weight reduction is a primary goal. Avoid tight clothing to help relieve discomfort. Patients will need to avoid leaning over or lying down immediately after meals and should sleep with the head of the bed elevated. Antacids help relieve the burning sensation. Large hiatal hernias or smaller sliding hernias may require surgical repair.

PROBLEMS OF THE STOMACH AND DUODENUM

Peptic Ulcer Disease

One in 10 Americans will be affected by PUD during their lives, and approximately 10% of patients seen in emergency departments with abdominal pain are diagnosed with PUD.[2]

An ulcer is the loss of tissue on the surface of the mucosa. In the GI tract, an ulcer extends through mucosa, submucosa, and often into the muscle layer. *Peptic ulcer* is the general term for an eroded mucosal lesion in the central portion of the GI tract. A peptic ulcer can occur in any area of the stomach exposed to pepsin. Areas affected include the lower portion of the esophagus, stomach, and first portion of the duodenum, called the *duodenal bulb*. Esophageal and gastric ulcers are less common. Most ulcers occur in the duodenal bulb, where gastric contents emptying into the duodenum through the pyloric valve are most concentrated. Gastric ulcers occur usually along the lesser curvature of the stomach. PUD itself is a benign disease, but ulcers do tend to recur. Gastric ulcers are more prone to develop into malignant disease. Weight loss is common in patients with gastric ulcers. Patients with duodenal ulcers may gain weight from frequent eating to counteract pain.

Peptic ulcer is caused by *Helicobacter pylori* in the stomach or intake of nonsteroidal antiinflammatory drugs (NSAIDs).[3] Nutrition or diet is not thought to play a significant role in the cause. *H. pylori* is a short, spiral-shaped, microaerophilic gram-negative bacillus (Figure 20-5) that attaches itself to gastric mucosa.[3] It is able to survive the acidic environment of the stomach by secreting enzymes to neutralize the acid. This allows *H. pylori* to find its way to the protective mucous lining of the stomach, and its spiral shape facilitates burrowing through the lining.[4]

Intake of aspirin or other NSAIDs such as ibuprofen (Motrin), naproxen (Naprosyn), and etodolac (Lodine) induce ulcer formation by interfering with formation of prostaglandins, the chemicals that help the mucosal lining resist caustic acid damage.[5] They irritate gastric mucosa and cause

---

BOX 20-1 MANAGEMENT OF GASTROESOPHAGEAL REFLUX DISEASE

Self-Care
- Over-the-counter (OTC) therapy
  - Antacids
  - Alginate/antacids
  - H_2-receptor antagonists

Lifestyle
- Stop smoking.
- Avoid alcohol, chocolate, fatty foods, large meals at night
- Refrain from lying down after meal.
- Elevate head of bed or use pillows.

Primary Care (Primary Care Physicians)
- Proton pump inhibitors (PPIs) or combination of alginate/antacid and acid suppressive therapy

Secondary Care (Specialists)
- Endoscopic examination
- PPIs

Data from Tytgat GN, McColl K, Tack J, et al: New algorithm for the treatment of gastro-esophageal reflux disease. *Aliment Pharmacol Ther* 27(3):249, 2008.

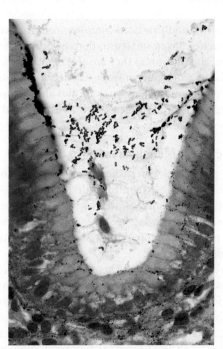

FIGURE 20-5 *Helicobacter pylori.* (From Kumar V, Abbas AK, Fausto N: *Robbins and Cotran pathologic basis of disease*, ed 7, Philadelphia, Pa., 2005, Saunders.)

KEY TERM
gastritis Inflammation of the stomach.

bleeding, erosion, and ulceration, especially with prolonged or excessive use. The NSAID group of drugs is so named to distinguish them from the corticosteroids, synthetic variants of the natural adrenal hormones. The NSAIDs include a dozen antiinflammatory drugs.

Clinical Symptoms

The basic symptoms of peptic ulcer are increased gastric tone and painful hunger contractions when the stomach is empty. In a duodenal ulcer, the amount and concentration of hydrochloric acid (HCl) are increased. In a gastric ulcer, the amount and concentration of HCl may be normal. Nutritional deficiencies are evident in low plasma protein levels, anemia, and loss of weight. Hemorrhage may be the first sign in some patients. Diagnosis is based on clinical findings, radiographs, or visualization by fiber-optic gastroscopy.

The primary goal of medical management for PUD is control of *H. pylori.* Additional supportive goals are to (1) alleviate symptoms, (2) promote healing, (3) prevent recurrences, and (4) prevent complications. In addition to general traditional measures, the rapidly expanding knowledge base and development of a number of new drugs have increased the physician's available management tools.

General Therapeutic Measures

Adequate rest, relaxation, and sleep have long been a foundation for general care of PUD to enhance the body's natural healing process. Positive stress-coping and relaxation skills, which help patients deal with personal psychosocial stressors, can be learned and practiced. Simple encouragement to talk about anxieties, anger, and frustrations helps to make patients feel better, and as soon as they are able, appropriate physical activity helps work out tensions. Habits that contribute to ulcer development, such as smoking and alcohol use, should be eliminated. Common drugs such as aspirin and NSAIDs should be avoided.

Pharmacologic Management

Current pharmacologic management of PUD includes a wider choice of drugs to control underlying physiologic cause and clinical symptoms, as well as to support healing. In various ways the following five types of drugs suppress gastric acid and pepsin secretion, protect mucosal tissue, buffer acid, and eliminate infection:

1. *H_2-receptor antagonists:* These agents, commonly called *H_2-blockers,* are popular drugs for controlling gastric acid secretion. They decrease HCl production by competing with histamine for receptor sites on parietal cells. Normally, histamine attaches to its specific cellular receptors (type H_2) on acid-producing parietal cells of gastric mucosa and mediates secretion of HCl. Thus the blocking action of these agents effectively controls acid and pepsin because inactive pepsinogen requires acid for activation. The four drugs in this classification have now been reclassified for OTC purchase: (1) cimetidine (Tagamet), (2) ranitidine (Zantac), (3) famotidine (Pepcid), and (4) nizatidine (Axid).

2. *PPIs:* This newer class of drugs, more potent than H_2-blockers, also suppresses gastric acid but by a different action. For example, prostaglandin analog, misoprostol, can be used with NSAIDs to prevent ulcer. This class of medication should not be used by pregnant women. Long-term use of PPIs may lead to hypomagnesemia, and it is recommended that serum magnesium levels should be monitored. In the parietal cells, the PPIs irreversibly inhibit a key enzyme, H^+/K^+-ATPase, that actively secretes hydrogen ions needed for HCl production. Without available H_2 ions, HCl cannot be made, and without acid, ulcers can heal rapidly. The U.S. Food and Drug Administration (FDA) has approved five drugs in this category: (1) lansoprazole (Prevacid), (2) omeprazole (Prilosec), (3) esomeprazole (Nexium), (4) rabeprazole (Aciphex), and (5) pantoprazole (Protonix). PPIs may interfere with liver metabolism of anticoagulants, diazepam (Valium), or phenytoin (Dilantin). Serum levels of these drugs should be monitored during concurrent therapy.

3. *Mucosal protectors:* Drugs of this type act as cytoprotective agents by helping the stomach heal itself. They produce a gel-like suspension that binds to the ulcer base and covers it and surrounding normal mucosal tissue to protect involved tissue from harm while it heals. This drug also forms complexes with pepsin that inactivates pepsin. An example of this type of drug is sucralfate (Carafate). These drugs are not as effective as the other options.

4. *Antacids:* These well-known substances counteract or neutralize acidity. They are safe and inexpensive to use. Two main types are (1) magnesium-aluminum compounds (Maalox, Mylanta) and (2) aluminum hydroxide (Basaljel, Amphojel). Aluminum-based preparations may cause constipation; magnesium-based preparations may cause diarrhea.

5. *Antibiotics:* Drugs of this type are used to control the *Helicobacter pylori* infection associated with PUD. Treatment using one or two antibiotics such as amoxicillin, tetracycline (not to be used for children younger than age 12), metronidazole, or clarithromycin is recommended for 10 days to 2 weeks, in conjunction with either ranitidine bismuth citrate, bismuth subsalicylate, or a PPI. The combination of acid suppression by the H_2-blocker or PPI with antibiotics helps alleviate ulcer-related symptoms (e.g., abdominal pain, nausea), heal inflammation, and may enhance efficacy of the antibiotics.[5] Currently the FDA has approved eight *H. pylori* treatment regimens (Box 20-2), although other combinations have been used effectively. Better eradication rates have been demonstrated using triple-therapy regimens rather than dual therapy, longer length of treatment (14 days instead of 10 days), or both. Major reasons for treatment failure are antibiotic resistance and patient noncompliance.[5]

Nutritional Management

Pharmacologic therapy is the treatment of choice for PUD. No evidence indicates that diet plays a significant role in treatment when compared with pharmacologic regimens.[6]

Dietary recommendations are formed from individual tolerance and should be considered supplemental to pharmacologic therapy. No conclusive evidence supports use of a traditional "bland" diet to decrease gastric acid secretion or increase the time it takes to heal ulcers.[2] In short, individuals with PUD should be encouraged to eat a healthy diet from foods they enjoy.

General nutritional therapeutic recommendations include the following[7]:

- Emphasize a balanced, nutritious diet.
- Limit the following foods and seasonings, and encourage avoidance of lifestyle habits known to increase acid secretion, inhibit healing, or both:
  - Caffeine (including coffee, tea, or decaffeinated coffee)
  - Black pepper
  - Chocolate
  - Foods that are irritating or not well tolerated
  - Alcohol
  - Eating less than 2 hours before bedtime

Personal Focus

Sound nutritional management plays an important supportive role in total medical care of persons with PUD. The individual must be the focus of treatment. The patient is not *an ulcer*; he or she is a person *with an ulcer*. The course of the disease is conditioned by the individuality of the patient and his or her life situation. The presence of the ulcer affects the patient's life and quality of life. In the long run a wide range of foods, attractive to the eye and the taste,

and regular, unhurried eating habits provide the best course of action (see the Case Study box, "The Patient with Peptic Ulcer Disease").

DISORDERS OF THE SMALL INTESTINE

Diarrhea and Malabsorption

Diarrhea

Diarrhea is not a disease; it is a symptom that can be attributed to many medical conditions (see the Perspectives in Practice box, "Nutritional Aspects of Diarrhea"). *Diarrhea* is defined as an increase in frequency of bowel movements compared with the usual pattern, an excess water content of stools affecting consistency or volume, or both. Diarrhea most directly involves the large intestine but may be caused by disease of the small intestine, pancreas, or gallbladder. General diarrhea may result from basic dietary excesses. Fermentation of sugars or excess fiber stimulation of intestinal muscle function may be involved.

Chronic diarrhea may occur as a result of GI tract motility dysfunction such as irritable bowel syndrome (IBS), malabsorption, metabolic disorders, food intolerances (e.g., lactose intolerance), food poisoning, infections, and human immunodeficiency virus (HIV) infection. In the case of lactose intolerance, the accumulated concentration of undigested lactose in the intestine, resulting from the lack of the enzyme lactase, creates increased osmotic pressure. This pressure effectively draws water into the gut and stimulates hypermotility, abdominal cramping, and diarrhea. Milk treated with lactase enzyme is tolerated by these persons without the difficulty encountered with regular milk. Secretory, osmotic, and inflammatory processes in the intestine result in increased losses of fluid and electrolytes from diarrhea.[8]

Malabsorption

In a normally functioning body, foods are digested and then nutrients are absorbed into the bloodstream, mostly from the small intestine. Malabsorption occurs either because a disorder interferes with how food is digested or because a disorder interferes with how nutrients are absorbed. Multiple causes of a malabsorption condition exist.[8] Symptoms of malabsorption include a change in bowel habits, apathy, fatigue, and a smooth surface on the lateral tongue. Some of these causes include the following:

- *Maldigestion problems:* pancreatic disorders, biliary disease, bacterial overgrowth, ileal disease (inflammatory bowel disease [IBD])
- *Intestinal mucosal changes:* mucosal surface alterations, intestinal surgery such as resections that shorten the bowel, lymphatic obstruction, intestinal stasis
- *Genetic disease:* cystic fibrosis (CF), with its complications of pancreatic insufficiency and lack of the pancreatic enzymes lipase, trypsin, and amylase
- *Intestinal enzyme deficiency:* lactose intolerance caused by lactase deficiency

The Patient with Peptic Ulcer Disease

Lowell is a 40-year-old businessman who was admitted to the city hospital 3 weeks ago after vomiting bright-red blood. A medical history revealed that a dull, gnawing pain in the upper abdomen began several months ago and has increased in severity during that time. It became more severe after his most recent out-of-state trip to one of his stores. Because the pain was usually accompanied by headaches, he took aspirin to help relieve it.

Initial hospital treatment consisted of blood transfusions, intravenous fluids and electrolytes, and vitamin C. Lowell continued to feel nauseated and weak, but he stopped vomiting. However, he passed several large, tarry stools during the first 24 hours. His initial nutrition assessment results included weight 68 kg (150 lb), height 175 cm (5 feet 9 inches), albumin 2.8 g/dL, prealbumin 14 mg/dL, transferrin 18% saturation value, hemoglobin (Hb) 11 g/dL, and hematocrit 35%. His medications included cimetidine, sucralfate, magnesium-aluminum hydroxide, and triple antibiotic therapy.

The patient began slowly to tolerate sips of clear liquids and then advanced to a regular diet as tolerated, showing continued improvement. Before he was discharged at the end of the second week, the registered dietitian (RD) discussed general nutritional needs with Lowell and his wife. He was advised to eat meals regularly in as relaxed a setting and manner as possible, eliminate his frequent between-meal snacks, and take his multivitamin supplement daily with his meals. In addition, general guidelines and a list of a few food-related items or habits to avoid were reviewed. He was also advised to stop smoking and to rest as much as possible before returning to work. His physician had also advised him to reduce his workload and scheduled a follow-up appointment in 1 week.

Lowell's wife accompanied him to the next appointment and reported she was pleased with his ability to put aside business duties and take more time to enjoy his family. Lowell stated his two teenage sons had been surprisingly supportive in assisting him in following the prescribed regimen, and he plans to make it his general habit.

Questions for Analysis

1. The radiographic diagnosis of Lowell's illness was a gastric ulcer in the antrum lesser curvature. What does this mean? Where do most ulcers occur? Why?
2. What factors contributed to Lowell's ulcer? What effect did each of them have?
3. Evaluate the results of Lowell's initial nutrition assessment data. How would you use this information in nutrition counseling?
4. Identify Lowell's basic nutritional needs. Outline a teaching plan based on these needs that you would use to help him with his new diet plan. How would you include his wife in formulating and implementing his nutrition care plan?
5. What role does vitamin C play in Lowell's therapy?
6. Why should Lowell give up coffee, cigarettes, and alcohol? What problems do you think he may encounter in trying to change these habits?

- *Cancer and its treatment:* absorbing surface effect of radiation and chemotherapy
- *Metabolic biochemical defects:* absorbing surface effects of pernicious anemia or gluten-induced enteropathy (celiac sprue)

Here we briefly review four of these malabsorptive conditions: (1) celiac sprue, (2) CF, (3) IBD, and (4) short-bowel syndrome (SBS).

Celiac Disease
Metabolic Defect

In 1889 a London physician named Gee observed a number of malnourished children having steatorrhea and distended abdomens. He gave the name *celiac* to the general clinical condition from the Greek word *kolia,* meaning belly or abdomen. It was not until the mid-1950s that the Dutch pediatrician Willem-Karel Dicke and his associates discovered the causative agent. Their tissue studies confirmed that the gliadin fraction of the protein gluten in wheat produced the fat malabsorption; further, what had been called *celiac disease (CD)* in children and *nontropical sprue* in adults was a single disease, which came to be called *celiac sprue.*[9] As currently used, the alternative terms *CD* and *gluten-sensitive enteropathy* are synonymous with celiac sprue. In all cases, such diseased tissues consistently show an eroded mucosal surface lacking the number and form of normal villi and having few microvilli, resulting in malabsorption of most nutrients (Figure 20-6). (For more information regarding genetic malabsorption diseases, see the Evidence-Based Practice box, "Food Intolerances from Genetic-Metabolic Disease," and the Focus on Culture box, "Did Your Ancestors Herd Dairy Cattle?")

Gluten molecules trigger an autoimmune and inflammatory response in the small intestine, causing the usually brushlike lining of the intestine to flatten, thereby becoming much less able to digest and absorb foods. Damage is reversed when gluten is removed from the diet. It is unclear why an immunologic response occurs when gluten is ingested by genetically predisposed persons.[10] The resulting malabsorption promotes malnutrition and severe debilitation.[8] Gluten is a protein present in some grains such as wheat, rye, and barley but not oats, rice, or corn.

CD occurs in roughly 1 in 133 persons in the United States, but only a small percentage of people with it have been diagnosed. CD, as a rule, commonly occurs in women, Caucasians and others of European ancestry, and first-degree relatives. It can occur at any age from infancy to late adulthood.[11]

Clinical Symptoms

Symptoms vary significantly from person to person. They may be intestinal or nonintestinal in nature, which makes diagnosis difficult. One person may present with diarrhea, another with constipation, and yet another with no stool elimination problems.[11] Children with CD most often display failure to thrive, with or without malabsorption. Adults most

PERSPECTIVES IN PRACTICE

Nutritional Aspects of Diarrhea

Gastrointestinal (GI) disease so often presents barriers to efficient nutrient absorption that nutritional deficiencies are planned for automatically. Unfortunately, many of these conditions also frequently lead to diarrhea, which results in further loss of fluids and electrolytes. As expected, replacement of these fluids is the initial and primary concern of therapy. However, different types of diarrhea also present other differences; control of type-specific problems requires different modes of treatment coordinated with treatment of the disease it accompanies. Before looking into possible treatment modes, three of the most common types of diarrhea should be examined: (1) watery, (2) fatty, and (3) small volume.

Watery diarrhea occurs when the amount of water and electrolytes moving into intestinal mucosa exceeds that amount absorbed into the bloodstream. This movement of water and electrolytes into the mucosa may be secretive or osmotic. If this movement of water and electrolytes into the mucosa is secretive, then it may be active or passive. Active movement occurs with excessive gastric hydrochloric acid (HCl) secretion or enterotoxin-induced infections such as cholera. Passive movement occurs with a rise in hydrostatic pressure that accompanies such infectious diseases as salmonellosis or tuberculosis, nonbacterial infections, fungal infections, renal failure, irradiation enteritis, and inflammatory bowel disease (IBD). Other conditions associated with watery diarrhea include hyperthyroidism, thyroid carcinoma, and hypermotility of the GI tract.

If this movement of water and electrolytes into the mucosa is osmotic, it will occur when nutrients are not absorbed because of intolerable levels of nonabsorbable particles present in intestinal chyme. Such particles include lactose (milk sugar) in individuals with lactase deficiency or gluten (a cereal protein found in wheat and rye and to a lesser degree in barley and oats) in persons with a reduced GI transit time caused by the removal of part of the intestinal tract.

Fatty diarrhea, or steatorrhea, occurs with maldigestion or malabsorption. Maldigestion involves a lack of enzymatic activity required to completely digest food, such as reduced pancreatic exocrine activity (release of intestinal enzymes from the pancreas) caused by pancreatic insufficiency. Malabsorption means digested materials do not make it across the intestinal mucosa to enter the bloodstream. This failure occurs in conditions in which the intestinal villi are destroyed, such as celiac disease (CD).

Small-volume diarrhea occurs mainly when the rectosigmoid area of the colon is irritated, such as in IBD (Crohn's disease or ulcerative colitis [UC]). It also occurs when inflammatory conditions affect areas adjacent to the colon, as in pelvic inflammatory disease, diverticulitis, appendicitis, or hemorrhagic ovarian cysts.

Metabolic consequences of each type of diarrhea are similar. Uncontrolled, they result in syncope, hypokalemia, acid-base imbalances, and hypovolemia, with resulting renal failure. They may also be accompanied by low levels of fat-soluble vitamins, vitamin B_{12}, or folic acid, or eventually lead to protein-energy malnutrition (PEM). In addition to these conditions, each type also manifests problems associated with the disorder they accompany. Workers with the Memorial Sloan-Kettering Cancer Center in New York and the Department of Medicine at Brooke Army Medical Center in Texas have developed recommendations for treating GI diseases associated with each type of diarrhea. These are summarized as follows, with the focus on the diarrheal aspects of disease:

- Watery diarrhea often accompanies inflammatory bowel conditions, such as Crohn's disease, for which nutrition therapy involves (1) increased protein and kcalories, (2) low fats and lactose, and (3) avoidance of foods that stimulate peristalsis. Thus secretive diarrhea, caused by microscopic colitis, is reduced by eliminating foods that may stimulate gastric acid secretion, and all types of watery diarrhea can be avoided by reducing the motility of the GI tract. In other conditions in which osmotic diarrhea occurs, such as dumping syndrome, this problem is prevented by giving fluids between meals to avoid any extreme difference in osmotic pressures on either side of the intestinal wall. Small, frequent meals also help prevent this problem, as well as painful distention.

- Steatorrhea frequently accompanies conditions associated with maldigestion such as chronic pancreatitis. Nutritional management of this disease involves (1) frequent meals high in protein and carbohydrates and low in fat; (2) use of medium-chain triglycerides (MCTs), which are more easily absorbed under adverse conditions; and (3) avoiding gastric stimulants, especially caffeine and alcohol. Steatorrhea also accompanies conditions of malabsorption, such as gluten-sensitive enteropathy. In addition to the nutritional management strategies listed, treating this type of diarrhea requires removal of products that damage the mucosal villi, including lactose and gluten, which is found in wheat, rye, barley, and oats, and food products and fillers such as hydrolyzed vegetable protein products. It sometimes requires restricting fat as well. In both cases, the primary concern is to monitor fats that would otherwise appear in the feces. As therapy progresses, fat content of the meal can be increased as tolerated to normal levels to improve palatability.

- Small-volume diarrhea may accompany diverticulosis of the colon. A high-residue diet is recommended to increase fecal bulk, thereby preventing diarrhea. To prevent flatulence and distention, fiber should be added to the diet gradually.

All types of diarrhea can result in malnutrition, primarily because of electrolyte and fluid losses. It is important to identify the type of diarrhea occurring with each patient; only then can an effective nutritional management strategy be designed to replace those losses, as well as to eliminate or prevent other nutrition-related problems that are possible for each case.

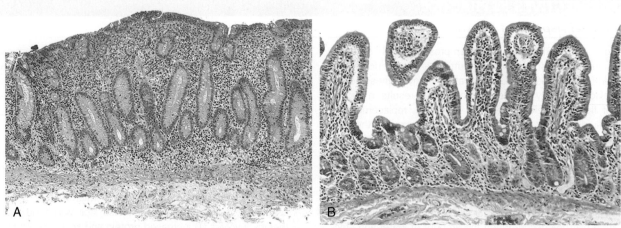

FIGURE 20-6 Comparison of normal intestinal villi and those in an individual with celiac disease (CD). **A,** Biopsy specimen of diseased mucosa shows diffuse severe atrophy and blunting of villi. **B,** Normal mucosal biopsy specimen. (From Kumar V, Abbas AK, Fausto N: *Robbins and Cotran pathologic basis of disease*, ed 7, Philadelphia, Pa., 2005, Saunders.)

EVIDENCE-BASED PRACTICE

Food Intolerances from Genetic-Metabolic Disease

Certain food intolerances may stem from underlying genetic disease that affects metabolism of one or more specific nutrients. Genetic disease results from the individual's specific gene inheritance. Genes in each cell control the metabolic functions of the cell. They regulate synthesis of approximately 1000 or more specific cell enzymes that control metabolism within the cell. A specific gene controls the synthesis of a specific enzyme. When that gene sequence is abnormal due to mutation, the cell is unable to make the enzyme. In turn, the specific metabolic reaction controlled by that specific missing enzyme cannot take place. Specific genetic disease caused by this metabolic block then manifests clinical symptoms connected with resulting abnormal metabolic products. As primary examples here, we look briefly at two such genetic diseases affecting food-nutrient intolerances: (1) phenylketonuria (PKU), which affects metabolism of amino acid and phenylalanine, leading to the need to limit certain protein foods; and (2) galactosemia, which affects carbohydrate metabolism, specifically food sources that contain lactose. Both are detected by newborn screening procedures that are mandatory by law.

Phenylketonuria

Phenylketonuria results from the missing cell enzyme phenylalanine hydroxylase, which metabolizes one of the essential amino acids, phenylalanine, to tyrosine, another nonessential amino acid. Phenylalanine then accumulates in the blood, and its alternate metabolites, the phenyl acids, are excreted in the urine. One of these urinary acids, phenylpyruvic acid, is a phenylketone; hence the name of the disease. Untreated, PKU can produce devastating effects, but present nutrition therapy can avoid these results. In past years, before current newborn screening laws and dietary treatment practices from birth, the most profound effect observed in persons with untreated PKU was severe mental retardation. The intelligence quotient (IQ) of affected persons was usually less than 50 and

often less than 20. Central nervous system (CNS) damage caused irritability, hyperactivity, convulsive seizures, and bizarre behavior.

PKU can now be well controlled by special nutrition therapy. After screening at birth, a special low-phenylalanine diet effectively controls serum phenylalanine levels so that they are maintained at appropriate amounts to prevent clinical symptoms and promote normal growth and development. Because phenylalanine is an essential amino acid necessary for growth, it cannot be totally removed from the diet. Blood levels of phenylalanine need to be constantly monitored, and the metabolic team nutritionist calculates the special diet for each infant and child to allow only a limited amount of phenylalanine that can be tolerated. In addition, without phenylalanine hydroxylase, tyrosine becomes essential amino acid for individuals with PKU. Based on extensive studies, guidelines for nutritional management of PKU are currently being used effectively to build lifetime habits; research now indicates that no safe age exists at which a child may discontinue the diet. This dietary management is built on two basic components: (1) a substitute for milk (a special medical food continued past infancy and childhood into adolescence and adulthood) and (2) guidelines for adding solid foods (both regular and special low-protein products) and then building continuing food habits.

Initial education and continuing support of parents is essential, because dietary management of PKU is the only known effective method of treatment and maintaining the diet becomes more difficult as the child grows older. Parents must understand and accept the necessity of the diet, and this requires patience, understanding, and continued reinforcement. The PKU team, together with parents, provides initial and continuing care so that the child with PKU will grow and develop normally. When PKU is diagnosed at birth, as a result of widespread screening programs, a child can have a healthy and happy life, instead of the profound disease consequences experienced in the past. Current practice of long-term

EVIDENCE-BASED PRACTICE

Food Intolerances from Genetic-Metabolic Disease—cont'd

nutritional management is especially critical for young women with PKU who are considering pregnancy. At least 6 months before becoming pregnant, women with PKU should meet with a metabolic team to discuss treatment and follow-up. It is possible for women with PKU to have normal children. However, maternal PKU presents the possibility of a potentially high-risk pregnancy if a low-phenylalanine diet is not strictly followed.

Galactosemia

This genetic disease affects carbohydrate metabolism so that the body cannot use the monosaccharide galactose. Three enzymes are responsible for conversion of galactose to glucose, and in galactosemia at least one of the enzymes is defective or missing. Milk, infants' first food, contains a large amount of the precursor lactose (milk sugar). When infants with galactosemia are given breast milk or regular infant formula, they vomit and have diarrhea. After galactose is initially combined with phosphate to begin metabolic conversion to glucose, it cannot proceed further in the infant with galactosemia. Galactose rapidly accumulates in the blood and in various body tissues. In the past, excess tissue accumulations of galactose caused rapid damage in the untreated infant. Clinical symptoms appeared soon after birth, and the child failed to thrive. Continued liver damage brought **jaundice**, an enlarged liver with **cirrhosis**, enlarged spleen, and ascites. Without treatment, death usually resulted from liver failure. If the infant survived, then continuing tissue damage and hypoglycemia in

the optic lens and the brain caused cataracts and mental retardation. Now, however, with newborn screening programs, infants with galactosemia are diagnosed at birth and started on special dietary management. With this vital nutrition therapy, children can grow and develop normally.

The main indirect source of dietary galactose is the lactose in milk. A galactose-free diet (free of all forms of milk and lactose) is observed, and the infant is fed a soy-based formula. Breast-feeding is not an option when this genetic condition is present. The body synthesizes the amount of galactose needed for body structures. As solid foods are added to the infant's diet at about 6 months of age, careful attention must be given to avoiding lactose from other food sources. Parents quickly learn to check labels carefully on all commercial products to detect any lactose or lactose-containing substances.

Websites of Interest
Galactosemia

National Organization for Rare Disorders: <www.rarediseases.org>.
Parents of Galactosemic Children, Inc.: <www.galactosemia.org>.

Phenylketonuria (PKU)

Children's PKU Network: <www.pkunetwork.org>.
National Coalition for PKU and Allied Disorders: <www.pku-allieddisorders.org>.
National PKU News: <www.pkunews.org>.

Data from Nelms MN, Sucher K, Long S: *Understanding nutrition therapy and pathophysiology,* Belmont, Calif., 2007, Wadsworth/Thomson Learning.

FOCUS ON CULTURE

Did Your Ancestors Herd Dairy Cattle?

Do you or anyone you know experience these symptoms—cramps, bloating, gas, diarrhea, nausea—anywhere from 30 minutes to 2 hours after consuming a food or beverage containing lactose? As you learned in Chapter 3, lactose is found in milk and some dairy products, and the enzyme lactase is necessary for us to digest lactose. Lack of this mucosal enzyme, lactase, results in a condition called *lactose intolerance.*

Humans are the only mammals that continue to drink milk past weaning. Most mammals produce lactase until they are weaned and stop drinking milk. Cessation of milk drinking and lactase production characterizes most of the world's population, especially those of Asian and African ancestry. For children older than 5 years, 90% to 95% of people of color (African Americans, Asians, Hispanics) are lactose intolerant, whereas only 20% to 25% of those of northern European descent do not tolerate dairy products. Lactose intolerance is usually referred to as a *disease* or *disorder.* Does this seem logical? Why is a trait found in 90% to 95% of the world's population abnormal? Perhaps lactose intolerance should be considered a normal adult condition.

Researchers from Cornell University believe lactose tolerance is the outcome of a genetic mutation that sustains

the functionality of lactase production into adulthood, allowing consumption of milk throughout life. This mutation occurs commonly among populations from Northern Europe, where raising cattle and other ruminant animals has been practiced for centuries because the environment made it safe and economical to do so.

It appears that the ability to produce lactase and absorb lactose is nutritionally beneficial for adults only if milk is consistently available. To test this theory, data were collected on adult lactose absorption and malabsorption from 270 indigenous African and Eurasian populations. Adult lactose malabsorption was found to be associated with extreme hot or cold climates (high and low latitudes). In addition to the geographic and climatic features of these regions that preclude the raising of dairy herds, historical evidence (pre-1900) indicates that nine deadly communicable cattle diseases occurred in these regions. The researchers concluded that areas of the world in which adult lactose malabsorption predominates are the same areas in which it is dangerous or impossible to sustain dairy herds. Thus the ability to digest lactose appears for the most part to be a genetic mutation.

Data from Bloom G, Sherman PW: Dairying barriers affect the distribution of lactose malabsorption. *Evol Hum Behav* 26(4):301, 2005.

frequently present with anemia caused by iron or folate deficiency (or both).[11] A partial listing of GI symptoms is summarized in Table 20-3.

Diagnosis

Individuals in the general population may not be identified by clinical symptoms, therefore remaining underdiagnosed, but screening remains controversial. Tissue transglutaminase antibodies (tTG-IgA) have been found to be a sensitive marker for CD.[11] Intestinal biopsy is then used to confirm diagnosis in patients with positive serologic tests. Depending on the degree of intestinal involvement, a complete blood count (CBC); levels of serum iron or ferritin, red cell folate, vitamin B_{12}, serum calcium, alkaline phosphatase, albumin, and β-carotene; and prothrombin time (PT) should be obtained in patients suspected of malabsorption problems.

Nutritional Management

The goal of nutritional management is to control intake of dietary gluten and prevent malnutrition. The diet is better defined as *low gluten* rather than *gluten free* because it is impossible to remove all gluten. Newer products labeled *gluten free* can contain wheat starch as a thickening agent, which cannot be recommended.[12] Wheat and rye are the main sources of glutenlike proteins; it is also present in oats and barley. Thus these four grains have always been eliminated from the diet. However, a growing body of evidence suggests that moderate amounts of oats may be safely used in diets of most adults with CD.[13] Corn and rice are usually the substitute grains used. Parents of children with CD need special instructions about food products to avoid, what constitutes a basic meal pattern, and recipes for food preparation. Careful label reading must be discussed, because many commercial products use the offending grains as thickeners or fillers, and parents' knowledge of food products that contain gluten is highly variable and influences the child's attitudes toward dietary compliance. Good dietary management varies according to the child's age, pathologic conditions, and clinical status. Generally, a dietary program based on the low-gluten diet should be followed (Box 20-3). In a small subgroup of patients, symptoms persist despite strict adherence to the diet. In rare instances, persons with such a refractory form of the disease respond only to parenteral nutrition (PN) support.

Cystic Fibrosis
Genetic-Metabolic Defect

Cystic fibrosis is inherited as an autosomal recessive trait in about 3% of the Caucasian population. It is the most common fatal genetic disease among Caucasians, occurring in about 1 in 3300 live Caucasian births, 1 in 15,300 African-American births, and 1 in 32,000 Asian-American births.[14] Approximately one third of CF cases in the United States involve adults. The leading characteristic of CF is hypersecretion of abnormal, thick mucus that obstructs exocrine glands and

TABLE 20-3	GASTROINTESTINAL SYMPTOMS ASSOCIATED WITH CELIAC DISEASE
SYMPTOM	**COMMENTS**
Abdominal pain	
Abdominal distention	Bloating, gas, indigestion
Constipation	
Decreased appetite	May also be increased or unchanged
Diarrhea	Chronic or occasional
Lactose intolerance	Common on diagnosis; usually resolves after treatment
Nausea and vomiting	
Steatorrhea	Stools that float, are foul smelling, bloody, or "fatty"
Weight loss	Unexplained (people can be overweight or normal weight on diagnosis)

Data from U.S. National Library of Medicine, National Institutes of Health: *Medline Plus A.D.A.M. medical encyclopedia: celiac disease-sprue,* Atlanta, Ga., 2005, A.D.A.M. Inc. from: <www.nlm.nih.gov/medlineplus/ency/article/000233.htm>. Retrieved May 14, 2014.

BOX 20-3 SAMPLE GLUTEN-FREE MENU

Breakfast
Denver omelet made with low-fat natural cheddar or Monterey Jack cheese and fresh vegetables
Rice cake (ingredient list should be checked to ascertain it is gluten free) topped with fruit jelly
Orange juice

Lunch
Tacos made with corn tortilla, black beans, fresh vegetables, low-fat natural cheese
Fresh green salad with oil and vinegar dressing
Homemade lemon/limeade

Evening Meal
Shrimp and fresh vegetable stir-fry in oil and spices
Brown rice or enriched white rice, plain
Sorbet
Cranberry juice/seltzer water spritzer

Snack
All-natural yogurt mixed with fresh peaches (or other fruit in season)

KEY TERMS
jaundice A syndrome characterized by hyperbilirubinemia and deposits of bile pigment in the skin, mucous membranes, and sclera, giving a yellow appearance to the patient.
cirrhosis Chronic liver disease, characterized by loss of functional cells, with fibrous and nodular regeneration.

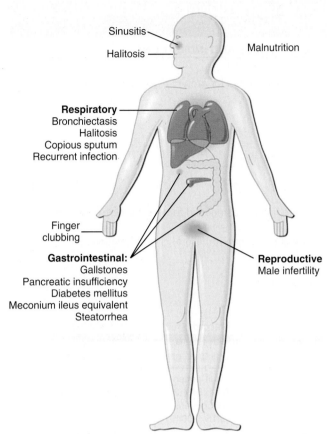

Sinusitis

Halitosis

Malnutrition

Respiratory
Bronchiectasis
Halitosis
Copious sputum
Recurrent infection

Finger
clubbing

Gastrointestinal:
Gallstones
Pancreatic insufficiency
Diabetes mellitus
Meconium ileus equivalent
Steatorrhea

Reproductive
Male infertility

FIGURE 20-7 Cystic fibrosis (CF). (From Axford JS, O'Callaghan CA: *Medicine,* ed 2, Malden, Mass., 2004, Blackwell Science.)

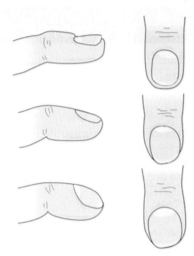

FIGURE 20-8 Clubbing of the fingers. (From Axford JS, O'Callaghan CA: *Medicine,* ed 2, Malden, Mass., 2004, Blackwell Science.)

ducts.[14] Therefore it can be classified as a *respiratory disease* or *GI disorder.*

The CF gene (found on chromosome 7q) is very large, and over 600 mutations that cause CF have been described.[14] The gene product is the cystic fibrosis transmembrane regulator (CFTR) protein, which regulates chloride transport and water flux across epithelial cells.[14] This results in an abnormally high concentration of sodium in perspiration and low water content in mucus.[14] CF primarily affects the pancreas, intestinal tract, sweat glands, and lungs; it causes infertility in male patients (Figure 20-7).[14]

Clinical Symptoms

Classic clinical symptoms of CF include the following effects in body organ systems[14]:

- Thick mucus in the lungs that accumulates and clogs air passages, damages epithelial tissue of these airways, and leads to chronic obstructive pulmonary disease (COPD) and frequent respiratory infections, both of which contribute to increased metabolism and increased energy-nutrient needs
- Pancreatic insufficiency caused by progressive clogging of pancreatic ducts and functional tissue degeneration, resulting in lack of normal pancreatic enzymes leading to

bulky, foul-smelling, oily stools (steatorrhea); progressive loss of functional insulin-producing beta cells in the islets of Langerhans', resulting in type 1 diabetes mellitus
- Malabsorption of undigested food nutrients and extensive malnutrition and stunted growth
- Excessive sweating in hot weather that may lead to dehydration and circulatory failure
- Biliary cirrhosis caused by progressive clogging of bile ducts producing biliary obstruction and functional liver tissue degeneration
- Inflammatory complications that may include arthritis, finger clubbing (Figure 20-8), or vasculitis
- Gallbladder disease, PUD, GERD, or episodes of partial intestinal obstruction
- Delayed puberty and maturity, probably the result of chronic malnutrition (men are typically infertile because the vas deferens fails to develop.)

Nutritional Management

The overall nutritional goal is to support normal nutrition and growth for all ages[15]:
- Unrestricted diet, including high-fat foods and additives
- Three meals and two to three snacks each day
- Vitamin supplementation
- Pancreatic enzymes
- Supplements and nutrient-dense nourishments may help
- Encouragement to consume whole grains, nuts, fruits, and vegetables for adequate vitamin and mineral intake
- Extra salt to replace that lost in sweat
- Adequate calcium, vitamin D, and vitamin K

Nutrition intervention is based on an initial and ongoing schedule for assessment, including anthropometrics, laboratory studies, and nutrition evaluation (Table 20-4). Related therapy is then outlined in five levels according to individual assessment results and nutrition care needs and actions (Table 20-5).

TABLE 20-4	BASIC NUTRITION ASSESSMENT FOR NUTRITIONAL MANAGEMENT OF CYSTIC FIBROSIS	
KEY ASSESSMENTS	**MONITORING SCHEDULE AND INDICATIONS**
Anthropometry	
Weight	Every 3 months or as needed for growth evaluation
Height (length)	
BMI (adults)	
Head circumference (until child is age 2)	
Midarm circumference	
Triceps skinfold	
Midarm muscle circumference (derived)*	
Biochemical Data	
CBC	Yearly routine care, interim as needed to detect deficiencies, iron status
TIBC, serum iron, ferritin	
Plasma/serum retinol, α-tocopherol	As indicated, weight loss, growth failure, clinical deterioration
Albumin, prealbumin	
Electrolytes, acid-base balance	Summer heat, prolonged fever
Random glucose	Annually to detect CFDM
Dietary Evaluation	
Dietary intake	As indicated, history and food records, full energy-nutrient analysis
Three-day fat balance study†	As indicated, weight loss, growth failure, clinical deterioration
Anticipatory guidance	Yearly, interim as needed according to growth or situational needs

Data from Hollander FM, De Roos NM, De Vries JH, et al: Assessment of nutritional status in adult patients with cystic fibrosis: whole-body bioimpedance vs body mass index, skinfolds, and leg-to-leg bioimpedance. *J Am Diet Assoc* 105(4):549, 2005; Ramsey BW, Farrell PM, Pencharz P: Nutritional assessment and management in cystic fibrosis: a consensus report—The Consensus Committee, *Am J Clin Nutr* 55:108, 1992; Yankaskas JR: Cystic fibrosis adult care: consensus conference report. *Chest* 125:1S, 2004.
BMI, Body mass index; *CBC,* complete blood count; *CFDM,* cystic fibrosis–related diabetes mellitus; *TIBC,* total iron-binding capacity.
*See Chapter 16 for equations.
†3-day food records for analysis of fat intake; stool collections for analysis of fat content and degree of malabsorption.

TABLE 20-5	LEVELS OF NUTRITION CARE FOR MANAGEMENT OF CYSTIC FIBROSIS	
LEVELS OF CARE	**PATIENT GROUPS**	**NUTRITION ACTIONS**
Level I—routine care	All	Diet counseling, food plans, enzyme replacement, vitamin supplements, nutrition education, exploration of problems
Level II—anticipatory guidance	Greater than 90% ideal weight-height index but at risk of energy imbalance; severe pancreatic insufficiency, frequent pulmonary infections, normal periods of rapid growth	Increased monitoring of dietary intake, complete energy-nutrient analysis, increased kcaloric density as needed; assess behavioral needs; provide counseling, nutrition education
Level III—supportive intervention	85% to 90% ideal weight-height index, decreased weight-growth velocity	Reinforce all previously mentioned actions, add oral supplements (energy-nutrient dense)
Level IV—rehabilitative care	Consistently less than 85% ideal weight-height index, nutritional and growth failure	All of the previously mentioned plus EN support by nasoenteric or enterostomy tube feeding (see Chapter 19)
Level V—resuscitative or palliative care	Less than 75% ideal weight-height index, progressive nutritional failure	All of the previously mentioned plus continuous enteral tube feedings or TPN (see Chapter 19)

Modified from Ramsey BW, Farrell PM, Pencharz P: Nutritional assessment and management in cystic fibrosis: a consensus report—The Consensus Committee. *Am J Clin Nutr* 55:108, 1992.
EN, Enteral nutrition; *TPN,* total parenteral nutrition.

Inflammatory Bowel Diseases
Nature and Incidence
The two most common forms of IBD are Crohn's disease and ulcerative colitis (UC).[16] Both conditions produce extended mucosal tissue lesions, although these lesions differ in extent and nature (Figure 20-9). However, they have been classified medically in a single group because they are similar in their clinical symptoms and management. Their causes remain unknown, although heredity, environment, and immune functions are thought to be contributing factors.[16] Incidence

TABLE 20-6   SIMILARITIES AND DIFFERENCES BETWEEN CROHN'S DISEASE AND ULCERATIVE COLITIS

MANIFESTATION	CROHN'S DISEASE	ULCERATIVE COLITIS
Cause	Unknown	Unknown
Genetics	Increased prevalence in first-degree relatives; NOD2 gene mutation on chromosome 16	Increased prevalence in first-degree relatives; susceptibility loci on chromosomes 2 and 6
Site of inflammation	Any part of the gastrointestinal (GI) tract	Rectum (and spreads proximally)
Mucosal layers affected		Epithelial
Abdominal pain	Common	Common
Diarrhea	Common	Common
Rectal bleeding	Sometimes	Common
Perforations	Common	Yes
Fibrosis, stricture, and fistulas	Common	No
Toxic megacolon	Rare	Common
Weight loss	Common	Common
Steatorrhea	Sometimes	No
Perianal disease	Common	No
Fever	Yes	No
Epidemiology	Developed countries, major age peak at ages 20-40, more common in women	Developed countries, major age peak at ages 20-40, more common in women
Relapses and remissions	Chronic	Usually no symptoms between attacks
Complications	Abscess, obstruction, fistulas, perianal disease, increased risk of colon cancer, malabsorption, kidney stones (oxalate and uric acid), gallstones	Many and varied including joint disorders, fatty liver, disorders of the eyes and skin
Prophylactic therapy	Not well established	Colonoscopy with multiple biopsies every 1-3 years
Prognosis	Recurrent morbidity throughout lives; risk of death approximately twice the general population	Mortality rate similar to general population

Data from Sartin JS: Gastrointestinal disorders. In Copstead LC, Banasik JL, editors: *Pathophysiology*, ed 4, St Louis, Mo., 2009, Saunders.

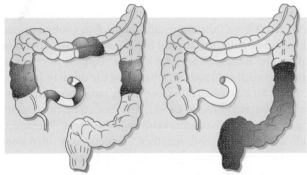

FIGURE 20-9 Crohn's disease *(left)* and ulcerative colitis (UC) *(right)*. Crohn's disease typically involves the small and large intestine in a segmental manner; UC generally starts in the rectum and progresses to involvement of varying lengths of the colon. (Modified from Cotran CS, Kumar V, Robbins SJ: *Robbins' pathologic basis of disease,* ed 4, Philadelphia, Pa., 1989, Saunders.)

of these diseases, especially Crohn's disease, has increased worldwide. Crohn's disease is particularly prevalent in industrialized areas of the world. It also appears among otherwise low-risk persons who move from rural to urban centers, with incidence being highest in people from 20 to 40 years of age and those of Jewish heritage.

Clinical Manifestations

Also called *regional enteritis* and *granulomatous colitis,* inflammation produced by Crohn's disease extends through all layers of the intestinal wall, most commonly in the proximal portion of the colon and less often the terminal ileum.[17] UC is an inflammatory disease of mucosal layers of the rectum and colon.[18] Similarities and differences between the two diseases are summarized in Table 20-6.

Medical Management

Because the cause of IBD is unknown, treatment is focused on alleviating and reducing inflammation. Similar drug therapies are used for Crohn's disease and UC: antibiotics, immunosuppressants, immunomodulators, and biologic therapies.[2,18] A small percentage of patients with UC require surgery.[18] Most common surgical procedures include total colectomy or ileostomy (Figure 20-10). Approximately 80% of patients with Crohn's disease will eventually require surgery. Fifty percent of these patients will require a second surgery within 10 years as a result of disease recurrence. Strictures often require minimal resection; colitis may require colectomy with ileorectal anastomosis or ileostomy. Abscesses are drained, and enteric fistulas are resected.[17,18]

Normal Anatomy   **Postcolectomy**

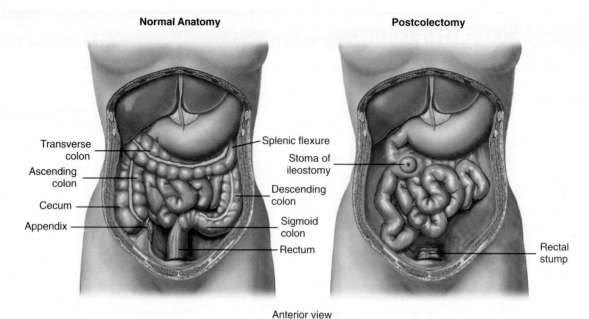

Anterior view

FIGURE 20-10 Colectomy (colon removal) with ileostomy. (Medical Illustration Copyright 2006 Nucleus Medical Art, All rights reserved. www.nucleusinc.com.)

Nutrition Therapy

Nutrition therapy centers on supporting the healing process and avoiding nutritional deficiency states and will be contingent on functional condition of the GI tract. Nutrition intervention depends on the functional status of the GI tract: extent of exacerbation, extent of diarrheal output, obstruction, surgery, and bleeding. When an oral diet cannot meet nutritional needs, enteral nutrition (EN) or PN is used[19]:

- Enteral feedings or total parenteral nutrition (TPN)
- Progression to low-fat, low-residue, high-protein, high-calorie, small, frequent meals
- Vitamin and mineral supplements: vitamin D, zinc, calcium, magnesium, folate, vitamin B_{12}, iron

Nutrition Therapy during Remission

Nutrition therapy in remission includes the following[19]:

- Tailor for the patient's current GI function
- Energy and protein at levels to maintain weight and replenish nutrient stores
- Avoid foods high in oxalate (see Appendix B)
- Increase antioxidant intake (see Chapter 6)
- Consider supplementation with omega-3 fatty acids and glutamine
- Use probiotics and prebiotics
- Diet as complete as possible

Short-Bowel Syndrome
Cause

Short bowel syndrome is a malabsorptive condition secondary to surgical removal of parts of the small intestine with extensive dysfunction of the remaining portion of the organ. Severity of malabsorption is contingent on the amount and location of bowel resection. Removal of the distal two thirds

of ileum and ileocecal valve often results in severe malnutrition because the ileocecal valve controls the transit time of intestinal contents. Removal often promotes a transit time too rapid for sufficient absorption of nutrients. Absorption of water, electrolytes, protein, fat, carbohydrates, vitamins, and minerals is significantly reduced when large portions of the small intestine are lost.[8,20]

Typically, in an adult the small intestine is 20 feet long, and the large intestine is 7 feet long. A general definition for SBS is a resection of more than 50% of the small intestine. Resections result from inherent conditions such as Crohn's disease or radiation enteritis, surgical bypass, or massive abdominal injury and trauma. They may also be required for vascular problems such as blood clots that cause the death of involved tissue or for extensive fistula formation, radiation injury, congenital abnormalities, or cancer. After resection, the remaining small intestine has remarkable ability to adapt.[2] Remaining villi may enlarge and lengthen, consequently increasing absorptive surface area of the remaining intestine. Nutrients must be ingested orally for this adaptive sequence to take place, and gradual increase in oral intake after resection could promote gradual recovery in absorptive capability. PN support may be necessary for the short term or indefinitely after surgical shortening of the gut.

KEY TERMS

probiotics Microbial foods or supplements that can be used to modify or reestablish intestinal flora and improve health of the host.

prebiotics Nondigestible food products that promote growth of symbiotic bacterial species already present in the colon.

Nutritional Management

Degrees of surgical resection create different problems, and nutrition therapy must be tailored to individual's remaining functional capacity. Initial nutritional needs are usually supplied by early EN or PN support (see Chapter 19). Frequent monitoring of the patient's responses to nutrition support, especially fluid and electrolyte balances and malnutrition signs, is essential. The patient is weaned from nutrition support to an oral diet as tolerated, accompanied by vitamin and mineral supplementation. Nutritional status should continue to be monitored. As adaptation progresses, early restriction of fat may be liberalized somewhat with moderate use of the more easily absorbed MCT oil to obtain needed kcalories.

Bowel Transplantation

Patients with complications such as recurrent sepsis, thrombosis of access sites, metabolic disorders, cholestasis, and hepatic dysfunction resulting from TPN failure may be considered candidates for intestine transplant, which may involve the entire small intestine or just a segment of it. Most intestine transplants are whole organ transplants and are often performed in combination with a liver transplant.

Patients who undergo small-bowel transplantation can have problems transitioning to oral nutrition. Furthermore, special feeding considerations should be taken into consideration during the initial phase after transplant when the graft begins to function (Table 20-7). Large amounts of fluids lost after surgery must be replaced to prevent dehydration. Oral rehydration solutions may be used, although intravenous fluids may be required to replace not only lost fluids but also magnesium, zinc, bicarbonate, potassium, and sodium. Fiber, pectin, paregoric, and loperamide may enhance intestinal absorption by slowing transit time.

DISORDERS OF THE LARGE INTESTINE

Flatulence

Everyone has it. Most believe they have too much, and everyone is embarrassed if they pass gas in the wrong place at the wrong time. History views flatulence with mixed reviews. Hippocrates professed, "Passing gas is necessary to well-being." The Roman Emperor Claudius decreed, "All Roman citizens shall be allowed to pass gas whenever necessary." Regrettably for flatulent Romans, Emperor Constantine later overturned this pronouncement.

Cause

Flatulence is the condition of having excessive stomach or intestinal gas. Gas in the gut is the result of swallowed air or production in the intestines. Air swallowing (aerophagia) is a common cause of gas in the stomach. Small amounts of air are swallowed when eating and drinking. Some people swallow additional air while they eat or drink rapidly, chew gum, smoke, or wear dentures that are too loose. Most swallowed air is expelled from the stomach by burping or belching. Residual gas moves into the small intestine and is partially absorbed. A small quantity of gas travels to the large intestine and is expelled through the rectum.

Gas is produced in the intestines when normal, harmless bacteria in the large intestine break down undigested foods humans cannot because of a lack of specific digestive enzymes. Gas in the intestines is made of primarily odorless vapors such as carbon dioxide (CO_2), oxygen, nitrogen, hydrogen, and sometimes methane. The unpleasant odor of flatulence is produced by bacteria in the large intestine that release small amounts of gases that contain sulfur. These gases eventually exit the body through the rectum. Hydrogen and CO_2 are produced after ingestion of certain fruits and vegetables containing indigestible carbohydrates and in those with

TABLE 20-7	GUIDELINES FOR INITIATING ENTERAL NUTRITION IN INTESTINE TRANSPLANT RECIPIENTS	
NUTRIENT	**GUIDELINE**	**COMMENT**
Carbohydrates	Concentrated sweets and hyperosmolar fruit juice may cause osmotic diarrhea.	Carbohydrate malabsorption and secondary lactase deficiency may increase luminal osmolarity and increase stomal output.
Fat	MCT or intravenous lipids short term.	Lacteals and lymphatics of small intestine are severed during organ retrieval causing fat malabsorption initially.
Glutamine	Long-chain fatty acid absorption may improve within 2-6 weeks as lacteals and lymphatics are regenerated.	Glutamine is a conditionally essential amino acid and fuel for enterocytes.
Bicarbonate	An enteral formula enriched with glutamine may theoretically improve absorptive function and mucosal structure after transplantation.	Bicarbonate losses from the ostomy are often increased.
Fluid	Supplement. Rehydration solutions may be helpful.	High intestinal losses are common.

Modified from Hasse JM: Nutrition assessment and support of organ transplant recipients. *J Parenter Enteral Nutr* 25:120, 2001. Reprinted with permission of SAGE Publications.
MCT, Medium-chain triglycerides.

TABLE 20-8   FOODS THAT MAY CAUSE GAS

CATEGORY		FOOD SOURCES
Sugars	Raffinose	Beans, cabbage, Brussels sprouts, broccoli, asparagus, other vegetables, whole grains
	Lactose	Milk, milk products (cheese, ice cream, processed foods)
	Fructose	Onions, artichokes, peas, wheat (fructose also used as a sweetener in some soft drinks and fruit drinks)
	Sorbitol	Fruits: apples, pears, peaches, prunes (sorbitol also used as an artificial sweetener in many dietetic foods and sugar-free candies and gums)
Starches		Potatoes, corn, noodles, wheat products (only starch that does not produce gas is rice)
Fiber	Soluble	Oat bran, beans, peas, most fruits
	Insoluble	Wheat bran, some vegetables

Modified from National Digestive Disease Information Clearinghouse (NDDIC), National Institute of Diabetes and Digestive and Kidney Diseases (NIDDK), National Institutes of Health (NIH): *Gas in the digestive tract*, NIH Pub No 08-883, Bethesda, Md., 2008, National Digestive Diseases Information Clearinghouse. from: <www.digestive.niddk.nih.gov/ddiseases/pubs/gas/>. Retrieved May 14, 2014.

malabsorption syndromes (CF, CD, pancreatic insufficiency). Large amounts of disaccharides pass into the colon and are fermented to hydrogen in those with lactose deficiency. Methane is produced in approximately one third of the population and is influenced minimally by food ingestion. The tendency to produce methane appears to be a familial trait.[21] Foods that produce gas in one person may not produce gas in another. Most foods that produce gas contain carbohydrates (Table 20-8); fats and proteins cause little gas.

Medical Management

The most common ways to reduce production of gas are to change the diet, take medications, and reduce the amount of air swallowed. The difficulty in suggesting dietary modification is individual tolerances. The quantity of gas produced by particular foods varies from person to person. Effective dietary change is typically the result of learning by way of trial and error.

Few well-controlled studies have demonstrated a clear-cut benefit from any drug,[22] but some OTC medicines are available to help reduce symptoms (Table 20-9). Although gas may be unpleasant and embarrassing, it is not life threatening. Education concerning causes, ways to reduce symptoms, and treatment help most people find relief.[22]

Irritable Bowel Syndrome
Cause

Sometimes called *spastic colon*, IBS is a recurring functional disorder typified by abdominal pain or discomfort with alternating diarrhea and constipation for which no organic explanation is available.[8] For those with IBS, the quantity of symptoms is not as important as quality of life. Work, social life, and even sexual intercourse can be disrupted by IBS.[8] IBS is an extremely common disorder, affecting up to 20% of the U.S. population, but most never seek medical attention.[2]

Clinical Symptoms

Manifestation of IBS may differ to a great extent from person to person. Some experience only diarrhea or constipation, whereas others experience an alternating pattern of both problems.[8] Some symptoms may be more marked than others. No physical findings or diagnostic tests confirm the diagnosis of IBS.[23] Diagnosis is determined by the presence of congruent symptoms and after ruling out organic diseases.[23] More than half of those diagnosed with IBS are female patients.

The symptom-based Rome III diagnostic criteria for IBS emphasize a clear-cut diagnosis instead of excluding other medical conditions.[23] These criteria are based on a detailed history, physical examination, and limited diagnostic tests, as well as presentation of a particular set of symptoms (for the last 3 months, with symptom onset at least 6 months before diagnosis) as follows[24]:

- Recurrent abdominal pain or discomfort* at least 3 days per month in the last 3 months associated with two or more of the following:
  - Improvement with defecation
  - Onset associated with a change in frequency of stool
  - Onset associated with a change in form (appearance) of stool
- The following other symptoms support, but are not essential, to the diagnosis of IBS:
  - More than three bowel movements per day or fewer than three bowel movements per week
  - Lumpy-hard or loose-watery stool form
  - Abnormal stool passage (straining, urgency, or feeling of incomplete evacuation)
  - Passage of mucus
  - Bloating or feeling of abdominal distention

Medical Management

Possibly the most helpful treatment intervention is to proffer assurance and a straightforward explanation of the functional nature of symptoms. Patients should be assured that their symptoms are real (i.e., not caused by stress or a psychologic or psychiatric disorder), although in some individuals stress can trigger or exacerbate symptoms of IBS.[24,25]

Discomfort means an uncomfortable sensation not described as pain.

TABLE 20-9	NONPRESCRIPTION MEDICATIONS USED TO TREAT FLATULENCE	
MEDICATION	**CLASSIFICATION**	**ACTION**

Simethicone
  Mylanta II
  Maalox II
  Di-Gel
	Antacid	Foaming agent that joins gas bubbles in the stomach, making gas more easily belched away; no effect on intestinal gas

Lactase
  Lactaid
  Lactrase
	Enzyme	Aids lactose digestion

Beano α-Galactosidase	Enzyme supplement	Contains sugar-digesting enzyme the body lacks to digest sugar in beans and many vegetables; has no effect on gas caused by lactose or fiber
Charcocaps	Activated charcoal	May produce relief from gas produced in colon

Data from National Digestive Disease Information Clearinghouse (NDDIC), National Institute of Diabetes and Digestive and Kidney Diseases (NIDDK), National Institutes of Health (NIH): *Gas in the digestive tract,* NIH Pub No 08-883, Bethesda, Md., 2008, NIH. from: <www.digestive.niddk.nih.gov/ddiseases/pubs/gas/>. Retrieved May 14, 2014; Maslar J, Kreplick LW: *Flatulence (gas),* Omaha, Neb., 2005, eMedicine Consumer Health. from: <www.emedicinehealth.com/Articles/5940-1.asp>. Retrieved May 14, 2014.

A chronic disorder, IBS can be treated but not cured. Therapy is directed at specific symptoms.[25] Antidiarrheal agents can decrease the motility and increase the consistency of stools for patients with diarrhea-predominant IBS. An α-adrenergic stimulating agent is sometimes used to treat diarrhea and abdominal pain by inhibiting norepinephrine activity. Other medications often used to treat IBS and assist in pain control are tricyclic antidepressants and selective serotonin reuptake inhibitors (SSRIs). Constipation-predominant IBS is often treated with bulking agents and osmotic laxatives. The newest medications for IBS are medications that work as 5-HT$_4$ receptor agonists and are effective in treating constipation-predominant IBS.[2]

Nutritional Management

Dietary triggers of IBS have not been established; however, dietary modification may provide symptomatic benefit. For some, a food diary in which food intake, symptoms, and activities are recorded may uncover dietary or psychosocial aspects that predispose symptoms. Malabsorption of lactose, fructose, and sorbitol can cause bloating, distention, flatulence, and diarrhea. An assortment of foods can trigger flatulence (see Table 20-8), which may cause pain and distention in some patients. To identify triggers, follow a low FODMAP (fermentable oligo-, di-, and monosaccharides and polyols) diet for 6 weeks and add high FODMAP food one at a time in small amounts to identify food that triggers the symptoms. Once identified, these foods can be limited to prevent "triggers." For a list of low FODMAP food choices, refer to Table 20-9.

For patients with constipation-predominant IBS, a high-fiber diet (20 to 30 g/day) may ease symptoms. Bran powder (1 tbsp two to three times daily with food or in 8 oz or more of liquid) provides the recommended amount. Some patients may report increased gas and distention from fiber supplementation with bran; therefore psyllium, methylcellulose, or polycarbophil are often better tolerated. For management of flatulence, refer to Table 20-10 for nonprescription medications and supplements.

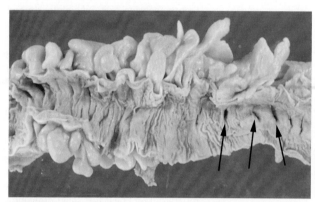

FIGURE 20-11 Diverticula. (From Lewis SM, Heitkemper M, Dirksen S: *Medical-surgical nursing: assessment and management of clinical problems,* ed 6, St Louis, Mo., 2004, Mosby.)

Diverticular Disease
Nature and Cause

A diverticulum is a small tubular sac that protrudes from a main canal or cavity in the body (Figure 20-11). Formation and presence of small diverticula protruding from the intestinal lumen, usually the colon, produce the condition *diverticulosis*. More often diverticulosis occurs in older adults. It develops at points of weakened musculature in the bowel wall, along the track of blood vessels entering the bowel from within. Direct cause is a progressive increase in pressure within the bowel from segmental circular muscle contractions that normally move the remaining food mass along and form the feces for elimination. When pressures become sufficiently high in one of these segments and dietary fiber is insufficient to maintain the necessary bulk for preventing high internal pressures within the colon, diverticula, small protrusions of the muscle layer, develop at that point. The condition causes no problem unless small diverticula become infected and inflamed from fecal irritation and colon bacteria. This diseased state is called *diverticulitis*. The commonly

TABLE 20-10 LOW FODMAP FOOD CHOICES

FOOD GROUP	FOODS TO EAT	FOODS TO LIMIT
Meats, poultry, fish, eggs	Beef, chicken, canned tuna, eggs, egg whites, fish, lamb, pork, shellfish, turkey, cold cuts	Foods made with high FODMAP fruits, sauces, or with HFCS
Dairy	Lactose-free dairy, small amounts of cream cheese, half and half, hard cheese (cheddar, Colby, parmesan, Swiss), mozzarella, sherbet	Buttermilk, chocolate, cottage cheese, ice cream, creamy/cheesy sauces, milk (from cow, sheep, or goat), sweetened condensed milk, evaporated milk, soft cheeses (brie, ricotta), sour cream, whipped cream, yogurt
Meat, nondairy alternatives	Almond milk, rice milk, rice milk ice cream, nuts, nut butters, seeds	Coconut milk, coconut cream, beans, black eyed peas, hummus, lentils, pistachios, soy products
Grains	Wheat-free grains/wheat-free flours (gluten-free grains are wheat free): bagels, breads, hot/cold cereals (corn flakes, Cheerios, cream of rice, grits, oats, etc.), crackers, noodles, pastas, quinoa, pancakes, pretzels, rice, tapioca, tortillas, waffles	Chicory root, inulin, grains with HFCS or made from wheat (terms for wheat: einkorn, emmer, kamut, spelt), wheat flours (terms for wheat flour: bromated, durum, enriched, farina, graham, semolina, white flours), flour tortillas, rye
Fruits	Bananas, berries, cantaloupe, grapes, grapefruit, honeydew, kiwi, kumquat, lemon, lime, mandarin orange, passion fruit, pineapple, rhubarb, tangerine	Avocado, apples, applesauce, apricots, dates, canned fruit, cherries, dried fruits, figs, guava, lychee, mango, nectarines, pears, papaya, peaches, plums, prunes, persimmon, watermelon
Vegetables	Bamboo shoots, bell peppers, bok choy, cucumbers, carrots, celery, corn, eggplant, lettuce, leafy greens, pumpkin, potatoes, squash (butternut, winter), yams, tomatoes, zucchini	Artichokes, asparagus, beets, leeks, broccoli, Brussels sprouts, cabbage, cauliflower, fennel, green beans, mushrooms, okra, snow peas, summer squash
Desserts	Any made with allowed foods	Any with HFCS or made with foods to limit
Beverages	Low FODMAP fruit/vegetable juices (limit to $\frac{1}{2}$ cup at a time), coffee, tea	Any with HFCS, high FODMAP fruit/vegetable juices, fortified wines (sherry, port)
Seasonings, condiments	Most spices and herbs, homemade broth, butter, chives, flaxseed, garlic flavored oil, garlic powder, olives, margarine, mayonnaise, onion powder, olive oil, pepper, salt, sugar, maple syrup without HFCS, mustard, low FODMAP salad dressings, soy sauce, marinara sauce (small amounts), vinegar, balsamic vinegar	HFCS, agave, chutneys, coconut, garlic, honey, jams, jellies, molasses, onions, pickle, relish, high FODMAP fruit/vegetable sauces, salad dressings made with high FODMAPs, artificial sweeteners: sorbitol, mannitol, isomalt, xylitol (cough drops, gums, mints)

Table from http://stanfordhospital.org/digestivehealth/nutrition/DH-Low-FODMAP-Diet-Handout.pdf, Stanford Hospitals and Clinics, August 2012.
FODMAP, Fermentable oligo-, di-, and monosaccharides and polyols; *HFCS,* high-fructose corn syrup.

used collective term covering diverticulosis and diverticulitis is *diverticular disease.*

Clinical Symptoms

As the inflammatory process grows, increased hypermotility and pressures from luminal segmentation cause pain. Pain and tenderness are usually localized in the lower left side of the abdomen and are accompanied by nausea, vomiting, distention, diarrhea, intestinal spasm, and fever. If the process continues, then intestinal obstruction or perforation may necessitate surgical intervention.

Nutritional Management

Diverticular disease is a common GI disorder among middle-aged persons and older adults. Aggressive nutrition therapy hastens recovery from an attack, shortens hospital stay, and reduces costs. Numerous studies and extensive clinical practice have demonstrated better management of chronic diverticular disease with an increased amount of dietary fiber than with old practices of restricting fiber. In acute episodes of

active disease, however, the amount of dietary fiber should be reduced. The relationship of dietary fiber and diverticular disease has been further reinforced by studies of populations, such as those in Japan, that have recently experienced the westernization of their culture. Chapter 3 provides an extended discussion of dietary fiber and its relation to health and disease. Historically, avoidance of nuts, seeds, and hulls has been recommended, but current literature indicates this is not required.[26-29]

Constipation

A common disorder, usually of short duration, constipation is characterized by retention of feces in the colon beyond normal emptying time. Americans spend a quarter of a billion dollars each year on laxatives for this problem. However, "regularity" of elimination is highly individual, and it is not necessary to have a bowel movement every day to be healthy. Usually this common, short-term problem results from various sources of nervous tension, worry, and changes in social setting. Such situations include vacations and travel with alterations in usual routines. In addition, it may be caused by prolonged use of laxatives or cathartics, low-fiber diets, inadequate fluid intake, or lack of exercise, all of which can contribute to a decreased intestinal muscle tone. Increasing activity and improving dietary intake to include adequate fiber (with a goal of 25 to 35 g/day) and fluid are usually sufficient strategies to remedy the situation. If chronic constipation persists, however, then agents that increase stool bulk may be necessary. These bulking agents include bran or more soluble forms of fiber. Taking laxatives or enemas on a regular basis should be avoided. The problem of constipation occurs in all age-groups but is almost epidemic in older adults. In all cases, a personalized approach to management of constipation is fundamental.

DISEASES OF THE GASTROINTESTINAL ACCESSORY ORGANS

The liver, the gallbladder, and the pancreas (Figure 20-12) are three major accessory organs that lie adjacent to the GI tract and produce important digestive agents that enter the intestine and aid in processing of food substances. Specific enzymes are produced for each of the major nutrients, and bile is added to assist in enzymatic digestion of fats. Diseases of these organs can easily affect GI function and cause problems in the normal handling of specific types of food.

Viral Hepatitis
Cause
Viral hepatitis (inflammation of the liver) is a major public health problem throughout the world, affecting hundreds of

millions of people. It causes considerable illness and death in human populations from acute infection or its effects, which may include chronic active hepatitis, cirrhosis, and primary liver cancer. During the past few years, knowledge of viruses that cause different types of hepatitis has grown rapidly. Currently, six unrelated human hepatitis viruses—A, B, C, D, and E—have been isolated and described. The two most common and well known are A and B, which serve as examples, as follows:

1. *Hepatitis A virus (HAV):* HAV is transmitted via the classic oral-fecal route through contaminated food and water. It is a prevalent infection worldwide, especially where overcrowding and poor hygiene or sanitation exists. An HAV vaccine has been developed that is far more effective than the former large and painful injection of gamma globulins, antibodies isolated from the blood. This vaccine protects travelers to developing countries, where the virus is endemic and may easily contaminate water and food.[30]

2. *Hepatitis B virus (HBV):* HBV is mainly spread via parenteral contact with infected blood or blood products, including contaminated needles, and sexual contact.[26] It has now been implicated worldwide as the major cause of chronic liver disease and associated liver cancer. HBV infection is closely related to the body's immune system. Approximately 10% to 20% of those who become infected with HBV become chronic carriers. Of this number, approximately 20% acquire chronic hepatitis that eventually progresses to cirrhosis and for some individuals, to liver cancer.[30] Universal immunization is recommended for persons of any age, but particularly for the following high-risk groups: male homosexuals, Alaska Natives,

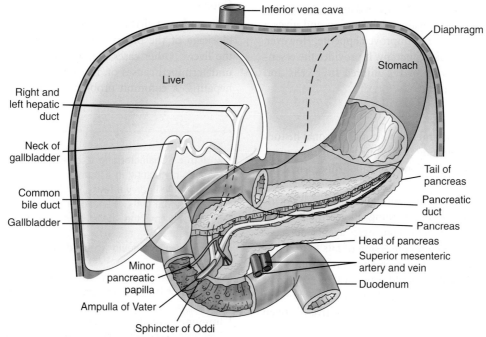

FIGURE 20-12 Liver, pancreas, and gallbladder. (From Copstead LE, Banasik JL: *Pathophysiology,* ed 4, Philadelphia, Pa., 2009, Saunders.)

immigrants from highly endemic areas, illicit drug users, domestic associates of HBV carriers, hemodialysis patients, residents of institutions, medical and dental personnel, patients needing frequent transfusions, and those planning to reside in high-risk areas (e.g., Far East and sub-Saharan Africa).[30]

Clinical Symptoms

Viral agents of hepatitis produce diffuse injury to liver cells, especially parenchymal cells. In milder cases, liver injury is largely reversible, but with increasing severity, more extensive necrosis occurs. In some cases, massive necrosis may lead to liver failure and death. A cardinal symptom of hepatitis is anorexia, which contributes to the risk of malnutrition. Varying clinical symptoms appear depending on the degree of liver injury. Jaundice, a major symptom, may or may not be obvious, depending on severity of the disease, and it can have nutritional and psychologic effects. In an outbreak of hepatitis, many infected persons may be nonicteric and thus go undiagnosed and untreated because jaundice has not developed sufficiently to be seen. Malnutrition and impaired immunocompetence contribute to spontaneous infections and continuing liver disease. General symptoms, in addition to anorexia, include malaise, weakness, nausea and vomiting, diarrhea, headache, fever, enlarged and tender liver, and enlarged spleen. When jaundice develops, it usually occurs for a preicteric period of 5 to 10 days, deepens for 1 to 2 weeks, then levels off and decreases. After this crisis point, a sufficient recovery of injured cells occurs, and a convalescence of 3 weeks to 3 months follows. Optimal care during this time is crucial to avoid relapse.

General Treatment

Bed rest is essential. Physical activity and exercise increases the severity and duration of the disease. A daily intake of 3000 to 3500 mL of fluid guards against dehydration and gives a general sense of well-being and improved appetite. However, optimal nutrition is the major therapy. It provides the essential foundation for recovery of the injured liver cells and overall return of strength.

Nutrition Therapy

A complete nutrition assessment and initial personal history provide the basis for planning care. Nutrition therapy principles relate to the liver's function in metabolizing each of the nutrients, as follows[31]:

- *Adequate protein:* Protein is essential for liver cell regeneration, as well as for maintaining all essential bodily functions. It also provides lipotropic agents such as methionine and choline for conversion of fats to lipoproteins and removal from the liver, thus preventing fatty infiltration. The daily diet should supply 1.0 to 1.2 g/kg of actual body weight (ABW) of high-quality protein. This amount is usually enough to achieve a positive nitrogen balance.
- *Low fat:* Less than 30% of calories should come from fat in case of steatorrhea.

- *Four to six small feedings:* To promote adequate intake and minimize loss of muscle, at least three meals and a bedtime snack are recommended.
- *Sodium:* If fluid retention is present, then limit sodium to 90 mEq/day (approximately 2000 mg).

Meals and Feedings

The problem of supplying a diet adequate to meet increased nutritional demands of a patient with an illness that makes food almost repellent calls for creativity and supportive encouragement. As the patient improves, appetizing and attractive food is needed. Because nutrition therapy is key to recovery, a major nutrition and nursing responsibility requires devising ways to encourage the increased amounts of food intake needed. The clinical dietitian and nursing staff should work together to achieve mutual goals planned for the patient. All staff attendants must observe appropriate precautions in handling patient trays to prevent spread of the infection.

Cirrhosis

Cirrhosis is the general term used for advanced stages of liver disease, regardless of the initial cause of the disease. Among all digestive diseases, cirrhosis of the liver, caused by chronic alcohol abuse, is the leading nonmalignant cause of death in the United States and most of the developed world. The majority of deaths occur among young and middle-aged adults. The French physician René Laënnec (1781-1826) first used the term *cirrhosis* (from the Greek word *kirrhos*, meaning orange-yellow) to describe the abnormal color and rough surface of the diseased liver. The cirrhotic liver is a firm, fibrous, dull-yellowish mass with orange nodules projecting from its surface (Figure 20-13).

Cause

Some forms of cirrhosis result from biliary obstruction, with blockage of the biliary ducts and accumulation of bile in the liver.[32] Other cases may result from liver necrosis from undetermined causes or, in some cases, from previous viral hepatitis. A common problem is fatty cirrhosis, associated

---

KEY TERMS

endemic Characterizing a disease of low morbidity that remains constantly in a human community but is clinically recognizable in only a few.

parenchymal cells Functional cells of an organ, as distinguished from the cells constituting its structure or framework.

necrosis Cell death caused by progressive enzyme breakdown.

icteric Alternative term for jaundice (*nonicteric* indicates absence of jaundice and *preicteric* indicates a state before development of icterus, or jaundice).

immunocompetence The ability or capacity to develop an immune response, that is, antibody production or cell-mediated immunity (or both), after exposure to antigen.

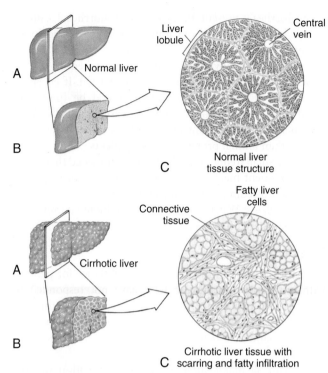

FIGURE 20-13 Comparison of normal liver and liver with cirrhotic changes. **A,** Anterior view of organ. **B,** Cross-section. **C,** Tissue structure. (Medical and Scientific Illustration.)

with the complicating factor of malnutrition. Continuing fatty infiltration causes cellular destruction and fibrotic tissue changes.

Clinical Symptoms

Early signs of cirrhosis include GI disturbances such as nausea, vomiting, loss of appetite, distention, and epigastric pain. In time, jaundice may appear, with increasing weakness, edema, ascites, and anemia from GI bleeding, iron deficiency, or hemorrhage. A specific macrocytic anemia from folic acid deficiency is also frequently observed. Steatorrhea is a common symptom. Major symptoms are caused by a basic protein deficiency and its multiple metabolic problems: (1) plasma protein levels fall, leading to failure of the capillary fluid shift mechanism (see Chapter 2), causing ascites; (2) lipotropic agents are not supplied for fat conversion to lipoproteins, and damaging fat accumulates in the liver tissue; (3) blood-clotting mechanisms are impaired because factors such as prothrombin and fibrinogen are not adequately produced; and (4) general tissue catabolism and negative nitrogen balance continue the overall degenerative process.

As the disease progresses, increasing fibrotic scar tissue impairs blood circulation through the liver, resulting in portal hypertension.[32] Contributing further to the problem is continuing ascites. Impaired portal circulation with increasing venous pressure may lead to esophageal varices, with danger of rupture and fatal massive hemorrhage.

Drug therapy includes use of broad-spectrum antibiotics to limit growth of intestinal bacteria and laxatives to speed

intestinal transit time, limiting the amount of time available for bacteria to produce ammonia in the GI tract. Lactulose, a synthetic derivative of lactose consisting of one molecule of galactose and one molecule of fructose, is a laxative that is used in the treatment of hepatic encephalopathy. Lactulose is ionized, cannot diffuse across the colon membrane, and is excreted in the stool. Lactulose can reduce blood ammonia levels by 25% to 50%. Diuretics may be given to reduce fluid retention and prevent ascites.

Nutrition Therapy

When alcoholism is an added underlying problem, treatment is difficult. Each patient requires supportive care. Therapy is usually aimed at correcting fluid and electrolyte problems and providing as much nutrition support as possible for hepatic repair. In any case, guidelines for nutrition therapy for cirrhosis of the liver should include the following principles[2,33]:

- *Energy:* 40 to 50 kcal/kg body weight. Fluid retention, if present, will affect the accuracy of estimating kcalorie needs. As muscle tissue is wasted, it is often replaced by fluid weight. An estimated dry weight (postparacentesis of ascites or well diuresed) should be used when feasible to estimate kcalorie needs.
- *Protein intake:* 1 to 1.5 g/kg body weight. Intake should be adequate to regenerate liver cells and prevent infections but not excessive to the point of aggravating ammonia buildup and inducing hepatic coma. Protein estimations should be based on dry weight whenever possible.
- *Sodium:* Intake is usually restricted to less than 2000 mg/day to help reduce fluid retention. A sodium intake level of less than 2000 mg/day is considered quite restrictive, and palatability of food is usually a problem. It may be necessary to liberalize the sodium restriction to improve intake.
- *Texture:* If esophageal varices develop, then it may be necessary to give soft foods that are smooth in texture to prevent the danger of rupture and hemorrhage.
- *Carbohydrate:* Adequate intake is needed to prevent catabolism of body protein for energy, which would further increase blood ammonia. Intestinal bacteria make ammonia from undigested proteins (proteins from shed mucosal cells, protein from GI tract bleed, and dietary proteins).
- *Fat:* Fat restriction should be less than 30% of calories (with or without MCT supplements) in patients with steatorrhea.
- *Vitamins and minerals:* The central role of the liver is to metabolize and store vitamins and minerals. Usually all people with advanced liver disease require supplementation of some vitamins, minerals, and trace elements. Nutrient supplementation is determined by monitoring serum levels and checking for clinical signs of deficiencies.
- *Alcohol:* To protect the liver from further injury, abstinence from alcohol is mandatory.
- *Personalized food plan:* Adequate intake is more likely, thus hastening recovery, if the food plan is developed based on

the likes and dislikes and real-life schedule of the patient. If appetite is a problem, then several small meals per day instead of full meals may be required.

- *Fluids:* Fluids should be encouraged unless ascites or edema is present. Water is the fluid of choice. Calorie-dense beverages such as juicelike drinks and soft drinks provide excess calories with little nutrient, often taking the place of nutrient-dense foods.

Hepatic Encephalopathy

The term *encephalopathy* refers to any disease or disorder that affects the brain, especially chronic degenerative conditions such as end-stage liver disease. Accumulation of toxic substances such as ammonia in the blood as a result of liver failure impairs consciousness and contributes to memory loss, personality change, tremors, seizures, stupor, and coma.

Cause

As cirrhotic changes continue in the liver, portal blood circulation diminishes and liver functions begin to fail. The normal liver has a major function of removing ammonia from blood by converting it to urea for excretion. The failing liver can no longer inactivate, detoxify substances, metabolize, or synthesize body compounds. A key factor involved in the progressive disease process is an elevated blood level of ammonia, and ammonia is one of the compounds that accumulate in the blood due to the liver's inability to convert it to urea. The resulting hepatic encephalopathy brings changes in consciousness, behavior, and neurologic status.

Clinical Symptoms

Typical response involves disorders of consciousness and alterations in motor function. Apathy, confusion, inappropriate behavior, and drowsiness is seen, progressing to coma. Speech may be slurred or monotonous. A coarse, flapping tremor known as *asterixis* is observed in the outstretched hands, caused by a sustained contraction of a group of muscles. Breath may have a fecal odor, called *fetor hepaticus.*

Basic Treatment Objectives

Fundamental objectives of treatment are twofold: (1) removal of sources of excess ammonia and (2) provision of nutrition support. Parenteral fluid and electrolytes are used to restore normal balances. Lactulose and neomycin may be used to control ammonia levels. Neomycin is an antibiotic that reduces the population of urea-splitting organisms within the bowel that produce ammonia.

Nutrition Therapy

General nutrition support for hepatic encephalopathy is based on the following five principles of dietary management[34]:

1. *Alcohol:* Abstinence is necessary.
2. *Energy:* Moderately high energy intake (25 to 40 kcal/kg) is needed to prevent breakdown of body tissue. Moderate fat intake of 30% of total kcal or less is encouraged unless steatorrhea is present. In the case of steatorrhea, fat intake can be reduced. Carbohydrates provide the majority of energy intake.
3. *Protein:* Generally protein intake is limited to 1.0 to 1.5 g/kg unless encephalopathy is associated. If encephalopathy is present, then protein should be limited to 60 g/day. Protein intake can be increased gradually as the patient improves. Plant protein seems to be better tolerated than animal protein by some patients.
4. *Meals:* Small frequent meals are better tolerated than large, less frequent meals. Soft foods that are low in fiber help prevent bleeding from esophageal varices.
5. *Supplements:* Water-soluble and fat-soluble vitamin supplements are often necessary.

Liver Transplantation

Liver transplantation is the treatment of choice for patients with end-stage liver disease who have not responded to conventional treatment. Patients being considered for liver transplantation undergo extensive physiologic and psychologic evaluations to detect possible contraindications to the procedure.[2]

As with all major surgery, aggressive nutrition support reduces risks. Careful pretransplantation nutrition assessment and support helps prepare the patient for the surgery. The general goal of posttransplant nutrition therapy is as follows[2]:

- *Energy:* 35-45 kcal/kg.
- *Protein:* 1.0-1.2 g/kg.
- *Other nutrients:* These are individualized based on the immunosuppressant drug regimen. (Complex carbohydrate should provide 50% to 60% of total kcalories. Use of corticosteroids results in the need for sodium to be restricted to 2 to 4 g/day. Cyclosporin and tacrolimus may require potassium restriction. Other minerals and electrolytes should be monitored.)
- *Vitamins:* Dietary Reference Intake (DRI) is provided to encourage proper wound healing.

Gallbladder Disease
Metabolic Function

The basic function of the gallbladder is to concentrate and store the bile produced in its initial watery solution by the liver. The liver secretes about 600 to 800 mL of bile per day, which the gallbladder normally concentrates fivefold to tenfold to accommodate this daily bile production in its small capacity of 40 to 70 mL. Presence of fat in the duodenum releases cholecystokinin (CCK) into the blood, which stimulates contraction of the gallbladder with release of concentrated bile into the common duct and then into the small intestine.

Cholecystitis and Cholelithiasis

The prefix *chole* of the two terms *cholecystitis* and *cholelithiasis* comes from the Greek word *chole,* which means bile. Thus cholecystitis is an inflammation of the gallbladder, and cholelithiasis is the formation of gallstones. Incidence of gallstones is associated with age, gender, and an assortment of medical factors (Box 20-4).

Inflammation of the gallbladder usually results from a low-grade chronic infection and may occur with or without gallstones. However, in 90% to 95% of patients, acute cholecystitis is associated with gallstones and is caused by the obstruction of the cystic duct by stones, resulting in acute inflammation of the organ. Gallstones can be classified into the following two main groups: (1) cholesterol stones and (2) pigment stones[35]:

1. *Cholesterol stones:* In the United States and most Western countries, more than 75% of gallstones are cholesterol stones. The infectious process produces changes in gallbladder mucosa, which affects its absorptive powers. The main ingredient of bile is cholesterol, which is insoluble in water. Normally, cholesterol is kept in solution by other ingredients in bile. However, when the absorbing mucosal tissue of the gallbladder is inflamed or infected, changes occur in the tissue. The absorptive powers of the gallbladder may be altered, affecting the solubility of the bile ingredients. Excess water or excess bile acid may be absorbed. Under these abnormal absorptive conditions, cholesterol may precipitate, forming gallstones of almost pure cholesterol.

2. *Pigment stones:* Black and brown pigment gallstones, although they differ in chemical composition and clinical features, are colored by the presence of bilirubin, the pigment in red blood cells. They are associated with chronic hemolysis in conditions such as sickle cell disease, thalassemia, cirrhosis, long-term TPN, and advancing age. Pigment stones are often found in bile ducts and may be related to a bacterial infection with *Escherichia coli.*

Clinical Symptoms

When inflammation, stones, or both are present in the gallbladder, contraction from the cholecystokinin-pancreozymin (CCK-PZ) mechanism causes pain, which is sometimes severe. Fullness, distention after eating, and particular difficulty with fatty foods are noted.

General Treatment

Surgical removal of the gallbladder, a cholecystectomy (Figure 20-14), is usually indicated. If the patient is obese, then some weight loss before surgery is advisable if surgery can be delayed. Supportive therapy is largely nutritional. Several

---

BOX 20-4	RISK FACTORS FOR GALLBLADDER DISEASE

- Female gender
- Ethnicity: Native American, particularly Pima Indians of North America
- High-cholesterol diet
- Use of oral contraceptives
- Obesity (body mass index [BMI] >30)
- Ileal resection or disease
- Diabetes mellitus
- Rapid weight loss (in obese persons)
- Positive family history
- Some medications (e.g., lipid-lowering agents)
- Gallbladder hypomobility

Data from Sartin JS: Alterations in function of the gallbladder and exocrine pancreas. In Copstead LC, Banasik JL, editors: *Pathophysiology,* ed 4, St Louis, Mo., 2009, Saunders.

Open Cholecystectomy
Removal of gallbladder through
open incision with lysis of adhesions

Laparoscopic Cholecystectomy
Not performed due to
excessive adhesions

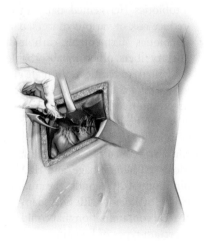
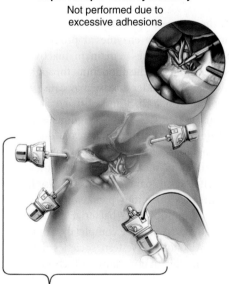

Laparoscopic instruments placed
through separate stab incisions

FIGURE 20-14 Open and laparoscopic cholecystectomy. (Medical Illustration Copyright 2006 Nucleus Medical Art, All rights reserved. www.nucleusinc.com.)

nonsurgical treatments for removing the stones, using chemical dissolution or mechanical stone fragmentation, have been developed. These methods provide effective alternatives to surgery in some cases.[35]

Nutrition Therapy

Basic principles of nutrition therapy for gallbladder disease include the following:

- *Fat:* Because dietary fat is the principal cause of contraction of the diseased organ and subsequent pain, it is poorly tolerated. Energy should come primarily from carbohydrates, especially during acute phases. Control of fat will also contribute to weight control, a primary goal because obesity and excess food intake have been repeatedly associated with the development of gallstones.
- *Energy content:* If weight loss is indicated, then recommended energy intake will be reduced according to need. Principles of weight management are discussed in Chapter 6. Usually such a diet will have a relatively low percentage of calories from fat, meeting the needs of the patient for fat moderation.
- *Cholesterol and "gas formers":* Two additional modifications usually found in traditional diets for gallbladder disease concern restriction of foods containing cholesterol and foods labeled *gas formers*. Neither modification has a valid rationale. The body synthesizes more cholesterol per day than is present in an average diet. Thus restriction of dietary cholesterol has little effect in reducing gallstone formation. Total dietary fat reduction is more important. As for the use of gas formers, such as legumes, cabbage, or fiber, blanket restriction seems unwarranted because food tolerances in any circumstances are highly individual.

Diseases of the Pancreas

Pancreatitis

Acute inflammation of the pancreas (pancreatitis) is caused by digestion of the organ tissues by enzymes it produces, principally trypsin. Normally, enzymes remain in inactive form until pancreatic secretions reach the duodenum through the common duct. However, gallbladder disease may cause a gallstone to enter the common bile duct and obstruct flow from the pancreas or cause a reflux of these secretions and bile from the common duct back into the pancreatic duct. This mixing of digestive materials activates powerful pancreatic enzymes within the gland. In such activated form, they begin their damaging effects on pancreatic tissue itself, causing acute pain. Sometimes infectious pancreatitis may occur as a complication of mumps or a bacterial disease. Mild or moderate pancreatitis may subside completely, but it has a tendency to recur. Alcohol in Western societies and malnutrition worldwide are the major causes of chronic pancreatitis.

General Treatment

Initial care consists of measures recommended for acute disease involving shock. These measures include intravenous feeding at first, replacement therapy of fluid and electrolytes, blood transfusions, antibiotics and pain medications, and gastric suction.

Nutrition Therapy

In early stages (i.e., acute pancreatitis), oral feedings are withheld because entry of food into the intestines stimulates pancreatic secretions and usually causes pain. Nutritional status is maintained by intravenous fluids or jejunal enteral feeding with peptide-based or elemental EN formulas. Most patients with pancreatitis are able to resume oral feeding in 2 to 5 days.[34]

PN is generally not recommended in pancreatitis unless a patient fails an enteral feeding trial. Pseudocysts, intestinal and pancreatic fistulas, pancreatic abscesses, and pancreatic ascites may make enteral feeding impossible.

▌HEALTH PROMOTION

A single layer of cells maintains a barrier between toxins and infections in the GI tract. At the same time, this same layer of cells absorbs macronutrients, micronutrients, and water and puts them into circulation. If that is not enough, then these cells also regulate bodily functions via hormonal and immunologic mechanisms. It is plain to see why we would want to keep this remarkable organ healthy.

In 1998, Hasler[36] summarized research that identified foods that provide several physiologic benefits. Among the findings are the following:

- Individuals who consume diets high in fruits and vegetables have only one half the cancer risk of those who consume very little of these foods.
- Intake of lycopene, the primary carotenoid found in tomatoes, is inversely associated with reduced risk of digestive tract cancer, among other cancers.
- Garlic and onions *might* offer a protective effect on cancers of the GI tract.
- Probiotics (fermented dairy products, such as yogurt) reduce risk of various cancers, particularly colon cancer.
- Prebiotics (fermentable carbohydrates such as starches, dietary fibers, other nonabsorbable sugars, sugar alcohols, and oligosaccharides) stimulate growth and activity of one or more of the "friendly" bacteria that live in the gut.

In addition to how we eat, how we live plays an important role in GI health. Strong evidence indicates that physical activity reduces risk of colon cancer by half. Physical activity might also reduce risk of cholelithiasis, constipation, diverticulosis, GI hemorrhage, and IBD.[37] Washing the hands for a minimum of 20 seconds (the amount of time it takes to sing "Happy Birthday") with hot, soapy water will reduce risk of oral-fecal contamination that could cause foodborne illnesses and certain types of hepatitis.

This information can be summed up very simply: Mom was right when she asked you to do the following:

- Eat your fruits and vegetables
- Go out and play (get plenty of physical activity)
- Wash your hands frequently and especially before eating

TO SUM UP

Nutrition therapy for GI disease is based on careful consideration of the following four major factors:

1. Secretory functions, providing chemical agents and environment necessary for digestion to occur
2. Neuromuscular functions required for motility and mechanical digestion
3. Absorptive functions, enhancing entry of nutrients into the circulatory system
4. Psychologic factors reflected by changes in GI function

Esophageal problems vary widely from simple dysphagia to serious diseases or obstruction. Nutrition therapy and mode of intake vary according to degree of dysfunction.

PUD is a common GI problem affecting millions of Americans. It is an erosion of the mucosal lining, mainly in the duodenal bulb and less commonly in the lower antrum portion of the stomach. PUD results in increased gastric tone and painful hunger contractions on an empty stomach, as well as nutrition problems such as low plasma protein levels, anemia, and weight loss. Current medical management consists of acid and infection control with a coordinated system of drugs, rest, and a regular diet (with few food and drink considerations) to supply essential nutrition support for tissue healing.

Intestinal diseases are classified as (1) *anatomic changes,* such as development of small tubular sacs branching off the main alimentary canal in diverticular disease; (2) *malabsorption,* from multiple maldigestive and malabsorptive conditions; (3) *IBD,* resulting from mucosal changes and infectious processes, as seen in UC and Crohn's disease; or (4) *SBS,* resulting from surgical resection of parts of the intestine. Nutrition therapy involves fluid and electrolyte replacement, modifications in the diet's protein and energy content and food texture, and increased vitamins and minerals, with continuous adjustment of the diet according to changes in toleration for specific foods. Allergic responses to common food allergens, as well as missing cell enzymes in genetic disease, may also contribute to GI and metabolic problems from related food intolerances.

Accessory organs to the GI tract—liver, gallbladder, and pancreas—have important functions related to digestion, absorption, and metabolism, and diseases of these organs interfere with the normal functions of the GI tract. Common liver disorders include hepatitis, usually caused by viral infection, and cirrhosis, an advanced liver disease leading to hepatic encephalopathy and progressive liver failure. The requirement of nutrient and energy levels vary with each condition.

Diseases of the gallbladder include cholecystitis, inflammation that interferes with the absorption of water and bile acids, and cholelithiasis, or gallstone formation. Treatment generally involves a reduced-fat diet and surgical removal of the gallbladder. Diseases of the pancreas include acute and chronic forms of pancreatitis, in which alcohol abuse can be a primary cause. Other causes include biliary disease, malnutrition, drug reactions, abdominal injury, and genetic predisposition. In acute pancreatitis, pain is severe because of pancreatic enzyme reflux with self-digestion of pancreatic tissue by its own enzymes. PN support is used to avoid enzyme stimulus, with gradual return to small, frequent meals as the attack subsides. In chronic pancreatitis, which is caused by alcoholism in Western societies and malnutrition worldwide, maldigestion from lack of enzymes because of pancreatic insufficiency creates nutrition problems. Nutrition care focuses on a nourishing diet with enzyme replacement and vitamin-mineral supplementation.

QUESTIONS FOR REVIEW

1. What is the basic principle of diet planning for patients with esophageal problems? Outline a general nutrition care plan for a patient with GERD complicated by a hiatal hernia.
2. In current practice, what are the basic principles of diet planning for patients with PUD? How do these principles differ from former traditional therapy?
3. Outline a course of nutritional management for a person with PUD, based on the current approaches to medical management. How would you plan nutrition education for continuing self-care and avoidance of recurrence?
4. Describe the cause, clinical signs, and treatment of each of the following intestinal diseases: malabsorption and diarrhea, IBD, diverticular disease, IBS, and constipation.
5. Compare the basics of food intolerances resulting from food allergy with those resulting from a specific genetic disease such as CF.
6. How are the major metabolic functions of the liver affected in liver disease? Give some examples.
7. What is the rationale for treatment in the spectrum of liver disease: hepatitis, cirrhosis, and hepatic encephalopathy?
8. Develop a 1-day food plan for a 45-year-old man, 183 cm (6 feet 1 inch) tall, weighing 90 kg (200 lb), with infectious hepatitis. Develop another plan for a similar patient with cirrhosis of the liver. What principles of diet therapy apply for each?
9. What are the principles of nutrition therapy for gallbladder disease? Write a 1-day meal plan for a 30-year-old woman, 165 cm (5 feet 6 inches) tall, weighing 81 kg (180 lb), who has an inflamed gallbladder with stones and is scheduled for a cholecystectomy.
10. Compare acute and chronic forms of pancreatitis in terms of cause, symptoms, and nutrition therapy. What role does special EN and PN support play in this therapy?

REFERENCES

1. Fisichella PM, Patti MG: *Achalasia*, Omaha, Neb., 2008, eMedicine.com, Inc. from: <www.emedecine.com>. Retrieved July 7, 2014.

2. Nelms MN, Sucher K, Long S: *Understanding nutrition therapy and pathophysiology*, Belmont, Calif., 2007, Wadsworth/Thomson Learning.

3. Blaser MJ: The bacteria behind ulcers. *Sci Am* 274(2):104, 1996.

4. Marchetti M, Arico B, Burroni D, et al: Development of a mouse model of *Helicobacter pylori* infection that mimics human disease. *Science* 267(5204):1655, 1995.

5. Division of Bacterial and Mycotic Disease, Centers for Disease Control and Prevention: *Helicobacter pylori and peptic ulcer disease*, Atlanta, Ga., 2005, Centers for Disease Control and Prevention. from: <www.cdc.gov/ulcer/>. Retrieved July 7, 2014.

6. Merck & Co, Inc.: *The Merck manual of diagnosis and therapy: Helicobacter pylori infection*, Whitehouse Station, N.J., 2007, Merck & Co, Inc. from: <www. merck.com>. Retrieved July 7, 2014.

7. American Dietetic Association: *Nutrition care manual: peptic ulcers: nutrition prescription*, Chicago, 2009, Author. from: <www.nutritioncaremanual.org>. Retrieved July 7, 2014.

8. Sartin JS: Gastrointestinal disorders. In Copstead LC, Banasik JL, editors: *Pathophysiology*, ed 4, Philadelphia, Pa., 2009, Saunders.

9. Trier JS: Celiac sprue. *N Engl J Med* 325(24):1709, 1991.

10. Beyer P: Medical nutrition therapy for lower gastrointestinal tract disorders. In Mahan LK, Escott-Stump S, editors: *Krause's food, nutrition, and diet therapy*, ed 12, Philadelphia, Pa., 2007, Saunders.

11. Mariné M, Fernández-Bañares F, Alsina M, et al: Impact of mass screening for gluten-sensitive enteropathy in working population. *World J Gastroenterol* 15(11):1331, 2009.

12. U.S. National Library of Medicine, National Institutes of Health: *Medline Plus medical encyclopedia: celiac disease— sprue*, Bethesda, Md., 2005, National Institutes of Health. from: <www.nlm.nih.gov/medlineplus/ency/ article/000233.htm>. Retrieved May 15, 2014.

13. Academy of Nutrition and Dietetics: *Nutrition care manual: celiac disease: nutrition care FAQs*, Chicago, 2009, from: <www.nutritioncaremanual.org>. Retrieved July 7, 2014.

14. Merck & Co, Inc.: *The Merck manual of diagnosis and therapy: cystic fibrosis*, Whitehouse Station, N.J., 2008, Merck & Co, Inc. from: <www.merck.com>. Retrieved July 7, 2014.

15. Academy of Nutrition and Dietetics: *Nutrition care manual: cystic fibrosis: nutrition intervention*, Chicago, 2009, from: <ww.nutritioncaremanual.org>. Retrieved July 7, 2014.

16. Merck & Co, Inc.: *The Merck manual of diagnosis and therapy: inflammatory bowel disease*, Whitehouse Station, N.J., 2007, Merck & Co, Inc. from: <www.merck.com>. Retrieved July 7, 2014.

17. Merck & Co, Inc.: *The Merck manual of diagnosis and therapy: Crohn's disease (regional enteritis; granulomatous ileitis or ileocolitis)*, Whitehouse Station, N.J., 2008, Merck & Co, Inc. from: <www.merck.com>. Retrieved July 7, 2014.

18. Merck & Co, Inc.: *The Merck manual of diagnosis and therapy: ulcerative colitis*, Whitehouse Station, NJ, 2008, Merck & Co, Inc. from: <www.merck.com>. Retrieved July 7, 2014.

19. Academy of Nutrition and Dietetics: *Nutrition care manual: Crohn's and ulcerative colitis: nutrition intervention*, Chicago, 2009. from: <www.nutritioncaremanual.org>. Retrieved July 7, 2014.

20. Merck & Co, Inc.: *The Merck manual of diagnosis and therapy: short bowel syndrome*, Whitehouse Station, NJ, 2008, Merck & Co, Inc. from: <www.merck.com>. Retrieved July 7, 2014.

21. Weseman RA: Adult small bowel transplantation. In Hasse JM, Blue LS, editors: *Comprehensive guide to transplant nutrition*, Chicago, 2002, American Dietetic Association.

22. Merck & Co, Inc.: *The Merck manual of diagnosis and therapy: gas-related complaints*, Whitehouse Station, NJ, 2007, Merck & Co, Inc. from: <www.merck.com>. Retrieved July 7, 2014.

23. Drossman DA: The functional gastrointestinal disorders and the Rome II process. *Gut* 45:1, 1999.

24. International Foundation for Functional Gastrointestinal Disorders: *About irritable bowel syndrome (IBS)*, Milwaukee, Wis., 1999-2010, International Foundation for Functional Gastrointestinal Disorders. from: <www.aboutibs.org>. Retrieved July 7, 2014.

25. Merck & Co, Inc.: *The Merck manual of diagnosis and therapy: irritable bowel syndrome*, Whitehouse Station, N.J., 2007, Merck & Co, Inc. from: <www.merck.com>. Rretrieved July 7, 2014.

26. Sheth AA, Longo W, Floch MH: Diverticular disease and diverticulitis. *Am J Gastroenterol* 103(6):1550, 2008.

27. Strate LL, Liu YL, Syngal S, et al: Nut, corn, and popcorn consumption and the incidence of diverticular disease. *JAMA* 300(8):907, 2008.

28. Eglash A, Lane CH: What is the most beneficial diet for patients with diverticulosis? *J Fam Pract* 55(9):813, 2006.

29. Jacobs DO: Diverticulitis. *N Engl J Med* 357(20):2057, 2007.

30. Merck & Co, Inc.: *The Merck manual of diagnosis and therapy: irritable bowel syndrome*, Whitehouse Station, N.J., 2007, Merck & Co, Inc. from: <www.merck.com>. Retrieved July 7, 2014.

31. Academy of Nutrition and Dietetics: *Nutrition care manual: hepatitis: nutrition prescription*, Chicago, 2009, from: <www.nutritioncaremanual.org>. Retrieved July 7, 2014.

32. Merck & Co, Inc.: *The Merck manual of diagnosis and therapy: cirrhosis*, Whitehouse Station, N.J., 2007, Merck & Co, Inc. from: <www.merck.com>. Retrieved July 7, 2014.

33. Academy of Nutrition and Dietetics: *Nutrition care manual: cirrhosis: nutrition prescription*, Chicago, 2009, from: <www.nutritioncaremanual.org>. Retrieved July 7, 2014.

34. Moore MC: *Pocket guide to nutrition assessment and care*, ed 6, St Louis, Mo., 2009, Mosby.

35. Sartin JS: Alterations in function of the gallbladder and exocrine pancreas. In Copstead LC, Banasik JL, editors: *Pathophysiology*, ed 4, Philadelphia, Pa., 2009, Saunders.

36. Hasler CM: Scientific status summary: functional foods— their role in disease prevention and health promotion. *Food Technol* 52(11):63, 1998.

37. Peters HPF, De Vries WR, Vanberge-Henegouw G, et al: Potential benefits and hazards of physical activity and exercise on the gastrointestinal tract. *Gut* 48:435, 2001.

FURTHER RESOURCES

Websites of Interest

Celiac Sprue
- Ask the Dietitian, Gluten and celiac sprue: www.dietitian.com/gluten.html.
- Celiac Disease Foundation: www.celiac.org.
- Celiac Sprue Association: www.csaceliacs.org.

Cirrhosis
- American Gastroenterological Association, Cirrhosis of the liver: www.gastro.org.
- American Liver Foundation: www.liverfoundation.org.
- National Institute of Diabetes and Digestive and Kidney Diseases: www.niddk.nih.gov.

Dysphagia
- Dysphagia Resource Center: www.dysphagia.com.
- Dysphagia-Dietcom: www.dysphagia-diet.com.
- Dysphagiaonline.com: www.dysphagiaonline.com.

Gastroesophageal Reflux Disease (GERD)
- About GERD: www.aboutgerd.org.
- American Gastroenterological Association: www.gastro.org.
- GERD Information Resource Center: www.gerd.com.

Celiac Disease (CD)
- Celiac Disease Foundation: www.celiac.org.
- Medline Plus, Celiac disease: www.nlm.nih.gov/medlineplus/celiacdisease.html.

- National Digestive Diseases Information, Celiac disease: www.digestive.niddk.nih.gov/ddiseases/pubs/celiac/.

Cystic Fibrosis (CF)
- Canadian Cystic Fibrosis Foundation: www.ccff.ca.
- Cystic Fibrosis Foundation: www.cff.org/home/.
- CysticFibrosis.com: www.cysticfibrosis.com.

Irritable Bowel Syndrome (IBS)
- About IBS: www.aboutibs.org
- Irritable Bowel Syndrome Self Help and Support Group: www.ibsgroup.org.

Pancreatitis
- eMedicine (search for pancreatitis for a number of resources): www.emedicine.com.
- National Institute of Diabetes and Digestive and Kidney Diseases: www.niddk.nih.gov
- Tummyhealth.com: www.tummyhealth.com.

Peptic Ulcer Disease
- National Institute of Diabetes and Digestive and Kidney Diseases: www.niddk.nih.gov.
- National Library of Medicine, *Helicobacter pylori* in Peptic Ulcer Disease: www.nlm.nih.gov/archive/20040830/pubs/cbm/pepulcer.html.

CHAPTER

21

Diseases of the Heart, Blood Vessels, and Lungs

Joyce Gilbert

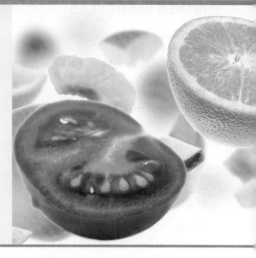

ⓔ EVOLVE WEBSITE

http://evolve.elsevier.com/Williams/essentials/

OUTLINE

Coronary Heart Disease
Essential Hypertension and Vascular Disease
Pulmonary Diseases

HEALTH PROMOTION
Added Food Factors in Coronary Heart Disease Therapy

In this chapter, we consider interrelated diseases of the circulatory system—heart, blood vessels, and lungs. In recent decades, these diseases of modern civilization have become the major causes of death of men and women in the United States and most other Western societies. One out of every three deaths is caused by heart disease; more than cancer, accidents, and acquired immunodeficiency syndrome (AIDS) combined. The magnitude of this overall health care problem is enormous.

CORONARY HEART DISEASE

Atherosclerosis

Underlying Disease Process

Atherosclerosis, the major arteriosclerosis disease and underlying pathologic process in coronary heart disease (CHD), is paramount in ongoing study in modern medicine. It is not a solitary disease entity but somewhat a pathologic progression that can involve vascular systems throughout the body, resulting in an extensive variety of clinical manifestations.[1]

An inflammatory process, the characteristic lesions involved are raised fibrous plaques (Figure 21-1) resulting from injury on the interior surface (intima) of blood vessels.[1] Once injury has occurred, plaques first appear as discrete lumps elevated above unaffected surrounding tissue and ranging in color from pearly gray to yellowish gray. Possible causes of injury are as follows[1]:

- Smoking
- Hypertension

- Diabetes
- Increased serum levels of low-density lipoprotein (LDL) cholesterol
- Decreases serum levels of high-density lipoprotein (HDL) cholesterol
- High levels of homocysteine
- Elevated C-reactive protein
- Increased serum fibrinogen
- Insulin resistance
- Oxidative stress
- Infection
- Periodontal disease

Additional risk factors are shown in Box 21-1 (see also the Focus on Culture box, "Is Cardiovascular Disease an Equal Opportunity Disease?").

About 90% of CHD patients have elevated levels of serum cholesterol, hypertension, smoke, or have diabetes.[2] The major risk factor for plaque development is a lipoprotein (LDL cholesterol) that carries cholesterol in the blood.[3] Oxidation of LDL cholesterol is the principal step in this process of atherogenesis. Inflammation with oxidative stress and activation of macrophages is the principal method of this step. The oxidized LDL cholesterol is toxic to the intima, initiates smooth muscle propagation, and triggers further immune and inflammatory responses causing formation of lesions called *fatty streaks*.[1]

This fatty degeneration and thickening narrow the vessel lumen and may allow a blood clot (or an embolus), to develop from its irritating presence. Eventually the clot may cut off

482

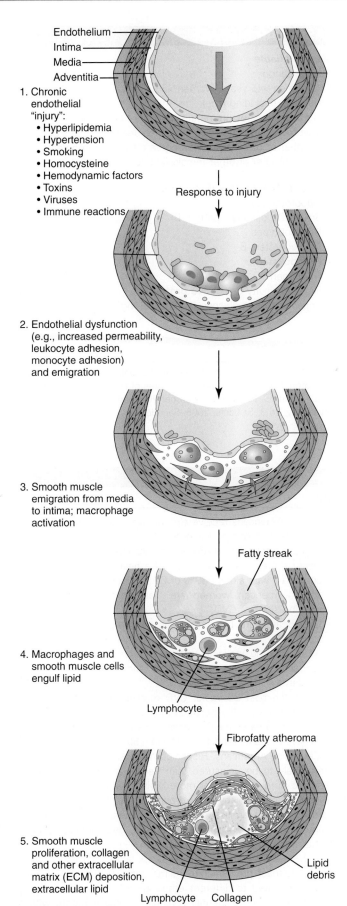

Endothelium
Intima
Media
Adventitia

1. Chronic
   endothelial
   "injury":
   • Hyperlipidemia
   • Hypertension
   • Smoking
   • Homocysteine
   • Hemodynamic factors
   • Toxins
   • Viruses
   • Immune reactions

Response to injury

2. Endothelial dysfunction
   (e.g., increased permeability,
   leukocyte adhesion,
   monocyte adhesion)
   and emigration

3. Smooth muscle
   emigration from media
   to intima; macrophage
   activation

Fatty streak

4. Macrophages and
   smooth muscle cells
   engulf lipid

Lymphocyte

Fibrofatty atheroma

5. Smooth muscle
   proliferation, collagen
   and other extracellular
   matrix (ECM) deposition,
   extracellular lipid

Lymphocyte   Collagen

Lipid
debris

FIGURE 21-1 Raised fibrous plaques. (From Kumar V, Cotran R, Robbins S: *Robbins basic pathology*, ed 7, Philadelphia, 2003, Saunders.)

blood flow in the involved artery. If the artery is a critical one, such as a major coronary vessel, then a heart attack occurs. Tissue area serviced by the involved artery is deprived of its vital oxygen and nutrient supply, a condition called *ischemia*, and the cells die. The localized area of dying or dead tissue is called an *infarct*. Because the artery involved supplies cardiac muscle, the *myocardium*, the result is called an *acute myocardial infarction (AMI)*. The two major coronary arteries, with their many branches, are so named because they lie across the brow of the heart muscle and resemble a crown (Figure 21-2). Figure 21-3 shows the anterior internal view of the normal human heart.

Cholesterol, Lipoproteins, and Lipids

Cholesterol is a soft, fatlike substance found in all cell membranes and blood and is a precursor of bile acids and steroid hormones. Cholesterol and triglycerides cannot dissolve in blood and must be transported to and from cells by individual components containing lipid and proteins (lipoproteins). The following five types of lipoproteins (Figure 21-4) are classified according to fat content and thus their density, with those having the highest fat content possessing the lowest density[4]:

1. Chylomicrons have the highest lipid content and lowest density and are composed mostly of dietary triglycerides, with a small amount of carrier protein. They accumulate in portal blood after a meal and are efficiently cleared from the blood by the specific enzyme lipoprotein lipase.

2. Very low-density lipoproteins (VLDLs) still carry a large lipid (triglyceride) content but include about 20%

KEY TERMS

atherosclerosis Common form of arteriosclerosis, characterized by the gradual formation—beginning in childhood in genetically predisposed individuals—of yellow cheeselike streaks of cholesterol and fatty material that develop into hardened plaques in the intima or inner lining of major blood vessels, such as coronary arteries, and eventually, in adulthood, cutting off blood supply to the tissue served by the vessels; the underlying pathologic process of coronary heart disease (CHD).

arteriosclerosis Blood vessel disease characterized by thickening and hardening of artery walls, with loss of functional elasticity, mainly affecting the intima (inner lining) of the arteries.

intima General term indicating an innermost part of a structure or vessel; inner layer of the blood vessel wall.

plaque Thickened deposits of fatty material, largely cholesterol, within the arterial wall that eventually may fill the lumen and cut off blood supply to the tissue served by the damaged vessel.

ischemia Deficiency of blood to a particular tissue, resulting from functional blood vessel constriction or actual obstruction of walls in atherosclerosis.

infarct An area of tissue necrosis caused by local ischemia, resulting from obstruction of blood circulation to that area.

BOX 21-1 MAJOR RISK FACTORS IN CARDIOVASCULAR DISEASE

Lipid Risk Factors

- Low-density lipoprotein (LDL) cholesterol >130 mg/dL
- High-density lipoprotein (HDL) cholesterol <40 mg/dL
- Total cholesterol >200 mg/dL
- Triglycerides >150 mg/dL

Nonlipid Risk Factors

Modifiable

- Tobacco smoke and exposure to tobacco smoke
- Hypertension (>140/90 mm Hg)
- Physical inactivity
- Obesity (body mass index [BMI] >30 kg/m^2) and overweight (BMI 25.0 to 29.9 kg/m^2)
- Diabetes mellitus
- Atherogenic diet (high intakes of saturated fats and cholesterol)
- Thrombogenic state
- Excessive alcohol consumption (>1 drink per day for women and >2 drinks per day for men)
- Individual response to stress and coping
- Some illegal drugs (cocaine and intravenous drug abuse)

Nonmodifiable

- Male gender
- Age (men >45 years, women >55 years)
- Heredity (including race)
- Family history of premature coronary heart disease (CHD) (myocardial infarction [MI] or sudden death <55 years of age in father or other male first-degree relative, or <65 years of age in mother or other female first-degree relative)

Probable Risk Factors (Emerging)

- Lipoprotein (a)
- Small LDL particles (pattern B)
- HDL subtypes
- Apolipoprotein B
- **Homocysteine**
- Fibrinogen
- High-sensitivity **C-reactive protein**
- Impaired fasting glucose (100 to 125 mg/dL)

Data from National Cholesterol Education Program (NCEP): *Third report of the NCEP Expert Panel on Detection, Evaluation, and Treatment of High Blood Cholesterol in Adults (Adult Treatment Panel III), full report,* Washington, D.C., 2002, National Institutes of Health, National Heart, Lung, and Blood Institute. from: <www.nhlbi.nih.gov/guidelines/cholesterol/atp3_rpt.htm>. Retrieved December 20, 2005; Banasik JL: Alterations in cardiac function. In Copstead LC, Banasik JL, editors: *Pathophysiology,* ed 3, St Louis, 2005, Saunders.

🌐 FOCUS ON CULTURE

Is Cardiovascular Disease an Equal Opportunity Disease?

"Race and ethnicity in the United States are associated with health status."

> Marian E. Gornick: Disparities in Medicare services: Potential causes, plausible explanations, and recommendations., *Health Care Financing Reviews,* 21(4):23, 2000.

The Pfizer Journal Panel[1] states the following:

The system of health care that exists in this country was developed at a time when life expectancy was short, diseases generally came on quickly and were all too frequently fatal, and patients needed lifesaving interventions at a relatively young age. The system has not changed, yet individuals who need health care now live a very long life, develop diseases that are chronic and disabling, and need prevention during a longer lifespan. One hundred million Americans have at least one chronic condition, and half of them have more. Among Americans older than age 65, 88% have one or more chronic illnesses, and one quarter of them have at least four conditions that should be treated.

After controlling for differences in age, health insurance status, disease severity, and other health problems, the following research findings might not be surprising but nonetheless are disheartening:

- African Americans, Hispanics, and other minorities on average have more underlying risk factors for cardiovascular disease (CVD), including hypertension, obesity, smoking, physical inactivity, higher level of body mass index (BMI), and low high-density lipoprotein (HDL) cholesterol.
- After minority patients develop CVD, they are less likely to receive higher-quality care and as a result are more likely to die.

- African Americans receive clot-reducing drugs after a heart attack less often than Caucasians.
- Approximately 18% of African-American patients have angioplasty surgery within 48 hours of a heart attack or stroke, compared with almost 30% of Caucasian patients.
- African-American women are "less familiar" with early warning signs of CVD.
- CVD deaths are highest among African Americans at all ages.
- All low-income and less-educated U.S. residents have higher mortality rates for heart disease and stroke than other residents.

During the past 30 years, CVD mortality rates have been decreasing across all racial and ethnic groups, but decline has been much greater for Caucasian Americans. African Americans have mortality rates for CVD about 50% higher than those of Caucasian Americans. Hispanic Americans are substantially more likely to be uninsured than Caucasian Americans, and Hispanic Americans are far more likely to lack a usual source of health care than any other group. Research has also found some immigrant families who assimilate into the United States, many of whom are Hispanic, experience deteriorating health status in subsequent generations.

So there is more to CVD than just risk factors. It may not be enough to teach prevention to the masses. Different life experiences attributed to different ethnic groups, as well as economic, time, and residential constraints, may compete with heart-healthy behaviors to increase risk of CVD. So if you are

⊕ FOCUS ON CULTURE

Is Cardiovascular Disease an Equal Opportunity Disease?—cont'd

a college student reading this information, then be thankful. You have just decreased your risk of CVD simply by being educated.

References

1. Pfizer Journal Panel, The quality of health care in the United States: building quality into the health care system. *Pfizer Journal* 9(9):1, 2005. from: <www.thepfizerjournal.com/default.asp?a=journal&n=tpj41>. Retrieved December 20, 2005.

Bibliography

Cook NL, Ayanian JZ, Orav EJ, et al: Differences in specialist consultations for cardiovascular disease by race, ethnicity, gender, insurance status, and site of primary care. *Circulation* 119:1–8, 2009. from: <circ.ahajournals.org>. Retrieved May 20, 2009.

De Lew N, Weinick RM: An overview: eliminating racial, ethnic, and SES disparities in health care. *Health Care Financ Rev* 21(4):1, 2000.

Gornick ME: Disparities in Medicare services: potential causes, plausible explanations, and recommendations. *Health Care Financ Rev* 21(4):23, 2000.

McWilliams JM, Meara E, Zaslavsky AM, et al: Differences in control of cardiovascular disease and diabetes by race, ethnicity, and education: U.S. trends from 1999 to 2006 and effects of Medicare coverage. *Ann Intern Med* 150:505, 2009.

The Henry J. Kaiser Family Foundation, Racial/ethnic differences in cardiac care: the weight of the evidence. *USAID Highlights* 2002. from: <http://www.kff.org/uninsured/20021009c-index.cfm>. Retrieved July 1, 2010.

Thomas AJ, Eberly LE, Smith GD, et al: Race/ethnicity, income, major risk factors, and cardiovascular disease mortality. *Am J Public Health* 95(8):1417, 2005.

Winkleby MA, Kraemer HC, Ahn DK, et al: Ethnic and socioeconomic differences in cardiovascular disease risk factors: findings for women from the Third National Health and Nutrition Examination Survey, 1988-1994. *JAMA* 280(23):1989, 1998.

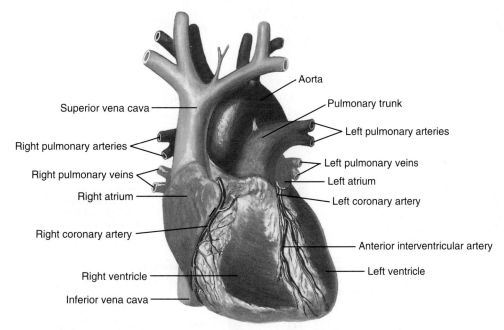

FIGURE 21-2 Coronary blood circulation. (From Seely RR, Stephens TD, Tate P: *Anatomy and physiology,* ed 3, St Louis, 1995, McGraw Hill.)

cholesterol. These lipoproteins are formed in the liver from endogenous fat sources.

3. Intermediate-density lipoproteins (IDLs) continue the delivery of endogenous triglycerides to cells and carry about 40% cholesterol.
4. LDLs carry, in addition to other lipids, about two thirds or more of total plasma cholesterol formed in blood serum from catabolism of VLDL. Because LDL carries cholesterol to cells for deposit in tissues, it is considered the main agent in elevated serum cholesterol levels, or the "bad" cholesterol.

KEY TERMS

homocysteine An amino acid produced in the human body; high serum homocysteine levels can damage the linings of the arteries and possibly make it easier for blood to clot. Most individuals with high homocysteine levels have low dietary intakes of folic acid, vitamin B_6, or vitamin B_{12}.

C-reactive protein A protein found in the blood; levels rise in response to inflammation.

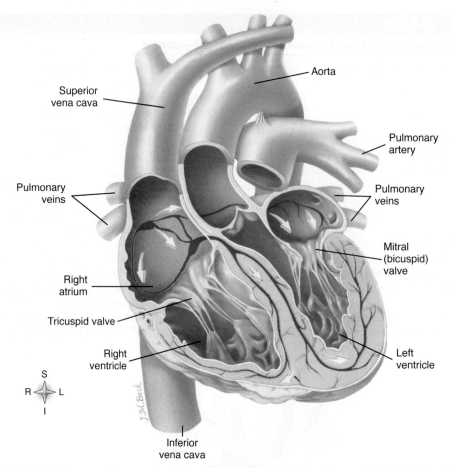

FIGURE 21-3 The normal human heart. Anterior internal view showing cardiac circulation. (From Thibodeau GA, Patton KT: *Anatomy and physiology,* ed 6, St Louis, 2007, Mosby.)

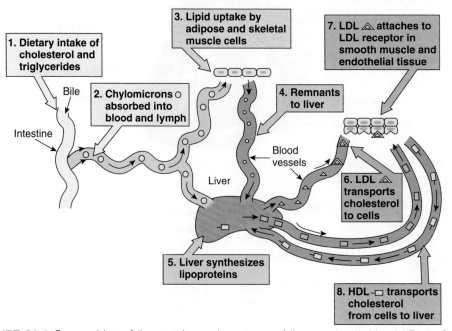

FIGURE 21-4 Composition of lipoproteins and transport of lipoproteins in blood. (From Gould BE: *Pathophysiology for the health professionals,* ed 3, Philadelphia, 2006, Saunders.)

TABLE 21-1   CHARACTERISTICS OF THE CLASSES OF LIPOPROTEINS

CHARACTERISTIC	CHYLOMICRONS	VERY LOW-DENSITY LIPOPROTEINS (VLDL)	INTERMEDIATE-DENSITY LIPOPROTEINS (IDL)	LOW-DENSITY LIPOPROTEINS (LDL)	HIGH-DENSITY LIPOPROTEINS (HDL)
Composition					
Triglycerides	85%, diet, exogenous	55%, endogenous	30%, endogenous	5%, endogenous	5%, endogenous
Cholesterol	5%	20%	40%	55%	20%
Phospholipid	3% to 6%	15% to 20%	20%	15% to 22%	25% to 30%
Protein	1% to 2%	5% to 10%	10%	20%	50%
Function	Transport dietary triglycerides to plasma and tissues, cells	Transport endogenous triglycerides to cells	Continue transport of endogenous triglycerides to cells	Transport cholesterol to peripheral cells	Transport free cholesterol from membranes to liver for catabolism
Place of Synthesis	Intestinal wall	Liver	Liver	Liver	Liver
Size and Density					
Description	Largest, lightest	Next largest, next lightest	Intermediate size, lighter	Smaller, heavier	Smaller, densest, heaviest
Density	0.095	0.095-1.006	1.00-1.03	1.019-1.063	1.063-1.210
Size in nanometers (nm)	80-1000	30-80	25-40	15-20	5-10

5. HDLs carry less total lipid and more carrier protein. They are formed in the liver from endogenous fat sources. Because HDL carries cholesterol from tissues to the liver for catabolism and excretion, higher serum levels of this "good" cholesterol form are considered protective against cardiovascular disease (CVD). A value of 60 mg/dL or more contributes definite protection and decreased risk.

The characteristics of these classes of lipoproteins are summarized in Table 21-1.

Functional Classification of Lipid Disorders

Current clinical practice is based on a useful functional classification that reveals two important factors: (1) recognition of genetic factors involved and (2) focus on the role of apolipoproteins in the course of lipoprotein formation, transport, or destruction. Both factors will be encountered in readings and in clinical work with patients. Thus the outline provided in this discussion is useful in understanding clinical problems involved and in counseling patients.

Apolipoproteins. The term *apolipoprotein* refers to a major protein part of a combined metabolic product, in this case a specific protein part of a combined lipid-protein molecule. For example, apolipoprotein B is a common attachment to LDL and serves two basic functions: (1) it aids transport of lipids in a water medium (i.e., blood), and (2) it transports lipids into cells for metabolic purposes. When apolipoprotein B-100, a single large protein molecule, attaches to one pole of the LDL, it provides a recognition site for LDL receptors on the cell, causing the entire LDL to be transported by pinocytosis into the cell for use in cell metabolism.[4] Various types of LDL have specific receptor sites for particular apolipoproteins to which the

apolipoprotein is attracted and that in large measure determine function.

Function. When lipoproteins are synthesized in the intestinal wall, liver, and blood serum, the protein component is made up of varying kinds of apolipoprotein parts. These genetically determined components influence the structure, receptor binding, and metabolism of lipoproteins. It is an apolipoprotein component that helps form special spherical droplets of lipid material for transport in the bloodstream (see Chapter 4). Apolipoprotein determination is currently a useful laboratory tool for identifying persons at high risk for CHD.[3]

Defects in Synthesis of Apolipoproteins. The current functional approach classifies lipid disorders into four major groups based on the underlying functional problem: (1) defects in apolipoprotein synthesis, (2) enzyme deficiencies, (3) LDL-receptor deficiency, and (4) other inherited hyperlipidemias.[3]

General Principles of Nutrition Therapy

Basic Guidelines. The National Cholesterol Education Program (NCEP) periodically publishes revised guidelines

---

KEY TERM

apolipoproteins   Separate protein compounds that attach to specific receptor sites on particular lipoproteins and activate certain functions, such as protein synthesis of a related enzyme. For example, apolipoprotein C-II is an apolipoprotein of high-density lipoprotein (HDL) and very low-density lipoprotein (VLDL) that functions to activate the enzyme lipoprotein lipase.

TABLE 21-2	ESSENTIAL COMPONENTS OF THERAPEUTIC LIFESTYLE CHANGES
COMPONENT	**RECOMMENDATION**
Nutrients that raise LDL	
Saturated fats	<7% of total energy intake
Dietary cholesterol	<200 mg/day
Therapeutic options for lowering LDL	
Plant stanols/sterols	2 g/day
Soluble fiber	10-25 g/day
Total energy (kilocalories)	Adjust total energy intake to maintain desirable body weight/prevent weight gain
Physical activity	Include enough moderate exercise to expend at least 200 kcal/day
Trans fats	Avoid
Limit sodium to 2400 mg per day	When indicated

Data from National Cholesterol Education Program (NCEP): *Third report of the NCEP Expert Panel on Detection, Evaluation, and Treatment of High Blood Cholesterol in Adults (Adult Treatment Panel III), full report,* Washington, D.C., 2002, National Institutes of Health, National Heart, Lung, and Blood Institute. from: <www.nhlbi.nih.gov/guidelines/cholesterol/atp3_rpt.htm>. Retrieved May 19, 2009; American Dietetic Association: *Nutrition care manual,* Chicago, 2005, American Dietetic Association. from: <www.nutritioncaremanual.org>. Retrieved May 19, 2009.
LDL, Low-density lipoprotein.

TABLE 21-3	NUTRIENT COMPOSITION OF THE THERAPEUTIC LIFESTYLE CHANGES DIET
COMPONENT	**RECOMMENDATION**
Polyunsaturated fat, including omega-3 fatty acids	Up to 10% total energy intake
Monounsaturated fat	Up to 20% total energy intake
Total fat	25% to 35% total energy intake*
Carbohydrate†	50% to 60% total energy intake
Dietary fiber	20-30 g/day
Protein	Approximately 15% total energy intake

Data from National Cholesterol Education Program (NCEP): *Third report of the NCEP Expert Panel on Detection, Evaluation, and Treatment of High Blood Cholesterol in Adults (Adult Treatment Panel III), full report,* Washington, D.C., 2002, National Institutes of Health, National Heart, Lung, and Blood Institute. from: <www.nhlbi.nih.gov/guidelines/cholesterol/atp3_rpt.htm>. Retrieved May 19, 2009; American Dietetic Association: *Nutrition care manual,* Chicago, 2005, American Dietetic Association. from: <www.nutritioncaremanual.org>. Retrieved May 19, 2009.
*Adult Treatment Panel III (ATP III) allows for increase of total fat to 35% total energy intake and reduction in carbohydrate to 50% for persons with the metabolic syndrome. Any increase in fat intake should be in the form of either polyunsaturated or monounsaturated fat.
†Carbohydrates should come primarily from foods rich in complex carbohydrates, including grains—especially whole grains—fruits, and vegetables.

for clinical management of high serum cholesterol. The Adult Treatment Panel I (ATP I) delineated strategy for primary prevention of CHD in persons with high levels of LDL cholesterol (160 mg/dL) or those with borderline-high LDL cholesterol (130 to 159 mg/dL) and two or more risk factors. The Adult Treatment Panel II (ATP II) substantiated these strategies and made further recommendations for intensive management of LDL cholesterol in persons with established CHD. A new lower LDL cholesterol of 100 mg/dL was established. The Adult Treatment Panel III (ATP III) report identified more intensive LDL-lowering therapy. The ATP III[3] suggests a comprehensive lifestyle approach to reducing risk for CHD called *therapeutic lifestyle changes (TLC)* and incorporates the following components[2,3]:

- Reduced intake of saturated fats and cholesterol
- Therapeutic dietary options to enhance the lowering of LDL (plant stanols and sterols and increased soluble fiber)
- Weight reduction
- Increased regular physical activity

Components of TLC are outlined in Table 21-2. The ATP III also suggests ranges for other macronutrients in the TLC Diet (Table 21-3).

Components of the Therapeutic Lifestyle Changes Diet

Saturated Fat and Cholesterol. In view of the fact that the major LDL-raising nutrient components are saturated fat and cholesterol, reducing saturated fat (less than 7% of total

energy intake) and cholesterol (less than 200 mg/day) in the diet is the foundation of the TLC Diet. The strongest nutritional influence on serum LDL cholesterol levels is saturated fats.[3] In fact, a "dose-response relationship" exists between saturated fats and LDL cholesterol levels. For every 1% increase in kilocalories (kcalories or kcal) from saturated fats as a percentage of total energy, serum LDL cholesterol increases approximately 2%. On the other hand, a 1% decrease in saturated fats will lower serum cholesterol by approximately 2%.[3] Although weight reduction by itself, even of a few pounds, will reduce LDL cholesterol levels, weight reduction attained using a kcalorie-controlled diet low in saturated fats and cholesterol will improve and maintain LDL cholesterol lowering. Although dietary cholesterol does not have the same influence as saturated fat on serum LDL cholesterol levels, high cholesterol intakes raise LDL cholesterol levels. Therefore reducing dietary cholesterol to less than 200 mg/day decreases serum LDL cholesterol in most persons.[3]

Monounsaturated Fat. The TLC Diet recommends substitution of monounsaturated fat for saturated fats at an intake level of up to 20% of total energy intake because monounsaturated fats lower LDL cholesterol levels relative to saturated fats without decreasing HDL cholesterol or triglyceride levels. It is recommended that plant oils and nuts be used because they are the best sources of monounsaturated fats.[3]

Polyunsaturated Fats. Polyunsaturated fats, in particular linoleic acid, reduce LDL cholesterol levels when used instead of saturated fats. However, they can also bring about small reductions in HDL cholesterol when compared side by side with monounsaturated fats. The TLC Diet recommends liquid vegetables oils, semiliquid margarines (soft, tub margarines), and other margarines low in trans fatty acids be used because they are the best sources of polyunsaturated fats; intakes can range up to 10% of total energy intake.[3]

Trans Fatty Acids. Two types of trans fatty acids exist: (1) those appearing naturally in foods (mostly meat products) and (2) those produced by the process of hydrogenation of unsaturated fats. Trans fats from partially hydrogenated fats are more harmful than naturally occurring trans fats,[5] raising serum LDL cholesterol and lowering serum HDL cholesterol.

Total Fat. In view of the fact that only saturated fats and trans fatty acids increase LDL cholesterol levels,[5] serum levels of LDL cholesterol are unrelated to total fat intake *per se*. For that reason, the ATP III suggests it is not crucial to limit total fat intake for the specific goal of reducing LDL cholesterol levels, provided saturated fats are decreased to goal levels.[2]

Carbohydrates. When saturated fats are replaced with carbohydrates, LDL cholesterol levels are reduced. On the other hand, very high intakes of carbohydrates (greater than 60% of total energy intake) are associated with a reduction in HDL cholesterol and an increase in serum triglyceride. Increasing soluble fiber intake can sometimes reduce these responses. On average, increasing soluble fiber to 10 to 25 g/day is accompanied by an approximately 5% reduction in LDL cholesterol.[2]

Protein. Despite the fact that dietary protein as a rule has an insignificant effect on serum LDL cholesterol level, replacing animal protein with plant-based protein has been reported to decrease LDL cholesterol.[2] This may be the result of plant-based foods providing good sources of proteins (legumes, dry beans, nuts, whole grains, and vegetables) containing less saturated fat than many animal proteins and no cholesterol. This is not to say animal proteins cannot be low in saturated fat and cholesterol. Fat-free and low-fat dairy products, egg whites, fish, skinless poultry, and lean cuts of beef and pork are also low in saturated fat and cholesterol. All foods of animal origin will contain cholesterol.

Further Dietary Options for Reducing LDL Cholesterol. Adding 5 to 10 g of soluble fiber (oats, barley, psyllium, pectin-rich fruit, and beans) per day is associated with approximately a 5% reduction in LDL cholesterol and is regarded as a therapeutic option to enhance reduction of LDL cholesterol. Plant sterols present an additional therapeutic option.[2] Daily intakes of 2 to 3 g plant stanol and sterol esters (isolated from soybean and tall pine tree oils) have been shown to lower LDL cholesterol by 6% to 15%.[2]

General Approach to Therapeutic Lifestyle Changes

The ATP III[2] suggests patients at risk for CHD or with CHD be referred to registered dietitians (RDs) or other qualified nutritionists for the duration of all stages of nutrition therapy

(NT). After 6 weeks of TLC, LDL cholesterol should be measured to evaluate response to TLC. If the LDL cholesterol target has been realized or an improvement in LDL lowering has occurred, then NT should be uninterrupted. If the goal has not been attained, then the physician can select from a number of alternatives. First, NT can be reexplained and reinforced. Next, therapeutic dietary options can be integrated into TLC. The response to NT should be assessed in an additional 6 weeks. If the LDL cholesterol target is achieved, then the current intensity of NT should be continued indefinitely. If downward movement is seen in LDL cholesterol measures, then thought should be given to continuing NT before adding LDL-lowering medications. If it looks unlikely the LDL target will be realized with NT, then medications should be considered.[2] The "Guide to Therapeutic Lifestyle Changes: Healthy Lifestyle Recommendations for a Healthy Heart" is shown in Box 21-2.

Drug Therapy

Although use of TLC will help many individuals attain their LDL cholesterol target goal, a segment of the population will need LDL-lowering medications to achieve the prescribed goal for LDL cholesterol. If treatment with TLC alone is unsuccessful after 3 months, then the ATP III recommends initiation of drug treatment. When drugs are used, however,

---

Metabolic syndrome is the name for a group of metabolic risk factors that increase risk for heart disease, type 2 diabetes, peripheral vascular disease (PVD), and stroke. Any one of these risk factors may develop, but they tend to occur together. Although no well-accepted criteria exist for diagnosis of metabolic syndrome, it is identified by the presence of at least three of the following:

- Abdominal obesity
  - Men: ≥40 inches (102 cm)
  - Women: ≥35 inches (88 cm)
- Elevated triglycerides (≥150 mg/dL)
- Reduced HDL cholesterol
  - Men: <40 mg/dL
  - Women: <50 mg/dL
- Elevated blood pressure (≥130/85 mm Hg)
- Elevated fasting blood glucose (≥100 mg/dL)

Data from American Heart Association: *Metabolic syndrome: information for professionals*, Dallas, Texas, 2009, American Heart Association. from: <www.americanheart.org/presenter.jhtml ?identifier=534>. Retrieved July 8, 2009; National Institutes of Health, National Heart, Lung, and Blood Institute: *Diseases and conditions index: metabolic syndrome*, Washington, D.C., 2010, National Institutes of Health, National Heart, Lung, and Blood Institute. From: <www.nhlbi.nih.gov/health/dci/Diseases/ms/ ms_whatis.html>. Retrieved July 8, 2009.

KEY TERM

trans fatty acids Fatty acids that have been hydrogenated to be used in margarine and in the food industry; have been shown to increase low-density lipoprotein (LDL) cholesterol and lower high-density lipoprotein (HDL) cholesterol.

BOX 21-2 GUIDE TO THERAPEUTIC LIFESTYLE CHANGES: HEALTHY LIFESTYLE RECOMMENDATIONS FOR A HEALTHY HEART

Food Items to Choose More Often

Breads and Cereals
- Six servings per day, adjusted to caloric needs
- Breads, cereals, especially whole grains; pasta; rice; potatoes; dry beans and peas; low-fat crackers and cookies

Vegetables
Three to five servings per day fresh, frozen, or canned, without added fat, sauce, or salt

Fruits
Two to four servings per day fresh, frozen, canned, dried

Dairy Products
Two to three servings per day fat-free, ½%, 1% milk, buttermilk, yogurt, cottage cheese, fat-free and low-fat cheese

Eggs
Fewer than two egg yolks per week; egg whites or egg substitute

Meat, Poultry, Fish
Five ounces per day
Lean-cut beef tenderloin, ground round, extra-lean hamburger; cold cuts made with lean meat or soy protein; skinless poultry; fish

Fats and Oils
Amount adjusted to caloric level: unsaturated oils; soft or liquid margarines and vegetable oil spreads; salad dressings, seeds, and nuts

Therapeutic Lifestyle Changes (TLC) Diet Options
Stanol/sterol-containing margarines; soluble-fiber food sources: barley, oats, psyllium, apples, bananas, berries, citrus fruits, nectarines, peaches, pears, plums, prunes, broccoli, Brussels sprouts, carrots, dry beans, soy products (tofu, miso)

Food Items to Choose Less Often

Breads and Cereals
- Many baked products, including doughnuts, biscuits, butter rolls, muffins, croissants, sweet rolls, Danish pastries, cakes, pies, coffee cakes, cookies
- Many grain-based snacks, including chips, cheese puffs, snack mix, regular crackers, buttered popcorn

Vegetables
Vegetables fried or prepared with butter, cheese, or cream sauce

Fruits
Fruits fried or served with butter or cream

Dairy Products
Whole milk, 2% milk, whole-milk yogurt, ice cream, cream, cheese

Eggs
Egg yolk, whole eggs

Meat, Poultry, Fish
Higher-fat meat cuts: ribs, T-bone steak, regular hamburger, bacon, sausage; cold cuts: salami, bologna, hot dogs; organ meats: liver, brains, sweetbreads; poultry with skin; fried meat; fried poultry; fried fish

Fats and Oils
Butter, shortening, stick margarine, chocolate, coconut

Recommendations for Weight Reduction

Weigh Regularly
Record weight, body mass index (BMI), and waist circumferences

Lose Weight Gradually
Goal: lose 10% of body weight in 6 months; lose ½ to 1 lb per week

Develop Healthy Eating Patterns
- Choose healthy foods (see "Food Items to Choose More Often").
- Reduce your intake of foods in "Food Items to Choose Less Often."
- Limit the number of eating occasions.
- Avoid second helpings.
- Identify and reduce hidden fat by reading food labels to choose products lower in saturated fat and calories, and ask about ingredients in ready-to-eat foods prepared away from home.
- Identify and reduce sources of excess carbohydrates such as fat-free and regular crackers, cookies and other desserts, snacks, and beverages that contain sugar.

Recommendations for Increased Physical Activity

Make Physical Activity Part of Daily Routines
- Reduce sedentary time.
- Walk or bike ride more and drive less.
- Take the stairs instead of an elevator.
- Get off the bus a few stops early and walk the remaining distance.
- Mow the lawn with a push mower, rake leaves, and work in a garden.
- Push a stroller.
- Clean your house.
- Do exercises or pedal a stationary bike while watching television.
- Play actively with your children.
- Take a brisk 10-minute walk or bike ride before work, during your work break, and after dinner.

Make Physical Activity Part of Exercise or Recreational Activities
- Walk or jog.
- Ride a bicycle or use an arm pedal bicycle.
- Swim or do water aerobics.
- Play basketball.
- Join a sports team.
- Play wheelchair sports.
- Play golf, pulling or carrying clubs.
- Go canoeing, cross-country skiing, or dancing.
- Take part in an exercise program at work, at home, at school, or at the gym.

Data from U.S. Department of Health and Human Services, Public Health Service, National Institutes of Health, National Heart, Lung, and Blood Institute: *Your guide to lowering your blood pressure with DASH,* NIH Pub No 06-4082, Bethesda, Md., 2006, U.S. Government Printing Office. from: <www.nhlbi.nih.gov>. Retrieved May 19, 2009.

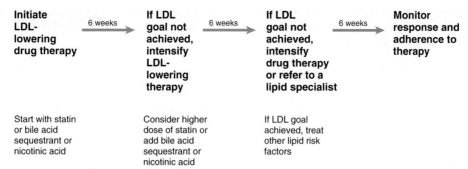

FIGURE 21-5 Progression of drug therapy. (From the National Cholesterol Education Program [NCEP]: *Third report of the NCEP Expert Panel on Detection, Evaluation, and Treatment of High Blood Cholesterol in Adults [Adult Treatment Panel III], full report,* Washington, D.C., 2001, National Institutes of Health, National Heart, Lung, and Blood Institute.)

TLC also should continue to be used concomitantly. NT affords further CHD risk reduction beyond drug efficacy.[2] The combined use of TLC and LDL cholesterol–lowering medications may include the following actions[5]:

- Intensive LDL lowering with TLC, including therapeutic dietary options
  - May prevent need for drugs
  - Can augment LDL-lowering medications
  - May allow for lower doses of medications
- Weight control plus increased physical activity
  - Reduces risk beyond LDL cholesterol lowering
  - Constitutes principal management of metabolic syndrome (see margin box above)
  - Raises HDL cholesterol
- Initiating TLC before medication consideration
  - For most people a trial of NT of about 3 months is advised before initiating drug therapy
  - Ineffective trials of NT exclusive of medications should not be protracted for indefinite period if the goals of therapy are not approached in reasonable time (medication should not be withheld if it is needed to reach targets in persons with high short-term or long-term CHD risk)
- Initiating drug therapy simultaneously with TLC
  - For severe hypercholesterolemia in which NT alone cannot attain LDL cholesterol targets
  - For those with CHD or CHD risk equivalents in whom NT alone will not attain LDL cholesterol targets

The general strategy for initiation and progression of drug therapy is outlined in Figure 21-5. (For information about particular herbs and supplements that affect the cardiovascular system, see the Complementary and Alternative Medicine [CAM] box, "It Does a Heart Good … or Does It?" and the Diet-Medications Interactions box, "Possible Interactions Between Cardiovascular Diseases and Natural Therapies.")

Acute Cardiovascular Disease: Myocardial Infarction
Medical Management

Initial medical treatment of myocardial infarction (MI), or heart attack, usually includes strong analgesics (usually morphine sulfate) for severe unremitting pain, oxygen therapy, intravenous nitroglycerin for ischemic discomfort, control of hypertension or management of pulmonary congestion, and aspirin to produce a rapid antithrombotic effect.[4] This protocol is sometimes referred to as *MONA* (morphine, oxygen, nitroglycerin, and aspirin).

Nutritional Management

In the initial acute phase of CVD, an MI requires close attention to dietary modifications. The basic clinical objective is cardiac rest to allow the healing process to begin. All care is directed toward this basic need for cardiac rest so that the damaged heart can be restored to normal functioning. In addition to TLC (see Table 21-3), sodium may be restricted to 2 to 4 g for hypertension or to control edema[2] (see the Case Study box, "The Patient with Myocardial Infarction").

Metabolic Syndrome

If the patient has metabolic syndrome, further attention must be given to the following[4]:
- Weight management
- Gradual increase in physical activity under physician's supervision
- Limiting alcohol intake

Chronic Coronary Heart Disease: Congestive Heart Failure

In chronic CHD a condition of congestive heart failure (CHF) may develop over time. Each year more than 550,000 new cases are diagnosed.[1] The progressively weakened heart muscle, the myocardium, is unable to maintain an adequate cardiac output to sustain normal blood circulation. Resulting fluid imbalances cause edema, especially pulmonary edema, to develop. This condition brings added problems in breathing called *respiratory distress* or *dyspnea,* which places added stress on the laboring heart. The most common cause of CHF is myocardial ischemia from coronary artery disease, hypertension, and cardiomyopathy. About half of CHF patients

---

KEY TERM
pulmonary edema   Accumulation of fluid in tissues of the lung.

COMPLEMENTARY AND ALTERNATIVE MEDICINE (CAM)

It Does a Heart Good ... or Does It?

Herbs are used by many to treat "what ails them." Although research is constantly being undertaken to test the efficacy of herbs, available information remains limited. The following table reviews the efficacy of herbal medicines that affect the cardiovascular system. In an effort to simplify the information, herbs are classified under the primary diseases they treat.

However, please keep in mind most herbal medicines have multiple, overlapping cardiovascular effects. It is also important to remember that herbs sold in the United States are not standardized doses or preparations; therefore no regulation exists regarding the safety of herbal products.

Cardiovascular Disorder	Commonly Used Herb/ Supplement	Efficacy of Herb/Supplement
Congestive heart failure (CHF)	Coenzyme Q10 (CoQ10) (mitoquinone, ubidecarenone, ubiquinone)	Reasonably good evidence supports use of CoQ10 as adjunct therapy; thought to work by improving efficiency of cardiac muscle
	Hawthorn (*Crataegus laevigata, C. monogyna, C. oxyacantha, C. pentagyna*)	No evidence hawthorn reduces CHF morbidity or mortality
	Carnitine	Improves myocardial contractility and relaxation and cardiac pump function in patients with ventricular dysfunction
	Taurine	Might be useful in adjuvant therapy in class II, III, and IV CHF
	Arginine	Might improve some CHF symptoms
	Creatine	Might improve skeletal muscle exercise tolerance in patients with CHF
	Vitamin B1 (thiamin)	Slight evidence that intravenous thiamin followed by oral supplementation could improve heart function in patients with CHF
	Vitamin E (α-tocopherol)	Ineffective for treatment of CHF
	Garlic (*Allium* spp., including *Allium sativum*)	Might mildly reduce blood pressure (approximately 10 mm Hg systolic and 5 mm Hg diastolic)
High blood pressure	CoQ10	Adjunctive treatment with 120 mg CoQ10 daily has been shown to reduce average blood pressure by about 9%; might prolong hypotensive effects of enalapril and nitrendipine without changing their maximal effect
	Fish oils (alternative names/supplement forms: docosahexaenoic acid [DHA], eicosapentaenoic acid [EPA], omega-3 fatty acids, omega-3 oils)	Might have slight antihypertensive effect
	Hawthorn	Might increase exercise tolerance
	Carnitine	Might increase exercise tolerance; decrease number of premature ventricular contractions (PVCs); might decrease need for some medications such as nitroglycerides, β-blockers, antihypertensives, diuretics, anticoagulants, antiarrhythmics, and hypolipidemics
	Inositol hexaniacinate (a form of niacin)	Might improve walking distance
	L-carnitine	Improves muscle energy use
	Mesoglycans	Might improve walking distance
	Policosanol	Improves walking distance
	Oxerutins	In combination with compression stockings, effective in reducing leg edema
	Diosmin/hesperidin (citrus bioflavonoids)	Significantly improves symptoms
	Butcher's broom (*Ruscus aculeatus*)	Improves symptoms of venous insufficiency
	Grape leaf	Dose-dependent improvements in symptoms
	Oligomeric proanthocyanidin complexes (OPCs)	Provide significant benefit in chronic venous insufficiency
	Gotu kola (*Centella asiatica*)	Dose-dependent improvements in symptoms
Angina pectoris	N-acetylcysteine (NAC) (modified form of the dietary amino acid cysteine)	Given in combination with nitroglycerin is more effective than either drug alone in preventing death, myocardial infarction (MI), or need for revascularization; unfortunately, combined treatment also associated with high rate of severe headache

🌸 COMPLEMENTARY AND ALTERNATIVE MEDICINE (CAM)

It Does a Heart Good ... or Does It?—cont'd

Cardiovascular Disorder	Commonly Used Herb/ Supplement	Efficacy of Herb/Supplement
Hypertension	Stevia	Might possess antihypertensive effects; considered safe when used at recommended doses
Peripheral vascular disease (PVD) (intermittent claudication)	Ginkgo (Ginkgo biloba)	Modest improvement in pain-free walking
Venous insufficiency	Horse chestnut (Aesculus hippocastanum)	Used in combination with compression stockings, useful treatment for pain, itching, leg fatigue, and feelings of tension in the legs

Bibliography

Bratman S, Girman AM: *Mosby's handbook of herbs and supplements and their therapeutic uses*, St Louis, 2003, Mosby.

Kuhn MA, Winston D: *Herbal therapy and supplements: a scientific and traditional approach*, Philadelphia, 2001, Lippincott Williams & Wilkins.

Springhouse Corporation: *Professional guide to complementary and alternative therapies*, Baltimore, Md., 2001, Springhouse.

🔖 DIET-MEDICATIONS INTERACTIONS

Possible Interactions Between Cardiovascular Diseases and Natural Therapies

Pharmaceutical Class	Natural Therapy	Interaction
Warfarin	Coenzyme Q_{10} (CoQ_{10})	Concurrent use could reduce effectiveness of drug; might increase excretion or metabolism of warfarin
Angiotensin-converting enzyme (ACE) inhibitors	Arginine, potassium	Possible hyperkalemia
	Dong quai (Angelica polymorpha sinensis), St. John's wort (Hypericum perforatum)	Possible increased risk of photosensitivity
	Iron	Mutual absorption interference; possible reduction of ACE inhibitor–induced cough
	Licorice (natural)	Antagonism of drug action
	Zinc	Correction of possible drug-induced depletion
Digitoxin, digoxin	Eleutherococcus (Siberian ginseng)	Interference with laboratory measurement of digoxin levels
	Hawthorn (Crataegus laevigata, C. monogyna, C. oxyacantha, C. pentagyna)	Might interfere with effects of digoxin or serum monitoring
	Horsetail, licorice (natural)	Possible hypokalemia leading to increased drug toxicity
	Magnesium	Absorption interference
	St. John's wort	Decreased serum levels of drug with possible rebound toxicity if herb is stopped
Loop diuretics	Dong quai, St. John's wort	Possible increased risk of photosensitivity
	Licorice (natural)	Potentiation of hypokalemic action of drug
Potassium-sparing diuretics	Arginine	Possible increased risk of hyperkalemia
	Licorice (natural)	Antagonism of drug action
	Magnesium	Risk of hypermagnesemia
	White willow (Salix alba)	Possible interference of salicylate content with spironolactone action
	Zinc	Excessive zinc levels with spironolactone
Thiazide diuretics	Calcium	Potential risk of hypercalcemia
	Dong quai, St. John's wort	Possible increased risk of photosensitivity
	Licorice (natural)	Potentiation of hypokalemic action of drug
Fluoroquinolones, tetracyclines	Calcium	Mutual absorption interference

Continued

DIET-MEDICATIONS INTERACTIONS

Possible Interactions Between Cardiovascular Diseases and Natural Therapies—cont'd

Pharmaceutical Class	Natural Therapy	Interaction
Levothyroxine	Calcium	Possible absorption interference
Calcium channel blockers (CCBs)	Combined high-dose calcium and vitamin D, grapefruit juice	Possible antagonism of drug action
Anticoagulant and antiplatelet agents	Fish oil	Possible increased risk of bleeding complications
	Vitamin C	Possible antagonism of drug action
	Garlic, ginkgo, high-dose vitamin E, policosanol	Possible increased risk of bleeding complications
	Horse chestnut, oligomeric proanthocyanidin complexes (OPCs)	Possible increased risk of bleeding complications
Amiloride	Magnesium	Possible hypermagnesemia
β-blockers	Calcium	Absorption interference
	Chromium	Increased high-density lipoprotein (HDL) levels
Nitrates	N-acetylcysteine (NAC)	Increase of headache side effects

Bibliography

Bratman S, Girman AM: *Mosby's handbook of herbs and supplements and their therapeutic uses*, St Louis, 2003, Mosby.

Kuhn MA, Winston D: *Herbal therapy and supplements: a scientific and traditional approach*, Philadelphia, 2001, Lippincott Williams & Wilkins.

Springhouse Corporation: *Professional guide to complementary and alternative therapies*, Baltimore, Md., 2001, Springhouse.

CASE STUDY

The Patient with Myocardial Infarction

Edward is a 37-year-old sedentary executive who was seen for an annual physical examination 6 months ago. He had no complaints other than feeling the "everyday pressures" of his job as a corporate attorney and head of the legal division. He admitted smoking two packs of cigarettes a day as a means of relieving stress.

Edward is 175 cm (5 feet 9 inches). At the time of his examination, he weighed 83 kg (185 lb). His blood pressure was 148/90 mm Hg, and his serum cholesterol level was 285 mg/dL. He was advised to quit smoking, exercise daily at a moderate pace, and lose 9 kg (20 lb).

Edward arrived in the hospital emergency department 3 months later complaining of severe chest pains and difficulty breathing. His wife reported that he had appeared pale that evening, had broken out into a cold sweat, and had vomited shortly after arriving home from work. Once regular breathing was restored by the emergency medical team and his pain subsided, a number of laboratory tests were ordered. These tests included serum glutamic-oxaloacetic transaminase (SGOT), lactate dehydrogenase (LDH), prothrombin time (PT), lipid panel plus high-density lipoprotein (HDL) cholesterol, sedimentation rate, coagulation times, fasting plasma glucose (FPG), blood urea nitrogen (BUN), and complete blood count (CBC). An electrocardiogram (ECG) was also ordered. The patient was then transferred to the coronary care unit for closer monitoring.

The following test results were elevated: SGOT, LDH, LDL, as well as total cholesterol, triglycerides, glucose, PT, white blood cell count, and sedimentation rate. HDL level was low. The ECG revealed an infarction of the posterior wall of the myocardium. The diagnosis was myocardial infarction (MI), with underlying familial hypercholesterolemia.

In consultation with the hospital's registered dietitian (RD), the cardiologist ordered a liquid diet, increasing it to a soft diet with low saturated fats 2 days later. The RD noted continued improvement in the patient's appetite accompanying recovery and recommended changing the diet order to the therapeutic lifestyle changes (TLC) diet.

One week later, Edward was discharged. During his convalescence, the RD and nurse met with him and his wife several times to discuss his continuing care at home. At each follow-up clinic visit with the physician and nutritionist, Edward showed good general recovery and enjoyment of his new modified fat and cholesterol food habits.

Questions for Analysis

1. What predisposing factors in Edward's lifestyle place him in the high-risk category for coronary heart disease (CHD)?
2. Why was moderate, consistent exercise originally recommended?
3. Explain the causes for Edward's initial symptoms.
4. How does each laboratory test ordered in the emergency department relate to cell metabolism? Why were the results elevated?
5. Explain the association between the final diet order and his lipid disorder.
6. What nondietary needs might Edward have while convalescing at home? What community agencies might be of assistance?

suffer diastolic dysfunction, whereas systolic function is preserved. This is more likely to develop in older adults, women, and those without history of MI.[1]

Etiology: Relationship to Sodium and Water

Fluid congestion of chronic heart disease relates to imbalances in the body's capillary fluid shift mechanism and its resulting hormonal effects, as follows:

- *Imbalance in capillary fluid shift mechanism:* As the heart fails to pump out returning blood fast enough, venous return is delayed. This causes a disproportionate amount of blood to accumulate in the vascular system working with the right side of the heart. Venous pressure rises, a sort of "backup" pressure effect, and overcomes the balance of filtration pressures necessary to maintain the normal capillary fluid shift mechanism (see Chapter 7). Fluid that would normally flow between interstitial spaces and blood vessels is held in the tissue spaces rather than recirculated.

- *Hormonal mechanisms:* Two hormonal mechanisms are involved in fluid balance in normal circulation. In this instance, both of the following contribute to cardiac edema:
  1. *Aldosterone mechanism:* This mechanism, described more completely by its full name, the *renin-angiotensin-aldosterone mechanism,* is normally a lifesaving sodium- and water-conserving mechanism that ensures essential fluid balances. In this case, however, it only compounds the edema problem. As the heart fails to propel blood circulation forward, deficient cardiac output effectively reduces blood flow through kidney nephrons. Decreased renal blood pressure triggers the renin-angiotensin system. Renin is an enzyme from the renal cortex that combines in blood with its substrate, angiotensinogen, which is produced in the liver, to produce in turn angiotensin I and II. Angiotensin II acts as a stimulant to the adrenal glands to produce aldosterone. This hormone in turn effects a reabsorption of sodium in an ion exchange with potassium in the distal tubules of the nephrons, and water reabsorption follows. Ordinarily this is a lifesaving mechanism to protect the body's vital water supply. In CHF, however, it only adds to the edema problem. The mechanism reacts as if the body's total fluid volume is reduced, when in truth the fluid is excessive; it is just that it is not in normal circulation but is being retained in the body's tissues.
  2. *Antidiuretic hormone (ADH) mechanism:* This water-conserving hormonal mechanism also adds to edema. Cardiac stress and reduced renal flow cause the release of ADH, also known as *vasopressin,* from the pituitary gland. ADH then stimulates still more water reabsorption in nephrons of the kidney, further increasing the problem of edema.

Increased Cellular Free Potassium

As reduced blood circulation depresses cell metabolism, cell protein is broken down and releases its bound potassium in the cell. As a result, the amount of free potassium inside the cell is increased, which increases intracellular osmotic pressure. Sodium ions in fluid surrounding the cell then also increase in number to balance increased osmotic pressure within the cell and to prevent cell dehydration. In time, the increased sodium outside the cell causes still more water retention.[6]

Nutritional Management

The basis for all care of the person with CHF is improving cardiac output while reducing the workload of the heart and minimizing congestive symptoms. Medical treatment involves oxygen therapy, decreased physical activity, and drug therapy with (1) diuretic and vasodilator agents to control fluid congestion in the lungs; (2) digitalis drugs to strengthen contractions of the heart muscle; and (3) sympathetic antagonists, angiotensin-converting enzyme (ACE) inhibitors, nitrate, and vasodilators to decrease workload of the heart.[7] Nutrition support involves the following[8]:

- *Sodium* is usually restricted to 2 g/day and may be adjusted upward to 3 g/day if necessary to promote food and nutrient intake.
- *Fluids* may be restricted to 1500 mL/day, if necessary.
- *Texture* may be modified to soft foods so that little physical effort is needed.
- *Meals* may be divided into smaller feedings to also decrease effort necessary for eating.
- *Alcohol* is generally limited to one drink per day. If alcohol is thought to be a causative factor in the heart disease, then abstinence is mandatory.

Cardiac Cachexia
Etiology

Sometimes with prolonged myocardial insufficiency and heart failure an extreme clinical condition of cardiac cachexia develops. Progressive, profound malnutrition results from an insufficient oxygen supply that cannot meet demands of red blood cell formation by bone marrow or energy needs for basic breathing. The enlarged, laboring heart is unable to maintain a sufficient blood supply to the body tissues, and nutrient delivery to cells is impaired. Edema, unpalatable sodium-restricted diets, drug reactions, and postoperative complications of cardiac surgery all worsen the anorexia and reduce food intake. In addition, the individual has probably become hypermetabolic and hypercatabolic. It should be no surprise that the incidence of nosocomial (hospital induced) cardiac cachexia is a common occurrence.

Nutrition Therapy

The goal is to help restore heart-lung function as much as possible and rebuild body tissue. Team care involving the

---

KEY TERMS

antidiuretic hormone (ADH) Water-conserving hormone from the posterior lobe of pituitary gland; causes resorption of water by kidney nephrons according to body need.

vasopressin Alternative name of antidiuretic hormone (ADH).

physician, clinical dietitian, nurse, patient, and family is essential. Nutrition support focuses on energy, nutrients, supplements, and feeding plan, as follows[4]:

- *Energy:* Sufficient kcalories are needed to cover basal energy needs, as well as energy for minimal activity and the hypermetabolism of severe CHF; more kcalories may be needed if major surgery is planned. Depending on the extent of malnutrition indicated by nutrition assessment, an increase of 30% to 50% of basal needs may be indicated.
- *Fluids:* Sufficient but not excessive fluid intake is needed, at a rate of about 0.5 mL/kcal/day or 1000 to 1500 mL/day.
- *Protein:* Approximately 1.0 to 1.5 g/kg body weight is needed to replace tissue losses and cover malabsorption.
- *Sodium:* Sodium restriction varies with individual status, usually in a range of 1 to 2 g/day, with attention to multiple alternate seasonings to enhance palatability of food.
- *Mineral-vitamin supplementation:* May need to supplement intake with folate, magnesium, thiamin, zinc, and iron depending on serum levels. Increasing vitamins E, B_6, B_{12}, and thiamin may be beneficial.
- *Feeding plan:* Small, frequent feedings are better tolerated. Large meals add to the risk of carbon dioxide (CO_2) accumulation and respiratory failure.
- *Enteral nutrition (EN) and parenteral nutrition (PN) support:* Tube feedings or PN may be appropriate. Several EN feeding formulas are available that have a low volume with a high density of kcalories. These are suitable for patients who require fluid restriction.

ESSENTIAL HYPERTENSION AND VASCULAR DISEASE

Hypertension

High blood pressure is one of the most prevalent vascular diseases worldwide. As the population ages, the prevalence of hypertension will increase. It is a major factor in the development of stroke, heart attack, heart failure, and kidney disease.[8] At least 95% of these individuals have **essential hypertension,** meaning its cause is unknown, although a strong familial predisposition exists, with its onset in young teenage years. It has often been called the *silent disease* because it carries no overt signs, but it can have serious implications if not treated and controlled.[9] The large United States study—Dietary Approaches to Stop Hypertension (DASH)—has clearly indicated that a diet rich in fruits, vegetables, and low-fat dairy foods and with reduced saturated and total fat can substantially lower blood pressure.[10] Individual treatment uses current antihypertensive drugs as needed.

Blood Pressure Controls

Arterial Pressure. As commonly measured, blood pressure is an indication of arterial pressure in vessels of the upper arm. This measure is obtained by an instrument for determining force of the pulse (Figure 21-6). This instrument is called a *sphygmomanometer,* from the Greek words *sphygmos* (meaning pulse), *manos* (meaning thin), and *metron*

(meaning measure). Pulse pressure is measured in millimeters of mercury (mm Hg) rise or in equivalent values read on gauges or digital indicators. The higher, or upper, value recorded is systolic pressure from contraction of the heart muscle. The lower value recorded is diastolic pressure, produced during the relaxation phase of the cardiac cycle.

Several factors contribute to maintaining fluid dynamics of normal blood pressure: (1) increased pressure on forward blood flow; (2) increased resistance from blood vessels through which the blood is flowing; and (3) increased viscosity of blood itself, making movement through vessels more difficult. Of these factors, increased viscosity is a rare event. Thus in discussing high blood pressure in general terms, we are dealing with the first two factors: (1) the pumping pressure of the heart muscle propelling blood forward and (2) resistance to this forward flow presented by blood vessel walls normally or by any abnormal added constriction or thickening.

Muscle Tone of Blood Vessel Walls. In hypertension, the body's finely tuned mechanisms designed to maintain fluid dynamics are not operating effectively. Normally these systems include several agents that act to variously dilate and constrict blood vessels to meet whatever need is present at a given time. In a person with hypertension, however, dilation or constriction of blood vessels does not occur in the normal manner. If not effectively treated, then uncontrolled elevated blood pressure results. Body systems that operate to help maintain normal blood pressure include (1) neuroendocrine functions of the sympathetic nervous system, mainly mediated by chemical neurotransmitters such as norepinephrine; (2) hormonal systems such as the renin-angiotensin-aldosterone mechanism and its vasopressor effect; and (3) enzyme systems such as the kallikrein-kinin mechanism (sometimes

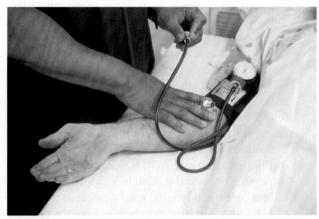

FIGURE 21-6 Monitoring blood pressure. (From Potter PA, Perry AG: *Basic nursing: essentials for practice,* ed 5, St Louis, 2003, Mosby.)

KEY TERM
essential hypertension An inherent form of hypertension with no specific discoverable cause and considered to be familial; also called *primary hypertension.*

TABLE 21-4   CLASSIFICATION OF BLOOD PRESSURE FOR ADULTS

BLOOD PRESSURE (BP) CLASSIFICATION	SYSTOLIC (in mm Hg)*	DIASTOLIC (in mm Hg)	LIFESTYLE MODIFICATION	INITIAL DRUG THERAPY	
				WITHOUT COMPELLING INDICATION	WITH COMPELLING INDICATION[†]
Normal[‡]	<120	and <80	Encourage	No antihypertensive drug indicated	None
Prehypertension	120-139	or 80-89	Yes	No antihypertensive drug indicated	Drug(s) for compelling indications[§]
Stage 1 hypertension[¶]	140-159	or 90-99	Yes	Thiazide-type diuretics for most; consider ACEI, ARB, BB, CCB, or combinations	Drug(s) for the compelling indications[§] Other antihypertensive drugs (diuretics, ACEI, ARB, BB, CCB) as needed
Stage 2 hypertension[¶]	>160	or >100	Yes	Two-drug combination for most[§]	

Data from National High Blood Pressure Program: *The seventh report of the Joint National Committee on Prevention, Detection, Evaluation, and Treatment of High Blood Pressure (JNC 7), National Institutes of Health, National Heart, Lung, and Blood Institutes,* NIH Pub No 04-5230, Washington, D.C., 2004, U.S. Government Printing Office. Available from: <http://www.nhlbi.nih.gov/guidelines/hypertension/jnc7full.htm>.

ACEI, Angiotensin-converting enzyme inhibitor; *ARB,* aldosterone receptor blocker; *BB,* β-blocker; *CCB,* calcium channel blocker.
*Treatment determined by highest blood pressure category.
[†]Heart failure, post-MI, high coronary disease risk, chronic kidney disease, recurrent stroke prevention.
[‡]Optimal blood pressure with respect to cardiovascular risk is less than 120/80 mm Hg. However, unusually low readings should be evaluated for clinical significance.
[§]Initial combined therapy should be used cautiously in those at risk for orthostatic hypotension.
[¶]Based on the average of two or more readings taken at each of two or more visits after initial screening.

operating with prostaglandins), which controls substances that act to dilate or constrict smooth muscle as needed.

Classifications of Blood Pressure

Hypertension is defined as systolic blood pressure of 140 mm Hg or higher, diastolic blood pressure of 90 mm Hg or higher or taking antihypertensive medication. The objective of identifying and treating hypertension is to reduce morbidity and mortality. For that reason, classification of adult (older than 18 years of age) blood pressure (Table 21-4) provides a mechanism for identifying high-risk individuals and provides guidelines for follow-up and treatment.[7]

Prevention and Treatment

The goal of prevention and management of hypertension is to reduce morbidity and mortality by the least intrusive means possible.[7] Lifestyle modifications (Table 21-5) offer the potential for preventing hypertension. They have been shown capable of lowering blood pressure and can reduce cardiovascular risk factors at minimal cost and risk.[7]

Nutritional Management of Hypertension

Taste for a given amount of salt with food is an acquired one, not a physiologic necessity. Sufficient sodium for the body's need is provided as a natural mineral in foods consumed. Some persons salt their foods heavily and thus form high salt taste levels. Others form lighter tastes by using smaller amounts. Common daily adult intakes of sodium range widely from about 2 to 4 g, with lighter tastes to as high as

10 to 12 g with heavier use. Salt (sodium chloride [NaCl]) intakes are about twice these amounts because sodium makes up about 40% of the NaCl molecule. The large amount of salt in the American diet, estimated to be about 6 to 15 g of sodium per day (260 to 656 mEq), is largely a result of the increased use of many processed food products. The main source of dietary sodium is food processing (about 75%). Approximately 10% to 11% occurs naturally in foods, about 15% is discretionary (half of which is contributed by table salt and half by cooking), and less than 1% comes from water.

Other nutrients that affect blood pressure are potassium and calcium. High potassium intake from food sources (see the Perspectives in Practice box, "Dietary Approaches to Stop Hypertension [DASH] Diet Pattern") such as fresh fruits and vegetables may protect against the development of hypertension and improve blood pressure control in those who do have hypertension.[7] Calcium in the form of low-fat dairy products (which are also low in saturated and total fat) is also recommended to reduce blood pressure. Moderate consumption of alcohol (equivalent to two drinks per day for men and one drink per day for women) is also known to reduce blood pressure.[7]

Cerebrovascular Accident

Arteriosclerotic vascular injury and hypertension may also affect blood vessels in the brain. A cerebrovascular accident (CVA), or stroke, occurs when a blood vessel carrying oxygen and nutrients to the brain ruptures (hemorrhagic stroke) or is clogged by a blood clot (ischemic stroke), interrupting

TABLE 21-5	LIFESTYLE MODIFICATIONS TO MANAGE HYPERTENSION*†	
SYSTOLIC BLOOD PRESSURE		**APPROXIMATE SBP**
MODIFICATION (RANGE)	**RECOMMENDATIONS**	**REDUCTION (RANGE)**
Weight reduction	Maintain normal body weight (BMI, 18.5-24.9 kg/m²).	5-20 mm Hg per 10-kg weight loss
Adapt DASH eating plan	Consume a diet rich in fruits and vegetables and low in fat.	8-14 mm Hg
Dietary sodium reduction	Reduce dietary sodium intake to no more than 2.4 g sodium or 6 g sodium chloride (NaCl).	2-8 mm Hg
Physical activity	Engage in regular aerobic physical activity such as brisk walking (at least 30 min per day, most days of the week).	4-9 mm Hg
Moderation of alcohol consumption	Limit consumption to no more than two drinks (1 oz or 30 mL ethanol [e.g., 24 oz beer, 10 oz wine, or 3 oz 80-proof whiskey]) per day in most men and to no more than one drink per day in women and lighter-weight persons.	2-4 mm Hg

Data from National High Blood Pressure Program: *The seventh report of the Joint National Committee on Prevention, Detection, Evaluation, and Treatment of High Blood Pressure, National Institutes of Health, National Heart, Lung, and Blood Institutes,* NIH Pub No 04-5230, Washington, D.C., 2004, U.S. Government Printing Office.
BMI, Body mass index; *DASH,* Dietary Approaches to Stop Hypertension.
*For overall cardiovascular risk reduction, stop smoking.
†The effects of implementing these modifications are dose and time dependent and could be increased for some individuals.

blood flow to an area of the brain. When any part of the brain does not receive blood and oxygen, nerve cells in the affected area die, resulting in loss of control of the abilities that area of the brain once controlled. During the past 20 years, with the declining U.S. early death rate from heart disease, stroke stands in third place as a leading cause of death of adults ages 25 to 65 years.[11] Nearly 170,000 Americans die annually of stroke, meaning someone in the United States experiences a stroke every 45 seconds.[2] Among all U.S. population groups, the incident rate for first stroke among African Americans is almost double that of European Americans.[12]

Four main types of stroke exist: two are caused by blood clots, and two are caused by ruptured blood vessels. Cerebral thrombosis and cerebral embolism account for approximately 70% to 80% of all strokes. Cerebral thrombosis, the most common stroke, occurs when a thrombus forms and blocks blood flow in an artery bringing blood to part of the brain. They usually occur at night or first thing in the morning when blood pressure is low. They are often preceded by a transient ischemic attack (TIA), or "ministroke." Cerebral embolism occurs when an embolus forms away from the brain, usually in the heart. The clot is carried in the bloodstream until it lodges in an artery leading to or in the brain and blocks the flow of blood.[2] A subarachnoid hemorrhage occurs when a blood vessel on the brain's surface ruptures and bleeds into the space between the brain and skull. A cerebral hemorrhage occurs when a defective artery in the brain bursts, flooding the surrounding tissue with blood.[2]

Nutrition Therapy

Paralysis and other problems may occur, depending on the site and extent of brain damage resulting from a stroke. Patients who experience left-sided CVA most commonly experience sight and hearing losses, including the ability to see where food is on plates or trays. Right-hemisphere, bilateral, or brainstem CVA causes significant problems with feeding and swallowing, in addition to speech problems.[7]

Dysphagia often occurs, and foods that cause choking or that are hard to manage should be avoided (dry or crisp foods, peanut butter, thinly pureed foods, raw vegetables, to mention a few). If the patient has problems with saliva production, then foods can be moistened with small amounts of liquid (au jus or gravy). Because thin liquids are often difficult to swallow, thickeners are used to make semisolid foods from soups, beverages, and juices.[7]

Peripheral Vascular Disease

Peripheral vascular disease (PVD) is characterized by narrowing of blood vessels in the legs and sometimes the arms. Blood flow is restricted and causes pain in affected area. Contributory risk factors include hypertension and diabetes mellitus. However, the greatest risk factor is cigarette smoking, which constricts blood vessels. More than 90% of patients with PVD are or were moderate to heavy smokers.

Symptoms and Complications

As arteries gradually narrow because of atherosclerosis (the most common cause), an aching, tired feeling occurs in leg muscles when walking. Resting the leg for a few minutes relieves pain, but it recurs shortly when walking is resumed. For this reason the symptom is called *intermittent claudication.* Sometimes a sudden arterial blockage occurs when a blood clot develops on the top of a plaque or a clot formed in the heart is carried to a peripheral artery and blocks it. The blockage causes sudden severe pain in the affected area, which becomes cold and either pale or blue and has no pulse. Movement and sensation are lost.

Dietary Approaches to Stop Hypertension (DASH) Diet Pattern

The following list indicates the number of recommended daily servings from each food group, with examples of food choices (based on the 2000-kcal reference diet). The number of servings may increase or decrease, depending on individual calorie needs, and can be found on the DASH website: www.nhlbi.nih.gov/health/public/heart/hbp/dash/.

Food Group	Daily Serving (Except Where Noted)	Serving Sizes	Examples and Notes	Significance to the Dash Diet Pattern
Grains and grain products	7-8	1 slice of bread 1 oz of dry cereal* ½ cup of cooked rice, pasta, or cereal	Whole wheat bread, English muffin, pita bread, bagel; cereals; grits; oatmeal	Major source of energy and fiber
Vegetables	4-5	1 cup of raw, leafy vegetables ½ cup of cooked vegetables 6 oz of vegetable juice	Tomatoes, potatoes, carrots, peas, squash, broccoli, turnip greens, collard greens, kale, spinach, artichokes, beans, sweet potatoes	Rich sources of potassium, magnesium, and fiber
Fruits	4-5	6 oz of fruit juice 1 medium fruit ¼ cup of dried fruit ½ cup of fresh, frozen, or canned fruit	Apricots, bananas, dates, grapes, oranges, orange juice, tangerines, strawberries, mangoes, melons, peaches, pineapple, prunes, raisins	Important sources of potassium, magnesium, and fiber
Low-fat or nonfat dairy foods	2-3	8 oz of milk 1 cup of yogurt 1½ oz of cheese	Fat-free or 1% milk, fat-free or low-fat buttermilk; nonfat or low-fat yogurt; part-nonfat mozzarella cheese, nonfat cheese	Major sources of calcium and protein
Meat, poultry, and fish	<2	3 oz of cooked meats, poultry, or fish	Select only lean meats; trim away visible fats; broil, roast, or boil, instead of frying; remove skin from chicken	Rich sources of protein and magnesium
Nuts, seeds, and legumes	4-5/wk	1½ oz or ½ cup of nuts ½ oz or 2 tbsp of seeds ½ cup of cooked legumes	Almonds, filberts, mixed nuts, peanuts, walnuts, sunflower seeds, kidney beans, lentils	Rich sources of energy, magnesium, potassium, protein, and fiber
Fats and oils†	2-3	1 tsp of soft margarine 1 tbsp of low-fat mayonnaise or salad dressing 2 tbsp of light salad dressing 1 tsp of vegetable oil	Soft margarine, low-fat mayonnaise, light salad dressing, vegetable oil (e.g., olive, corn, canola, safflower)	DASH has 27% of calories as fat, including that in or added to foods
Sweets	5/wk	1 tbsp of sugar 1 tbsp of jelly or jam ½ oz of jelly beans 8 oz of lemonade	Maple syrup, sugar, jelly, jam; fruit-flavored gelatin, jelly beans, fruit punch, sorbet, ices, hard candy	Sweets should be low in fat

*Equals ½ to ¼ cup, depending on cereal type. Check the product's nutrition label.
†Fat content changes serving counts for fats and oils. For example, 1 tbsp of regular salad dressing equals 1 serving; 1 tbsp of low-fat dressing equals ½ serving; 1 tbsp of fat-free dressing equals 0 servings.

Strategies for Adopting DASH
Dietary changes are best achieved through small changes in food selections. Use this list of tips as a way to initiate discussion and dietary compliance to reduce hypertension among your clients.

Tips on Eating the DASH Way
- Change gradually.
- If you now eat one or two vegetables a day, then add a serving at lunch and another at dinner.
- If you do not eat fruit now or have only juice at breakfast, then add a serving to your meals or have it as a snack.

- Gradually increase your use of fat-free and low-fat dairy products to three servings a day. For example, drink milk with lunch or dinner instead of soda, sugar-sweetened tea, or alcohol. Choose low-fat (1%) or fat-free (skim) dairy products to reduce your intake of saturated fat, total fat, cholesterol, and kcalories.
- Read food labels on margarines and salad dressings, and choose those lowest in unsaturated fat. Some margarines are now trans-fat free.
- Treat meat as one part of the whole meal instead of the focus.

Continued

Dietary Approaches to Stop Hypertension (DASH) Diet Pattern—cont'd

- Limit meat to 6 oz a day (two servings), which is all that is needed (3 to 4 oz is about the size of a deck of cards).
- If you now eat large portions of meat, cut them back gradually, by one half or one third at each meal.
- Include two or more vegetarian-style (meatless) meals each week.
- Increase servings of vegetables, rice, pasta, and dry beans at meals. Try casseroles, pasta, and stir-fry dishes that have less meat and more vegetables, grains, and dry beans.
- Use fruit or other foods low in saturated fat, cholesterol, and kcalories as desserts and snacks.
- Fruits and other low-fat foods offer great taste and variety. Use fruits canned in their own juices. Fresh fruits require little or no preparation. Dried fruits are a good choice to carry with you or to have ready in the car.
- Try these snacks ideas: unsalted pretzels or nuts mixed with raisins, graham crackers, low-fat and fat-free yogurt and frozen yogurt, popcorn with no salt or butter added, and raw vegetables.

Try these additional tips:
- Choose whole grain foods to get added nutrients such as minerals and fiber. For example, choose whole wheat bread and whole grain cereals.
- If you have trouble digesting dairy products, then try taking lactase enzyme pills or drops (available at drugs and grocery stores) with the dairy foods or buy lactose-free milk or milk with lactase enzyme added to it.
- Use fresh, frozen, or no-salt-added canned vegetables.

Bibliography

U.S. Department of Health and Human Services, Public Health Service, National Institutes of Health, National Heart, Lung, and Blood Institute: *Your guide to lowering your blood pressure with DASH*, NIH Pub No 06-4082. Bethesda, Md., 2006, U.S. Government Printing Office. from: <www.nhlbi.nih.gov>. Retrieved May 19, 2009.

Treatment

By far the most important treatment for the patient is to stop smoking. As with coronary vessels, surgery on diseased vessels is sometimes required: (1) arterial reconstructive surgery to bypass them, (2) endarterectomy to remove obstructing fatty deposits on inner linings, or (3) balloon angioplasty to widen vessels. Drug therapy may include antiplatelet or anticoagulant agents to prevent blood clotting. NT consists of regular fat and cholesterol modifications described for CHD. Exercise is also important. The person should walk every day with medical clearance, gradually increasing to about 1 hour, stopping whenever intermittent pain occurs and resuming when it stops. Regular inspection of feet, daily washing and stocking change, good-fitting shoes to avoid pressure, and scrupulous foot care (ideally by a podiatrist) are essential to prevent infection.

PULMONARY DISEASES

Chronic Obstructive Pulmonary Disease
Clinical Characteristics
Progressive CHF contributes to lung disease and risk of respiratory failure. Malnutrition is common with the debilitating condition of chronic obstructive pulmonary disease (COPD). This term describes a group of disorders in which airflow in the lungs is limited and respiratory failure develops. Chronic bronchitis and emphysema are two main interrelated COPD conditions. Malnutrition usually accompanies COPD, and its presence increases illness and death rates associated with the disease process. Anorexia and significant weight loss reflect a growing inability to maintain adequate nutritional status, which in turn severely compromises pulmonary function.

Progression of the disease process, with its increasing shortness of breath, prevents the person from living a normal life, and prognosis is poor. Eventually, in progressive respiratory failure, the patient becomes dependent on a mechanical respirator and controlled oxygen supply. A poor prognosis is associated with a compromised nutritional status in these patients.

Nutritional Management
Respiratory failure is actually a failure of pulmonary exchange of oxygen and CO_2. Thus its common manifestations are hypoxemia, deficient oxygenation of blood, and hypercapnia, excess CO_2 in the blood. Patients with COPD have increased energy requirements, which will vary for each individual. Requirements for carbohydrate, protein, and fat will be determined by the underlying lung disease, oxygen therapy, medications, weight status, and any acute fluid fluctuations.[4] A balanced proportion of protein (15% to 20%

KEY TERMS
dysphagia Difficulty in swallowing, commonly associated with obstructive or motor disorders of the esophagus.
intermittent claudication A symptomatic pattern of peripheral vascular disease (PVD), characterized by the absence of pain or discomfort in a limb, usually the legs, when at rest, which is followed by pain and weakness when walking, intensifying until walking becomes impossible, and then disappearing again after a rest period; seen in occlusive arterial disease.
hypoxemia Deficient oxygenation of the blood, resulting in hypoxia, reduced oxygen supply to tissue.
hypercapnia Excess carbon dioxide (CO_2) in the blood.

total kcalories) with fat (30% to 45% total kcalories) and carbohydrate (40% to 55% total kcalories) is necessary to maintain appropriate respiratory quotient (RQ) from substrate use.[4] Although it is important not to overfeed patients with COPD (especially too much carbohydrate), these patients often have difficulty taking in sufficient amounts of food because of fatigue (food preparation, shortness of breath, the act of eating) and lose weight. Commonly, other coexisting diseases (CVD, diabetes mellitus, renal disease, or cancer) may be present, thereby influencing total amount and kind of carbohydrate, protein, and fat prescribed.[4]

Pneumonia

The term *pneumonia* comes from the Greek word *pneuma*, meaning breath. It is an acute inflammation of the lung caused by an infectious agent and can stem from three sources: (1) aspiration of normal bacterial flora, gastric contents, or both in oropharyngeal secretions; (2) inhalation of contaminants (e.g., virus); or (3) contamination from systemic circulation. A common disorder, community-acquired pneumonia is the most lethal infectious disease in the United States and the sixth leading cause of death.[13]

Symptoms

Generally the immune response—cough with or without sputum production, sneezing, and mucociliary clearance (pulmonary defense mechanisms)—guard against pneumonia.[13] Community-acquired pneumonia is usually bacterial in origin and produces exudate that is hard to expectorate. Viral pneumonia does not produce exudate.[13] Hospital-acquired, or nosocomial, pneumonia develops in up to 5% of hospitalized patients.[13] Nosocomial pneumonia and community-based pneumonia are caused by different pathogens. Aspiration of infected pharyngeal or gastric secretions delivers bacteria straight to the lungs. This is promoted by exogenous factors such as contamination by dirty hands and equipment, treatment with broad-spectrum antibiotics that promote emergence of drug-resistant organisms, and patient factors such as malnutrition, smoking, preexisting lung disease, advanced age, swallowing disorders, and chest or upper abdominal surgery. Signs and symptoms are nonspecific; however, fever, purulent sputum, and leukocytosis are present in most patients.[13]

Treatment

Sputum and blood specimens are cultured before antibiotic treatment. The usual treatment is with a broad-spectrum penicillin antibiotic. Erythromycin may be added if the presence of an atypical organism is suspected. Oxygen therapy is often used, and in severe cases the patient may be ventilated. Nosocomial pneumonia is treated more aggressively with broad-spectrum antibiotics and tailored to a specific clinical setting because of the high mortality rate.[13]

Nutritional Management

Sufficient fluids (3 to 3.5 L) should be given daily if not contraindicated. Frequent small meals may be better tolerated.

A multivitamin and mineral supplement may be beneficial, and fiber should be encouraged to avoid constipation. Adequate fruit and fruit juice intake will supply necessary potassium.[7]

Tuberculosis

Tuberculosis (TB), caused by *Mycobacterium tuberculosis*, is one of the world's more widespread and deadly diseases. It occurs disproportionately among disadvantaged populations such as the malnourished, the homeless, and those living in overcrowded and substandard housing. *M. tuberculosis* is an airborne disease, and strains resistant to one or more first-line antituberculosis drugs are increasing.[13]

Symptoms

Typical symptoms of TB are malaise, anorexia, weight loss, fever, and night sweats. Chronic cough is the most universal pulmonary symptom. It may be dry at first but becomes productive of purulent sputum as the disease progresses. More often than not, the sputum is blood streaked. Patients appear chronically ill and malnourished.[3,11]

Treatment

The basic goals of TB treatment are as follows[13]:
- Administer multiple drugs to which organisms are susceptible.
- Add at least two new antitubercular agents to a regimen when treatment failure is suspected.
- Provide the safest, most effective therapy in the shortest period of time.
- Ensure adherence to therapy.

Nonadherence (because of adverse drug reaction) to treatment is a major cause of treatment failure, continued transmission of TB, and development of drug resistance. Hospitalization for initial therapy of TB is not necessary for most patients,[13] but hospitalization has increased because of increasing resistance of the organism to treatment and an increasing number of cases.[4]

Nutritional Management

The objective of nutritional management is to maintain weight or prevent weight loss. If febrile, then patients will be hypermetabolic. A well-balanced diet with liberal amounts of protein and adequate kcalories is usually necessary. Ensure the patient is consuming adequate amounts of calcium, iron, vitamin C, and B-complex vitamins.[4]

HEALTH PROMOTION
ADDED FOOD FACTORS IN CORONARY HEART DISEASE THERAPY

The primary focus of NT for CHD is on control of lipid factors, including cholesterol and saturated fats. Two other food factors, however, play a different role. In varying ways they help to protect us from the development of CHD.[3]

Dietary Fiber

Studies indicate water-soluble types of dietary fiber have significant cholesterol-lowering effect. Soluble fiber includes gums, pectin, certain hemicelluloses, and the body's storage polysaccharide, glycogen. Foods rich in soluble fiber include oat bran and dried beans, with additional amounts in barley and fruits. Oat bran, for example, contains a primary water-soluble gum, β-glucan, which is a lipid-lowering agent. Soluble dietary fiber has the following properties:

- Delays gastric emptying
- Slows intestinal transit time
- Slows glucose absorption
- Is fermented in the colon into short-chain fatty acids that may inhibit liver cholesterol synthesis and help clear LDL cholesterol

On the other hand, insoluble dietary fiber—cellulose, lignin, and many hemicelluloses—found in vegetables, wheat, and most other grains does not have these lipid-lowering effects. Thus an increased use of soluble fiber food sources, especially oat bran and legumes, would have beneficial effects.

Omega-3 Fatty Acids

Studies indicate omega-3 fatty acids, eicosapentaenoic acid (EPA) and docosahexaenoic acid (DHA) (see Chapter 4), found mostly in seafood and marine oils, also have protective functions. They can do the following:

- Change pattern of plasma fatty acids to alter platelet activity and reduce platelet aggregation that causes blood clotting, thus lowering the risk of coronary thrombosis
- Decrease the synthesis of VLDL
- Increase antiinflammatory effects

It would seem, then, factors in foods such as oats, dried beans, and fatty fish would provide valuable lipid-lowering additions to our diets.

> **KEY TERM**
> **hyperlipoproteinemia** Elevated level of lipoproteins in the blood.

TO SUM UP

CHD remains the leading cause of death in the United States. Atherosclerosis, its underlying pathologic process, involves the formation of plaque, a fatty substance that builds up along the interior surfaces of blood vessels, interfering with blood flow and damaging blood vessels. If this buildup becomes severe, then it cuts off blood supplies of oxygen and nutrients to tissue cells, which in turn begin to die. When this occurs in a coronary artery, the result is an MI, or heart attack. When it occurs in a brain vessel, the result is a CVA, or stroke.

Risk for atherosclerosis increases with the amount and type of blood lipids (lipoproteins) available. The apolipoprotein portion of lipoproteins is an important genetically determined part of the disease process. Elevated serum LDL cholesterol level is a primary factor in atherosclerosis development.

Initial dietary recommendations for acute CVD (heart attack) include caloric restriction, soft-textured foods, and small, frequent meals to reduce the metabolic demands of digestion, absorption, and metabolism of foods and their nutrients. Maintenance of a lean body weight is important. Persons with chronic CHD (e.g., CHF) and those with essential hypertension benefit from weight management, exercise, and sodium restriction to overcome cardiac edema and to help control elevated blood pressure.

Current dietary recommendations to help prevent CHD involve maintaining a healthy weight; limiting fats to 25% to 30% of all kcalories, with the majority being unsaturated food forms; limiting sodium intake to 2 to 3 g/day; and increasing exercise.

Concerted efforts are needed to combat development of cardiac cachexia in progressive heart failure. In addition, atherosclerotic plaques may occur in the extremities, usually the legs, causing PVD and the pain of intermittent claudication when walking. Progressive respiratory failure interferes with normal exchange of blood gases, oxygen and CO_2, and results in COPD, for which changed ratios of the fuel macronutrients are sometimes indicated.

QUESTIONS FOR REVIEW

1. Which types of hyperlipoproteinemia occur most often? Identify lipids that are elevated in each case, as well as predisposing factors. Describe the types of diet recommended for each.
2. Identify four dietary recommendations that should be made for the person with a heart attack. Describe how each recommendation helps recovery.
3. What dietary changes can the average American make to reduce saturated fats and to substitute polyunsaturated fats?
4. What does the term *essential hypertension* mean? Why would weight management and sodium restriction contribute to its control?
5. Outline NT for cardiac cachexia and discuss the rationale for each aspect of the feeding plan.
6. Discuss the cause and treatment of PVD.
7. Outline NT for COPD, and discuss the rationale for the fuel macronutrient adjustments.

REFERENCES

1. Brashers VL: Alterations of cardiovascular function. In McCance KL, Huether SE, editors: *Pathophysiology: the biologic basis for disease in adults and children*, ed 3, St Louis, 2006, Mosby.
2. American Heart Association: *Heart disease and stroke statistics*, Dallas, Texas, 2009, American Heart Association. from: <www.americanheart.org>. Retrieved May 16, 2009.
3. National Cholesterol Education Program (NCEP): *Third report of the NCEP Expert Panel on Detection, Evaluation, and Treatment of High Blood Cholesterol in Adults (Adult Treatment Panel III), full report*, Washington, D.C., 2002, National Institutes of Health, National Heart, Lung, and Blood Institute. from: <www.nhlbi.nih.gov/guidelines/cholesterol/atp3_rpt.htm>. Retrieved May 14, 2009.
4. Mahan LK, Escott-Stump S, editors: *Krause's food & nutrition therapy*, ed 12, St Louis, 2008, Saunders.
5. Mozaffarian D, Katan MB, Ascherio A, et al: Trans fatty acids and cardiovascular disease. *N Engl J Med* 354(15):1601, 2006.
6. Banasik JL: Alterations in cardiac function. In Copstead LC, Banasik JL, editors: *Pathophysiology*, ed 3, St Louis, 2005, Saunders.
7. Banasik JL: Heart failure and dysrhythmias: common sequelae of cardiac diseases. In Copstead LC, Banasik JL, editors: *Pathophysiology*, ed 3, St Louis, 2005, Saunders.
8. Antman EM, Anbe DT, Armstrong PW, et al: ACC/AHA guidelines for the management of patients with ST-elevation myocardial infarction—executive summary: a report of the ACC/AHA Task Force on Practice Guidelines (Committee to Revise the 1999 Guidelines on the Management of Patients With Acute Myocardial Infarction). *Circulation* 110:588, 2004.
9. National High Blood Pressure Program: *The seventh report of the Joint National Committee on Prevention, Detection, Evaluation, and Treatment of High Blood Pressure, National Institutes of Health, National Heart, Lung, and Blood Institutes*, Washington, D.C., 2004, U.S. Government Printing Office. NIH Pub No 04-5230.
10. Sachs FN, Svetkey LP, Vollmer WM, et al: Effects on blood pressure of reduced dietary sodium and the Dietary Approaches to Stop Hypertension (DASH). *N Engl J Med* 344:3, 2001.
11. National Center for Health Statistics, Centers for Disease Control and Prevention: *Stroke/cerebrovascular disease*, Hyattsville, Md., 2009, Centers for Disease Control and Prevention. from: <www.cdc.gov/nchs/fastats/stroke.htm>. Retrieved May 18, 2009.
12. American Heart Association: *Stroke statistics*, Dallas, Texas, 2005, American Heart Association. from: <www.americanheart.org>. Retrieved August 8, 2009.
13. Schumann L: Restrictive pulmonary disorders. In Copstead LC, Banasik JL, editors: *Pathophysiology*, ed 3, St Louis, 2005, Saunders.

FURTHER RESOURCES

Websites of Interest

- American Heart Association: www.americanheart.org. *[Information for health professionals and consumers regarding cardiovascular diseases and stroke.]*
- Centers for Disease Control and Prevention. Health Topic: Heart Disease: http://www.cdc.gov/heartdisease/index.htm. *[This website provides credible and reliable health information for consumers, health professionals, policy makers, and the media.]*
- MedlinePlus, Heart Diseases: www.nlm.nih.gov/medlineplus/heartdiseases.html. *[This is the National Institutes of Health website for consumers. It is produced by the National Library of Medicine to provide reliable, up-to-date health information about diseases, conditions, and wellness issues.]*
- Womenshealth.gov. Heart Health and Stroke: http://www.womenshealth.gov/heart-stroke/heart-disease-stroke-prevention/index.cfm. *[The Office of Women's Health is housed in the U.S. Department of Health and Human Services to promote health equity for women and girls through sex/gender-specific approaches.]*
- World Health Organization (WHO). Cardiovascular Diseases: www.who.int/cardiovascular_diseases/en/. *[Part of the United Nations, WHO is responsible for providing leadership on global health matters.]*

Diabetes Mellitus

Joyce Gilbert

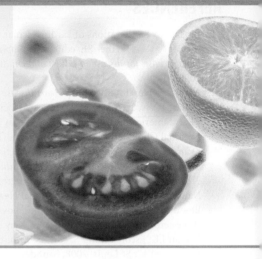

EVOLVE WEBSITE

http://evolve.elsevier.com/Williams/essentials/

OUTLINE

Nature of Diabetes
General Management of Diabetes
Rationale for Diabetes Nutrition Therapy
Implementing Nutrition Therapy

Issues Related to Medical Therapy
Management of Diabetes Nutrition Therapy
Diabetes Education Program
HEALTH PROMOTION

In this chapter of our continuing clinical nutrition series, we look at the problem of diabetes. We seek to understand its nature and how it can be managed to maintain good health and avoid complications.

Diabetes is a serious, costly, and increasingly common chronic disease. In the United States, 25.86 million people (8.3% of the population) have diabetes. An estimated 18.8 million Americans have diagnosed diabetes, and an additional 7 million have undiagnosed diabetes. Approximately 1.9 million new cases of diabetes are diagnosed each year.[1] Diabetes can be diagnosed on the basis of two fasting glucose readings of 126 mg/dL or higher or a random glucose level of 200 mg/dL or higher and symptoms such as polyuria, polydipsia, and unexplained weight loss.[2]

Although elevation of blood glucose level is the hallmark characteristic of diabetes, it is a group of metabolic disorders resulting from a defect in insulin secretion, insulin action, or both. These defects interfere with normal cellular uptake of glucose and use of glucose within cells. Restoring normal metabolic function is the goal in the early diagnosis and treatment of diabetes. Restoration of normal metabolism can prevent many of the short-term complications such as hyperglycemia and hypoglycemia and the longer-term microvascular, macrovascular, and neurologic complications that affect multiple body systems.

Direct and indirect health costs of diabetes were estimated to be $245 billion in 2012 in the United States (or more than

1 out of every 5 health care dollars).[3] The death rate among middle-aged people with diabetes is double the death rate of those who do not have diabetes. Diabetes causes preventable complications that can be life threatening, including heart disease. Lifestyle changes can delay the progression of diabetes, as can controlling blood glucose, lipids, and blood pressure.

NATURE OF DIABETES

History

The metabolic disease we know today as *diabetes mellitus* has been with us for a long time. Ancient records describe its devastating effects as observed by early healers. In the first century AD, the Greek physician Aretaeus wrote of a malady in which the body "ate its own flesh" and gave off large quantities of urine. He gave it the name *diabetes,* from the Greek word meaning *siphon* or *to pass through.* Much later, in the seventeenth century, the word *mellitus,* from the Latin word for *honey,* was added because of the sweet nature of the urine. This addition also distinguished it from **diabetes insipidus** (*insipid,* meaning tasteless, or not sweet), another disorder, although uncommon, in which the passage of copious amounts of urine had been observed. Today, use of the single name diabetes always means diabetes mellitus.

As medical knowledge began to grow, early clinicians—such as Rollo in England and Bouchardat in France—observed that diabetes became less severe in overweight patients who lost weight. Later another French physician, Lancereaux, and his students described two kinds of diabetes: (1) *diabète gras* ("fat diabetes") and (2) *diabète maigre* ("thin diabetes").[4] All of these observations preceded any knowledge about **insulin** or any relation to the pancreas. During these times, which have aptly been called the *diabetic dark ages,* individuals with diabetes had short lives and were maintained on a variety of semistarvation diets.[5]

Later, evidence began to point to the pancreas as a primary organ involved in the disease process. Paul Langerhans (1847-1888), a young German medical student, found special clusters—or islets—of cells scattered throughout the human pancreas that were different from the rest of the tissue. Although their function was still unknown, these special islet cells were named for their young discoverer: the islets of Langerhans. Research at that time focused on the pancreas. Finally, in 1921 and 1922 a University of Toronto team discovered and successfully used the controlling agent from the "island cells," naming it *insulin* for its source.[6]

Classification

The American Diabetes Association classifies diabetes into the four categories[2]:

1. Type 1 diabetes (T1DM), formerly called insulin-dependent diabetes mellitus
2. Type 2 diabetes (T2DM), formerly called non-insulin-dependent diabetes mellitus
3. Gestational diabetes mellitus (GDM)
4. Other specific types

The terms *insulin-dependent diabetes mellitus* (IDDM) and *non-insulin-dependent diabetes mellitus* (NIDDM), should no longer be used because they are confusing and have often resulted in classifying patients based on treatment rather than cause of their diabetes.[2]

T1DM is characterized by sudden, severe insulin deficiency requiring insulin therapy to prevent ketoacidosis, coma, and death. T1DM generally appears during childhood or adolescence and accounts for 5% to 10% of the cases of diabetes. However, T1DM can occur at any age, and almost half of new cases are diagnosed after 20 years of age. Two forms of T1DM exist: (1) immune-mediated diabetes and (2) idiopathic diabetes. Immune-mediated diabetes results from a cellular-mediated autoimmune destruction of the beta cells of the pancreas.[7] Idiopathic diabetes has no known cause.

The onset of T1DM is often rapid, accompanied by classic symptoms of weight loss and increased urination and thirst, especially if a viral infection or other stress increases the need for insulin. Onset may be less acute, or a "honeymoon period" of 6 to 12 months may occur in which the diabetes may appear to be "cured" after an initial acute onset and initiation of insulin therapy. Destruction of the beta cells in the pancreas and loss of insulin production are usually gradual, accounting for the honeymoon period after insulin therapy restores normal glucose and metabolic stress is resolved.

T2DM is associated with insulin resistance and obesity combined with inadequate insulin produced in the pancre-atic beta cells to compensate for the insulin resistance or an insulin secretory defect with insulin resistance.[2] T2DM accounts for 90% to 95% of all cases of diabetes, and symptoms may include poor wound healing, blurred vision, or recurrent gum or bladder infections. Many individuals are not symptomatic, and the diabetes may be detected as the result of a routine blood test. Obesity and physical inactivity are strong risk factors for T2DM.[8-10] A large waist circumference is considered to be a biomarker for insulin resistance and the metabolic syndrome associated with diabetes, hypertension, and dyslipidemia (typically low high-density cholesterol and elevated triglyceride levels).[11] Although T2DM is associated with insulin resistance and is typically diagnosed after 40 years of age, it is occurring in epidemic proportions in younger populations, including children and adolescents. Most children diagnosed with T2DM have a family history of T2DM, are overweight or obese, are insulin resistant, or have physical signs of insulin resistance such as acanthosis nigricans.[10] Undiagnosed, these young people may be at early risk for cardiovascular disease (CVD).[10] Current testing criteria and diabetes risk factors to help identify T2DM before the onset of complications has been developed by the American Academy of Pediatrics and the American Dietetic Association (ADA).[11]

GDM is defined as carbohydrate intolerance of variable severity with onset or first recognition during pregnancy. GDM develops in 2% to 5% of all pregnancies, and 30% to 40% of women with GDM are likely to develop T2DM.[12] In T2DM and GDM, a relative insulin deficiency exists because the pancreas fails to produce the level of insulin needed to compensate for insulin resistance.

Other specific types of diabetes include genetic defects of the beta cell, genetic defects in insulin action, disease of the exocrine pancreas, endocrinopathies, and other uncommon forms of immune-mediated diabetes.[2]

Recently, the American Diabetes Association identified an intermediate classification of individuals whose glucose levels

---

KEY TERMS

diabetes insipidus   A condition of the pituitary gland and insufficiency of one of its hormones, vasopressin (antidiuretic hormone); characterized by a copious output of a nonsweet urine, great thirst, and sometimes a large appetite. However, in diabetes insipidus these symptoms result from a specific injury to the pituitary gland, not a collection of metabolic disorders as in diabetes mellitus. The injured pituitary gland produces less vasopressin, a hormone that normally helps the kidneys reabsorb adequate water.

insulin   Hormone formed in the beta cells of the islets of Langerhans in the pancreas. It is secreted when blood glucose and amino acid levels rise and assists their entry into body cells. It also promotes glycogenesis and conversion of glucose into fat and inhibits lipolysis and gluconeogenesis (protein breakdown). Commercial insulin is manufactured from pigs and cows; new "artificial" human insulin products have recently been made available.

do not meet the criteria, but are still considered high risk for developing diabetes.[2] This category consists of individuals diagnosed with *prediabetes*. If cross-sectional data were applied to the 2007 U.S. population, about 57 million adults (20 years or older) in the United States are estimated to have had prediabetes in 2007.[1] People are considered to have prediabetes if they have impaired fasting glucose (IFG) or impaired glucose tolerance (IGT); some people have both conditions.[1] IFG is identified through fasting blood glucose, and IGT is identified by an oral glucose tolerance test (OGTT).[11] Formerly called *borderline diabetes*, IFG, IGT, and prediabetes are associated with metabolic syndrome that includes abdominal obesity, dyslipidemia (high triglycerides, low high-density lipoprotein [HDL] cholesterol, or both), and hypertension.[1] Research has shown lifestyle interventions can reduce the rate of progression to T2DM.[13,14] Table 22-1 outlines criteria used to diagnose diabetes.

Contributing Causes
Genetics

For some time, early insulin assay tests developed to measure level of insulin activity in blood found insulin-like activity in diabetes to be two or three times normal insulin levels. It is now evident that diabetes is a syndrome with multiple forms, resulting from (1) lack of insulin or (2) insulin resistance (or from both).[2]

Diabetes has long been associated with body weight, since the early observations of differences in "fat diabetes" and "thin diabetes."[4] Current research has reinforced the relation of overweight state to development of T2DM. Obesity can increase circulating insulin levels, which will ultimately lead to increased insulin resistance. In addition, individuals with a family history may have mutations on genes that control insulin production or may inherit insulin resistance not directly related to obesity. Thus multiple genetic mutations may interact to increase the risk of T2DM.

Environmental Role: "Thrifty Gene"

Environmental factors apparently play a role in unmasking the underlying genetic susceptibility—a "thrifty" diabetic genotype that probably developed during primitive times. This theory indicates diabetes may be associated with past genetic modifications for survival during varying periods of food availability. Gene mutations and the thrifty trait associated with T2DM facilitated more efficient use of limited food during times of difficult survival conditions. As food supplies became more plentiful, negative aspects of the thrifty trait began to appear. Such is indeed the case, for example, with the experience of Pima Indians in Arizona, as earlier studies and recent archeological excavations have indicated.[15] In earlier times, this group ate a limited diet mainly of carbohydrate foods harvested through heavy physical labor in a primitive agricultural climate. Now, however, with the "progress" of civilization, the Pimas have become obese, and half of the adults have T2DM (the highest reported rate of this type of diabetes in the world). Native Americans develop diabetes at almost three times the rate of Caucasians. This same pattern is seen among populations of now-urbanized Pacific Islanders, South Asians, Asian Indians, and Creoles, although less is known about the exact numbers.[8,9] Other at-risk populations include Hispanic and Latino Americans, who are 1.5 times as likely to develop diabetes as Caucasians, and African Americans, who develop diabetes at 1.6 times the rate of Caucasians.[1] Thus evidence suggests that these groups have a genetic susceptibility to T2DM (diabetic genotype) and that the disease is triggered by environmental factors, including obesity (see the Focus on Culture box, "Type 2 Diabetes: An Equal Opportunity Disease?"). Several specific genes involved in energy metabolism are thought to increase the risk for developing obesity, T2DM, or both. As we commonly observe, lifestyle (dietary and physical activity habits) can interact with genetics in the development of T2DM.

Symptoms

Symptoms of T1DM in its uncontrolled state include the following:
- Increased thirst (polydipsia)
- Increased urination (polyuria)
- Increased hunger (polyphagia)
- Weight loss (more common with T1DM)
- Fruity smell to breath (symptom of ketoacidosis)
- Fatigue or weakness

These symptoms occur because in an insulin-deficient state, blood glucose levels and renal filtration of glucose are increased beyond the kidney's threshold for reabsorption; as the level of glucose excreted increases, urine volume increases. Without adequate glucose use, fat mobilization increases, and an increased breakdown of fat leads to excess ketone formation.

T2DM may be asymptomatic, or symptoms may be more subtle and may include the following:
- Poor wound healing or recurrent infections
- Blurred vision (result of effects of hyperglycemia on shape of the cornea, which is returned to normal after glucose levels are stabilized)
- Skin irritation or infection
- Recurrent gum or bladder infections

Classic symptoms of diabetes are the result of short-term effects of hyperglycemia. These symptoms are reversible if blood glucose levels are returned to a normal or near-normal level.

Metabolic Pattern of Diabetes
Overall Energy Balance and Energy Nutrients

Because initial symptoms of glycosuria and hyperglycemia are related to excess glucose, historically diabetes was called a *disease of carbohydrate metabolism*. However, as more becomes known about the intimate interrelationships of carbohydrate, fat, and protein metabolism, we view it in more general terms. It is a metabolic disorder resulting from lack of insulin (absolute, partial, or unavailable) affecting more or less each basic energy nutrient. It is especially related to metabolism of the two fuels in the body's overall energy system: (1) carbohydrate and (2) fat.

TABLE 22-1 CRITERIA FOR DIAGNOSING DIABETES

DIABETES TYPE	FORMER TERMS	ETIOLOGY	CRITERIA
Type 1 diabetes (T1DM)*: immune-mediated or idiopathic	Insulin-dependent diabetes mellitus (IDDM), type I diabetes, juvenile-onset diabetes, ketosis-prone diabetes, brittle diabetes	Beta cell destruction, usually leading to absolute insulin deficiency	Symptoms[†] of diabetes mellitus and casual plasma glucose ≤200 mg/dL (*casual* is defined as any time of day without regard to last meal)
			or
Type 2 diabetes (T2DM) (adults)	Non-insulin-dependent diabetes mellitus (NIDDM), type II diabetes, adult-onset diabetes, maturity-onset diabetes, ketosis-resistant diabetes, stable diabetes	Insulin resistance with insulin secretory defect	Fasting plasma glucose (FPG) ≤126 mg/dL (*fasting* is defined as no kcalorie intake for at least 8 hr)
			or
			2-hr postprandial plasma glucose (PPG) ≤200 mg/dL during oral glucose tolerance test (OGTT) (performed as described by the World Health Organization [WHO] using glucose load containing the equivalent of 75 g anhydrous glucose dissolved in water)
T2DM (children)			Overweight (body mass index [BMI] >85th percentile for age and gender, weight for height >85th percentile, or weight >120% of ideal for height) *plus* Any two of the following: • Family history of T2DM in first- or second-degree relative • Native American, African American, Latino, Asian American, Pacific Islander • Signs of insulin resistance or conditions associated with insulin resistance (acanthosis nigricans, hypertension, dyslipidemia, or polycystic ovary syndrome [PCOS])
Gestational diabetes (GDM)			One-step approach: diagnostic OGTT Two-step approach: initial screening to measure plasma or serum glucose concentration 1 hr after 50 g oral glucose load (glucose challenge test [GCT]) and perform diagnostic OGTT on those women exceeding glucose threshold value on GCT (glucose threshold >140 mg/dL identifies >80% of women with GDM)
Impaired glucose tolerance (IGT)	Borderline diabetes, chemical diabetes		2-hr PPG >140 mg/dL and <200 mg/dL

Data from American Diabetes Association: Standards of medical care in diabetes—2008. *Diabetes Care* 31(Suppl 1):S12, 2008, with permission from The American Diabetes Association.

*Patients with any form of diabetes may require insulin treatment at some stage of their disease. Such use of insulin does not classify the patient as having T1DM.

[†]Symptoms include polyuria, polydipsia, and unexplained weight loss.

⊕ FOCUS ON CULTURE

Type 2 Diabetes: An Equal Opportunity Disease?

Type 2 diabetes (T2DM) occurs disproportionately in people of color throughout the United States. Rates of T2DM are two to six times higher in Native Americans, Alaska Natives, African Americans, and Hispanic Americans than in the non-Hispanic Caucasian population. In addition, people of color experience onset at an earlier age, and their complications are harsher. Although the cause for these ethnic disparities has not been identified, it is hypothesized that the differences may lie in the interaction of inherent susceptibility and modifiable risk factors such as physical inactivity and poor diet.

Ethnic Group	Prevalence (Ages 20+)	Additional Information
Non-Hispanic Caucasians	6.6%	
Native Americans	16.5% of the population: 6.0% among Alaska Natives, 29.3% among Native Americans	Diagnosis 2.2 times more likely than Caucasians Pima tribe has highest rate of diabetes in the world: 50% Complications of diabetes are major causes of death and health problems in most Native American populations
African Americans	11.8%	Diagnosis 1.6 times more likely; 25% between ages 65 and 74 have diabetes; 1 in 4 women older than age 55 has diabetes
Latinos/Hispanics	10.4%	Diagnosis 1.5 times more likely Approximately 11.9% of Mexican Americans have diabetes Approximately 12.6% of Puerto Rican Americans have diabetes Approximately 8.2% of Cuban Americans have diabetes

Bibliography

Brown TL: Ethnic populations. In Ross TA, Boucher JL, O'Connell BS, editors: *American Dietetic Association guide to diabetes medical nutrition therapy and education*, Chicago, 2005, American Dietetic Association.

Centers for Disease Control and Prevention: *National diabetes fact sheet: general information and national estimates on diabetes in the United States, 2007*, Atlanta, Ga., 2008, U.S. Department of Health and Human Services, Centers for Disease Control and Prevention. from: <www.cdc.gov/diabetes/pubs/pdf/ndfs_2007.pdf>. Retrieved July 13, 2010.

Normal Blood Glucose Control

Control of blood glucose level within its normal range of 70 to 120 mg/dL (3.9 to 6.7 mmol/L) is vital to normal overall fuel metabolism and other metabolic functions. A knowledge of factors involved in maintaining a normal blood glucose level is essential to understanding the impairment of these factors (see Chapters 3 and 4). An overview of these normal balancing controls is illustrated in Figure 22-1.

Sources of Blood Glucose

Two sources of blood glucose ensure a constant supply of this primary body fuel: (1) diet, energy nutrients in our food (i.e., dietary carbohydrate, protein, fat), and (2) glycogen, the backup source from constant turnover of "stored" liver glycogen by a process called glycogenolysis.

Uses of Blood Glucose

To prevent continued rise of blood glucose above the normal range, excess glucose is converted to other substances based on need. These include the following: (1) glycogenesis, conversion of glucose to glycogen for storage in liver and muscle; (2) lipogenesis, conversion of glucose to fat and storage in adipose tissue; and (3) glycolysis, cell oxidation of glucose for energy.

Pancreatic Hormonal Controls

The following three types of islet cells scattered in clusters throughout the pancreas (islets of Langerhans) provide hormones closely integrated in the regulation of blood glucose levels.

1. *Alpha cells:* Arranged around the outer rim of the islets are alpha cells, one to two cells thick, making up about 30% of the total cells. These cells synthesize glucagon.
2. *Beta cells:* The largest portion of islets is occupied by beta cells filling the central zone or about 60% of the gland. These primary cells synthesize insulin.
3. *Delta cells:* Interspersed between alpha and beta cells, or occasionally between alpha cells alone, are delta cells, the remaining 10% of total cells. These cells synthesize somatostatin.

This specific arrangement of human islet cells is illustrated in Figure 22-2.

Interrelated Hormone Functions

Juncture points of the three types of islet cells act as sensors of blood glucose concentration and its rate of change. They constantly adjust and balance the rate of secretion of insulin, glucagon, and somatostatin to match whatever conditions

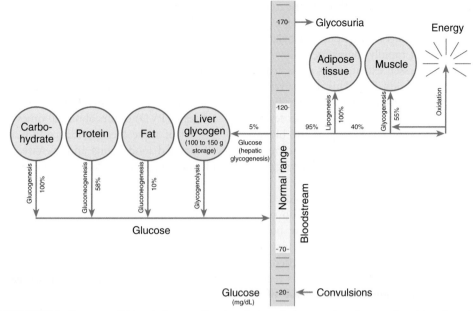

FIGURE 22-1 Sources of blood glucose (food and stored glycogen) and normal routes of control.

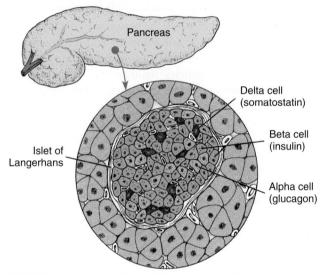

FIGURE 22-2 Islets of Langerhans, located in the pancreas.

prevail at any time. Each of the following three hormones has specific interbalanced functions:

1. *Insulin:* Although the precise mechanisms are not entirely clear in every case, insulin has a profound effect on glucose control. It functions extensively in the metabolism of all three energy nutrients, as follows:
   - Insulin facilitates transport of glucose through cell membranes by way of special insulin receptors. These receptors are located on the membrane of insulin-sensitive cells, including those in adipose tissue, muscle tissue, and monocytes. These insulin receptors mediate all metabolic effects of insulin. Research has shown that cells of obese persons with diabetes have fewer than the normal number of insulin receptors. Weight loss in

obese individuals and physical exercise increase the number of these receptors. The insulin receptor also appears to control several metabolic steps within the cell.
   - Insulin enhances conversion of glucose to glycogen and its consequent storage in the liver (glycogenesis). Insulin also, then, inhibits the breakdown of glycogen to glucose and its release into the body.
   - Insulin stimulates conversion of glucose to fat (lipogenesis) for storage as adipose tissue.
   - Insulin inhibits fat breakdown (lipolysis) and the breakdown of protein.
   - Insulin promotes uptake of amino acids by skeletal muscles, thus increasing protein synthesis.

KEY TERMS

glycogenolysis Production of blood glucose from liver glycogen.

glycogenesis Synthesis of glycogen from blood glucose.

lipogenesis Synthesis of fat from blood glucose.

glycolysis Cell oxidation of glucose for energy.

glucagon A polypeptide hormone secreted by the alpha cells of the pancreatic islets of Langerhans in response to hypoglycemia; has an opposite balancing effect to that of insulin, raising the blood sugar, and thus is used as a quick-acting antidote for the hypoglycemic reaction of insulin. It stimulates the breakdown of glycogen (glycogenolysis) in the liver by activating the liver enzyme phosphorylase and thus raises blood sugar levels during fasting states to ensure adequate levels for normal nerve and brain function.

somatostatin A hormone formed in the delta cells of the pancreatic islets of Langerhans and the hypothalamus. It is a balancing factor in the maintenance of normal blood glucose levels by inhibiting insulin and glucagon production in the pancreas as needed.

- Insulin influences glucose oxidation through the main glycolytic pathway.

2. *Glucagon:* The hormone glucagon functions as a balancing antagonist to insulin. It rapidly causes breakdown of liver glycogen and, to a lesser extent, fatty acids from adipose tissue to serve as body fuel. This action raises blood glucose levels to protect the brain and other body tissues. It helps maintain normal blood glucose levels during fasting hours of sleep. A lowering of the blood glucose concentration, increased amino acid concentrations, or sympathetic nervous system stimulation triggers glucagon secretion.

3. *Somatostatin:* Although pancreatic islet delta cells are the major source of somatostatin, this hormone is also synthesized and secreted in different regions of the body, including the hypothalamus. It acts in balance with insulin and glucose to inhibit their interactions as needed to maintain normal blood glucose levels. It also helps regulate blood glucose levels by inhibiting the release of a number of other hormones as needed.

Metabolic Changes in Diabetes

In uncontrolled diabetes, insulin is lacking to facilitate operation of normal blood glucose controls; abnormal metabolic changes occur, as follows, that affect glucose, fat, and protein and account for symptoms of diabetes:

- *Glucose:* Blood glucose cannot be oxidized properly through the main glycolytic pathway in the cell to furnish energy (see Chapter 8), and a lack of insulin allows the breakdown of hepatic glycogen and the release of glucose; therefore glucose builds up in the blood (hyperglycemia).
- *Fat:* Formation of fat (lipogenesis) is curtailed, and fat breakdown (lipolysis) increases. This leads to excess formation and accumulation of ketones (ketoacidosis). Appearance of the major ketone, acetone, in urine indicates development of ketoacidosis.
- *Protein:* Tissue protein is also broken down in an effort to secure energy. This causes weight loss and nitrogen excretion in the urine.

GENERAL MANAGEMENT OF DIABETES

Treatment Goals: Basic Objectives

The diabetes care team—the physician, dietitian, nurse, and person with diabetes—are guided by the following three basic objectives:

1. *Maintain optimal nutrition:* The first objective is to fulfill the basic nutritional requirement for health, growth and development, and a desirable body weight.
2. *Prevent hypoglycemia or hyperglycemia:* This second objective is designed to keep the person relatively free of hypoglycemia or insulin reaction, which requires immediate countermeasures, and hyperglycemia, which, if untreated, contributes to more serious ketoacidosis or diabetic coma.
3. *Prevent complications:* The third objective recognizes the increased risk a person with diabetes faces for developing complications that reflect the damaging effects of chronic diabetes on the tissues of small and large blood vessels and peripheral nerves. These damages may occur in tissues such as eyes (**retinopathy**), nerves (**neuropathy**), and kidneys (**nephropathy**). In addition, coronary artery disease occurs in persons with diabetes about four times as often as in the general population. Peripheral vascular disease (PVD) occurs about 40 times as often.

In all of these areas, evidence indicates that consistent, well-planned food habits and exercise, balanced as needed with early aggressive insulin therapy, can significantly help normalize metabolism and thereby reduce risks of these potentially serious complications.[16]

This aggressive insulin therapy consists of multiple daily injections or continuous subcutaneous infusion by an insulin pump (Figure 22-3). Self-monitoring of blood glucose (SMBG) levels is used to guide decisions to improve glycemic control. The added cardiovascular risk associated with diabetes is reflected in having blood pressure and lipid goals for diabetes management that are similar to those used in treating individuals who have diagnosed CVD (Table 22-2).

Self-Care Role of the Person with Diabetes

To effectively control diabetes, the person with diabetes must play a central role. Daily self-discipline and informed self-care, supported by a skilled and sensitive health care team, are required for sound diabetes management. Ultimately, all persons with diabetes must treat themselves. This is especially true with the stricter normal blood glucose control currently being used, with frequent SMBG and multiple insulin injections or an insulin infusion pump. Thus even greater need now exists for comprehensive diabetes education programs that encourage self-monitoring and self-care responsibility. Diabetes-related issues also need to be addressed as an integral component of primary care. Weight, activity, variety, and excess are themes that are relevant for assessing basic needs and providing basic recommendations.

KEY TERMS

retinopathy   Noninflammatory disease of the retina—the visual tissue of the eye—characterized by microaneurysms, intraretinal hemorrhages, waxy yellow exudates, "cotton wool" patches, and macular edema; a complication of diabetes that may lead to proliferation of fibrous tissue, retinal detachment, and blindness.

neuropathy   General term for functional and pathologic changes in the peripheral nervous system; in diabetes, a chronic sensory condition affecting mainly the nerves of the legs, marked by numbness from sensory impairment, loss of tendon reflexes, severe pain, weakness, and wasting of muscles involved.

nephropathy   Disease of the kidneys; in diabetes, renal damage associated with functional and pathologic changes in the nephrons, which can lead to glomerulosclerosis and chronic renal failure.

TABLE 22-2	METABOLIC GOALS IN DIABETES MANAGEMENT		
INDICATOR	**NORMAL VALUE**	**GOAL**	**ADDITIONAL ACTION SUGGESTED***
Plasma values (mg/dL)			
Average preprandial glucose	<110	90-130	>90/<150
Average bedtime glucose	<120	110-150	>110/<180
Whole blood values†(mg/dL)			
Average preprandial glucose	<100	80-120	>80/<140
Average bedtime glucose	<110	100-140	>100/<160
Hemoglobin A_{1c} (HbA_{1c}) (%)	<6	<7	<8
Low-density lipoprotein (LDL) cholesterol		<100 mg/dL	
High-density lipoprotein (HDL) cholesterol		Men: >55 mg/dL	
		Women: >55 mg/dL	
Triglycerides		<150 mg/dL	
Blood pressure		<130/80 mm Hg	

Data from American Diabetes Association: Standards of medical care in diabetes—2008. *Diabetes Care* 31(Suppl 1):S12, 2008, with permission from The American Diabetes Association.
*Depends on individual patient circumstances.
†Measurement of capillary blood glucose.

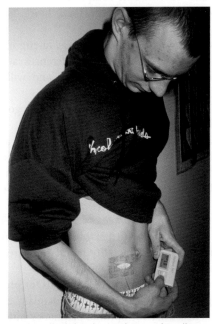

FIGURE 22-3 Insulin injecting using an insulin pump. (From Peckenpaugh NJ: *Nutrition essentials and diet therapy*, ed 11, St Louis, 2010, Saunders.)

RATIONALE FOR DIABETES NUTRITION THERAPY

Nutrition therapy (NT) for diabetes is multifaceted. Physicians and nurses can no longer rely on preprinted diet sheets to assume they are providing nutrition care for patients.[17] No standard American Diabetes Association or diabetic diet exists. The American Diabetes Association does not sanction any single meal plan or specific percentages of nutrients.[18] It is essential that persons with diabetes are assessed by a registered dietitian (RD) to determine an appropriate nutrition prescription and plan for self-management education.[11] In addition, diet orders such as *no sugar added, no*

concentrated sweets, low sugar, and *liberal diabetic* are not considered suitable because they do not reflect diabetes nutritional recommendations and pointlessly restrict sucrose. Such meal plans support the erroneous concept that simply limiting sucrose-sweetened foods will enhance blood glucose control.[18]

Nutrition therapy should be individualized, taking usual eating habits and other lifestyle factors into consideration.[19] Consistency within an eating pattern will result in better glycemic control than abiding by an arbitrary eating style. Nutrition recommendations are the same for individuals with diabetes as for the general population in regard to total fat, saturated fat, cholesterol, fiber, vitamins, and minerals. Recommendations for protein, carbohydrates, sucrose, and alcohol are modified, depending on the nature of diabetes in relation to carbohydrate metabolism or effects of complications.[17]

Type 1 Diabetes Mellitus

Recognizing the need for a more comprehensive program of care of diabetes, based on the individual metabolic balance concept and designed to help delay or avoid life-threatening complications of this chronic disease, a national U.S. clinical research study supported by the National Institutes of Health was organized. The Diabetes Control and Complications Trial (DCCT)[16] involved 1441 subjects in 29 clinical centers across the country for approximately 10 years. The study was designed to compare the effects of intensive insulin therapy aimed at achieving blood glucose levels as close as possible to the normal nondiabetic range with effects of conventional therapy on early microvascular complications of T1DM. The DCCT demonstrated that lowering hemoglobin A_{1c} (HbA_{1c}) from 9% to 7% in the intensively treated group reduced the risk of the development or progression of eye, kidney, and neurologic complications by 50% to 75%.[11,20] Dietary strategies played an important role in achieving control in the intensively treated group.[21] Reduction in complications was linearly related to improvement in glycemic control, indicating risk reduction can be achieved even if intensification of treatment fails to achieve a near-normal HbA$_{1c}$.[17,22] The adverse effects of intensive therapy included a twofold to threefold increase in severe hypoglycemia and a weight gain of 10 lb (4.5 kg).[16] Initial weight was considerably higher, but providing consultation about overeating to prevent or treat hypoglycemia appears to attenuate the weight gain.

Type 2 Diabetes Mellitus

The United Kingdom Prospective Diabetes Study (UKPDS) evaluated the effects of treatments to improve glycemic control and cardiovascular risk factors in individuals with newly diagnosed diabetes. Glycemic control and cardiovascular risk reduction therapies reduced rates of macrovascular and microvascular complications. The UKPDS confirmed DCCT findings with respect to preventing microvascular complications of diabetes and provided evidence that a comprehensive risk reduction approach could also reduce macrovascular complications.[23-26] The major cause of morbidity and mortality in persons with diabetes is CVD. T2DM and its common coexisting conditions (e.g., hypertension, dyslipidemia) are considered to be independent risk factors for macrovascular disease.[11]

Gestational Diabetes Mellitus

For women with preexisting diabetes or GDM, risks of fetal abnormalities and mortality are increased in the presence of hyperglycemia. Maternal insulin does not cross the placenta, but glucose does, causing the fetus's pancreas to increase insulin production if the mother becomes hyperglycemic. This increased production of insulin causes **macrosomia**, which is the most typical characteristic of babies born to women with diabetes. Other problems such as hyperinsulinemia and hyperglycemia may occur.[27] Therefore every effort should be made to control blood glucose levels.[11] All women with GDM should receive counseling by an RD when possible.[28] Individualized medical nutrition therapy (MNT), contingent on maternal weight and height, should include provision of adequate kilocalories (kcalories or kcal) and nutrients to meet the needs of the pregnancy and be consistent with established maternal blood glucose goals.[28] At the start, SMBG should be planned four times a day (fasting and 1 or 2 hours postprandial). Frequency can be decreased once glycemic control is established. Blood glucose goals during pregnancy are as follows[28]:

- *Fasting:* ≤105 mg/dL
- *1-hour postprandial:* ≤155 mg/dL
- *2-hours postprandial:* ≤130 mg/dL

IMPLEMENTING NUTRITION THERAPY

Nutrition intervention is governed by consideration of treatment goals and lifestyle changes the person with diabetes is ready to make, preferably to predetermined energy levels and percentages of carbohydrates, protein, and fat. The objective of NT is to support and facilitate individual lifestyle and

behavior changes that will lead to improved glycemic control. Cultural and ethnic preferences should be taken into consideration, and individuals with diabetes should be included in the decision-making process.[17]

Current nutrition principles and recommendations focus on lifestyle goals and strategies for treatment of diabetes. For the first time, the 2002 evidence-based nutrition recommendations purposely address lifestyle approaches to diabetes prevention, because MNT for treating and managing diabetes may not necessarily be the same for preventing or delaying onset of diabetes.[17] Goals of NT that apply to all persons with diabetes are as follows[17]:

- Attain and maintain optimal metabolic outcomes.
  - Blood glucose levels in the normal (or near-normal) range
  - Lipid and lipoprotein profiles that reduce risk for macrovascular diseases
  - Blood pressure levels that reduce risk for vascular disease
- Prevent and treat chronic complications.
- Improve health through healthy food choices and physical activity.
- Address individual nutritional needs, taking into consideration personal and cultural preferences and lifestyle while respecting individuals' wishes and willingness to change.

Additional, more specific medical nutrition goals include the following[17]:

- *Youth with T1DM:* NT goals for children and adolescents with T1DM should ensure provision of sufficient energy for normal growth and development. Insulin regimens should be integrated into usual eating and physical activity habits.
- *T2DM in children and adolescents:* Goals for NT for children and adolescents with T2DM should facilitate changes in eating and physical activity habits to decrease insulin resistance and enhance metabolic status.
- *Pregnant and lactating women:* NT goals for pregnant and lactating women should provide adequate energy and nutrients necessary for optimal pregnancy outcomes.
- *Older adults:* Nutritional and psychosocial needs of an aging individual should be provided in NT goals.
- *Individuals treated with insulin or insulin secretagogues:* Self-management education for treatment and prevention of hypoglycemia, acute illness, and exercise-related blood glucose problems should be included in MNT goals for individuals treated with insulin or insulin secretagogues.
- *Individuals at risk for diabetes:* For those at risk for developing diabetes, physical activity should be encouraged and food choices that facilitate moderate weight loss (or at least prevent weight gain) should be promoted.

In addition, any medications a person has been prescribed should be considered as well; certain foods and drinks may

> **KEY TERM**
> **macrosomia** Unusually large size.

DIET-MEDICATIONS INTERACTIONS

Interactions with Diabetes Drugs

Drug Class	Drug Names	Interactions/Instructions
α-Glucosidase inhibitor agents	Acarbose: Precose Miglitol: Glyset	Take with first bite of main meal Limit alcohol
Biguanide agents	Metformin: Glucophage Metformin and glibenclamide: Glucovance, Glucophage, Glyburide	Take with meals to decrease GI distress May cause anorexia
DPP-4 inhibitors	Sitagliptin: Januvia Saxagliptin: Onglyza	Does not cause hypoglycemia when used as a single agent Increases insulin release after meals; lowers glucagon release
Insulin and related agents	Insulin mixtures, intermediate acting, long acting, rapid acting, short acting	May increase weight Should use alcohol with caution and under advice from physician (alcohol increases hypoglycemic effect of insulin) Large weight gain increases insulin needs
Meglitinide agents (nonsulfonylurea insulin releasers)	Nateglinide: Starlix Repaglinide: Prandin	Take 15-30 min before meals May increase weight Tooth disorders Nausea/vomiting Diarrhea/constipation Limit alcohol May increase risk of hypoglycemia in malnutrition
Sulfonylurea agents	Acetohexamide: Dymelor Tolazamide: Tolinase Tolbutamide: Orinase Chlorpropamide: Diabinese	Take with first meal of the day Nausea Avoid alcohol Increased risk of hypoglycemia in geriatric or malnourished patients
Sulfonylurea agents— second generation	Glimepiride: Amaryl Glyburide: DiaBeta, Micronase, Glynase PresTabs	Take 30 min before first meal of the day Hyperglycemia with high doses of nicotinic acid May increase or decrease appetite Increased weight Dyspepsia, nausea Constipation/diarrhea Avoid alcohol Possible hypoglycemia in geriatric or malnourished patients
Thiazolidinedione agents	Pioglitazone: Actos Rosiglitazone: Avandia	Take once a day without regard to food Increased weight
Pramlintide agent	Symlin	Used with insulin, an increased risk of insulin-induced severe hypoglycemia, particularly in patients with T1DM; seen usually within 3 hours of injection
Exenatide	Byetta	Hypoglycemia can occur when combined with sulfonylureas, or Byetta combined with metformin and a sulfonylurea

GI, gastrointestinal; T1DM, type 1 diabetes.

Bibliography

American Diabetes Association: *Living with diabetes: what are my options?* Alexandria, Va., 2010, American Diabetes Association. from: <http://www.diabetes.org/living-with-diabetes/treatment-and-care/medication/oral-medications/what-are-my-options.html>. Retrieved July 13, 2010.

Drugs A-Z: *Rancho*, Santa Fe, Calif., 2005, RxList. from: <www.rxlist.com>. Retrieved May 24, 2009.

Pronsky ZM: *Food medication interactions*, ed 16, Birchrunville, Pa., 2010, Food-Medication Interactions.

interfere with them (see the Diet-Medications Interactions box, "Interactions with Diabetes Drugs").

ISSUES RELATED TO MEDICAL THERAPY

Blood Glucose Control

Insulin Therapy

The management goal for persons with T1DM is to maintain a normal blood glucose level as closely as possible. Strong evidence from the DCCT, as well as accumulating practice experience, indicates that maintaining such a "normoglycemic" state helps prevent the chronic complications of long-term uncontrolled hyperglycemia.[29] To achieve this goal, more intensive insulin therapy with the different types of insulin now available is being used. Insulin is increasingly being used as adjunctive therapy in T2DM.

Types of Insulin. A number of insulin preparations are available for therapeutic use, and new ones are constantly being developed to meet medical care needs for individual patients and market changes. Individual responses to insulin types is highly variable. According to time of action, they are as follows:

1. *Rapid-acting insulins:* These insulins have various names (e.g., Humulin R, Semilente, Velosulin R), depending on the manufacturer. Rapid-acting insulins have their onset of action within approximately ½ hour after injection and stay in the body for less than 5 hours. This type of insulin peaks about 2 hours after injection. Human insulin analog, Humalog (generic name, insulin lispro), has the shortest time-action curve of any insulin currently available. Short-acting insulins have their onset of action in ½ to 1 hour and have a 6- to 8-hour duration. Short-acting insulins peak around 3 hours. A number of variables influence absorption rate, such as site of injection, physical activity, skin temperature, and any circulating antiinsulin antibodies. The effect on blood glucose can be detected in about 1 hour, peaks at 4 to 6 hours, and lasts about 12 to 16 hours.

2. *Intermediate-acting insulins:* These insulins include Humulin L, Lente, NPH, Insulatard N, and Insulatard. Effect is detected in about 2 hours, peaks at about 11 hours, and lasts about 20 to 29 hours.

3. *Long-acting insulins:* These insulins include Humulin U. Its duration is somewhat longer than that of intermediate-acting insulins. It can be difficult to use because basal insulin is difficult to predict or control when the insulin peaks. Insulin glargine rDNA, which was first released in 2001, is a recombinant deoxyribonucleic acid (rDNA) insulin analog specifically formulated to provide a long, flat response. However, insulin glargine rDNA (trade name, Lantus) cannot be mixed with other insulins, and two injections are needed to combine the action with a short-acting insulin. It is a long-acting insulin that works slowly over 24 hours and may not be used in combination with another type of insulin or an oral hypoglycemic medication to keep blood glucose regulated. Treatment algorithms are developed to adjust insulin on the basis of lifestyle and SMBG.

The process of intensifying T1DM management occurs in several stages. The initial dose of insulin is usually calculated based on current body weight with 0.5 to 0.6 units of insulin/kg/day, with approximately half being for basal needs and half being as boluses for meals. During this initial phase a consistent carbohydrate intake is needed to identify a blood glucose pattern. Next, the client can move on to more complex planning using monitoring results to achieve better glycemic control and a more flexible lifestyle. Bolus requirement varies widely, but the initial dose is often estimated to provide 1 unit of short-acting insulin per 15 g of carbohydrate. Gradually the client learns to adjust insulin for changes in food or activity using a ratio of carbohydrate intake to insulin dose. A similar approach is used for insulin therapy in other forms of diabetes. In the treatment of T2DM, insulin may be used alone or in conjunction with an oral agent.

Insulin and Exercise Balance. Exercise benefits all persons with diabetes through its action in increasing the

TABLE 22-3	MEAL-PLANNING GUIDE FOR ACTIVE PEOPLE WITH TYPE 1 DIABETES MELLITUS
EXCHANGE NEEDS	**SAMPLE MENUS**
Moderate Activity	
30 Minutes	
1 bread *or*	1 bran muffin *or*
1 fruit	1 small orange
1 Hour	
2 bread + 1 meat *or*	Tuna sandwich *or*
2 fruit + 1 milk	½ cup fruit salad + 1 cup milk
Strenuous Activity	
30 Minutes	
2 fruit *or*	1 small banana *or*
1 bread + 1 fat	½ bagel + 1 tsp cream cheese
1 Hour	
2 bread + 1 meat + 1 milk *or*	Meat and cheese sandwich + 1 cup milk *or*
2 bread + 2 meat + 2 fruit	Hamburger + 1 cup orange juice

number of insulin receptors on muscle cells, thus increasing insulin efficiency. However, physical activity must be regular to be effective. A detailed history of personal activity and exercise habits provides information that is needed to help a client plan a wise program of regular moderate exercise. Guidelines for extra food to cover periods of heavier exercise, athletic practice, or competition can be included (Table 22-3).

Insulin Delivery Systems. Intensive insulin therapy for maintaining more normal blood glucose control requires multiple injections of rapid-acting insulin, alone or in combination with basal intermediate-acting insulin. This is accomplished either by regular injection with disposal syringes or with an insulin pump. The pump is not for everyone, but for many, using an insulin pump to achieve a basal insulin infusion and bolus insulin for meals has made life easier. It is a small device that is easily worn on the belt with a subcutaneous needle in the abdomen and buttons the wearer pushes to obtain a fixed programmed flow of insulin in balance with food intake. Frequent monitoring is needed to adjust insulin dose with either multiple injections or the insulin pump.

Oral Antidiabetic Drugs

Five classes of oral antidiabetic drugs are used to treat hyperglycemia in T2DM: (1) sulfonylurea, (2) biguanide, (3) thiazolidinedione, (4) meglitinide, and (5) α-glucosidase inhibitor. When lifestyle changes alone cannot normalize metabolism, MNT should help optimize metabolic control and reduce potential medication side effects. Table 22-4

TABLE 22-4	**MEDICATIONS USED TO TREAT DIABETES**				
DRUG CLASS	**DRUG NAMES**	**ACTION**	**TARGET ORGANS**	**SIDE EFFECTS**	**HOW TAKEN**
α-Glucosidase inhibitor agents	Acarbose: Precose Miglitol: Glyset	Delays absorption of glucose from GI tract	Small intestine	Excess flatulence, diarrhea (particularly after high-carbohydrate meal), abdominal pain; may interfere with iron absorption	Must be taken with meals three times/day
Biguanide agents	Metformin: Glucophage	Decreases hepatic glucose production and intestinal glucose absorption; improves insulin sensitivity	Liver, small intestine, and peripheral tissues	Less likely to gain weight; may lose weight; anorexia, nausea, diarrhea, metallic taste; may reduce absorption of vitamin B_{12} and folic acid; rarely suitable for adults <80 yr	Take with first main meal
Insulin and related agents	Insulin mixtures: Humulin 50/50, Humulin 70/30, Novolin 70/30	Exogenous insulin preparations	Cells	Hypoglycemia, fatigue, hunger, nausea, muscular weakness or trembling, headache, sweating, blurred vision, fainting, weight gain, skin irritation	Subcutaneous injection
	Intermediate acting: Humulin L, Humulin N, Iletin II Lente, Iletin II NPH, Novolin L, Novolin N	Exogenous insulin preparations		Hypoglycemia, fatigue, hunger, nausea, muscular weakness or trembling, headache, sweating, blurred vision, fainting, weight gain, skin irritation	Subcutaneous injection
	Long acting: Humulin U, Lantus (insulin glargine)	Exogenous insulin preparations		Hypoglycemia, fatigue, hunger, nausea, muscular weakness or trembling, headache, sweating, blurred vision, fainting, weight gain, skin irritation	Subcutaneous injection
	Rapid acting: Humalog, insulin lispro, insulin aspart	Exogenous insulin preparations		Hypoglycemia, fatigue, hunger, nausea, muscular weakness or trembling, headache, sweating, blurred vision, fainting, weight gain, skin irritation	Subcutaneous injection, intramuscular or intravenous in special situations
	Short acting: Humulin R, Iletin II Regular, Novolin R, Novolin BR	Exogenous insulin preparations		Hypoglycemia, fatigue, hunger, nausea, muscular weakness or trembling, headache, sweating, blurred vision, fainting, weight gain, skin irritation	Subcutaneous injection, intramuscular or intravenous in special situations
Meglitinide agents (nonsulfonylurea insulin releasers)	Nateglinide: Starlix Repaglinide: Prandin	Stimulates secretion of insulin	Pancreatic beta cells	Hypoglycemia and weight gain; repaglinide (Prandin) has a slightly increased risk for cardiac events	Take with meals

Continued

DRUG CLASS	DRUG NAMES	ACTION	TARGET ORGANS	SIDE EFFECTS	HOW TAKEN
Sulfonylurea agents—first generation	Acetohexamide: Dymelor Tolazamide: Tolinase Tolbutamide: Orinase Chlorpropamide: Diabinese	Stimulates secretion of insulin	Pancreatic beta cells	Hypoglycemia and weight gain; tolbutamide may be associated with cardiovascular complications; chlorpropamide (Diabinese) can cause hyponatremia and should not be used by women who are pregnant, who are nursing, or those individuals allergic to sulfa drugs; sulfonylurea interacts with many other drugs (prescription, OTC, and alternative); Diabinese: avoid alcohol	Take before or with meals
Sulfonylurea agents—second generation	Glimepiride: Amaryl Glyburide: DiaBeta, Micronase, Glynase PresTabs				
Thiazolidinedione agents	Pioglitazone: Actos Rosiglitazone: Avandia	Improves insulin sensitivity	Activates genes involved with fat synthesis and carbohydrate metabolism	Possible liver damage, weight gain, mild anemia	Once or twice daily

Data from Nelms MN, Sucher K, Lacey L, Long S: *Nutrition therapy and pathophysiology,* ed 2, Belmont, Calif., 2010, Thomson Cengage; Mahan LK, Escott-Stump S, editors: *Krause's food & nutrition therapy,* ed 12, St Louis, 2008, Saunders.
GI, Gastrointestinal; *OTC,* over the counter.

provides a brief review of insulin and oral antidiabetic drugs (see the Complementary and Alternative Medicine [CAM] box, "Herbs and Supplements Commonly Used in Diabetes Mellitus").

Insulin is often used in T2DM as adjunctive therapy when oral agents are not achieving glycemic control. A nighttime dose of insulin is commonly used to help reduce fasting glucose levels, especially if fasting levels are 13.9 mmol/L (250 mg/dL) or higher. Insulin therapy is also commonly used as adjunctive therapy when glycemic control is not achieved with oral agent monotherapy or combination therapy.

Adjunctive Therapies

Two new injectable drugs have been approved by the U.S. Food and Drug Administration (FDA). Exenatide (Byetta) is first in its class of drugs for treatment of T2DM for patients taking metformin, a sulfonylurea, or a combination of metformin and a sulfonylurea. This class of drugs is referred to as *incretin mimetics.* Isolated from the saliva of Gila monsters, exenatide works to lower blood glucose levels by increasing insulin secretion. It only has this effect in the presence of

elevated blood glucose levels; therefore it does not tend to increase risk of hypoglycemia on its own.

Pramlintide (Symlin) is a synthetic form of the hormone amylin. Amylin and insulin are produced by the beta cells in the pancreas. Amylin, insulin, and glucagon work together to maintain normal blood glucose levels. Pramlintide injections taken with meals modestly improve HbA$_{1c}$ levels by slowing gastric emptying rate without altering overall absorption of nutrients. In addition, pramlintide suppresses glucagon secretion from the liver and regulates food intake because of centrally mediated modulation of appetite.

Testing Methods for Monitoring Results

Frequent testing of blood glucose levels is necessary for successful **tight control** of T1DM and to reduce risk of complications.

KEY TERM

tight control   Keeping blood glucose levels as close to normal as possible.

COMPLEMENTARY AND ALTERNATIVE MEDICINE (CAM)

Herbs and Supplements Commonly Used in Diabetes Mellitus

Herb/ Supplement	Common Uses	Efficacy	Safety	Drug-Herb Interactions	Interaction
Chromium	Glycemic control	Improved glycemic control	No adverse effects reported	Hyperglycemic agents and any other agent used for glycemic control	Possible risk of hypoglycemia
Cinnamon (*Cinnamomum verum*)	Glycemic control	Increases use of endogenous insulin	Large amounts increase heart rate and intestinal motility, followed by sleepiness and depression As a spice, long-term use safe	None known	
Ginseng (*Panax ginseng*)	Glycemic control	Improved glycemic control	Possible overstimulation and insomnia	Hyperglycemic agents and any other agent used for glycemic control	Possible risk of hypoglycemia
				May enhance effect of stimulants, antibiotics, MAOIs	Estrogenic effects of ginseng may cause vaginal bleeding and breast nodules
				Antagonism of warfarin; might falsely elevate digoxin levels	
				Increases alcohol clearance; might decrease diuretic effect of furosemide	
				Might potentiate effects of hormones and anabolic steroid therapies	
Evening primrose oil (*Oenothera biennis*)	Peripheral neuropathy	May be helpful	No adverse effects reported	Phenothiazines	Might increase risk of seizures
Lipoic acid	Neuropathy	Slight evidence intravenous lipoic acid can reduce symptoms of peripheral neuropathy in the short term Evidence for oral lipoic acid inadequate	No adverse reactions documented	Some concern that lipoic acid potentiates the effects of insulin, but this has not been documented in formal studies	None noted
Vanadium	Glycemic control	May improve glycemic control	Usually well tolerated, but GI disturbances can occur Studies suggest excess is toxic (hepatotoxicity, nephrotoxicity, teratogenicity, and developmental/reproductive toxicity)	Might cause hypoglycemia if used in conjunction with an effective antidiabetic regimen	None noted

GI, Gastrointestinal; *MAOIs,* monoamine oxidase inhibitors.

Bibliography

Bratman S, Girman AM: *Mosby's handbook of herbs and supplements and their therapeutic uses,* St Louis, 2003, Mosby.

Contributors and Consultants: *Professional guide to complementary and alternative therapies,* Springhouse, Pa., 2001, Springhouse.

Kuhn MA, Winston D: *Herbal therapy and supplements: a scientific and traditional approach,* Philadelphia, 2001, Lippincott Williams & Wilkins.

Self-Monitoring of Blood Glucose. For insulin doses to be administered in sufficient time intervals and amounts to maintain normal blood glucose, close monitoring of immediate blood glucose levels is mandatory. Small, lightweight, easy-to-use, hand-sized meters, easily carried in pockets and handbags, are available for convenient use. A reagent test strip is inserted into the blood glucose meter, a drop of capillary blood from the finger obtained with an automatic lancer is placed on the reagent test strip, and a digital reading of the blood glucose level appears on the meter. The frequency of monitoring varies according to need for control and goal of care. More frequent self-monitoring is indicated for unstable forms of diabetes, persons using insulin pumps, and those who want close control and freedom of movement. Usually two to eight before- and after-meal tests are performed daily. During pregnancy, postprandial monitoring is performed at 1 hour after meals. Glucose goals are lower during pregnancy because of the dilution effect of having increased blood volume.

Glycated Hemoglobin. The most common glycated hemoglobin (Hb) test is the HbA$_{1c}$. Glycated Hb molecules are relatively stable within the red blood cell. During the 120-day life of the red blood cell, glucose molecules attach themselves to Hb. This irreversible glycosylation of Hb depends on the concentration of blood glucose. The glycosylation of proteins in various body systems appears to play a role in the development of diabetic complications. The greater the level of circulating glucose is during the life of the red blood cells, the greater is the concentration of glycohemoglobin. Thus measurement of HbA$_{1c}$ relates to the level of blood glucose during a longer period. It provides an effective tool for evaluating the long-term management of diabetes and degree of control.[11] Because glucose attaches to Hb during the life of the red blood cell, the test gives an accumulated history of glucose levels across time, providing an effective management tool for evaluating progress and making decisions about treatment changes. Obtaining an HbA$_{1c}$ level every 6 to 8 weeks can be used to monitor the overall glucose control.

Physical Activity Habits

In counseling clients with diabetes, a detailed history of personal activity and physical exercise habits should be discussed. This information is then used as a basis for planning a wise program of regular moderate exercise. Guidelines for extra food to cover periods of heavier exercise or athletic practice and competition are included (see Table 22-3). Self-monitoring is a regular procedure now used by most persons with T1DM and T2DM. It is a helpful means of determining the balance needed at any point in time between exercise, insulin, and food.

Gestational Diabetes

Occasionally the stress of pregnancy may bring about GDM, which is a form of glucose intolerance that has onset during pregnancy and is resolved on parturition.[30] Risk of fetal abnormalities and mortality are increased in the presence of hyperglycemia; therefore every effort should be made to control blood glucose levels. All women with GDM should receive nutrition counseling by a RD when possible.[28]

Changes that take place during pregnancy greatly affect insulin use. Some hormones and enzymes produced by the placenta are antagonistic to insulin, thus reducing its effectiveness. Maternal insulin does not cross the placenta, but glucose does, causing the fetal pancreas to increase insulin production if maternal blood glucose levels get too high. Increased production of insulin causes the most predictable characteristic of infants born to women with diabetes, macrosomia, in addition to other problems such as respiratory difficulties, hypocalcemia, hypoglycemia, hypokalemia, and jaundice.[27]

Individualization of NT based on maternal weight and height is recommended.[28] MNT should include the provision of adequate kcalories and nutrients to meet pregnancy needs and should be consistent with accepted maternal blood glucose goals.[28] SMBG provides important information about the effect of food on blood glucose levels. At the beginning of the pregnancy, minimal daily SMBG should be planned four times a day (fasting, and 1 or 2 hours after each meal). Blood glucose goals during pregnancy are fasting, less than 105 mg/dL; 1-hour postprandial, 155 mg/dL; and 2-hour postprandial, less than 130 mg/dL.[28] The frequency of SMBG may be decreased once blood glucose control is established. However, some monitoring should continue throughout pregnancy.

Recommended weight gains and nutrient requirements are the same as for established pregnancy guidelines, as follows[27]:

- Underweight (body mass index [BMI] less than 18.5): 28 to 40 lb
- Normal/healthy weight (BMI 18.5 to 24.9): 25 to 35 lb
- Overweight (BMI 25 to 29.9): 15 to 25 lb
- Obesity (class 1) (BMI 30 to 34.9): less than 15 lb
- Obesity (class 2) (BMI 35 to 39.9): not available
- Obesity (class 3) (BMI greater than 40): not available

No kcalorie modifications are needed for the first trimester.[17] During the second and third trimesters, increased energy intake of approximately 180 kcal/day is suggested.[27] High-quality protein should be increased by 25 g/day. As with any pregnancy, 600 mcg/day of folic acid is recommended for prevention of neural tube defects (NTDs) and other congenital abnormalities.[27] Alcohol consumption is not recommended in any amount.

Kcaloric restriction must be considered with care. A minimum of 1700 to 1800 kcal/day of carefully selected foods has been shown to prevent ketosis. Intakes less than this level are not advised.[28] Weight gain goals are established using prepregnancy BMI. Weight gain should still occur even if patients have gained substantial weight before the onset of GDM. Each patient with GDM should be evaluated individually by an RD, their care plans should be fine-tuned, and patient education should be provided as required to realize weight goals.

Impaired Fasting Glucose and Impaired Glucose Tolerance

The terms *IFG* and *IGT* refer to a metabolic stage somewhere between normal glucose homeostasis and overt diabetes. Although not clinical entities in their own right, these conditions are risk factors for future diabetes and CVD.[2,11] Lifestyle interventions should be consistent with current guidelines for overweight and obesity and address cardiovascular risk factors and common concomitant conditions. The Da Qing IGT and Diabetes Study provided preliminary evidence that diet and exercise intervention can lower the conversion to overt diabetes during the 6-year period.[14] The Finnish Diabetes Prevention Study demonstrated that a lifestyle change program could reduce the risk for developing T2DM by 58% during a 3-year period.[13] In the United States, the Diabetes Prevention Program (DPP) has confirmed the findings of the Finnish trial in a highly diverse American population with IGT. The DPP addressed how an intensive diet and exercise intervention compares with metformin in a three-arm randomized clinical trial that uses placebo as the third arm.

MANAGEMENT OF DIABETES NUTRITION THERAPY

Counseling Process in Nutrition Therapy for Diabetes

NT for diabetes is highly individualized. The American Diabetes Association recommendations clearly state that no single diabetic or American Diabetes Association diet exists. Today the recommended diet is a dietary prescription based on individual nutrition assessment and treatment goals.[19] This model emphasizes actions of the diabetes team clinical dietitian in an individualized, integrated four-point approach: (1) assessment, (2) goal setting, (3) nutrition intervention, and (4) evaluation, as follows[31]:

1. *Assessment:* The first step involves a comprehensive assessment of the client's background. It includes clinical information, medical and lifestyle data such as personal SMBG, and dietary history. Interview follow-up tools such as questionnaires and food records assess general food patterns and nutrient intake.
2. *Nutrition diagnosis:* The second step identifies and labels problems the client may have.
3. *Nutrition intervention:* The third step guides the client in selecting and using the most appropriate meal-planning guide from the number that are now available, based on individual needs for knowledge and skills to change or maintain eating habits and daily living practices.
4. *Monitoring and evaluation:* Together the client and dietitian evaluate goals and nutrition intervention, as well as ongoing clinical data, to help the client succeed at the established individual program. They then make any desired adjustments, and the dietitian provides continuing counseling and education as needed.

Diabetes Meal-Planning Tools

Since the DCCT, growing emphasis has been placed on selecting a planning approach that meets the needs of each client from a wide array of meal-planning guides. Regardless of the diabetes NT management tool, the first vital principle in working with persons who have diabetes is to begin where they are physically, mentally, and emotionally. Any food-planning process must focus first on the unique individual rather than on the case or disease. Numerous planning approaches are used by skilled and sensitive clinical dietitians who tailor their actions to the person's learning needs and abilities, as well as his or her nutritional needs, personal needs, and lifestyle issues. The use of the exchange lists as a dietary management tool is widespread; they are outlined on the Evolve website.

Carbohydrate Counting

Carbohydrate counting is one of the most commonly used methods of meal planning. Research shows carbohydrate is the primary nutrient affecting postprandial blood glucose level and consequently insulin requirements.[21,22] Carbohydrate quantity and distribution can affect metabolic control.[22] Carbohydrate counting can help people with diabetes become more aware of carbohydrate content of the foods they eat and consistency of food consumption at meals and when snacking.[19]

At an advanced level, carbohydrate counting is a tool that allows the person with diabetes to focus on adjustment of foods, medication, and activity based on patterns from daily food intake records and blood glucose records.[19] To use carbohydrate counting effectively, the dietetic professional and person with diabetes must have a good understanding of intensive insulin therapy.[22]

Carbohydrate content can be measured in grams of carbohydrate or servings: one carbohydrate serving equals 15 g carbohydrate. Most people find it easier to count the number of carbohydrate servings consumed rather than keeping track of grams of carbohydrate consumed.[22] Box 22-1 provides a brief outline of carbohydrate content of foods to equal one serving of carbohydrate.

Planning for Special Needs

Sick Days. When general illness occurs, food and insulin amounts must be adjusted accordingly. Texture may be modified as needed to use easily digested and absorbed liquid foods while still maintaining as many as possible glucose equivalents of the usual food plan.

Physical Activity. For any strenuous physical activity, the client with T1DM must make special advanced plans. This is particularly true of a young person with diabetes who is engaging in athletic practice or competition. Energy demands of exercise are discussed in Chapter 14.

Travel. When a trip is planned, the clinical dietitian must confer with the client to guide food choices according to what will be available. SMBG levels, insulin therapy equipment, and making food plans are just as important on a trip as they are at home. The traveler always needs to plan ahead with the health care team (see the Perspectives in Practice box, "Travel and Illness: 'Real-Life' Situations").

Dining Out. Provide similar guidelines and suggestions for various situations when the client eats meals away from home. As a general rule, the plan must be made ahead of time; therefore accommodations for what is eaten at home before and after the restaurant meal will reflect the continuing balance needs of the day. Have the client get the menu ahead of time. Many restaurants are willing to fax their menus, or they may be available on websites.

Stress. Any form of emotional stress is reflected in variations of diabetes control.[22] These variations are caused by hormonal responses that act as antagonists to insulin. The clinical dietitian must help the client learn and practice a variety of useful stress reduction activities.

DIABETES EDUCATION PROGRAM

Goal: Person-Centered Self-Care

In past years the traditional medical model has guided diabetes education in its methods, language, and the respective roles assumed. Professionals have viewed themselves as having major authoritative roles and have assigned to the person with diabetes the more passive role of patient. With notable exceptions in certain places, this model has been followed in most cases. However, with the increasing movement toward changing roles of practitioners and consumers in the health care system, persons with diabetes are assuming a more active voice in planning and conducting their own care. Several barriers in our traditional system stem from three sources: (1) our culture, (2) our health care delivery system, and (3) our professional training habits. Essentially, much of the core problem focuses on communication. For example, a list of words we use too commonly that may be objectionable to persons with diabetes, along with the preferred language, include the following:

- Diabetic used as a noun: The word *diabetic* is an adjective and should not be used alone as a noun. Instead, use the phrase *person with diabetes*.
- Compliance: The word *compliance* raises red flags in minds of persons with diabetes. It is a purely medical term and connotes an authoritative physician position. Instead, the word *adherence* should be used, which has been adopted by national committees and associations working in the field of diabetes. The word *adherence* indicates placement of more decision-making responsibility on the person with diabetes to determine courses of action in varying situations, which is, of course, the necessity.
- Patient: Instead of *patient*, the phrase *person with diabetes* should be used. Persons with diabetes are patients only when they are in the hospital or seeing a physician for an illness.
- Cheating: A particularly abusive word in the minds of many persons with diabetes, especially parents of children and young people with diabetes, is the word *cheating*, because it suggests dishonesty or failure to live up to an external code. By and large, persons with diabetes do not cheat. They may kid themselves, or they may be inaccurate in their reporting, but they do not cheat. Instead phrases such as *having difficulty* or *having a problem with* should be used.

Contents: Tools for Self-Care

A plan for diabetes education must recognize the need for building self-sufficiency and responsibility within persons with diabetes and their families. It should provide practical guidelines that build on necessary skills that a person with diabetes must have for the best possible control, as well as additional surrounding factors related to life situations and

PERSPECTIVES IN PRACTICE

Travel and Illness: "Real-Life" Situations

People do not stop living their lives just because they have diabetes. They still travel, and they still catch colds, influenza, and other common illnesses. Special considerations to all areas of diabetes management will enhance safe traveling, as well as the traveler's health. What kind of information does the person with diabetes need to know when traveling or if he or she becomes too ill to eat? The following are a few helpful hints you may want to offer clients for these situations.

Traveling Safely with Diabetes
General Tips

1. Ensure that you have sufficient medication (insulin or oral glucose-lowering medication) for the entire trip.
2. Carry some form of medical identification that includes the type of diabetes you have, name, address, telephone number, emergency contact information, medications taken, physician's name and phone number, and additional relevant medical conditions. Preferably, this information should be worn on a necklace or bracelet (rather than carrying it in a wallet or purse).
3. Take extra snacks such as cereal bars, vanilla wafers, peanut butter crackers, or glucose tablets or gel.
4. Always keep insulin cool, especially when vacationing in warm climates.
5. Keep some money available for food purchases if necessary. Change for vending machines may not always be available.
6. Always carry blood glucose monitoring equipment. Blood glucose levels should be checked before beginning a trip, as well as every 2 hours. An extra check should be done whenever symptoms of hypoglycemia occur, even if recent blood glucose checks were acceptable.
7. Walking around and stretching every 2 to 4 hours helps stimulate circulation.
8. Whenever possible, travel with a companion.
9. Wear comfortable shoes.
10. Plan for time zone changes. Meal schedules may need to be revised to balance with insulin activity pattern.
11. If traveling abroad, learn to say the following in the local language: "I have diabetes. Please give me something sweet to drink."
12. If travel is frequent, contact a registered dietitian (RD) or diabetes educator for ideas for healthful, portable meals and snacks.

Driving Tips

1. If diabetes medications have the potential to cause hypoglycemia, medications and meals will need to be scheduled during a long trip.
2. If diabetes medications have the potential to cause hypoglycemia, food should be eaten before leaving home or snacks should be taken in the automobile. Traffic may not be conducive to stopping at a favorite store or restaurant for a quick meal or snack.
3. Keep nonperishable, carbohydrate-containing foods in the automobile in case flat tires, traffic jams, or breakdowns occur. Handy, premeasured carbohydrate amounts may be beneficial to avoid overeating or undereating. Replenish the food supply as needed to avoid running out at inopportune times.
4. Always carry blood glucose monitoring equipment when driving. Blood glucose levels should be checked before the trip begins, as well as every 2 hours while driving. An extra check should be done if symptoms of hypoglycemia occur (even if recent blood glucose checks have been acceptable).
5. An extra glucose meter should not be kept in an automobile. Internal automobile temperatures can get very hot and very cold. Strips and meters exposed to extreme temperatures may not be accurate or function properly.
6. High blood glucose levels may cause the following symptoms that can affect driving:
   - Fatigue related to the body's inability to use glucose for energy
   - Increased urination, causing preoccupation, repeated stops, and a delay in arriving at destination
   - Blurry vision, which may impair ability to see road signs clearly; blurry vision may be especially problematic at night or while driving in rain or snow
   - Numbness or tingling in hands or feet, which may impair ability to steer, accelerate, and stop the vehicle
7. Prompt attention to hypoglycemia and treatment is necessary to prevent mental confusion and even losing consciousness. When blood glucose is low, the first organ affected is the brain. Keep appropriate sources of carbohydrates available in the automobile.
8. If driving hours at a time, it is important to stop the automobile, get out and stretch, and walk around every 2 to 4 hours.
9. Wear medical identification. Law enforcement officers may not be familiar with diabetes or symptoms of hypoglycemia or hyperglycemia. They can mistake impaired awareness and judgment for drunkenness.
10. Whenever possible, drive with a friend.
11. If driving for several hours, set an alarm as a reminder for blood glucose checks, meals, and even times to stretch and walk.
12. Visual disturbances can occur with either hyperglycemia or hypoglycemia.
13. If driving long distances, take twice as many diabetes supplies as thought to be needed. Be aware of all medicines taken (prescription and over-the-counter [OTC] medications).
14. Always carry money for toll booths, parking fees, and telephone calls. Consider keeping a cell phone to call for assistance.

Flying Tips

1. Call ahead to airlines to advise them that you have diabetes and supplies you may need.
2. Carry a copy of your physician's prescription for insulin and other medications.
3. Carry a letter from the physician explaining the need to carry syringes/injection devices and insulin.
4. If problems are encountered, request to speak to a manager or supervisor.

Continued

PERSPECTIVES IN PRACTICE

Travel and Illness: "Real-Life" Situations—cont'd

5. Carry insulin onto the aircraft. Insulin should not be packed in luggage that will be stored in the hold of an airplane. Low temperatures can damage the insulin.
6. Notify the Transportation Security Administration (TSA) representative that you have diabetes and are carrying your supplies with you. The following are allowed through the checkpoint once screened:
   - Insulin and insulin-loaded dispensing products clearly marked and labeled
   - Unlimited number of unused syringes when accompanied by insulin or other injectable medication
   - Lancets, blood glucose meters, blood glucose meter test strips, alcohol swabs, meter-testing solutions
   - Insulin pump and supplies
   - Glucagon emergency kit clearly identified and labeled
   - Urine ketone test strips
   - Unlimited number of used syringes when transported in sharps disposal container or other similar hard-surfaced container

Sick Day Survival

1. Keep taking diabetes medications even if solid foods cannot be eaten.
2. For insulin users the physician may prescribe extra doses or increased amounts of insulin during an illness.
3. Blood glucose should be tested and recorded every 4 hours.
4. Test for ketones in urine if blood glucose level stays at or greater than 240 mg/dL for at least 4 hours.
5. Try to use regular meal plan and diet, but if that is not possible, soft foods or liquids can be consumed to take the place of carbohydrates usually eaten. Some easily digested foods to replace one serving (15 g) of carbohydrate include the following:
   - ⅓ to ½ cup fruit juice
   - ½ cup regular soft drink
   - ½ cup regular gelatin
   - ½ cup hot cereal
   - ½ cup vanilla ice cream
   - 1 cup broth-based soup
6. To prevent dehydration, sip 3 to 6 oz of noncaffeinated, sugar-free beverages or water every hour. Sugar-free fluids may be alternated with liquids containing sugar to help control blood glucose levels.
7. Keep a thermometer on hand to determine body temperature.
8. When buying OTC medicines, choose one that is sugar free. In addition to the word *sugar* on labels, *dextrose, fructose, lactose, sorbitol, mannitol, xylitol,* and *honey* indicate that a product contains sugar.
9. OTC cold medications containing epinephrine-like compounds (including ephedrine, pseudoephedrine, phenylpropanolamine, phenylephrine, and epinephrine) can raise blood glucose levels and should only be used with a physician's approval.
10. *Planning ahead:* Keep the following items on hand in case of colds, influenza, or other kinds of illnesses:
    - Thermometer
    - Urine test strips for ketones (check expiration date periodically)
    - Approved OTC cold and influenza medicines
    - Syringes or prescription for them (if insulin is not usually taken but is part of a sick day plan)
    - Short-acting insulin (keep refrigerated)
    - Extra prescriptions for all medications usually taken (or have on file at pharmacy)
    - Nonperishable foods such as noncaffeinated soft drinks (regular and diet), regular gelatin, Popsicles, sport drinks, saltines, and canned fruit juices
11. Call the physician if any of the following occurs:
    - Vomiting for several hours
    - Diarrhea recurring within 6 hours
    - Difficulty breathing
    - Blood glucose levels greater than 240 mg/dL for 24 hours if using oral medications; blood glucose levels greater than 240 mg/dL for two consecutive tests (4 hours apart) after taking supplemental insulin
    - Blood glucose levels less than 60 mg/dL
    - Moderate to large amounts of ketones in urine and no improvement after at least 12 hours
    - Signs of dehydration such as dry skin or mouth, sunken eyes, or weight loss
    - Sickness that continues from 12 to 48 hours without improvement
    - Increased fatigue
    - Stomach or chest pain
    - Temperature that stays at higher than 101° F
    - Acute loss of vision
12. When calling your physician, he or she will want to know your blood glucose levels and urine ketone levels, how long the illness has lasted, what medicines have been taken, temperature, how much you have had to eat or drink, and other symptoms that have been experienced.
13. If it is necessary to go to the emergency department, the staff should be informed that you have diabetes.

In summary, in all cases the client must be advised to (1) maintain a steady intake of food every day, (2) replace the carbohydrate value of solid foods with that of liquid or soft foods as needed, (3) monitor blood and urine frequently for sugar and ketone levels, and (4) contact the physician if the illness lasts more than a day or so.

Bibliography

American Diabetes Association: *Traveling with diabetes supplies,* Alexandria, Va., 2006, American Diabetes Association. from: <www.diabetes.org/advocacy-and-legalresources/discrimination/public_accommodation/travel.jsp>. Retrieved May 23, 2009.

Diabetes Mall: FAA regulations for diabetes supplies. *Diabetes News* 2001. from: <www.diabetesnet.com/news/news100701.php>. Retrieved May 23, 2009.

National Diabetes Information Clearinghouse: *What I need to know about eating and diabetes,* Bethesda, Md., 2003, National Institute of Diabetes and Digestive and Kidney Diseases, National Institutes of Health. NIH Pub No 03-5043.

CASE STUDY
The Woman with Type 2 Diabetes Mellitus

Angela is a 35-year-old woman diagnosed 2 years ago with type 2 diabetes mellitus (T2DM). She has three children whose birth weights were in the range of 4.5 to 5 kg (10 to 11 lb). The children, now teenagers, show no signs of diabetes, and their weights are reported to be within normal limits despite their mother's fondness for cooking. Her husband, an underpaid construction worker, is slightly overweight.

Approximately 6 months ago, Angela was seen with a complaint of a series of infections that lasted longer than usual during the past 2 months. At that time she was measured as 165 cm (5 feet 5 inches) and 71 kg (156 lb). Her glucose tolerance test was positive. She was seen for follow-up twice during the next month, each time showing hyperglycemia and glycosuria. At the second follow-up, an oral antidiabetic medication was prescribed, and she was referred for medical nutrition therapy (MNT).

Angela did not keep this appointment or her subsequent medical appointment. She was not seen again until 1 month ago, when she arrived at the emergency department with ketoacidosis. She responded well to treatment and was placed on a 1200-kcal diet and a mixture of intermediate- and rapid-acting insulin given in two injections a day. Her discharge plan included a referral for a MNT consultation session and diabetes education classes.

Questions for Analysis
1. What factors do you think contributed to the ketoacidosis?
2. What relation do these factors have to diabetes control?
3. Why did Angela first appear to have T2DM?
4. Assume that Angela administers insulin before breakfast and before the evening meal. What additional information is necessary to develop an individualized meal plan?
5. Identify any personal factors that may affect Angela's adherence to her treatment plan. Do you anticipate any problems?
6. If so, then how would you attempt to help her solve them?
7. Outline a diabetes education plan for Angela.

psychosocial needs. Content areas include needs in relation to the nature of diabetes, nutrition and basic meal planning, insulin (or oral medication) effects and how to regulate them, monitoring of blood glucose, how to deal with illness, and, if relevant, urine ketones (see the Case Study box, "The Woman with Type 2 Diabetes Mellitus").

Educational Materials: Person-Centered Standards

A broad, confusing array of diabetes education materials are available. Some are excellent, and some should be discarded. Whatever is used should measure up to several basic person-centered requirements by doing the following:
- Give the intended receiver credit for having some intelligence and wanting new information.
- Inform persons fully and completely, giving both sides when experts disagree (as they surely do on occasion).
- Appeal to various levels of audience, ranging from basic to sophisticated.
- Never be patronizing, dehumanizing, or childish.

HEALTH PROMOTION
Nutrition Questions from Persons with Diabetes

Persons with diabetes have many questions about their diets, especially when they are newly diagnosed and anxieties are high. They do not want just a yes-or-no answer. For any diet item of concern, they want to know if it can be used. If use of the diet item should be limited, then they want to know why this is so and exactly how often they can use it.

Alcohol and Diabetes: Do They Mix?
Questions about alcohol and various sweeteners are common. People with diabetes should follow the same sensible drinking guidelines as people without diabetes, as follows[17,32,33]:
- Use alcohol only in moderation (one drink/day for women, two drinks/day for men).
  - One drink = 12 oz regular beer, 5 oz wine, or $1\frac{1}{2}$ oz of 80-proof distilled spirits (whiskey, scotch, rye, vodka, brandy, cognac, rum).
- Never drink alcohol on an empty stomach.
- Some medications may not mix with alcohol; check with physician or pharmacist.
- Never drink and drive.
- Never drink if pregnant or trying to become pregnant.
- Above all, use common sense.

Having diabetes should not prevent consumption of alcohol; however, some considerations must be made. Alcoholic beverages, depending on amount and type, can cause hyperglycemia and hypoglycemia. Alcohol moves very quickly from the stomach into the bloodstream; it does not require digestion or metabolism. Approximately 30 to 90 minutes after an alcoholic drink is consumed, alcohol in the bloodstream is at its highest concentration. Because the liver plays the biggest role in removing alcohol from the blood, it stops making glucose while cleansing alcohol from the body. If blood glucose levels are falling during the same time, then hypoglycemia can occur very quickly. Those who take insulin or oral hypoglycemic agents should also be aware that these can lower blood glucose levels. This is why two shots of whiskey on an empty stomach lowers blood sugar dramatically.

Alcoholic beverages can be high in kcalories (and low in food value) and can raise blood glucose, especially if mixed with sweet mixers, fruit juices, or ice cream. Two ounces of 90-proof alcohol contain almost 200 kcal. Wine coolers, liqueurs, and port wines are also high in sugar and kcalories. This can interfere with weight loss goals and practicing tight control. Alcohol also increases serum cholesterol levels, although this effect is transient. In addition, it can lead to hyperlipoproteinemia, with high triglyceride levels in susceptible individuals, including persons with diabetes, when it is excessive. Alcohol can also make neuropathy and retinopathy worse.

For clients who choose to use alcohol, they should ask themselves the following three basic questions:

1. Is my diabetes under control?
2. Does my health care provider agree that I am free from any health problems that alcohol can make worse (e.g., high blood pressure, neuropathy)?
3. Do I know how alcohol can affect me and my diabetes?

If the answer to all three questions is *yes,* then the client can have an occasional drink. In addition to the sensible drinking guidelines listed earlier, the following recommendations should also be considered:

- Discuss the use of alcohol with your physician or dietitian.
- Drink with caution, and carry identification.
- Choose drinking buddies wisely. (Make sure at least one friend or trusted companion knows that you have diabetes and is aware of what should be done in case of hypoglycemia.)
- Have a snack before going to bed to prevent hypoglycemia during sleep.
- Do not drink if you are practicing tight control (because alcohol impairs judgment); have neuropathy, hypertriglyceridemia, or hypertension; or are taking Diabinese (which causes nausea, flushing, headache, or dizziness when mixed with alcohol); or Glucophage (which can cause lactic acidosis).
- Always sip alcoholic drinks slowly.
- If you are a man and taking insulin, you can include two alcoholic beverages in addition to your regular meal plan. If you are a woman taking insulin, then you can include one alcoholic beverage. Do not omit food in exchange for an alcoholic drink.
- If you are not taking insulin (and watching your weight), you can substitute alcohol for fat choices and in some cases extra starch choices (sweet wines, sweet vermouth, and wine coolers).

Can I Use Fructose in My Diabetic Diet?

How would you answer this question from your diabetic client? Fructose has been touted as a sweetener for persons with diabetes because it is a naturally occurring sugar that is as much as 1.0 to 1.5 times as sweet as sucrose. However, can the person with diabetes use it safely?

Although fructose as a sweetener is not for all persons with diabetes, generally you can reply, "Yes, but with qualifications." The following should be considered:

- Advertising claims promoting fructose are sometimes so misleading that many consumers mistakenly believe that it can be used as a "free" food. However, fructose has the same nutritive value as other sugars—4 kcal/g. Persons with T1DM should especially be instructed to use fructose as carefully as they use any other food with a caloric and carbohydrate value.
- The quantity must be limited. If used, then the maximum amount is 75 g/day.
- Consumption of fructose in large amounts may have adverse effects on plasma lipids. It may also cause loose stools and gas when consumed in amounts greater than approximately 25 g/serving.
- The sweetness of fructose varies with temperature, acidity, and dilution. It has been used satisfactorily in some cooked desserts. However, with high temperatures, a rise in pH, and increased concentration of solution, its sweetness is reduced.

▌TO SUM UP

Whatever methods or materials we use, one central fact remains: The person who has diabetes is the most important and a fully equal member of the diabetes care team. Interdisciplinary approaches and strategies that involve this recognition can be developed.

Diabetes mellitus is a syndrome composed of many metabolic disorders collectively characterized by hyperglycemia and other symptoms. Treatment relies heavily on a basic type of therapy—a carefully controlled diet. Diabetes is classified in four categories: (1) *T1DM,* (2) *T2DM,* (3) *GDM,* and (4) *prediabetes.*

Blood glucose levels are controlled primarily by hormones of pancreatic islet cells: insulin, which facilitates passage of glucose through cell membranes via special membrane receptors; glucagon, which ensures adequate levels of glucose to prevent hypoglycemia; and somatostatin, which controls the actions of insulin and glucagon to maintain normal blood glucose levels. Diabetes results from inadequate insulin secretion or insulin resistance from too few receptor sites. Symptoms range from polydipsia, polyuria, polyphagia, and signs of abnormal energy metabolism to fluid and electrolyte imbalances, acidosis, and coma in seriously uncontrolled conditions.

Approximately 5% to 10% of all persons with diabetes have T1DM, which often develops during childhood or adolescence. Treatment involves blood glucose self-monitoring, insulin administration, and regular meals and exercise to balance insulin activity. T2DM occurs mostly in adults, particularly those who are overweight. Acidosis is rare. Treatment consists of weight management and exercise. The food plan for both types of diabetes should be low in saturated fats and cholesterol to reduce cardiovascular risk. Moderate regular exercise increases efficiency of insulin and aids in weight management. GDM occurs in 2% to 5% of all pregnancies.

QUESTIONS FOR REVIEW

1. Describe the major characteristics of T1DM and T2DM. Explain how these characteristics influence differences in NT. List and describe medications used to control these conditions.

2. Identify and explain symptoms of uncontrolled diabetes mellitus.

3. Describe three major complications of uncontrolled diabetes. What therapy is used in the DCCT designed to achieve and maintain normal blood glucose levels and help avoid these complications?

4. Glenn just found out that he has diabetes mellitus. He is a sedentary, 45-year-old man who is 170 cm (5 feet 8 inches) tall and weighs 94 kg (210 lb). No medications were prescribed for him. What is his BMI? If he decides to drink, then how much alcohol could be allowed and how should he fit it into his diet? Defend your answer. Glenn wants to help his children reduce their chances of developing diabetes. What advice would you offer?

REFERENCES

1. Centers for Disease Control and Prevention: *National diabetes fact sheet: general information and national estimates on diabetes in the United States, 2010,* Atlanta, Ga., 2011, U.S. Department of Health and Human Services, Centers for Disease Control and Prevention. from: <http://www.cdc.gov/DIABETES/pubs/pdf/ndfs_2011.pdf>. Retrieved March 20, 2013.

2. American Diabetes Association: Diagnosis and classification of diabetes mellitus. *Diabetes Care* 33(Suppl 1):S62, 2010.

3. American Diabetes Association: *The cost of diabetes,* Alexandria, Va., 2012, American Diabetes Association. from: <http://www.diabetes.org/advocate/resources/cost-of-diabetes.html>. Retrieved March 20, 2013.

4. Whitehouse FW: Classification and pathogenesis of the diabetes syndrome: a historical perspective. *J Am Diet Assoc* 81(3):243, 1982.

5. Nestle M: A case of diabetes mellitus. *N Engl J Med* 81:127, 1982.

6. Bliss M: *The discovery of insulin,* Chicago, 1982, University of Chicago Press.

7. Atkinson MA, Eisenbarth GS: Type 1 diabetes: new perspectives on disease pathogenesis and treatment. *Lancet* 358(9277):221, 2001.

8. McKeigue PM, Shah B, Marmot MG: Relation of central obesity and insulin resistance with high diabetes prevalence and cardiovascular risk in South Asians. *Lancet* 337:382, 1991.

9. Dowse GK, Zimmet PZ, Gareeboo H, et al: Abdominal obesity and physical inactivity as risk factors for NIDDM and impaired glucose tolerance in Indian, Creole, and Chinese Mauritians. *Diabetes Care* 14(4):271, 1991.

10. National Diabetes Education Program: *Overview of diabetes in children and adolescents,* Washington, D.C., June 2011, U.S. Department of Health and Human Services. from: <www.ndep.nih.gov/diabetes/youth/youth_FS.htm#IdentifyingType2>. Retrieved March 21, 2013.

11. American Diabetes Association: Standards of medical care in diabetes—2011. *Diabetes Care* 34(Suppl 1):S11, 2011.

12. Dabelea D, Snell-Bergeon JK, Heartsfield CL, et al: Increasing prevalence of gestational diabetes mellitus (GDM) over time and by birth cohort. *Diabetes Care* 28:579, 2005.

13. Tuomilehto J, Lindstrom J, Eriksson JG, et al: Prevention of type 2 diabetes mellitus by changes in lifestyle among subjects with impaired glucose tolerance. *N Engl J Med* 344:1343–1350, 2001.

14. Pan XR, Li GW, Hu YH, et al: Effects of diet and exercise in preventing NIDDM in people with impaired glucose tolerance: the Da Qing IGT and Diabetes Study. *Diabetes Care* 20:537, 1997.

15. Wendorf M, Goldfine ID: Archeology of NIDDM—excavation of the thrifty genotype. *Diabetes* 40:161, 1991.

16. Diabetes Control and Complications Trial Research Group: The effect of intensive treatment of diabetes on the development and progression of long-term complications in insulin-dependent diabetes mellitus. *N Engl J Med* 329:977, 1993.

17. Franz MJ, Bantle JP, Beebe CA, et al: Evidence-based nutrition principles and recommendations for the treatment and prevention of diabetes and related complications. *Diabetes Care* 25:148, 2002.

18. American Diabetes Association: Translation of the diabetes nutrition recommendations for health care institutions. *Diabetes Care* 25(Suppl):S61, 2002.

19. American Diabetes Association: Nutrition recommendations and interventions for diabetes. *Diabetes Care* 31(Suppl):S61, 2008.

20. American Diabetes Association: Implications of the Diabetes Control and Complications Trial (position statement). *Diabetes Care* 25:S25, 2002.

21. Delahanty LM, Halford BN: The role of diet behaviors in achieving improved glycemic control in intensively treated patients in the Diabetes Control and Complications Trial. *Diabetes Care* 16:1453, 1993.

22. Harris MI, Eastman RC: Is there a glycemic threshold for mortality risk? *Diabetes Care* 21:331, 1998.

23. The Oxford Center for Diabetes, Endocrinology and Metabolism Diabetes Trials Unit: *UK prospective diabetes study,* Oxford, England, 1998, Oxford Center for Diabetes, Endocrinology and Metabolism. from: <http://www.dtu.ox.ac.uk/ukpds_trial/index.php>. Retrieved January 17, 2006.

24. Murray P, Chune GW, Raghavan VA: Legacy effects from DCCT and UKPDS: what they mean and implications for future diabetes trials. *Curr Atheroscler Rep* 12(6):432, 2010.

25. Ousman Y, Sharma M: The irrefutable importance of glycemic control. *Clin Diabetes* 19:71, 2001.

26. American Diabetes Association: Implications of the United Kingdom Prospective Diabetes Study (position statement). *Diabetes Care* 25:S28, 2002.

27. Thomas AM, Gutierrez YM: *American Dietetic Association guide to gestational diabetes mellitus,* Chicago, 2005, American Dietetic Association.

28. American Diabetes Association: Gestational diabetes mellitus (position statement). *Diabetes Care* 27(Suppl):88S, 2004.

29. Anderson EJ, Richardson M, Castle G, et al: The DCCT Research Group: nutrition interventions for the intensive therapy in the Diabetes Control and Complications Trial. *J Am Diet Assoc* 93(7):768, 1993.

30. Buchanan TA, Xiang A, Kjos SL, et al: What is gestational diabetes? *Diabetes Care* 30(Suppl 2):S105, 2007.

31. Ross TA, Boucher JL, O'Connell BS: *American Dietetic Association guide to diabetes medical nutrition therapy and education*, Chicago, 2005, American Dietetic Association.

32. American Diabetes Association: *Alcohol*, Alexandria, Va., 2010, American Diabetes Association. from: <http://www.diabetes.org/food-and-fitness/food/what-can-i-eat/alcohol.html>. Retrieved July 13, 2010.

33. Joslin Diabetes Center: *Managing diabetes: fitting alcohol into your meal plan*, Boston, 2006, Joslin Diabetes Center. from: <http://www.joslin.org/info/Fitting_Alcohol_Into_Your_Meal_Plan.html>. Retrieved May 29, 2009.

FURTHER READINGS AND RESOURCES

Websites of Interest

- American Association of Diabetes Educators (AADE). As a multidisciplinary organization of health professionals who teach about diabetes, the AADE and its website provide information about the scope of practice and standards related to diabetes education; the website also has information and AADE publications: www.aadenet.org.

- American Diabetes Association. The American Diabetes Association publishes many health professional and client materials in addition to its scientific journals; in an annual supplement to *Diabetes Care,* the American Diabetes Association reissues its practice guidelines that address a wide array of clinical issues, including nutrition; these guidelines can be downloaded from the American Diabetes Association website free of charge; local information about American Diabetes Association activities can be obtained from either the website or toll-free telephone number; diabetes self-management educational programs that are reviewed and receive American Diabetes Association "recognition" are covered by Medicare and other third-party payers: www.diabetes.org; 1-800-DIABETES.

- Centers for Disease Control and Prevention, National Center for Chronic Disease Prevention and Health Promotion, Diabetes Public Health Resource. This site has information about the Diabetes Control Program in each state and diabetes-related statistics such as the rise in the prevalence and incidence of diabetes; the National Diabetes Fact Sheet *CDC Information* is available as a downloadable file: www.cdc.gov/diabetes; 1-877-CDC-DIAB.

- Diabetes Care and Education (DCE) Practice Group of the Academy of Nutrition and Dietetics. The DCE publishes *On the Cutting Edge*, a theme-centered newsletter on timely topics related to nutrition and diabetes; educational materials developed by the DCE are available for purchase from the Academy of Nutrition and Dietetics; the DCE website provides information about the Medicare MNT benefits for persons with diabetes, Health Care Financing Administration (HFCA) rules for American Diabetes Association Education Recognition Programs reimbursement, and Current Procedural Terminology (CPT) codes for MNT; the website also provides information about the DCE publications and e-mail listserv: www.dce.org www.eatright.org.

- National Diabetes Education Program (NDEP). The NDEP is a federally sponsored initiative that involves public and private partnerships to improve the treatment and outcomes for people with diabetes through a variety of activities; the NDEP publications include a newsletter, materials for people with diabetes (in several languages), materials for health care providers, materials for organizations, and media kits; single copies of most materials are available free of charge or can be downloaded from the NDEP website: www.ndep.nih.gov; 1-800-860-8747.

- National Institutes of Diabetes and Digestive and Kidney Diseases (NIDDK), National Diabetes Information Clearinghouse (NDIC). The NIDDK website provides information about its diabetes-related clinical trials and other research programs, a directory of diabetes organizations, health education programs, and diabetes-related topics; downloadable files include *Diabetes Dateline,* a NIDDK newsletter; client education materials; and information for health professionals; the NIDDK website also includes the National Diabetes Information Clearinghouse, which disseminates information about online and print materials and provides access to database searches for diabetes-related references: www.niddk.nih.gov.

Renal Disease

Joyce Gilbert

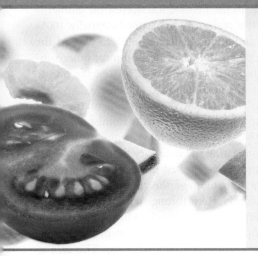

This chapter reviews basic kidney function and pathophysiology of kidney diseases. Nutrition assessment methodology and nutritional recommendations for chronic kidney disease (CKD), maintenance dialysis therapy, postrenal transplantation, acute renal failure (ARF), renal stones, and urinary tract infection (UTI) are discussed.

BASIC KIDNEY FUNCTION

The main functions of the kidney are excretory, regulatory, and endocrine. The excretory function serves to remove potentially toxic metabolic waste products such as urea, the major end product of protein metabolism, from the blood. The regulatory function controls electrolyte, acid-base, and fluid balance. The result is maintenance of proper serum concentrations of sodium, potassium, calcium, phosphorus, chloride, bicarbonate, and hydrogen ions. The endocrine functions include conversion of the biologically inactive form of vitamin D (25-hydroxycholecalciferol) to the biologically active vitamin D (1,25-dihydroxycholecalciferol), synthesis of erythropoietin (needed for red blood cell production in the bone marrow), and synthesis and release of renin, which regulates systemic blood pressure.[1]

These functions are accomplished by the unique architecture of the nephron, the basic functioning unit of the kidney. Each human adult kidney consists of approximately 1 million nephrons (Figure 23-1). The key structures of the nephron are the glomerulus and the tubules.

KEY TERM

nephron Microscopic anatomic and functional unit of the kidney that selectively filters and resorbs essential blood factors, secretes hydrogen ions as needed for maintaining acid-base balance, and then resorbs water to protect body fluids and forms and excretes a concentrated urine for elimination of wastes. The nephron includes the renal corpuscle (glomerulus), the proximal convoluted tubule, the loop of Henle, the distal convoluted tubule, and the collecting tubule, which empties the urine into the renal medulla. The urine passes into the papilla and then to the pelvis of the kidney. Urine is formed by filtration of blood in the glomerulus and by the selective reabsorption and secretion of solutes by cells that constitute the walls of the renal tubes. Approximately 1 million nephrons exist in each kidney.

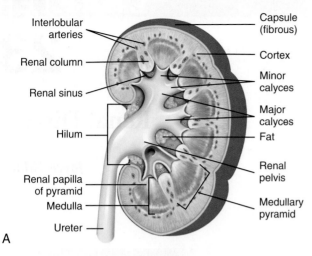

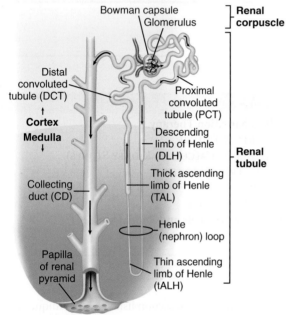

FIGURE 23-1 A, Kidney structure. **B,** Components of nephron. (From Thibodeau GA, Patton KT: *Anatomy & physiology,* ed 7, St Louis, 2010, Mosby.)

Glomerulus

At the head of each nephron, blood enters in a single capillary and then branches into a group of collateral capillaries. This tuft of collateral capillaries is held closely together in a cup-shaped membrane. This cup-shaped capsule is named *Bowman's capsule* for the young English physician Sir William Bowman. In 1843 Bowman established the basis of plasma filtration and consequent urine secretion from the interrelationship of blood-filled glomeruli and enveloping membrane. The filtrate formed here is cell free and virtually protein free.

Tubules

Continuous with the base of Bowman's capsule, nephron tubules wind in a series of convolutions toward their terminal in the renal pelvis. The following list details specific reabsorption functions performed by the four sections of the tubule:

1. *Proximal tubule:* In the first section nearest the glomerulus, major nutrient reabsorption occurs. Essentially, 100% of the glucose and amino acids and 80% to 85% of the water, sodium, potassium, chloride, and most other substances are reabsorbed. Only 15% to 30% of the filtrate remains to enter the next section.
2. *Loop of Henle:* This narrowed midsection of the renal tubule is named for the German anatomist Friedrich Henle, who in 1845 first demonstrated its unique structure and function in creating the necessary fluid pressures for ultimately forming concentrated urine. At this narrowed midsection, the thin loop of the tubule dips into the central renal **medulla**. Here, through a balanced system of water and sodium exchange through sodium pumps in the limbs of the loop (the countercurrent system), important fluid density is created surrounding the loop. This area of increased density in the central part of the kidney is important to concentrate urine through osmotic pressure because the lower collecting tubule later passes through this same area of the kidney.
3. *Distal tubule:* This latter portion of tubule functions primarily in providing acid-base balance through secretion of ionized hydrogen. It also conserves sodium by reabsorbing it under the influence of the hormones aldosterone and vasopressin (also called *antidiuretic hormone* [ADH]).
4. *Collecting tubule:* In this final widened section of the tubule, filtrate is concentrated to save water and form urine for excretion. Water is absorbed under the influence of pituitary hormone vasopressin (ADH) and osmotic pressure of the denser surrounding fluid in this central part of the kidney. The resulting volume of urine, now concentrated and excreted, is only 0.5% to 1% of the original water and solutes filtered at the beginning in Bowman's capsule.

It is through these specialized anatomic components that the kidney serves to maintain homeostasis of the body's internal environment.[1]

CHRONIC KIDNEY DISEASE

Chronic kidney disease (CKD) is a syndrome in which progressive, irreversible losses of excretory, endocrine, and metabolic capacities of the kidney occur as a result of kidney damage (Table 23-1). Determination of renal function requires evaluation of glomerular filtration rate (GFR), which is accomplished through clearance tests. Clearance tests measure the rate at which substances are cleared from the plasma by the glomerulus. In clinical practice, GFR is best approximated by using prediction equations and factoring in serum creatinine concentration, age, gender, race, and body size. Recommended prediction equations for adults are the Modification of Diet in Renal Disease (MDRD) study and Cockcroft-Gault equations.[2] A normal GFR is 125 mL/min/1.73 m². As kidney disease progresses, the GFR falls. Chronic renal failure progresses slowly over time and may include periods during which kidney function remains stable. However, once the disease progresses to stage 5 kidney failure, continuance of life requires initiation of maintenance **dialysis** therapy or subsequent kidney transplantation[3] (see the Case Study box, "The Patient with Chronic Renal Failure").

CKD is a public health problem. The incidence and prevalence of end-stage renal disease (ESRD) have increased 20% to 25% in the United States during the past decade.[4] Of the group being treated by dialysis, 97 per million were older than age 70, compared with 2.1 per million who were children[3] (see the Focus on Culture box, "Kidney Failure: Another Equal Opportunity Disease?"). The total cost for the CKD problem continues to increase.

The most common causes of CKD are diabetic nephropathy and hypertension. Other common causes of kidney failure include **glomerulonephritis**, cystic kidney disease, and urologic disease.[4] Table 23-1 outlines the stages of chronic kidney disease.

PATHOPHYSIOLOGY OF GLOMERULAR DISEASE

The majority of nondiabetic glomerular diseases are the result of immune-mediated mechanisms. Although renal injury induced by antibody alone is known to occur, the mechanisms involved in renal injury that results from antigen-antibody complex formation are better understood. Antigen-antibody complex formation occurs as a result of antibody reacting either to circulating antigens or to native kidney antigens expressed on renal cell membranes. Immune complex deposition may occur within the glomerular basement membrane (GBM), between the GBM and epithelial cell (subepithelial), between the GBM and endothelial cell (subendothelial), or within the mesangial matrix. The pattern of immune complex deposition within the glomerulus is helpful diagnostically because different diseases have characteristic patterns.[4,5] For example, membranous nephropathy is characterized in part by subepithelial immune complex deposition (Figures 23-2 and 23-3).

TABLE 23-1   STAGES OF CHRONIC KIDNEY DISEASE*

STAGE	DESCRIPTION	GFR RANGE (mL/min/1.73 m²)
1	Kidney damage with normal or ↑ GFR	≥90
2	Kidney damage with mild ↓ GRF	60-89
3	Moderate ↓ GFR	30-59
4	Severe ↓ GFR	15-29
5	Kidney failure	<15 (or dialysis)

Modified from National Kidney Foundation: K/DOQI clinical practice guidelines for chronic kidney disease: evaluation, classification and stratification. *Am J Kidney Dis* 39(Suppl 1):S1, 2002.
CKD, Chronic kidney disease; *GFR*, glomerular filtration rate.
*CKD is defined as either kidney damage or GFR <60 mL/min/1.73 m² for ≥3 months. Kidney damage is defined as pathologic abnormalities or markers of damage, including abnormalities in blood or urine tests or imaging studies.

Deposition of immune complexes leads to activation of the **complement** system, which mediates injury through inflammatory or noninflammatory mechanisms. Chemotactic complement components formed as products of the activated complement cascade result in the migration of inflammatory cells into glomeruli. These cells, which include platelets, macrophages, and polymorphonuclear neutrophils (leukocytes), all produce products that are either directly cytotoxic or serve as mediators for further cell or matrix injury (e.g., proteases, reactive oxygen species, lipid mediators, cytokines). When subepithelial immune complexes activate complement, a noninflammatory mechanism is responsible for glomerular injury.[6]

TREATMENT OF CHRONIC KIDNEY DISEASE

The approach to treatment of CKD has shifted focus from diagnosis and treatment of established kidney diseases to detection and treatment at much earlier stages.[3] The clinical course of this disease can be significantly improved if specific interventions are instituted early in development of the disease. These include annual screening for microalbuminuria (greater than 30 mg/day or 20 mcg/min of albumin in the urine); improving glycemic control; aggressive antihypertensive therapy with angiotensin-converting enzymes or angiotensin receptor blockers; and lifestyle modifications that include weight loss, reduction in salt and alcohol intake, and exercise.[7]

Less traditional interventions that have been explored for their beneficial effects on renal disease include nutrients such as amino acids and carbohydrates. A class of nutrients that continues to be investigated for potential benefits on progression of renal disease is omega-3 fatty acids (see the Health Promotion section later in this chapter).

Through its initiative, *K/DOQI: Kidney Disease Outcomes Quality Initiative*, the National Kidney Foundation recently published clinical practice guidelines for evaluation, classification, and stratification of CKD.[3] A main rationale for development of these clinical guidelines was the accumulation of evidence that adverse effects of CKD, including kidney failure, cardiovascular disease (CVD), and premature death can be prevented or delayed by earlier testing and treatment of CKD.[3]

K/DOQI guidelines for CKD recommend that during health evaluations all individuals be evaluated as to whether they are at increased risk of having or developing renal disease. Individuals are to be considered at risk if they have diabetes, hypertension, autoimmune diseases, systemic infections, exposure to drugs or procedures associated with acute decline in kidney function, recovery from acute kidney failure, are older than 60 years of age, have a family history of kidney disease, or reduced kidney mass.[3] Table 23-1 identifies the stages of disease and associates each stage with a level of GFR. As the GFR falls below 60 mL/min/1.73 m², nutrition intervention becomes an important component of medical care.

CASE STUDY

The Patient with Chronic Renal Failure

Mr. Steinberg is 45 years old, married, and works as a city planner for a large municipal government. He cited a recent history of nausea, anorexia, **hematuria**, and swollen ankles during a physical examination. His wife reported that he had been tiring more easily than usual during the past year. A history of prior illnesses proved negative, except for a severe case of influenza with sore throat 10 years before during an epidemic when he was stationed with the Army overseas. Tests were ordered, and the patient was advised to return in 1 week for review of the test results (and sooner if any changes in his symptoms were noted).

Mr. Steinberg did return, with additional symptoms of headaches and occasionally blurred vision. At that time his blood pressure was 160/98 mm Hg, his temperature was 37.5° C (99.6° F), and he had lost 4 kg (8¾ lb). Laboratory tests showed albumin and red and white blood cells in the urine, with an elevated **blood urea nitrogen (BUN)**; a phenolsulfonphthalein (PSP) test indicated a reduced filtration rate. The diagnosis was chronic renal failure.

The physician discussed the diagnosis and its serious prognosis with Mr. and Mrs. Steinberg, giving them the benefits and disadvantages of **hemodialysis** and kidney transplantation. Antihypertensive medication was prescribed along with other drugs to minimize discomfort.

During the following weeks Mr. Steinberg continued to lose weight, had increasing joint pain, and became anemic. He found it increasingly difficult to maintain his hectic schedule of frequent meetings, conferences, and public speeches because of gastrointestinal (GI) bleeding, increasing nausea, and occasional muscle spasms. Small mouth sores made eating very difficult.

Finally, the Steinbergs informed the physician of their decision to accept the kidney transplant as a means of controlling the disease process. They were referred to the registered dietitian (RD) for renal diet counseling to control protein, sodium, potassium, phosphate, and fluids, as well as to ensure adequate kilocalorie (kcalories or kcal) intake. After discussing these needs for nutritional maintenance before surgery, the RD helped them develop a meal plan based on Mr. Steinberg's food preferences. Food selection and preparation were discussed in detail, with many ideas for building in as much variety and taste appeal as possible.

The Steinbergs' follow-up with the food plan was excellent. One month later the laboratory values were almost normal, blood pressures averaged 140/88 mm Hg, the headaches and blurred vision had virtually disappeared, and Mr. Steinberg had gained 3.2 kg (7 lb) of his lost weight. The nutrient supplements, including the amino acid analogs, were taken each day as instructed.

Fortunately a kidney donor was soon found, and with the aid of drug control of immune responses the transplant surgery was apparently a success. Mr. Steinberg convalesced well at home, kept all follow-up visits with the health care team, and has continued to be asymptomatic 1 year after surgery.

Questions for Analysis

1. Identify a metabolic imbalance caused by chronic renal failure that may account for each symptom presented by Mr. Steinberg.
2. What factors affect the amount of protein needed by persons with chronic renal failure? What amounts are usually used? Why? What are the amino acid analogs used with the low-protein diet, and why are they used?
3. What factors affect the amount of sodium needed by persons with chronic renal failure? How much is usually recommended?
4. Why is it important to control potassium levels? How much is recommended? What clinical signs presented by Mr. Steinberg may indicate that he had not been getting enough potassium?
5. Why is control of phosphate important in the diet for chronic renal failure? What additional means may be used to control it?
6. What factors affect fluid balance in chronic renal failure? How much is usually allowed?
7. Outline a general teaching plan you would use to instruct the Steinbergs about the presurgical and postsurgical dietary needs.

KEY TERMS
medulla Inner tissue substance of the kidney.
hematuria The abnormal presence of blood in the urine.
blood urea nitrogen (BUN) The nitrogen component of urea in the blood; a measure of kidney function; elevated levels of BUN indicate a disorder of kidney function.
hemodialysis Removal of certain elements from the blood according to their rates of diffusion through a semipermeable membrane (e.g., by a hemodialysis machine).
dialysis Process of separating crystalloids and colloids in solution by the difference in their rates of diffusion through a semipermeable membrane; crystalloids pass through readily, and colloids pass through only very slowly or not at all.

KEY TERMS
glomerulonephritis A form of nephritis affecting the capillary loops in an acute short-term infection. It may progress to a more serious chronic condition leading to irreversible renal failure.
complement A complex series of enzymatic proteins occurring in normal serum that interact to combine with and augment (fill out, complete) the antigen-antibody complex of the body's immune system, producing lysis when the antigen is an intact cell; composed of 11 discrete proteins or functioning components, activated by the immunoglobulin factors IgG and IgM.

FOCUS ON CULTURE

Kidney Failure: Another Equal Opportunity Disease?

Of the millions of Americans currently living with kidney disease, a disproportionate number are African American. This reflects an incidence rate fourfold greater than that of their European-American counterparts and is most commonly attributed to increased prevalence of high blood pressure, diabetes, and a familial history of the disease. However, not only are African Americans at an increased risk for developing kidney disease but also they seem to acquire it earlier in life, with almost half not knowing they have the condition until dialysis is required.

This is a startling realization, considering early interventions can limit damage done to the kidneys. Later diagnosis of kidney disease can result in increased rates of chronic problems, dialysis dependency, and need for transplantation. The difficulty is that relatively few African Americans receive screening or intervention. Adding to the problem, with diabetes being the primary risk factor for kidney disease, one third of the cases of diabetes among African Americans go undiagnosed, demonstrating the need for further screening.

According to the National Kidney Foundation, African Americans represent 13% of the American population but make up 35% of those on kidney transplant waiting lists. Consequently, although an increased kidney transplant demand exists for African Americans, a moderately low donorship rate is seen from this group, compounding the problem.

The following five primary reasons influence low African-American kidney donorship:

1. Lack of transplant awareness
2. Religious myths and misconceptions
3. Distrust of the medical community
4. Fear of premature declaration of death after signing a donor card
5. Fear of potential preference for races other than African Americans

Whether the increased rate of kidney disease in African Americans stems from lack of awareness, lack of health care, or genetic factors, the fact remains that African Americans possess many risk factors affecting renal health. Screenings and education about blood glucose and blood pressure control at a younger age, along with lifestyle and medication interventions, have been shown to have dramatic results in kidney health. Unfortunately, only a small percentage actually receives these screenings or treatment. This problem is a major one that is made all the more disheartening by the unnecessary suffering involved. It is hoped that with increased attention brought to kidney disease, the incidence rate in the African-American population will decline.

Bibliography

Freedman B, Spray BJ, Tuttle AB, et al: The familial risk of end-stage renal disease in African Americans. *Am J Kidney Dis* 21(4):387, 1993.

National Kidney Foundation: Diabetes, chronic kidney disease and special populations, New York. Available at: <http://www.kidney.org/professionals/tools/diabetesandckd.cfm>.

National Kidney and Urologic Diseases Information Clearinghouse, National Institute of Diabetes and Digestive and Kidney Diseases, National Institutes of Health: Strategic plan on minority health disparities, Bethesda, Md.. Available at: <http://www2.niddk.nih.gov/AboutNIDDK/ReportsAndStrategicPlanning/Strategic_Plan_Minority_Health_Disparities.htm>.

Reif M, Hall P: *Kidney failure among African Americans*, Cincinnati, Ohio, 2001, NetWellness. from: <www.netwellness.org/healthtopics/kidney/faq2.cfm>. Retrieved June 19, 2009.

Tarver-Carr M, Powe NR, Eberhardt MS, et al: Excess risk of chronic kidney disease among African-American versus white subjects in the United States: a population-based study of potential explanatory factors. *J Am Soc Nephrol* 13:2363, 2002.

NUTRITION ASSESSMENT OF PATIENTS WITH CHRONIC KIDNEY DISEASE

Malnutrition is a significant comorbidity of CKD, including patients on hemodialysis or **peritoneal dialysis** therapy.[5] Life-threatening malnutrition is present in 5% to 10% of patients, and moderate malnutrition is present in an additional 20% to 40%.[8] Factors contributing to malnutrition in patients with renal failure are listed in Box 23-1.

Evaluating and monitoring nutritional status are vital components of nutrition care of patients with kidney disease. The high prevalence of malnutrition, large number of aberrations in normal metabolism, and complications including anorexia and catabolism all indicate the need for consistent monitoring. Nutrition assessment is best completed by a registered dietitian (RD) who has received special training in renal nutrition care.

When completing a nutrition assessment, an array of indexes, each representing a specific data category, are measured independently and then evaluated collectively to ascertain the nutritional status of the renal patient. Table 23-2 lists the data categories that encompass the nutrition assessment of the renal patient. Specific indexes used to evaluate biochemical values are listed in Table 23-3. Following is a review of indexes most commonly measured from each data category.[9]

History and Physical Examination

Medical History

The medical record should include information concerning comorbid conditions, medications, past hospitalizations, weight history, socioeconomic status, and functional status, as well as information from the physical examination. Any major organ or GI diseases, surgeries, or previous symptoms

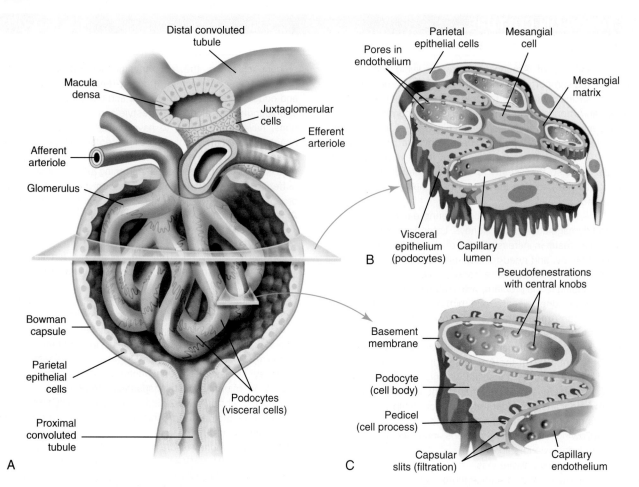

FIGURE 23-2 Anatomy of the glomerulus and juxtaglomerular apparatus. **A,** Longitudinal cross-section of glomerulus and juxtaglomerular apparatus. **B,** Horizontal cross-section of glomerulus. **C,** Enlargement of glomerular capillary filtration membrane. (From McCance K, Huether S: *Pathophysiology: the biologic basis for disease in adults and children,* ed 5, St Louis, 2006, Mosby.)

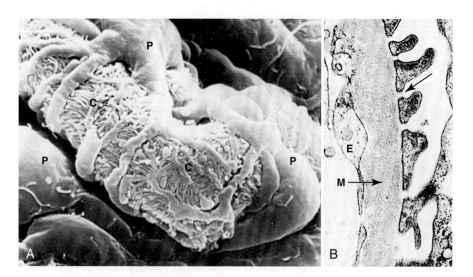

FIGURE 23-3 Glomerular capillary. **A,** Scanning electron micrograph of normal glomerular capillary *(C)* enclosed by podocytes *(P)* with primary processes and interdigitating foot processes. **B,** Glomerular capillary wall showing foot processes of endothelial podocytes *(F),* filtration slit membrane *(arrow),* basement membrane *(M),* and fenestrated endothelium *(E)* (magnification, ×40,000). (From Kissane JM, editor: *Anderson's pathology,* ed 9, St Louis, 1990, Mosby.)

of malabsorption or other digestive problems, including nausea, vomiting, and diarrhea, should be noted. Impairment in fluid and electrolyte balance, hypertension and hypotension, proteinuria, and any previous symptoms of uremia that affect appetite, food intake, digestion, or nutritional status should also be noted.

Psychosocial History

A psychosocial history evaluates a patient's mental status, as well as factors regarding economics, education level, physical home environment, food shopping and preparation capabilities, and available support systems. The goal is to create an individualized intervention the patient or patient's support system can understand and apply. Factors that might compromise nutritional status include depression or improper food preparation and storage equipment. This component of the assessment process helps identify patients requiring social services to assist with economic needs or special services to provide regular access to food and medications.

Demographics

Information on age, marital status, gender, and ethnicity is needed to assess nutritional status. Many reference standards used to classify clinical indexes adjust for gender and age. Knowledge of ethnicity affects the ability to individualize nutrition therapy; marital status helps identify support systems.

BOX 23-1	FACTORS CONTRIBUTING TO THE PRESENCE OF MALNUTRITION IN PATIENTS WITH CHRONIC RENAL FAILURE

1. Anorexia as a result of the following:
   - Nausea, emesis, medications
   - Uremia/uremic state of metabolism
   - Underdialysis
   - Accumulation of uremic toxins not completely removed by dialysis
2. Metabolic acidosis
3. Endocrine disorders (insulin resistance, **hyperparathyroidism**, impaired response to insulin-like growth factor I)
4. Comorbidity (infections, intercurrent illnesses)
5. Reduced nutrient intake
6. Dialysis related to the following:
   - Inadequate dose of dialysate
   - Catabolism (bioincompatible membrane)
   - Loss of amino acids and protein to the dialysate
   - Dialysate reused with bleach
7. Psychosocial
   - Depression
   - Inability to purchase or prepare food adequately
   - Loss of or poorly fitting dentures

Data from Wolfson M: Causes, manifestations, and assessment of malnutrition in chronic renal failure. In Kopple JD, Massry SG, editors: *Nutrition management of renal disease*, ed 2, Philadelphia, 2004, Lippincott Williams & Wilkins.

Physical Activity

Assessment of the patient's physical capabilities is needed to maintain activities of daily living (ADLs) and proper level of physical exercise for psychologic and physical therapeutics. The following questionnaires have been validated for the purpose of measuring physical activity and physical functioning in the ESRD patient population: the Stanford 7-Day Physical Activity Recall, Physical Activity Scale for the Elderly, Human Activity Profile, and Medical Outcomes Study Short-Form 36-Item Questionnaire.

Current Medical and Surgical Issues

Identification of nutritional implications of medical and surgical problems is imperative for the nutrition assessment procedure. For the patient with chronic, progressive disease, this requires acknowledgment of any newly diagnosed medical and surgical illnesses.

Diet and Food Intake

This category relies on subjective patient reporting to evaluate qualitative and quantitative aspects of food intake. One of the most useful outputs from this category is calculation of nutrient intake. Other outputs include information related to past and current food intake (qualitative and quantitative), eating patterns, and specific food preferences. This information allows an approximation of the diet's adequacy. It also helps to identify nutrient factors that may be contributing to medical problems. Qualitative data are essential for formulation of individual diet therapy, including meal plans and menus.

Diet History

Nutrition history is usually obtained at the initial meeting. It is an all-inclusive collection of some objective, but primarily subjective, information concerning the patient's food consumption, such as aversions, allergies, preferences, and intake. Information on previous and current diet intake assists in devising interventions to improve diet or devising an acceptable therapeutic meal plan. The most commonly used tools to obtain food intake information differ in approach to data collection, retrospective versus prospective, and whether the information is a qualitative description of intake versus a quantitative one.

KEY TERMS

peritoneal dialysis Dialysis through the peritoneum into and out of the peritoneal cavity.

hyperparathyroidism Abnormally increased activity of the parathyroid gland, resulting in excessive secretion of parathyroid hormone (PTH), which usually helps regulate serum calcium levels in balance with vitamin D hormone; excess secretion occurs when the serum calcium level falls below normal, as in chronic renal disease or in vitamin D deficiency.

TABLE 23-2   NUTRITION ASSESSMENT PARAMETERS IN CHRONIC KIDNEY DISEASE

PARAMETER	WHAT IT MEASURES	COMPONENTS
History and physical examination	Past and present nutritional status; areas that should be addressed when developing a plan of care	Review of medical record Patient, family, and/or caregiver interview Psychosocial history Ability to obtain, prepare, ingest, and enjoy food Mental status Educational level Functional status Person responsible for shopping/preparing food Patient's functional status (activities of daily living) Diet histories: usual food intake, food intake patterns, and factors affecting intake Religious/cultural beliefs Use of supplements and alternative or complementary therapies Past diet restrictions (and education) Patient's ability to chew, swallow, taste, and smell foods Changes in appetite and eating pattern Food preferences, allergies, and intolerances Use of alcohol Practice of pica
Anthropometric assessment	Weight status; nutritional status; distribution of body fat, lean muscle mass, and bone	Body weight (can be difficult to determine because of fluid retention) Estimated dry weight or edema-free body weight Hemodialysis: weight postdialysis Peritoneal dialysis: weight after drainage of dialysate with peritoneum empty Interdialytic weight gains Fluid gains between hemodialysis treatments Height Initial measurement essential Recumbent bed height, arm span, or knee height may be used if patient cannot stand Estimation of frame size Body mass index Estimate of body composition Skinfold thicknesses
Energy and nutrient requirements	Must be individually assessed based on type of dialysis, cause of kidney disease, and other comorbidities	Kcalories per kg formulas
Subjective global assessment	Useful measure of protein-energy nutritional status in maintenance dialysis patients	4-item, 7-point scale Medical history Weight change during previous 6 months Dietary intake Gastrointestinal symptoms Physical examination Visual assessment of subcutaneous tissue and muscle mass
Biochemical parameters	Monitored on ongoing basis to assess nutritional status	See Table 23-3

Data from Barbá PD, Goode JL: Nutrition assessment in chronic kidney disease. In Byham-Gray L, Wiesen K, editors: *A clinical guide to nutrition care in kidney disease,* Chicago, 2004, American Dietetic Association.

Food Record. A food record provides qualitative and approximate quantitative food intake information that is best collected prospectively. The minimal time recommended for data collection is 3 days; a reasonable maximum is 5 days. The patient should provide intake information for weekends and weekdays so that variability can be determined. For the dialysis patient, it is strongly recommended the food record include intake for days on which dialysis takes place, as well as those on which it does not, in addition to a weekend versus weekday pattern. A difference in food intake between dialysis and nondialysis days has been noted in the type and amount of food selected.

TABLE 23-3   BIOCHEMICAL PARAMETERS FOR ASSESSING NUTRITIONAL STATUS

PARAMETER	SUBSTANCE	NORMAL RANGE	CKD RANGE
Visceral protein stores	Albumin	3.5-5.0 g/dL	WNL for laboratory or >4.0 g/dL
	Prealbumin (transthyretin)	15-36 mg/dL	>30 mg/dL
	Transferrin	Female subjects: 15%-50%	WNL
		Male subjects: 20%-50%	
	C-reactive protein (CRP)	0.8 mg/dL	2-15 mg/dL
Static (somatic) protein reserves	Serum creatinine	Female subjects: 0.5-1.1 mg/dL	2-15 mg/dL
		Male subjects: 0.6-1.2 mg/dL	
Other estimates of protein reserves	Nitrogen balance		
Fluid, electrolyte, and acid-base status	Sodium	135-145 mEq/L	WNL
	Potassium	3.5-5.0 mEq/L	3.5-6.0 mEq/L
	Calcium	WNL for laboratory	Normal: 8.4-10.2 mg/dL; preferably at low end of normal (8.4-9.5 mg/dL)
	Phosphorus	3.0-4.5 mg/dL	3.5-5.5 mg/dL
	CO_2	23-29 mEq/L	22-25 mEq/L
	Glucose	70-105 mg/dL	WNL <200 nonfasting before dialysis; intake has influence
Indirect indices of renal function and dialysis adequacy	Serum creatinine	Female subjects: 0.5-1.1 mg/dL	2-15 mg/dL
		Male subjects: 0.6-1.2 mg/dL	
	Blood urea nitrogen (BUN)	10-20 mg/dL	60-80 mg/dL in anuric; well dialyzed and eating adequate protein
	Kt/V (hemodialysis)	N/A	1.2
	Kt/V (peritoneal dialysis)	N/A	2.0-2.2
Anemia	Hemoglobin (Hb)	Female subjects: 12-16 g/dL	Variable: 11-12 g/dL
		Male subjects: 14-18 g/dL	
	Ferritin	Female subjects: 10-150 mg/mL	≥100 mg/mL, but no known benefit >800 mg/mL
		Male subjects: 12-300 mg/mL	
	Serum iron	Female subjects: 50-170 mcg/dL	WNL
		Male subjects: 60-175 mcg/dL	
Hyperlipidemia	Serum cholesterol	<200 mg	WNL <150 mg; evaluate for nutrient deficit
	Triglycerides	Female subjects: 35-135 mg/dL	WNL <200 mg/dL
		Male subjects: 40-160 mg/dL	
Renal osteodystrophy	Calcium	WNL for laboratory	Normal: 8.4-10.2 mg/dL; preferably at low end of normal (8.4-9.5 mg/dL)
	Alkaline phosphatase	30-85 U/mL	WNL for laboratory
	Parathyroid hormone (PHT) (i) intact	10-65 pg/mL	150-300 pg/mL
	Biointact (third generation)	60-140 pg/mL	80-160 pg/mL

Data from Barbá PD, Goode JL: Nutrition assessment in chronic kidney disease. In Byham-Gray L, Wiesen K, editors: *A clinical guide to nutrition care in kidney disease,* Chicago, 2004, American Dietetic Association; Wilkens KG: Medical nutrition therapy for renal disorders. In Mahan LK, Escott-Stump S, editors: *Krause's food & nutrition therapy,* ed 12, St Louis, 2008, Saunders.
CKD, Chronic kidney disease; *WNL,* within normal limits.

The patient should be provided with instructions on how to approximate food portion sizes and servings of fluid to ensure accurate reporting. Use of food models is very helpful. The food record should include time of day of any intake (meals and snacks), names of foods eaten, approximate amount of food ingested, method of preparation, and special recipes or steps taken in the food preparation. The same instructions apply to fluid intake. Brand names are requested when available.

Some patients find it is more convenient to record food intake at the end of the day. This is an inferior method because the data collection becomes retrospective and more subject to error. Calculation of intake of total protein, protein quality, carbohydrate, fat, fatty acid classes, and other selected nutrients is best completed by a computerized nutrient analysis program.

24-Hour Food Recall. The 24-hour food recall is an interactive tool in which the clinician assists the patient in remembering qualitative and quantitative food intake via prompting. The clinician can sit with a patient during dialysis and slowly help the patient recall the previous day's intake of food and fluid. Food models or drawings can be used to help the patient identify portion size. One 24-hour recall, however, does not provide sufficient information to ascertain total food intake.

A variation of the 24-hour recall for a dialysis patient is to meet with the patient during three consecutive treatments, or at least four sessions within a 2-week period, and obtain one 24-hour recall at each visit. Effort should be made to obtain a recall for a weekend day, a dialysis day, and a non-dialysis day. To obtain a total food intake on a dialysis day, the practitioner can ask the patient what he or she had to eat so far that day and record it. The patient or family member can finish recording for the rest of the day, or the clinician can meet with the patient at the next session to help him or her recall what was eaten for the rest of that day. Calling the patient's home on a daily basis to obtain the needed information is an option but is not practical.

Food Frequency Questionnaires. Food frequency questionnaires (FFQs) approximate nutrient intake by identifying periodicity of intake of specific foods within food groups that are significant sources of a particular nutrient or nutrients (e.g., dairy products are a good source of calcium, vitamin D, and protein). A food frequency consists of listing foods according to group, such as vegetables, fruits, dairy, protein, and so forth. The patient is questioned as to how often he or she eats this food per day, per week, and per month. An approximation of adequacy of intake of specific nutrients can be calculated from the results.

Biochemical Values

Serum biochemical values are used to assess and monitor nutritional status over time. Selected serum values pertain to visceral protein stores, static protein reserves, overall protein nutriture, immune competence, iron stores, as well as vitamin, mineral, and trace element status. In addition to these components, nutrition assessment involves evaluating fluid, electrolyte, and acid-base status; renal function; dialysis adequacy for the patient receiving replacement therapy; serum lipid levels; and bone health.

Visceral Protein Stores

Serum Albumin. Albumin, the most abundant plasma protein, functions to maintain plasma oncotic pressure and serves as a major carrier protein for drugs, hormones, enzymes, and trace elements. Clinically significant hypoalbuminemia occurs with different types of malnutrition besides kidney disease (e.g., protein-energy kwashiorkor, uncomplicated) in children and adults. In these conditions, hypoalbuminemia usually indicates other metabolic derangements, as well as a poor prognosis. From these observations, serum albumin became a part of routine nutrition assessment of the hospitalized patient and subsequently the renal patient.

Although serum albumin levels have been used extensively in clinical practice, research studies, and nutritional surveys to assess nutritional status of the CKD population, reliability and sensitivity of this parameter have been questioned. Concerns are independent of conditions that change serum albumin as a marker of visceral protein stores. Use of albumin for assessment purposes has been criticized because of its long half-life, averaging 14 to 20 days, and large body pool, 4 to 5 mg/kg, making albumin slow to respond to changes in visceral protein stores. It is therefore a late marker of malnutrition.

Prealbumin (Thyroxine-Binding Prealbumin, Transthyretin). Prealbumin is a carrier protein for retinol-binding protein (RBP) and thus has a major role in transport of thyroxine. Its short half-life of 2 to 3 days and its small body pool make it more sensitive than albumin to changes in protein status. This was the first visceral protein found to be low in healthy children who were eating marginal amounts of protein. In primates, prealbumin reflects overall nitrogen balance during starvation and refeeding. Decreases in serum levels occur independently of nutritional status when acute metabolic stress is seen, including trauma, minor stress, and inflammation. Serum concentration has also been observed to decrease in liver disease and with iron supplementation. Prealbumin can be useful as a nutritional marker after acute metabolic stress.

The low molecular weight of prealbumin (approximately 54,980 daltons) precludes its use as a marker of nutritional status in patients with CKD who have a decreased GFR. Prealbumin levels have been reported to be elevated in the euvolemic patient with chronic renal failure. In hemodialysis patients, high levels have been observed and are attributed to decreased renal catabolism. A decline in the proportion of circulating free prealbumin versus that complexed with RBP may explain the diminished catabolism and therefore the elevated levels. A concentration of less than 30 mg/dL (normal range, 10 to 40 mg/dL) may indicate malnutrition in the hemodialysis patient and has recently been associated with an increased risk of death. These studies indicate prealbumin level may serve as a better nutrition assessment tool and predictor of patient outcome than the traditionally used serum albumin in the dialysis population.

Transferrin (Siderophilin). The main function of transferrin is to bind ferrous iron and to transport iron to the bone marrow. Its half-life of 8 to 10 days and small body pool enable it to respond more rapidly to short-term changes in protein status, compared with albumin. Its value is influenced

---

KEY TERM

proteinuria The presence of an excess of serum proteins, such as albumin, in the urine.

by iron pool status and needs to be assessed in conjunction with this value.

C-Reactive Protein. C-Reactive protein (CRP) mirrors the acute-phase response to inflammation. Increases are regulated by the rise in circulating cytokines and tumor necrosis factor-α (TNF-α), very powerful determinants of albumin levels in CKD patients.

Body Weight

Initial assessment of body weight and monitoring of weight change over time represent critical components of the nutrition assessment process. Weight loss in excess of 5% to 10%, depending on the patient's overall nutritional status, or substandard weight for height should be considered a risk factor for malnutrition. Interrelationships between weight loss over time and outcome in the renal patient population have not yet been reported.

Body mass index (BMI), current weight, usual weight, ideal body weight (IBW), percentage usual weight, percentage IBW, and, particularly, percentage weight change over a defined time period are important parameters of body weight.

A database or sheet in the patient's chart committed to record body weight is recommended for every patient.

ALTERED NUTRIENT REQUIREMENTS WITH CHRONIC KIDNEY DISEASE

Nutrition intervention for patients with CKD includes modifications for sodium, fluid, potassium, phosphorus, calcium, vitamin D, iron, calories, and protein. Although global recommendations are available, nutrition care must be individualized based on serum chemistry levels, fluid balance, and nutritional status. These concerns are addressed in the following discussion (see the Diet-Medications Interactions box, "Common Drugs Used for Renal Disorders and Potential Food-Drug Interactions").

Sodium and Potassium

As kidney function declines, the ability of the nephrons to maintain sodium balance through sodium excretion diminishes. However, an adaptive mechanism results in undamaged nephrons being able to excrete an increased percentage of

---

🔖 DIET-MEDICATIONS INTERACTIONS

Common Drugs Used for Renal Disorders and Potential Food-Drug Interactions

DRUGS	POTENTIAL FOOD-DRUG INTERACTIONS, SIDE EFFECTS, AND RECOMMENDATIONS
Pyelonephritis and Urinary Tract Infections	
Ceftriaxone and gentamicin	Sufficient water and fluids should be consumed
	Monitor glucose changes in persons with diabetes mellitus
	Avoid use with alcohol
Sulfisoxazole (Gantrisin)	Can deplete folacin and vitamin K
Trimethoprim (Trimpex), trimethoprim/sulfamethoxazole (Bactrim, Septra, Cotrim)	May cause diarrhea, gastrointestinal (GI) distress, stomatitis
Nitrofurantoin (Furadantin, Macrodantin)	Sufficient fluid intake necessary
Quinolones: ofloxacin (Floxin), norfloxacin (Noroxin), ciprofloxacin (Cipro), trovafloxacin (Trovan)	Should be taken with food or milk
	Adequate dietary protein is necessary
	Nausea, vomiting, anorexia are common
	Milk, yogurt, and calcium supplements should be avoided when taking Cipro; caffeine intake should be limited
	Floxin should be taken separately from vitamin supplements; nausea is one side effect
Urolithiasis/Nephrolithiasis (Kidney Stones)	
Allopurinol (Zyloprim) and probenecid (usually used instead of or in conjunction with purine-restricted diet)	Drink 10-12 glasses of fluid daily
	Avoid concomitant intake of vitamin C supplements
	Patient should maintain alkaline urine
	Side effects include nausea, vomiting, diarrhea, abdominal pain
Thiazide diuretics	Increase intake of high-potassium foods
	Control sodium intake
	Increase magnesium intake
	Dry mouth or gastrointestinal (GI) distress may occur
d-Penicillamine	Requires vitamin B_6 and zinc supplementation
	Increase fluid intake with cystinuria
	Take 1 to 2 hours before/after meals
	Stomatitis, diarrhea, nausea, vomiting, abdominal pain may occur
Demerol and similar medications	Dry mouth, constipation, nausea, vomiting can occur

Continued

🖊 DIET-MEDICATIONS INTERACTIONS

Common Drugs Used for Renal Disorders and Potential Food-Drug Interactions—cont'd

DRUGS	POTENTIAL FOOD-DRUG INTERACTIONS, SIDE EFFECTS, AND RECOMMENDATIONS
Acute Renal Failure	
Exchange resins (Kayexalate)	Take separately from calcium and antacids by several hours
Sorbitol	Bloating, flatulence, diarrhea may occur
Chronic Kidney Disease	
Phosphate binders: calcium acetate or calcium carbonate	Nausea/vomiting may occur
Ergocalciferol (vitamin D analog)	Additional water necessary to prevent constipation
	Monitor fluids carefully if urine output decreased
	Avoid long-term use
Recombinant human erythropoietin (r-HuEPO)	Iron supplements necessary
	Do not take iron supplement at same time as calcium
Hemodialysis	
Kayexalate	Take separately from calcium supplements or antacids
Transplantation (patients are usually on three to four of the five drugs listed following)	
Corticosteroids (prednisone, Solu-Cortef)	Increased catabolism of proteins
	Negative nitrogen balance
	Hyperphagia
	Ulcers
	Decreased glucose tolerance
	Sodium and fluid retention
	Impaired calcium absorption and osteoporosis
	Cushing's syndrome
	Obesity
	Muscle wasting
	Increased gastric secretion
Cyclosporine	Nausea, vomiting, diarrhea
	Hyperlipidemia and hyperkalemia may occur
	Elevated glucose and lipids
Immunosuppressants (Muromonab, Orthoclone [OKT3], antithymocyte globulin [ATG])	Nausea, anorexia, diarrhea, vomiting
Azathioprine (Imuran)	Fever
	Stomatitis
	Leukopenia, thrombocytopenia
	Oral and esophageal sores
	Macrocytic anemia
	Pancreatitis
	Vomiting, diarrhea
	Folate supplementation may be needed
	Dietary modifications (liquid or soft diet, use of oral supplements) may be needed
Tacrolimus (Prograf, FK506)	GI distress, nausea, vomiting, diarrhea
	Hyperglycemia

Data from Escott-Stump S: *Nutrition and diagnosis-related care,* ed 6, Philadelphia, 2007, Lippincott Williams & Wilkins.

filtered sodium, with the effect being a decrease in the fractional reabsorption and an increase in fractional excretion of sodium by renal tubules. As GFR falls to 10 mL/min, a sodium restriction of 2 to 3 g may be required to maintain sodium and fluid balance. Clinical symptoms of excessive sodium intake include shortness of breath, hypertension, congestive heart failure (CHF), and edema.

Kidney regulation of potassium balance is obtained by renal excretion of potassium in an amount equal to that absorbed by the gastrointestinal (GI) tract. Potassium balance is dependent on the ability of the tubules to continue to secrete potassium into the ultrafiltrate. This ability will decrease as kidney failure progresses. As serum potassium levels increase to more than 5.0 mg/dL, dietary potassium restriction to approximately 3 to 4 g/day may be needed.[10]

Phosphorus, Calcium, and Vitamin D

The consequence of abnormalities of calcium, phosphorus, and vitamin D metabolism seen in CKD is development of bone diseases, which are referred to as *renal osteodystrophy*. Diagnoses include osteoporosis, osteosclerosis, osteomalacia, and osteitis fibrosa. The healthy kidney filters about 7 g of

TABLE 23-4	RECOMMENDED DIETARY NUTRIENT INTAKE FOR PATIENTS WITH CHRONIC KIDNEY DISEASE			
NUTRIENT	**STAGES 1 AND 2**	**STAGE 3**	**STAGE 4**	**STAGE 5**
Protein (g/kg/day)	0.75	0.75	0.6	0.6-0.75
Energy (kcal/kg/day)	Based on energy expenditure	Based on energy expenditure	30-35 kcal/kg/day	30-35 kcal/kg/day
Sodium (mg/day)	1-4 g/day, depending on comorbidities	1-4 g/day, depending on comorbidities	1-4 g/day, depending on comorbidities	1-4 g/day, depending on comorbidities
Potassium (mEq/day)	Usually no restriction unless serum level high	Usually no restriction unless serum level high	Usually no restriction unless serum level high	Usually no restriction unless serum level high
Phosphorus (mg/kg/day)	Monitor and restrict if serum levels >4.6	8-12 mg/g protein or 800-1000 mg/day	8-12 mg/g protein or 800-1000 mg/day	8-12 mg/g protein or 800-1000 mg/day
Calcium (mg/day)	1.2-1.5 mg/day; serum calcium should be maintained on lower end	1.2-1.5 mg/day; serum calcium should be maintained on lower end	Same as stages 1-3, but not to exceed 2000 mg/day	Same as stages 1-3, but not to exceed 2000 mg/day
Vitamins and minerals	Dietary Reference Intakes (DRIs) for all	DRIs for B complex and C vitamins; individualize vitamin D, zinc, and iron	DRIs for B complex and C vitamins; individualize vitamin D, zinc, and iron	DRIs for B complex and C vitamins; individualize vitamin D, zinc, and iron

Modified from Fedje L, Karalis M: Nutrition management in early stages of chronic kidney failure. In Byham-Gray L, Stover J, Wiesen K, editors: *A clinical guide to nutrition care in kidney disease, ed 2,* Chicago, 2013, Academy of Nutrition and Dietetics. Copyright Academy of Nutrition and Dietetics. Reprinted with permission.

phosphorus per day, of which 80% to 90% is reabsorbed by the renal tubules and the remaining 10% is excreted into urine. Phosphorus balance can be maintained until the GFR falls below 20 mL/min. At that point, phosphorus accumulation occurs in the serum. In addition, conversion of vitamin D to the active form 1,25-dihydrocholecalciferol is diminished, resulting in low serum calcium levels and elevated parathyroid hormone (PTH) levels. Dietary intervention for bone disease management is dietary phosphorus restriction to 8 to 12 mg of phosphorus per kilogram of body weight per day. In addition to dietary phosphate restriction, most patients require oral calcium, oral or intravenous vitamin D, or vitamin D analogs (or a combination of these therapies). Serum PTH, calcium, and phosphorus levels must be monitored closely to avoid excesses and deficiencies that can exacerbate the bone disease.[10]

Iron

Because of the diminished ability of the failing kidney to synthesize adequate amounts of erythropoietin, most patients with chronic renal failure develop anemia if left untreated. Recommended levels for hematocrit are 33% to 36%; for hemoglobin (Hb), 11 to 12 g/dL. These target levels are accomplished through administration of recombinant human erythropoietin (r-HuEPO) and 10 to 18 mg oral iron. Doses are individualized. If left untreated, then adverse clinical events can occur, including increased mortality rates, malnutrition, angina, cardiac enlargement, and impaired immunologic response.

Calories and Protein

K/DOQI guidelines for CKD recommend 0.6 g protein per kilogram of body weight per day when GFR is less than

25 mL/min and the patient is not on dialysis. For individuals who do not want to observe this diet or are unable to maintain adequate caloric intake, a diet providing protein in the amount of 0.75 g/kg/day should be considered. At this same level of GFR, caloric intake for patients younger than 60 years is recommended to be 35 kcal/kg/day; for those 60 years or older, 30 to 35 kcal/kg/day.[11] Other diet recommendations that integrate current data concerning protein, calories, fatty acids, vitamins, and minerals until additional data are available are listed in Table 23-4.

MEDICAL NUTRITION THERAPY

Chronic Kidney Disease Stages 1 to 4

Nutrition goals for CKD stages 1 to 4 should center on comorbid states (diabetes, hypertension, and hyperlipidemia) and slowing development of potential CVD[3,11]:

- Protein: 0.60 to 0.75 g/kg of body weight, 50% or greater high biologic value (HBV) protein
- Energy: 35 kcal/kg of body weight for younger than 60 years of age; 30 to 35 kcal/kg of body weight for older than 60 years of age
- Sodium: 1 to 3 g/day
- Potassium: usually unrestricted unless serum level is high
- Phosphorus: 800 to 1000 mg/day when serum phosphorus is greater than 4.6 mg/dL or parathyroid hormone (PTH) is elevated

---

KEY TERM

osteodystrophy Defective bone formation.

- Calcium 1.0 g/day to 1.5 g/day, not to exceed 2 g/day with binder load
- Fluid: no restriction
- Vitamins/minerals: Daily Reference Intakes (DRIs) for B complex and vitamin C; individualize vitamin D, iron, and zinc

Chronic Kidney Disease Stage 5

A patient requiring maintenance hemodialysis usually requires two or three treatments per week, with each treatment lasting $2\frac{1}{2}$ to 5 hours. During treatment the patient's blood circulates through the dialysis solution in an artificial kidney (the dialyzer), maintaining normal blood levels of life-sustaining substances the patient's own kidneys can no longer accomplish. An alternative form of peritoneal dialysis is practical for long-term ambulatory therapy at home.

The diet of a patient on kidney dialysis is a vital aspect of maintaining biochemical control. Several basic objectives govern each individually tailored diet, designed to (1) maintain adequate protein and calorie intake, (2) prevent dehydration or fluid overload, (3) maintain normal serum potassium and sodium blood levels, and (4) maintain acceptable phosphate and calcium levels[3,11]:

- Protein: 1.2 g/kg or more of body weight, 50% or greater HBV protein (at least 50% of dietary protein should come from HBV protein [meats, poultry, game, fish, eggs, soy, and dairy])
- Energy: 35 kcal/kg of body weight for patients younger than 60 years old; 30 to 35 kcal/kg of body weight for patients older than 60 years old
- Sodium: 1 to 3 g/day
- Potassium: 2 to 3 g/day; adjust based on serum levels
- Phosphorus: 800 to 1000 mg/day when serum phosphorus is greater than 5.5 mg/dL or PTH is elevated
- Calcium: 2 g/day or less; include binder load
- Fluid: urine output +1000 cc
- Vitamins/minerals:
  - Vitamin C: 60 to 100 mg/day
  - Vitamin B$_6$: 2 mg/day
  - Folate: 1 mg/day
  - Vitamin B$_{12}$: 3 mcg/day
  - DRIs for all other water-soluble vitamins
  - Vitamin E: 15 IU/day
  - Zinc: 15 mg/day
  - Iron and vitamin D: individualize

Stage 5: Peritoneal Dialysis

An alternative form of dialysis, peritoneal dialysis, allows dialysate solutions to flow directly through a catheter port established through the abdominal wall into the abdominal cavity. The solution is typically a dextrose-salt solution. High osmolality of the solution causes waste materials to diffuse across the saclike **peritoneum** lining the abdominal cavity (see the Perspectives in Practice box, "Peritoneal Dialysis"). Then this dialysate collection of waste materials flows back into the dialysate bag for disposal. The peritoneal membrane serves as the filtering mechanism.[12]

Two main types of peritoneal dialysis exist:
1. Continuous ambulatory peritoneal dialysis (CAPD), in which a dialysis solution in a plastic pouch is infused and drained via gravity each day (24 hours), five times at 4-hour intervals
2. Continuous cyclic peritoneal dialysis (CCPD), in which three or four machine-delivered exchanges are given at night, about 3 hours each, leaving about 2 L of dialysate solution in the peritoneal cavity for 12 to 15 hours during the day

Nutritional concerns specific to peritoneal dialysis involve calories contributed by the dialysate, which are usually 1.5%, 2.5%, or 4.25% dextrose in 1.5 to 2 L of solution, and the concern that fluid and potassium intake can be liberalized compared with hemodialysis because of the enhanced clearance of potassium.

- Protein: 1.2 to 1.3 g/kg or more of body weight, 50% or greater HBV
- Energy: 35 kcal/kg of body weight for patients younger than 60 years old; 30 to 35 kcal/kg of body weight for patients older than 60 years old, including dialysate calories
- Sodium: 2 to 4 g/day; monitor fluid balance
- Potassium: 3 to 4 g/day; adjust to serum levels
- Phosphorus: 800 to 1000 mg/day when serum phosphorus is more than 5.5 mg/dL or PTH is elevated
- Calcium: 2 g/day or less; include binder load
- Fluid: maintain balance
- Vitamins/minerals:
  - Vitamin C: 60 to 100 mg/day
  - Vitamin B$_6$: 2 mg/day
  - Folate: 1 mg/day
  - Vitamin B$_{12}$: 3 mcg/day
  - Vitamin B$_{12}$: may need 1.5 to 2 mg/day because of dialysis losses
  - DRIs for all other B vitamins
  - Vitamin E: 15 IU/day
  - Zinc: 15 mg/day
  - Iron and vitamin D: individualize

Table 23-5 summarizes dietary recommendations for patients receiving hemodialysis and peritoneal dialysis.

Kidney Transplantation

Nutritional care of kidney transplant recipients is divided into three phases: (1) pretransplantation, (2) acute posttransplantation, and (3) chronic posttransplantation. Pretransplant nutrition concerns are based on current renal replacement therapy, if any, along with assessment of nutritional status.[13]

KEY TERM

peritoneum A strong smooth surface—a serous membrane—lining the abdominal and pelvic walls and the undersurface of the diaphragm, forming a sac that encloses the body's vital visceral organs within the peritoneal cavity.

PERSPECTIVES IN PRACTICE

Peritoneal Dialysis

A variety of types of peritoneal dialysis exist; the two main types are continuous ambulatory peritoneal dialysis (CAPD) and continuous cyclic peritoneal dialysis (CCPD). The choice of which type of peritoneal dialysis to perform depends on lifestyle and clinical considerations, much the same way the decision to choose hemodialysis or peritoneal dialysis is made. CAPD is an ambulatory dialysis procedure that introduces dialysate directly into the peritoneal cavity. Solutes and water flow across the peritoneal membrane into dialysate fluid. This is accomplished by attaching a disposable bag containing dialysate to a catheter permanently inserted into the peritoneal cavity, waiting an individually prescribed amount of time (i.e., "dwell time") for solution exchange, and then lowering the bag to allow the force of gravity to cause the waste-containing fluid to drain into it. When the bag is empty, it can be folded around the waist or tucked into a pocket, allowing the user mobility.

The exchange takes place via osmosis and diffusion, with the rate being determined in part by the amount of dextrose in the solution. The most common dialysate solutions are 1.5%, 2.5%, or 4.25% dextrose in 1.5 to 2 L of solution. The actual rate of solute transport, type and number of peritoneal dialysis exchanges, and solution dwell times vary among patients. Each patient is prescribed an individualized dialysis prescription that includes the number and type of dialysate solutions to use each day and the length of dwell times. A method to determine membrane function and the optimal peritoneal dialysis method for each patient is the peritoneal equilibration test. Peritoneal solute and solvent movement rates vary among patients and over time can vary even within the same patient. Therefore clinical monitoring of dialysis adequacy is important. Patients using CAPD as a renal replacement therapy have better mobility than those on hemodialysis. In addition, they typically have a more liberal diet in regard to dietary potassium, phosphorus, and total fluid intake due in large part to the more continuous nature of the therapy. Protein requirement is increased and can be a challenge for some patients. Table 23-5 lists the nutritional recommendations for patients on peritoneal dialysis. Special nutrient considerations are as follows:

- *Protein and amino acid* losses average 5 to 15 g/24 hours; amino acid losses average 3 g/day (see Table 23-5 for protein requirements).
- *Potassium* requirements depend on the number of solution exchanges, whether the patient has any residual renal function, and the individual clearance characteristics of the patient's peritoneal membrane. On average, potassium recommendation is 3 to 4 g/day. Some patients will require potassium supplementation.
- *Phosphorus-binding antacids* are not as needed because of improved control of phosphorus blood levels with CAPD use.
- *Dietary sodium* is usually restricted to 2 to 4 g/day. The recommendation must be individualized in accordance to the patient's fluid status, blood pressure, and thirst.
- *Fluid* requirements depend on weight, blood pressure, and residual renal function.

CAPD poses nutrition-related problems related to weight gain from the dialysate and, on the other end of the spectrum, anorexia because of glucose absorption from the dialysate.

One method available to calculate glucose absorption in an individualized manner is the D/D_0 formula: grams of glucose absorbed.

$$\text{Glucose (g)} = (1 - D/D_0)\, x_i,$$

where D_0 is initial dextrose in the dialysate at zero hours (g); D is remaining dextrose in the dialysate after an appropriate dwell time (g); D/D_0 is the fraction of glucose remaining in the dialysate; and x_i is initial glucose instilled:

- 13 g/L for 1.5% dextrose
- 22 g/L for 2.5% dextrose
- 38 g/L for 4.25% dextrose

In addition to posing possible weight management problems, extra dextrose can lead to elevated triglycerides and low-density lipoprotein (LDL) levels and depressed levels of protective high-density lipoproteins (HDLs), thus increasing risk of coronary heart disease in long-term users.

Nutritionists and nurses who counsel patients being transferred from hemodialysis to a CAPD regimen may find that patients need guidance in adjusting to their new diet. The following guidelines may be helpful:

- Increase potassium intake by eating a wide variety of fruits and vegetables each day.
- Encourage liberal fluid intake to prevent dehydration.
- Encourage complex carbohydrates while avoiding overindulging in concentrated sweets to help control triglyceride and HDL levels.
- Maintain lean body weight by incorporating the kcalories provided by the dialysate into the total meal plan (to be calculated and explained to the patient by the renal dietitian).

Bibliography

National Kidney Foundation: K/DOQI clinical practice guidelines for nutrition in chronic renal failure. *Am J Kidney Dis* 35(Suppl 2):S9, 2000.

National Kidney Foundation: Kidney disease outcomes quality initiative (K/DOQI): practice guidelines for peritoneal dialysis adequacy. *Am J Kidney Dis* 37(Suppl 1):S55, 2001.

Passadakis T, Vagemezis V, Oreopoulos D: Peritoneal dialysis: better than, equal to, or worse than hemodialysis? Data worth knowing before choosing a dialysis modality. *Perit Dial Int* 21:25, 2001.

Theofilou P: Quality of life in patients undergoing hemodialysis or peritoneal dialysis treatment. *J Clin Med Res* 3(3):132–138, 2011.

Valderrabano F, Lopez-Gomez J: Quality of life in end-stage renal disease patients. *Am J Kidney Dis* 38(3):443, 2001.

Wiggins K: *Guidelines for nutrition care of renal patients*, ed 3, Chicago, 2002, American Dietetic Association.

TABLE 23-5	NUTRITIONAL RECOMMENDATIONS FOR PATIENTS ON HEMODIALYSIS AND PERITONEAL DIALYSIS THERAPY	
NUTRIENT	**HEMODIALYSIS**	**PERITONEAL DIALYSIS**
Protein (g/kg)*	1.2 average weight (50% HBV)	1.2-1.3 SBW or adjusted BW (>50% HBV)
Energy (kcal/kg)*	30 kcal/kg if <60 years of age and 30-35 kcal/kg if >60 years of age or obese	30-35 if >60 years of age and 35 if <60 years of age
If patient <90% or >115% of median standard weight, use aBW$_{ef}$		
Phosphorus	800-1000 mg/day or <17 mg/kg IBW or SBW	800-1000 mg or 10-15 mg phosphorus/g protein
Sodium	2-4 g if fluid output ≥1 L	
	2 g if fluid output ≤1 L	2-4 g
	2 g if anuria	
Potassium	40 mg/kg IBW or SBW	2-4 g (considered consistent with unrestricted diet)
Fluid	2 L if fluid output ≥1 L	1-3 L/day
	1-1.5 L if fluid output ≤1 L	
	1 L if anuria	
Calcium	Individualized	<2000 mg including diet and binders

Data from Biesecker R, Stuart N: Nutrition management of the adult hemodialysis patient. In Byham-Gray L, Wiesen K, editors: *A clinical guide to nutrition care in kidney disease*, Chicago, 2004, American Dietetic Association; McCann L: Nutrition management of the adult peritoneal dialysis patient. In Byham-Gray L, Wiesen K, editors: *A clinical guide to nutrition care in kidney disease*, Chicago, 2004, American Dietetic Association.
BW, Body weight; *BW$_{ef}$*, edema-free body weight; *HBV*, high biologic value; *IBW*, ideal body weight; *SBW*, standard body weight.
*For continuous ambulatory peritoneal dialysis (CAPD) and automated peritoneal dialysis (APD) include dialysate calories.

TABLE 23-6	NUTRITIONAL GUIDELINES FOR ADULT KIDNEY TRANSPLANT RECIPIENTS	
NUTRIENT	**ACUTE PERIOD**	**CHRONIC PERIOD**
Protein	1.3-2 g/kg[a]	0.8-1 g/kg; limit with chronic graft dysfunction
Energy	30-35 kcal/kg[a] or BEE × 1.3 (may increase with postoperative complications)	Adjust calories to maintain desirable body weight
Carbohydrates	Limit simple carbohydrate intake with elevated blood glucose levels and/or unwanted weight gain	Emphasize complex carbohydrate intake and distribution
Fat	Remainder of calories	Emphasize PUFA and MUFA
Potassium	2-4 g if hyperkalemic	Unrestricted unless hyperkalemic
Sodium	Restrict if blood pressure/fluid status dictates	2-4 g with hypertension and/or edema
Calcium	1200-1500 mg	1200-1500 mg
Phosphorus	DRIs; may need supplementation to normalize serum levels	DRIs[b]
Fluids	Limited only by graft function (generally unrestricted)	Limited only by graft function (generally unrestricted)

From Cochran CC, Kent PS: Nutrition management of the renal transplant patient. In Byham-Gray L, Stover J, Wiesen K, editors: *A clinical guide to nutrition care in kidney disease*, ed 2, Chicago, 2013, Academy of Nutrition and Dietetics. Copyright Academy of Nutrition and Dietetics. Reprinted with permission.
BEE, Basal energy expenditure; *DRIs*, Dietary Reference Intakes; *MUFA*, monounsaturated fatty acids; *PUFA*, polyunsaturated fatty acids.
[a]Based on standard or adjusted body weight.
[b]Due to lack of research, no specific recommendations are available for this population. Currently the DRI is used as guideline.

The nutritional challenges of the acute posttransplant period are most often related to posttransplantation medications (see the Evidence-Based Practice box, "Kidney Transplantation"). Hyperlipidemia, weight gain, and abnormal blood glucose levels can result, often because of side effects of the antirejection medications such as corticosteroids and cyclosporine A.[14] Foodborne infections can be life-threatening for transplant patients receiving immunosuppressive medications; therefore food safety education should be routinely included.

During the chronic posttransplant period, overnutrition may lead to complications such as obesity, dyslipidemias,

diabetes mellitus, and hypertension. Nutritional goals are to provide adequate nutrition, prevent infection, and manage long-term nutritional complications.[13] A summation of nutritional guidelines for this patient group is provided in Table 23-6.

ACUTE RENAL FAILURE

The catabolic acute renal failure (ARF) patient, most frequently encountered in the intensive care setting, presents a management challenge to the entire team of physicians, nurses, dietitians, respiratory therapists, dialysis staff,

Kidney Transplantation

Thousands of patients await transplantation every year. Others cannot consider a transplant because of medical or psychosocial issues (or because of both). Overall, kidney transplantation remains the treatment of choice for the majority of patients with CKD. Advances in solid organ transplantation and immunosuppressive therapy have resulted in improved patient survival and improved viability of transplanted kidneys.

Nearly 50% of all kidney transplant recipients will be alive with a successful functioning transplant 10 years after transplantation. One-year cadaver kidney success rates are 89%, and 5-year success rates are 65%. In comparison, success rates for recipients of living donor kidneys are 97% at 1 year and 78% at 5 years. A patient who is trouble free for the first 3 months after the transplantation has an excellent prognosis. Most common causes of death after the first year are cardiovascular disease (CVD), infection, and cancer.

The patient who receives a kidney transplant has a challenging first year. Visits to the transplant team occur an average of two or three times per week during the first month and once per week for up to 3 months after the surgery. Visits then drop to once monthly during the first year if no problems occur. After the first year it is recommended that patients have their laboratory parameters monitored every 1 to 2 months.

Medication regimens are challenging for the transplant recipient. Immunosuppressive agents, lipid-lowering drugs, antihypertensives, and hypoglycemic agents are needed for quite some time. Significant side effects can occur from these medicines, and adherence to the rigid medication schedule is critical for successful allograft survival. Medical problems that can develop during the first year include infections such as cytomegalovirus, hyperlipidemia, bone disease, diabetes, CVD, hypertension, and dental problems. Weight gain as a side effect of medications can also become a problem (see Table 23-6 for nutritional recommendations for the kidney transplant recipient).

Morbidity and mortality rates for kidney transplantation are clinically significant. These statistics should improve as advances in the technology of the surgery and pharmacologic management occur over time. Not every patient will medically qualify for transplantation, and every candidate must be assessed for his or her ability to meet the demands of the posttransplantation period. In addition, evidence suggests that living kidney donors have survival similar to nondonors, and their risk of CKD is not increased.

In the future, perhaps the availability of organs for transplantation will be increased by improvements in living-related surgeries, development of artificial organs, and most optimistically, finding a cure for progressive kidney disease.

Bibliography

2001 Annual report: End Stage Renal Disease Clinical Performance Measures Project. *Am J Kidney Dis* 39(Suppl 2):S1, 2002.

Baiardi F, Degli Esposti E, Cocchi R, et al: Effects of clinical and individual variables on quality of life in chronic renal failure patients. *J Nephrol* 15(1):61, 2002.

Braun WE: Update on kidney transplantation: increasing clinical success, expanding waiting lists. *Cleve Clin J Med* 69(6):501, 2002.

Ibrahim HN, Foley R, Tan L, et al: Long-term consequences of kidney donation. *N Engl J Med* 360(5):459, 2009.

Matas AJ, Halbert RJ, Barr ML, et al: Life satisfaction and adverse effects in renal transplant recipients: a longitudinal analysis. *Clin Transplant* 16(2):113, 2002.

pharmacists, and other technicians. These patients are in negative nitrogen balance and generate much urea resulting from the catabolic process. Infection is a major threat, and it aggravates the existing malnutrition.

Disease Process

Renal failure may occur acutely with sudden shutdown of renal function after some metabolic insult or traumatic injury to normal kidneys. It is typically characterized by retention of nitrogenous waste products, fluid overload, acid-base disturbances, electrolyte imbalance, and hemodynamic instability. ARF is linked with major in-hospital morbidity and mortality.[15] Immediate and continuing nutrition support is essential.

ARF may have various causes: (1) severe injury such as extensive burns or crushing injuries that cause widespread tissue destruction; (2) infectious diseases such as peritonitis; (3) traumatic shock after surgery on the abdominal aorta; (4) toxic agents in the environment such as carbon tetrachloride or poisonous mushrooms; or (5) immunologic drug reactions such as penicillin reaction in allergic or sensitive persons.[15]

Clinical Symptoms

The major sign of ARF is oliguria (diminished urine output) often accompanied by proteinuria or hematuria. This diminished urine output is brought on by underlying tissue problems that characterize ARF. Usually blockage of tubules is seen, caused by cellular debris from tissue trauma or urinary failure with backup retention of filtrate materials.[15]

Oliguria

Diminished urinary output is a cardinal symptom, often with proteinuria or hematuria accompanying the small output. Water balance becomes a crucial factor. The course of the disease is usually divided into an oliguric phase followed by a diuretic phase. The urinary output during the oliguric phase varies from as little as 20 to 200 mL/day.

KEY TERM

oliguria Secretion of a very small amount of urine in relation to fluid intake.

Anorexia, Nausea, and Lethargy

During this initial phase of ARF, the patient may be lethargic and anorectic and experience nausea and vomiting. Blood pressure elevation and signs of uremia may be present. Oral intake is usually difficult in this catabolic period.[15]

Increasing Serum Urea Nitrogen and Creatinine Levels

During the initial catabolic period after injury, surgery, or some other metabolic dysfunction, the serum urea nitrogen level increases along with the creatinine level. These increases result from tissue breakdown of muscle mass. Blood potassium, phosphate, and sulfate levels also increase, and sodium, calcium, and bicarbonate levels decrease.[15]

Basic Treatment Goals

Treatment must be individualized, adjusted according to the progression of the illness, the type of treatment being used, and the patient's response. In general, however, basic therapy objectives are as follows[15]:

- Reduce and minimize protein breakdown
- Prevent protein catabolism, and minimize uremic toxicity
- Prevent dehydration or overhydration
- Correct acidosis carefully
- Correct electrolyte depletions, and avoid excesses
- Control fluid and electrolyte losses from vomiting and diarrhea
- Maintain optimal nutritional status
- Maintain appetite, general morale, and sense of well-being
- Control complications—hypertension, bone pain, nervous system problems

Nutritional Requirements for Patients with Acute Renal Failure

The nutrition requirements for the ARF patient are directly influenced by the type of renal replacement therapy (if any), nutritional and metabolic status, and degree of hypercatabolism. Current recommendations for protein and calories for this patient population are defined in the following discussion.

When energy requirements cannot be measured directly, calorie requirements can usually be met by providing 25 to 35 kcal/kg IBW, reserving the upper limit of the range for patients who are severely catabolic and whose nitrogen balance does not improve at lower intakes.[15] Protein sources containing essential and nonessential amino acids should be provided. For patients whose ARF is expected to resolve in a few days and who are not catabolic and will not need dialysis, 0.8 to 1.2 g/kg body weight of protein is recommended. The patient's nutritional and metabolic status and renal diagnosis determine the exact dose. For patients who are catabolic, receiving acute hemodialysis, or both, the recommendation is 1.2 to 1.5 g/kg body weight of protein.[15]

Total fluid intake for any patient depends on the amount of residual renal function (i.e., if the patient is oliguric or anuric) and fluid and sodium status. In general, fluid intake can be calculated by adding 500 mL (for insensible losses) to the 24-hour urine output. During diuresis, fluids should be increased to prevent dehydration.[15]

Although the diet should be as liberal as possible to support sufficient intake, nutrient needs should be frequently reevaluated because requirements may change as a consequence of resumption of kidney function, use of dialysis, and anabolism. Sodium needs may increase to restore losses from diuresis, but the general recommendation is 2 to 3 g per day. Potassium requirements depend on lab values and the degree of hyperkalemia. In general, 2 to 3 g/day is suggested, but requirements may possibly increase with dialysis, restoration of kidney function, and anabolism. Phosphate binders may be necessary, along with a restriction of 8 to 15 mg/kg body weight per day. Requirements may increase with daily dialysis, return of kidney function, and anabolism.[15]

UROLITHIASIS (CALCULI OR KIDNEY STONES)

Disease Process

Kidney stone disease is an ancient medical problem. Records of its incidence have appeared in medical documents since the days of Hippocrates. It continues to be a prevalent health problem. Multiple stone attacks affect 12% of American men and 5% of women during their lifetimes.[16]

Kidney stone disease appears to be chronic and recurrent. Calculi form when excessive amounts of reasonably insoluble salts are found in the urine or when inadequate fluid intake creates highly concentrated urine. When any solid substance forms, sediment continues to build up. The salts that form crystals can grow to form stones.[16] Immobility can also cause calculi because of stasis of urine and ensuing chemical alterations.[16,17] The existence of stones typically becomes evident only when they obstruct the flow of urine.[17]

Although the basic cause of kidney stones remains unknown, many factors contribute directly or indirectly to their formation. These factors relate to the nature of the urine itself or to conditions of the urinary tract environment. The risk for urinary calculi development is affected by a number of factors, including age, gender, race, geographic location, seasonal factors, fluid intake, diet, and occupation. Geographic locations affect stone formation as the result of indirect factors such as average temperature, humidity, and rainfall, and their influence on fluid and dietary patterns.[16] According to the concentration of urinary constituents, roughly 75% of major stones formed are calcium stones. The rest consist chiefly of uric acid, struvite, or cystine (Figure 23-4).[17]

Major Types of Stones
Calcium Stones

Calcium stones are composed of calcium compounds, usually calcium oxalate, calcium carbonate, or calcium phosphate. Calcium stones form as a result of hypercalciuria that can

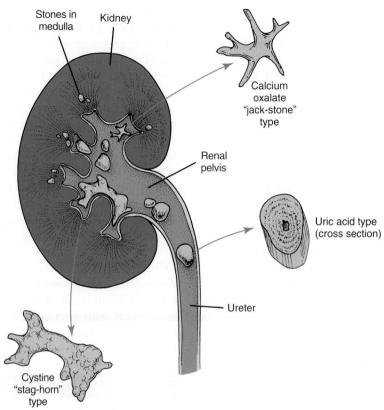

FIGURE 23-4 Renal stones in kidney, pelvis, and ureter.

result from alkaline urine, inadequate fluid intake, high levels of dietary oxalate (see Appendix B), prolonged immobilization, or parathyroid tumor.[16,17] Oxalates occur naturally only in a few food sources, and individual absorption and excretion rates influence availability. Only eight foods cause a significant increase in urinary oxalate excretion: (1) spinach, (2) rhubarb, (3) beets, (4) nuts, (5) chocolate, (6) tea, (7) wheat bran, and (8) strawberries. Nutrition therapy for individuals prone to stone formation may be limited to restriction of these eight foods, with results monitored by laboratory analysis of urine composition.

- *Animal protein:* A diet high in animal protein, such as the typical American diet, has been linked to increased excretions of calcium, oxalate, and urate. A vegetarian type of diet has been recommended by some investigators as a wise choice for persons prone to stone formation.
- *Dietary fiber:* Added dietary fiber has been found to reduce risk factors for stone formation, especially calcium stones.

Struvite Stones

Next to calcium stones in frequency are struvite stones, composed of a single compound—magnesium ammonium phosphate ($MgNH_4PO_4$). These are often called *infection stones* because they are associated with UTIs. The offending organism in the infection is *Proteus mirabilis.* This is a urea-splitting bacterium that contains urease, an enzyme that hydrolyzes urea to ammonia. Thus urinary pH becomes alkaline. In the ammonia-rich environment, struvite precipitates

and forms large, "staghorn" stones.[16] Surgical removal is usually indicated.

Uric Acid Stones

Excess uric acid excretion may be caused by an impairment in intermediary metabolism of purine, as occurs in gout. Cancer chemotherapy may also cause urine to be acidic, which aids in hyperuricemia.

Cystine Stones

A hereditary metabolic defect in renal tubular reabsorption of the amino acid cystine causes this substance to accumulate in urine. This condition is called *cystinuria.* Because this is a genetic disorder, it is characterized by early onset and a positive family history. This is one of the most common metabolic disorders associated with kidney stones in children before puberty.

Clinical Symptoms

Severe pain and numerous urinary symptoms may result, with general weakness and sometimes fever. Laboratory examination of urine and chemical analysis of any stone passed help determine treatment.

General Treatment
Fluid Intake

Large fluid intake produces a more dilute urine and is a foundation of therapy. Dilute urine helps to prevent concentration of stone constituents.

Urinary pH

An attempt to control solubility factor is made by changing urinary pH to an increased acidity or alkalinity, depending on the chemical composition of the stone formed. An exception is calcium oxalate stones because solubility of calcium oxalate in urine is not pH dependent. Conversely, however, calcium phosphate is soluble in an acid urine.

Stone Composition

When possible, dietary constituents of the stone are controlled to reduce the amount of the substance available for precipitation.

Binding Agents

Materials that bind stone elements and prevent their absorption in the intestine cause fecal excretion. For example, sodium phytate is used to bind calcium, and aluminum gels are used to bind phosphate. Glycine and calcium have a similar effect on oxalates.

Alternative Remedies

A number of herbs are also used to help prevent the development of kidney stones (see the Complementary and Alternative Medicine [CAM] box, "Common Herbal Treatments for Kidney Stones").

Nutrition Therapy

Manipulation of single nutritional components is usually not effective. General nutrition recommendations for kidney stones entail the following[18]:

- Protein: not to exceed the DRI of 0.8-1.0 g/kg body weight/day
- Calcium: should not be restricted; intake should be balanced throughout the day
- Fluids: 12-16 cups to produce urine volume to more than 2.5 L/day
- Oxalate: less than 40-50 mg/day
- Sodium: decrease intake to 2300 (100 mEq) to 3450 (250 mEq) mg/day
- Energy: level to maintain healthy weight
- Vitamin and mineral supplements: vitamin C should be restricted to DRI; B vitamins have not been shown to be harmful

URINARY TRACT INFECTION

Disease Process

The term *UTI* refers to a wide variety of clinical infections in which a significant number of microorganisms are present in any portion of the urinary tract. A common form is cystitis, an inflammation of the bladder that is very prevalent in young women. At least 20% of women experience a UTI during their lifetime, of which the vast majority are cases of uncomplicated cystitis.[16,17] The condition is called *recurrent UTI* if three or more bouts are experienced in 1 year.

The majority of cases are caused by aerobic members of the fecal flora, especially *Escherichia coli*. The presence of these organisms in urine is termed *bacteriuria*. Urine produced by the normal kidney is sterile and remains so as it travels to the bladder. In UTIs, however, the normal urethra has microbial flora; therefore any voided urine generally contains many bacteria. Bacteriuria is present when the quantity of organisms is more than 100,000/mL of urine. The female anatomy is more conducive to entry of these bacteria into the urinary tract. Recurrent cystitis occurs mostly in young and otherwise healthy women who have infections that usually correspond with sexual activity and continued diaphragm use. In most cases, simply changing to another birth control method will solve the problem. Cystitis is characterized by frequent voiding and burning on urination.

Treatment

Although regular consumption of cranberry juice can help prevent UTIs, it is not effective for treatment. Intake of adequate fluids helps to produce a dilute urine. It is important to control a UTI, because UTIs are a risk factor in stone formation.

RESOURCES

The renal diet is complex and presents a challenge to practitioners and even more so to patients. A basic resource, the National Renal Diet educational series, provides valuable guides. These standardized guidelines for nutrition intervention and patient education in renal disease have been developed by the collaborative work of renal dietitians from the Academy of Nutrition and Dietetics Renal Dietitians Dietetic Practice Group and the National Kidney Foundation Council on Renal Nutrition. The *Professional Guide* can be used in conjunction with other guides from the Academy of Nutrition and Dietetics for the care of renal disease patients. Because dietary management must be tailored to the stage of the disease and method of treatment, the series of materials contains a professional guide and six client booklets, each designed with special food lists to meet specific needs of the various renal disease requirements. These Academy of Nutrition and Dietetics resources give the practitioner a comprehensive basis for individualizing dietary instructions and provide the patient and family with a practical guide for everyday decisions and plans for food choices.

The Council on Renal Nutrition of the National Kidney Foundation is an expert resource for information. Membership includes a subscription to the *Journal of Renal Nutrition*, a quarterly publication geared toward nutritionists, scientists, and physicians interested and working in the fields of nephrology and renal nutrition. (For contact information, see the Websites of Interest section at the end of this chapter.)

Nutritional status and care have been documented to have important roles in patient outcomes; therefore interest in renal nutrition and the number of online resources have substantially increased. (See the Websites of Interest section for a listing of websites that provide excellent information and

COMPLEMENTARY AND ALTERNATIVE MEDICINE (CAM)

Common Herbal Treatments for Kidney Stones

Patients interested in complementary and alternative medicine may also be interested in knowing low fluid intake greatly increases risk of developing all types of kidney stones.

HERB	EFFICACY	SIDE EFFECTS AND/OR RISKS	DRUG INTERACTION
Citrate	Might help prevent oxalate and acid stones by binding with calcium in urine, reducing the amount of calcium available to form calcium oxalate stones. It also alkalizes urine, inhibiting development of calcium oxalate and uric acid stones.		Increases serum levels of ephedra, flecainide, mecamylamine, and methamphetamine. Decreases serum levels of lithium, methotrexate, salicylates, sulfonylureas, and tetracyclines. Hyperkalemia can occur when taking ACE inhibitors and potassium-sparing diuretics.
Calcium	Calcium supplements might slightly increase kidney stone risk, whereas dietary calcium reduces risk of kidney stones.	Increased intakes are associated with increased risk of prostate cancer.	Concurrent use of calcium with pheasant's eye (Adonis vernalis) increases risk of cardiac toxicity. CCBs can be affected by combinations of calcium supplements and high doses of vitamin D. Might decrease blood level of atenolol (β-blocker) and possibly other β-blockers. Interferes with absorption of tetracyclines and levothyroxine. Excess intake can interfere with absorption of iron, zinc, magnesium, iodine, manganese, and copper.
Magnesium (magnesium oxide or magnesium hydroxide)	No strong evidence that magnesium prevents calcium oxalate stones.	Should not be taken by those with severe heart or kidney disease without consultation with a health care provider.	Might decrease absorption of psyllium.
Vitamin B₆ (pyridoxamine)	Weak evidence indicates that vitamin B₆ might help prevent calcium oxalate stones.	Vitamin B₆ deficiency increases the amount of oxalate in urine. Large doses may cause nausea, vomiting, and potential risk of neurotoxicity.	None were found.
GLA (omega-6 oils, omega-6 fatty acids, evening primrose oil, black currant oil, borage oil)	No evidence is available.	No adverse effects have been noted.	Increases bleeding time when used with anticoagulant therapy. GLA is synergistic with paclitaxel.

ACE, Angiotensin-converting enzyme; *CCBs,* calcium channel blockers; *GLA,* γ-linolenic acid.

Bibliography
Bratman S, Girman AM: *Mosby's handbook of herbs and supplements and their therapeutic uses,* St Louis, 2003, Mosby.

Herr SM: *Herb-drug interaction handbook,* ed 2, Nassau, NY, 2002, Church Street Books.

links to other sites pertaining to renal nutrition and nephrology.)

HEALTH PROMOTION

OMEGA-3 FATTY ACIDS AND RENAL DISEASE

Despite countless research efforts, the mechanisms responsible for the progressive nature of renal disease remain elusive. Historically, nutrition science has been an inherent component of research directed toward identifying nutrient manipulations that ameliorate kidney disease, metabolic abnormalities associated with chronic renal insufficiency, and mechanisms by which nutrients modulate factors involved in promoting exacerbation of existing disease. In all of these research areas, dietary protein, phosphorus, and caloric deprivation have been more widely studied than other nutrients. However, more recently, research interest has become directed toward dietary essential fatty acids (EFAs). This shift is in response to a growing body of evidence indicating that fatty

acid substitution of cell membrane phospholipids modulates biochemical pathways implicated in the pathophysiology of progressive kidney disease and CVD, which are so prominent in the renal patient population.

It has been demonstrated that altering the availability of EFAs can influence the natural course of several important diseases in the mammalian organism. For example, epidemiologic studies of the Dutch, Japanese, and native Greenland Eskimo populations attribute their low incidence of heart disease to a fish diet high in omega-3 fatty acids. Beneficial observations have included an improved lipid profile, prolonged survival, and improved renal function.

Dietary EFAs are direct precursors to the biologically diverse and potent class of compounds called *eicosanoids*. EFAs can also modulate cellular production of interleukins (ILs). Several chronic inflammatory and renal diseases are characterized in part by an overproduction of eicosanoids and ILs. These facts suggest manipulation of dietary fatty acids might contribute a therapeutic influence by altering proinflammatory and other activated pathways in disease processes.

TO SUM UP

Through its unique functional units, the nephrons, the kidneys act as a filtration system, reabsorbing substances the body needs, secreting additional hydrogen ions to maintain a proper pH balance in the blood, and excreting unnecessary materials in a concentrated urine.

Renal function may be impaired by a variety of conditions. These include inflammatory and degenerative diseases, infection and obstruction, chronic diseases such as hypertension and diabetes, environmental agents such as insecticides and solvents and other toxic substances, and some medications and trauma. Some clinical conditions that affect structure

and function include glomerulonephritis, ARF and chronic renal failure, renal calculi, and UTIs.

Stage 5 of CKD is treated by dialysis—hemodialysis or peritoneal dialysis—and kidney transplantation. The diet for CKD needs to include ample calories and protein with restrictions for GFR of less than 25 mL/min/1.73 m^2 only if the patient is able to maintain adequate caloric intake. Dialysis patients must be monitored closely for calories, protein, fluid, and electrolyte balance. All of the diets need to be individualized to ensure overall nutritional adequacy and adherence. Monitoring of nutritional status is important for all patients.

QUESTIONS FOR REVIEW

1. For each of the following conditions, outline nutritional components of therapy, explaining effect of each on kidney function: glomerulonephritis, ARF (renal insufficiency), and chronic renal failure.
2. Identify four clinical conditions that impair renal function. Give an example of each, describing its effect on various structures in the kidney.
3. List nutritional factors that must be monitored in individuals undergoing renal dialysis.

4. Summarize the rationale and nutrient recommendations for patients who have received a renal transplant.
5. Outline nutrition therapy used for patients with various types of kidney stones. Describe each type of stone and explain the rationale for each aspect of therapy.
6. For what condition is a UTI a predisposing factor? What general nutrition principles are recommended in the treatment of such infections?

REFERENCES

1. Huether SE: Structure and function of the renal and urologic systems. In Huether SE, McCance KL, editors: *Understanding pathophysiology*, ed 4, St Louis, 2008, Mosby.
2. National Kidney Foundation: K/DOQI clinical practice guidelines and clinical practice recommendations for diabetes and chronic kidney disease. *Am J Kidney Dis* 49(Suppl 2):S12, 2007.
3. National Kidney Foundation: K/DOQI clinical practice guidelines for chronic kidney disease: evaluation, classification and stratification. *Am J Kidney Dis* 39(Suppl 1):S1, 2002.
4. U.S. Renal Data System: *USRDS 2008 Annual Report: Atlas of chronic kidney disease and end-stage renal disease in the United States*, Bethesda, Md., 2008, National Institutes of Health, National Institute of Diabetes and Digestive and Kidney Diseases.

5. Beekley MD: Update on nutrition and chronic kidney disease. In *Medscape Nephrology, Chronic Kidney Disease Expert Column*, 2007. from: <www.medscape.com>. Retrieved June 2, 2009.

6. Gray M, Huether SE, Forshee BA: Alterations of renal and urinary tract function. In McCance KL, Huether SE, editors: *Pathophysiology. The biologic basis for disease in adults and children*, ed 5, St Louis, 2006, Saunders.

7. American Diabetes Association: Diabetic nephropathy. *Diabetes Care* 25(Suppl 1):S85, 2002.

8. Kalantar-Zadeh K, Kopple J: Malnutrition as a risk factor for morbidity and mortality in maintenance patients. In Kopple J, Massry S, editors: *Nutritional management of renal disease*, Philadelphia, 2004, Lippincott Williams & Wilkins.

9. Barbá PD, Goode JL: Nutrition assessment in chronic kidney disease. In Byham-Gray L, Wiesen K, editors: *A clinical guide to nutrition care in kidney disease*, Chicago, 2004, American Dietetic Association.

10. Fedje L, Karalis M: Nutrition management in early stages of chronic kidney failure. In Byham-Gray L, Wiesen K, editors: *A clinical guide to nutrition care in kidney disease*, Chicago, 2004, American Dietetic Association.

11. National Kidney Foundation: K/DOQI clinical practice guidelines for nutrition in chronic renal failure. *Am J Kidney Dis* 35(Suppl 2):S9, 2000.

12. Biesecker R, Stuart N: Nutrition management of the adult hemodialysis patient. In Byham-Gray L, Wiesen K, editors: *A clinical guide to nutrition care in kidney disease*, Chicago, 2004, American Dietetic Association.

13. Cochran CC, Kent PS: Nutrition management of the renal transplant patient. In Byham-Gray L, Wiesen K, editors: *A clinical guide to nutrition care in kidney disease*, Chicago, 2004, American Dietetic Association.

14. Weil SE: Nutrition in the kidney transplant recipient. In Danovitch GM, editor: *Handbook of kidney transplantation*, ed 5, Philadelphia, 2010, Lippincott, Williams & Wilkins.

15. Bickford A, Schatz SR: Nutrition management in acute renal failure. In Byham-Gray L, Wiesen K, editors: *A clinical guide to nutrition care in kidney disease*, Chicago, 2004, American Dietetic Association.

16. Huether SE, Gray M: Alterations of renal and urinary tract functions. In Huether SE, McCance KL, editors: *Understanding pathophysiology*, ed 4, St Louis, 2008, Mosby.

17. Gould BE: *Pathophysiology for the health professions*, ed 3, St Louis, 2006, Mosby.

18. American Dietetic Association: *Nutrition care manual. Celiac disease: nutrition care FAQs*, Chicago, 2009, Author. from: <www.nutritioncaremanual.org>. Retrieved June 11, 2009.

FURTHER RESOURCES

Websites of Interest

- Academy of Nutrition and Dietetics. The website of the world's largest food and nutrition professionals organization provides information regarding nutrition and health through research, education, and advocacy: www.eatright.org.
- *American Journal of Kidney Diseases.* This is the website of the official journal of the National Kidney Foundation: www.ajkd.org.
- Da Vita. Provider of dialysis services and education for patients with CKD: www.davita.com.
- Hypertension, Dialysis and Clinical Nephrology (HDCN). Provides up-to-date, selected information on renal disorders and their treatment: www.hdcn.com.
- *Journal of the American Society of Nephrology:* www.jasn.org.
- *Journal of Renal Nutrition.* This site also provides links to the homepage of the National Kidney Foundation and the Council on Renal Nutrition: www.jrnjournal.org.
- National Kidney Foundation: www.kidney.org
- Nephrology News and Issues Online (NephrOnline): www.nephronline.com.

Acquired Immunodeficiency Syndrome (AIDS)

Adriana Campa, Irene Hatsu, and Marianna K. Baum

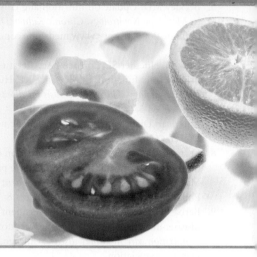

The human immunodeficiency virus (HIV) and its end stage, acquired immunodeficiency syndrome (AIDS), are nutrition-related conditions.[1] Nutrition status and nutrition interventions are critical in the care of people living with HIV. Several international studies have shown that mild to moderate malnutrition impairs the immune response and increases the severity and mortality of infections.[2-4] Although the advent of potent combined antiretroviral therapy (cART) has not provided a permanent cure, it has transformed HIV into a manageable, chronic disease. As a consequence, nutrition interventions in those living with HIV are rapidly evolving to tailor nutrition support to the special needs created by the stages of the infection and its treatment.

EVOLUTION OF HIV AND THE AIDS EPIDEMIC

HIV/AIDS is a pandemic that has claimed more than 25 million lives globally since the first case was reported in June 1981, including over 619,000 in the United States.[5] There are 33.4 million people living with HIV/AIDS worldwide, and approximately 1.2 million in this country. The incidence of new cases in the United States is approximately 50,000 annually. Homosexual men (61% of new cases in 2010), drug users, and minorities account for most U.S. new cases.[5] Approximately 97% of the cases of HIV/AIDS are found in low- and middle-income countries, especially in sub-Saharan Africa, with the number of new cases increasing in Asia.[6]

On June 30, 2013, the World Health Organization (WHO) revised their HIV treatment guidelines by recommending starting antiretroviral therapy (ART) at a CD4 cell count of 500 cells/μL or less. Simultaneously, the treatment progress update issued by WHO, the *Joint United Nations Programme on HIV/AIDS* (UNAIDS), and the United Nations Children's Fund (UNICEF) identified challenges in providing access to treatment for all eligible persons, as many of the most affected countries have limited resources to attain this standard.[7,8]

In addition to causing disease and death, the pandemic impacts families, communities, and the economic development of countries. Many of the regions hardest hit by HIV are limited-resource countries with high prevalence of other infectious diseases, food insecurity, and social and political problems. The most common method of transmission in the rest of the world is by heterosexual contact. HIV is a blood-borne virus transmitted by direct contact with infected body fluids via unprotected heterosexual and homosexual intercourse, through intravenous needle sharing, and from mother to child during pregnancy, delivery, and breastfeeding. Worldwide, approximately half of all persons living with HIV/AIDS are women who acquire HIV mainly via heterosexual contact.[6]

The epidemic of HIV/AIDS has transformed our perception of public health, research, cultural attitudes, and social behaviors.[9] The incidence of new cases has decreased, and prevention has helped to reduce HIV prevalence rates in several countries. In addition, the number of people with

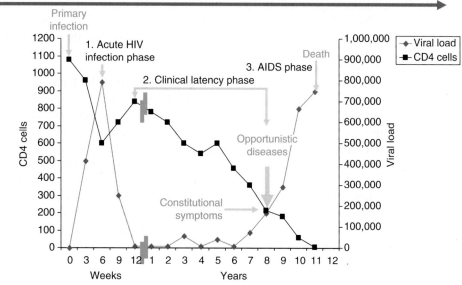

FIGURE 24-1 Phases of HIV disease progression. (Adapted from Pantaleo G, Graziosi C, Fauci AS: New concepts in the immunopathogenesis of human immunodeficiency virus infection. *New Engl J Med* 328[5]:327-335,1993.)

HIV receiving treatment in resource-poor countries has increased since 2002.[5]

Disease Progression

As shown in Figure 24-1, HIV infection has several phases.[10] The Centers for Disease Control and Prevention and the World Health Organization have developed several classification systems that define four clinical stages using CD4 cell counts and clinical conditions for stages 2, 3, and 4.[11] For easier understanding, we have defined disease progression in three major phases: (1) acute infection, (2) asymptomatic and latency, and (3) AIDS. The acute stage occurs when the virus is transmitted and enters the bloodstream. From that moment on, the infection becomes a progressive disease, with the condition worsening over time. Without proper treatment, infected persons are likely to advance to AIDS, the final stage of the disease. The rate of progression is different depending on the characteristics of the host (exposure to infection, nutritional status, access to care, etc.) and the virus (HIV subtypes, superinfections, resistance to treatment, etc.).

Acute Infection Stage

The genetic information of HIV, a retrovirus, is in the form of ribonucleic acid (RNA). HIV uses a reverse transcriptase enzyme to change RNA into double-stranded deoxyribonucleic acid (DNA) (Figure 24-2). The new DNA is inserted by integrase, another viral enzyme, into the infected cell's genetic material. When the new DNA is activated, the viral information is translated, causing a sequence of cellular events that end with cell death, and the dead cell sheds infectious HIV particles called virions. If the cell remains dormant, then the viral genetic material may remain dormant for years, which

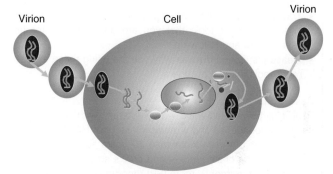

FIGURE 24-2 HIV life cycle.

makes HIV difficult to cure.[12] Although the acute stage of HIV infection may vary, typically it lasts for 3 to 6 weeks after the primary infection. Most individuals experience varying nonspecific symptoms of fatigue, sore throat, muscle pain, fever, night sweats, and enlarged lymph nodes.[12,13] The process of developing antibodies to HIV is called *seroconversion,* and it may last days or weeks. Subsequent HIV testing by enzyme-linked immunosorbent assay (ELISA) becomes positive.

Asymptomatic Stage (Latency)

Following the acute stage, HIV enters a period of inactivity or latency. An extended asymptomatic period usually continues for the next 10 to 12 years. However, this seemingly inactive period of relative wellness can be deceiving. Antibodies typically appear within 4 to 7 weeks after infection through blood products but may remain seronegative for 6 to 14 months after sexual transmission. This phase between infection and manifestation of antibody is referred to as the *window period.*[12] During the asymptomatic stage of infection, viral replication continues and cellular destruction takes place in many tissues and organs of the body. The virus continues to proliferate during this phase.[13] During this protracted phase, many individuals will still not exhibit clinical signs of the infection, whereas others have generalized enlarged lymph nodes[14] and may present clinical manifestations of CDC clinical stages 2 and 3.[11] Viral replication appears to be reduced during this time. CD4 cell count decreases slowly, resulting in a weaker immune response.[13]

Final Stage (AIDS)

This is the last stage of the HIV infection, which is characterized by severe damage to the immune system and immune failure. CD4 cell count is 200 cells/μL or lower. Opportunistic infections and AIDS-defining conditions manifest in

this stage with numerous serious complications such as gastrointestinal (GI) effects and neurologic effects such as AIDS dementia. (See the Case Study box "HIV in an Adult").

Diagnosis of HIV Infection
Testing Procedures[15]

HIV infection is diagnosed by detection of the virus or by the detection of specific antibodies, as is done in the routine screening of blood and blood products for transfusion and in most epidemiologic studies. The recommended procedure for virus detection is a two-step process. The first step is ELISA screening. Second, suspected positive samples from the ELISA screening are followed with Western blot testing for confirmation. Both tests are highly sensitive and specific, and both are used to confirm the results before informing the

---

CASE STUDY

HIV in an Adult

Nutritional Assessment:

- Please do a complete nutritional assessment and develop a treatment and follow-up plan for the patient described below.
- You also need to identify and describe the nutritional indices and assessment tools that you are going to use for his assessment and follow-up.
- Please justify and discuss why you are using these assessment tools instead of others.

Case Study

Paul is a 58-year-old male Army veteran, with a history of cocaine dependence and a medical history of HIV since 1993. He was a heroin user more than 10 years ago, while in the Army. Paul is a chain smoker and drinks socially. The patient came to the emergency room (ER) reporting depressed mood, thoughts of worthlessness, helplessness, and low self-esteem for the past 2 months previous to the ER visit. He also stated that he lost approximately 25 pounds in the past 3 months. His height is 6 feet 2 inches, and his weight is 155 lb. The laboratory values for this visit are in the table below. He admitted that he has been neglecting his care, not taking his antiretroviral medication, which consists of one tablet of Atripla daily. He also reports to be unable to sleep for more than 3 hours per night. He admitted that he felt so "down" that last night he binged on crack cocaine. The patient also described severe difficulties with his family and friends. He left his wife 2 months ago after an argument. He described insomnia and nightmares for 3 to 4 weeks, describing that he witnessed his friend being murdered in a drug-related affair. He also described multiple losses, including the death of his older daughter (the oldest of four daughters) to AIDS in 2006. He was arrested in 2008 for assault. He has a history of multiple suicide attempts by hanging and overdose of psychiatric medications while in jail. He missed his last health care appointment 3 months ago. The patient finished high school and has been working on and off as a security officer. He is currently unemployed. Paul is presently on Supplemental Security Income benefits for disabled

adults. He is not receiving Supplemental Nutrition Assistance Program (SNAP) *benefits.*

Height	188 cm
Weight	70.4 kg
Usual weight	81.9 kg
Percentage weight loss	14%
Body weight (percentage of usual)	86%
Triceps skinfold	<25th percentile
Midarm muscle circumference	<25th percentile
CD4+ cell count	118 cells/μL
Viral load	3.2 log copies/mL
Serum potassium	3.1 mEq/dL
Blood glucose	70 mg/dL
Blood urea nitrogen (BUN)	32 mg/dL
Creatinine	0.4 mg/dL
Serum albumin	2.8 mg/dL
Serum osmolality	325 mOsm/kg
Calculated basal energy expenditure (BEE)	2450 kcal/day

Questions for Analysis

1. Is Paul's HIV infection under control? Is his adherence to medication adequate?
2. Is he involved in risky behaviors for transmitting the disease?
3. Based on laboratory and anthropometric data, does Paul appear to be malnourished? Please support your response with evidence.
4. Assess Paul's food security and access to food. What type of assessment could help you determine this?
5. What are the acute or immediate nutrition goals? What about long-term goals?
6. What nutritional information will Paul need based upon his ART regimen?
7. What type of referrals or follow-up is Paul going to need to prevent further nutritional depletion?

individual. Because a positive test is such a personal and life-changing event, most experienced physicians caring for HIV-infected patients repeat all positive tests again, even when they have been confirmed by Western blotting, before informing the individual.

There are enzyme immunoassay (EIA) tests that use other body fluids to look for antibodies to HIV. These tests work in a similar manner to the standard blood ELISA tests and require a confirmatory Western blot in the same fluid. These new tests include the oral fluid (not saliva) test that is collected from the mouth using a special collection device and the urine tests. The sensitivity and specificity (accuracy) of the urine tests are somewhat less than that of the blood and oral fluid tests.[15]

Rapid HIV Testing

Rapid tests have also been developed. The CDC has published guidelines for their use, training, and counseling. These tests use blood from venipuncture, finger-stick, or oral fluids, producing results in 20 minutes. As the previously described tests, they need a confirmatory Western blot test.[16]

Home Testing Kits

This type of test was first licensed in 1997. Currently only the Home Access HIV-1 Test SystemExternal Link is approved by the U.S. Food and Drug Administration. This is not a true home test, but a home collection kit, which can be found in most drug stores. The collection procedure involves pricking a finger with a device, depositing blood drops from the pricked finger on a special card, and then mailing the card in to be tested at a licensed laboratory. The kit provides an identification number to use when contacting the laboratory for the results. Callers may speak to a counselor before taking the test, while waiting for the test result, and when the results are given. All individuals who receive a positive test result are provided referrals for a follow-up confirmatory test, as well as information and resources on treatment and support services.[15,17]

RNA Viral Assays

Viral load assays are used to assess prognosis, determine the need for and type of combination antiretroviral therapy (cART) to use, and monitor the effectiveness of the treatment. RNA tests look for genetic material of the virus and can be used in screening the blood supply and for detection of very early cases of the infection when ELISA tests are unable to detect antibodies to HIV.[15]

Clinical Symptoms and Illnesses

Early clinical symptoms that may follow initial exposure to the virus add further confirmation to the HIV-seropositive testing procedures. Initial symptoms and possible associated diseases that characterize later HIV stages have been generally described earlier in discussion of basic disease progression. Some examples of these common opportunistic infections that manifest depending on CD4$^+$ cell count range are listed in Table 24-1.

TABLE 24-1	COMMON INFECTIOUS COMPLICATIONS OF AIDS
MICROORGANISM	**NUTRITIONAL IMPLICATIONS**
Parasites	
Pneumocystis carinii	Dyspnea, fever, weight loss
Toxoplasma gondii	Fever
Cryptosporidium	Malabsorption, diarrhea
Isospora belli	Diarrhea
Microspora	Malabsorption, diarrhea
Entamoeba histolytica	Diarrhea
Giardia lamblia	Diarrhea
Acanthamoeba	Meningoencephalitis
Bacteria	
Campylobacter	Abdominal pain, cramping, bloody diarrhea, fever
Legionella	Fever
Listeria monocytogenes	Fever
Mycobacterium-avium-intracellulare	Fever, weight loss, diarrhea, malabsorption
Salmonella	Diarrhea, bacteremia
Shigella	Abdominal pain, bloody diarrhea, fever
Fungi	
Aspergillus	Fungemia, fevers, weight loss
Candida albicans	Thrush, stomatitis, esophagitis, nausea
Cryptococcus neoformans	Fever, nausea, vomiting
Histoplasma capsulatum	Fever, weight loss, dysphagia
Viruses	
Cytomegalovirus	Esophagitis, colitis, diarrhea
Herpes simplex virus	Ulcerative mucocutaneous lesions, stomatitis, esophagitis, pneumonia
Epstein-Barr virus	Oral hairy leukoplakia
Hepatitis B	Nausea, vomiting, fever
Herpes zoster	Mucocutaneous lesions

Data from the Academy of Nutrition and Dietetics: *Manual of clinical dietetics*, ed 6, Chicago, 2000, Academy of Nutrition and Dietetics; Gold JWM: HIV-1 infection: diagnosis and management. *Med Clin North Am* 76(1):1, 1992; Bernard EM, Sepkowitz KA, Telzak EE, et al: Pneumocystosis. *Med Clin North Am* 76(1):107, 1992; and Ralten DJ: Nutrition and HIV infection: a review and evaluation of the extent of knowledge of the relationship between nutrition and HIV infection. *Nutr Clin Pract* 6(3):1S, 1991.

MEDICAL MANAGEMENT

With the advent of antiretroviral treatments in 1996, HIV became a chronic disease. The treatment regimen for HIV is cART. The standard combination includes nucleoside reverse transcriptase inhibitors (NRTIs), protease inhibitors (PIs), and non-nucleoside reverse transcriptase inhibitors (NNRTIs). New families of ART are now being used, such as fusion inhibitors and the HIV integrase strand transfer inhibitors that are to be used when the first lines of ART fail to control the viral load.[18] Although resistant viral strains to these medications have been recognized, the death rate from AIDS-related diseases has been significantly decreased with ART.[19]

Combination ART is used to achieve long-term viral suppression (measured by HIV viral load) and immunologic restoration (measured by CD4+ T-cell count) as a means to decrease HIV-related morbidity and mortality and improve quality of life. This is frequently complicated because retroviruses incorporate into the genetic material of the host and may not be removed by ART. Therefore medications to manage HIV are typically prescribed for the lifetime of the infected individual. Furthermore, HIV may hide in "sanctuaries" that are body regions where the cART may not be active such as the central nervous system (CNS).[19]

Indications for starting ART were updated in February 2013, with recommendations to start ART at CD4+ T-cell count less than 500 cells/mm³ to reduce risk of disease progression and to prevent transmission of HIV.[20] Antiretroviral therapy is recommended for pregnant women, those with HIV-associated nephropathy, and individuals coinfected with hepatitis B virus (HBV) regardless of CD4+ T-cell count.[19] Adherence to this drug regimen can be demanding for the HIV-infected individual and health care providers. It is critical to assess the patient's commitment to ART adherence because of its importance for successful therapy, and the patient's understanding of the benefits and risks of treatment. Furthermore, dosing convenience, drug safety profiles, viral genetic testing, and drug-drug interactions ought to be considered for the selection of treatment for each individual. On the whole, ART toxicities can be common and should be evaluated and compared to the benefits of favorable virologic and immunologic responses.[20]

Classes of Drugs

More than 20 antiretroviral agents, from five classes of drugs, exist[20]:

- Nucleoside/nucleotide reverse transcriptase inhibitors (NRTIs)
- Non-nucleoside reverse transcriptase inhibitors (NNRTIs)
- Protease inhibitors (PIs)
- Entry inhibitors (fusion and C-C chemokine receptor type 5 [CCR5] entry inhibitors)
- Integrase inhibitors

Although many of these drugs are available as fixed-dose combinations, the majority are formulated as individual medications. This makes treatment regimens easier, lessens pill burden, and increases patient medication compliance.[20] Many side effects occur from these drugs, which may contribute to noncompliance with drug regimens as listed in Table 24-2.

TABLE 24-2   ANTIRETROVIRAL DRUGS USED TO TREAT HIV/AIDS AND POTENTIAL ADVERSE NUTRITIONAL CONSEQUENCES

Multi-Class Combination Products

BRAND NAME	GENERIC NAME	MANUFACTURER NAME	POTENTIAL ADVERSE NUTRITIONAL CONSEQUENCES
Atripla	efavirenz, emtricitabine and tenofovir disoproxil fumarate	Bristol-Myers Squibb and Gilead Sciences	It should be taken on an empty stomach, long-term intake associated with reduced bone density. Common GI reactions to tenofovir are diarrhea, nausea.
Complera	emtricitabine, rilpivirine, and tenofovir disoproxil fumarate	Gilead Sciences	Take with meal. Although uncommon, it has been associated with abdominal fullness, flatulence, indigestion, lack of appetite, diarrhea, nausea, and vomiting. Potential redistribution of body fat. It contains tenofovir, and its long-term intake has been associated with reduced bone density.
Stribild	elvitegravir, cobicistat, emtricitabine, tenofovir disoproxil fumarate	Gilead Sciences	Nausea and diarrhea.

Nucleoside Reverse Transcriptase Inhibitors (NRTIs)*

BRAND NAME	GENERIC NAME	MANUFACTURER NAME	POTENTIAL ADVERSE NUTRITIONAL CONSEQUENCES
Combivir	lamivudine and zidovudine	GlaxoSmithKline	Take without regard to meals; constipation, taste alterations possible; macrocytic anemia or neutropenia possible. Uncommon side effects are abdominal pain, nausea, vomiting.
Emtriva	emtricitabine, FTC	Gilead Sciences	Take without regard to meals; snacks may reduce GI upset.

TABLE 24-2   ANTIRETROVIRAL DRUGS USED TO TREAT HIV/AIDS AND POTENTIAL ADVERSE NUTRITIONAL CONSEQUENCES—cont'd

BRAND NAME	GENERIC NAME	MANUFACTURER NAME	POTENTIAL ADVERSE NUTRITIONAL CONSEQUENCES
Epivir	lamivudine, 3TC	GlaxoSmithKline	Take without regard to meals; snacks may reduce GI upset.
Epzicom	abacavir and lamivudine	GlaxoSmithKline	Take without regard to meals; snacks may reduce gastrointestinal (GI) upset; alcohol can increase drug levels; nausea, vomiting, diarrhea, and loss of appetite possible.
Hivid	zalcitabine, dideoxycytidine, ddC (no longer marketed)	Hoffmann-La Roche	Take without regard to meals; vomiting, stomach/abdominal pain, oral lesions, constipation, or persistent nausea may occur; rare chance of pancreatitis.
Retrovir	zidovudine, azidothymidine, AZT, ZDV	GlaxoSmithKline	Take without regard to meals; constipation, taste alterations possible; macrocytic anemia or neutropenia possible.
Trizivir	abacavir, zidovudine, and lamivudine	GlaxoSmithKline	Take without regard to meals; snacks may reduce GI upset; alcohol can increase drug levels; nausea, vomiting, diarrhea, and loss of appetite possible.
Truvada	tenofovir disoproxil fumarate and emtricitabine	Gilead Sciences	Take without regard to meals; diarrhea, nausea, vomiting, and flatulence possible.
Videx EC	enteric-coated didanosine, ddI EC	Bristol Myers-Squibb	Take 30 min before or 2 hr after meal; do not mix with acidic liquid (e.g., grapefruit juice, oranges, other citrus; tomatoes or tomato juice); do not take antacids with magnesium or aluminum within 2 hr; nausea possible.
Videx	didanosine, dideoxyinosine, ddI	Bristol Myers-Squibb	
Viread	tenofovir disoproxil fumarate, TDF	Gilead Sciences	Take without regard to meals; diarrhea, nausea, vomiting, and flatulence possible.
Zerit	stavudine, d4T	Bristol Myers-Squibb	Take without regard to meals; snacks may limit GI upset; mouth/esophageal ulcers possible.
Ziagen	abacavir sulfate, ABC	GlaxoSmithKline	Take without regard to meals; snacks may reduce GI upset; alcohol can increase drug levels; nausea, vomiting, diarrhea, and loss of appetite possible.

Non-Nucleoside Reverse Transcriptase Inhibitors (NNRTIs)*

BRAND NAME	GENERIC NAME	MANUFACTURER NAME	POTENTIAL ADVERSE NUTRITIONAL CONSEQUENCES
Edurant	rilpivirine	Tibotec Therapeutics	Take with meal, a protein drink alone does not replace a meal. Although uncommon, it has been associated with abdominal fullness, flatulence, indigestion, lack of appetite, nausea and vomiting.
Intelence	etravirine	Tibotec Therapeutics	Take after a meal; nausea possible.
Rescriptor	delavirdine, DLV	Pfizer	Take without regard to meals; avoid St. John's wort; constipation, diarrhea, dry mouth, and flatulence possible; decreased appetite possible.
Sustiva	efavirenz, EFV	Bristol Myers-Squibb	High-fat/high-calorie meals increase peak plasma concentrations; take on empty stomach; take at bedtime to decrease adverse effects; taste alterations, potential loss of appetite, and flatulence possible.
Viramune (Immediate Release)	nevirapine, NVP	Boehringer Ingelheim	Take without regard to meals; snacks may limit GI upset; nausea and loss of appetite possible
Viramune XR (Extended Release)	nevirapine, NVP	Boehringer Ingelheim	

Continued

TABLE 24-2	ANTIRETROVIRAL DRUGS USED TO TREAT HIV/AIDS AND POTENTIAL ADVERSE NUTRITIONAL CONSEQUENCES—cont'd

Protease Inhibitors (PIs)[†]

BRAND NAME	GENERIC NAME	MANUFACTURER NAME	POTENTIAL ADVERSE NUTRITIONAL CONSEQUENCES
Agenerase	amprenavir, APV (no longer marketed)	GlaxoSmithKline	Take on empty stomach; low fat limits GI upset (avoid high fat meals); avoid grapefruit juice; increase fluid intake; avoid taking antacids within 2 hr; nausea, vomiting, gas, and diarrhea possible.
Aptivus	tipranavir, TPV	Boehringer Ingelheim	Take with a fatty meal.
Crixivan	indinavir, IDV	Merck	Avoid grapefruit juice; avoid St. John's wort; *(unboosted)* take 2 hr before or 2 hr after meals; take on empty stomach, but if not tolerated may take with nonfat milk; eat low-fat meals and light snacks; *(ritonavir [RTV] boosted)* timing of food intake not a consideration; loss of appetite, nausea, and metallic taste possible.
Invirase	saquinavir mesylate, SQV	Hoffmann-La Roche	Take within 2 hr of a meal; GI intolerance, nausea, and diarrhea possible.
Kaletra	lopinavir and ritonavir, LPV/RTV	Abbott Laboratories	Time of food not a consideration; nausea, vomiting, and diarrhea possible.
Lexiva	fosamprenavir calcium, FOS-APV	GlaxoSmithKline	Take without regard to meals; diarrhea, nausea, and vomiting possible.
Norvir	ritonavir, RTV	Abbott Laboratories	Take with food if possible (may improve tolerability); nausea, vomiting, diarrhea, and taste changes possible.
Prezista	darunavir	Tibotec, Inc.	Take with food; diarrhea and nausea are possible.
Reyataz	atazanavir sulfate, ATV	Bristol-Myers Squibb	Take with food; avoid taking simultaneously with antacids or H_2 blockers.
Viracept	nelfinavir mesylate, NFV	Agouron Pharmaceuticals	Diarrhea is possible.

Fusion Inhibitors[‡]

BRAND NAME	GENERIC NAME	MANUFACTURER NAME	POTENTIAL ADVERSE NUTRITIONAL CONSEQUENCES
Fuzeon	enfuvirtide, T-20	Hoffmann-La Roche & Trimeris	Not applicable. It is a subcutaneous application.

Entry Inhibitors: CCR5 Co-Receptor Antagonist[§]

BRAND NAME	GENERIC NAME	MANUFACTURER NAME	POTENTIAL ADVERSE NUTRITIONAL CONSEQUENCES
Selzentry	maraviroc	Pfizer	No food effect; take with or without food; abdominal pain possible.

HIV Integrase Strand Transfer Inhibitors[‖]

BRAND NAME	GENERIC NAME	MANUFACTURER NAME	POTENTIAL ADVERSE NUTRITIONAL CONSEQUENCES
Isentress	raltegravir	Merck & Co., Inc.	Take with or without food; nausea and diarrhea possible.
Tivicay	dolutegravir	GlaxoSmithKline	Take 2 hr before or 6 hr after taking cation-containing antacids or laxatives, sucralfate, oral iron supplements, oral calcium supplements, or buffered medications. Body fat redistribution is possible.

Data from Dong KR, Mangili A: Highly active antiretroviral therapy (HAART). In Hendricks KM, Dong KR, Gerrior JL, editors: *Nutrition management of HIV and AIDS*, Chicago, 2009, Academy of Nutrition and Dietetics; Panel on Antiretroviral Guidelines for the use of antiretroviral agents in HIV-1-infected adults and adolescents, Washington, DC, 2008, Department of Health and Human Services; Keithley JK, Swanson B: *Nursing guidelines: HIV and nutrition*, ANAC, Ohio. <http//www. nursesinaidscare.org>. Accessed October 19, 2013.
*Nucleoside/nucleotide reverse transcriptase inhibitors (NRTIs) and non-nucleoside reverse transcriptase inhibitors (NNRTIs) prevent reverse transcriptase from making more copies of the human immunodeficiency virus (HIV) genome.
†Protease inhibitors (PIs) prevent protease from breaking apart long strands of viral proteins to make the smaller, active proteins HIV needs to reproduce.
‡Fusion inhibitors are specific types of entry inhibitors chat prevent fusion between HIV's outer envelope and the cell's outer membrane.
§Entry Inhibitors—CCR5 co-receptor antagonists are chemokine receptor antagonists; they are the first antiretrovirals to bind a cellular protein of the host.
‖Integrase inhibitors prevent integrase from inserting HIV's genetic material into an infected cell's genetic material.

NUTRITION THERAPY

Basic Role of Nutrition in the HIV Disease Process

Infections in general create an environment that leads to reduction in nutrient intake and absorption, as well as an increase in the utilization and requirement for nutrients.[21,22] HIV infection is associated with the destruction of the immune system. As a result, it is critical to maintain adequate nutritional status in HIV-infected individuals. The disease, in combination with underlying or consequent malnutrition, creates a vicious cycle that aggravates disease progression and affects chances of survival.[23] Poor nutritional status may accelerate disease progression and lead to poor outcomes. Additionally, HIV infection impairs nutrient intake, digestion, absorption, and utilization, leading to weight loss, nutrient deficiencies, and compromised immune function and competence, as well as susceptibility to infections.[22,23]

In people living with HIV, clinical symptoms and treatment side effects such as loss of appetite, nausea and vomiting may lead to reduction in food and nutrient intake.[24-26] This contributes to weight loss and nutrient deficiency even in asymptomatic patients.[24,27] Weight loss has been persistent among people who are infected with HIV even in the era of ART.[27] In addition to inadequate intake, diarrhea and malabsorption of macronutrients and micronutrients are also common during HIV infection. These conditions are exacerbated by infections from pathogens like *Cryptosporidium* and *cytomegalovirus*. When fat malabsorption is present, it may cause decreased bioavailability or deficiency of fat-soluble vitamins.[23] Even among asymptomatic patients, HIV infection can lead to intestinal defects like permeability and epithelial damage.[23,28,29] The infection can also alter the body's ability to metabolize and store nutrients such as carbohydrates,[24] proteins, and fats by altering the effect of enzymes and hormones needed for their metabolism. HIV infection may impair the production of enzymes and transport proteins in the gastrointestinal tract that are needed for nutrient digestion and absorption.[22]

Poor nutritional status impairs immune function either directly or indirectly. Directly, nutritional deficiency can interfere with the primary activity of the lymphoid system such as during immune cell triggering, interaction, and differentiation. Indirectly, it can affect other metabolic and cellular processes needed for immune regulation.[30] Several micronutrients are necessary for proper immune function. Vitamin A is important for the growth and function of T and B cells, antibody responses, as well as for the maintenance of the epithelial integrity of the respiratory and gastrointestinal tract.[23] Vitamin E is essential for the function of T, B, and phagocytic cells.[31] It also acts as an antioxidant protecting vitamin A and fats from oxidation.[22] Zinc and selenium are important nutrients for the immune system, acting as antioxidants, with involvement in the development of cell-mediated and nonspecific immunity as well as vitamin A transport.[22] Several other vitamins and minerals play a role in immune function, either at the physical barrier (skin/mucosal) level, cellular immunity level, or antibody production level.[32] Vitamins B_6, B_{12}, C, D, folic acid, iron, and copper all work to enhance the protective activities of immune cells. With the exception of vitamin C and iron, the rest of the nutrients work to support antibody production.[32] Nutritional deficiency during HIV infection could result in increased levels of prooxidants, leading to oxidative stress, which may hasten HIV replication through nuclear factor κB (NF-κB), a transcriptional promoter of proteins involved in HIV transcription.[23] It can also result in immunosuppression, which may affect viral expression and replication and ultimately disease progression and death. Factors that could contribute to poor nutrition include inadequate nutrient intake and absorption, poor appetite, metabolic problems, chronic infection and limited food availability, among others.[22]

HIV-infected individuals are more susceptible to infections because of compromised immunity. Chronic HIV infection also increases the nutritional requirements of those infected above those who are uninfected.[23,33,34] ART medications can also affect energy expenditure, contributing to higher caloric needs.[34] HIV-infected individuals who are asymptomatic require on average 10% more energy intake than what is recommended for noninfected healthy individuals for the same age and sex.[33] This requirement increases to 20% to 30% during the symptomatic phase. Increased energy requirement, among other nutrient needs, has made optimal nutrition critical for managing the HIV infection.[35]

Nutritional Status During HIV Infection

Nutritional status, defined by *Mosby's Medical Dictionary* as the "extent to which nutrients are available to meet metabolic needs,"[36] is a good predictor of morbidity and mortality in the course of HIV infection.[37,38] There are several indicators used in measuring nutritional status such as anthropometric measures (weight, height, body mass index [BMI], and body composition), biochemical measures (such as serum levels of nutrients), clinical measures (such as hemoglobin, hematocrit, and serum albumin), and dietary intake of nutrients. The impact that an infection has on nutritional status is dependent on the baseline nutritional status, as well as the nature and severity level of the infection.[39] During HIV infection, higher mortality rates are predicted by poor nutritional status, even when treatment is initiated.[40,41] When compared to noninfected individuals, HIV-infected patients have lower serum concentration of nutrients and were more susceptible to nutritional deficiencies.[42-45]

Early HIV studies reported a severe impact of the disease on nutritional status before the era of ART. Malnutrition, often associated with low serum levels of micronutrients, was common regardless of the socioeconomic status of the population infected, and serum nutrient deficiencies were associated with disease progression.[23,44,46] Review articles that examined the prevalence and impact of micronutrient deficiency in HIV patients in the pre-ART era reported deficiencies in vitamins A, C, E, B_{12}, zinc, and selenium.[23,47,48] Vitamin B_6, and vitamin D deficiencies were also reported in HIV patients prior to ART use.[44,49] Since the advent of ART use, morbidity and mortality in HIV-infected individuals has declined; however, poor nutritional status is still being reported among some populations.[41,50]

Studies conducted in developed countries among HIV patients receiving ART report conflicting results on micronutrient status, even when supplementation was sometimes provided.[51-58] Some studies found significant differences in serum concentrations of α-tocopherol, α- and β-carotene, vitamin B_{12}, and folate between those receiving ART and controls.[53,55,58] Other cross-sectional and longitudinal studies found no differences in vitamins A and E,[54,55] B_6 and folate,[52] selenium, zinc, iron, and copper between those receiving ART and controls.[51,54] One study found those who received ART to have lower plasma concentration of vitamin A compared to controls.[56] A recent study reported 77% of HIV-infected study participants to be malnourished. It is unclear, however, whether these individuals were receiving ART treatment or not.[59]

Most studies investigating micronutrient status in HIV-infected individuals used serum or plasma measures.[23,46] These measures have some limitation because they may not be sensitive indicators of micronutrient status,[23] and most of these micronutrients are acute-phase reactants and will vary in body compartments during an infection.[46] HIV-infected individuals are susceptible to opportunistic infections; hence, unless other infections were accounted and controlled for in these studies, the results might have limitations. A consistent body of literature exists that supports a strong relationship between HIV infection and poor nutritional status.[46] Most evidence supports that this relationship is a reciprocal, vicious and deadly cycle, in which malnutrition and HIV infection advance each other.[22,23]

Weight loss is another indicator of nutritional status, and it has been linked to adverse outcomes during HIV infection.[60] Although ART treatment improved survival rates, weight loss (even as low as 5%) continued to be an independent predictor of morbidity and mortality in this population up until the early years of the Millennium, when ART was available and reports of increased overweight/obesity started to emerge among the population.[27,61] In 2000, the Nutrition for Healthy Living (NFHL) found 13% of its 633 participants to have wasting at the time of enrollment to the study.[38] At follow-up visits, 18% and 21% had, respectively, lost more than 10% and more than 5% of their body weight, with 8% having a BMI of less than 20.38 kg/m². The weight loss observed in this group occurred in patients successfully treated with ART, in those for whom ART treatment failed, and also in ART-naïve patients.[50] The weight loss was also found to be a combination of fat and lean body mass loss, depending on initial body weight and etiology of weight loss,[62] that is, whether it was a result of abnormalities in intake or altered metabolism.[27]

The NFHL also reported overweight in its cohort to be between 33% to 40% in men and 27% to 34% in women. Among this same cohort, obesity rates were 6% to 13% in men and 21% to 29% in women.[63,64] Other studies have also reported increasing overweight and obesity rates among HIV-infected individuals, with several studies reporting higher prevalence of overweight and obesity compared to wasting in the study populations.[65-68] It appears that overweight/obesity is being reported at diagnosis, with continued weight gain during HIV infection. One author suggests this to be a reflection of improved health status in this population, even as the trend mirrors what is being observed in the general public.[67] With between 46% and 60% overweight/obesity rates being reported in certain HIV-infected populations, obesity, and not weight loss or wasting, seems to be the new nutritional concern for this population, especially when coronary heart disease is on the rise in the ART-treated individuals.[67,68] Lack of access to nutritious foods, metabolic abnormalities, and illicit drug use, all of which can aggravate weight loss and the catabolic nature of the HIV disease are still common; hence, it is important not to completely rule out weight loss as a nutrition concern in this population.[69-78] The new epidemic of overweight and obesity may be attributed to unhealthy eating habits, excessive caloric and fat intake, and treatment-related metabolic alterations especially with lipid metabolism.[64,79-83]

Several studies have reported on issues of dietary and nutrient intake of HIV-infected individuals.[84-90] Caloric and fat over-consumption seems to be a consistent theme in developed areas.[84,85,87-89] In low-income settings, the opposite problem exists, with numerous studies reporting inadequate nutrient intake to be common among HIV-infected people, especially in those regions where ART is still not widely available.[24,91,92] In resource-adequate areas, low intakes have been reported in HIV-infected sociodemographic groups such as women, drug abusers and minorities at risk for health care disparities and adverse clinical outcomes.[25,91,93] On the other hand, adequate nutrient consumption is found in HIV-infected men who are educated, high-income earners, and users of supplements.[86,87] Two studies found nutrient intake among these economically advantaged HIV-infected individuals to be higher than that reported by HIV noninfected populations.[86,93] Some studies that have investigated biochemical markers such as hemoglobin, hematocrit, and albumin among HIV-infected people have consistently reported these parameters as low in this population.[59,84,89,90,94-96] Most of the studies, however, have been conducted in low-resource areas. A multicenter study, conducted among women in North America, reported low albumin levels in those infected with HIV and concluded that baseline albumin level independently predicted mortality in this group, with a 48% mortality rate in the lowest serum albumin category compared to 11% in the highest category.[97]

In summary, the impact that an infection has on nutritional status is dependent on the nutritional status at the onset of the infection, as well as the nature and severity of the infection. In HIV infection, the literature is consistent in demonstrating a strong relationship between HIV infection and poor nutritional status. Most evidence supports that this relationship is a reciprocal, vicious, and deadly cycle, in which malnutrition and HIV infection advance each other. In the

United States, where ART is available, and HIV has become a manageable disease, the nutritional care has shifted its emphasis from preventing wasting toward preventing obesity, hyperlipidemias, and other long-term complications of treatment as described in Box 24-1.

Food Insecurity Among HIV-Infected Persons

In 2011, more than 50 million individuals lived in households that experienced food insecurity.[98] According to the U.S. Department of Agriculture (USDA), these included 17.9 million households, 11 million of which experienced low food security and 5.7% of which experienced very low food security.[98] Several studies have evaluated the prevalence of food insecurity among people infected with HIV, and their reports suggest that the prevalence is higher than those recorded at the national level, especially in resource-adequate settings. One study[61] found that 81% of HIV-infected adults surveyed in Miami who experienced wasting were food insecure, while another study conducted in Miami and Atlanta among a similar population reported 34% food insufficiency.[99] In British Columbia, 48% of HIV-positive study participants were reported to be food insecure,[72] while another study conducted in the same province, but among HIV-infected intravenous drug users, had a food insecurity prevalence of 64%.[100] Among homeless and marginally housed HIV-infected individuals in San Francisco,[75] it was estimated that 49% had food insecurity. Another study involving HIV-infected patients from eight veterans' clinics, in the Veteran Aging Cohort Study, reported that 24% of participants receiving ART treatment were food insecure.[101]

Food insecurity needs to be addressed because it has been found to contribute to HIV transmission, especially among food-insecure women responsible for their households.[102,103] Food insecurity also impacts HIV transmission by compromising nutritional status, and consequently, immunologic status.[104] Inadequate nutrient intake may affect the mucosal integrity of the genitalia and gastrointestinal tract, leading to increased risk of HIV transmission. Compromised nutritional status has been associated with mother-to-child transmissions in resource-constrained settings.[105,106]

Food insecurity interferes with HIV-related care and services.[106-110] A recent study found food insecurity to be associated with missed clinic visits, with 17% of study participants having to give up ART treatment, while 30% and 32% did not access outpatient and inpatient treatment, respectively, because of competing demands for food.[77] HIV-infected persons who are food insecure, especially those with low socioeconomic status and limited resources, frequently need to choose between receiving HIV-related services or food procurement.[106,108]

ART for HIV infection is most effective when adherence to treatment is greater than 95%.[111] Studies conducted in developed countries and resource-limited settings have identified that food-insecure HIV-infected individuals are less likely to adhere to treatment, compared to their food-secure counterparts.[75,112] Adherence to treatment, however, increased among those who received food assistance, stressing the importance of food assistance among low-income HIV-infected patients.[113-115]

During the nutritional assessment and care of the HIV patient, it is important to ask questions on food insecurity, and refer the patient to the community and government programs, such as SNAP and food pantries, that provide a food security net for these patients who are at very high nutritional risk.

Nutrition Assessment

A thorough initial nutrition assessment for people living with HIV is important for the continuing nutrition care that follows. A registered dietitian (RD) should perform an assessment that provides the necessary information for planning and individualizing the nutritional support for the HIV-infected person. The nutritional assessment should establish rapport between the patient and the provider, creating a human context within which this continuum of nutritional care and support is provided. The basic nutrition assessment will provide a practical guide for HIV-infected patients, using the framework of the Nutrition Care Process[116] and these four steps: (1) nutrition assessment and reassessment, (2) nutrition diagnosis, (3) nutrition intervention, and (4) nutrition monitoring and evaluation.

The Components of the Nutrition, Clinical and Biochemical Assessments
Components of Nutritional Assessment

- **Diet Intake Assessment**
  - Usual intake, current intake, restrictions, modifications (use 24-hour recall and food diaries)
  - Ethnic and cultural food practices
  - Limitations in food access, food preparation, or both
  - Food intolerances, allergies, or both
  - Use of macronutrient or micronutrient supplements (or use of both)
  - Alcohol intake
  - Patient's goals for improving his or her intake
  - Use of fraudulent nutrition products or fads
- Psychosocial issues and comorbidities related to nutrition
  - Living situation, personal support
  - Food environment, types of meals, eating assistance needed
  - History of eating disorders or body image concerns
  - Housing status
- Food insecurities
  - Access to safe food and water
  - Comorbidities related to the disease and treatment
  - Other related comorbidities
- Medications related to the disease and/or comorbidities

Components of Clinical Assessment[116]

- Medical history
- Physical parameters related to nutrition care
- Physical activity level

BOX 24-1   NUTRITION-RELATED COMPLICATIONS OF AIDS AND NUTRITIONAL CARE

Nutrition-Related Complications of AIDS

Wasting/Rapid Weight Loss due to:

- Reduced intake
- Excessive nutrient losses due to vomit, diarrhea, or malabsorption
- Hypermetabolism
- Adverse gastrointestinal (GI) reactions to treatment

Nutritional Anemias

- Microcytic anemia/iron deficiency
- Macrocytic anemia/folate or vitamin B_{12} deficiency

Insulin Resistance

Lipodystrophy/Lipoatrophy

Loss of peripheral fat, in the face, arms, legs and/or buttocks, and an accumulation of central fat in the intraabdominal area, upper back (buffalo hump), and/or breasts

Hyperlipidemias:

- Triglyceridemias
- Total and low-density lipoprotein cholesterolemia

Sore Mouth/Throat, Stomatitis

Diarrhea

HIV Dementia

Nutrition Care and Recommendations

- Recommend a high-calorie (35 kcal/kg), high-protein (1.5 to 2 g/kg) diet with snacks between meals
- Oral high-calorie or protein supplement if extra calories/protein needed
- The physician may prescribe appetite stimulants if needed (Megace, Marinol, etc.)

Iron deficiency anemia:

- Daily oral iron supplements and recommend iron-rich foods, such as meat, fish, poultry, beans, dried fruits and fortified grains, cereals, and energy bars. Also good sources of vitamin C (orange juice, cantaloupe slices) at every meal
- Avoid iron-binding foods such as tea, coffee, or milk with meals or supplements.

Folate or vitamin B_{12} deficiency anemia:

- Oral folate supplements
- IM or SQ injections of vitamin B_{12}
- A high-protein diet (1.5 g/kg); meats, eggs, and milk products are rich in vitamin B_{12}
- Fresh fruits, and vegetables and their juices
- Monitor insulin resistance by measuring blood sugar, triglycerides, and Hgb_{A1c} if fasting glucose levels are consistently elevated, and adjust the diet accordingly
- Diabetic diet if needed
- A healthy diet using the MyPlate recommendations and an exercise regimen similar to those recommended for uninfected individuals
- Caloric intake should be adjusted to achieve and maintain a healthy body weight

The National Cholesterol Education Program (NCEP) Therapeutic Lifestyle Changes (TLC) diet

For a complete description of this diet, please access the National Heart, Lung, and Blood Institute website at http://www.nhlbi.nih.gov/guidelines/cholesterol/index.htm

- Eat cold foods such as ice creams, Popsicles, and Italian ices
- Moisten foods by adding gravies or sauces or soaking in liquids; prefer soft foods
- Avoid hard foods, and acidic, spicy, hot foods or beverages
- Avoid beverages that irritate or stimulate motility such as drinks that contain alcohol, and carbonated or caffeinated beverages
- Eat easy-to-digest foods, such as canned peaches, cooked carrots, baked chicken, turkey, or fish
- Avoid lactose-containing products such as milk and its products
- Avoid gassy foods
- Eat binding foods such as bananas, rice, applesauce, tea, toast, and gummy bears
- Replace fluid and electrolytes with electrolyte-containing foods and fluids
- Use safety strategies for food handling, storage, and preparation, as well as strategies for eating safely in restaurants and traveling abroad; see Box 24-2

The care of a caregiver, who actively supports the nutritional care of the patient, is essential to maintain adequate nutritional status, adherence to medication, and prevent HIV disease progression

Data from Keithley JK, Swanson B: *Nursing guidelines: HIV and nutrition*, ANAC, Ohio. <http//www. nursesinaidscare.org>. Accessed October 19, 2013; U.S. Food and Drug Administration: *Protecting and promoting your health. Antiretroviral drugs used in the treatment of HIV infection*, <http://www.fda.gov/ForConsumers/byAudience/ForPatientAdvocates/HIVandAIDSActivities/ucm118915.htm>. Updated August 20, 2013. Accessed October 19, 2013.

- Existing nutrition-related issues:
  - Hepatitis
  - Diabetes
  - Oral health issues
  - Bone disorders
- Family history of nutrition-related issues
- Weight history
- Usual level of physical activity
- GI complications
- Medications:
  - Potential food and drug interactions
  - Nutrition-related adverse effects
- Use of any complementary therapies (see the Complementary and Alternative Medicine [CAM] box, "Are Persons with HIV and AIDS Vulnerable to Nutritional Quackery?")
- Presence of opportunistic infections that may affect intake or metabolism
- Anthropometric measurements
  - Weight
  - Body mass index (BMI)
  - Subcutaneous fat stores

Components of the Biochemical Assessment

- Albumin
- Complete blood count

 COMPLEMENTARY AND ALTERNATIVE MEDICINE (CAM)

Are Persons with HIV and AIDS Vulnerable to Nutritional Quackery?[116]

People with chronic diseases, such as acquired immunodeficiency syndrome (AIDS), who lack curative therapy and have poor prognoses are susceptible to claims of unproved therapies and nutrition quackery. The following questionable practices are some of the nutritional quackery being touted as treatments for human immunodeficiency virus (HIV) infection.

Megadoses of Nutrients

Large doses of vitamins A and C, selenium, and zinc have been recommended to restore cell-mediated immunity by increasing T-cell number and activity. The value of such large doses has not been established in controlled clinical studies. In fact, the opposite is true; megadoses of these nutrients can be dangerous. Chronic intakes of vitamin A in excess of 25,000 IU/day can be toxic, especially to the liver. Doses of vitamin C greater than 2000 mg can cause diarrhea, nausea, and gastrointestinal (GI) upset; increase the risk of kidney stones; and cause a urine test to test falsely positive for diabetes. Chronic intakes of excess zinc, as little as 25 mg/day, can cause GI distress, nausea, and impaired immune function. Selenium is also toxic in high (>400 mcg daily) chronic doses. In a review of the literature on HIV and micronutrients, Campa and Baum found evidence that micronutrient supplementation at nutritional doses is beneficial in people living with HIV.[117]

- Glucose
- Serum iron
- Electrolytes
- Vitamin levels
- Blood lipids
- Renal function
- Liver enzyme levels

GOALS OF NUTRITION THERAPY

Adequate nutritional status is associated with survival in individuals with HIV.[118] Nutrition interventions have been shown to reduce morbidity, improve health outcomes, reduce cost, and shorten hospital stays. Goals of nutrition intervention include the following:

- Early assessment and treatment of conditions leading to malnutrition
- Maintenance of nutrition status
  - Weight
  - Protein stores
- Management of comorbid conditions
  - Obesity
  - Diabetes
  - Hyperlipidemia
- Management of nutrition-related sideeffects from HIV or disease treatment

Nutrient Requirements

Adequate intake of nutrients is critical in restoring and maintaining health. The benefits of providing adequate amounts of energy, protein, fat, and micronutrients for people living with HIV are well-described in the literature[1]; the optimal amounts of each nutrient to improve disease outcomes, however, need more research.[117]

Energy

Individuals' energy needs will vary depending on numerous factors, including nutrient malabsorption, altered metabolism, nutrient depletion, severity of disease, and opportunistic infections. Adequate energy intake is important to prevent weight loss and loss of lean body mass. Care should be taken to estimate recommendations for daily energy intake, although no standard level of energy intake has been established.[1]

Protein

A diet that offers a protein intake ranging from 1.2 to 2.0 g protein/kg body weight may be beneficial for people living with HIV who have suffered wasting due to HIV progression, secondary opportunistic infections, and/or severe socioeconomic conditions. For those patients early in the disease who are asymptomatic, the Dietary Reference Intakes (DRIs) or 0.8 g protein/kg body weight may be adequate. Although high biologic value protein is desirable, a balanced combination of animal and vegetarian sources of protein may be used. Strict vegetarians should eat an extensive variety of foods to achieve sufficient intake of essential amino acids. In general, vegetarians will benefit from additional protein (1 g protein/kg/day), calorie, iron, and vitamin B_{12} supplementation.

Fat

Fat requirements of individuals with HIV do not seem to be different from the general population. Some medications, therapies for HIV, symptoms of infections (i.e., diarrhea), and malabsorption syndromes will possibly necessitate modification in the timing, quality, and type of fat intake for some persons. It is crucial to work with each individual closely to determine his or her needs.

Micronutrients

Currently, the complete function of micronutrients in treatment of HIV is not completely known. However, individuals are sure to benefit from a varied diet rich in micronutrients.

Food and Water Safety

The compromised immune system of individuals with AIDS puts them at great risk for foodborne (Box 24-2) or waterborne (Box 24-3) illnesses. Fortunately, nearly all cases of foodborne and waterborne illnesses can be reduced or prevented with appropriate safety measures including safe food handling and use of safe water sources (see Box 24-1). It is essential for the RD to stress food and water safety in nutrition counseling for individuals living with HIV, their significant others, and their caretakers.

According to the Centers for Disease Control and Prevention (CDC), boiling municipal tap water and use of bottled water are not essential unless a local public health department has issued notice that public drinking water is not safe for individuals living with HIV. Box 24-2 outlines precautions of particular importance for individuals living in areas without a municipal water source. Ice and fountain drinks in restaurants are often made from municipal water and should be avoided if safety of the water is unknown. Food and water sanitation may not be adequate when traveling abroad. Guidelines for choosing safer beverages are outlined in Box 24-4.

Antiretroviral Therapy–Associated Metabolic and Body Composition Changes

Although ART has revolutionized medical treatment of HIV and AIDS and reduced incidence of malnutrition and infections, its adverse effects continue to be a major obstacle to patient compliance and a limiting factor that drives the cost-benefit ratio for pharmacologic therapy. Lipodystrophy and its related fat distribution complications have become the major nutrition issues in patients being treated with PIs. Lipodystrophy syndrome consists of changes in body shape that are caused by abnormal redistribution of fat. Fat accumulates in the abdominal area (truncal and visceral obesity), in the axillary pads, and in the dorsocervical pads ("buffalo

---

BOX 24-2 FOOD SAFETY PRECAUTIONS FOR INDIVIDUALS LIVING WITH HIV

Purchasing Food
- Do not eat food that has passed the expiration date or purchase past the "sell by" date.
- Make sure all dairy products (including cheeses) and juices have been pasteurized or made with pasteurized ingredients.
- When shopping, put packaged meat, poultry, and fish in separate plastic bags to ensure juices do not drip on other foods.
- Do not purchase food that has been displayed in unsafe or unclean conditions (e.g., meat that has been unrefrigerated or cooked shrimp that is displayed with raw shrimp).
- Do not purchase cans that are dented, leaking, or bulging.

Preparing and Serving Food
- Wash hands with warm soapy water before and after preparing and eating foods. Also wash hands before and after using the bathroom, handling pets, or changing diapers.
- Wash counter surfaces, cutting boards, can openers, and utensils with hot soapy water before and after use. Sanitize kitchen surfaces, using a commercial sanitizing product or a mixture of 1 teaspoon of chlorine bleach per 1 quart of water.
- Avoid cross-contamination of foods, using separate cutting boards for cooked and uncooked foods.
- Do not eat raw or undercooked meat, eggs, poultry, fish, or shellfish. (This includes hotdogs, types of sushi and

sashimi that contain raw fish, and foods that contain raw eggs.)
- Use an appropriate food thermometer to ensure that all foods reach the proper internal temperature before serving.

Storing Foods
- Store raw meat, poultry, and seafood in separate containers on the bottom shelf of the refrigerator
- Freeze fresh meat, poultry, and seafood that you do not plan to use within a few days. Do not refreeze previously frozen foods and thawed foods, especially meat, poultry, and seafood.
- Use refrigerator and freezer thermometers to ensure foods are stored at appropriate temperatures (freezer at 0° F and refrigerator at 40° F).

Eating Out
- Choose "well done" meats, fish, and poultry. Make sure they are served hot.
- Avoid raw or undercooked eggs. Order fried eggs cooked "hard" and avoid eggs that are "sunny-side-up." Scrambled eggs should not be runny.
- If you aren't sure about the ingredients in a dish or how it is cooked, ask your wait staff before you order.
- Avoid open salad bars in public places.

Reprinted with permission from Vining L: General nutrition issues for healthy living with HIV infection. In Hendricks KM, Dong KR, Gerrior JL, editors: *Nutrition management of HIV and AIDS*, Chicago, 2009, American Dietetic Association.

BOX 24-3   EXTRA PRECAUTIONS TO ENSURE SAFE WATER

Persons living with HIV should avoid drinking water straight from lakes, rivers, streams, springs, or the ocean. Current recommendations from the Centers for Disease Control and Prevention (CDC) state the following:

- Because it might not be possible to be sure if tap water is safe, it is advisable to avoid tap water, including water or ice from a refrigerator ice maker, which is made with tap water.
- Always check with the local health department and water utility to see if they have issued any special notices for people with HIV about tap water.
- You may also wish to boil or filter your water, or drink bottled water.
- Drinks made at a fountain might not be safe because they are made with tap water.
- If you choose to boil or filter your water or drink only bottled water, do this all the time, not just at home.
- Boiling is the best way to kill germs in your water. Heat your water at a rolling boil for 1 minute. After the boiled water cools, put it in a clean bottle or pitcher with a lid and store it in the refrigerator. Use the water for drinking, cooking, or making ice.
- Water bottles and ice trays should be cleaned with soap and water before use. Don't touch the inside of them after cleaning. If you can, clean your water bottles and ice trays yourself.

BOX 24-4   CHOOSING SAFER BEVERAGES

Safer Beverages
- Carbonated beverages ("sodas") that come in cans or bottles (check seal to ensure safety)
- Fruit drinks that come in cans or bottles (check seal to ensure safety)
- Steaming hot tea or coffee
- Pasteurized milk and other dairy products
- Pasteurized juices

Beverages That May Not Be Safe
- Fountain drinks or drinks served over ice
- Drinks made by mixing frozen concentrate with water
- Iced tea or coffee
- Unpasteurized milk and other dairy products
- Fresh fruit juices (e.g., unpasteurized cider, fresh-squeezed orange juice)

Reprinted with permission from Vining L: General nutrition issues for healthy living with HIV infection. In Hendricks KM, Dong KR, Gerrior JL, editors: *Nutrition management of HIV and AIDS*, Chicago, 2009, Academy of Nutrition and Dietetics. Data from Centers for Disease Control and Prevention: *Safe food and water*, <http://www.cdc.gov/hiv/resources/brochures/food.htm>. Accessed July 15, 2013; Keithley JK, Swanson B: *Nursing guidelines: HIV and nutrition*, ANAC, Ohio. <http//www. nursesinaidscare.org>. Accessed October 19, 2013.

---

hump") but decreases in the legs, arms, and nasolabial and cheek pads.[118,119] Lipodystrophy, although not life threatening, can cause varying degrees of depression, anxiety, social withdrawal, and low self-esteem, which can ultimately lead to poor medication compliance.[1] Many patients discontinue therapy, risking progression of HIV infection. ART can also cause hyperlipidemia (especially hypertriglyceridemia and hypercholesterolemia) and insulin resistance, which can significantly increase the risk of developing cardiovascular disease (CVD). This is a major concern and potentially a major deterrent to early or continuous therapy. Overall, the risk of myocardial infarction (MI) in HIV-infected patients taking PIs appears to be twofold to threefold greater than in the general population.[120] Persons on ART are also at increased risk of developing diabetes, hypertension, and osteoporosis.

Obtaining baseline anthropometrics (waist-hip ratio, bioelectric impedance analysis, skinfold measurements) and serial measurements (i.e., at each clinic visit) is important for monitoring changes in body composition. In addition, baseline measurements of triglycerides, total cholesterol and lipoproteins (high-density lipoprotein [HDL], low-density lipoprotein [LDL], very low-density lipoprotein [VLDL]), blood glucose, and blood pressure should be obtained (also at each clinic visit to monitor for changes). Diet, exercise, and pharmacologic agents are useful in the treatment of lipodystrophy syndrome. Patients with abnormal LDL, HDL, and total cholesterol levels may benefit from observing the therapeutic lifestyle changes (TLC) diet, which emphasizes grains, cereals, legumes, fruits, vegetables, lean meats, poultry, fish, and low-fat dairy products. Diet-resistant hyperlipidemia may need to be controlled with lipid-lowering agents. Currently researchers are trying to determine which drugs can be used safely and effectively in persons on anti-HIV drugs. Individuals with insulin resistance and hyperglycemia will need counseling for carbohydrate counting and may benefit from a tailored diabetic diet. An individual with hypertriglyceridemia will need to limit intake of simple carbohydrates and alcohol. Exercise, especially weight training, may help prevent muscle wasting in the arms, legs, and buttocks, whereas aerobic exercise may help control abdominal visceral fat accumulation. Clinical trials are ongoing to determine actual benefits (see Box 24-1).

Use of Anabolic Agents in HIV and AIDS

The use of anabolic agents has been recommended as an effective way of improving gains in lean body mass. Anabolic agents such as oxandrolone and nandrolone decanoate are known to promote protein anabolism and are generally safe when taken as prescribed.[121] Recombinant human growth hormone (rhGH) (trade name Serostim) is the most extensively studied anabolic agent; it has also been shown to significantly improve lean body mass and nitrogen balance in treatment of HIV/AIDS wasting.[122] Human growth hormone therapy may help control some of the body composition changes seen in some individuals with lipodystrophy. However, many potential side effects exist for anabolic agents, including gynecomastia, testicular atrophy and decreased fertility, salt retention, lipid and carbohydrate abnormalities, and acne. Resistance or weight training have shown benefits in people living with HIV, and they have been found safe and effective for maintaining and improving lean body mass in infected people who are physically able to exercise.[123]

Nutrition Counseling, Education, and Supportive Strategies

Professionals and patients must be involved throughout the progressive course of the disease, because the patient's wishes and needs are ultimately paramount in various treatments and decisions about care. The goal of nutrition counseling is to make the fewest possible changes in the person's lifestyle and food patterns to promote optimal nutritional status while providing comfort and quality of life. In this person-centered care process, several counseling principles are particularly pertinent:

- *Motivation:* Changed behavior in any area requires motivation, desire, and ability to achieve one's goals. Until the patient perceives food patterns and behaviors as appropriate goals, it is best to wait for a better time and begin with establishing a general supportive climate in which to continue working together. Any specific obstacle raised by the patient, such as time, physical limitations, money, or increased anxiety, can be met with related suggestions for the patient to consider. Priorities among needs should be recognized in the care plan, and items should be introduced according to order of importance and immediacy of the patient's nutrition problems.
- *Justification:* Any diet or food behavior change, with possible benefits and risks, must be clearly explained to the patient. The reason *why* something is being done is important to everyone. Understanding may increase compliance.
- *Provider-patient agreement:* In the best interests of all concerned, the patient and health care provider must agree to changes. Any change should be structured around daily routines and include caregivers. The nutrition counselor should provide any needed information and encouragement throughout the process.
- *Manageable steps:* All information given and actions agreed on should proceed in manageable steps, as small as necessary, in order of complexity and difficulty. Information overload can discourage anyone, and the particular stress load at any point can be intolerable for the patient. At such points of stress, patients are more vulnerable to the lure of unproved HIV/AIDS therapies.

Special Considerations for Children with AIDS[1]

Malnutrition, particularly inadequate calories and protein, and dehydration are serious issues in children with AIDS. In adults, the disease affects nutritional status. In children, not only is nutritional status affected but also growth and development can be significantly impaired, resulting in growth failure. A strong relationship exists between early nutritional status—poor growth, cachexia, poor oral intake, taste changes, decreased absorption of nutrients, and increased energy expenditure—and mortality risk; poor nutritional status increases mortality.

Nutrition assessments should be performed routinely in all children with AIDS so that any problems can be identified and treated as they occur and nutritional deficits can be minimized. As with adults, assessments should include evaluation of anthropometrics, visceral protein stores, red blood cell indexes, and electrolytes. In addition, growth assessment should be performed as frequently as needed, or following the standard pediatric schedule to monitor growth curves. Appetite, intake, and feeding ability should also be assessed. Developmental delays related to the disease can also increase the risk for developing failure to thrive.

Providing adequate calories to maintain linear growth and support weight gain can be difficult as a result of chronic infections, fever, and medications. The CDC revised the criteria for pregnant women, infants, and children in July 2012, and issued the following recommendation for the postnatal management of the HIV-exposed neonate[124]:

- A complete blood count and differential should be performed on newborns as a baseline evaluation.
- Decisions about the timing of subsequent monitoring of hematologic parameters in infants depend on baseline hematologic values, gestational age at birth, clinical condition of the infants, the zidovudine dose being administered, receipt of other antiretroviral drugs and concomitant medications, and maternal antepartum ART.
- If hematologic abnormalities are identified in infants receiving prophylaxis, decisions on whether to continue infant antiretroviral prophylaxis need to be individualized. Consultation with an expert in pediatric HIV infection is advised if early discontinuation of prophylaxis is considered.
- Some experts recommend more intensive monitoring of hematologic and serum chemistry and liver function assays at birth and when diagnostic HIV polymerase chain reaction tests are obtained in infants exposed to combination ARV drug regimens *in utero* or during the neonatal period.
- A recheck of hemoglobin and neutrophil counts is recommended 4 weeks after initiation of prophylaxis for infants who receive combination zidovudine/lamivudine-containing ARV prophylaxis regimens.
- Routine measurement of serum lactate is not recommended. However, measurement can be considered if an infant develops severe clinical symptoms of unknown etiology (particularly neurologic symptoms).
- Virologic tests are required to diagnose HIV infection in infants younger than 18 months of age and should be performed within the first 14 to 21 days of life, at 1 to 2 months, and at 4 to 6 months of age.

- To prevent *Pneumocystis jirovecii* pneumonia (PJP), all infants born to women with HIV infection should begin PJP prophylaxis at ages 4 to 6 weeks, after completing their ARV prophylaxis regimen, unless there is adequate test information to presumptively exclude HIV infection (see USPHS/IDSA Guidelines for the Prevention and Treatment of Opportunistic Infections in HIV-Exposed and Infected Children at http://aidsinfo.nih.gov/guidelines).
- Health care providers should routinely inquire about pre-mastication of foods fed to infants, instruct HIV-infected caregivers to avoid this practice, and should advise on safer feeding options.

Diarrhea and malabsorption in the infected child can result in dehydration, which can be very serious in infants and young children, and the onset may occur suddenly.[1] To prevent dehydration, offer Popsicles, Jell-O, juices, and other beverages frequently. Oral rehydration fluids, such as Pedialyte, will also help to replace electrolytes lost with acute or chronic diarrhea.

The following list contains suggestions to provide supplemental calories and nutrient intake[1]:

- Use a calorie-dense formula (24 to 27 kcal/oz) for infants. Add glucose polymers or medium-chain triglycerides (MCTs) to formulas, or reduce the amount of water added to powdered formulas to boost calories.
- Try liquid medical nutritional supplements, such as PediaSure, to provide supplemental calories.
- Add fats such as butter, margarine, or mayonnaise to foods to boost calories.
- Encourage nutrient-dense snacks such as raisins and peanuts or peanut butter.
- For the older, lactose-tolerant child, add skim milk powder to whole milk to boost calories and proteins.

- Make adjustments in diet consistency and temperatures to overcome eating difficulties associated with disease complications and any other eating problems.
- For lactose-intolerant children with AIDS, use soy-based infant formulas instead of milk.
- Add Lactaid (the enzyme lactase) to milk for better tolerance and digestion.
- Use low-lactose dairy foods such as yogurt and mild cheddar cheese, if tolerated.

Vitamin and mineral supplements in amounts one or two times the Recommended Dietary Allowance (RDA) may ensure adequate intake of these nutrients and contribute to meeting increased requirements that occur during hypermetabolic states. Attention should also be given to drug-nutrient interactions and other effects of these drugs on nutritional status.

Caregivers need to be particularly careful about food safety and sanitation. Safe food preparation is as important for children as it is for adults with HIV/AIDS, and the same food safety guidelines also apply.

Proper procedures and sanitary formula preparation must be followed for infants being bottle-fed. Infants should not be put to bed with a bottle of milk or juice, because they are easily contaminated. Unpasteurized milk and milk products should never be given, because they may be a source of *Salmonella* and other microorganisms that can cause intestinal infections.

Children should never be fed any food directly from a jar to avoid possible bacterial contamination of the remaining food from the child's mouth. Fruits and vegetables should be peeled or cooked, and meat, chicken, and fish should be well cooked. All utensils and dishes should be washed in a dishwasher or in hot, soapy water.

▌ TO SUM UP

The viral evolution and current worldwide spread of HIV infection have reached epidemic proportions and are still growing. Disease progression follows three distinct stages (1) HIV acute infection; (2) asymptomatic (latency) stage and (3) final full-blown AIDS, with complicating diseases leading to death. This overall disease progression from initial infection to death lasts about 10 to 12 years or in some cases even longer. The Public Health Service and the CDC are responsible for monitoring the disease and providing leadership in research and treatment development, based on collaborative information exchange with scientists worldwide.

During the initial decade of the epidemic in the 1980s, scientists learned the nature and life cycle of the new mutation of HIV, as well as its transmission modes and population groups at risk. Development of diagnostic-testing procedures has enabled population surveillance, individual detection of disease, and personal care to proceed. The important role of nutrition support in the personal care of HIV-infected individuals has become evident.

Medical management of HIV infection, which is without a vaccine or cure, involves supportive treatment of associated illnesses and complicating diseases coupled with administration of ART. In the terminal HIV stage, the virus eventually gains sufficient strength to destroy white blood cells of the host's immune system and death follows.

Nutritional management focuses on providing personal individual nutrition support to address the nutrition-related diseases associated with HIV itself, its complications, and its long-term treatment, as well as the aging of people living with HIV. The process of nutrition care involves performing a comprehensive nutrition, clinical, and biochemical assessment, which includes evaluation of personal needs, planning care with each patient and his or her caregivers, and meeting practical food needs. Throughout the nutrition care process, nutrition counseling, education, and strategic services, it is also important to provide or refer the patient and caregivers to psychosocial support. Although HIV/AIDS cannot be cured with nutrition, appropriate individualized nutritional support can prolong life.

QUESTIONS FOR REVIEW

1. Describe the evolutionary history of HIV and its current worldwide epidemic spread. How is it transmitted, and why do you think it has spread so rapidly? Identify major population groups at risk.

2. Describe the nature of HIV and its action in the human body. What is a retrovirus?

3. Describe the progression of HIV infection in terms of its stages of development from initial infection to death.

4. Identify the drugs currently used in the medical management of HIV/AIDS, and describe any associated actions, side effects, or toxicities that may relate to dietary management.

5. Discuss the causes of HIV wasting and its medical and nutrition therapies.

6. Outline the basic parts of a comprehensive initial nutrition assessment of a patient with HIV/AIDS.

7. Describe the general process of planning nutrition care based on patient assessment information and the main types of nutrition problems in patients with HIV/AIDS. Devise a related plan of action for each type of problem. Can you give an example of how you might follow up to determine which parts of your plan worked and which parts did not work? List any adjustments that should be made to your original nutrition care plan based on that follow-up.

REFERENCES

1. Fields-Gardner C, Campa A: American Dietetic Association. Position of the American Dietetic Association: Nutrition Intervention and Human Immunodeficiency Virus Infection. *J Am Diet Assoc* 110(7):1105–1119, 2010.

2. Tomkins A: Malnutrition, morbidity and mortality in children and their mothers. *Proc Nutr Soc* 59(1):135–146, 2000.

3. Caulfield LE, de Onis M, Blössner M, et al: Undernutrition as an underlying cause of child deaths associated with diarrhea, pneumonia, malaria, and measles. *Am J Clin Nutr* 80(1):193–198, 2004.

4. Blössner M, de Onis M: *Malnutrition: quantifying the impact at national and local levels*, Geneva, 2005, WHO.

5. AIDS.gov: *HIV/AIDS Basics.* <http://aids.gov/hiv-aids-basics/hiv-aids-101/statistics/index.html>. Reviewed June 6, 2012. Accessed May 17, 2013.

6. World Health Organization: Data and Statistics. Annex 8. HIV and AIDS statistics by WHO and UNICEF regions, 2010. <http://www.who.int/hiv/data/en/>. Accessed July 5, 2013.

7. Piot P, Quinn TC: Response to the AIDS pandemic—a global health model. *N Engl J Med* 368(23):2210–2218, 2013.

8. World Health Organization: WHO issues new HIV recommendations calling for earlier treatment, 2013. <http://www.who.int/mediacentre/news/releases/2013/new_hiv_recommendations_20130630/en/index.html>. Accessed July 3, 2013.

9. Brandt AM: How AIDS invented global health. *N Engl J Med* 368(23):2149–2152, 2013.

10. Pantaleo G, Graziosi C, Fauci AS: New concepts in the immunopathogenesis of human immunodeficiency virus infection. *N Engl J Med* 328(5):327–335, 1993.

11. HIV Classification: *CDC and WHO Staging Systems,* <http://hab.hrsa.gov/deliverhivaidscare/clinicalguide11/cg-205_hiv_classification.html>. Accessed July 9, 2013.

12. Rote NS: Hypersensitivities, infection, and immune efficiencies. In Huether SE, McCance KL, editors: *Understanding pathophysiology*, ed 4, St Louis, 2008, Mosby.

13. Rote NS: Alterations in immunity and inflammation. In McCance KL, Huether SE, editors: *Pathophysiology: the biologic basis for disease in adults and children*, ed 5, St Louis, 2006, Mosby.

14. Gould BE: *Pathophysiology for the health professions*, ed 3, St Louis, 2006, Mosby.

15. Centers for Disease Control and Prevention: *National HIV and STD Testing Resources, HIV Testing*: <http://hivtest.cdc.gov/faq.aspx#tested>. Accessed July 11, 2013.

16. Centers for Disease Control and Prevention: *Division of HIV/AIDS Prevention. National Center for HIV/AIDS, Viral Hepatitis, STD, and TB Prevention, Rapid HIV testing.* Last modified July 27, 2012: <http://www.cdc.gov/hiv/topics/testing/rapid/index.htm>. Accessed July 11, 2013.

17. U.S. Department of Health and Human Services. U.S. Food and Drug Administration: <http://www.fda.gov/Biologics BloodVaccines/BloodBloodProducts/ApprovedProducts/LicensedProductsBLAs/BloodDonorScreening/InfectiousDisease/UCM080466>. Accessed July 15, 2013.

18. HIV and AIDS Activities: Antiretroviral drugs used in the treatment of HIV infection.

19. Dong KR, Mangili A: Highly active antiretroviral therapy (HAART). In Hendricks KM, Dong KR, Gerrior JL, editors: *Nutrition management of HIV and AIDS*, Chicago, 2009, American Dietetic Association.

20. *Guidelines for the use of antiretroviral agents in HIV-1 in adults and adolescents.* <aidsinfo.nih.gov/contentfiles/lvguidelines/adultandadolescentgl.pdf>. Accessed July 15, 2013.

21. Katona P, Katona-Apte J: The Interaction between Nutrition and Infection. *Clin Infect Dis* 46(10):1582–1588, 2008.

22. Piwoz E, Preble E: *HIV/AIDS and nutrition: a review of the literature and recommendations for nutritional care and support in sub-Saharan Africa*, Washington, DC, 2000, Academy for Educational Development [AED], Support for Analysis and Research in Africa Project [SARA].

23. Semba RD, Tang AM: Micronutrients and the pathogenesis of human immunodeficiency virus infection. *Br J Nutr* 81(03):181–189, 1999.

24. McCorkindale C, Dybevik K, Coulston AM, et al: Nutritional status of HIV-infected patients during the early disease stages. *J Am Diet Assoc* 90(9):1236–1241, 1990.

25. Kim JH, Spiegelman D, Rimm E, et al: The correlates of dietary intake among HIV-positive adults. *Am J Clin Nutr* 74(6):852–861, 2001.

26. Baum M, Cassetti L, Bonvehi P, et al: Inadequate dietary intake and altered nutrition status in early HIV-1 infection. *Nutrition* 10(1):16–20, 1994.

27. Mangili A, Murman DH, Zampini AM, et al: Nutrition and HIV infection: review of weight loss and wasting in the era of highly active antiretroviral therapy from the nutrition for healthy living cohort. *Clin Infect Dis* 42(6):836–842, 2006.

28. Babameto G, Kotler DP: Malnutrition in HIV infection. *Gastroenterol Clin North Am* 26(2):393–415, 1997.

29. Keating J, Bjarnason I, Somasundaram S, et al: Intestinal absorptive capacity, intestinal permeability and jejunal histology in HIV and their relation to diarrhoea. *Gut* 37(5):623–629, 1995.

30. Cunningham-Rundles S: Effects of nutritional status on immunological function. *Am J Clin Nutr* 35(5):1202–1210, 1982.

31. Meydani SN, Beharka AA: Recent developments in vitamin E and immune response. *Nutr Rev* 56(1 Pt 2):S49–S58, 1998.

32. Maggini S, Wintergerst ES, Beveridge S, et al: Selected vitamins and trace elements support immune function by strengthening epithelial barriers and cellular and humoral immune responses. *Br J Nutr* 98(1):S29–S35, 2007.

33. WHO: *Nutrient requirements for people living with HIV/AIDS: report of a technical consultation*, Geneva, 2003, WHO.

34. Shevitz AH, Knox TA, Spiegelman D, et al: Elevated resting energy expenditure among HIV-seropositive persons receiving highly active antiretroviral therapy. *AIDS* 13(11):1351–1357, 1999.

35. FANTA: *Food assistance programming in the context of HIV. Food and Nutrition Technical Assistance (FANTA) Project and World Food Programme (WFP)*, Washington, DC, 2007, FANTA Project, Academy for Educational Development.

36. *Mosby's medical dictionary*, ed 8, 2009, Elsevier Inc.

37. Melchior J-C, Niyongabo T, Henzel D, et al: Malnutrition and wasting, immunodepression, and chronic inflammation as independent predictors of survival in HIV-infected patients. *Nutr* 15(11–12):865–869, 1999.

38. Chlebowski RT, Grosvenor MB, Bernhard NH, et al: Nutritional status, gastrointestinal dysfunction, and survival in patients with AIDS. *Am J Gastroenterol* 84(10):1288–1293, 1989.

39. Scrimshaw NS: Effect of infection on nutritional status. *Proc Natl Sci Counc Repub China B* 16(1):46–64, 1992.

40. Liu E, Spiegelman D, Semu H, et al: Nutritional status and mortality among HIV-infected patients receiving antiretroviral therapy in Tanzania. *J Infect Dis* 204(2):282–290, 2011.

41. Koethe JR, Heimburger DC: Nutritional aspects of HIV-associated wasting in sub-Saharan Africa. *Am J Clin Nutr* 91(4):1138S–1142S, 2010.

42. Semba RD, Shah N, Strathdee SA, et al: High prevalence of iron deficiency and anemia among female injection drug users with and without HIV infection. *J Acquir Immune Defic Syndr* 29(2):142–144, 2002.

43. Periquet BA, Jammes NM, Lambert WE, et al: Micronutrient levels in HIV-1-infected children. *AIDS* 9(8):887–893, 1995.

44. Beach RS, Mantero-Atienza E, Shor-Posner G, et al: Specific nutrient abnormalities in asymptomatic HIV-1 infection. *AIDS* 6(7):701–708, 1992.

45. Lacey CJ, Murphy ME, Sanderson MJ, et al: Antioxidant-micronutrients and HIV infection. *Int J STD AIDS* 7(7):485–489, 1996.

46. Tang AM, Lanzillotti J, Hendricks K, et al: Micronutrients: current issues for HIV care providers. *AIDS* 19(9):847–861, 2005.

47. Tang AM, Smit E: Selected vitamins in HIV infection: a review. *AIDS Patient Care STDS* 12(4):263–273, 1998.

48. Baum MK: Role of Micronutrients in HIV-infected intravenous drug users. *J Acquir Immune Defic Syndr* 25:S49–S52, 2000.

49. Haug CJ, Aukrust P, Haug E, et al: Severe deficiency of 1,25-dihydroxyvitamin D_3 in human immunodeficiency virus infection: association with immunological hyperactivity and only minor changes in calcium homeostasis. *J Clin Endocrinol Metab* 83(11):3832–3838, 1998.

50. Wanke CA, Silva M, Knox TA, et al: Weight Loss and Wasting Remain Common Complications in Individuals Infected with Human Immunodeficiency Virus in the Era of Highly Active Antiretroviral Therapy. *Clin Infect Dis* 31(3):803–805, 2000.

51. Batterham M, Gold J, Naidoo D, et al: A preliminary open label dose comparison using an antioxidant regimen to determine the effect on viral load and oxidative stress in men with HIV/AIDS. *Eur J Clin Nutr* 55(2):107–114, 2001.

52. Look MP, Riezler R, Berthold HK, et al: Decrease of elevated N,N-dimethylglycine and N-methylglycine in human immunodeficiency virus infection during short-term highly active antiretroviral therapy. *Metabolism* 50(11):1275–1281, 2001.

53. Remacha AF, Cadafalch J, Sardà P, et al: Vitamin B-12 metabolism in HIV-infected patients in the age of highly active antiretroviral therapy: role of homocysteine in assessing vitamin B-12 status. *Am J Clin Nutr* 77(2):420–424, 2003.

54. Rousseau MC, Molines C, Moreau J, et al: Influence of highly active antiretroviral therapy on micronutrient profiles in HIV-infected patients. *Ann Nutr Metab* 44(5–6):212–216, 2000.

55. Tang AM, Smit E, Semba RD, et al: Improved antioxidant status among HIV-infected injecting drug users on potent antiretroviral therapy. *J Acquir Immune Defic Syndr* 23(4):321–326, 2000.

56. Toma E, Devost D, Lan NC, et al: HIV-protease inhibitors alter retinoic acid synthesis. *AIDS* 15(15):1979–1984, 2001.

57. Wellinghausen N, Kern WV, Jochle W, et al: Zinc serum level in human immunodeficiency virus-infected patients in relation to immunological status. *Biol Trace Elem Res* 73(2):139–149, 2000.

58. Woods MN, Tang AM, Forrester J, et al: Effect of dietary intake and protease inhibitors on serum vitamin B_{12} levels in a cohort of human immunodeficiency virus—positive patients. *Clin Infect Dis* 37(Suppl 2):S124–S131, 2003.

59. Khalili H, Soudbakhsh A, Hajiabdolbaghi M, et al: Nutritional status and serum zinc and selenium levels in Iranian HIV infected individuals. *BMC Infect Dis* 8:165, 2008.

60. Wheeler DA, Gibert CL, Launer CA, et al: Weight loss as a predictor of survival and disease progression in HIV infection. *J Acquir Immune Defic Syndr* 18(1):80–85, 1998.

61. Campa A, Zhifang Y, Lai S, et al: HIV-related wasting in HIV-infected drug users in the era of highly active antiretroviral therapy clinic. *Infect Dis* 41(8):1179–1185, 2005.

62. Tang AM, Forrester J, Spiegelman D, et al: Weight loss and survival in HIV-positive patients in the era of highly active antiretroviral therapy. *J Acquir Immune Defic Syndr* 31(2):230–236, 2002.

63. Hendricks KM, Willis K, Houser R, et al: Obesity in HIV-infection: dietary correlates. *J Am Coll Nutr* 25(4):321–331, 2006.

64. Shevitz AH, Knox TA: Nutrition in the era of highly active antiretroviral therapy. *Clin Infect Dis* 32(12):1769–1775, 2001.

65. Amorosa V, Synnestvedt M, Gross R, et al: A tale of 2 epidemics: the intersection between obesity and HIV infection in Philadelphia. *J Acquir Immune Defic Syndr* 39(5):557–561, 2005.

66. Crum-Cianflone N, Roediger MP, Eberly L, et al: Increasing rates of obesity among HIV-infected persons during the HIV epidemic. *PLoS One* 5(4):e10106, 2010.

67. Crum-Cianflone N, Tejidor R, Medina S, et al: Obesity among patients with HIV: the latest epidemic. *AIDS Patient Care STDS* 22(12):925–930, 2008.

68. Hodgson LM, Ghattas H, Pritchitt H, et al: Wasting and obesity in HIV outpatients. *AIDS* 15(17):2341–2342, 2001.

69. Campa A, Yang Z, Sales S, et al: Inadequate food and micronutrient intake in HIV⁺ drug users. International conference on AIDS, Barcelona, Spain, 2002.

70. Anema A, Weiser SD, Fernandes KA, et al: High prevalence of food insecurity among HIV-infected individuals receiving HAART in a resource-rich setting. *AIDS Care* 23(2):221–230, 2011.

71. Quach LA, Wanke CA, Schmid CH, et al: Drug use and other risk factors related to lower body mass index among HIV-infected individuals. *Drug Alcohol Depend* 95(1–2):30–36, 2008.

72. Normen L, Chan K, Braitstein P, et al: Food insecurity and hunger are prevalent among HIV-positive individuals in British Columbia, Canada. *J Nutr* 135(4):820–825, 2005.

73. Vogenthaler N, Hadley C, Rodriguez A, et al: Depressive symptoms and food insufficiency among HIV-infected crack users in Atlanta and Miami. *AIDS Behav* 15(7):1520–1526, 2011.

74. Weiser S, Bangsberg D, Kegeles S, et al: Food insecurity among homeless and marginally housed individuals living with HIV/AIDS in San Francisco. *AIDS Behav* 13(5):841–848, 2009.

75. Weiser S, Frongillo E, Ragland K, et al: Food insecurity is associated with incomplete HIV RNA suppression among homeless and marginally housed HIV-infected individuals in San Francisco. *J Gen Intern Med* 24(1):14–20, 2009.

76. Weiser SD, Fernandes KA, Brandson EK, et al: The association between food insecurity and mortality among HIV-infected individuals on HAART. *J Acquir Immune Defic Syndr* 52(3):342–349, 2009.

77. Weiser SD, Tsai AC, Gupta R, et al: Food insecurity is associated with morbidity and patterns of healthcare utilization among HIV-infected individuals in a resource-poor setting. *AIDS* 26(1):67–75, 2012.

78. Baum MK, Jayaweera DT, Duan R, et al: Quality of life, symptomatology and healthcare utilization in HIV/HCV co-infected drug users in Miami. *J Addict Dis* 27(2):37–48, 2008.

79. Dorey-Stein Z, Amorosa VK, Kostman JR, et al: Severe weight gain, lipodystrophy, dyslipidemia, and obstructive sleep apnea in a human immunodeficiency virus-infected patient following highly active antiretroviral therapy. *J Cardiometab Syndr* 3(2):111–114, 2008.

80. Grinspoon S: Insulin resistance in the HIV-lipodystrophy syndrome. *Trends Endocrinol Metab* 12(9):413–419, 2001.

81. Batterham MJ, Garsia R, Greenop PA: Dietary intake, serum lipids, insulin resistance and body composition in the era of highly active antiretroviral therapy. Diet FRS Study. *AIDS* 14(12):1839–1843, 2000.

82. Jaime PC, Florindo AA, Latorre Mdo R, et al: Central obesity and dietary intake in HIV/AIDS patients. *Rev Saude Publica* 40(4):634–640, 2006.

83. Joy T, Keogh HM, Hadigan C, et al: Dietary fat intake and relationship to serum lipid levels in HIV-infected patients with metabolic abnormalities in the HAART era. *AIDS* 21(12):1591–1600, 2007.

84. Chlebowski RT, Grosvenor M, Lillington L, et al: Dietary intake and counseling, weight maintenance, and the course of HIV infection. *J Am Diet Assoc* 95(4):428–435, 1995.

85. Hendricks KM, Dong KR, Tang AM, et al: High-fiber diet in HIV-positive men is associated with lower risk of developing fat deposition. *Am J Clin Nutr* 78(4):790–795, 2003.

86. Hendricks KM, Mwamburi DM, Newby P, et al: Dietary patterns and health and nutrition outcomes in men living with HIV infection. *Am J Clin Nutr* 88(6):1584–1592, 2008.

87. Hendricks KM, Sansavero M, Houser RF, et al: Dietary supplement use and nutrient intake in HIV-infected persons. *AIDS Read* 17(4):211–216, 2007.

88. Smit E, Graham NMH, Tang A, et al: Dietary intake of community-based HIV-1 seropositive and seronegative injecting drug users. *Nutrition* 12(7–8):496–501, 1996.

89. Swaminathan S, Padmapriyadarsini C, Sukumar B, et al: Nutritional status of persons with HIV infection, persons with HIV infection and tuberculosis, and HIV-negative individuals from Southern India. *Clin Infect Dis* 46(6):946–949, 2008.

90. Vorster HH, Kruger A, Margetts BM, et al: The nutritional status of asymptomatic HIV-infected Africans: directions for dietary intervention. *Public Health Nutr* 7(08):1055–1064, 2004.

91. Luder E, Godfrey E, Godbold J, et al: Assessment of nutritional, clinical, and immunologic status of HIV-infected, inner-city patients with multiple risk factors. *J Am Diet Assoc* 95(6):655–660, 1995.

92. Chlebowski RT, Grosvenor M, Kruger S, et al: Dietary intake in HIV infection: relative caloric deficiency in patients with AIDS. *Int Conf AIDS* 5:467, 1989. (abstract no. Th.B.P.307).

93. Woods MN, Spiegelman D, Knox TA, et al: Nutrient intake and body weight in a large HIV cohort that includes women and minorities. *J Am Diet Assoc* 102(2):203–211, 2002.

94. Steenkamp L, Dannhauser A, Walsh D, et al: Nutritional, immune, micronutrient and health status of HIV-infected children in care centres in Mangaung, South Africa. *J Clin Nutr* 22(3):131–136, 2009.

95. Dusingize J-C, Hoover DR, Shi Q, et al: Association of serum albumin with markers of nutritional status among HIV-infected and uninfected Rwandan women. *PLoS One* 7(4):e35079, 2012.

96. Graham SM, Baeten JM, Richardson BA, et al: A decrease in albumin in early HIV type 1 infection predicts subsequent disease progression. *AIDS Res Hum Retroviruses* 23(10):1197–1200, 2007.

97. Feldman JG, Burns DN, Gange SJ, et al: Serum albumin as a predictor of survival in HIV-infected women in the Women's Interagency HIV Study. *AIDS* 14(7):863–870, 2000.

98. Food Security in the US: 2012, Economic Research Service. USDA. <http://www.ers.usda.gov/topics/food-nutrition-assistance/food-security-in-the-us.aspx>. Accessed on July 12, 2013.

99. Vogenthaler NS, Hadley C, Lewis SJ, et al: Food insufficiency among HIV-infected crack-cocaine users in Atlanta and Miami. *Public Health Nutr* 15:1–7, 2010.

100. Anema A, Kerr T, Weiser SD, et al: Prevalence and correlates of self-reported hunger among HIV$^+$ and HIV$^-$ injection drug users in Canada, 5th International AIDS Society Conference on HIV Pathogenesis and Treatment, Cape Town, South Africa, 2009.

101. Wang E, McGinnis K, Fiellin D, et al: Food insecurity is associated with poor virologic response among HIV-infected patients receiving antiretroviral medications. *J Gen Intern Med* 26(9):1012–1018, 2011.

102. Dunkle KL, Jewkes RK, Brown HC, et al: Transactional sex among women in Soweto, South Africa: prevalence, risk factors and association with HIV infection. *Soc Sci Med* 59(8):1581–1592, 2004.

103. Oyefara JL: Food insecurity, HIV/AIDS pandemic and sexual behaviour of female commercial sex workers in Lagos metropolis, Nigeria. *Sahara J* 4(2):626–635, 2007.

104. Gillespie S, Kadiyala S, Greener R: Is poverty or wealth driving HIV transmission? *AIDS* 21(7):S5–S16, 2007.

105. Gillespie S, Kadiyala S, International Food Policy Research I: *HIV/AIDS and food and nutrition security: from evidence to action*, Washington, DC, 2005, IFPRI.

106. Anema A, Vogenthaler N, Frongillo E, et al: Food insecurity and HIV/AIDS: current knowledge, gaps, and research priorities. *Curr HIV/AIDS Rep* 6:224–231, 2009.

107. Mshana GH, Wamoyi J, Busza J, et al: Barriers to accessing antiretroviral therapy in Kisesa, Tanzania: a qualitative study of early rural referrals to the national program. *AIDS Patient Care STDS* 20(9):649–657, 2006.

108. Tuller DM, Bangsberg DR, Senkungu J, et al: Transportation costs impede sustained adherence and access to HAART in a clinic population in southwestern Uganda: a qualitative study. *AIDS Behav* 14(4):778–784, 2010.

109. Unge C, Johansson A, Zachariah R, et al: Reasons for unsatisfactory acceptance of antiretroviral treatment in the urban Kibera slum, Kenya. *AIDS Care* 20(2):146–149, 2008.

110. Wig N, Bhatt SP, Sakhuja A, et al: Dietary adequacy in Asian Indians with HIV. *AIDS Care* 20(3):370–375, 2008.

111. Ramirez Garcia P, Cote JK: Factors affecting adherence to antiretroviral therapy in people living with HIV/AIDS. *J Assoc Nurses AIDS Care* 14(4):37–45, 2003.

112. Olupot-Olupot P, Katawera A, Cooper C, et al: Adherence to antiretroviral therapy among a conflict-affected population in Northeastern Uganda: a qualitative study. *AIDS* 22(14):1882–1884, 2008.

113. Cantrell RA, Sinkala M, Megazinni K, et al: A pilot study of food supplementation to improve adherence to antiretroviral therapy among food-insecure adults in Lusaka, Zambia. *J Acquir Immune Def Syndr* 49(2):190–195, 2008.

114. Byron E, Gillespie S, Nangami M: Integrating nutrition security with treatment of people living with HIV: lessons from Kenya. *Food Nutr Bull* 29(2):87–97, 2008.

115. Tirivayi N, Koethe JR, Groot W: Clinic-based food assistance is associated with increased medication adherence among HIV-infected adults on long-term antiretroviral therapy in Zambia. *J AIDS Clin Res* 3(7):24, 2012.

116. Academy of Nutrition and Dietetics: *Resources for Health Practitioners*, <http://www.eatright.org/HealthProfessionals/content.aspx?id=7077>. Accessed July 15, 2013.

117. Campa A, Baum MK: Micronutrients and HIV-infection. *HIV Therapy* 4(4):437–469, 2010.

118. Kotler DP: Lipodystrophy—it just gets more complicated. *Paper presented at the Eighth Annual Conference on Retroviruses and Opportunistic Infections*, Chicago, February 6, 1991.

119. Scerola D, Di Matteo A, Uberti F, et al: Reversal of cachexia in patient treated with potent antiviral therapy. *AIDS Read* 10(6):365, 2000.

120. Loss JC: The use of anabolic agents in HIV disease. *Support Line* 3:1999.

121. Schambelan M, Mulligan K, Grunfeld C: Recombinant growth hormone in patients with HIV-associated wasting: a randomized, placebo-controlled trial. *Ann Intern Med* 125:873, 1996.

122. FDC Reports: Serono Serostim required on state Medicaid formularies, HCFA says. *FDC Reports, vol 66*, Chevy Chase, Md, 1999.

123. Fillipas S, Cherry CL, Cicuttini F, et al: The effects of exercise training on metabolic and morphological outcomes for people living with HIV: a systematic review of randomised controlled trials. *HIV Clin Trials* 11(5):270–282, 2010.

124. Panel on Antiretroviral Therapy and Medical Management of HIV-Infected Children: *Guidelines for the Use of Antiretroviral Agents in Pediatric HIV Infection*. Available at: <http://aidsinfo.nih.gov/contentfiles/lvguidelines/pediatricguidelines.pdf>. Accessed July 15, 2013.

Cancer

Beth Kunkel

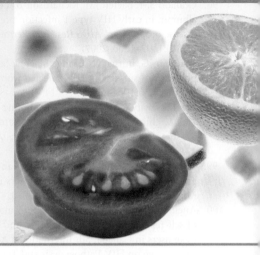

OUTLINE

Process of Cancer Development
Carcinogens and Cancer Prevention
Public Health Guidelines for Cancer Risk Reduction
Cancer-Related Health Disparities
Population-Based Screening Recommendations for
   Cancers
Postdiagnostic Staging of Cancers

Practice Guidelines for Treatment of Cancers
Treatment of Cancer
Medical Nutrition Therapy for Patients with Cancer
Alterations in Nutritional Status Associated with
   Neoplastic Disease Process
Complementary and Alternative Medicine (CAM)

This chapter focuses on cancers, which, as a group of diseases, are among the prevalent diseases in the world. We examine the nature of the cancer process, associated risk factors, and treatments with a focus on the role of nutrition.

Here we look at nutrition and cancer in two basic areas: (1) the role of nutrition in cancer development and risk reduction and (2) the role of nutrition in cancer therapy and rehabilitation. Cancer development and its prevention are discussed in relation to the interplay of environment, the body's defense system, and nutritional factors that govern each. Nutrition support has a significant role in medical therapy during both the treatment and posttreatment phases of cancer management in the effectiveness of therapy and quality of life. To understand these nutritional relationships, we must understand the nature of cancer as a growth process.

PROCESS OF CANCER DEVELOPMENT

According to the National Cancer Institute of the National Institutes of Health, the term *cancer* refers to a category of diseases in which abnormal cells divide without control and are able to invade other tissues. Cancer cells can spread to other parts of the body through the blood and lymph systems.

Cancer is, thus, a generic term encompassing more than 100 different types of conditions. Most cancers are named for the organ or type of cell in which they start; for example, cancer that begins in the colon is called *colon cancer*; cancer that begins in melanocytes of the skin is called *melanoma*.

Cancer types can be categorized as follows:
- Carcinoma—cancer that begins in the skin or in tissues that line or cover internal organs. There are a number of subtypes of carcinoma, including adenocarcinoma, basal cell carcinoma, squamous cell carcinoma, and transitional cell carcinoma.
- Sarcoma—cancer that begins in bone, cartilage, fat, muscle, blood vessels, or other connective or supportive tissue.
- Leukemia—cancer that starts in blood-forming tissue such as the bone marrow and causes large numbers of abnormal blood cells to be produced and enter the blood.
- Lymphoma and myeloma—cancers that begin in the cells of the immune system.
- Central nervous system cancers—cancers that begin in the tissues of the brain and spinal cord.[1]

Cancer Cell

Almost every time a cell divides, the DNA is replicated without error; this allows living organisms to grow and sustain themselves throughout their normal life span. However, there are occasional mutations that occur during DNA replication that either may be of no physiologic significance or may produce aberrations in the synthesis of various proteins and/or in phases of the cell cycle. These disruptions can have a host of implications for the organism, including the transformation of a normal cell into a cell with the capacity for the abnormal growth that results in cancers. Defining and categorizing these disruptions in the cell cycle is an area of intense scientific inquiry that has yielded significant insights over the past 3 or 4 decades.

It was once thought that cancer resulted from a single mutation or group of mutations that allowed for unregulated cell growth. In fact, it is now generally understood that cancers develop through a series of four distinct steps: (1) initiation, (2) promotion, (3) development, and (4) progression.[2]

Most errors in DNA replication are repaired by "DNA repair genes" prior to cell division and thus have minimal physiologic significance. In other instances, after cell division, some mutations trigger synthesis of various **tumor suppression genes** such as p53, which lead to cellular suicide or **apoptosis** of the mutated cell. These types of mutations may also have minimal physiologic significance. However, in certain heritable cancers, such as heritable colon cancers and melanomas, there is an inherited mutation that suppresses expression of one or more of the tumor suppressor genes. This mutation increases the probability of developing cancers resulting from an event that would normally result in apoptosis of the mutated cell.

In other instances that may result in the development of cancer cells, there is no change in DNA sequence, but posttranscriptional and/or posttranslational modifications in DNA do not occur normally. These modifications typically involve DNA methylation or in formation of **chromatin** or **histones**. Many of these types of modifications are under environmental control, and, hence, potentially reversible. The emerging science of **epigenetics** focuses on the environmental control of these posttranscriptional and/or posttranslational modifications in gene expression and in DNA modification and chromatin structure.[3,4]

In still other instances, regions of mutated DNA, or **oncogenes**, code for the expression of proteins that leads to abnormal cell growth or division. These mutations may involve genes that (1) activate/deactivate carcinogens, (2) govern normal cell cycle, (3) govern cell senescence, (4) govern cell signaling, and (5) govern cell differentiation.

Thus, these mutations result in a deregulation of some facet of cellular function. For example, some mutations disrupt cell signaling pathways by leading to overproduction of growth factors, cytokines, and proteases. The resulting cells produce larger volumes of these compounds and, therefore, affect normal neighboring cells through a variety of impacts on the cellular microenvironment. These impacts may be termed the *invasion metastasis cascade* and consist of the following critical steps: (1) local invasion, (2) the invasion of blood vessels, (3) transport of the cancer cell through the blood to a distant site, (4) escape of the cancer cell from the blood to tissue, and (5) adaptation of the relocated cancer cell to the new local environment that allows for its continued growth. The tumor microenvironment is critical in achieving these cascading steps.[5]

Regardless of the mechanism by which cells are mutated, their abnormal growth may result in neoplasms (literally new growth). These neoplasms are categorized as either benign, which lack the ability to spread to other tissues, or malignant, which possess the ability to spread to other tissues. Malignant neoplasms can spread to other tissues by direct or indirect invasion. In direct invasion, the neoplasms grow so large that they enter adjacent tissues or crowd the tissue so as to render

---

KEY TERMS

lymph   The clear fluid that travels through the lymphatic system and carries cells that help fight infections and other diseases. Also called *lymphatic fluid*.

melanocyte   A cell in the skin and eyes that produces and contains the pigment called melanin.

adenocarcinoma   Cancer that begins in glandular (secretory) cells. Glandular cells are found in tissue that lines certain internal organs and makes and releases substances in the body, such as mucus, digestive juices, or other fluids. Most cancers of the breast, pancreas, lung, prostate, and colon are adenocarcinomas.

basal cell carcinoma   Cancer that begins in the lower part of the epidermis (the outer layer of the skin). It may appear as a small white or flesh-colored bump that grows slowly and may bleed. Basal cell carcinomas are usually found on areas of the body exposed to the sun. Basal cell carcinomas rarely metastasize (spread) to other parts of the body. They are the most common form of skin cancer. Also called basal cell cancer.

squamous cell carcinoma   Cancer that begins in squamous cells. Squamous cells are thin, flat cells that look like fish scales, and are found in the tissue that forms the surface of the skin, the lining of the hollow organs of the body, and the lining of the respiratory and digestive tracts. Most cancers of the anus, cervix, head and neck, and vagina are squamous cell carcinomas. Also called *epidermoid carcinoma*.

transitional cell carcinoma   Cancer that begins in the transitional cells. Transitional cells are cells that vary in shape depending on whether the tissue is being stretched. Transitional cells may be stretched without breaking apart. They line hollow organs such as the bladder.

cancer   A malignant cellular tumor with properties of tissue invasion and spreading to other parts of the body.

immune system   A complex network of cells, tissues, organs, and the substances they make that helps the body fight infections and other diseases. The immune system includes white blood cells and organs and tissues of the lymph system, such as the thymus, spleen, tonsils, lymph nodes, lymph vessels, and bone marrow.

it less effective. The indirect spread of neoplasms occurs when neoplastic cells enter the blood or lymphatic system and invade other tissues. These neoplastic cells retain the original mutation as they reproduce in their new host tissue. Therefore, they retain the name of the original tissue. For example, a bone sarcoma (osteosarcoma) that has spread to the liver is termed a *hepatic osteosarcoma*, while a carcinoma that originated in the liver (hepatic carcinoma) and has spread to the bone is termed a *hepatic carcinoma of the bone*.

CARCINOGENS AND CANCER PREVENTION

Diet and Epigenetics

Understanding the fundamental biochemical and physiologic processes that underlie development of cancers is key to designing preventive and treatment strategies. Developments and refinements in the sciences of genetics, epigenetics, proteomics, metabolomics, and other related sciences are elucidating specific cellular alterations that may lead to neoplastic growth in some instances and not in others. While still in their developmental phases, these areas of science hold great promise for improving evidence-based diagnostic and treatment protocols and refinement of public health recommendations. In particular, the results of epigenetic research are to allow greater understanding of the role of environmental factors, such as radiation, naturally occurring and synthetic chemicals, diet, infections, and occupation on the etiology of different forms of cancers.[6]

Researchers in epigenetics have identified several dietary constituents that may function as natural chemopreventive agents by influencing the activity or expression of DNA methyltransferases and histone-modifying enzymes. Some of these chemopreventive agents include the following:

- Micronutrients (folate, retinoic acid, and selenium compounds)
- Butyrate
- Polyphenols from green tea, apples, coffee, black raspberries, and other dietary sources
- Genistein and soy isoflavones
- Curcumin
- Resveratrol
- Dihydrocoumarin
- Nordihydroguaiaretic acid (NDGA)
- Lycopene
- Anacardic acid
- Garcinol
- Constituents of *Allium* species and cruciferous vegetables, including indol-3-carbinol (I3C), diindolylmethane (DIM), sulforaphane, phenylethyl isothiocyanate (PEITC), phenylhexyl isothiocyanate (PHI), diallyldisulfide (DADS) and its metabolite allyl mercaptan (AM)
- Cambinol
- Relatively unexplored modulators of histone lysine methylation (chaetocin, polyamine analogs)

So far, data on humans are limited, but advances in technology will allow exploration of nutriepigenomics at a genome-wide level to better understand the importance of epigenetic mechanisms for gene regulation in cancer chemoprevention.[7]

An example of the potential for understanding the role of nutrition in epigenetics is illustrated by a series of studies conducted using experimental animals. In these studies, rodents were fed diets deficient in methionine, choline, folate, and/or vitamin B_{12}, which are the micronutrients involved in methyl group metabolism. Deficiencies in these nutrients resulted in hypomethylation of DNA and an increased incidence of hepatocarcinoma in rodents. Assays revealed lower levels of S-adenosyl methionine, aberrant levels of DNA-methyltransferases, methyl CpG binding proteins, histone methyltransferase protein expression, and histone posttranslational modification.[8]

Radiation

Exposure to radiation may lead to DNA alterations through a variety of mechanisms that are not yet fully understood. Such radiation damage may be ionizing, such as from X-rays, radioactive materials, and atomic exhausts or wastes, or it may be nonionizing, such as from sunlight. Ultraviolet radiation in sunlight is one of the most prominent sources of environmental carcinogens. It is highly genotoxic but does not penetrate the skin. The common forms of skin cancers—basal cell carcinoma and squamous cell carcinoma—are

---

KEY TERMS

tumor suppression gene A type of gene that makes a protein called a *tumor suppressor protein* that helps control cell growth. Mutations (changes in DNA) in tumor suppressor genes may lead to cancer. Also called *antioncogene*.

apoptosis A type of cell death in which a series of molecular steps in a cell lead to its death. This is one method the body uses to get rid of unneeded or abnormal cells. The process of apoptosis may be blocked in cancer cells. Also called *programmed cell death*.

chromatin The combination of DNA and proteins that make up the contents of the nucleus of a cell. The primary functions of chromatin are to (1) package DNA into a smaller volume to fit in the cell, (2) strengthen the DNA to allow mitosis, (3) prevent DNA damage, and (4) control gene expression and DNA replication. The primary protein components of chromatin are histones that compact the DNA.

histone A type of protein found in chromosomes. Histones bind to DNA, help give chromosomes their shape, and help control the activity of genes.

epigenetics The study of how age and exposure to environmental factors, such as diet, exercise, drugs, and chemicals, may cause changes in the way genes are switched on and off without changing the actual DNA sequence. These changes can affect a person's risk of disease and may be passed from parents to their children.

oncogene A gene that is a mutated (changed) form of a gene involved in normal cell growth. Oncogenes may cause the growth of cancer cells. Mutations in genes that become oncogenes can be inherited or caused by being exposed to substances in the environment that cause cancer.

From: www.cancer.gov/dictionary.

TABLE 25-1 AMERICAN CANCER SOCIETY GUIDELINES FOR INDIVIDUAL CHOICES ON NUTRITION AND PHYSICAL ACTIVITY

GUIDELINE	TARGETS
Achieve and maintain a healthy weight throughout life	• Be as lean as possible throughout life without being underweight. • Avoid excess weight gain at all ages. For those who are overweight or obese, losing even a small amount of weight has health benefits and is a good place to start. • Get regular physical activity and limit intake of high-calorie foods and drinks as keys to help maintain a healthy weight.
Be physically active	• **Adults:** Get at least 150 min of moderate intensity or 75 min of vigorous intensity activity each week (or a combination of these), preferably spread throughout the week. • **Children and teens:** Get at least 1 hr of moderate or vigorous intensity activity each day, with vigorous activity on at least 3 days each week. • Limit sedentary behavior such as sitting, lying down, watching TV, and other forms of screen-based entertainment. • Doing some physical activity above usual activities, no matter what one's level of activity, can have many health benefits.
Eat a healthy diet, with an emphasis on plant foods	• Choose foods and drinks in amounts that help you get to and maintain a healthy weight. • Limit how much processed meat and red meat you eat. • Eat at least 2½ cups of vegetables and fruits each day. • Choose whole grains instead of refined grain products.
If you drink alcohol, limit your intake	• Drink no more than 1 drink per day for women or 2 per day for men.

From American Cancer Society. Guidelines for Nutrition and Physical Activity for Cancer Prevention. Available at: http://www.cancer.org/healthy/eathealthygetactive/acsguidelinesonnutritionphysicalactivityforcancerprevention/acs-guidelines-on-nutrition-and-physical-activity-for-cancer-prevention-intro. Accessed September 2013.

easily cured by surgical removal. However, a far more lethal form of skin cancer, malignant melanoma, occurs in skin cells that produce the pigment melanin.

Viruses

Viruses may be thought of as a major risk factor for cancer development. A virus contains a small chromosome, DNA or RNA, with a relatively small number of genes, usually fewer than five and never more than several hundred. Generally, when viruses produce disease, they act as parasites, taking over the cell to replicate themselves. Numerous oncogenic viruses have been identified that are capable of producing tumors only in hosts in which the virus can replicate. They transform cells by integrating a DNA copy of the virus (termed a *provirus*) into the host cell genome. Recognized examples of viral-associated cancers include the following:

- Human papillomavirus (HPV) and cervical cancer[9]
- Retroviruses and certain breast and skin cancers[10]
- Epstein-Barr virus and certain lymphomas
- Hepatitis B and C and hepatocellular carcinoma
- Human immunodeficiency virus (HIV) and Kaposi's sarcoma[11]

PUBLIC HEALTH GUIDELINES FOR CANCER RISK REDUCTION

The American Cancer Society (ACS) has published guidelines for nutrition and physical activity to reduce the risk of developing cancers (Table 25-1). These guidelines emphasize individual choices that may reduce the risk of developing cancers, and include maintaining an appropriate weight and eating a diet rich in fruits and vegetables. These guidelines provide general guidance for population-based strategies for reducing the risk of developing cancers based on the available science. As advances in genetic research continue, some of these strategies may be modified to address risks for specific population groups.

In addition to the individual choice guidelines, the ACS also recommends that public, private, and community organizations work together at national, state, and local levels to apply policy and environmental changes that (1) increase access to affordable, healthy foods in communities, places of work, and schools, and decrease access to and marketing of foods and drinks of low nutritional value, particularly to youth, and (2) provide safe, enjoyable, and accessible environments for physical activity in schools and workplaces, and for transportation and recreation in communities.

Another set of public health guidelines for reducing cancer risk, morbidity, and mortality are provided through the Healthy People 2020 program. Healthy People 2020 provides science-based, 10-year national objectives designed to improve health of Americans. One topic area within those objectives addresses cancers. Table 25-2 lists the 20 objectives related to cancer and the target set to be achieved by 2020. The Healthy People 2020 objectives focus on reducing the incidence of common forms of cancers and improving rates

TABLE 25-2   HEALTHY PEOPLE 2020 CANCER OBJECTIVES AND PROGRESS

GOAL	TARGET
Reduce overall cancer death rate	10% improvement
Reduce lung cancer death rate	10 % improvement
Reduce female breast cancer death rate	10% improvement
Reduce the death rate from cancer of the uterine cervix	10% improvement
Reduce colorectal cancer death rate	15% improvement
Reduce oropharyngeal cancer death rate	10% improvement
Reduce prostate cancer death rate	10% improvement
Reduce melanoma cancer death rate	10% improvement
Reduce invasive colorectal cancer	15% improvement
Reduce invasive uterine cervical cancer	10% improvement
Reduce late stage female breast cancer	5% improvement
Increase the number of central, population-based registries from the 50 states and the District of Columbia that capture case information on at least 95% of the expected number of reportable cancers	Total coverage
Increase the proportion of cancer survivors who are living 5 years or longer after diagnosis	10% improvement
Increase mental and physical health-related quality of life among cancer survivors	
Increase the proportion of women who receive a cervical cancer screening based on the most recent guidelines	10% improvement
Increase the proportion of adults who receive a colorectal cancer screening based on the most recent guidelines	26% improvement
Increase the proportion of women who receive breast cancer screening based on the most recent guidelines	10% improvement
Increase the proportion of adults who were counseled about cancer screening consistent with the most recent guidelines	10% improvement
Increase the proportion of men who have discussed the advantages and disadvantages of the prostate-specific antigen (PSA) test to screen for prostate cancer with their health care provider	10% improvement
Increase the proportion of persons who participate in behaviors that reduce their exposure to harmful ultraviolet (UV) irradiation and avoid sunburn	

From U.S. Department of Health and Human Services. Healthy People 2020, Goals and Objectives for Cancer. from: http://healthypeople.gov/2020/topicsobjectives2020/objectiveslist.aspx?topicId=5. Accessed September 2013.

of screening and not specifically on lifestyle alterations that may reduce risk; however, public health interventions to reduce risk aid in achieving these objectives. In the *2011/2012 Cancer Trends Progress Report*, the National Cancer Institute (NCI), one of the National Institutes of Health, cited progress toward the major cancer-related Healthy People targets. Their conclusions are as follows:

- The rate of cancer incidence has declined since 1998.
- Death rates for the four most common cancers (prostate, female breast, lung, and colorectal), as well as for all cancers combined, have continued to decline.
- Death rates are increasing for cancer of the pancreas, liver, intrahepatic bile duct, and corpus uteri and unspecified uterus.
- Length of cancer survival has increased for all cancers combined. For all sites, the proportion of people surviving 5 years from diagnosis in 2003 (most recent year with 5-year follow-up) was 66.7 percent.
- Incidence rates of some cancers are rising, including melanoma of the skin, non-Hodgkin lymphoma, leukemia, childhood cancer, cancers of the kidney and renal pelvis, thyroid, pancreas, liver and intrahepatic bile duct, testis, myeloma, and esophagus.

- Lung cancer incidence rates in women continue to rise but less rapidly.
- Cancer treatment spending continues to rise along with total health care spending.
- Unexplained cancer-related health disparities remain among population subgroups. For example, African Americans have elevated rates of both new cancers and cancer deaths.
- Pap test use has declined from 81% in 2000 to 74% in 2010. Mammography rates have decreased from 69% in 2000 to 67% in 2010. Screening rates for colorectal cancer have increased from 52% in 2008 to 59% in 2010.[12]

CANCER-RELATED HEALTH DISPARITIES

Despite overall reductions in incidence of many of the most prevalent types of cancers and increased rates of survival, improvements do not affect all population groups equally. The decreased incidences are probably associated with early detection of precancerous tissue. That is, there are disparities. The NCI defines "cancer health disparities" as "differences in the incidence, prevalence, mortality, and burden of cancer and related adverse health conditions that exist among specific population groups in the United States" (http://crchd.cancer.gov/disparities/defined.html).

These disparities are highlighted in the *2011/2012 Cancer Trends Progress Report*.[12] African-American populations have a higher incidence of both new cancers and deaths from cancer than Caucasians. Other minority populations, such as Latinos, Native Americans, and Asian/Pacific Islanders experience disproportionately higher rates of specific forms of cancers. For example, African Americans have a higher incidence and death rate from colorectal cancer than any other racial or ethnic group. Asian/Pacific Islanders have the highest incidence of stomach cancer of any of the racial or ethnic groups in the United States and are more than twice as likely to die from stomach cancer as Caucasians.

Higher rates of incidence of specific cancers within certain racial and ethnic groups may suggest a genetic association; however, there are many complex and interrelated factors that contribute to these disparities in cancer incidence and death among these groups. The most obvious factors are associated with health care coverage and socioeconomic status.

Socioeconomic status is most often based on a person's income, education level, occupation, and other factors, such as social status in the community. It is the major predictor of access to education and health insurance, employment in certain occupations, and living conditions that are associated with the risks of developing and surviving cancer. These predictors may be positive or negative. For example, lower socioeconomic status is associated with living conditions and employment in occupations where exposure to environmental toxins is more common. Socioeconomic status also appears to play a major role in influencing the prevalence of behavioral risk factors for cancer, such as tobacco smoking, physical inactivity, obesity, and excessive alcohol intake, as well as in following cancer screening recommendations. In addition to socioeconomic status, financial, physical and cultural beliefs may be barriers that prevent individuals or groups from obtaining effective health care.

In addition to the interactions among race, ethnicity, and socioeconomic status on the incidence of cancers, people from medically underserved populations are more likely to be diagnosed with late-stage diseases, in part because of lack of access to or knowledge of early screening tests. These late stage cancers might have been treated more effectively or cured if diagnosed earlier.[13] An example of the effects of combinations of all these factors on morbidity and mortality from cancers among people in developing countries is discussed in the Focus on Culture box, "Cancers in Developing Countries."

POPULATION-BASED SCREENING RECOMMENDATIONS FOR CANCERS

Among the reasons for the decreased incidence of cancer, particularly late stage cancers, is widespread use of screening tests for several of the most commonly diagnosed cancers. Early detection of cancer increases the probability of successful treatment. Detection and treatment of precancerous lesions before becoming malignant may also be achieved through effective implementation of screening tests. Among the most commonly used screening tests are

- Mammography (for breast cancer)
- Pap test (for cervical cancer)
- Fecal occult blood test (for colorectal cancer)
- Colorectal endoscopy or colonoscopy (for colorectal cancer)
- Prostate specific antigen (PSA) (for prostate cancer)

The U.S. Preventive Services Task Force (USPSTF) issues evidence-based guidelines for screening for cervical, colorectal, and breast cancers. These guidelines are regularly updated and provide resources for administration of these screening tools among population groups based on age, family history, race, and presence of risk factors. The most current recommendations may be accessed at the USPSTF website: http://www.uspreventiveservicestaskforce.org/recommendations.htm.

POSTDIAGNOSTIC STAGING OF CANCERS

Cancers can be diagnosed at several points in their development as a result of screening tests or other types of physical or clinical examinations. Many malignancies are confirmed microscopically, since malignant cells have a distinctive microscopic appearance. These include abnormalities in cell shape and size, variation in nuclear size and shape, incomplete cellular differentiation, loss of normal tissue organization, and a poorly defined tumor boundary.

After cancer has been diagnosed, physicians conduct a series of tests to determine the progression of the disease. These tests may be clinical or pathologic. Clinical tests include physical examinations; imaging tests, such as computed tomography (CT) or positron emission tomography (PET) scans and magnetic resonance imaging (MRI) scans; blood tests; and biopsies. Pathologic tests are primarily conducted on tissues removed during surgery to remove the tumor and associated tissues, such as lymph nodes. The results of both clinical and pathologic tests are used to answer questions about size of the tumor, its spread to nearby lymph nodes, and the extent to which it may have metastasized to other tissues.

Based on results of these tests, the cancer is assigned a "stage." The most commonly used staging system is the TNM system, in which *T* refers to tumor size, *N* refers to lymph node involvement, and *M* refers to metastasis. Each section also includes levels; for example, a T4, N0, M0 tumor would be large (T4) but with no lymph node involvement (N0) or metastasis (M0).

Other staging systems are used for some specific types of cancers. Stages can be as a number (0, I, II, III, or IV), in which lower numbers reflect more localized growth. Stages may also be identified with terms, such as *carcinoma in situ, localized, regional,* or *distant.* In this system, carcinoma in situ

Cancers in Developing Countries

While cancers are widely thought to be diseases of affluence among the developed countries, there is increasing recognition of the prevalence of cancers in developing countries. According to 2008 WHO statistics, cancer causes approximately 7.9 million deaths worldwide each year. About 70% of these deaths, or 5.5 million, occur in the developing world. This number is projected to increase to 6.7 million in 2015 and 8.9 million in 2030. In contrast, cancer deaths in wealthy countries are expected to remain fairly stable over the next 20 years.

There are many global trends that contribute to this increased incidence in cancers in the developing world, including population aging, rapid unplanned urbanization, and globalization of unhealthy lifestyles. It is estimated that 40% of all cancers worldwide, including those in developing countries, are preventable. For example, increased urbanization and globalization of unhealthy lifestyles contribute to the development of preventable cancers associated with increased exposure to carcinogens through tobacco use, unhealthy diets, and environmental pollutants.

Public health programs have been very successful in addressing deaths from communicable diseases, according to reports from the UN Millennium Development Goals (MDGs) project. Infant and childhood mortality has declined from 90 deaths per 1000 live births in 1990 to 48 in 2012; deaths from malaria have declined by 26% since 2001; and deaths from tuberculosis have declined by 41% since 1991. Rates of infections with HIV have decreased by 21% since 2001. These successes contribute to a rise in the proportion of populations who are adults, and at an increased risk of developing cancers.

The disease burden that results from cancers is significant in developing countries. In some African countries, only 20% of patients survive cancers, such as cervical cancer, that are highly curable in developed countries. On average, 70% of cancer patients in developing countries are diagnosed at a late stage of illness, when treatment is no longer effective and the only possible intervention is palliative care. Even basic palliative care, such as pain management, fails to reach more than 5 million terminally ill cancer patients every year.

This disease burden can be expressed in terms of an almost total lack of response capacity. Throughout the developing world, most health systems are designed to cope with episodes of communicable diseases. They have demonstrated an increasing capacity for effectiveness in this area as measured by achievement in meeting the MDGs. Most developing countries do not have the capacity—measured as financial resources, facilities, equipment, technology, infrastructure, staff, or training—to address care for cancers. In large parts of Africa, treatments such as surgery, radiotherapy, and chemotherapy are largely unavailable. For example, according to the director-general of the World Health Organization (WHO), in 2010, 30 countries did not have a single radiation therapy machine.

In most developing countries, the capacity for the basic components of cancer control could be built upon the evidence base and technology from developed countries. Basic components of cancer control—public education, prevention, early detection, diagnosis and treatment, and palliative care—could be incorporated into other disease prevention programs utilizing some of the strategies that have been effective in meeting the MDG targets.

Bibliography

Cancer Control: Knowledge into Action: WHO Guide for Effective Programmes. Diagnosis and Treatment. 2008. from: <http://www.who.int/cancer/modules/9789241547406/en/index.html>. Accessed Sept. 20, 2013.

Chan M: Cancer in developing countries: facing the challenge. from: <http://www.who.int/dg/speeches/2010/iaea_forum_20100921/en/index.html>.

United Nations Millennium Development Goals. from: <http://www.un.org/millenniumgoals/>. Accessed Sept. 22, 2013.

refers to a highly localized area of dysplasia for which there is no evidence of spreading, while distant refers to cancers that have metastasized to areas of the body distant from their original location.

PRACTICE GUIDELINES FOR TREATMENT OF CANCERS

The health care team for patients with cancer includes oncologists, nurses, dietetics professionals, and other support personnel. Since there are more than 300 different forms of cancers, each with different treatment options depending on the stage of the cancer, it is difficult to generalize about treatments. Over the past decade, with the increased emphasis on evidence-based practice, professional organizations have established practice guidelines. Practice guidelines are developed through a process that includes a systematic literature review on the effectiveness of specific outcomes of specific interventions. After this systematic review, guidelines are developed based on the strength of the evidence for that particular intervention.

Professional organizations that have developed practice guidelines for treatment of various types of cancer include the National Comprehensive Cancer Network (http://www.nccn.org/professionals/physician_gls/f_guidelines.asp) and the American Society of Clinical Oncology (http://www.asco.org/institute-quality/guidelines). The Academy of Nutrition and Dietetics (AND) has practice guidelines for various aspects of oncology nutrition, such as appropriate methods to estimate Resting Energy Expenditure (REE) and use of parenteral nutrition (http://andevidencelibrary.com).

These guidelines are updated regularly and should be reviewed by health care professionals as part of designing treatment protocols for all patients.

TREATMENT OF CANCER

Just as knowledge of the epigenetics of cancer is changing rapidly, so too are treatments. However, most current cancer therapy takes four major forms: (1) surgery, (2) radiation, (3) chemotherapy, and (4) biological therapy. Each of these treatment modalities entail physiologic and psychologic stresses, including damage to cell DNA structure, changes in normal body function, and alterations in quality of life. Nutrition support seeks to alleviate these problems and to enhance the potential success of cancer therapy.

Surgery

Diagnosis of certain cancers in early stages of development allows for surgical removal of operable tumors as a major treatment of a large number of patients with cancer. Surgical treatment may also be used with other forms of therapy for removal of single metastases or for prevention and alleviation of symptoms.

Radiation Therapy

Radiation therapy damages DNA; therefore, cell division and growth are impaired. Its effectiveness in treatments of cancer is predicated on its ability to limit neoplastic cell growth. Radiotherapy may be used alone or in conjunction with other therapies for curative and palliative care. Radiation used in cancer therapy may employ either external radiation beams or internal isotopes (brachytherapy).

- In external beam radiation therapy, radiation emitted from a linear accelerator is directed at a highly specific treatment site. This type of radiation frequently causes nutrition-related side effects and changes in quality of life.
- In brachytherapy, highly radioactive isotopes, such as cobalt 60, are placed directly into or next to the tumor to deliver a localized dose. Nutritional side effects do not generally occur from this type of radiotherapy.[14]

Chemotherapy

Chemotherapy refers to the use of chemical agents as a treatment for cancer. It may be used as the only form of treatment, but is typically used in conjunction with surgery, radiation therapy, or biological therapy. Chemotherapy can be administered as follows:

- To decrease size of a tumor before surgery or radiation therapy. This is called *neoadjuvant chemotherapy*.
- To destroy cancer cells that may remain after surgery or radiation therapy. This is called *adjuvant chemotherapy*.
- To work synergistically with radiation therapy and biological therapy.
   In general, the effectiveness of chemotherapeutic agents is greater when tumor burden is less. Tumor burden may be less because of early detection or initial treatment by surgery or

radiation. Selection and dosage of chemotherapeutic agents is based on the type of cancer and the evidence-based practice guidelines that have been developed for use by physicians. The agents may be administered singly or in combination and are frequently given serially in dosages designed to halt growth of the neoplastic cells. These repeated series of chemotherapy treatments are known as "rounds," and side effects of the treatments may increase in intensity with sequential rounds of treatments.

Mode of Action

Chemotherapeutic agents are effective because they disrupt normal cellular processes responsible for cell growth and reproduction. Some agents interfere with DNA synthesis. Others disrupt DNA structure and RNA replication. Others prevent mitosis, cause hormonal imbalances, or disrupt protein synthesis by limiting the availability of specific amino acids. This diversity in mode of action provides a basis for classifying chemotherapeutic agents, as follows:
- Alkaloid agents—inhibit microtubule function
- Alkylating agents—chemically alter cellular DNA
- Antibiotic agents—prevent normal DNA functions
- Antimetabolite agents—block cell division by imitating purines or pyrimidines
- Enzymal agents—prevent normal functions of DNA
- Hormonal agents—damage cell division[15]

Chemotherapy Administration

Chemotherapy may be administered in several ways, as follows:
- Injection—chemotherapeutic agent is given intramuscularly or subcutaneously
- Intraarterial (IA)—chemotherapeutic agent is given directly into the artery that is feeding the cancer
- Intraperitoneal (IP)—chemotherapeutic agent is given directly into the peritoneal cavity
- Intravenous (IV)—chemotherapeutic agent is given directly into a vein
- Topically—chemotherapeutic is rubbed directly onto the skin
- Orally—chemotherapeutic agent is given as pills, capsules, or liquids

Biological Therapy

Advances in cell biology and physiology as well as epigenetics have led to development of specific biological, or targeted, therapies for treatment of cancers. Targeted therapies are transforming cancer treatments by facilitating discovery of therapeutic targets within cancer cells and designing treatments that selectively interfere with them.

Forms of biological therapies include antibodies, vaccines, and small molecules that traverse the cell membrane. These treatments are often used in combination with chemotherapy or as adjuvant therapy with surgery or radiation. These therapies affect primarily or exclusively the neoplastic cell and thus limit the collateral damage to other rapidly dividing cells associated with chemotherapeutic agents.

An excellent tutorial on targeted therapies is available through the National Cancer Institute at http://www.cancer.gov/cancertopics/understandingcancer/targetedtherapies/htmlcourse.

MEDICAL NUTRITION THERAPY FOR PATIENTS WITH CANCER

Nutrition care for persons with cancer should follow the Nutrition Care Process (NCP) as outlined by the AND.[16] The NCP has four basic sequential, but interrelated, steps:

1. *Nutrition assessment* is a systematic approach to collect, record, and interpret relevant data from patients, clients, family members, caregivers, and other individuals and groups. Nutrition assessment is an ongoing, dynamic process that involves initial data collection as well as continual reassessment and analysis of the patient's or client's status compared to specified criteria.
2. *Nutrition diagnosis* is a food and nutrition professional's identification and labeling of an existing nutrition problem that the food and nutrition professional is responsible for treating independently.
3. *Nutrition intervention* is a purposefully planned action(s) designed with the intent of changing a nutrition-related behavior, risk factor, environmental condition, or aspect of health status. Nutrition intervention consists of two interrelated components: planning and intervention. The nutrition intervention is typically directed toward resolving the nutrition diagnosis or the nutrition etiology. Less often, it is directed at relieving signs and symptoms.
4. *Nutrition monitoring and evaluation* identifies the amount of progress made and whether goals or expected outcomes are being met. Nutrition monitoring and evaluation identifies outcomes relevant to the nutrition diagnosis and intervention plans and goals.

For each of these steps, the plan should include specific, measurable outcomes.

Development of an effective nutrition care plan for persons with cancer will necessarily require collaboration with other members of the health care team and caregivers, periodic monitoring, and a holistic approach to patient management. Many of the common signs and symptoms associated with cancer care are related to quality of life and activities of daily living and, therefore, impact food behaviors and nutrient intake (see the Case Study box, "Patient with Cancer").

Nutritional Needs of Cancer Patients

Patients with cancer typically have increased needs for energy, protein, vitamins and minerals, and fluid based on the disease itself and its treatment. Individual needs and food tolerances vary, but general guidelines are the same.

Energy

Increased energy needs of cancer patients may result from either a disease-induced hypermetabolic state or tissue-healing requirements or both. Calculation of energy needs

---

CASE STUDY

Patient with Cancer

As a dietitian working with a medical oncology practice, you received a referral for Yolande, a 45-year-old mother of four who has been diagnosed with Stage 1 triple negative breast cancer. She has had a lumpectomy and the sentinel lymph node biopsy was negative. She weighs 125 lb and is 62 inches tall; results of her lab tests are unremarkable. Her recommended course of treatment includes six rounds of chemotherapy conducted over the next 3 months followed by 4 weeks of radiation therapy.

Yolande is originally from Haiti and works full time as a fulfillment clerk for an online shopping business. Her husband works 50 hours a week in construction. The two older children are in elementary school and the two younger children are in full-time day care.

Questions for Analysis

1. Outline components of the initial nutrition assessment of this client. What additional information might you need to conduct a thorough nutrition assessment?
2. Develop a nutrition diagnostic statement that follows the pattern of the Nutrition Care Process.
3. Describe the appropriate nutrition intervention, including planning and implementation steps.
4. Develop a plan for monitoring and evaluation.

After three rounds of chemotherapy, Yolande has maintained her weight and does not report significant issues with nausea. However, she reports increasing fatigue and an intolerance to intense smells during food preparation. Develop an appropriate modification to her nutrition care plan.

---

follows determination of the REE and additional needs for activity and tissue healing, in accordance with practice guidelines for the type of cancer. Macronutrient composition should be apportioned to allow sufficient protein for tissue healing and maintenance. Generally, carbohydrates comprise the majority of the calorie intake, with fat providing about 30% of the total calories. Overfeeding must be avoided to minimize the risk of "refeeding syndrome."

Protein

Tissue protein synthesis, a necessary component of healing and rehabilitation, requires essential amino acids and nitrogen. Efficient protein use, which depends on an optimum protein-to-calorie ratio, promotes wound repair and tissue maintenance and prevents tissue catabolism. A protein intake of about 0.8 to 1.2 g/kg/day is adequate for most patients with cancer. In some instances, such as cachexia, protein supplementation may be necessary.

Vitamins and Minerals

Adequate intakes of vitamins and minerals are important for normal tissue function and healing and for maintenance of immune function. However, there is insufficient evidence to suggest efficacy of use of vitamin or mineral supplements (see the discussion on complementary and alternative medicine [CAM]. Key vitamins and minerals control protein and energy metabolism through their roles in cell enzyme systems. Increased dietary consumption of vegetables and fruits is the best way to obtain these vitamins and minerals.

Fluids

Most adults require approximately 35 mL/kg, or between 1500 and 2000 mL, of water each day. Adequate fluid intake is important to replace gastrointestinal (GI) losses or losses caused by infection and fever, and to aid in renal excretion of metabolic breakdown products from destroyed cancer cells and medications.

Medical Nutrition Therapy of the Surgery Oncology Patient

One factor in successful surgical outcomes is adequate nutritional status of the patient; this is especially true of patients with cancer because their general condition may be weakened. Working with the patient to obtain optimal nutritional status preoperatively and providing appropriate nutrition support postoperatively are fundamental to the healing process.

Development of nutrition interventions that include provision of adequate nutrient intake to facilitate healing, including energy, protein and micronutrients, is important both preoperatively and postoperatively. Additionally, postoperative care may involve diet modification, particularly for those patients whose treatment involves surgery on some component of the GI system. For these patients, there may be specific challenges with normal eating, digestion, and absorption of nutrients that necessitate modifications in nutrient content, texture, and/or timing of eating. These challenges are characteristic of the portion of the GI tract involved rather than to the cancer itself, as seen in the following:

- *Head and neck surgery,* or resections in the oropharyngeal area, will affect ability to consume foods. During the healing process, individuals may require diets with texture modifications or, in some instances, modifications in the feeding modality such as placement of feeding tubes. Depending on the nature of the surgery, long-term adjustments in texture and/or feeding modality may be necessary.
- *Gastric or intestinal resections* may result in numerous problems related to digestion and absorption of nutrients. During the healing process, modifications in macronutrient composition of the diet and in timing of feedings may be necessary. Depending on the nature of the surgery, long-term adjustments in macronutrient composition of the diet and in timing of feeding may be necessary. Particular attention should be paid to nutritional status for fat-soluble nutrients, fluid, and electrolytes.
- *Pancreatectomy* causes loss of digestive enzymes with ensuing malabsorption and weight loss; it also induces insulin-dependent diabetes mellitus.

Medical Nutrition Therapy of the Radiation Oncology Patient

Not all patients who receive radiation therapy will experience nutrition-related side effects (Table 25-3). Those who receive radiation treatments to the head and neck region, to parts of the GI tract, or to other organs within the abdominal cavity are most likely to experience nutrition-related signs and symptoms. Current practice guidelines from the AND include strong evidence for both pretreatment evaluation and ongoing medical nutrition therapy (MNT) for patients with head and neck cancers undergoing radiation therapy.[17] MNT has been demonstrated to improve calorie and protein intake, maintain anthropometric measures, and improve quality of life for these patients.

- *Head and neck* radiation therapy typically affects oral mucosa and salivary secretions, as well as the esophagus, influencing taste sensations and sensitivity to food temperature and texture. Common side effects include mucositis, xerostomia, hypogeusia, and dysnomia (alteration in or loss of smell). MNT may include modification in texture and temperature of the diet. Additionally, modifications in appearance and aroma of foods may assist with management of anorexia and hypogeusia. For treatments that impact salivary secretions, treatments to stimulate saliva production include medications and inclusion of foods such as chewing gums and hard candies that stimulate saliva production. These treatments may mitigate impact on oral mucosa and dentition.
- *Abdominal cavity* radiation therapy may produce denuded bowel mucosa and loss of villi with tissue edema and congestion; vascular changes occur as a result of intimal thickening, thrombosis, ulcer formation, or inflammation. In the intestinal wall, fibrosis, stenosis, necrosis, or ulceration may occur. Modifications in macronutrient composition and timing of feedings may be necessary. Particular attention should be given to nutritional status for fat-soluble nutrients, fluids, and electrolytes.

In addition to these specific impacts on nutritional status, fatigue is very common among radiation oncology patients. This general fatigue may impact the patient's appetite or ability to prepare and consume food. The level of fatigue typically increases with duration of the radiation treatments and may significantly impact the patient's quality of life. Fortunately, the fatigue typically resolves following treatment.

Medical Nutrition Therapy of the Chemotherapy Patient

The impact of chemotherapeutic agents on rapidly reproducing normal cells is most apparent in cells of the bone marrow, GI tract, and hair follicles, and accounts for many of the side effects of chemotherapy with implications for MNT.

- *Bone marrow effects* include interference with production of red and white blood cells and platelets. While there are medications that stimulate production of these cell types,

TABLE 25-3	DIETARY MODIFICATIONS FOR NUTRITION-RELATED SIDE EFFECTS OF CANCER
SIDE EFFECT	**SUGGESTED DIETARY MODIFICATIONS**
Anorexia	Provide small, frequent meals.
	Offer high-calorie, high-protein, nutrient-dense foods.
	Encourage consumption of the highest-calorie, highest-protein foods first.
	Avoid foods with offensive odors.
	Encourage favorite foods.
Altered perception of taste and odor	Maximize use of herbs and seasonings to enhance flavor of foods.
	If the flavor and aroma of red meats are offensive, avoid these foods and use alternative protein-rich foods such as chicken, fish, cheese, eggs, and milk.
	Serve cold foods and beverages more often than hot foods and beverages.
	Vary appearance (i.e., color, texture) of foods.
	Prepare and serve food in glass or porcelain rather than metal pans or dishes.
Stomatitis and mucositis	Provide foods in liquid, semisolid, or pureed form.
	Avoid tart, citric, or acidic foods and beverages.
	Avoid extremes in temperature.
	Avoid excessively seasoned and spicy foods.
	Avoid dry, coarse foods; serve foods with sauces or gravies.
	Encourage foods that melt or are liquid or soft textured at room temperature.
	Avoid carbonated beverages.
Xerostomia	Moisten foods with sauces, gravies, liquid, melted butter, mayonnaise, or yogurt.
	Encourage naturally soft, moist foods.
	Encourage sipping of liquids throughout the day.
	Avoid alcohol.
Dysphagia	Provide foods in liquid, semisolid, or pureed form.
	Maximize calorie and protein density of food as much as possible.
	Use commercially available liquid nutritional supplements.
Nausea and vomiting	Give small, frequent meals.
	Give dry foods without added fats or sauces, such as dry toast.
	Give liquids only between meals.
	Avoid greasy, fried, high-fat foods.
	Avoid foods with strong odors.
Diarrhea	Provide small, frequent meals.
	Encourage plenty of liquids to prevent dehydration.
	Avoid greasy, fried, high-fat foods.
	Consider limiting dietary lactose if these foods exacerbate symptoms.
	Avoid high-fiber foods.
	Avoid gassy, cruciferous vegetables, such as broccoli and cauliflower.
	Avoid caffeine.

Data from Dobbin M, Harmuller VW: Suggested management of nutrition-related symptoms. In MacCallum PD, Polisena CG, editors: *The clinical guide to oncology nutrition,* Chicago, 2000, American Dietetic Association.

patients may benefit from modifications in diet to increase intake of vitamins and minerals involved in blood cell and platelet formation. Additional concerns associated with leukopenia include increased risk of foodborne infections. MNT for these patients might include the use of a neutropenic diet, in which foods identified by the FDA in the U.S. Food Code as "potentially hazardous"[18] and other foods likely to have a high microbial count, such as raw fruits and vegetables, are restricted.

- *GI effects* include nausea and vomiting, stomatitis, anorexia, ulcers, and diarrhea. Nausea and vomiting is a common side effect of chemotherapy, affecting over 50% of patients at some point in their treatment.

Chemotherapy-induced emesis (CIE) is managed with increasing effectiveness by following practice guidelines on use of antiemetic medications tailored for the emetogenic potential of chemotherapeutic agents.[19] Malabsorption and fluid and electrolyte imbalances may result from inadequate control of CIE and should be monitored by the registered dietitian (RD). In addition to the direct physical effects of CIE, it also significantly impacts quality of life.

Other GI effects may include postgastrectomy "dumping" syndrome, general diarrhea, constipation, flatulence, or specific lactose intolerance or surgery responses, such as those that occur with intestinal resections and various ostomies.

Helpful guidance for patients with colostomies, ileostomies, or ileoanal reservoirs is necessary.

In addition to MNT approaches to managing symptoms associated with GI distress, such as alterations in macronutrient composition and timing of feeding, nutrition professionals should also recognize the impact of these symptoms on quality of life.

ALTERATIONS IN NUTRITIONAL STATUS ASSOCIATED WITH NEOPLASTIC DISEASE PROCESS

Malnutrition is the most common secondary diagnosis in patients with cancer and is a prognostic indicator for poor response to cancer therapy and shortened survival time. The disease process itself may be associated with three basic systemic effects—(1) anorexia, (2) altered metabolic state, and (3) negative nitrogen balance—which are often accompanied by a continuing weight loss. These effects may vary widely with individual patients, according to type and stage of the disease, from mild, scarcely discernible responses to the extreme forms of debilitating cachexia seen in advanced disease, and they are estimated to cause more than 50% of the cancer deaths.[20]

Anorexia associated with cancers is frequently accompanied by depression or discomfort during normal eating. This contributes to a limited nutrient intake at a time when the disease process causes an increased metabolic rate and nutrient demand. The weight loss associated with anorexia may contribute to development of cachexia, a severe wasting process.

Cachexia is not a local effect but rather arises from systemic metabolic effects, the etiology of which is not clearly understood. This extreme weight loss and weakness are associated with abnormalities in fat, muscle, and glucose metabolism, mediated in part by natural body defense substances such as tumor necrosis factor and cytokines.[20] Not all patients who develop cachexia will respond to medical nutrition therapy.

COMPLEMENTARY AND ALTERNATIVE MEDICINE (CAM)

Patients who face treatments for cancers may choose to incorporate some form of complementary medicine as a component of their treatment. The National Center for Complementary and Alternative Medicine (NCCAM) of the NCI defines complementary and alternative medicine as treatments that are not currently considered to be part of conventional medicine. In general, *complementary medicine* refers to treatments that are used in conjunction with conventional medicine, and *alternative medicine* refers to treatments that are used as an alternative to conventional medicine. Another term, which is sometimes used interchangeably with CAM, is *integrative medicine*. NCCAM defines integrative medicine

as treatment that combines conventional medicine with CAM therapies that have been reported to be safe and effective after being studied in patients. It is important that CAM therapies that are incorporated into care processes be those for which safety and effectiveness have been studied or those which are very unlikely to cause any harm, such as relaxation and various spiritual practices.

Four of 10 adults who participated in the 2007 National Health Interview Survey reported using CAM therapy in the past 12 months, with the most commonly used treatments being natural products and deep breathing exercises.[21] Similarly, about 4 in 10 cancer survivors reported using complementary therapies such as prayer, faith and spiritual practice, relaxation, and nutritional supplements, including vitamins.[22] There is limited evidence to suggest benefits from use of various botanical supplements, vitamin supplements, mineral supplements, or antioxidants as a component of cancer treatment. Similarly, there is concern, but limited evidence, that use of these supplements may interfere with the efficacy of various cancer treatments, particularly chemotherapeutic agents.[23]

The Society for Integrative Oncology has developed practice guidelines designed to assist health care professionals to make evidence-based decisions on various aspects with integrative oncology. These guidelines, presented in Table 25-4, have recommendations for the clinical encounter and for various treatment modalities. The recommendations are also evaluated based on benefits versus risks/burdens and the strength of the recommendation. These guidelines, like those of other professional organizations, are reviewed on a regular basis and updated to reflect changes in the evidence base. These recommendations support the limited evidence available for effectiveness of nutritional supplements in cancer prevention, treatment, or survivorship.

KEY TERM

cachexia Loss of body weight and muscle mass, and weakness that may occur in patients with cancer, AIDS, or other chronic diseases.
From: www.cancer.gov/dictionary.

KEY TERMS

complementary and alternative medicine (CAM) A group of different medical and health care systems, practices, and products that are not presently considered to be part of conventional medicine. Complementary medicine is used together with conventional medicine. Alternative medicine is used in place of conventional medicine.

integrative medicine A system of treatment that combines conventional medicine with CAM therapies that have been reported to be safe and effective after being studied in patients. In practice, many CAM therapies used in along with conventional medicine have not yet been well tested.

From: http://www.cancer.gov/cancertopics/pdq/cam/cam-cancer-treatment/patient/page2.

TABLE 25-4   PRACTICE GUIDELINES FOR INTEGRATIVE ONCOLOGY

CATEGORY	RECOMMENDATION	BENEFITS AND RISKS	IMPLICATIONS
The clinical encounter	Inquire about the use of complementary and alternative therapies as a routine part of initial evaluations of cancer patients.	Benefits clearly outweigh risks or burdens	Strong recommendation; may change when higher-quality evidence is available
The clinical encounter	All patients with cancer should receive guidance about the advantages and limitations of complementary therapies in an open, evidence-based, and patient-centered manner by a qualified professional. Patients should be fully informed of the treatment approach, the nature of the specific therapies, potential risks/benefits, and realistic expectations.	Benefits clearly outweigh risks or burdens	Strong recommendation; may change when higher-quality evidence is available
Mind-body medicine	Mind-body modalities are recommended as part of a multidisciplinary approach to reduce anxiety, mood disturbance, and chronic pain and improve quality of life.	Benefits clearly outweigh risks or burdens	Strong recommendation; can apply to most patients in most circumstances without reservation
Mind-body medicine	Support groups, supportive/expressive therapy, cognitive-behavioral therapy, and cognitive-behavioral stress management are recommended as part of a multidisciplinary approach to reduce anxiety, mood disturbance, chronic pain, and improve quality of life.	Benefits clearly outweigh risks or burdens	Strong recommendation; can apply to most patients in most circumstances without reservation
Touch therapy	For cancer patients experiencing anxiety or pain, massage therapy delivered by an oncology-trained massage therapist is recommended as part of multimodality treatment.	Benefits clearly outweigh risks or burdens	Strong recommendation; may change when higher-quality evidence is available
Touch therapy	The application of deep or intense pressure is not recommended near cancer lesions or enlarged lymph nodes, radiation field sites, medical devices (such as indwelling intravenous catheters), or anatomic distortions such as postoperative changes or in patients with a bleeding tendency.	Benefits closely balanced with risks and burden	Weak recommendation; best action may differ depending on circumstances or patients' or societal values
Physical therapy	Regular physical activities can play many positive roles in cancer care. Patients should be referred to a qualified exercise specialist for guidelines on physical activity to promote basic health.	Benefits clearly outweigh risks or burdens	Strong recommendation; can apply to most patients in most circumstances without reservation
Energy therapy	Therapies based on a philosophy of bioenergy fields are safe and may provide some benefit for reducing stress and enhancing quality of life. There is limited evidence as to their efficacy for symptom management, including reducing pain and fatigue.	Benefits clearly outweigh risks or burdens	Strong recommendation; can apply to most patients in most circumstances without reservation
Acupuncture	Acupuncture is recommended as a complementary therapy when pain is poorly controlled, when nausea and vomiting associated with chemotherapy or surgical anesthesia are poorly controlled, or when the side effects from other modalities are clinically significant.	Benefits clearly outweigh risks or burdens	Strong recommendation; can apply to most patients in most circumstances without reservation

TABLE 25-4	PRACTICE GUIDELINES FOR INTEGRATIVE ONCOLOGY—cont'd		
CATEGORY	**RECOMMENDATION**	**BENEFITS AND RISKS**	**IMPLICATIONS**
Acupuncture	Acupuncture is recommended as a complementary therapy for radiation-induced xerostomia.	Benefits clearly outweigh risks or burdens	Strong recommendation; can apply to most patients in most circumstances without reservation
Acupuncture	Acupuncture does not appear to be more effective than sham acupuncture for treatment of vasomotor symptoms (hot flashes) in postmenopausal women in general. In patients experiencing severe symptoms not amenable to pharmacologic treatment, however, a trial of acupuncture treatment can be considered.	Benefits clearly outweigh risks or burdens	Strong recommendation; can apply to most patients in most circumstances without reservation
Acupuncture	For patients who do not stop smoking despite use of other options or those suffering from symptoms such as cancer-related dyspnea, cancer-related fatigue, chemotherapy-induced neuropathy, or postthoracotomy pain, a trial of acupuncture may be helpful, but more clinical studies of acupuncture are warranted.	Uncertainty in estimates of benefits, risks, and burden; may be closely balanced	Very weak recommendations; other alternatives may be equally reasonable
Acupuncture	Acupuncture should be performed only by qualified practitioners and used cautiously in patients with bleeding tendencies.	Benefits clearly outweigh risks or burdens	Strong recommendation; may change when higher-quality evidence is available
Diet and nutritional supplements	Research in diet and cancer prevention is based mainly on studies of populations consuming dietary components in whole-food form, with secure food supplies and access to a variety of food and drinks. Therefore, nutritional adequacy should be met by selecting a wide variety of foods; dietary supplements are usually unnecessary.	Benefits clearly outweigh risks or burdens	Strong recommendation; can apply to most patients in most circumstances without reservation
Diet and nutritional supplements	It is recommended that patients be advised regarding proper nutrition to promote basic health.	Benefits clearly outweigh risks or burdens	Strong recommendation; can apply to most patients in most circumstances without reservation
Diet and nutritional supplements	Based on a current review of the literature, specific dietary supplements are not recommended for cancer prevention.	Benefits clearly outweigh risks or burdens	Strong recommendation; can apply to most patients in most circumstances without reservation
Diet and nutritional supplements	Evaluation of patients' use of dietary supplements prior to the start of cancer treatment is recommended. Also recommended are referral of cancer patients to trained professionals for guidelines on diets, nutritional supplementation, promotion of optimum nutritional status, management of tumor- and treatment-related symptoms, satisfaction of increased nutritional needs, and correction of any nutritional deficits while on active treatment.	Benefits clearly outweigh risks or burdens	Strong recommendation; can apply to most patients in most circumstances without reservation

Continued

TABLE 25-4	PRACTICE GUIDELINES FOR INTEGRATIVE ONCOLOGY—cont'd		
CATEGORY	RECOMMENDATION	BENEFITS AND RISKS	IMPLICATIONS
Diet and nutritional supplements	It is recommended that dietary supplements, including botanicals and megadoses of vitamins and minerals, be evaluated for possible side effects and potential interaction with other drugs. Those that are likely to interact adversely with other drugs, including chemotherapeutic agents, should not be used concurrently with immunotherapy, chemotherapy, or radiation or prior to surgery.	Benefits clearly outweigh risks or burdens	Strong recommendation; can apply to most patients in most circumstances without reservation
Diet and nutritional supplements	For cancer patients who wish to use nutritional supplements, including botanicals for purported antitumor effects, it is recommended that they consult a trained professional. During the consultation, the professional should provide support, discuss realistic expectations, and explore potential benefits and risks. It is recommended that use of those agents occur only in the context of clinical trials, recognized nutritional guidelines, clinical evaluation of the risk/benefit ratio based on available evidence, and close monitoring of adverse effects.	Benefits clearly outweigh risks or burdens	Strong recommendation; may change when higher-quality evidence is available
Diet and nutritional supplements	As with nutritional supplementation during treatment, survivors should be evaluated for supplement use and referred to a trained professional for evaluation to meet specific nutritional needs and to correct nutritional deficits as indicated. For older cancer survivors, nutritional supplementation may reduce nutrient inadequacies, although survivors who use supplements are usually the least likely to need them.	Benefits closely balanced with risks and burden	Weak recommendation; best action may differ depending on circumstances or patients' or societal values

Data from Deng GE, Frenkel M, Cohen L, et al: Evidence-based clinical practice guidelines for integrative oncology: complementary therapies and botanicals. *J Soc Integr Oncol* 7(3):85, 2009.

TO SUM UP

Cancer is a term applied to abnormal, malignant growths in various body tissue sites. The cancerous cell is derived from a normal cell that loses control over cell reproduction through a variety of mechanisms, including mutation, carcinogens, radiation, and oncogenic viruses. It is also influenced by many epidemiologic factors such as diet, alcohol use, and smoking, as well as physical and psychologic stress factors.

Cancer therapy consists primarily of surgery, radiation, and chemotherapy. Medical nutrition therapy for the patient with cancer should be highly individualized and depends on the response of each body system to the disease and to the treatment itself. It should carefully follow the nutrition care process and be based on current practice guidelines. Since the course of treatment for cancers spans several months, regular monitoring and evaluation may be needed to ensure optimal nutrition care.

QUESTIONS FOR REVIEW

1. What is cancer? What may be roles of DNA methylation and apoptosis in development of cancers?
2. List and describe the rationale and mode of action of the types of therapies used to treat cancer.
3. Outline the general procedure for the nutritional management of a patient with cancer.

REFERENCES

1. National Cancer Institute: *What Is Cancer?* from: <http://www.cancer.gov/cancertopics/cancerlibrary/what-is-cancer>.
2. Reif AE, Hearen T: Consensus on synergism between cigarette smoke and other environmental carcinogens in the causation of lung cancer. *Adv Cancer Res* 76:161, 1999.
3. Bollati V, Baccarelli A: Environmental epigenetics. *Heredity (Edinb)* 105:105, 2010.
4. Shen H, Laird PW: Interplay between the cancer genome and epigenome. *Cell* 153:38, 2013.
5. Mbeunkui F, Johann DJ Jr: Cancer and the tumor microenvironment: a review of an essential relationship. *Cancer Chemther Pharmacol* 63:571, 2009.
6. Wild CP: Environmental exposure in cancer epidemiology. *Mutagenesis* 24:117, 2009.
7. Gerhauser C: Cancer chemoprevention and nutriepigenetics: state of the art and future challenges. *Top Curr Chem* 329:73, 2013.
8. Jang H, Shin H: Current trends in the development and application of molecular technologies for cancer epigenetics. *World J Gastroenterol* 19:1030, 2013.
9. Franco EL, Duarte-Franco E, Ferenczy A: Cervical cancer: epidemiology, prevention and the role of human papillomavirus infection. *CMAJ* 164:1017, 2001.
10. Sourvinos G, Tsatsanis C, Spandidos DA: Mechanisms of retrovirus-induced oncogenesis. *Folia Biol* 46:226, 2000.
11. Shih WL, Fang CT, Chen PJ: Anti-viral treatment and cancer control. *Recent Results Cancer Res* 193:269, 2014.
12. *Cancer Trends Progress Report—2011/2012 Update, National Cancer Institute*, Bethesda, Md., 2012, NIH, DHHS, from: <http://progressreport.cancer.gov>.
13. National Cancer Institute Fact Sheet: *Cancer Health Disparities*, 2013. from: <http://www.cancer.gov/cancertopics/factsheet/disparities/cancer-health-disparities>.
14. National Cancer Institute Fact Sheet: *Radiation Therapy and Cancer*, 2010. from: <http://www.cancer.gov/cancertopics/factsheet/Therapy/radiation>.
15. MedIndia Network for Health: *Chemotherapy Drugs.* from: <http://www.medindia.net/Patients/PatientInfo/chemotherapy-drugs-classification.htm>.
16. Writing Group of the Nutrition Care Process/Standardized Language Committee: Nutrition Care Process and Model Part I: The 2008 Update. *J Am Diet Assoc* 108:1113, 2008.
17. Academy of Nutrition and Dietetics: *Oncology Evidence Based Nutrition Practice Guidelines.* from: <http://andevidencelibrary.com/topic.cfm?cat=3250>. Accessed September 2013.
18. Food and Drug Administration: *US Food Code*, 2009. from: <http://www.fda.gov/Food/GuidanceRegulation/RetailFoodProtection/FoodCode/ucm186464.htm>.
19. Basch E, Prestrud AA, Hesketh, PJ, et al: Antiemetics: ASCO Clinical Practice Guideline Update. *J Clin Oncol* 29:4189, 2012.
20. National Cancer Institute: *Nutrition in Cancer Care PDQ.* from: <http://www.cancer.gov/cancertopics/pdq/supportivecare/nutrition/HealthProfessional>. Accessed September 2013.
21. Barnes PM, Bloom B, Nahin RL: Complementary and alternative medicine use among adults and children: United States, 2007. *Natl Health Stat Report* 12:1, 2009.
22. Gansler T, Kaw C, Crammer C, et al: A population-based study of prevalence of complementary methods use by cancer survivors: a report from the American Cancer Society's studies of cancer survivors. *Cancer* 113:1048, 2008.
23. National Cancer Institute: *Cancer and CAM: What the Science Says.* from: <http://nccam.nih.gov/health/providers/digest/cancer-science.htm?nav=gsa>. Accessed September 2013.

ADDITIONAL RESOURCES

American Cancer Society: <www.cancer.org/>.
[Excellent resource for the public and medical personnel.]
Breastcancer.org: <www.breastcancer.org/>.
[This nonprofit organization's website provides reliable, complete, and up-to-date information about breast cancer.]
MD Anderson Cancer Center (University of Texas): <www.mdanderson.org/>.
[One of the world's most-respected medical centers devoted entirely to care of cancer patients, research, and cancer prevention.]
National Cancer Institute: <www.cancer.gov/>.
[Part of the National Institutes of Health (NIH), this is the principal government agency for cancer research and training.]
OncoLink (University of Pennsylvania): <www.oncolink.com/>.
[Founded by Penn cancer specialists to help cancer patients, families, health care professionals, and the general public.]
WebMD: <www.webmd.com/diseases_and_conditions/cancer.htm>.
[Part of the WebMD medical information network, Cancer Health Center provided information regarding cancer.]

APPENDIXES

Body Mass Index: Obesity Values (Second of Two BMI Tables)*

BMI	36	37	38	39	40	41	42	43	44	45	46	47	48	49	50	51	52	53	54
HEIGHT (INCHES)					**BODY WEIGHT (POUNDS)**													
58	172	177	181	186	191	196	201	205	210	215	220	224	229	234	239	244	248	253	258
59	178	183	188	193	198	203	208	212	217	222	227	232	237	242	247	252	257	262	267
60	184	189	194	199	204	209	215	220	225	230	235	240	245	250	255	261	266	271	276
61	190	195	201	206	211	217	222	227	232	238	243	248	254	259	264	269	275	280	285
62	196	202	207	213	218	224	229	235	240	246	251	256	262	267	273	278	284	289	295
63	203	208	214	220	225	231	237	242	248	254	259	265	270	278	282	287	293	299	304
64	209	215	221	227	232	238	244	250	256	262	267	273	279	285	291	296	302	308	314
65	216	222	228	234	240	246	252	258	264	270	276	282	288	294	300	306	312	318	324
66	223	229	235	241	247	253	260	266	272	278	284	291	297	303	309	315	322	328	334
67	230	236	242	249	255	261	268	274	280	287	293	299	306	312	319	325	331	338	344
68	236	243	249	256	262	269	276	282	289	295	302	308	315	322	328	335	341	348	354
69	243	250	257	263	270	277	284	291	297	304	311	318	324	331	338	345	351	358	365
70	250	257	264	271	278	285	292	299	306	313	320	327	334	341	348	355	362	369	376
71	257	265	272	279	286	293	301	308	315	322	329	338	343	351	358	365	372	379	386
72	265	272	279	287	294	302	309	316	324	331	338	346	353	361	368	375	383	390	397
73	272	280	288	295	302	310	318	325	333	340	348	355	363	371	378	386	393	401	408
74	280	287	295	303	311	319	326	334	342	350	358	365	373	381	389	396	404	412	420
75	287	295	303	311	319	327	335	343	351	359	367	375	383	391	399	407	415	423	431
76	295	304	312	320	328	336	344	353	361	369	377	385	394	402	410	418	426	435	443

From National Heart, Lung, and Blood Institute, National Institute of Diabetes and Digestive and Kidney Disease: Appendix V: Body mass index chart (chart 2), *Clinical guidelines on the identification, evaluation, and treatment of overweight and obesity in adults. The Evidence Report,* NIH Pub No 98-4083, Bethesda, Md., 1998, National Institutes of Health.

To use the table, find the appropriate height in the left-hand column. Move across to a given weight. The number at the top of the column is the BMI of that height and weight. Pounds have been rounded off.

*NOTE: For lower body mass index values, see Table 8-5.

B

Food Sources of Oxalates

FRUITS

- Berries, all
- Concord grapes
- Currants
- Figs
- Fruit cocktail
- Plums
- Rhubarb
- Tangerines

VEGETABLES

- Baked beans
- Beans, green and wax
- Beet greens
- Beets
- Celery
- Chard, Swiss
- Chives
- Collards
- Eggplant
- Endive
- Kale
- Leeks
- Mustard greens
- Okra
- Peppers, green
- Rutabagas
- Spinach
- Squash, summer
- Sweet potatoes
- Tomato soup
- Tomatoes
- Vegetable soup

NUTS

- Almonds
- Cashews
- Peanut butter
- Peanuts

BEVERAGES

- Chocolate
- Cocoa
- Draft beer
- Tea

OTHER

- Grits
- Soy products
- Tofu
- Wheat germ

Calculation Aids and Conversion Tables*

In 1799 a group of French scientists set up the metric system of weights and measures. Today, with refinements over years of usage, it is called the *Système International d'Unités* (SI) and is used in most countries throughout the world. The United States continues to follow the British/American system of weights and measures. Given below are a few conversion factors to help you make these transitions in your necessary calculations.

METRIC SYSTEM OF MEASUREMENT

Similar to our monetary system, this is a simple decimal system based on units of 10. It is uniform and used internationally.

Weight Units

1 kilogram (kg) = 1000 grams (gm or g)
1 g = 1000 milligrams (mg)
1 mg = 1000 micrograms (mcg or µg)

Length Units

1 meter (m) = 100 centimeters (cm)
1000 m = 1 kilometer (km)

Volume Units

1 liter (L) = 1000 milliliters (mL)
1 mL = 1 cubic centimeter (cc)

Temperature Units

The Celsius (C) scale is based on 100 equal units between 0° C (freezing point of water) and 100° C (boiling point of water). This scale is used entirely in all scientific work.

Energy Units

Kilocalorie (kcal) = Amount of energy required to raise 1 kg water 1° C

Kilojoule (kJ) = Amount of energy required to move 1 kg mass 1 m by a force of 1 newton
1 kcal = 4.184 kJ

BRITISH/AMERICAN SYSTEM OF MEASUREMENT

Our customary system is made up of units having no uniform relationships. It is not a decimal system but rather a collection of different units brought together in usage and language over time. It is predominantly used in the United States.

Weight Units

1 pound (lb) = 16 ounces (oz)

Length Units

1 foot (ft) = 12 inches (in)
1 yard (yd) = 3 feet (ft)

Volume Units

3 teaspoons (tsp) = 1 tablespoon (Tbsp)
16 Tbsp = 1 cup
1 cup = 8 fluid ounces (fl oz)
4 cups = 1 quart (qt)
5 cups = 1 imperial quart (qt), Canada

Temperature Units

The Fahrenheit (F) scale is based on 180 equal units between 32° F (freezing point of water) and 212° F (boiling point of water) at standard atmospheric pressure.

CONVERSIONS BETWEEN MEASUREMENT SYSTEMS

Weight

1 oz = 28.35 g
2.2 lb = 1 kg

---

*Differences in Canadian measurements are indicated as needed.

Length

1 in = 2.54 cm
1 ft = 30.48 cm
39.37 in = 1 m

Volume

1.06 qt = 1 L
0.85 imperial qt = 1 L (Canada)

Temperature

Boiling point of water: 100°C; 212°F
Body temperature: 37°C; 98.6°F
Freezing point of water: 0°C; 32°F

Interconversion Formulas

Fahrenheit temperature (°F) = 9/5 (°C) + 32
Celsius temperature (°C) = 5/9 (°F − 32)

Approximate Metric Conversions

WHEN YOU KNOW	MULTIPLY BY	TO FIND
Weight		
Ounces	28	Grams
Pounds	0.45	Kilograms
Length		
Inches	2.54	Centimeters
Feet	30.48	Centimeters
Volume		
Teaspoons	5	Milliliters
Tablespoons	15	Milliliters
Fluid ounces	30	Milliliters
Cups	0.24	Liters
Pints	0.47	Liters
Quarts	0.95	Liters

Cultural Dietary Patterns and Religious Dietary Practices

Only foods that are specifically associated with these cultural groups are noted. Individuals may also consume typical American foods, as dietary adaptations are common. Assumptions of dietary patterns cannot be made, but knowledge of these unique foods provides a common understanding of the range of possible food choices.

CULTURAL DIETARY PATTERNS

CULTURE	BREAD, CEREAL, RICE, AND PASTA GROUP	VEGETABLE GROUP	FRUIT GROUP	MILK, YOGURT, AND CHEESE GROUP	MEAT, POULTRY, FISH, DRY BEANS, EGGS, AND NUTS GROUP	FATS, OILS, AND SWEETS GROUP
Native American	Blue corn flour (ground dried blue corn kernels) used to make corn bread; mush dumplings; fruit dumplings (walakshi); fry bread (deep-fried biscuit dough); ground sweet acorns; hominy; tortillas; wheat and rye products; wild rice	Artichokes, cacti, chili peppers, mushrooms, nettles, onions, potatoes, pumpkins, squash, sweet potatoes, tomatoes, wild greens, turnips, and yucca	Dried wild berries, cherries, and grapes; berries, elderberries, persimmons, plums, and rhubarb	None in traditional diet	Bear, buffalo, deer, elk, moose, rabbit, and squirrel Duck, goose, quail, and wild turkey A variety of fish, legumes, nuts, and seeds	Tallow and lard Maple sugar and pine sugar
Northern European	Barley, hops, oat, rice, rye, and wheat products	Artichokes, asparagus, beets, Brussels sprouts, cabbage, carrots, cauliflower, celery, cucumbers, eggplant, fennel, green peppers, kale, leeks, mushrooms, olives, onions, peas, potatoes, radishes, spinach, turnips, and watercress	Apples, apricots, cherries, currants, gooseberries, grapes, lemons, melons, oranges, peaches, pears, plums, prunes, raspberries, rhubarb, and strawberries	Cheese (made from cow, sheep, or goat milk), cream, milk, sour cream, and yogurt	Beef, lamb, oxtail, pork, rabbit, veal, and venison Chicken, duck, goose, pheasant, pigeon, quail, and turkey A wide variety of fish, legumes, and nuts	Butter, lard, margarine, olive oil, vegetable oil, and salt pork Honey and sugar
Southern European	Cornmeal, rice, and wheat products	Arugula, artichokes, asparagus, broccoli, cabbage, cardoon, cauliflower, celery, chicory, cucumbers, eggplant, endive, escarole, fennel, kale, kohlrabi, mushrooms, mustard greens, olives, pimentos, potatoes, radicchio, Swiss chard, turnips, and zucchini	Apples, apricots, bananas, cherries, citron, dates, figs, grapefruit, grapes, lemons, medlars, oranges, peaches, pears, pineapples, prunes, pomegranates, quinces, raisins, and tangerines	Cheese (made from cow, sheep, buffalo, or goat milk), and milk	Beef, goat, lamb, pork, and veal Chicken, duck, goose, pigeon, turkey, and woodcock A variety of fish, shellfish, legumes, and nuts	Butter, lard, olive oil, and vegetable oil Honey and sugar

	Grains/Breads	Vegetables	Fruits	Dairy	Meats/Protein	Fats/Sweets
Central European and Russian	Barley, buckwheat, corn, millet, oats, potato starch, rice, rye, and wheat products	Asparagus, beets, Brussels sprouts, cabbage, carrots, cauliflower, celery, chard, cucumbers, eggplant, endive, kohlrabi, leeks, mushrooms, olives, onions, parsnips, peppers, potatoes, radishes, sorrel, spinach, and turnips	Apples, apricots, a variety of berries, currants, dates, grapes, grapefruit, lemons, melons, oranges, peaches, pears, plums, prunes, quinces, raisins, rhubarb, and strawberries	Buttermilk, cheese, cream, milk, sour cream, and yogurt	Beef, boar, hare, lamb, pork, sausage, veal, and venison; Chicken, Cornish hen, duck, goose, grouse, partridge, pheasant, quail, squab, and turkey; A variety of fish, shellfish, legumes, and nuts	Butter, bacon, chicken fat, flaxseed oil, lard, olive oil, salt pork, and vegetable oil; Honey, sugar, and molasses
African American (southern United States)	Biscuits; corn bread as spoon bread, cornpone, hush puppies, or grits; and rice	Broccoli, cabbage, corn; leafy greens including dandelion greens, kale, mustard greens, collard greens, and turnip greens; okra, pumpkins, potatoes, spinach, squash, sweet potatoes, tomatoes, and yams	Apples, bananas, berries, fruit juices, peaches, and watermelon	Buttermilk and some cheese	Beef; pork and pork products including scrapple (cornmeal and pork), chitterlings (pork intestines), bacon, pigs feet and ears; Fried meats and poultry, organ meats (kidney, liver, tongue, and tripe); Fish (catfish, crawfish, salmon, shrimp, and tuna); A variety of legumes and nuts	Butter and lard; Honey, molasses, and sugar
Mexican	Corn (tortillas, masa harina), wheat, and rice products; sweet bread	Cactus (nopales), calabaza criolla, chili peppers, corn, jicama, onions, peas, plantains, squash (chayote, pumpkins, etc.), tomatillos, tomatoes, yams, and yucca root (cassava or manioc)	Avocados, bananas, cactus fruit, carambola, casimiroa, cherimoya, coconuts, granadilla, guanabana, guava, lemons, limes, mamey, mangoes, melons, oranges, papayas, pineapples, strawberries, sugar cane, and zapote	Cheese, flan, sour cream, and milk	Beef, goat, and pork; Chicken and turkey; Firm-fleshed fish, shrimp, and a variety of legumes	Bacon fat, lard (manteca), salt pork, and dairy cream; Sugar and panocha (raw brown cane sugar)

Continued

CULTURAL DIETARY PATTERNS—cont'd

CULTURE	BREAD, CEREAL, RICE, AND PASTA GROUP	VEGETABLE GROUP	FRUIT GROUP	MILK, YOGURT, AND CHEESE GROUP	MEAT, POULTRY, FISH, DRY BEANS, EGGS, AND NUTS GROUP	FATS, OILS, AND SWEETS GROUP
Central American	Corn (tamales, tortillas), rice, and wheat products	Asparagus, beets, cabbage, calabaza, chayote, chili peppers, corn, cucumbers, eggplant, hearts of palm, leeks, loroco flowers, onions, pacaya buds, plantains, pumpkins, spinach, sweet peppers, tomatillos, watercress, yams, yucca, and yucca flowers	Apples, avocados, bananas, breadfruit, cherimoya, coconuts, grapes, guava, mamey, mangoes, nances, oranges, papayas, passion fruit, pejibaye, pineapples, prunes, raisins, tamarind, tangerines, and zapote	Cheese, cream, and milk	Beef, iguana, lizard, pork, and venison Chicken, duck, and turkey A variety of fish, shellfish, and legumes	Butter, lard, vegetable oils, and shortening Honey, sugar, and sugar syrup
Caribbean Islands	Cassava bread; cornmeal (surrulitos); oatmeal; rice; and wheat products	Arracacha, arrowroot, black-eyed peas, cabbage, calabaza, callaloo, cassava, chili peppers, corn, cucumbers, eggplant, malangas, okra, onions, palm hearts, peppers, radishes, spinach, squash, sweet potatoes, taro, and yams	Acerola cherries, akee, avocados, bananas, breadfruit, caimito, cherimoya, citron, coconuts, cocoplum, gooseberries, granadilla, grapefruit, guanabana, guava, jackfruit, kumquats, lemons, limes, mamey, mangoes, oranges, papayas, pineapples, plantains, pomegranates, raisins, sapodilla, sugar cane, and tamarind	Cheese and milk	Beef, goat, and pork Chicken and turkey A variety of fish, shellfish, and legumes	Butter, coconut oil (used as a fat), lard, and olive oil Sugar cane products
Cuban and Puerto Rican	Rice; starchy green bananas, usually fried (plantains)	Beets, breadfruit, chayote, chili peppers, eggplant, onions, tubers (yucca), white yams (boniato)	Coconuts, guava, mangoes, oranges (sweet and sour), prunes and mango paste	Flan, hard cheese (queso de mano)	Chicken, fish (all kinds and preparations, including smoked, salted, canned, and fresh), shellfish, legumes (all kinds, especially black beans), pork (fried), sausage (chorizo), calf brain, beef tongue	Olive and peanut oil, lard Coconut (used as a sweetener)

South American	Amaranth (corn, rice, quinoa) and wheat products	Ahipa, arracacha, calabaza, cassava, green peppers, hearts of palm, kale, okra, oca, onions, rosella, squash, sweet potatoes, yacon, and yams	Avocados, abiu, acerola, apples, bananas, caimito, casimiroa, cherimoya, feijoa, guava, grapes, jackfruit, jabitocaba, lemons, limes, lulo, mammea, mangoes, melons, olives, oranges, palm fruits, papaya, passion fruit, peaches, pineapples, pitanga, quinces, sapote, and strawberries	Cheese and milk	Beef, frog, goat, guinea pig, llama, mutton, pork, and rabbit; Chicken, duck, and turkey; A variety of fish, shellfish, and nuts	Palm oil, olive oil, and butter; Sugar cane, brown sugar, and honey
Chinese	Rice and related products (flour, cakes, and noodles); noodles made from barley, corn, and millet; wheat and related products (breads, noodles, spaghetti, stuffed noodles [won ton] and filled buns [bowl])	Bamboo shoots; cabbage (napa); celery; Chinese turnips (lo bok); dried day lilies; dry fungus (Black Judas's ear); leafy green vegetables, including kale, cress, mustard greens (gai choy), chard (bok choy), amaranth greens (yin choy), wolfberry leaves (gou gay), and Chinese broccoli (gai lan); eggplant; lotus tubers; okra; snow peas; stir-fried vegetables (chow yuk); taro roots; white radish (daikon); yams; and yam beans	Apples, bananas, custard apples, coconuts, dates, longan, figs, grapes, kumquats, limes, litchi, mangoes, muskmelons, oranges, papayas, passion fruit, peaches, persimmons, pineapples, plums, pomegranates, pomelos, tangerines, and watermelon	Milk (cow, buffalo, and soy)	Beef, lamb, and pork; Chicken, duck, quail, squab; A large variety of fish and shellfish, in addition to legumes and nuts	Lard; peanut, soy, sesame, and rice oil; Honey, rice or barley malt, palm sugar, sorghum sugar, and dehydrated cane juice

Continued

CULTURAL DIETARY PATTERNS—cont'd

CULTURE	BREAD, CEREAL, RICE, AND PASTA GROUP	VEGETABLE GROUP	FRUIT GROUP	MILK, YOGURT, AND CHEESE GROUP	MEAT, POULTRY, FISH, DRY BEANS, EGGS, AND NUTS GROUP	FATS, OILS, AND SWEETS GROUP
Japanese	Rice and rice products, rice flour (mochiko), noodles (comen/soba), buckwheat, and millet	Artichokes, asparagus, bamboo shoots (takenoko), burdock (gobo), cabbage (napa), eggplant, horseradish (wasabi), mizuna, mushrooms (shiitake, matsutake, nameko), Japanese parsley (seri), lotus root (renkon), pickled cabbage (kimchee), pickled vegetables, seaweed (laver, nori, wakame, kombu), snow peas, spinach, sweet potatoes, vegetable soup (mizutaki), watercress, white radish (daikon)	Asian pear (nashi), apricots, bananas, cherries, figs, grapefruit (yuzu), kumquats, lemons, limes, persimmons, pineapples, plums, strawberry, and tangerines (mikan)	Milk, butter, and ice cream	Beef, deer, lamb, pork, rabbit, and veal Fish and shellfish, including dried fish with bones, raw fish (sashimi), and fish cake (kamaboko) A variety of poultry (chicken, duck, goose, turkey) Legumes (black beans, red beans, soybeans [as tofu, fermented soybean, and sprouts])	Lard; soy, sesame, rapeseed, and rice oil Honey and sugar
Korean	Barley, buckwheat, millet, rice, and wheat products	Bamboo shoots, bean sprouts, beets, cabbage, chives, chrysanthemum leaves, cucumbers, eggplant, fern, green onions, green peppers, leeks, lotus root, mushrooms, onions, perilla, seaweed, spinach, sweet potatoes, turnips, water chestnuts, watercress, and white radishes	Apples, Asian pears, cherries, dates, grapes, melons, oranges, pears, persimmons, plums, and tangerines	Very little, if any, consumption	Beef, oxtail, pork, chicken, pheasant A variety of fish, shellfish, legumes, and nuts	Sesame oil and vegetable oil Honey and sugar
Filipino	Noodles, rice, rice flour (mochiko), stuffed noodles (won ton), white bread (pan de sal)	Amaranth, bamboo shoots, beets, burdock root, cassava, Chinese celery, dark green leafy vegetables (malunggay and saluyot), eggplant, garlic, green peppers, hearts of palm, hyacinth bean, kamias, leek, mushrooms, okra, onions, sweet potatoes (camotes), turnips, and root crop (gabi)	Apples, avocados, bananas, bitter melons (ampalaya), breadfruit, coconuts, guava, jackfruit, limes, mangoes, papayas, pod fruit (tamarind), pomelos, rambutan, rhubarb, star fruit, tangelos (naranghita), and watermelon	White cheese, evaporated cow or goat milk, and soymilk	Beef, carabao, goat, pork, monkey, organ meats, and rabbit Fish, dried fish (dilis), egg roll (lumpia), fish sauce (alamang and bagoong) Legumes such as mung beans, bean sprouts, and chickpeas; soybean curd (tofu)	Coconut oil (used as a fat), lard, and vegetable oil Brown and white sugar, coconut (used as a sweetener), and honey

	Grains	Vegetables	Fruits	Dairy	Meat/Protein	Fats and Sweets
Pacific Islanders	Rice and wheat products	Arrowroot, bitter melons, burdock root, cabbage, carrots, cassava, daikon, eggplant, ferns, green peppers, horseradish, jute, kohlrabi, leeks, lotus root, mustard greens, green onions, seaweed, spinach, squash, sweet potatoes, taro, water chestnuts, and yams	Acerola cherries, apples, apricots, avocados, bananas, breadfruit, coconuts, guava, jackfruit, kumquats, litchis, loquat, mangoes, melons, papayas, passion fruit, peaches, pears, pineapples, plums, prunes, strawberries, and tamarind	Very little, if any, consumption	Beef, pork, chicken, duck, squab, and turkey A variety of fish, shellfish, and legumes	Butter, coconut oil, lard, sesame oil, and vegetable oil Sugar
South Asian	Rice, wheat, buckwheat, corn, millet, and sorghum products	Agathi flowers, amaranth, artichokes, bamboo shoots, beets, bitter melons, Brussels sprouts, cabbage, collard greens, cucumbers, drumstick plant, eggplant, lotus root, manioc, mushrooms, okra, pandanus, plantain flowers, sago palm, spinach, squash, turnips, water chestnuts, water lilies, and yams	Apples, apricots, avocados, bananas, coconuts, dates, figs, grapes, guava, jackfruit, limes, litchis, loquats, mangoes, melon, nongus, oranges, papayas, peaches, pears, persimmons, pineapples, plums, pomegranates, pomelos, star fruit, sugar cane, tangerines, and watermelon	Milk (evaporated and fermented products), cheese, and milk-based desserts	Beef, goat, mutton, pork, chicken, duck A variety of fish, seafood, legumes, and nuts	Coconut oil, ghee, mustard oil, peanut oil, sesame seed oil, and sunflower oil Sugar cane, jaggery, and molasses Chicken fat
Jewish (both cultural and religious customs)	Bagel, buckwheat groats (kasha), dumplings made with matzo meal (matzo balls or knaidelach), egg bread (challah), noodle or potato pudding (kugel), crepe filled with farmer cheese and/ or fruit (blintzes), unleavened bread or large crackers made with wheat flour and water (matzo)	Potato pancakes (latkes); vegetable stew made with sweet potatoes, carrots, prunes, and sometimes brisket (tzimmes); beet soup (borscht)			A mixture of fish formed into balls and poached (gefilte fish); smoked salmon (lox)	

RELIGIOUS DIETARY PRACTICES

	SEVENTH-DAY ADVENTIST	BUDDHIST	EASTERN ORTHODOX	HINDU	JEWISH	MORMON	MUSLIM	ROMAN CATHOLIC
Beef		Avoided by most devout		Prohibited or strongly discouraged				
Pork	Prohibited or strongly discouraged	Avoided by most devout		Avoided by most devout	Prohibited or strongly discouraged		Prohibited or strongly discouraged	
All meat	Avoided by most devout	Avoided by most devout	Permitted but some restrictions apply	Avoided by most devout	Permitted but some restrictions apply		Permitted but some restrictions apply	Permitted but some restrictions apply
Eggs/dairy	Permitted but avoided at some observances	Permitted but avoided at some observances	Permitted but some restrictions apply	Permitted but avoided at some observances	Permitted but some restrictions apply			
Fish	Avoided by most devout	Avoided by most devout	Permitted but some restrictions apply	Permitted but some restrictions apply	Permitted but some restrictions apply			
Shellfish	Prohibited or strongly discouraged	Avoided by most devout	Permitted but avoided at some observances	Permitted but some restrictions apply	Prohibited or strongly discouraged			
Meat and dairy at the same meal					Prohibited or strongly discouraged			
Leavened foods					Permitted but some restrictions apply			
Ritual slaughter of animals					Practiced		Practiced	
Alcohol	Prohibited or strongly discouraged			Avoided by most devout		Prohibited or strongly discouraged	Prohibited or strongly discouraged	
Caffeine	Prohibited or strongly discouraged					Prohibited or strongly discouraged	Prohibited or strongly discouraged	Avoided by most devout

Compiled by Staci Nix for *Williams' basic nutrition & diet therapy*, ed 12, St Louis, Mo., 2005, Mosby. Modified from Kittler PG, Sucher KP: *Food and culture*, ed 4, Belmont, Calif., 2004, Brooks/Cole, a division of Thomson Learning (www.thomsonrights.com).

Federal Food Assistance Programs

Programs described below are funded by the U.S. government with state allocations based on population, numbers of eligible participants, and other factors. States may be required to provide some degree of match in support of the statewide program.

Supplemental Nutrition Assistance Program (SNAP) (formerly the food stamp program)

Type of Program: Entitlement program.

Supervising Agency: United States Department of Agriculture.

Population Served: Individuals and families with incomes falling within 130% of the federal poverty line and assets not exceeding federal guidelines. SNAP eligibility and benefits take into consideration household income, household size, housing costs, total assets, and work registration requirements. Eligibility requirements and benefits are adjusted annually.

Benefits Provided/Nutrition Standards: SNAP benefits increase the amount of money participants have available to spend for food. Recipients receive electronic debit cards (also known as EBT or electronic benefit transfer cards). At the time of purchase funds are transferred from the client's account to the retailer's account. SNAP benefits can be used to buy most foods, as well as seeds and plants for raising food for the household, although there are exceptions.

The following items cannot be purchased using SNAP benefits:

- Hot, ready-to-eat foods
- Foods that will be eaten in the store
- Vitamin or mineral supplements, or medicines
- Pet foods
- Nonfood items such as soap, cleaning supplies, paper products, toothpaste, or cosmetics
- Tobacco items
- Alcoholic beverages

The average monthly SNAP benefit is about $133 per person and about $275 per household.

Number Served: More than 47 million people are served by SNAP benefits. Nearly half (45%) are children under the age of 18, and about 9% are age 60 or older. Fifty-six percent of SNAP households with children are single-adult households.

Availability of Nutrition Education: Most states offer nutrition education in conjunction with their SNAP program, but not all families are reached, and participation is voluntary. See discussion of the Supplemental Nutrition Assistance Program-Education Program (SNAP-Ed) later.

The Emergency Food Assistance Program (TEFAP)

Type of Program: States are required to set and enforce income eligibility requirements for distribution of food for home use; persons receiving meals are considered to be low-income.

Supervising Agency: United States Department of Agriculture with state oversight on the local level.

Population Served: Individuals and families must meet income guidelines (usually falling at or below the federal poverty line). Food is distributed to individuals and families through local food pantries and may be made available to school meal programs, meal programs for older adults, soup kitchens and emergency feeding locations, or child care facilities.

Benefits Provided/Nutrition Standards: Specific foods available for distribution are subject to market conditions but may include meat, poultry, or fish; canned fruits and vegetables; fruit juice; dried eggs; dried beans; pasta; milk; cheese; cereals; and soups.

Number Served: More than 840 million pounds of food can be distributed annually.

Availability of Nutrition Education: No formal mandate; may be provided at facilities or locations serving meals or distributing food.

CHILD NUTRITION PROGRAMS

National School Lunch Program

Type of Program: Serves all children of school age who choose to participate. Free lunches are provided to children whose family income falls at or below 130% of the federal poverty level, and lunches are available at a reduced cost of no more than 40 cents to children whose family incomes fall between 130% and 185% of the federal poverty level. Programs can choose to receive either commodity foods or cash reimbursement, based on the number of students served.

Supervising Agency: United States Department of Agriculture.

Population Served: Children in public schools, nonprofit private schools, and residential child care programs.

Benefits Provided/Nutrition Regulations: Nutritionally balanced lunches provide one third of the dietary reference intakes (DRIs) for protein, vitamin A, vitamin C, iron, and calcium. New standards limit the number of kcalories served in an effort to combat child obesity, and mandate increased servings of vegetables and fruits and the use of whole grains to comply with recommendations of the *Dietary Guidelines for Americans*. (For details, see the table "Nutrition Standards for School Meal Programs" later.)

Number Served: More than 100,000 schools and child care institutions offer a school lunch program, and meals are served to 31 million children every school day. Since the program's inception in 1946, it has served over 224 billion meals.

Availability of Nutrition Education: Team Nutrition, a comprehensive nutrition education program developed to support the National School Lunch Program, contains integrated activities for the school classroom, lunchroom, and after-school setting that promote healthy food choices, portion control, and physical activity.

National School Breakfast Program

Type of Program: Serves all children of school age who choose to participate. Free breakfasts are provided to children whose family income falls at or below 130% of the poverty level, and breakfasts are available at a reduced cost to children whose family income falls between 130% and 185% of the poverty level. Children receiving the reduced price pay no more than 30 cents.

Supervising Agency: United States Department of Agriculture.

Population Served: Children in public schools, nonprofit private schools, and residential child care programs.

Benefits Provided/Nutrition Regulations: Breakfast must provide one fourth of the DRIs for protein, calcium, iron, vitamin A, and vitamin C. New standards control kcalories and promote healthy eating according to the *Dietary Guidelines for Americans*. (For details, see the table "Nutrition Standards for School Meal Programs.")

Number Served: More than 89,000 schools offer a breakfast program, and about 13 million children receive a daily breakfast; over 10 million children obtain their breakfast at a free or reduced price.

Availability of Nutrition Education: See National School Lunch Program above.

Summer Food Service Program

Type of Program: Entitlement program where available.

Supervising Agency: United States Department of Agriculture.

Population Served: Children meeting income eligibility guidelines.

Benefits Provided/Nutrition Regulations: Provides breakfast and/or a noon meal during summer vacation periods for children who depend on school meal programs for a significant portion of their nutrient intake. Meals must meet the same nutrition standards in place for the school breakfast and lunch programs. Summer meals are usually offered as part of a summer school or camp experience sponsored by a local school district, recreation department, or other government or nonprofit community agency.

Number Served: Nearly 2.5 million children participate daily.

Availability of Nutrition Education: May be offered as part of the educational or recreational program.

School Milk Program

Type of Program: Available to all children in participating schools or child care facilities.

Supervising Agency: United States Department of Agriculture.

Population Served: Children in schools or child care facilities or summer camps that do not offer a breakfast or lunch program.

Benefits Provided/Nutrition Regulations: Participating schools or programs are reimbursed for the milk provided free to children meeting income guidelines or sold to children at a nominal cost. Milk must be pasteurized, fortified with vitamins A and D according to FDA standards, and be fat free or low fat (1% fat).

Number Served: More than 4100 schools and child care facilities participate, serving 61 million half-pints of milk annually.

Availability of Nutrition Education: Unknown.

Child and Adult Care Food Program (CACFP)

Type of Program: Available to all children and adults in participating programs and facilities.

Supervising Agency: United States Department of Agriculture.

Population Served: Child care programs serving children up to 12 years of age, adult day care programs serving persons age 60 and over, or day programs caring for individuals who are chronically impaired or disabled. Such settings include Head Start, other child care and adult day care centers, after-school programs, recreation centers, and emergency shelters caring for children.

Benefits Provided/Nutrition Regulations: Cash reimbursements to the program or facility providing meals are based on the recipients' eligibility for free or reduced-price meals. Children and adults are eligible to receive two meals and one snack each day, with an additional meal or snack if care exceeds 8 hours.

Number Served: 3.3 million children and 120,000 adults.

Availability of Nutrition Education: May be offered as part of a recreational or educational program.

Special Supplemental Nutrition Program for Women, Infants, and Children (WIC)

Type of Program: Participation is based on both income and medical or nutritional risk. Income eligibility (at or below 185% of the federal poverty line) does not ensure benefits: only those judged to be at medical or nutritional risk may participate to the extent that resources are available.

Supervising Agency: United States Department of Agriculture; local programs are administered through state health departments.

Population Served: Women falling within income guidelines who are pregnant, postpartum, or breast-feeding, and infants and children up to 5 years of age, who are found to be at nutritional risk. Postpartum mothers can receive supplementary food for 6 months, and breast-feeding mothers can receive supplementary food for 12 months.

Eligibility must be determined by a health professional using the following criteria:

1. *Medically based risk:* anemia; underweight; overweight; poor prior pregnancy outcome; or history of pregnancy complications.
2. *Dietary risk:* mothers, infants, or children with nutrient deficiencies or nutrition-related medical conditions; inappropriate nutrition/feeding practices; or diets that fail to meet the *Dietary Guidelines for Americans.*

Benefits Provided/Nutrition Regulations: Participants receive vouchers or electronic debit cards to purchase designated foods that are rich sources of protein, calcium, iron, vitamin A, and vitamin C. Specific types and amounts of food are provided in the food packages for different categories of recipients according to age or condition. Vouchers or debit cards may be used to purchase fresh fruits and vegetables at local farmers' markets. Food packages have been adjusted to comply more closely with the *Dietary Guidelines for Americans.*

Approved WIC Foods:

Infants
- Iron-fortified infant formula
- Iron-fortified infant cereal
- Baby food fruits and vegetables
- Baby food meat

Women and Children
- Vitamin C–rich fruit juice (unsweetened; fruit drinks not allowed)
- Vitamin C–rich vegetable juice (unsweetened)
- Eggs
- Milk (soy beverages, cheese, and tofu are also available)
- Cheese
- Iron-fortified breakfast cereal (may not contain more than 6 gm sucrose/sugar per 1 oz of dry cereal; whole grain preferred)
- Whole wheat bread (brown rice, oatmeal, and soft corn or whole wheat tortillas, and whole grain barley are also available)
- Peanut butter
- Dried or canned legumes
- Canned fish (light tuna, salmon, sardines, and mackerel)
- Fruits and vegetables (fresh, frozen, canned, dried; no added sugar, fats, or oils)

(The regulatory requirements for WIC food packages and the alternative choices available can be found at http://www.fns.usda.gov/wic/benefitsandservices/foodpkg.htm.)

Number Served: Of the 8.9 million individuals who receive monthly benefits, 4.7 million are children, 2.1 million are infants, and 2.1 million are women.

Availability of Nutrition Education: Public health nutritionists provide nutrition counseling at every WIC visit, and nutrition education is offered to individuals and groups. WIC also provides health screening and referrals to other indicated medical or social services.

WIC has been shown to be cost-effective in (1) reducing the number of premature and very low-birth-weight infants, (2) reducing health care expenditures within the first 60 days after birth, and (3) lowering the number of preschool children with iron-deficiency anemia.

NUTRITION PROGRAM FOR THE ELDERLY/ NUTRITION SERVICES INCENTIVE PROGRAM

Type of Program: Available to all persons 60 years of age or over regardless of income, although the program targets those with greatest social or economic needs, including low-income older adults, minority older adults, those residing in rural areas with limited access to services, and those at high risk of institutionalization. Participants are encouraged to make a donation to help meet the cost of the meals provided. Growing transportation needs are putting a strain on nutrition program budgets. The Nutrition Services Incentive Program was developed to provide additional funding to be used for food only.

Supervising Agency: Administration on Aging, United States Department of Health and Human Services.

Population Served: Congregate meals are offered at noon in community centers, churches, senior housing, or similar locations with familiarity and easy access for the aging population. Meals are home delivered for those who cannot leave their homes as a result of illness, disability, or a dependent family member; certification for home-delivered meals must be renewed every 6 months by a health or social services professional.

Benefits Provided/Nutrition Regulations: A hot meal is served on weekdays at noon at congregate meal sites; delivered meals may include a cold lunch for the evening meal or cold breakfast for the following day. As the costs of daily home delivery continue to rise, programs have experimented with weekly delivery of several frozen meals that can be defrosted and reheated as needed. Unfortunately, occasional delivery of several frozen meals takes away the social aspect of a daily visitor, important to a homebound or isolated senior. Meals should provide at least one third of the DRIs for all nutrients as defined for persons above age 50 and conform to the *Dietary Guidelines for Americans* in total fat, percent saturated fat, and sodium.

Number Served: More than 3 million older adults receive meals regularly.

Availability of Nutrition Education: May be offered as part of the educational or recreational program at congregate sites.

EXPANDED FOOD AND NUTRITION EDUCATION PROGRAM (EFNEP)/ SUPPLEMENTAL NUTRITION ASSISTANCE PROGRAM-EDUCATION (SNAP-Ed)

Type of Program: Services are directed toward individuals and families falling within the federal poverty guidelines and/ or receiving SNAP benefits, but SNAP recipients are not required to participate.

Supervising Agency: United States Department of Agriculture.

Population Served: Families with children, older adults, and youth. Individuals are recruited through neighborhood contacts, local welfare agencies, and the Special Supplemental Nutrition Program for Women, Infants, and Children.

Nutritional Regulations: EFNEP and SNAP-Ed do not provide actual food but support limited-resource families through education, thereby helping them to obtain the knowledge and skills necessary for making healthy food choices and using their food dollars wisely. Programs are delivered to both youth and adults by Cooperative Extension agents, paraprofessionals, and volunteers. Paraprofessionals are indigenous to the communities and populations they serve.

Number Served: Over 480,000 youth and 130,000 adults are reached by EFNEP each year, with an indirect effect on an additional 400,000 family members.

Availability of Nutrition Education: An experiential series of lessons offers hands-on opportunities to develop skills in food preparation, food safety, food budgeting and management, and wise shopping. Group classes, media methods, one-on-one instruction, and educational mailings are used to reach various audiences. The EFNEP reporting system indicates that 85% of adults improve their food management practices (e.g., planning meals and shopping more wisely), and 95% increase their daily fruit and vegetable intakes by 1 cup; nearly 60% of youth improve their food preparation and food safety skills.

NUTRITION STANDARDS FOR SCHOOL MEAL PROGRAMS

Meal Pattern	BREAKFAST MEAL PATTERN			LUNCH MEAL PATTERN		
	GRADES K–5	GRADES 6-8	GRADES 9-12	GRADES K–5	GRADES 6-8	GRADES 9-12
Meal Pattern	Amount of Food Per Week (Minimum Per Day)					
Fruits (cups)*	5 (1)	5 (1)	5 (1)	2½ (½)	2½ (½)	5 (1)
Vegetables (cups)*	0	0	0	3¾ (¾)	3¾ (¾)	5 (1)
Dark Green	0	0	0	½	½	½
Red/Orange	0	0	0	¾	¾	1¼
Beans/Peas (Legumes)	0	0	0	½	½	½
Starchy	0	0	0	½	½	½
Other†	0	0	0	½	½	¾
Additional Veg to Reach Total	0	0	0	1	1	1½
Grains (oz eq)*,‡	7-10 (1)	8-10 (1)	9-10 (1)	8-9 (1)	8-10 (1)	10-12 (2)
Meat/Meat Alternates (oz eq)*	0	0	0	8-10 (1)	9-10 (1)	10-12 (2)
Fluid Milk (cups)§	5 (1)	5 (1)	5 (1)	5 (1)	5 (1)	5 (1)

OTHER SPECIFICATIONS: DAILY AMOUNT BASED ON THE AVERAGE FOR THE WEEK

Minimum/Maximum kcal‖	350-500	400-550	450-600	550-650	600-700	750-850
Saturated fat (% of total kcal)	<10	<10	<10	<10	<10	<10
Sodium (mg)	≤430	≤470	≤500	≤640	≤710	≤740
Trans fat	Nutrition label must indicate zero grams of trans fat per serving					

*See Table 1-3 footnotes for definitions of specific foods included in each of these groups; serving equivalents can be found in Table 1-2.
†Can be met with additional amounts from the Dark Green, Red/Orange, or Legumes groups.
‡At least half of the grains offered must be whole grains.
§Fluid milk must be low fat (1% milk fat or less) or fat free; can be flavored or unflavored.
‖Foods of minimal nutritional value are not allowed.

Page numbers followed by "f" indicate
figures, "t" indicate tables, and "b"
indicate boxes.

603